THE SURGICAL REVIEW
AN INTEGRATED BASIC AND CLINICAL SCIENCE STUDY GUIDE

THE SURGICAL REVIEW
AN INTEGRATED BASIC AND CLINICAL SCIENCE STUDY GUIDE

EDITED BY

Daniel Kreisel, M.D.
Alexander S. Krupnick, M.D.
Larry R. Kaiser, M.D.

LIPPINCOTT WILLIAMS & WILKINS
A **Wolters Kluwer** Company
Philadelphia · Baltimore · New York · London
Buenos Aires · Hong Kong · Sydney · Tokyo

Acquisitions Editor: Lisa McAllister
Developmental Editor: Alexandra T. Anderson
Production Editor: Frank Aversa
Manufacturing Manager: Colin J. Warnock
Cover Designer: Patricia Gast
Compositor: Lippincott Williams & Wilkins, Desktop Division
Printer: Edwards Brothers

© 2001 by LIPPINCOTT WILLIAMS & WILKINS
530 Walnut Street
Philadelphia, PA 19106 USA
LWW.com

All rights reserved. This book is protected by copyright. No part of this book may be reproduced in any form or by any means, including photocopying, or utilized by any information storage and retrieval system without written permission from the copyright owner, except for brief quotations embodied in critical articles and reviews. Materials appearing in this book prepared by individuals as part of their official duties as U.S. government employees are not covered by the above-mentioned copyright.

Cover: The Agnew Clinic (1889), by Thomas Eakins, courtesy of the University of Pennsylvania School of Medicine.

Printed in the USA

Library of Congress Cataloging-in-Publication Data

The surgical review : an integrated basic and clinical science study guide / edited by Daniel Kreisel, Alexander S. Krupnick, and Larry R. Kaiser.
    p. ; cm.
  Includes bibliographical references and index.
  ISBN 0-7817-2801-0 (alk. paper)
   1. Surgery--Examinations, questions, etc. I. Kreisel, Daniel. II. Krupnick, Alexander S. III. Kaiser, Larry R.
   [DNLM: 1. Surgery. 2. Surgical Procedures, Operative--methods. WO 100 S9628 2000]
  RD37.2.S9749 2000
  617'.0076--dc21
                                                                                          00-055876

Care has been taken to confirm the accuracy of the information presented and to describe generally accepted practices. However, the authors, editors, and publisher are not responsible for errors or omissions or for any consequences from application of the information in this book and make no warranty, expressed or implied, with respect to the currency, completeness, or accuracy of the contents of the publication. Application of this information in a particular situation remains the professional responsibility of the practitioner.

The authors, editors, and publisher have exerted every effort to ensure that drug selection and dosage set forth in this text are in accordance with current recommendations and practice at the time of publication. However, in view of ongoing research, changes in government regulations, and the constant flow of information relating to drug therapy and drug reactions, the reader is urged to check the package insert for each drug for any change in indications and dosage and for added warnings and precautions. This is particularly important when the recommended agent is a new or infrequently employed drug.

Some drugs and medical devices presented in this publication have Food and Drug Administration (FDA) clearance for limited use in restricted research settings. It is the responsibility of the health care provider to ascertain the FDA status of each drug or device planned for use in their clinical practice.

To our wives Fritzi and Shauna, our parents, and Max, future Chief of Surgery.
D.K., A.S.K.

To Clyde F. Barker, surgical scholar and mentor to a generation of surgical residents.
L.R.K.

Contents

Contributing Authors ix

Foreword xiii

Preface xv

SECTION I: BODY AS A WHOLE

1. Neurosurgery 3
   G. Timothy Reiter and Kevin D. Judy

2. Immunology and Transplantation 37
   Daniel Kreisel and Bruce R. Rosengard

3. Surgical Infections and Antimicrobial Agents 59
   Sarah Bouchard and Harry L. Anderson III

4. Tumor Biology 69
   Isabelle Bedrosian and Brian J. Czerniecki

5. Melanoma, Sarcoma, Lymphoma, and the Spleen 91
   Mark B. Faries and Francis R. Spitz

6. Wound Healing 110
   Alexander S. Krupnick and N. Scott Adzick

7. Burn Injury and Management 123
   Alexander S. Krupnick and N. Scott Adzick

8. Anesthesia 139
   Michael B. Rodricks and C. William Hanson III

9. Fluids, Electrolytes, Shock, Trauma Resuscitation 148
   Vicente H. Gracias, Brian S. King, and Patrick M. Reilly

10. Hernias 159
    Robert A. Larson and Jo Buyske

11. Statistics and Epidemiology 174
    Alphonso Brown and Rudolf N. Staroscik

SECTION II: GASTROINTESTINAL SYSTEM

12. The Esophagus 185
    Michael Lanuti and Joseph S. Friedberg

13. The Stomach and Duodenum 197
    Jagajan J. Karmacharya and Jon B. Morris

14. The Small Bowel 211
    Samantha K. Hendren and Noel N. Williams

15. The Colon, Rectum, and Anus 235
    Edward Y. Woo and John L. Rombeau

16. Hepatobiliary System 256
    Allan S. Stewart and James F. Markman

17. Nutrition, Digestion, and Absorption 272
    Wilson Y. Szeto and Gordon P. Buzby

SECTION III: CARDIOVASCULAR AND RESPIRATORY SYSTEMS

18. Hemostasis and Thrombosis 295
    T. Sloane Guy and L. Henry Edmunds

19. Cardiovascular Physiology 304
    Frank W. Bowen and Robert C. Gorman

20. Cardiovascular Pathophysiology and Treatment 314
    Howard K. Song and Timothy J. Gardner

21. Vascular Disease and Vascular Surgery 333
    David G. Neschis and Michael A. Golden

22. Pulmonary Physiology 355
    Eric S. Lambright and Joseph B. Shrager

23. Thoracic Pathophysiology and Malignancies 365
    Seth D. Force and Larry R. Kaiser

SECTION IV: GENITOURINARY SYSTEM, HEAD AND NECK, AND MUSCULOSKELETAL SYSTEM

24. Genitourinary System 385
    Jonathan Masoudi and Keith N. Van Arsdalen

25. Female Reproductive System 402
    Sally Y. Segel and Sara J. Marder

26. Otorhinolaryngology 418
    Steven J. Wall and Ara A. Chalian

27. Orthopedic Surgery 440
    George Yeh and John L. Esterhai, Jr.

SECTION V: ENDOCRINE SYSTEM

28. Thyroid, Parathyroid, and Adrenal Glands 469
Todd W. Bauer, David Maron, Eugene A. Choi, and Douglas L. Fraker

29. The Pancreas 492
Patrick K. Kim and Ernest F. Rosato

30. The Breast 504
Subhasis Chatterjee and Linda S. Callans

Subject Index 523

Contributing Authors

N. Scott Adzick, M.D.
C. Everett Koop Professor of
　Pediatric Surgery
Surgeon-in-Chief
The Children's Hospital of Philadelphia
34th Street & Civic Center Boulevard
Philadelphia, Pennsylvania 19104

Harry L. Anderson III, M.D.
Assistant Professor of Surgery, Surgical
　Critical Care
Hospital of the University of Pennsylvania
3400 Spruce Street
Philadelphia, Pennsylvania 19104

Todd W. Bauer, M.D.
Resident in Surgery
Hospital of the University of Pennsylvania
3400 Spruce Street
Philadelphia, Pennsylvania 19104

Isabelle Bedrosian, M.D.
Resident in Surgery
Hospital of the University of Pennsylvania
3400 Spruce Street
Philadelphia, Pennsylvania 19104

Sarah Bouchard, M.D.
Research Fellow in Pediatric Surgery
The Children's Hospital of Philadelphia
34th Street & Civic Center Boulevard
Philadelphia, Pennsylvania 19104

Frank W. Bowen, M.D.
Resident in Surgery
Hospital of the University of Pennsylvania
3400 Spruce Street
Philadelphia, Pennsylvania 19104

Alphonso Brown, M.D.
Fellow in Gastroenterology
Hospital of the University of Pennsylvania
3400 Spruce Street
Philadelphia, Pennsylvania 19104

Jo Buyske, M.D.
Assistant Professor of Surgery
Hospital of the University of Pennsylvania;
Chief of Surgery
Presbyterian Hospital
3400 Spruce Street
Philadelphia, Pennsylvania 19104

Gordon P. Buzby, M.D.
Associate Professor of Surgery
Hospital of the University of Pennsylvania
3400 Spruce Street
Philadelphia, Pennsylvania 19104

Linda S. Callans, M.D.
Assistant Professor of Surgery
Hospital of the University of Pennsylvania
3400 Spruce Street
Philadelphia, Pennsylvania 19104

Ara A. Chalian, M.D.
Assistant Professor of Otorhinolaryngology
Hospital of the University of Pennsylvania
3400 Spruce Street
Philadelphia, Pennsylvania 19104

Subhasis Chatterjee, M.D.
Resident in Surgery
Hospital of the University of Pennsylvania
3400 Spruce Street
Philadelphia, Pennsylvania 19104

Eugene A. Choi, M.D.
Research Fellow
Harrison Department of Surgical Research
Hospital of the University of Pennsylvania
3400 Spruce Street
Philadelphia, Pennsylvania 19104

Brian J. Czerniecki, M.D., Ph.D.
Assistant Professor of Surgery
Division of Surgical Oncology
Hospital of the University of Pennsylvania
3400 Spruce Street
Philadelphia, Pennsylvania 19104

L. Henry Edmunds, M.D.
The Julian Johnson Professor of Surgery
Division of Cardiothoracic Surgery
Hospital of the University of Pennsylvania
3400 Spruce Street
Philadelphia, Pennsylvania 19104

John L. Esterhai, Jr., M.D.
Associate Professor of Orthopaedic Surgery
Hospital of the University of Pennsylvania
3400 Spruce Street
Philadelphia, Pennsylvania 19104

Mark B. Faries, M.D.
Resident in Surgery
Hospital of the University of Pennsylvania
3400 Spruce Street
Philadelphia, Pennsylvania 19104

Seth D. Force, M.D.
Resident in Surgery
Hospital of the University of Pennsylvania
3400 Spruce Street
Philadelphia, Pennsylvania 19104

Douglas L. Fraker, M.D.
Jonathan E. Rhoads Associate Professor of Surgical Science
Chief, Division of Surgical Oncology
Hospital of the University of Pennsylvania
3400 Spruce Street
Philadelphia, Pennsylvania 19104

Joseph S. Friedberg, M.D.
Assistant Professor of Surgery
Section of Thoracic Surgery
Hospital of the University of Pennsylvania
3400 Spruce Street
Philadelphia, Pennsylvania 19104

Timothy J. Gardner, M.D.
William M. Measey Professor of Surgery
Chief, Cardiothoracic Surgery
Hospital of the University of Pennsylvania
3400 Spruce Street
Philadelphia, Pennsylvania 19104

Michael A. Golden, M.D.
Associate Professor of Surgery
Division of Vascular Surgery
Hospital of the University of Pennsylvania
3400 Spruce Street
Philadelphia, Pennsylvania 19104

Robert C. Gorman, M.D.
Assistant Professor of Surgery
Division of Cardiothoracic Surgery
Hospital of the University of Pennsylvania
3400 Spruce Street
Philadelphia, Pennsylvania 19104

Vicente H. Gracias, M.D.
Assistant Professor of Surgery
Division of Trauma and Critical Care
Hospital of the University of Pennsylvania
3400 Spruce Street
Philadelphia, Pennsylvania 19104

T. Sloane Guy, M.D.
Resident in Surgery
Hospital of the University of Pennsylvania
3400 Spruce Street
Philadelphia, Pennsylvania 19104

C. William Hanson III, M.D.
Assistant Professor of Anesthesia
Hospital of the University of Pennsylvania
3400 Spruce Street
Philadelphia, Pennsylvania 19104

Samantha K. Hendren, M.D.
Resident in Surgery
Hospital of the University of Pennsylvania
3400 Spruce Street
Philadelphia, Pennsylvania 19104

Kevin D. Judy, M.D.
Assistant Professor of Neurological Surgery
Hospital of the University of Pennsylvania
3400 Spruce Street
Philadelphia, Pennsylvania 19104

Larry R. Kaiser, M.D.
Eldridge L. Eliason Professor of Surgery
Director, Section of General Thoracic Surgery
Hospital of the University of Pennsylvania
3400 Spruce Street
Philadelphia, Pennsylvania 19104

Jagajan J. Karmacharya, M.D., F.R.C.S.
Research Fellow
Department of Plastic Surgery
The Children's Hospital of Philadelphia
34th Street & Civic Center Boulevard
Philadelphia, Pennsylvania 19104

Patrick K. Kim, M.D.
Resident in Surgery
Hospital of the University of Pennsylvania
3400 Spruce Street
Philadelphia, Pennsylvania 19104

Brian S. King, M.D.
Fellow in Trauma Surgery and Surgical Critical Care
Hospital of the University of Pennsylvania
3400 Spruce Street
Philadelphia, Pennsylvania 19104

Daniel Kreisel, M.D.
Resident in Surgery
Hospital of the University of Pennsylvania
3400 Spruce Street
Philadelphia, Pennsylvania 19104

Alexander Sasha Krupnick, M.D.
Resident in Surgery
Hospital of the University of Pennsylvania
3400 Spruce Street
Philadelphia, Pennsylvania 19104

Eric S. Lambright, M.D.
Resident in Surgery
Hospital of the University of Pennsylvania
3400 Spruce Street
Philadelphia, Pennsylvania 19104

Michael Lanuti, M.D.
Resident in Surgery
Hospital of the University of Pennsylvania
3400 Spruce Street
Philadelphia, Pennsylvania 19104

Robert A. Larson, M.D.
Resident in Surgery
Hospital of the University of Pennsylvania
3400 Spruce Street
Philadelphia, Pennsylvania 19104

Sara J. Marder, M.D.
Assistant Professor of Gynecology
Hospital of the University of Pennsylvania
3400 Spruce Street
Philadelphia, Pennsylvania 19104

James F. Markman, M.D., Ph.D.
Assistant Professor of Surgery
Hospital of the University of Pennsylvania
3400 Spruce Street
Philadelphia, Pennsylvania 19104

David Maron, M.D.
Research Fellow
Harrison Department of Surgical Research
Hospital of the University of Pennsylvania
3400 Spruce Street
Philadelphia, Pennsylvania 19104

Jonathan Masoudi, M.D.
Chief Resident in Urology
Hospital of the University of Pennsylvania
3400 Spruce Street
Philadelphia, Pennsylvania 19104

Jon B. Morris, M.D.
Associate Professor of Surgery
Associate Dean of Clinical Education
Hospital of the University of Pennsylvania
3400 Spruce Street
Philadelphia, Pennsylvania 19104

David G. Neschis, M.D.
Fellow in Vascular Surgery
Hospital of the University of Pennsylvania
3400 Spruce Street
Philadelphia, Pennsylvania 19104

Patrick M. Reilly, M.D.
Assistant Professor of Surgery
Division of Trauma and Critical Care
Hospital of the University of Pennsylvania
3400 Spruce Street
Philadelphia, Pennsylvania 19104

G. Timothy Reiter, M.D.
Resident in Neurological Surgery
Hospital of the University of Pennsylvania
3400 Spruce Street
Philadelphia, Pennsylvania 19104

Michael B. Rodricks, M.D.
Fellow in Anesthesia, Critical Care Medicine
Hospital of the University of Pennsylvania
3400 Spruce Street
Philadelphia, Pennsylvania 19104

John L. Rombeau, M.D.
Professor of Surgery
Hospital of the University of Pennsylvania
3400 Spruce Street
Philadelphia, Pennsylvania 19104

Ernest F. Rosato, M.D.
Profesor of Surgery
Chief, Gastrointestinal Surgery
Hospital of the University of Pennsylvania
3400 Spruce Street
Philadelphia, Pennsylvania 19104

Bruce R. Rosengard, M.D.
Assistant Professor of Surgery
Division of Cardiothoracic Surgery
Hospital of the University of Pennsylvania
3400 Spruce Street
Philadelphia, Pennsylvania 19104

Sally Y. Segel, M.D.
Fellow in Maternal-Fetal Medicine
Hospital of the University of Pennsylvania
3400 Spruce Street
Philadelphia, Pennsylvania 19104

Joseph B. Shrager, M.D.
Assistant Professor of Surgery
Section of Thoracic Surgery
Hospital of the University of Pennsylvania
3400 Spruce Street
Philadelphia, Pennsylvania 19104

Howard K. Song, M.D.
Resident in Surgery
Hospital of the University of Pennsylvania
3400 Spruce Street
Philadelphia, Pennsylvania 19104

Francis R. Spitz, M.D.
Assistant Professor of Surgery
Hospital of the University of Pennsylvania
3400 Spruce Street
Philadelphia, Pennsylvania 19104

Rudolf N. Staroscik, M.D., M.S.C.E.
Assistant Professor of Surgery
Hospital of the University of Pennsylvania
3400 Spruce Street
Philadelphia, Pennsylvania 19104

Allan S. Stewart, M.D.
Resident in Surgery
Hospital of the University of Pennsylvania
3400 Spruce Street
Philadelphia, Pennsylvania 19104

Wilson Y. Szeto, M.D.
Resident in Surgery
Hospital of the University of Pennsylvania
3400 Spruce Street
Philadelphia, Pennsylvania 19104

Keith N. Van Arsdalen, M.D.
Professor of Urology
Hospital of the University of Pennsylvania
3400 Spruce Street
Philadelphia, Pennsylvania 19104

Steven J. Wall, M.D., Ph.D.
Resident in Otorhinolaryngology, Head and
    Neck Surgery
Hospital of the University of Pennsylvania
3400 Spruce Street
Philadelphia, Pennsylvania 19104

Noel N. Williams, M.D.
Assistant Professor of Surgery
Hospital of the University of Pennsylvania
3400 Spruce Street
Philadelphia, Pennsylvania 19104

Edward Y. Woo, M.D.
Resident in Surgery
Hospital of the University of Pennsylvania
3400 Spruce Street
Philadelphia, Pennsylvania 19104

George Yeh, M.D.
Resident in Orthopaedic Surgery
Hospital of the University of Pennsylvania
3400 Spruce Street
Philadelphia, Pennsylvania 19104

Foreword

This book represents the culmination of a resident-initiated effort. Dan Kreisel and Sasha Krupnick came to me with the idea for this book, having recognized that no single source existed for review and preparation for the Surgery In-Training examination. Despite the fact that the Residency Review Committee mandates a course in surgical basic science, tremendous variation exists in the quality and scope of these courses. *The Surgical Review*, organized based on the format of the American Board of Surgery In-Training examination, can serve as the basis for the academic portion of the Surgery Residency. Each chapter has been prepared by a resident and a University of Pennsylvania faculty member to summarize the knowledge underlying each aspect of the surgical curriculum. As I read through the chapters, in my role as Executive Editor of the book, I was struck by their outstanding readability. The depth and breadth of the material covered in the book should also prove useful for practicing surgeons who wish to review for the Recertification Examination in Surgery.

I would be remiss in not pointing out the incredible effort put forth by Lisa McAllister and Alexandra Anderson at Lippincott Williams & Wilkins. My colleagues and I are extremely grateful for all they have done to make this book a reality. Finally, I would like to recognize Dr. Clyde F. Barker, the Chairman of Surgery at the University of Pennsylvania for the last 18 years, who has been a guiding force for countless residents and medical students and whose efforts have allowed the department to become one of the finest in the world. Dr. Barker continues to serve as an outstanding role model to all who are involved in academic surgery: an outstanding researcher, clinician, and educator.

Larry R. Kaiser, M.D.
Philadelphia

Preface

Approximately 8,000 surgical residents take the American Board of Surgery In-Training/Surgical Basic Science Examination (ABSITE), and 1,300 general surgeons prepare for the written American Board of Surgery examination every year. Despite these numbers, no single study guide has been available that covers the broad basic science and clinical knowledge base required to complete these examinations successfully. Studying for these tests has always been an arduous and frustrating task, requiring an extensive review of both basic and clinical science in a limited amount of time; as well as the surgical subspecialties that are heavily emphasized on the ABSITE. Such information may be unknown to a general surgeon and usually is not included in the standard general surgery teaching curriculum. Junior residents and interns in general surgery who have never taken the In-Service Examination usually express the frustration of not knowing the specific areas on which they need to concentrate.

The Surgical Review addresses this frustration by presenting a complete compilation of surgical basic science and clinical knowledge required to prepare successfully for the American Board of Surgery In-Service Training Examination and the Surgical Board Exam. The book is organized based on the format of the ABSITE: basic science and clinical aspects of general surgery, as well as surgical subspecialties, are covered in a concise and comprehensive manner. Each chapter is written by a senior resident who has taken the In-Service Examination numerous times, and by a University of Pennsylvania faculty member considered an expert in the field.

Each chapter presents a topic in an easy-to-read, "predigested" format so that even the busiest surgical resident or intern can prepare for the In-Service Examination within one or two months simply by reading one chapter per day, or every other day. Although *The Surgical Review* is a comprehensive text and is meant to be read from cover to cover, those wishing to do so can focus on only specific topics. Because the knowledge base covered in this book represents all surgery-based examinations, it offers the ideal review opportunity for practicing physicians recertifying in general surgery, as well as for senior medical students studying for the USMLE.

We thank Lisa McAllister and Alexandra Anderson at Lippincott Williams & Wilkins for their tremendous effort and assistance during the process of writing this book. We also thank Dr. Clyde Barker, who has exerted tremendous effort to foster an academic environment at the University of Pennsylvania, and Dr. Larry Kaiser, who serves as a role model for a new generation of academic surgeons. Their enthusiasm and dedication to resident education have made this project possible.

Daniel Kreisel, M.D.
Alexander S. Krupnick, M.D.

THE SURGICAL REVIEW
AN INTEGRATED BASIC AND CLINICAL SCIENCE STUDY GUIDE

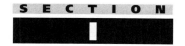

BODY AS A WHOLE

1

NEUROSURGERY

G. TIMOTHY REITER AND KEVIN D. JUDY

In the beginning of the 20th century most neurosurgical procedures were still performed by the general surgeon. Harvey Cushing first recognized the need for a surgeon dedicated solely to this field and defined neurosurgery as a distinct subspecialty. Although the broad knowledge base of neuroanatomy, neurophysiology, and neuropathophysiology necessary for a complete understanding of this field is constantly evolving, familiarity with these concepts is a must for all physicians.

MICROSCOPIC ANATOMY

The central nervous system (CNS) is composed of neurons and supporting neuroglial cells. The *neuron* is the functional unit in the CNS. It has a cell body, one axon, and multiple dendrites. The *axon* carries an impulse away from the cell body. A bundle of axons is a nerve fiber. *Dendrites* are neuronal cell processes that carry impulses to the cell body.

Neuroglial cells, such as astrocytes, oligodendrocytes, ependymocytes, and microglia, surround and support the neurons. *Astrocytes* contain gliofilaments made of glial fibrous acidic protein. These filaments are rigid and provide physical support to the CNS. Astrocytes have foot processes that surround capillaries and contribute to the blood–brain barrier (BBB). *Gliosis* is the overgrowth of the cytoplasmic processes of astrocytes in an injured area of the CNS, similar to a scar. *Oligodendrocytes* produce and maintain myelin in the CNS, while in the peripheral nervous system (PNS), *Schwann cells* produce and maintain myelin. Each oligodendrocyte can myelinate many axons in the CNS; however, each Schwann cell can only myelinate one axon in the PNS. *Ependymocytes* form the simple cuboidal epithelial lining of the ventricular system. Resting *microglial cells* are present within gray and white matter of the CNS and are analogous to the resident macrophages found in other tissues of the body. They are able to transform into phagocytic cells within the CNS. A mass of neuronal cell bodies and supporting glial cells is referred to as *gray matter*. Many axons traveling together with their supporting glial cells are called *white matter*.

The BBB is primarily formed at the level of the capillaries. It consists of three layers: the vascular endothelium with tight junctions between cells, a basal lamina, and the perivascular foot processes of astrocytes that encircle the capillaries. The functional component of the BBB is the tight junctions between the endothelial cells, which impede many substances from moving into the CNS from the bloodstream. Substances can cross the BBB by diffusion, carrier-mediated transport, or energy requiring active transport. With disease and after injury, the BBB can break down, making it more permeable. The neurohypophysis (posterior pituitary), median eminence, pineal gland, organum vasculosum of the lamina terminalis, subfornical organ, subcommissural organ, and area postrema all lack a BBB and are called the *circumventricular organs*.

Action potentials (APs) are signals transmitted along axons. In the resting state, the inside of the neuron has a net negative charge, while the extracellular fluid has a net positive charge. This creates an electrical gradient across the cell membrane, which normally equals -70 mV and is called the *resting membrane potential*. It is produced by the sodium pump, which actively transports potassium into the cell and sodium out of the cell using one molecule of adenosine triphosphate (ATP) for every three sodium ions exchanged. This produces a high intracellular concentration of potassium compared to the extracellular fluid and a high extracellular concentration of sodium compared to the intracellular fluid. Excitation of the neuron may be due to chemical or mechanical stimuli. At a certain threshold, voltage-gated sodium channels are opened and an AP is initiated by the large influx of sodium into the cell. Sodium moves into the cell down its concentration and electrical gradient. This process is termed *depolarization,* because the membrane potential becomes positive. The AP is transmitted down the axon by the sequential depolarization of the membrane. Myelin encircles some of the axons and acts like an insulator around an electric wire. The voltage-gated sodium channels are only located at intermittent gaps in the myelin sheath called *nodes of Ranvier*. This lets the AP propagate much faster down the axon and is referred to as a saltatory conduction. A myelinated axon can conduct an AP at a rate of up to 120 m per second, while an unmyelinated axon can conduct an AP at a rate of up to only 2 m per second.

Neurons communicate with one another through synapses, which are the gaps between the end bulb of the axon of one neuron and the cell body of another neuron. Most synapses in humans are chemical synapses. *Chemical synapses* have neurotransmitters stored in synaptic vesicles located at the end bulbs of axons. Neurotransmitters are released from the presynaptic membrane and travel across the gap to the postsynaptic membrane where they bind to receptors. If an excitatory neurotransmitter binds to a receptor on the postsynaptic membrane, the membrane potential becomes less negative. If enough excitatory neurotransmitters bind to the postsynaptic membrane, it reaches its threshold, and it is depolarized producing an AP. If an inhibitory neurotransmitter is released and binds to a receptor on the postsynaptic membrane, the membrane potential becomes more negative, called *hyperpolarization*. It is more difficult to generate an AP in a hyperpolarized neuron.

ANATOMY

The scalp consists of five layers. From superficial to deep, there is the skin, then a layer of connective tissue. Underneath the connective tissue is the galea aponeurotica (galea). The large blood vessels of the scalp are located in the connective tissue layer just above the galea. With lacerations through the galea, it retracts, which decreases the bleeding from these vessels. When surgically repairing the scalp, a deep layer of sutures is needed to approximate the galea. Below the galea is a layer of loose connective tissue and below that is the periosteum of the skull. A subgaleal hematoma forms from bleeding into the loose connective tissue layer underneath the galea and most commonly occurs in children after traumatic injuries.

The skull is a protective bony case for the brain. It is composed of multiple bones including the frontal, nasal, lacrimal, parietal, sphenoid, temporal, ethmoid, and occipital. The junction between the frontal and parietal bones is the coronal suture, the junction between the two parietal bones is the sagittal suture, and the junction between the parietal and occipital bones is the lambdoid suture. The pterion is the area where the frontal, parietal, temporal, and sphenoid bones come together on the side of the skull forming an *H*.

The spinal cord is surrounded by the bony vertebral column. There are seven cervical vertebrae, twelve thoracic vertebrae, five lumbar vertebrae, five sacral vertebrae, which are fused, and four coccygeal vertebrae, which are also fused. This makes a total of 33 vertebrae (Fig. 1-1). Each

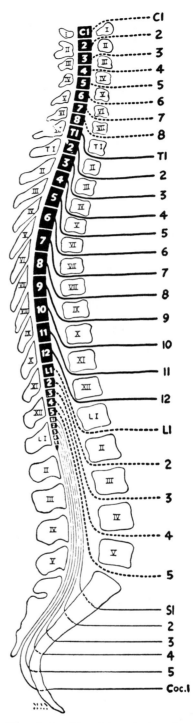

FIGURE 1-1. The relationship of the spinal cord segments to the vertebrae and spinal roots to the intervertebral foramina. (From Carpenter, Sutin. *Human neuroanatomy*. Baltimore: Williams & Wilkins, 1983, with permission.)

vertebra, except C-1, has a body, paired pedicles, paired transverse processes, paired laminae, and a spinous process. C-1 through C-6 have bilateral transverse foramina through which the vertebral arteries pass. C-1 is called the *atlas* and C-2 is called the *axis*. The odontoid process, also called the *dens,* is a superiorly projecting process that comes off the body of the axis. It articulates with the atlas and allows for rotation of the head. Between the vertebral bodies are intervertebral disks. They consist of a fibrous outer ring, called the *annulus fibrosis,* and an inner elastic portion, called the *nucleus pulposus.* The disk has a limited blood supply, often making it a nidus for infectious processes. Most rotation occurs in the upper cervical and lumbar spine while most flexion and extension occurs in the lower cervical and lumbar spine.

The meninges form a cover over the brain and spinal cord and consist of three layers: the dura matter, the arachnoid membrane, and the pia matter. The dura matter is the outermost layer and is composed of two layers around the brain, but only one layer around the spinal cord. Around the brain, there is an outer periosteal layer and inner meningeal layer of dura, which mostly lie adjacent to each other but separate at certain locations to form the venous dural sinuses. The meningeal layer of the dura has several reflections that form partitions. These include the *falx cerebri,* which separates the cerebral hemispheres, the tentorium cerebelli (tentorium), which separates the occipital lobe and temporal lobe from the cerebellum and brainstem, the diaphragma sellae through which the pituitary stalk passes, and the falx cerebelli, which separates the hemispheres of the cerebellum.

Inside the dura is the thin, delicate arachnoid membrane, which for the most part follows the inner dural surface. Between the dura matter and arachnoid membrane is the subdural space. Inside the arachnoid membrane is the pia matter, which lies on the surface of the brain and spinal cord. Between the arachnoid membrane and the pia matter is the subarachnoid space. At the base of the brain, these spaces are substantial, are filled with cerebrospinal fluid (CSF), are called the *basal cisterns,* and on computed tomography (CT) of the brain are seen surrounding the brainstem. Major arteries, including the circle of Willis, are located in the subarachnoid space. The arachnoid membrane and pia matter collectively are called the *leptomeninges.*

The right and left cerebral hemispheres consist of gray matter on the surface of the gyri, white matter below the gyri, and deep central neuronal masses called the *basal ganglia.* On the cerebral surface are multiple gyri and sulci. Each hemisphere is divided into a frontal, parietal, temporal, and occipital lobe. The central sulcus (of Rolando) separates the frontal lobe from the parietal lobe. The lateral fissure (of Sylvius) separates the temporal lobe from the frontal and parietal lobes (Fig. 1-2). The parieto-occipital sulcus, seen on the medial surface of the hemisphere, separates the parietal lobe from the occipital lobe. The lobes of the brain are located in different fossae. The anterior cranial fossa contains the frontal lobes. The middle cranial fossa

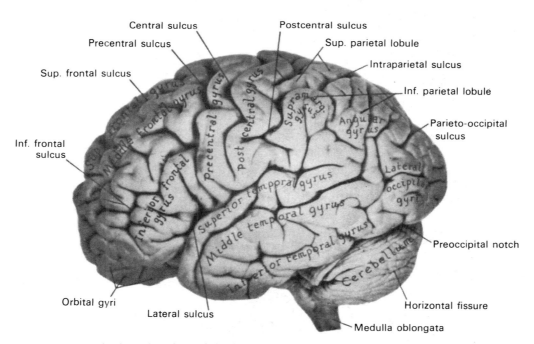

FIGURE 1-2. The lateral surface of the brain. (From Carpenter, Sutin. *Human neuroanatomy.* Baltimore: Williams & Wilkins, 1983, with permission.)

contains the temporal lobe. The posterior cranial fossa contains the cerebellum and the brainstem. Specific functions can be assigned to different lobes of the brain. The frontal lobes are involved in personality, emotion, and the planning and execution of movement. The parietal lobes process sensory information. The occipital lobes are concerned with vision. The dominant temporal lobe (usually the left side) contains the language areas of the brain. The basal ganglia is comprised of the caudate nucleus, the putamen, the globus pallidus, and the amygdaloid nuclear complex. The caudate, putamen, and globus pallidus are called the *corpus striatum* and they play an important role in the motor system. The putamen and globus pallidus together are called the lentiform nuclei. Diseases of the basal ganglia are characterized by disorders of movement, which include involuntary movements (Huntington chorea) or the inability to initiate movements (Parkinson disease).

Blood to the brain is supplied by the paired internal carotid arteries and by the paired vertebral arteries. The vertebral arteries come together to form the basilar artery, which lies on the anterior surface of the brainstem. The internal carotid arteries and basilar artery form an anastomotic loop called the *circle of Willis*, which is located at the base of the brain just anterior to the brainstem. Each internal carotid artery bifurcates into an anterior cerebral artery and a middle cerebral artery. The basilar artery bifurcates into the paired posterior cerebral arteries. Communicating arteries join the carotid and basilar arteries to form the circle of Willis. The anterior communicating artery connects the left and right anterior cerebral arteries. The paired posterior communicating arteries join the internal carotid artery to the posterior cerebral artery on the same side (Fig. 1-3). The internal carotid arteries and their branches supply the frontal, parietal, and most of the temporal lobes. The basilar artery and its branches supply the brainstem, the cerebellum, the occipital lobes, and the inferior temporal lobes. Eighty percent of the blood flow to the brain is supplied by the internal carotid arteries.

The *venous anatomy* of the brain consists of a deep and a superficial system of drainage. The superficial system is composed of superficial veins on the convexity of the cortex, which drain into the superior sagittal sinus. The deep system drains into the internal cerebral veins, which join to form the great cerebral vein (of Galen). It becomes the straight (rectus) sinus, which runs along the midline of the tentorium. The systems meet at the confluens sinuum (Torcular herophili), where the superior sagittal sinus joins the rectus sinus. The paired transverse sinuses carry blood from the confluens sinuum to the sigmoid sinuses, which become the internal jugular veins (Fig. 1-4).

Within the brain are CSF-filled spaces called *ventricles*. There are a pair of lateral ventricles, a midline third ventricle, and a midline fourth ventricle. Each lateral ventricle connects to the third ventricle through the interventricular

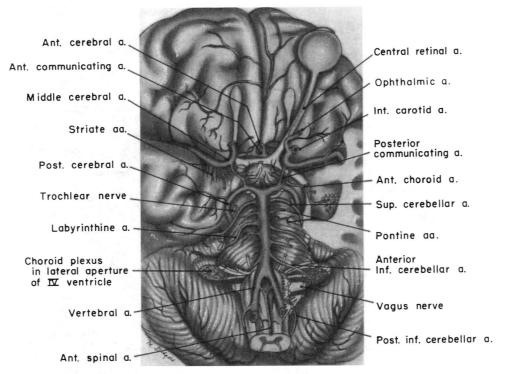

FIGURE 1-3. The ventral surface of the brain illustrating the arterial anatomy. (From Carpenter. *Core text of neuroanatomy.* Baltimore: Williams & Wilkins, 1991, with permission.)

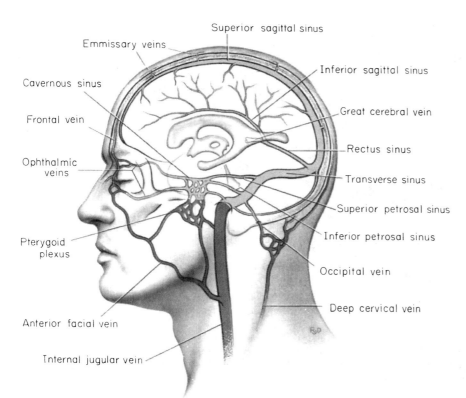

FIGURE 1-4. The venous drainage of the brain. (From Carpenter. *Core text of neuroanatomy.* Baltimore: Williams & Wilkins, 1991, with permission.)

foramen (of Monro). The third ventricle connects to the fourth ventricle through the cerebral (sylvian) aqueduct. The fourth ventricle connects to the subarachnoid space around the brainstem by the midline foramen of Magendie and the paired lateral foramina of Luschka. CSF is produced by the choroid plexus, which is found in all of the ventricles. In general, the flow of CSF goes from the lateral ventricles to the third ventricle and then to the fourth ventricle. From here, it enters the subarachnoid space surrounding the brain and the spinal cord (Fig. 1-5). CSF passes from the subarachnoid space to the venous system through the arachnoid villi (granulations), which are located in the walls of the dural sinuses. This is a dynamic system in that the choroid plexus makes about 500 mL of CSF per day, but only about 150 mL of CSF is present within the CNS at one moment.

The cerebellum is located dorsal to the brainstem and below the tentorium in the posterior fossa. It is divided into a midline portion called the *vermis* and two lateral hemispheres. It has three paired connections to the brainstem: the superior cerebellar peduncles go to the midbrain, the middle cerebellar peduncles go to the pons, and the inferior cerebellar peduncles go to the medulla. The paired deep cerebellar nuclei lie within the cerebellar white matter. From medial to lateral, they are the fastigial, globose, emboliform, and dentate nuclei.

The brainstem is divided into four parts (Fig. 1-6). From rostral to caudal, these are the diencephalon, the midbrain (mesencephalon), the pons (metencephalon), and the medulla oblongata (myelencephalon). The largest subdivision of the diencephalon is the thalamus. Both sensory input to the cerebrum and motor output from the cerebrum pass through the thalamus. The midbrain is the smallest division of the brainstem. It is divided into the tectum, the tegmentum, and the crura cerebri. The substantia nigra lies between the crura cerebri and the tegmentum and has efferent and afferent connections with the basal ganglia. Loss of dopaminergic neurons in the substantia nigra is seen in Parkinson disease. The pons consists of a large ventral part containing descending motor fibers and the pontine nuclei that project to the cerebellum via the middle cerebellar peduncle and a smaller dorsal portion in which the pontine reticular formation and various cranial nerve nuclei are located. Anteriorly, the basilar artery runs on the surface of the pons in the basilar sulcus. The medulla is the most caudal portion of the brainstem, which inferiorly becomes the spinal cord. It can be divided into the dorsal medullary reticular formation, which is associated with arousal and wakefulness, and the ventral medullary pyramids, which contain the motor output from the cerebrum. Dorsal to the medulla and the pons lies the fourth ventricle.

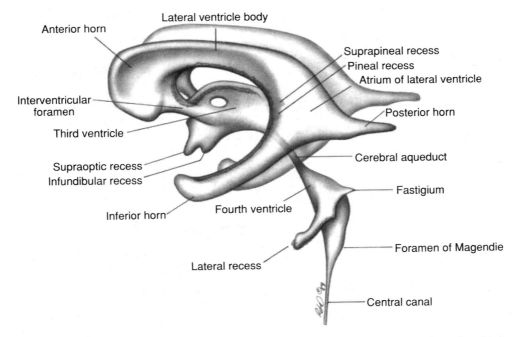

FIGURE 1-5. The ventricular system of the brain. Cerebrospinal fluid flow is from lateral to third to fourth ventricle. (From Carpenter. *Core text of neuroanatomy*. Baltimore: Williams & Wilkins, 1991, with permission.)

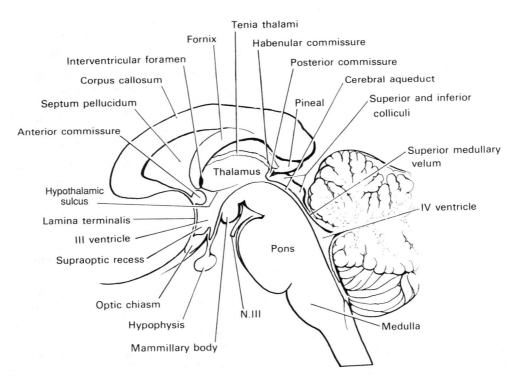

FIGURE 1-6. The brainstem in a midsagittal section. (From Carpenter, Sutin. *Human neurosanatomy*. Baltimore: Williams & Wilkins, 1983, with permission.)

At the base of the brain, anterior to the brainstem, and just posterior to the optic chiasm is the *hypophysis* (pituitary gland). The *infundibulum* (stalk of the hypophysis) descends from the inferior surface of the hypothalamus, passes through the *diaphragma sellae* (a dural reflection with a hole in the middle), and enters the *sella turcica,* where it becomes the hypophysis. The hypophysis is divided into an anterior and a posterior lobe. The hypothalamus communicates with the *adenohypophysis* (anterior lobe) by a portal system of blood vessels. Adrenocorticotropic hormone (ACTH), thyrotropin, prolactin, growth hormone, follicle-stimulating hormone, and luteinizing hormone are produced in the adenohypophysis and released into the bloodstream under the control of releasing hormones from the hypothalamus. The hypothalamus also contains neurons that project axons to the neurohypophysis (posterior hypophysis). These axons transport hormones, such as antidiuretic hormone (vasopressin) and oxytocin, which are made in the hypothalamus, to the posterior hypophysis, where they are released into the bloodstream (Fig. 1-7).

The spinal cord is the continuation of the brainstem as it passes through the foramen magnum and the cord ends as the conus medullaris around the L-1 vertebral body. The spinal cord and bony spinal column start out the same length, but during development, the bony spinal column outgrows the cord and the lumbar and sacral nerve roots must travel caudally in the spinal canal before they reach their respective vertebral body and exit to the periphery. The collection of spinal roots that travel inferiorly within the spinal canal below the conus medullaris is called the *cauda equina.* The filum terminale is a condensation of pia matter that extends inferiorly from the conus medullaris and becomes the coccygeal ligament, which attaches to the coccyx. The thecal sac refers to the dural tube within the spinal canal. The denticulate ligaments arise laterally from the pia matter between the ventral and dorsal spinal roots and attach to the adjacent dura matter. Their function is to stabilize the spinal cord.

The spinal cord has eight pairs of cervical roots, twelve pairs of thoracic roots, five pairs of lumbar roots, five pairs of sacral roots, and one pair of coccygeal roots. The cervical roots exit over the pedicle of the same numbered vertebra, with the eighth cervical root exiting over the first thoracic pedicle. The thoracic and lumbar roots exit below the pedicle of the same numbered vertebral body (Fig. 1-1). The spinal roots leave the spinal cord as an anterolateral ventral

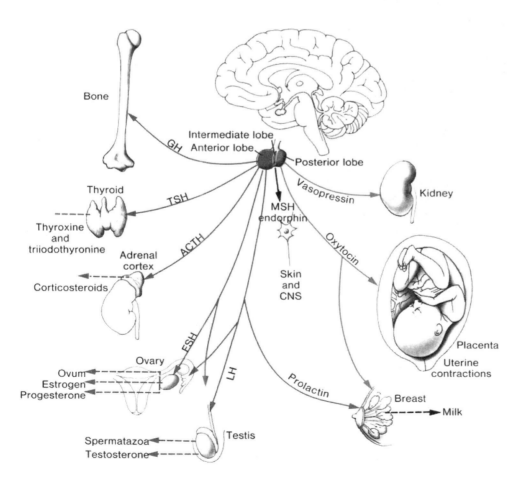

FIGURE 1-7. The actions of the pituitary hormones on their target organs. (From Carpenter, Sutin. *Human neuroanatomy.* Baltimore: Williams & Wilkins, 1983, with permission.)

root (motor) and a posterolateral dorsal root (sensory). These unite in the intervertebral (neural) foramina to form the spinal nerve. The spinal nerve is composed of afferent sensory fibers and efferent motor fibers. Sensory fibers, from the periphery, enter the spinal nerve, travel to the dorsal root ganglion located in the intervertebral foramen, become the dorsal root, and enter the spinal cord. The white matter of the spinal cord, which is mostly composed of axons, is located peripherally. Some major tracts within the spinal cord are the lateral corticospinal tract, the lateral spinothalamic tract, and the posterior columns. The centrally located anterior and posterior horns of the spinal cord contain the gray matter, which contains neuronal cell bodies.

The arterial blood supply of the spinal cord comes from the anterior and posterior spinal arteries, which are all branches of the vertebral arteries. As the anterior and posterior spinal arteries descend along the spinal cord, they receive additional feeding branches from multiple radicular arteries. In the neck, the radicular arteries are branches of the vertebral arteries and the thyrocervical trunks. In the thorax, the radicular arteries branch from the intercostal arteries, and in the low back, the radicular arteries are branches of lumbar arteries. An important radicular artery is the artery of Adamkiewicz, which usually arises on the left side between T-10 and L-2. It supplies the lower thoracic spinal cord and conus medullaris (Fig. 1-8). Damage to the arterial system of the spinal cord causes ischemia of the spinal cord and results in a stroke, which may cause paralysis, sensory loss, or loss of bowel and bladder function. A spinal cord stroke may occur during the repair of a thoracic or abdominal aortic aneurysm if a radicular artery, which feeds the spinal cord, is compromised. A strategy to avoid spinal cord ischemia includes the preoperative placement of a lumbar drain to decrease the intraspinal pressure and therefore increase intraspinal blood flow during the procedure.

FUNCTIONAL ORGANIZATION

The motor system is located anteriorly or ventrally in most parts of the CNS and it is composed of efferent fibers that carry impulses from the CNS to the periphery. The upper motor neuron (UMN) is a pyramidal neuron with its cell body in the precentral gyrus of the frontal lobe. The *motor homunculus* is a representation of the body in the primary motor area located in the precentral gyrus (Fig. 1-9). The axon of the UMN travels through the genu (muscles of the face) or posterior limb (muscles of the body) of the internal

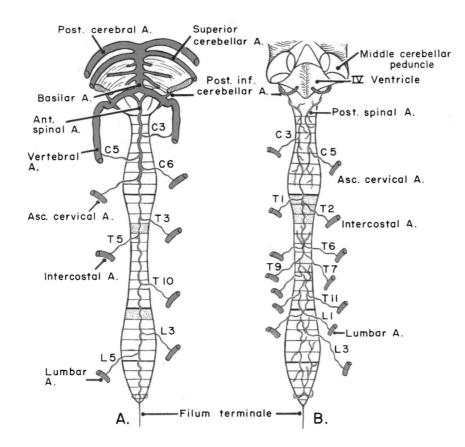

FIGURE 1-8. The arterial supply to the spinal cord. The watershed zones are stippled. A, anterior view; B, posterior view. (From Carpenter. *Core text of neuroanatomy.* Baltimore: Williams & Wilkins, 1991, with permission.)

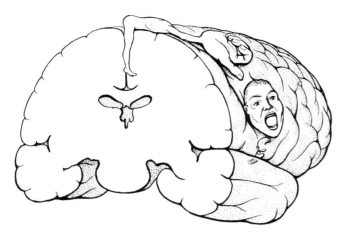

FIGURE 1-9. The sensory or motor homunculus. The representation of the body in the precentral (motor) or postcentral (sensory) gyri. (From Carpenter. *Core text of neuroanatomy.* Baltimore: Williams & Wilkins, 1991, with permission.)

capsule, down the crura cerebri, through the medullary pyramids, where the axon crosses over to the contralateral side (decussation of the pyramids), and finally down the lateral corticospinal tract in the spinal cord. The UMN axon synapses on the lower motor neuron (LMN) cell body (anterior horn cell) in the anterior horn of the spinal cord. The LMN sends its axon ipsilaterally to the motor end plate of the muscle it innervates. The ventral roots of the spinal cord are composed of LMN axons. If a UMN is damaged, its inhibitory effect on the LMN is lost and the LMN becomes hyperactive, resulting in a spastic paralysis. When the LMN is damaged, the muscle loses its innervation, resulting in a flaccid paralysis.

The sensory system is located, for the most part, in the posterior or dorsal portion of the CNS. It is composed of afferent fibers, which carry information from peripheral receptors to the CNS. The postcentral gyrus, within the parietal lobe, contains the primary somesthetic areas. The secondary somesthetic areas lie adjacent to the primary areas. The sensory homunculus is a representation of the body in the somatosensory cortex (Fig. 1-9). The cortical sensory areas receive input from the ventral posterior nuclei of the thalamus, which relays impulses from the posterior columns, spinothalamic tract (body), and trigeminothalamic tract (face). The paired posterior columns contain afferent fibers that transmit information regarding kinesthetic sense (position and movement) and tactile sense (touch and pressure). In the spinal cord, the posterior columns are divided into the fasciculus gracilis, which contains afferent fibers from the leg, and the fasciculus cuneatus, which contains afferent fibers from the arm. The fibers of the posterior columns enter the spinal cord and ascend, without crossing the midline, to the nucleus cuneatus and nucleus gracilis, both of which are located in the medulla. Fibers from the nucleus cuneatus and nucleus gracilis cross the midline in the medulla and ascend in the contralateral medial lemniscus to the thalamus. The paired lateral spinothalamic tracts are formed by afferent pain and temperature fibers from peripheral receptors. These fibers synapse in the dorsal root ganglia and then enter the spinal cord as the dorsal roots. The lateral spinothalamic tract crosses in the anterior white commissure of the spinal cord within two to three levels after entering the cord and ascends in the contralateral half of the spinal cord. The trigeminothalamic tract carries pain and temperature fibers from receptors in the face.

The input to the visual system is light entering the eye. The image of an object is represented on the retina upside down and backwards. Therefore, the superior temporal (lateral) visual field of one eye is represented on the inferior nasal (medial) portion of the retina of the same eye. The retinal fibers travel in the optic nerves (cranial nerve II) to the optic chiasm. Here, the fibers from temporal halves of visual fields (the nasal halves of the retinas) cross, but the fibers from the nasal halves of the visual fields (temporal half of the retina) do not cross. The fibers then leave the chiasm and form the optic tracts. The temporal half of the visual field of one eye and the nasal half of the visual field of the other eye travel together in one optic tract. In other words, the left half of the visual field of both eyes is in the right optic tract and the right half of the visual field of both eyes is in the left optic tract. The optic tracts travel to the lateral geniculate bodies of the thalamus. The optic radiations leave the thalamus and travel to the occipital lobes. The primary visual area is in the calcarine sulcus of the occipital lobe. Stereoscopic vision first occurs in the occipital cortex. In general, only lesions between the retina and the chiasm can produce a unilateral visual loss. Lesions between the chiasm and the occipital lobes produce ipsilateral visual-field deficits in both eyes, called a *homonymous hemianopsia*. The closer the lesion is to the occipital lobe, the more congruent are the field cuts of the homonymous hemianopsia (Fig. 1-10).

Other brainstem structures concerned with vision include the superior colliculus and the Edinger-Westphal nucleus. The superior colliculus receives visual input from the retina and sends impulses indirectly to the motor neurons of the upper spinal cord (*tectospinal tract*) involved in reflex head and neck movements initiated by visual stimuli. The Edinger-Westphal nucleus supplies the parasympathetic fibers to the constrictor muscle fibers in the iris. The sympathetic fibers to the dilator muscle fibers in the iris come from the superior cervical ganglion. The movement of the eyes are controlled by the extraocular muscles. The oculomotor nerve (cranial nerve III) innervates the superior rectus, the medial rectus, the inferior rectus, the inferior oblique, and the levator palpebrae muscles. It carries parasympathetic fibers to the ciliary muscle and the sphincter muscle of the pupil. The trochlear nerve (cranial

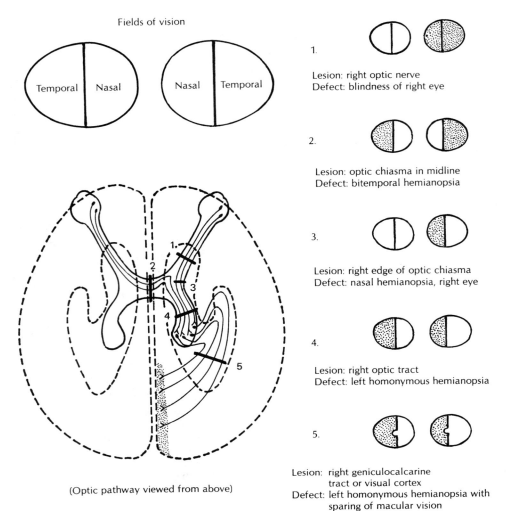

FIGURE 1-10. Visual deficits caused by lesions at different points along the visual pathway. (From Barr and Kiernan. *The Human Nervous System.* Philadelphia: JB Lippincott Co, 1993, with permission.)

nerve IV) supplies the superior oblique muscle. The abducens nerve (cranial nerve VI) supplies the lateral rectus muscle.

The input to the auditory system is sound that travels as a wave to the ear. The sound wave causes movement of the tympanic membrane, which transmits the impulse to the bones in the middle ear (malleus, incus, and stapes). The impulse is converted to a fluid wave in the perilymph of the cochlea. Hair cells in the cochlea transform the fluid wave into an electrical impulse that travels down the cochlear nerve (a division of cranial nerve VIII). In the brainstem, the cochlear nerve fibers synapse in the inferior colliculus. From here, projections go to the medial geniculate body of the thalamus and then to the transverse gyrus of Heschl located in the temporal lobe. Each temporal lobe receives input from both ears.

The language areas of the brain are involved in the comprehension and production of speech. The area involved in comprehension of speech is the *Wernicke area,* which is an auditory area located in the temporal lobe of the dominant hemisphere. The area involved in production of speech is the *Broca area,* which is a motor area in the frontal lobe of the dominant hemisphere. Named patterns of aphasia include Wernicke aphasia, Broca aphasia, global aphasia, and conduction aphasia. *Wernicke aphasia* is a problem with the comprehension of speech. The patient can speak fluently, but the sentences produced have no meaning and do not make sense. *Broca aphasia* is a motor aphasia in which the patient can comprehend speech but cannot produce speech and is not fluent. The speech muscles are not paralyzed, but they cannot be coordinated to produce meaningful speech (apraxia). A *global aphasia* is a lesion destroying almost all of the language areas, leaving patients unable to speak, comprehend, read, write, or repeat what is said to them. A *conduction aphasia* is when the connection between Broca and Wernicke areas is disrupted. The most striking feature of a conduction aphasia is the difficulty patients have repeating what is said to them.

The autonomic nervous system (ANS) is divided into the sympathetic nervous system and the parasympathetic nervous system. The fibers of the autonomic nervous system run in the lateral portions of the spinal cord. The sympathetic and the parasympathetic nervous systems both innervate smooth muscle, cardiac muscle, and numerous glands in the body. The *sympathetic nervous system* is a global activating system concerned with fight or flight reactions, and the *parasympathetic nervous system* is a more precise regulator of bodily functions and homeostasis. The ANS is not under voluntary control and its input is not required for the viscera to function. Both these systems are able to change the activity of the viscera and carry sensory information from the viscera to the CNS.

NEURORADIOLOGY

Plain x-rays, CT, and magnetic resonance imaging (MRI) are frequently used diagnostic studies in neurosurgery. Anteroposterior, lateral, and oblique plain films show bony detail of the skull and spinal column and can demonstrate traumatic and degenerative disease. CT is more sensitive than plain films for fractures, but CT is also more expensive and time consuming.

A *CT scan* displays a true image of CNS structures. The x-ray beam of a CT scanner is rotated around the patient's body to develop a 2-dimensional image. The various tissues of the body attenuate radiation differently, due to different tissue densities, and are assigned different values of Hounsfield units (HU), named after Godfrey Hounsfield who developed CT for clinical use. Each point (pixel) within an axial slice of the body gets a value based on its attenuation of the x-ray beam. Tissue attenuation spans between +1,000 HU, signifying total attenuation, and -1,000 HU, signifying no attenuation. Water is assigned the value of 0 HU and air is assigned the value of -1,000 HU. Fat has a value between -40 and -100 HU. White and gray matter have similar densities, with values between 30 and 50 HU. Calcified structures (bone) have values of around 150 HU.

A gray scale is used to view the images. The endpoints (black and white on the image) can be chosen anywhere between +1,000 and -1,000 HU. The width of the window is the difference between these endpoints. The window level is the center value of the chosen range. The smaller the window, the greater the difference in shades of gray between two similar HU values within that window. The drawback of a small window is that more tissue lies outside of the chosen window and that tissue is either black or white. Differently windowed images are sensitive to particular processes. Common window algorithms include brain windows, subdural windows, and bone windows. A *brain window* is a narrow window that allows differentiation of white and gray matter, even though they have similar HU values. For example, a brain window width may be chosen to be 100 HU with its center at 50 HU. This makes the endpoints of the gray scale 0 HU and 100 HU. If the difference between gray and white matter is 20 HU, this is a difference of 20% of the total window width and a 20% difference in the shade of gray between the gray and white matter. Unfortunately, bony detail is lost because it usually lies outside of this window. To see bony detail, a wider window (*bone window*) is used. A width of 2,000 HU centered at 500 HU may be chosen. White and gray matter signals are still 20 HU apart, but this is only a 1% difference in this window, making them virtually the same shade of gray. A *subdural window* is an intermediate window between brain and bone windows that helps differentiate acute blood from bone (Fig. 1-11).

When tissue attenuates very little radiation (low HU value), it is referred to as *hypodense* and appears dark gray to black on a CT image. Tissue and fluid with a high water content will be hypodense in relation to normal brain tissue on CT. Examples are areas of brain edema and the ventricu-

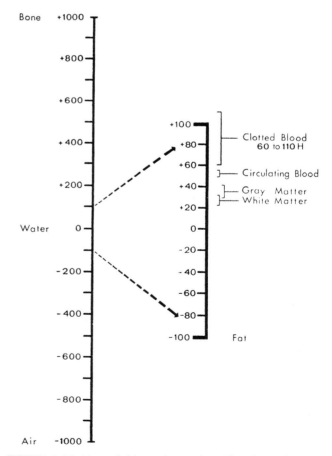

FIGURE 1-11. Hounsfield number scale with values of certain body tissues. This determines the appearance of the tissue on computed tomographic scan. (From Taveras. *Neuroradiology.* Baltimore: Williams & Wilkins, 1996, with permission.)

lar system, which is filled with CSF. Other hypodense substances are air and fat. When a tissue attenuates a significant amount of radiation (high HU value), it is referred to as *hyperdense* and appears bright or white on the CT image. Hyperdense substances include bone, acute blood, and iodinated contrast. Very dense tissue may also appear hyperdense to normal brain tissue but not as hyperdense as bone. An example is a highly cellular tumor such as a medulloblastoma.

When intravenous (i.v.) contrast is given, an area where the blood–brain barrier has broken down will appear white, which is referred to as an *area of enhancement*. Some enhancing chronic processes include tumors, infections, and abscesses. Enhancement occurs from the breakdown of the blood–brain barrier and not from increased vascularity, although contrast will opacity the lumen of a large vessel. With the correct timing, the vessels of the circle of Willis can be imaged while contrast is passing through them and reconstructed in three dimensions, which is called *CT angiography*.

CT is good for imaging acute processes necessitating an emergent neuroradiological evaluation such as a hemorrhage from a trauma, a brain tumor, a stroke, or an aneurysm and for bony pathology such as vertebral fractures. Acute hemorrhage is hyperdense to normal brain tissue on CT when viewed using brain windows. In an emergent situation, i.v. contrast is not given because acute hemorrhage can be confused with an area of enhancement. One acute process not well imaged by CT is an ischemic stroke. An infarcted area of the brain will be hypodense on CT after 6 to 12 hours. The scan is still useful in this situation to rule out a hemorrhage. When a stroke becomes hypodense on CT, it involves both the gray matter on the surface of the brain and the white matter below it. This is due to cytotoxic edema resulting in increased intracellular water and cell death. An abscess or metastatic tumor usually appears as a sharply demarcated ring-enhancing mass surrounded by white matter edema on CT. A primary brain tumor usually shows less distinct margins and irregular enhancement compared to an abscess or metastatic tumor.

MRI is another method of imaging the CNS. Tissues are described as having different intensities (CT, density; MRI, intensity). A tissue is described as *hypointense* (darker), *isointense* (the same), or *hyperintense* (brighter) to a reference tissue. MRI images can be acquired in the axial, coronal, and sagittal planes. The lumen of a large vessel will appear as a flow void (black). Different sequences are used to evaluate different tissues and processes. A T1-weighted sequence demonstrates good anatomic detail of soft tissues. With this sequence, tissue and fluid with a high water content are hypointense (edema, CSF). Fat is hyperintense. T1-weighted scans are done with and without gadolinium, an i.v. contrast agent, to look for areas where the blood–brain barrier has broken down. These areas will appear hyperintense and are referred to as *areas of enhancement*. A T2-weighted sequence is sensitive to focal changes in tissue water content, which is of value in differentiating normal brain tissue from abnormal tissue. In this sequence, tissue and fluid with a high water content are hyperintense (edema, CSF). Magnetic resonance angiography (MRA) can be used to evaluate the blood flow in the extracranial carotid arteries and in the arteries of the circle of Willis. Blood vessels are imaged in multiple planes with the surrounding soft tissue removed from the image. *Magnetic resonance venography* (MRV) is used to evaluate the blood flow in the cerebral venous sinuses.

Chronic processes not needing an emergent neuroradiological evaluation are better evaluated by MRI. These include tumors of the brain and spinal cord, congenital abnormalities, vascular malformations, degenerative disk disease of the spine, and inflammatory processes of the CNS such as multiple sclerosis. MRI is also superior in imaging soft tissue at the base of skull, which includes the sellar (pituitary) region and the posterior fossa. The enhancement patterns on MRI are similar to what is seen on CT.

Today, angiography and myelography are rarely performed in the initial diagnostic workup of a neurosurgical patient. Instead, they are used to gain additional information once the diagnosis is made. *Angiography* is used in the head, neck, and spine. It is an invasive procedure and cerebral angiography carries a risk of stroke from 0.5% to 3%. Most commonly, cerebral angiography is used to evaluate a patient with a nontraumatic subarachnoid hemorrhage (SAH) or a patient suspected of having a carotid stenosis, carotid dissection, traumatic arterial injury, arteriovenous malformation (AVM), or vasculitis. Therapeutic procedures can be performed during angiography and include the coiling of an aneurysm, the embolization of a vessel that is bleeding, the embolization of a vessel that is pathologic (e.g., a feeding artery of an AVM), the thrombolysis of an acute ischemic stroke, and the stenting of a carotid stenosis.

Myelography of the spine is an invasive procedure that is used less often today, because MRI has become the primary mode of imaging the spinal cord. CT has enhanced the utility of myelography by adding axial images obtained in a postmyelogram CT. There are still occasions when a myelogram can add important information by showing excellent detail of spinal column anatomy in relation to the outline of the spinal cord and roots within the thecal sac. Two clinical situations when myelography is useful include diffuse disease of the subarachnoid space, such as tumor seeding and arachnoiditis, and a complex spinal case in which the patient has had previous surgery or has had a nondiagnostic CT and MRI.

BASIC PROCEDURES

Basic intracranial procedures include burr holes, intracranial pressure (ICP) monitoring, ventriculostomy, stereotactic biopsy, craniectomy, craniotomy, and insertion of a ventriculoperitoneal shunt. *Burr holes* are drilled in the skull to gain access to the epidural and subdural space and are used as a starting point for a craniectomy or craniotomy. They are also used to drain chronic subdural hematomas (SDHs). An *ICP monitor* (bolt) is passed through a hole in the skull into the subarachnoid space, subdural space, epidural space, or into the substance of the brain. It can measure the ICP and record the ICP waveform, but it cannot be used to drain CSF. A *ventriculostomy* is a catheter placed through a hole in the skull, through the brain, and into the ventricular system. It can be used to measure the ICP, record the ICP waveform, and therapeutically drain CSF to lower the ICP. A *stereotactic biopsy* can be done under CT or MRI guidance. It can be used to obtain tissue diagnosis in a patient with an unresectable intracranial mass or masses or for drainage of a brain abscess. A *craniectomy* is performed by removing a portion of bone to gain intracranial access and not replacing that piece of bone at the end of the operation. A *craniectomy* may be performed to relieve elevated intracranial pressure in a case of traumatic head injury with severe brain swelling. Leaving the bone off gives the brain room to expand. A *craniotomy* is performed by removing a portion of the skull to gain intracranial access and replacing that portion of bone at the end of the operation. A *ventriculoperitoneal shunt* is a catheter that connects the ventricular system to the peritoneal cavity. The flow of CSF in the shunt is regulated by a pressure-responsive one-way valve. Flow of CSF is only allowed to go from the ventricle to the peritoneum. A shunt is used to treat hydrocephalus.

Basic spinal procedures include posterior and anterior approaches. The posterior approaches provide access to the dorsal and lateral aspects of the thecal sac and include laminectomy and microdiskectomy. A *laminectomy* is done through a midline incision in the back parallel to the spinal axis. The lamina are exposed and then removed to expose the posterior aspect of the thecal sac. A *microdiskectomy* is done for a ruptured lumbar disk. The ruptured disk is approached from a small midline incision on the back. A portion of the lamina on the side of the ruptured disk usually needs to be removed to gain access to the space around the thecal sac where the fragment of disk is located. An anterior approach to the spine provides exposure of the vertebral bodies, intervertebral disks, and anterior aspect of the thecal sac. Removal of the entire vertebral body, called a *corpectomy*, can be done from an anterior approach in the cervical, thoracic, and lumbar spine. An *anterior cervical diskectomy* is the removal of an intervertebral disk in the cervical spine. Discectomies in the thoracic and lumbar spine can also be accomplished with an anterior approach. After removal of a vertebral body and disk, a piece of bone, usually fibula or iliac crest, is placed in the defect, which is referred to as a *fusion*.

ABNORMALITIES OF THE CSF SPACES

Hydrocephalus is an increase in the total amount of CSF in the ventricular system resulting either from the restriction of the bulk flow of CSF or from the overproduction of CSF. As a result, the ventricular system dilates and the ICP increases. When the bulk flow of CSF is disturbed, either noncommunicating or communicating hydrocephalus results. Noncommunicating, also called *internal* or *obstructive*, hydrocephalus results from an obstruction within one of the ventricles, the foramen, or the aqueduct. The ventricular system proximal to the obstruction becomes dilated. Most frequently, the obstruction occurs where the ventricular system is narrow, such as in the aqueduct of Sylvius, the foramina of Monro, or the outlets of the fourth ventricle (the foramina of Luschka and Magendie). Obstructions are created by tumors, intraventricular clots, parasites, and various other mass lesions. Communicating hydrocephalus, also referred to as *external hydrocephalus*, results when there is an impediment to CSF flow in the subarachnoid space, a failure of adequate resorption of CSF, or the overproduction of CSF. Dilation of the entire ventricular system occurs. Communicating hydrocephalus may occur after meningitis, and it is caused by the blockage of CSF flow within the basal cisterns, part of the subarachnoid space. After an SAH, communicating hydrocephalus is caused by inadequate resorption of CSF at the arachnoid granulations. Communicating hydrocephalus can also occur after trauma, encephalitis, and intraventricular hemorrhage. Hydrocephalus, caused by the overproduction of CSF, may occur with a choroid plexus papilloma or carcinoma.

Hydrocephalus may be present at birth. A hydrocephalic newborn is seen in three to four per 1,000 live births. Hydrocephalus may also develop after a child is born. Infants, between birth and 2 years of age, frequently develop hydrocephalus secondary to a congenital lesion. Two congenital malformations associated with hydrocephalus are the Chiari II malformation and the Dandy-Walker malformation. The Chiari II malformation is described further in the congenital malformations section. The *Dandy-Walker syndrome* is noncommunicating hydrocephalus, a posterior fossa cyst, and cerebellar dysgenesis. The posterior fossa cyst is in communication with the fourth ventricle, but the normal outflow of the fourth ventricle, the foramina of Magendie and Luschka, are atretic. Other lesions that cause noncommunicating hydrocephalus in infants include aqueductal atresia or stenosis, developmental cysts, encephaloceles, neoplasms, arachnoid cysts, and vascular abnormalities such as a vein of Galen aneurysm. In a hydrocephalic infant with open cranial sutures, the skull expands along with the ventricles and the infant develops a large head (macrocrania) and widened cranial sutures. Without dysgenesis of the brain, there are no early neurological symptoms. As the ventricles expand

and the ICP increases, the superficial scalp veins become prominent and the anterior fontanelle bulges. Neurological signs of increased ICP include papilledema and bilateral abducens palsies, which result in a loss of lateral gaze. With long-standing elevated ICP, optic atrophy occurs, resulting in visual deterioration and the child develops a spastic paralysis of the lower extremities secondary to the lower extremity motor fibers being stretched over the enlarged lateral ventricles. The infant may develop *Parinaud syndrome,* which is paralysis of upward gaze (setting sun sign), paralysis of accommodation, and the failure of the pupils to react to light. In hydrocephalic infants, transillumination of the head is possible because the skull is mainly filled with CSF.

In children older than 2 years, frequent causes of hydrocephalus include brain tumors, meningitis, intracerebral hemorrhage, and aqueductal stenosis. In this age-group, the presentation is often acute because the cranial sutures are closed. Symptoms include headache, vomiting, and lethargy. With acute hydrocephalus, progression to unresponsiveness and even death may be rapid. With chronic hydrocephalus, a slow progressive onset of symptoms from the elevated ICP occurs. The parents may complain of slowed cognitive function, behavior changes, or deteriorating school performance. In addition, the child may suffer from endocrine or hypothalamic disorders. In adults, hydrocephalus generally has an insidious onset. Common causes include infectious meningitis, ventriculitis, late onset aqueductal stenosis, intraventricular hemorrhage, SAH, and neoplasm. The elderly can develop normal pressure hydrocephalus in which the patient has large ventricles, but the ICP is not elevated. Normal pressure hydrocephalus is characterized by a triad of symptoms: ataxia, urinary incontinence, and progressive cognitive decline (dementia). It can be diagnosed by clinical improvement of a patient after a high-volume lumbar puncture (LP).

When imaging hydrocephalic patients with MRI or CT, enlarged ventricles are seen. The tissue surrounding the frontal horns of the lateral ventricles may be hypodense, a process called *transependymal flow* of CSF. In these areas, CSF is being forced through the ventricular walls by the increased intraventricular pressure. The temporal horns of the lateral ventricles are prominent and the third ventricle is more rounded than usual (Fig. 1-12).

Acute hydrocephalus is an emergency and is treated with a ventriculostomy or *ventriculoperitoneal shunt.* Chronic hydrocephalus is treated with a shunt. The ventricular portion can be inserted either through a frontal or parietal burr hole. The distal end of a shunt can be placed in the peritoneum (ventriculoperitoneal shunt), the pleura (ventriculopleural), or the right atrium of the heart (ventriculoatrial). Most shunts are inserted on the right side of the head, to avoid the dominant hemisphere. After the insertion of a shunt, children must be followed closely for motor development, intellectual function, and ventricular

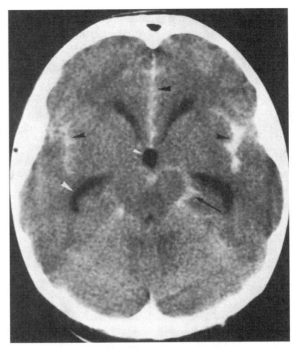

FIGURE 1-12. A noncontrast computed tomographic scan of the brain. Early hydrocephalus is demonstrated by the prominence of the temporal horns of the lateral ventricles and a rounded third ventricle. Subarachnoid hemorrhage is present in both sylvian (lateral) fissures and the interhemispheric fissure. (From Greenfield. *Surgery:* scientific principles and practice. Philadelphia: JB Lippincott Co, 1993, with permission.)

size. Complications of shunt placement include infections, malfunctions of the hardware, and perforation of abdominal viscera. An alternative way to treat communicating hydrocephalus is insertion of a *lumboperitoneal shunt.* The catheter is inserted into the thecal sac of the lumbar spine, and CSF is drained into the peritoneal cavity. Whenever possible, the underlying cause of the hydrocephalus should be treated.

An *arachnoid cyst* is a CSF-filled cavity not in continuity with the ventricular system. They are congenital lesions commonly found in the temporal fossa and are frequently asymptomatic. When they do present with neurological symptoms, it usually occurs in childhood. They can act as mass lesions causing signs of increased ICP (headache, vomiting, lethargy) or focal signs (hemiparesis, aphasia).

In the spinal cord, a cystic dilation within the parenchyma of the cord filled with CSF is called a *syrinx. Syringomyelia* is a syrinx lined by glial tissue within the substance of the spinal cord. *Hydromyelia* is a dilation of the central canal of the spinal cord and is lined by ependymal tissue, like the ventricular system. Hydromyelia is commonly seen with Chiari malformations. Both syringomyelia and hydromyelia may be asymptomatic or they may cause weakness, sensory loss, or myelopathy.

CONGENITAL MALFORMATIONS

Two percent of infants are born with a congenital abnormality and 60% of these involve the CNS. Most of the CNS defects occur during the closure of the dorsal midline structures. Normally, the neural groove closes in the midline to form the neural tube. At each end of the newly formed neural tube are openings called the *anterior* and *posterior neuropores*. The anterior neuropore normally closes before the posterior neuropore. The neural tube becomes encircled in bone and is covered by skin. Defects occurring at the posterior end of the neural tube cause spinal dysraphism and defects occurring at the anterior end of the neural tube cause cranial dysraphism. *Spinal dysraphism* is the failure of ectodermal and mesodermal midline structures to fuse. Abnormal closure of the neural groove, failure of bony fusion, and maldevelopment of the ectoderm are all possible. *Spina bifida* is the failure of the bony structures to fuse in the midline. When the spinal cord is not affected, it is usually not symptomatic and is found incidentally. Spinal dysraphism can be divided into occult spinal dysraphism and open spinal dysraphism.

Open spinal dysraphism (spina bifida aperta or spina bifida cystica) occurs when the bone and overlying skin fail to fuse in the midline, allowing meninges and sometimes neural tissue to herniate out through the defect. Two forms of open spinal dysraphism are meningocele and myelomeningocele. When the neural tissue is not involved and only CSF-filled meninges (dura) herniates through the defect in the bone and skin, it is called a *meningocele*. Even though the spinal cord is not involved, one-third of affected neonates still have a neurological deficit. Surgical treatment involves excision of the meningocele, closure of the dura in a watertight manner over the posterior defect, and closure of the skin defect.

When bone, dura, and neural tissue all fail to fuse, the malformation is called a *myelomeningocele,* which is the most common CNS birth defect. There is incomplete closure of the posterior neuropore, resulting in a mass of unfused neural tissue to protrude from the back of the neonate. Unfortunately, there is complete motor, sensory, and autonomic failure below the lesion, which includes the loss of bowel and bladder function. Families who have had a child with a myelomeningocele or who have a close relative who has had a child with a myelomeningocele, particularly if it is a maternal relative, are at a greater risk of having a child with a myelomeningocele. A mother deficient in folic acid is also at a greater risk of having an affected child. Because the neural tube closes at 3 to 4 weeks gestation, frequently before a pregnancy is confirmed, women planning to become pregnant should take a dietary supplement with folic acid. A myelomeningocele is fixed as soon as possible after birth (usually within 36 hours) to prevent infection (meningitis). In utero repair is currently being investigated. The operative goals are to preserve as much neural tissue as possible, to release the tethering of the spinal cord by the surrounding soft tissue, and to achieve a watertight dural closure.

Almost all neonates with a myelomeningocele have a *Chiari II* (Arnold-Chiari) *malformation* and hydrocephalus. The Chiari II malformation is manifested by the caudal displacement of cerebellar vermis, fourth ventricle, and medulla through the plane of the foramen magnum. It is also associated with supratentorial abnormalities, such as hydrocephalus and microgyria, and myelodysplasia (developmental abnormalities of the spinal cord). The *Chiari I malformation* has a lesser degree of brain herniation than the Chiari II malformation. Only the cerebellar tonsils are displaced caudally through the plane of the foramen magnum.

Myeloschisis is similar to a myelomeningocele, but the exposed neural tissue is uncovered by meninges (dura). It is a more severe, but less common, defect than a myelomeningocele. The unfused spinal cord lies on the surface of the back uncovered by meninges or skin. Most commonly, this occurs in the thoracolumbar region, resulting in paraplegia and absence of bladder function. It is also associated with a Chiari II malformation and hydrocephalus. It is treated in a similar manner as a myelomeningocele.

When a spinal dysraphic condition is covered by skin, making it not obvious on gross inspection of the back, it is usually found later in life and is referred to as *occult spinal dysraphism* (spina bifida occulta). Lipomyelomeningocele, split cord malformation, and neurenteric cysts are all forms of occult spinal dysraphism. *Lipomyelomeningocele* is a subcutaneous lipoma that extends through a defect in the dura and blends with the substance of the spinal cord or attaches to the conus medullaris. A *split cord malformation* is the presence of two hemicords in one or two dural sacs separated by a septum within the spinal canal. *Neurenteric cysts* are rests of endodermal tissue in the CNS. Affected infants commonly present with midline cutaneous stigma or a malformation of the foot or leg. The midline cutaneous stigmata may be a tuft of hair, a capillary hemangioma, a subcutaneous mass, a rudimentary appendage, or an atretic meningocele, which is a small discolored area of thinned skin. A midline tuft of hair on the back over the thoracolumbar region is almost always associated with some form of spina bifida occulta. Older children and adults more commonly present with pain, progressive neurological dysfunction, or scoliosis. Neurological deficits include bladder dysfunction and weakness of the lower extremities. Diagnosis is made by MRI. Treatment includes early surgery before the progression of any neurological deficits.

A *congenital dermal sinus* is a dysraphic condition that begins as an opening in the skin and continues as an epithelial lined tract that can end outside of the dura or extend through it. They can be found anywhere along the neural axis but are most commonly found in the lumbosacral region. A dermal sinus can be associated with recurrent bouts of meningitis, a meningitis from an unusual organism, or a meningitis from a mixture of organisms. An opening in the skin over the coccyx, in the intergluteal cleft, is not a congenital dermal sinus. Instead, it is a coccygeal pit, which is benign and requires no further workup.

Tethering of the spinal cord is associated with spinal dysraphism. A *tethered cord* is tightly attached to a surrounding nonneural structure, causing the spinal cord to be abnormally stretched as the child grows, which may result in a neurological deficit. A tethered cord needs to be released at the same time the spinal dysraphic state is repaired.

Cranial dysraphism results from the failure of the anterior end of the neural tube to close properly, which occurs much less commonly than spinal dysraphism. *Anencephaly* is the failure of anterior neuropore to close and is not compatible with life. An *encephalocele* is a midline skull defect with a cystic protrusion of the meninges and brain, which is usually covered by skin and frequently associated with hydrocephalus.

TRAUMA

The pathophysiology of head injury is divided into a primary and secondary phase. The primary injury occurs at the time of the traumatic event, consists of the irreversible damage suffered by neurons and axons in the brain, and cannot be changed by subsequent treatments. Following the primary injury, a secondary injury to the brain may occur. Therapeutic intervention is targeted at preventing or minimizing secondary injury to the brain. Mechanisms of secondary injury include metabolic abnormalities, hypoxia, and hypovolemia. These can be caused by hypoventilation, blood loss, hypotension, and endocrine disturbances such as diabetes insipidus. Ischemia can lead to cell death causing cytotoxic edema and an increase in ICP. The goal of treatment is to prevent secondary injury by supporting the blood pressure and controlling the ICP.

The evaluation of a traumatically injured patient, whether there is a suspected head or spinal cord injury (SCI), proceeds with a rapid clinical assessment, starting with the ABCs of ATLS. After the patient is stabilized, an efficient neurological history and exam, including the determination of the Glasgow Coma Scale (GCS), is performed (Table 1-1). Prehospital personnel should be asked whether an awake patient had any loss of consciousness before reaching the hospital. The examination should include the evaluation of the size and function of the pupils, noting whether the patient is awake or can be aroused easily, whether the patient follows commands, whether the patient is confused, and whether he or she has any pain in the head, neck, or back. All four extremities should be evaluated for motor function and sensation. If the patient is unresponsive or does not follow commands, movement of the extremities can be produced by painful central stimuli

TABLE 1-1. THE GLASGOW COMA SCALE

Parameter	Response	Score
Eye opening	Spontaneous	4
	To voice	3
	To pain	2
	None	1
Motor response	Follows commands	6
	Localizes to pain	5
	Withdraws from pain	4
	Flexor posturing to pain	3
	Extensor posturing to pain	2
	None	1
Verbal response	Oriented	5
	Confused	4
	Inappropriate words	3
	Incomprehensible sounds	2
	None	1
	Total	15

(e.g., sternal rub). Any eye opening or verbal response produced by a painful stimulus applied to an unresponsive patient should be noted. Initial radiological evaluation consists of a lateral cervical spine film and a head CT.

Head injury can be stratified by severity into mild, moderate, and severe. A mild head injury (GCS 13 to 15) usually does not result in any significant primary brain injury. There may be a transient loss of consciousness, commonly referred to as a *concussion*. Other common symptoms of mild head injury are headache, nausea, lethargy, and at times restlessness. Management includes a CT scan of the head, which is positive for a hemorrhage less than 10% of the time, and x-rays of the cervical spine, because neck injuries are commonly associated with head injuries. The patient may be admitted to the hospital for observation and frequent neurological exams. A patient with a moderate head injury (GCS 9 to 12) usually presents lethargic and possibly combative. The initial evaluation includes a lateral cervical spine film and a CT scan of the head. The patient is admitted to the hospital for observation and frequent neurological checks. About 10% of moderately head-injured patients will have a discrete lesion on CT scan. A patient with a severe head injury presents with a GCS of 8 or less. Such a patient is not awake and needs to be intubated for protection of the airway. If possible, a neurological examination should be performed before the patient is sedated and paralyzed for intubation. A lateral cervical spine film and a CT scan of the head should be part of the initial evaluation. Up to 40% of those with a severe head injury have a large epidural, subdural, or intraparenchymal hematoma (IPH) on CT scan and need an emergent craniotomy to evacuate the clot and stop the bleeding.

A traumatic head injury may result in a scalp laceration, skull fracture, epidural hematoma (EDH), SDH, or IPH. A *scalp laceration* may hemorrhage profusely. As long as there is not an adjacent skull fracture, the initial management includes holding pressure on the edges of the laceration to decrease the bleeding. As soon as possible, the wound should be debrided and irrigated. Scalp lacerations through the galea should be closed in two layers. First, the galea needs to be approximated, then the overlying skin is approximated.

Skull fractures can be classified into different types. A skull fracture with the overlying skin intact is a *closed fracture*. If the skin is disrupted, it is an open (compound) fracture and the patient is at risk for a CNS infection. If a fracture extends into a sinus or a mastoid air cell, it is considered *open*. A *linear fracture* has a single fracture line. A *stellate fracture* has several fracture lines radiating out from a central point. If there is fragmentation of the bone, it is a *comminuted fracture*. A *diastatic fracture*, which is more common in young children, extends into and causes separation of a suture. If the outer table of at least one edge of a fracture fragment lies below the normal anatomic level of the inner table of the adjacent skull, it is a depressed skull fracture.

The treatment of skull fractures depends on the type, where they are located, and the presence of any associated pathology. Most closed skull fractures that are not depressed require no specific treatment. If the fracture line crosses a vascular channel, e.g., the middle meningeal artery in the temporal bone or the sagittal sinus at the vertex of the skull, it can be associated with an EDH or SDH. Large hematomas need to be surgically removed. Open fractures are treated in the operating room with debridement, irrigation, and closure of the galea and skin. A dural laceration may be seen with a comminuted skull fracture and needs to be repaired. A depressed skull fracture requires surgery to elevate the fragments if it is causing a neurological deficit, is an open fracture, is associated with a CSF leak, or is depressed greater than the thickness of the skull (generally 8 to 10 mm). However, a depressed skull fracture over a dural sinus may be dangerous to elevate and these indications do not apply.

Basilar skull fractures have distinct clinical presentations, can cause cranial nerve palsies, and commonly have associated CSF leaks. Fractures in the floor of the anterior cranial fossa frequently produce raccoon eyes (periorbital ecchymosis). *Battle sign* (ecchymosis behind the ear) is associated with a fracture in the petrous portion of the temporal bone, which forms the floor of the middle cranial fossa. A facial nerve palsy can occur with a fracture of the temporal bone. Facial weakness may begin immediately if the nerve has been lacerated by the fracture or may be delayed if the facial nerve has only been contused. A contused nerve will progressively swell and become compressed within its bony canal. If a basilar skull fracture extends into a paranasal sinus or mastoid air cell, a traumatic CSF leak is possible. Fluid may drain from the nose (CSF rhinorrhea) or ear (CSF otorrhea) or may drain down the back of the throat. Antibiotics are not routinely given by neurosurgeons for traumatic CSF leaks because they usually seal spontaneously in 7 to 10 days and infectious complications are uncommon. Traumatic CSF leaks are initially treated with elevation of the head—to decrease the ICP—and observation. If the leak fails to stop after 7 to 10 days, a lumbar drain may be placed or a surgical repair can be undertaken.

An EDH arises between the inner table of the skull and the dura. It does not cross suture lines, because the dura is tightly attached to the inner surface of the skull at the suture lines, and therefore has a characteristic convex shape. An EDH is a high-pressure bleed from a lacerated epidural artery. The most common source is a lacerated middle meningeal artery or one of its branches, which results in a temporal EDH. Less commonly, an EDH can also occur after a tear in the wall of a venous sinus secondary to depressed skull fracture. The classic, but uncommon, scenario of a patient with an EDH involves a victim with an initial brief loss of consciousness immediately after the accident, followed by a lucid interval and then a progressive decrease in the level of consciousness. More commonly, patients only have a progressive decrease in their level of consciousness. Focal signs, such as a hemiparesis, are often associated with this injury (Fig. 1-13).

An SDH arises between the dura and arachnoid membrane. It is caused by the laceration of a subdural bridging vein that runs from the cortex to the dura, which results in a low-pressure venous hemorrhage. An SDH is crescent shaped over the surface of the cerebral hemisphere and is bounded by the falx cerebri and tentorium (dural reflections). An SDH may also be caused by a tear in the subdural wall of a venous sinus or the extension of an IPH into the subdural space. SDHs are often subdivided by the length of time they have been present into acute, subacute, and chronic. An *acute SDH* is found at the time of injury. Treatment for small asymptomatic acute SDH is observation, frequent neurological exams, and a follow-up CT scan of the brain to ensure the hemorrhage is not enlarging. Treatment for a large, symptomatic, acute SDH entails an emergent craniotomy to evacuate the clot and stop the bleeding. An acute SDH is often associated with a severe head injury, and even after the evacuation of the hematoma, a patient may have a residual neurological deficit from the widespread neuronal injury (Fig. 1-14). A *subacute SDH* occurs after a minor blow to the head. The symptoms begin a few days to weeks after the injury and include headache, progressive lethargy, hemiparesis, or double vision (cranial nerve VI nerve palsy). Treatment entails drainage of the subacute SDH by burr holes if it is liquid or a craniotomy if it is an organized clot. Postoperative patients usually recover well. A *chronic SDH* also occurs after a minor blow to the head. Often, the patient does not remember the injury. A chronic SDH is believed to start as a small SDH, which slowly becomes encased in fibrous membrane. It then liquefies and gradually enlarges. With increasing size, headache, lethargy, and focal neurological deficits can

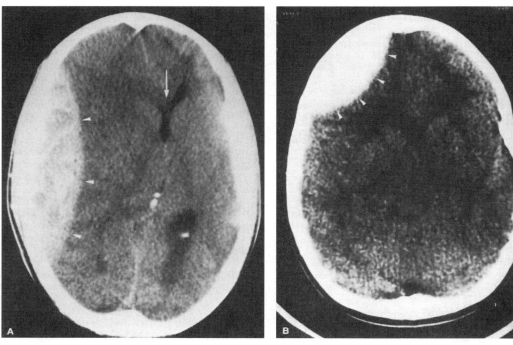

FIGURE 1-13. Two noncontrast computed tomographic scans of the brain. **A:** A large epidural hematoma with marked midline shift. **B:** A smaller epidural hematoma. Note the lenticular shape of both. (From Greenfield. *Surgery:* scientific principles and practice. Philadelphia: JB Lippincott Co, 1993, with permission.)

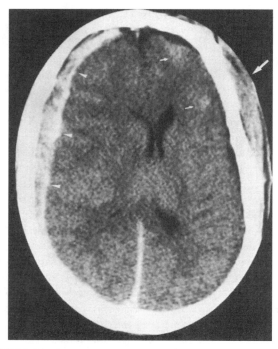

FIGURE 1-14. A noncontrast computed tomographic scan of the brain. An acute subdural hematoma with marked midline shift. Note the crescent shape. (From Greenfield. *Surgery:* scientific principles and practice. Philadelphia: JB Lippincott Co, 1993, with permission.)

occur. Papilledema, from increased ICP, may be seen on ophthalmologic examination. Chronic SDHs are commonly seen in infants and the elderly. A subdural hygroma presents as a chronic SDH but occurs secondary to a tear in arachnoid membrane. This allows CSF to flow into the subdural space from the subarachnoid space. Burr holes can be used to drain the hygroma fluid from the subdural space.

Other forms of traumatic intracranial hemorrhage include an intraparenchymal hematoma and a traumatic SAH. An IPH results from tearing intraparenchymal capillaries. It is associated with a cerebral contusion and subarachnoid hemorrhage. A *traumatic* SAH occurs when a vessel in the subarachnoid space is damaged and bleeds. Trauma is the most common cause of all SAHs (the most common cause of a nontraumatic SAH is rupture of a cerebral aneurysm).

Diffuse axonal injury (DAI) is commonly seen with severe blunt head trauma. In DAI, many axons within the brain are injured as a result of shearing forces. DAI is best diagnosed on MRI, which shows multiple hemorrhages in deep white matter structures such as the corpus callosum and hemorrhages within the brainstem.

In 1995, the Brain Trauma Foundation published the *Guidelines for the Management of Severe Head Injury,* which outlines how to manage a patient with a GCS between 3 and 8. This is an evidence-based approach to head injury management with each recommendation assigned a degree of certainty. The three degrees of certainty are standards, guidelines, and options, which reflect a high, moderate, and unclear degree of clinical certainty of the management principle. The following is a summary of these guidelines.

The guidelines make recommendations about blood pressure and oxygenation goals during the initial resuscitation of a patient with a head injury. There is not a standard of treatment due to insufficient data, but there is a guideline that recommends maintaining a systolic blood pressure of greater than 90 mm Hg and a PaO_2 of greater than 60 mm Hg. The option presented is to keep the mean arterial pressure greater than 90 mm Hg so that the cerebral perfusion pressure (CPP) is maintained above 70 mm Hg. The CPP is calculated by subtracting the ICP from the mean arterial pressure (MAP), or mathematically, CPP = MAP − ICP and MAP = (2DBP + SPB)/3, where *DBP* is the diastolic blood pressure and SBP is the systolic blood pressure.

The best method for ICP monitoring, the indications for ICP monitoring, when to treat elevated ICP, and when to treat a low CPP are all addressed. The best way to monitor ICP is with a ventricular catheter, when possible, because it is the most accurate method and can be used to lower ICP by the drainage of CSF. There is no standard for when to monitor ICP, but there are guidelines. Any patient with a GCS of 3 to 8 after cardiopulmonary resuscitation and an abnormal CT scan of the head showing a contusion, hematoma, edema, or swelling of the brain should be monitored. In a patient with a GCS of 3 to 8 and a normal CT scan of the head, monitoring is indicated if they are more than 40 years old, are decerebrate or decorticate posturing, or have a systolic blood pressure less than 90 mm Hg. The treatment of elevated ICP is also not governed by a standard, but a guideline of treating ICP above 20 to 25 mm Hg is recommended. The options of corroborating the ICP treatment threshold with the clinical examination and CPP measurement and maintaining the CPP at or above 70 mm Hg are presented.

The topic of hyperventilation in the head-injured patient is governed by recommendations of what not to do. The standard of treatment is that a severely head-injured patient should not be hyperventilated below a $PaCO_2$ of 25 mm Hg for a prolonged period of time. The recommended treatment guideline is a severely head injured patient should not be hyperventilated below a $PaCO_2$ of 35 mm Hg for the first 24 hours after the injury. Two options are as follows: brief periods of hyperventilation can be used with acute neurological deterioration and hyperventilation therapy may be instituted with jugular venous oxygen saturation and cerebral blood flow monitoring.

The use of mannitol and high-dose barbiturate therapy in the severely head-injured patient is addressed. There is not enough data to outline standards for the use of either of these drugs. The guideline concerning the use of mannitol states that it is an effective means of lowering elevated ICP in a severely head-injured patient at a dose between 0.25 to 1 g per kilogram of body weight. Mannitol is probably most effective if given in intermittent boluses rather than an i.v. drip. The options for mannitol use are as follows: It can be used emergently before ICP monitoring is instituted if there are signs of transtentorial herniation not secondary to systemic pathology and hypovolemia is avoided. In a patient at risk for renal failure, the serum osmolality should be kept below 320 mOsmol, and the patient being treated with mannitol needs to have a Foley catheter. The guideline set fourth for the use of high-dose barbiturate therapy (pentobarbital coma) states it can be used in a severely head-injured patient with elevated ICP refractory to other methods of management but hemodynamically stable and with the possibility of making a meaningful recovery.

The use of both glucocorticoids and antiseizure drugs are governed by standards. The standard recommendation for glucocorticoid therapy after severe head injury is not to use them. The standard concerning antiseizure drugs after severe head injury is their prophylactic use does not prevent late posttraumatic seizures. There is not a guideline for antiseizure drugs, but the option of using them to prevent early posttraumatic seizures is given. When phenytoin is given prophylactically, it should be given for 7 days after the injury then discontinued unless the patient develops a seizure disorder.

Finally, a critical pathway for treatment of the severely head-injured patient is outlined. The expert opinions of the committee members who wrote the *Guidelines for the Management of Severe Head Injury* are used to formulate this pathway. Early management interventions to minimize ICP include elevating the head of the patient, repositioning the neck into a neutral position to improve the venous drainage from the brain, treating hyperthermia aggressively, beginning prophylactic treatment against seizures, sedating the patient with or without pharmacological paralysis, avoiding hypoxia, and resuscitating the volume status of the patient. If the patient has ICP elevations after the institution of the above therapies and has a ventriculostomy, intermittent drainage of CSF should be used to lower the ICP. If this does not work or the patient does not have a ventriculostomy, mannitol should be used. The patient can also be ventilated to keep the $PaCO_2$ at 35 mm Hg or just above this level. If using mannitol, the serum osmolality should be kept below 320 mOsmol. If all of this is unsuccessful, further hyperventilation directed by jugular venous saturation measurements or cerebral blood flow monitoring should be considered. If all of this fails, second-tier therapy, such as high-dose barbiturate therapy should be considered. It must be remembered that an acute elevation in ICP could also be due to a newly developed hemorrhage. Therefore, a low threshold to repeat the CT scan of the head should be maintained.

The outcome after head injury depends on several factors. The potential for recovery is inversely proportional to age and proportional to the GCS on admission. Other determinants of poor outcome include elevated ICP that is refractory to surgical and medical management, abnormal brainstem reflexes on initial examination, preexisting illnesses, penetrating trauma (especially gunshot wounds), intracranial hemorrhage, SDH, delay in treatment, multiple system trauma, and systemic insults, which include acidosis, hypoxia, and hypotension. When a patient has both an SDH and an IPH, he or she has a very poor prognosis.

There are several mechanisms of supratentorial brain herniation that can occur with elevated ICP. One important mechanism is transtentorial (central) herniation, which presents with the classic triad of lethargy that progresses to unresponsiveness (coma), a fixed and dilated ipsilateral pupil, and a contralateral hemiplegia. With increased ICP, *Cushing triad* is seen, which consists of hypertension, bradycardia, and respiratory irregularity. If unsuccessfully treated, transtentorial herniation results in death. Another form of brain herniation is *uncal herniation*, which is similar to transtentorial herniation, but a decrease in consciousness occurs late and decorticate posturing rarely occurs. *Subfalcine herniation* is the forced displacement of a cingulate gyrus under the falx and to the contralateral side. *Infratentorial herniation* of the cerebellum can involve the upward movement of the cerebellum into the supratentorial compartment or the downward herniation of the cerebellar tonsils.

Patients with loss of brain function are declared braindead. They must meet strict criteria on physical examination and diagnostic tests. During testing for brain death, a patient must have an adequate blood pressure, an adequate body temperature, and cannot be pharmacologically impaired. A brain-death examination includes a neurological test of the brainstem reflexes, an apnea test, and a confirmatory study showing no blood flow to the brain (cerebral angiography, cerebral radionuclide angiogram).

Finally, it is important to remember that intracranial hemorrhage can be the cause, not the result, of a traumatic injury. For example, a patient may suffer an intracranial bleed from an aneurysm or an AVM and then fall or be involved in an automobile accident. In these situations, the location of hemorrhage may give a clue to the etiology.

All trauma patients are initially assumed to have an unstable spinal column and are treated with spinal precautions. The patient is placed on a backboard in a rigid cervical collar. When moved, the patient is logrolled. On initial clinical assessment, any tenderness of the neck or back is noted. On neurological examination, sensation and voluntary motor strength in all extremities is evaluated, along with perianal sensation and voluntary contraction of the external anal sphincter. X-rays of the cervical spine are done, which include a lateral view showing the skull base to the top of the T-1 vertebral body, anteroposterior view, and odontoid view. Additional radiographs of the thoracic and lumbar spine can be done to view areas that are tender, have palpable deformities, or are involved in penetrating trauma. Thoracic and lumbar spine films are also obtained if the patient has a neurological deficit. An area of the spine suspicious for a fracture can be further evaluated with a CT scan including reconstructed sagittal and coronal images. An acute disk rupture or an epidural hematoma can also be seen on CT. The x-ray and CT findings need to be correlated to the neurological examination. In a patient with a spinal cord injury (SCI), a discrepancy between the radiological level and the neurological level needs to be further evaluated in an emergent manner. An MRI can evaluate the spinal cord and look for compressive lesions away from the site of bony injury, which may require emergent surgery if associated with progressive neurological deficits. In a patient without any neurological deficits or bony fractures, ligamentous injury must be ruled out because this could make the cervical spine unstable. Lateral flexion and extension cervical spine x-rays in the awake, nonimpaired patient show instability if there is movement between the vertebral bodies. Flexion and extension films should not be done if palpation or movement of the neck is painful. When this is the case, the patient should be kept in a hard cervical collar until the resolution of his or her neck pain (at least a week) and then flexion extension x-rays should be performed. Neck pain may cause neck muscle spasms, which could mask instability.

Neck fractures can be divided into upper (C1-2) and subaxial (C3-7) cervical spine fractures. Injuries of the upper cervical spine include atlanto-occipital dislocations, Jefferson fractures, hangman's fractures, and odontoid fractures. *Atlanto-occipital dislocation* occurs when the ligaments that hold the skull to the spinal column are disrupted. Often, this is a fatal cervical spine injury because of a respiratory arrest. A *Jefferson fracture* consists of bilateral fractures through the arches of C-1, which usually results from axial compression. This fracture usually makes the patient's cervical spine unstable, but the patient commonly does not have any neurological deficits. It is treated with immobilization of the neck. A *hangman's fracture* consists of bilateral fractures through the pars interarticularis of C-2. The pars interarticularis is the junction of the pedicle and lamina in the ring of C-2. Classically, with judicial hangings, it is caused by hyperextension and distraction of the neck (therefore, during a hanging, the noose needs to be anterior to the neck to cause this fracture), but it is more commonly caused by hyperextension and axial loading of the neck as a result of a motor vehicle accident. Often, there is anterior subluxation (traumatic spondylolisthesis) of C-2 on C-3. The patient's cervical spine with an isolated hangman's fracture is usually stable and neurological deficits are infrequent. Hangman's fractures are also treated with immobilization of the neck. The most common fracture of C-2 is an odontoid fracture (dens). *Odontoid fractures* are classified into three types. A type I fracture is through the odontoid process and it does not involve the junction of the odontoid process with the body of C-2. This is a rare fracture that is usually unstable and may need surgical treatment. A type II fracture is through the base of the odontoid process at its junction with the body of C-2. This is the most common odontoid fracture and usually makes the patient's cervical spine unstable. Most type II fractures in adults can be treated with halo immobilization, but in certain instances, surgical fusion is needed. A type III fracture extends through the odontoid process into the body of C-2 (Fig. 1-15). The cervical spine of the patient is usually stable and the patient is treated by immobilizing the neck.

Subaxial cervical spine injuries include subluxations, locked facets, teardrop fractures, and clay shoveler's fractures. Subluxation of one vertebral body on another is caused by a flexion injury to the cervical spine. A horizontal subluxation of greater than 3.5 mm or angular subluxation of greater than 11 degrees on a lateral cervical spine film indicates ligamentous instability. Locked facets can be either unilateral or bilateral. Both are a severe form of subluxation and are caused by flexion injuries. The initial treatment of locked facets is to emergently put the patient in traction (Gardner-Wells tongs) to reduce the dislocation and realign the spinal column. Usually, 10 lb of traction for each cervical level above the dislocation is the maximum amount of weight applied. Frequent neurological examinations need to be performed during the application of traction and the procedure should be aborted with any neurological deterioration. In addition, frequent x-rays to evaluate the degree of reduction and alignment of the spinal column should be checked. When traction is unsuccessful or there is neurological deterioration, surgical reduction is indicated. A teardrop fracture results from hyperflexion of the neck and is named because of its appearance on x-ray. A lateral cervical spine film will show a small bone chip anterior and inferior to the fractured vertebral body. This vertebral body is usually wedged anteriorly and a fragment of it is posteriorly displaced into the spinal canal (Fig. 1-15). A teardrop fracture makes the patient's cervical spine unstable and the patient is frequently quadriplegic. Surgical stabilization of the cervical spine is needed.

Fractures at the thoracolumbar junction are seen with traumatic injuries and the possibility of spinal instability needs to be addressed. A three-column model has been proposed by Denis, which divides the structural components of the thoracolumbar spinal column into an anterior, middle, and posterior column. The anterior column consists of the anterior longitudinal ligament and the anterior two thirds of the vertebral body. The middle column consists of the posterior one third of the vertebral body and the posterior longitudinal ligament. The posterior column contains the posterior elements, the facet joints, and the associated ligaments (Fig. 1-16). When two or more of these columns are injured, the spine is considered unstable. Instability alone is not an indication for surgery. Most thoracolumbar fractures without neurological deficits can be treated with bed rest and if unstable immobilized in a clamshell orthosis.

The timing of surgery with spinal fractures remains a controversial topic. Some general guidelines of when early surgery is appropriate for traumatic injuries of the cervical, thoracic, and lumbar spine include progressive neurological deterioration, severe compression of the spinal cord seen on MRI or CT and consistent neurological deficits, an open wound that requires debridement, and the need for early mobilization and rehabilitation. The goals of surgical intervention are to decompress the neural structures, correct the alignment of the bony elements, and stabilize the spinal column.

SCI can be associated with a fracture of the vertebral column, a herniation of an intervertebral disk, a ligamentous

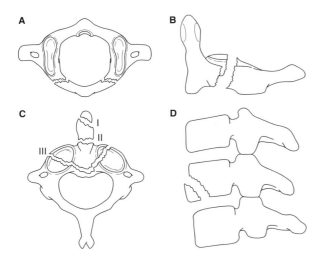

FIGURE 1-15. Cervical spine fractures. **A:** A Jefferson fracture. Superior view of the atlas (C-1). **B:** A hangman's fracture. Lateral view of the axis (C-2). **C:** The three types of odontoid fractures. Superior view of the axis (C-2). **D:** A teardrop fracture. Lateral view of the lower cervical spine.

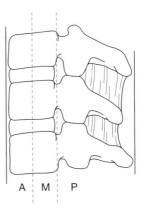

FIGURE 1-16. The three-column model of the thoracolumbar spine. Lateral view. A, anterior column; M, middle column; P, posterior column.

injury of the spine, or a penetrating traumatic injury. Head injury is commonly associated with SCI. Lesions at C-3 or above are associated with respiratory failure. A patient with lesions between C-4 and C-6 suffer from borderline respiratory function and commonly have insufficient tidal volumes. If the level of injury is above T-5, the patient can go into neurogenic shock. The output of the sympathetic nervous system to the body is cut off, which leads to the loss of vascular tone and hypotension. Because the parasympathetic output is now unopposed, the patient becomes bradycardiac. Other common systemic problems associated with SCI include an ileus of the gastrointestinal (GI) tract and bladder distention, which can cause compression of the pelvic veins and impede the venous return to the heart. With a complete SCI, a patient will acutely go into *spinal shock*, which is characterized by a flaccid paralysis and loss of spinal reflexes below the level of the lesion. It occurs due to the loss of supraspinal excitatory input to the injured portion of the cord and lasts on average from 3 to 4 weeks. After this period, the patient gradually gets increased muscle tone with hyperactive reflexes.

SCI can be divided into complete and incomplete injuries. A *complete injury* has a total loss of motor, sensory, and autonomic function below the level of the injury. This includes the loss of motor and sensory function in the lowest sacral segment (S4-5), which consists of perianal sensation and voluntary external anal sphincter contraction. An *incomplete injury* has sparing of some sensory or motor function below the level of injury, which needs to include sparing of sensory function in the lowest sacral segment (perianal sensation). Incomplete SCIs have a better prognosis for neurological recovery than complete SCIs.

Several classic patterns of incomplete SCI are described. The *Brown-Sequard syndrome* occurs with an anatomical or functional hemisection of the spinal cord. Clinically, the patient has an ipsilateral motor paralysis, ipsilateral loss of light touch, ipsilateral loss of position sense, and contralateral loss of pain and temperature sensation. A patient with *central cord syndrome* has a more profound weakness of the upper extremities, particularly affecting fine finger movements in the hand, than the lower extremities. Both the motor (corticospinal) and the pain and temperature (spinothalamic) tracts are affected. Frequently, it is seen after an elderly individual, with a narrow spinal canal from cervical spondylosis, suffers a face-first fall, causing the neck to hyperextend. It is also seen in people with a congenitally narrow cervical spinal canal. The *anterior spinal artery syndrome* is caused by the occlusion of the anterior spinal artery, resulting in an infarction of the anterior and lateral funiculi of the spinal cord. Clinically, it presents with a bilateral motor paralysis, from infarction of the corticospinal tracts, and a bilateral loss of pain temperature sensation, from infarction of the spinothalamic tracts, below the level of the injury. The dorsal columns, which carry position sense and light touch, are not affected. An acute disk rupture may cause anterior spinal artery syndrome by directly compressing the anterior spinal artery.

A patient with a traumatic SCI is given high-dose corticosteroids. They have been shown to improve the neurological recovery after a blunt injury to the spinal cord. The dosing regime is an initial i.v. bolus of methylprednisolone at 30 mg/kg over 15 minutes followed by a 45-minute pause. Then a continuous i.v. infusion of 5.4 mg/kg per minute is given for 24 or 48 hours. If steroids are administered within 3 hours of the injury, they should be given for a total of 24 hours. If steroids are initiated between 3 and 8 hours after the injury, then a total of 48 hours should be given. If begun more than 8 hours after the injury, steroids have not been proven beneficial. In addition, high-dose steroids have not been shown to improve neurological outcome after an injury to the cauda equina or after a penetrating injury to the spinal cord. Proposed beneficial mechanisms of high-dose steroids include the inhibition of lipid peroxidation and the augmentation of blood flow to the injured portion of the spinal cord.

In the United States, *child abuse* is the most frequent cause of severe head injuries in infants less than 1 year of age. Either a blow to the infant's head, even with a soft object, or shaking the infant can have catastrophic results. In toddlers, a significant proportion of hospitalizations for traumatic injuries are the result of abuse. Any suspected case of child abuse needs to be reported immediately to a child abuse investigation team. When the child is medically stable, a skeletal survey can be done to look for long bone or rib fractures at different stages of healing. This may indicate previous abusive episodes.

PERIPHERAL NERVE INJURY

Seddon and Sunderland both set up classification schemes for peripheral nerve injury. Seddon stratified injuries into three tiers: neuropraxia, axonotmesis, and neurotmesis. *Neurapraxia* is the transient loss of function because of a local conduction block. The motor fibers are affected more often than the sensory fibers and the autonomic fibers are usually spared. The neurological deficit is frequently incomplete and there is little, if any, muscle atrophy. If demyelination of large fibers occurs, the recovery time may be prolonged. Surgery is not indicated. Recovery can occur within hours but most commonly occurs within 6 to 8 weeks. Anatomic continuity and electrical conductivity are preserved. Neuropraxia usually occurs after a mild traction or compression injury.

In *axonotmesis*, the axon and its myelin sheath are disrupted. The connective tissue stroma is preserved and the portion of the axon distal to the injury undergoes *wallerian degeneration*. The result is complete motor, sensory, and autonomic paralysis, along with progressive muscle atrophy. Surgery is not indicated, because a path for distal nerve regeneration is still present within the intact connective tissue stroma. The nerve will regrow at a rate of about 1 mm per day or 1 inch per month. Recovery is usually good and occurs in the order of innervation from proximal to distal. This type of injury is often caused by a stretch injury or a prolonged compressive injury.

Neurotmesis is the complete disruption of all components of a nerve, making spontaneous recovery impossible. The axons, myelin sheaths, and connective tissue stroma are all disrupted and the portion of the axons distal to the injury undergo wallerian degeneration. Neurotmesis can result from transection of a nerve or a severe crush, traction, or ischemic injury that causes massive internal disruption of a nerve, even though it may still be in continuity. Complete muscle, sensory, and autonomic paralysis result and are accompanied by progressive muscle atrophy. If untreated, scar tissue blocks the nerve from regenerating and may cause a painful *neuroma,* which is a mass of misdirected axons. Even with surgery, recovery is usually incomplete.

The Sunderland classification has five degrees of injury. *First-degree injury* is a reversible local conduction block, similar to neuropraxia. *Second-degree injury* is a disruption of the axon and myelin sheath only, equivalent to axonotmesis. *Third degree injury* is the disruption of the axons, myelin sheaths, and endoneurium, but the fascicular pattern of the nerve is preserved. If it is a mild injury, it is similar to axonotmesis. If it is a severe injury, it is similar to neurotmesis. In *fourth-degree injuries,* the fascicular pattern of the nerve is disrupted, but the epineurium is still intact. *Fifth-degree injury* is the transection of the nerve. Both fourth-degree and fifth-degree injuries are equivalent to neurotmesis.

Part of the clinical examination in a patient with a peripheral nerve injury is eliciting *Tinel sign,* which is useful for following regrowth of nerves. By lightly tapping over a regenerating nerve, the patient will experience tingling paresthesia in the cutaneous distribution of the regenerating nerve. The point at which this is first elicited is the most distal point of small fiber regeneration. This point will move distally along the extremity as the nerve regenerates. Helpful clinical tests in the evaluation of a peripheral nerve injury include plain films and electromyography (EMG). When a peripheral nerve injury is diagnosed, plain films to rule out a foreign body or fracture should be done. EMG evaluates the electrical activity in muscles. Immediately after a normal muscle is denervated, EMG results will be normal. A few weeks after the injury, changes consistent with denervation, such as fibrillation potentials and the absence of voluntary action potentials, will be seen on EMG. Early reinnervation changes include a decrease in the amount of fibrillation potentials and nascent polyphasic potentials. However, EMG reinnervation changes do not guarantee recovery.

Treatment of peripheral nerve injuries depends on the continuity of the nerve and the type of wound. A nerve in continuity that has lost function distal to an injury should initially be observed for spontaneous recovery. If its recovery is taking longer than expected, an external neurolysis, freeing the nerve from surrounding scar tissue, may be indicated. If there is no evidence of recovery after several weeks, the injured portion of the nerve can be excised and the cut ends repaired with an end-to-end anastomosis with or without a graft. If the injured nerve is not in continuity, the type of wound needs to be considered. If the nerve was sharply cut and the wound is relatively clean, the nerve can be immediately repaired with an end-to-end anastomosis. If the wound is dirty or there is extensive tissue damage, a secondary repair a few weeks after injury is indicated. A surgically repaired nerve should not be under any tension. To keep tension at a minimum after the operation, the joints of the extremity can be flexed, the nerve can be freed from local attachments, and a nerve graft may be used. A *nerve graft* is simply a conduit for distal regeneration of a nerve when a gap in the nerve needs to be bridged. Commonly, the sural nerve is used as a graft. Bad *prognostic factors* in a peripheral nerve injury include an associated bony fracture, older age, proximal nerve injury, extensive neural tissue loss, and associated soft tissue injury. A worse prognosis is also seen with injuries to nerves that have mixed sensory and motor function and in injured extremities with severe muscle denervation. If a nerve graft is used, the additional suture line worsens the prognosis.

Injury to a peripheral nerve can also be secondary to chronic compression. The most frequent example in the upper extremity is *carpal tunnel syndrome,* which is median nerve entrapment within the carpal tunnel of the wrist. Other structures that pass through the carpal tunnel include the tendons of the flexor digitorum profundus and superficialis muscles. The patient with carpal tunnel syndrome complains of paresthesia and loss of sensation in the radial half of the palm, the thumb, the index finger, the middle finger, and radial half of the ring finger. In more severe cases, weakness of the first and second lumbrical, opponens pollicis, abductor pollicis brevis, and flexor pollicis brevis muscles may occur. Surgical treatment consists of dividing the transverse carpal ligament to relieve the compression. A *tardy ulnar palsy* is the compression of the ulnar nerve at the elbow.

Causalgia is a rare syndrome of burning pain, autonomic dysfunction, and trophic changes in an extremity after a major peripheral nerve injury. Symptoms begin in the distribution of the affected nerve and progress to involve the entire limb. The syndrome begins as a swollen limb with erythema that is very sensitive to tactile stimulation and may exhibit hyperhidrosis. The extremity later becomes pale, cool, and atrophic. *Reflex sympathetic dystrophy* is similar to causalgia but does not involve a major peripheral nerve injury. In both of these, the affected limb is not used due to the constant burning pain that may intensify with touch or movement of the limb. The limb eventually becomes useless. The joint creases disappear, the skin becomes smooth, and the bones become osteopenic. Treatments include a *sympathectomy* or a transcutaneous peripheral nerve stimulator.

VASCULAR DISORDERS

An intracranial hemorrhage is a common reason for a neurosurgical consultation and can take the form of a subarachnoid hemorrhage, intraventricular hemorrhage, intraparenchymal hematoma (IPH), subdural hematoma (SDH), epidural hematoma, or a combination of these. Some nontraumatic lesions that cause intracranial bleeding are cerebral aneurysms, arteriovenous malformations (AVM)s, hypertensive arteriopathy, and amyloid angiopathy. The patient with an intracranial hemorrhage may present with various symptoms and signs including headache, lethargy, photophobia, stiff neck, or a focal neurological deficit such as a hemiparesis or cranial nerve palsy. When a nontraumatic intracranial hemorrhage is suspected, an emergent CT scan of the head should be done. The etiology of the bleed can often be postulated based on its location.

Cerebral aneurysms (Berry aneurysms) are the most common cause of nontraumatic SAH, accounting for 75% to 80% of it (trauma is the most common cause of all SAHs). Cerebral aneurysms form where the vessel wall is abnormal because of a congenital defect or a degenerative change, which results in a thin-walled outpouching of the artery wall. This usually occurs at a point where an artery is branching off its parent artery close to the circle of Willis and the aneurysm is named for the branching vessel at its origin. The wall of an aneurysm lacks an internal elastic lamina and muscularis layer. Only the intimal layer and adventitia of the artery form the dome of aneurysm. Eighty five percent of cerebral aneurysms occur in the anterior (carotid) circulation and the most common locations are at the origin of the anterior communicating artery, the origin of the posterior communicating artery, and the bifurcation of the middle cerebral artery. Other locations for anterior circulation aneurysms include the carotid bifurcation and the origin of the anterior choroidal artery. Locations of posterior circulation aneurysms include the basilar artery bifurcation, the origin of the posterior inferior cerebellar artery, and the vertebrobasilar junction.

An *unruptured cerebral aneurysm* is discovered incidentally on CT, MRI, or angiography done for an unrelated reason or may present with symptoms of local mass effect. A symptomatic unruptured posterior communicating artery aneurysm may compress the oculomotor nerve and cause an ipsilateral third nerve palsy. Giant cerebral aneurysms, larger than 2.5 cm, can present as intracerebral mass lesions, which may present like a tumor.

Cerebral aneurysms most commonly present after they rupture and produce an SAH. The peak ages for rupture of a cerebral aneurysm are between 55 and 60 years, but they do occur in younger adults. Clinically, a patient complains of the sudden onset of an explosive headache, which is described as the worst headache of his or her life. With the onset of the headache, there is a change in the level of consciousness, due to the transient elevation of the ICP, which may be limited to transient confusion or could result in prolonged unresponsiveness (coma). Nausea and vomiting, seizures, and focal deficits may accompany the sudden headache. Blood in the subarachnoid space causes a sterile meningitis, which results in a stiff neck, photophobia, and a low-grade fever. The headache lasts for days, until the subarachnoid blood is cleared. The hemorrhage may occur during sleep or physical stress. It may be the cause of a fall or motor vehicle accident, so an SAH in a distribution similar to an aneurysmal bleed in a trauma patient warrants further workup. Recognizing the signs and symptoms of an aneurysmal SAH is important because approximately one-third of patients have a *sentinel bleed,* which is a small warning bleed, days to weeks before a large SAH. If recognized early, a catastrophic hemorrhage can be prevented. Unfortunately, a sentinel bleed is not always recognized. About 10% of patients die before reaching the hospital.

A patient with an SAH from an aneurysm is graded based on the most recent clinical examination using the *Hunt-Hess grading scale. Grade 0* corresponds to a patient with an unruptured aneurysm. Grades 1 to 5 describe patients with ruptured cerebral aneurysms. *Grade 1* is assigned to a patient with a mild headache and mild nuchal rigidity. *Grade 2* corresponds to a patient with a moderate to severe headache and nuchal rigidity. These patients may also have a cranial nerve palsy. *Grade 3* is a lethargic or confused patient who may have mild focal neurological deficit. *Grade 4* patients are unresponsive (comatose) and may have a moderate to severe hemiparesis. *Grade 5* corresponds to an unresponsive patient with decerebrate posturing.

The initial diagnostic study for a patient with a suspected SAH is a CT scan of the head. Subarachnoid blood may be seen in the sylvian fissures, the basal cisterns, or the interhemispheric fissure (Fig. 1-12). An intracerebral hematoma or an SDH may also occur with ruptured aneurysm when the powerful jet of blood dissects into the parenchyma of the brain or the subdural space. If there is a high clinical suspicion of an SAH, but the CT scan does not show any subarachnoid blood and does not demonstrate a mass intracranial lesion, an *LP* is indicated. If the CSF is *xanthochromatic* or if it is bloody and does not clear as it is drained into successive collection tubes, the patient has suffered an SAH. When an SAH has occurred, four-vessel (bilateral carotid and bilateral vertebral arteries) cerebral arteriography is performed to look for an aneurysm. Seventy-five to eighty percent of patients with nontraumatic SAH will be found to have a ruptured aneurysm. About 20% of these patients will have multiple cerebral aneurysms. Much less commonly, a patient will have an AVM associated with an aneurysm. In about 15% of patients with a nontraumatic SAH, no cause will be found.

The goals of treatment are to prevent rebleeding, which is the greatest cause of morbidity and mortality in the first few days after an aneurysmal rupture, and to minimize the risk of vasospasm. All patients with a ruptured cerebral aneurysm are admitted to the intensive care unit (ICU) and measures to prevent rebleeding are instituted. These include strict bed rest with head elevation, systolic blood pressure controlled (usually below 150 mm Hg), and minimal stimulation. Frequent neurological examinations are performed by the nursing staff. Medications administered to the patient may include an anticonvulsant (phenytoin) and a calcium channel blocker (nimodipine), which has been shown to help prevent vasospasm. Corticosteroids may be given in the perioperative period.

Further treatment depends on the Hunt-Hess grade of the patient. To prevent rebleeding in grade 1, 2, and 3 patients, early surgery is performed to place a clip across the neck of the aneurysm and exclude it from the cerebral circulation. *Surgical clipping* of the aneurysm is done within 72 hours of the bleed to avoid the high-risk period for vasospasm. If a patient has gone into vasospasm, the brain does not tolerate surgery well. Grade 4 and 5 patients may have hydrocephalus secondary to the SAH and treating this with an emergent ventriculostomy may allow the patient to wake up, improve his or her Hunt-Hess grade, and undergo surgery. Grade 4 and 5 patients who do not improve are medically managed. In a Hunt-Hess grade 4 or 5 patient or a patient with a preexisting medical condition, which makes surgery riskier, a ruptured aneurysm can be thrombosed by the endovascular placement of coiled wires into its dome. A microcatheter is passed from the femoral artery into the aneurysm and detachable coils are placed within the aneurysm. The coils promote clots to form within the aneurysm, isolating it from the circulation.

During postbleed days 3 and 14, *vasospasm* is the major cause of morbidity and mortality. It is an idiopathic narrowing of the intracranial vessels, which most commonly occurs after aneurysmal SAH and it may last for 3 to 4 weeks. Vasospasm is seen on over 50% of arteriograms from patients with aneurysmal SAH, but only about 30% of patients with aneurysmal SAH are symptomatic from it. Decreased blood flow in the narrowed vessels causes focal ischemia of the brain and focal neurological deficits, such as aphasia and hemiparesis. Treatment (triple-H therapy) is aimed at increasing the cerebral blood flow by increasing the systemic blood volume (*hypervolemia*), increasing the systemic blood pressure (*hypertension*), and decreasing the rheology of the blood (*hemodilution*). The goal hematocrit to optimize the rheological properties of blood and not sacrifice oxygen-carrying capacity is 30%. If medical management fails, vessels in spasm can be treated with endovascular techniques, such as the direct intraarterial injection of papaverine and arterial balloon dilation. Unsuccessfully treated symptomatic vasospasm leads to an ischemic stroke and even death.

Other types of aneurysms that affect the cerebral circulation are mycotic, traumatic, and fusiform atherosclerotic aneurysms. Aneurysms secondary to infection or trauma are usually located more distally on the cerebral vasculature. *Mycotic aneurysms* are caused by bacterial or fungal infections. They may occur as a complication of infectious endocarditis when an infectious embolus enters the cerebral circulation. The embolus usually travels into a distal branch of the middle cerebral artery, because it receives the greatest percentage of blood flow to the brain of all cerebral arteries, and gets stuck. The local infectious and inflammatory processes create the aneurysm. *Traumatic aneurysms* occur at distal locations in the cerebral vasculature usually near a fixed structure such as the falx cerebri. A traumatic pericallosal aneurysm is thought to be created by the relatively mobile pericallosal artery being torn by the immobile falx. *Fusiform atherosclerotic aneurysms* occur in the proximal internal carotid artery and in the vertebrobasilar complex. They are difficult lesions to treat, because they are a dilation of the entire circumference of the vessel wall. An extracranial to intracranial arterial bypass procedure (*EC–IC bypass*) may be valuable in treating these lesions when symptomatic. Several variations of this operation are performed, including connecting the superficial temporal artery to the middle cerebral artery or using a vein graft to connect the extracranial internal carotid or vertebral artery to an intracranial artery such as the middle cerebral artery.

An extradural ophthalmic artery aneurysm may form if the ophthalmic artery branches off of the internal carotid artery within the cavernous sinus before it enters the dura. If this aneurysm ruptures, it hemorrhages into the cavernous sinus, which results in a carotid-cavernous fistula (CC fistula). This is a direct arterial-to-venous shunt. A CC fistula may also occur with a traumatic injury of the intracavernous carotid artery. If a CC fistula has a high flow or is causing visual deterioration, it is treated by endovascular balloon occlusion.

An *AVM* is a congenital abnormality consisting of a collection of abnormal vessels. By definition, there is a direct arterial-to-venous connection without intervening capillaries and therefore a decreased resistance to blood flow compared to normal brain. An AVM frequently presents in the third or fourth decade of life either ruptured or unruptured. Common symptoms of an *unruptured AVM* include headaches, seizures, or progressive neurological deficits, which may be secondary to ischemia created by the AVM stealing blood from the adjacent normal cortex due to its lower resistance to blood flow than normal brain (*steal syndrome*). Focal deficits may also occur from the mass effect of the dilated vessels of the AVM on the surrounding brain. An unruptured AVM is believed to have a risk of hemorrhage of about 1% per year. A patient with a *ruptured AVM* may present with a headache, loss of consciousness, seizure, or focal neurological deficit. On CT of the head, a ruptured AVM commonly produces an intracerebral hematoma within the parenchyma of the brain. Less frequently, intraventricular hemorrhage or SAH may occur. The hematoma is most commonly located within a cerebral hemisphere.

The goal of acute treatment is to help the patient survive the initial hemorrhage. Large life-threatening hematomas causing unresponsiveness (coma) and impending herniation need to be evacuated emergently. Awake and responsive patients can be observed in the ICU, because a previously ruptured AVM has a hemorrhage rate of about 5% per year, with no substantial increase in this rate during the period immediately following a bleed. After the patient recovers from the bleed, cerebral angiography and MRI of the head are used to define the anatomy of the AVM. On angiography, a nidus of abnormal vessels is seen, early draining veins are seen, and in about 10%, an aneurysm is seen on a feeding artery. On MRI, abnormal flow voids are seen. Depending on the location and extent of the AVM, it may be possible to surgically resect the lesion. Endovascular embolization of the feeding arteries may be done preoperatively during the angiogram. Rarely, embolization may totally obliterate the AVM. Stereotactic radiosurgery is used for smaller AVMs, particularly when they are deep within the brain. It takes 6 months to 2 years for the AVM to be obliterated after radiosurgery and unfortunately the risk of rebleeding is not decreased during this time.

Another entity that presents with an intracerebral hematoma is a *hypertensive hemorrhage*. Patients usually have a long-standing history of hypertension and the presenting signs and symptoms depend on where the bleed occurs. Most commonly, the hemorrhage begins in the putamen or external capsule when a deep perforating artery, which has undergone chronic degenerative hypertensive–related changes, ruptures. Other common sites of origin for the hemorrhage are the thalamus, cerebellum, and brainstem. Less frequently, a lobar hemorrhage in the cerebral cortex may be associated with hypertension. A patient who has bled into the putamen, external capsule, or thalamus presents with a progressive focal neurological deficit and progressive lethargy. A headache may or may not be associated with the bleed. On examination, the patient has one or more of the following symptoms and signs: a contralateral hemiparesis, a contralateral hemisensory loss, or a contralateral hemianopsia. A hemorrhage in this location is usually caused by the rupture of a lenticulostriate or thalamoperforating artery. A patient who suffers a cerebellar hypertensive hemorrhage complains of the sudden onset of a headache, nausea and vomiting, and dizziness. Ataxia may be found on examination. The hematoma may directly compress the brainstem, resulting in the loss of upward gaze and progressive lethargy until the patient is unresponsive. A hypertensive hemorrhage in the pons results from the rupture of a pontine artery, a branch off the basilar artery.

Unfortunately, these are almost always fatal. The patient usually presents unresponsive and quadriparetic and has pinpoint pupils.

A hypertensive hemorrhage is diagnosed on an emergent noncontrast CT of the head by the location of the hematoma. Intraventricular hemorrhage may accompany the intraparenchymal clot and both may cause hydrocephalus. Coagulation studies should be ordered emergently, including a platelet count, a prothrombin time, and a partial prothrombin time. If abnormal, platelets or clotting factors should be given. For supratentorial hematomas, surgical evacuation is reserved for large, life-threatening clots that have not already neurologically devastated the patient. For cerebellar hematomas, immediate treatment is required consisting of an emergent suboccipital craniectomy and evacuation of the hematoma. Surgery is not needed to stop the hemorrhage or prevent further hemorrhages. Once the patient has bled, blood pressure control is important to prevent another hemorrhage. If the patient survives the bleed and is not neurologically devastated, the prognosis is good. The hematoma frequently dissects along axonal planes and causes minimal tissue destruction. Some of the initial neurological deficits may be secondary to edema and to direct compression of surrounding cortex by the hematoma. These deficits will improve as the hematoma resolves. The best treatment for a hypertensive hemorrhage is to prevent it from occurring by controlling chronic hypertension.

Another vascular disorder of the brain is *ischemic cerebrovascular disease*. Ischemic strokes most commonly occur in the distribution of the carotid arteries, because they are responsible for about 80% of the blood supply to the brain. Ischemic events can be classified according to their duration into transient ischemic attacks, reversible ischemic neurological deficits, and completed strokes. A *transient ischemic attack* (TIA) usually lasts less than 30 minutes but by definition can last up to 24 hours. Complete neurological recovery always occurs. A TIA of the retina is called *amaurosis fugax,* which is described by patients as a shade being pulled down or up across one eye causing the transient loss of vision. A TIA of the brain may cause a transient hemiparesis, hemisensory deficit, or aphasia. A *reversible ischemic neurological deficit* (RIND) lasts 24 hours to 3 days. Again, full recovery of neurological function occurs. A *completed stroke* is when a neurological deficit associated with brain ischemia lasts longer than 3 days.

A stroke can be caused by the formation of a thrombus in a large cerebral artery or the passage of an embolus into a cerebral arteriole. When an occlusive or nonocclusive thrombus forms in a large artery, the blood flow to a portion of the brain may be cut off or decreased below a critical threshold and ischemia results. Most commonly, this is caused by thrombus superimposed on a vessel lumen narrowed by atherosclerosis. The region of the brain supplied by the occluded artery depends entirely on collateral flow from other cerebral vessels. If there is adequate collateral blood supply to the region in jeopardy, no ischemia results. If not, this region becomes ischemic and a neurological deficit may occur. A frequent extracranial site of atherosclerotic disease is the carotid bifurcation and origin of the internal carotid artery. Intracranial atherosclerosis commonly occurs in the carotid siphon, in the distal internal carotid artery, and in the proximal middle cerebral artery. Complete cutoff of the blood supply to an area of the brain results from the embolic occlusion of a cerebral arteriole. An embolus may originate from an atherosclerotic ulceration at the carotid bifurcation, a mural thrombus in the heart, or a valvular lesion in the heart. Heart-derived emboli are associated with atrial fibrillation and myocardial infarctions. Emboli most frequently pass into the middle cerebral arteries. Clinically, the patient presents with a focal, sometimes progressive, neurological deficit and may be lethargic.

The best treatment is prevention. Risk factors need to be identified and treated or modified. Risk factors for ischemic stroke include hypertension, diabetes, hypercholesterolemia, obesity, smoking, and a family history of stroke. Medical treatment of ischemic cerebrovascular disease includes antiplatelet therapy and anticoagulation. Surgical treatment may compliment medical therapy and consists of carotid endarterectomy for common carotid and proximal internal carotid artery atherosclerotic disease. Multiple randomized trials have shown a benefit in recently symptomatic patients with a significant carotid stenosis contralateral to their symptoms, as long as the patient has not had a recent major stroke or does not have any comorbid medical conditions that would greatly increase the risk of surgery. In asymptomatic patients, several randomized studies have also shown a benefit for carotid artery endarterectomy. It is important to note that in these studies, most patients were white men. When selecting a patient for surgery, it is important to rule out, with cerebral angiography or MRA, more distal stenotic lesions in the internal carotid artery, which may be the cause of the ischemic symptoms.

Carotid endarterectomy can be done using local anesthesia, to allow for frequent neurological examinations, or general anesthesia, utilizing electroencephalogram (EEG) monitoring. If the neurological examination of the patient or the EEG changes while the carotid artery is clamped, a temporary shunt from the common carotid artery to the internal carotid artery is needed during the surgery. The shunt is a plastic tube that the surgeon is able to work around to remove the plaque. When releasing the arteries, the clamp on the common carotid artery is released first, then the external carotid is opened (so any emboli dislodged by the restoration of blood flow will enter the external carotid circulation), and finally the internal carotid is released. An acceptable mortality rate for carotid artery endarterectomy is 1%, with an acceptable morbidity rate between 1% and 5%.

When the internal carotid artery stenosis is higher up in the neck, it is inaccessible to an endarterectomy procedure. With this and other surgically inaccessible ischemic cerebrovascular disease, a microvascular bypass from the external carotid artery to the internal carotid artery (EC–IC bypass) may be helpful.

The spinal cord is affected by the same vascular disorders that affect the brain; however, they occur much less commonly.

TUMORS

Brain tumors account for about 10% of all neoplasms and can be either primary CNS tumors or metastases. *Primary tumors* arise from various cells in the cortex, the coverings of the brain, and the pituitary gland. *Metastatic tumors* can spread by local extension or through the blood, lymph, or CSF. The location of brain tumors varies with age. In adults, about 70% of brain tumors are supratentorial (located above the tentorium cerebelli). The most common brain tumor in adults is a metastatic lesion. In children, about 70% of brain tumors are infratentorial (in the posterior fossa) and account for 15% to 20% of all childhood tumors. In fact, brain tumors are the second most common childhood cancer in overall prevalence (leukemia is the most common) and the most common solid tumor of childhood.

A brain tumor may present with signs and symptoms of increased ICP, a focal deficit, or a seizure. The increased ICP is a result of the tumor adding tissue mass within the skull. The modified *Monro-Kellie* hypothesis states that the skull is a nonexpansile structure that can only hold a finite volume of blood, brain, CSF, and any abnormal components (tumor, hematoma, etc.). If the amount of one of these increase, the amount of a different one must decrease. Therefore, elevated ICP results when mechanisms compensating for the additional volume from the tumor are overwhelmed. Adding to the increased ICP is any associated edema, hydrocephalus, or tumor hemorrhage. Symptoms of increased ICP include chronic headaches—which are worse upon awakening in the morning, worse with dependent head positions, and exacerbated during straining—nausea or vomiting, and personality changes, which include lack of motivation and apathy. Elevated ICP is also associated with slowed cognitive function and will lead to progressive lethargy and eventually unresponsiveness. The signs of increased ICP include papilledema and a unilateral or bilateral abducens (cranial nerve IV) palsy. Because of the long intracranial course of the abducens nerve, it can be compressed by the elevated ICP and is referred to as a *false localizing sign*. Patients with brain tumors also present with neurological deficits. With supratentorial tumors, deficits include a monoparesis, hemiparesis, hemisensory deficit, visual deficit, aphasia, and cranial nerve palsies. With infratentorial tumors, neurological deficits include ataxia, nystagmus, and cranial nerve palsies.

A patient with a supratentorial brain tumor may present with a seizure, either partial or generalized. A partial seizure may be a *simple partial seizure* with focal motor or sensory symptoms but no loss of consciousness, a *complex partial seizure* with some alteration of consciousness and an associated automatism, or a *partial seizure with secondary generalization,* which is a seizure that begins focally and progresses to involve the entire body, including a loss of consciousness. A *generalized seizure* starts on both sides of the body simultaneously and consciousness is lost at the onset. A brain tumor should be suspected in any patient over 20 years old who has his or her first idiopathic seizure.

Patients with suspected intracranial masses are best evaluated with a CT or MRI of the head. With an acute presentation—e.g., a new onset seizure, progressive neurological deficit, or lethargy—an unenhanced CT is indicted because it is a quick way to look for large lesions with mass effect or acute hemorrhage, which may be life threatening. If the patient is wide awake and there is no sense of urgency, an MRI with and without contrast can be done, which is a more sensitive imaging modality for the soft tissues in the CNS.

Primary brain tumors can be divided into tumors that are derived from elements normally present in the CNS and tumors that are derived from embryonic remnants. The tumors that arise from cells normally found in the CNS can be divided into tumors that arise from neural tube derivatives (astrocytomas, glioblastomas, oligodendrogliomas, ependymomas, choroid plexus papillomas), tumors that arise from neurons (medulloblastomas, gangliomas), tumors that arise from neural crest derivatives (meningiomas, acoustic neuromas), and tumors that arise from other cells present in the CNS (primary CNS lymphoma, hemangioblastomas, glomus jugulare tumors, pituitary adenomas). Tumors that are derived from embryonic remnants include craniopharyngiomas, germinomas, teratomas, epidermoids, and dermoids.

Glioma is a general term for any tumor arising from a stromal cell of the CNS, which is a derivative of the neural tube. A glioma frequently has indistinct borders and infiltrates the surrounding brain by spreading along white matter tracts. However, a glioma will rarely metastasize outside of the CNS but may spread to other areas within the CNS through the CSF. Over time, a glioma may transform from a benign tumor into a malignant tumor. Types of gliomas include low-grade astrocytomas, anaplastic astrocytomas, glioblastomas, oligodendrogliomas, ependymomas, and choroid plexus papillomas.

Low-grade astrocytomas tend to grow slowly and cause mild symptoms for several years before they are diagnosed, and they most commonly present in people between the ages of 30 and 50 years. On MRI or CT, a low-intensity or low-density supratentorial mass is seen that may or may not enhance. Histological sections show brain parenchyma that is more cellular than normal, with infiltration of the surrounding brain. Treatment consists of surgical resection and for more aggressive tumors, postoperative external beam radiation therapy. The 5-year survival rate has been reported to be up to 50%. Low-grade astrocytomas commonly transform into high-grade anaplastic astrocytomas and glioblastomas.

Anaplastic astrocytomas (AAs) are high-grade lesions that are more cellular and have a more rapid growth rate than low-grade astrocytomas. They commonly present in 45 to 65 year olds. On MRI or CT, a hypointense or hypodense mass, which usually enhances, is seen. Pathologic section shows increased cellularity and infiltration of the surrounding brain. The cells have more malignant characteristics than low-grade astrocytomas including nuclear pleomorphism, bizarre-looking nuclei, and mitoses. Treatment is surgical resection, if possible, and postoperative external beam radiation. If the lesion is not amenable to resection, a stereotactic biopsy can be done for diagnosis. Average survival is about 2 years.

The most malignant glioma is the *glioblastoma multiforme* (GBMs, glioblastomas), which is a form of astrocytoma. GBMs are the most common primary intracranial tumor. The peak age of occurrence is between 50 and 70 years old. The diagnosis is based on the histological characteristics of the tumor, which include nuclear pleomorphism, mitoses, necrosis, pseudopalisading of cells around the necrotic areas, and neovascularization with endothelial cell proliferation. GBMs are often associated with tumor hemorrhage. Treatment is surgical resection, if possible, or a stereotactic biopsy for diagnosis. This is followed by external beam radiation and chemotherapy. Average survival is less than 1 year. A subset of GBMs or AAs are called *butterfly gliomas* because they invade the corpus callosum and involve both cerebral hemispheres. These tumors are unresectable and have a poor prognosis.

A benign subset of astrocytomas are the *pilocytic astrocytomas,* which occur mainly in children and adolescents. A common location of this tumor is within the cerebellum and a complete resection can result in a cure. Cerebellar pilocytic astrocytomas have a favorable prognosis, with a 10-year survival rate of 80%. Unfortunately, pilocytic astrocytomas also occur around the third ventricle and in the brainstem. Tumors in these locations are difficult to completely resect without devastating neurological consequences and are therefore difficult to cure. A much lower 5-year survival rate of 15% to 30% is associated with these tumors. Pilocytic astrocytomas may also originate in the optic nerve and are called *optic nerve gliomas.* A complete resection is possible, with unilateral optic nerve involvement, which may be curative. Unfortunately, optic nerve gliomas may invade the optic chiasm or hypothalamus, making total resection impossible.

Oligodendrogliomas are derived from the cells that produce and maintain myelin in the CNS (oligodendrocytes).

They occur much less frequently than astrocytomas, making up about 5% of gliomas. Oligodendrogliomas are slow-growing neoplasms that usually present with seizures. Most commonly, they occur in 40 to 50 year olds and they are rare in children. On MRI or CT, they are almost always supratentorial, usually located in the frontal lobe, commonly have areas of calcification, and usually enhance with the administration of i.v. contrast. Microscopically, they usually appear benign with cells that resemble "fried eggs," but anaplastic features are possible. In up to one-third of cases, neoplastic oligodendrocytes are mixed with neoplastic astrocytes or ependymal cells, called a *mixed glioma.* Treatment consists of surgical resection. With an incomplete resection or for a tumor with malignant histology, postoperative external beam radiation is added. The 5-year survival rate for oligodendrogliomas (not including mixed gliomas) is 50% to 80%, with a 20-year survival rate of around 6%.

Ependymocytes, which line the ventricular system, are the cell of origin of *ependymomas,* which comprise about 5% of gliomas. The peak incidence occurs in childhood when two thirds of ependymomas are located in the posterior fossa, usually growing in the floor of the fourth ventricle. When they occur in adults, they are usually supratentorial and about one-half are intraventricular. They may cause hydrocephalus, from obstruction to the flow of CSF, and may metastasize through the CSF. On MRI or CT, they appear as enhancing well-circumscribed masses. Treatment consists of surgical resection; however, they frequently recur, resulting in a 5-year survival rate of about 50%.

Choroid plexus papillomas are tumors that arise from the cells that produce CSF. They occur within the ventricular system and are benign. Hydrocephalus, classically considered to be secondary to the overproduction of CSF but also probably due to intraventricular tumor hemorrhage, is commonly associated, and a patient may present because of elevated ICP. When malignant, which is rare, they are *choroid plexus carcinomas.* In children, choroid plexus papillomas frequently are located in the left lateral ventricle, and in adults, they are frequently located in the fourth ventricle. This is opposite to the usual supratentorial brain tumor location in adults and infratentorial location in children. Treatment consists of surgical resection.

Medulloblastomas, also referred to as *primitive neural ectoderm tumors* (PNETs), originate from primitive bipotential cells of the cerebellum. About two thirds of PNETs occur in children and adolescents and they are rare in people older than 40 years. In addition, 20% of childhood brain tumors are PNETs. Commonly, medulloblastomas present with signs of increased ICP and signs of cerebellar dysfunction, which include ataxia and nystagmus. PNETs are usually located in the vermis of the cerebellum, which forms the roof of the fourth ventricle (as opposed to ependymomas, which are located in the floor of the fourth ventricle). In patients over the age of 15, they may occur in the cerebellar hemispheres. PNETs are very cellular, malignant lesions that can metastasize through the CSF, but they rarely metastasize outside of the CNS. After diagnosis but before surgical manipulation of the tumor, the CSF should be checked for malignant cells. With gross total resection and craniospinal radiation therapy, the 5-year survival rate is about 75%. Chemotherapy may also be used, particularly with recurrent tumors and in young children not able to be irradiated. If gross total resection is not possible, the 5-year survival rate is much lower.

Meningiomas account for about 17% of intracranial tumors. They are benign extraaxial primary CNS tumors that arise from cells of the arachnoid granulations located within the meninges. Women are more frequently affected than men and progesterone receptors and estrogen receptors have been found on meningioma cells. Meningiomas are most commonly diagnosed in patients between the ages of 30 and 60 years. The common locations for meningiomas are as follows: the convexity of the cerebral hemisphere, parasagittal, the floor of the anterior cranial fossa (olfactory groove), the sphenoid wing, the clivus, the falx cerebri, the posterior fossa, the tuberculum sellae, and the middle cranial fossa. Usually, they indent the brain but do not invade it; however, they may invade the adjacent bone. On MRI or CT, they brightly enhance with i.v. contrast administration and may have a dural tail, which is the enhancing portion of thickened dura adjacent to the tumor. Treatment involves surgical resection of the tumor and the involved dura. Meningiomas have a good long-term prognosis and low recurrence rate. Rarely, a meningioma will be atypical or malignant. The prognosis is worse for atypical or malignant meningiomas, which recur more frequently.

Acoustic neuromas are tumors composed of Schwann cells most often arising from the vestibular portion of the eighth cranial nerve (more properly called *acoustic schwannomas*). Adult women are most frequently affected. Acoustic neuromas commonly present with hearing loss or cerebellar dysfunction. Facial numbness, from compression of the facial nerve as it exits the brainstem, and obstructive hydrocephalus, from brainstem compression, may also occur. Acoustic neuromas are benign lesions, which may be cured with a complete resection. The surgery is made challenging by the important neural structures adjacent to the tumor in the cerebellopontine angle, which include the brainstem and the facial nerve (cranial nerve VII). The preservation of hearing and facial nerve function is directly related to the size of the tumor. *Neurofibromatosis type II* is associated with bilateral acoustic neuromas. Schwannomas may also grow on other sensory cranial nerves, including the trigeminal nerve.

Primary CNS lymphomas are increasing in incidence. Frequently, they are related to immunosuppression associated with organ transplantation and acquired immunodeficiency syndrome. They may have single or in about one fourth of cases multiple foci. Most commonly, they are of B-cell origin and are radiosensitive. Treatment includes stereotactic biopsy for diagnosis, radiation, and steroids.

Hemangioblastomas are benign tumors that arise from vascular cells. They are uncommon, making up about 1% of intracranial tumors. In adults, they are the most common primary intraaxial tumor within the posterior fossa. They most frequently present in the fourth decade of life. Hemangioblastomas are usually located in the cerebellum and present with cerebellar dysfunction and hydrocephalus. Less commonly, they are located in the brainstem, spinal cord, or cerebral hemisphere. On MRI or CT, they may appear as a large cyst with a brightly enhancing mural nodule, or less frequently, they may be solid tumors that brightly enhance. *Polycythemia,* from a hematopoietic factor released from the tumor, is often present in a patient with a hemangioblastoma. Complete surgical resection is curative for an isolated lesion. They have a good prognosis with about an 80% survival rate at 10 years. The combination of CNS hemangioblastomas, retinal angiomatosis, renal and pancreatic cysts, and renal cell carcinoma is called *von Hippel Lindau disease,* which is localized to a mutation on the short arm of chromosome 3 and has an autosomal dominant inheritance pattern.

Pituitary adenomas are benign tumors that arise from the anterior lobe of the pituitary gland (hypophysis). They most commonly present in patients between the ages of 20 and 40 years. They can be divided into microadenomas, measuring less than 1 cm in diameter, and macroadenomas, measuring greater than 1 cm in diameter. Microadenomas are discovered because of symptoms directly related to the tumor overproducing one or more pituitary hormones. Common presentations include amenorrhea and galactorrhea from prolactin overproduction by a prolactinoma, acromegaly from growth hormone excess, and Cushing disease from overproduction of ACTH. *Macroadenomas* do not produce any active pituitary hormones. Instead, they become symptomatic by compressing surrounding structures, causing visual loss, hypopituitarism, and hyperprolactinemia. They also may cause headaches. The stereotypical field cut associated with a macroadenoma is a bitemporal hemianopsia from the compression of the medial portions of both optic nerves just anterior to the optic chiasm. *Hyperprolactinemia* is caused by the tumor compressing the pituitary stalk, which blocks dopamine (released from the hypothalamus) from traveling through the stalk to the posterior lobe of the pituitary gland, where it normally inhibits the production of prolactin. Most microadenomas and masses located in the sella are treated surgically using a transsphenoidal approach through the nose and sphenoid sinus. Prolactinomas also can be treated medically with dopamine agonists, such as bromocriptine. For large macroadenomas with significant suprasellar extension, resection of the tumor can also be accomplished through a craniotomy. Overall, the prognosis is good.

Metastatic brain tumors are the most common brain tumor in adults. They arise from a lung tumor 35% of the time, breast tumor 20%, malignant melanoma 10%, kidney tumor 10%, and GI tumor 5% of the time. Testicular cancer may also metastasize to the brain. They most commonly affect older adults. Signs and symptoms of lesions in the cerebral hemispheres include headache, a change in mental status, seizures, and neurological deficits. Cerebellar lesions may cause ataxia, nystagmus, and vomiting. On CT or MRI, metastatic lesions are located at the junction between the gray and white matter and extensive vasogenic edema is seen in the white matter surrounding the tumor. Treatment includes corticosteroids, which effectively decrease the amount of vasogenic edema and have been shown to prolong survival. Surgical treatment includes either a biopsy for diagnosis in a patient with multiple lesions or a craniotomy for resection of a single lesion in a patient with an expected survival of at least 4 months. In carefully selected patients, multiple metastatic lesions may all be resected. Whole brain radiation therapy is used postoperatively and in nonsurgical patients expected to survive at least a couple months. A single session of focused radiation, known as *stereotactc radiosurgery,* is now being used for multiple small metastatic lesions. The prognosis depends on the type of primary tumor, with median survival times in the 1- to 2-year range. Metastatic lesions also occur within the dura, skull, and posterior pituitary gland.

Meningeal carcinomatosis is metastatic spread of a systemic cancer to the leptomeninges. This most commonly occurs with childhood leukemia, adult lymphoma, breast cancer, lung cancer, and melanoma. Presenting signs may include a cranial nerve palsy, radiculopathy, obstructive hydrocephalus, and meningeal signs (headache, stiff neck, photophobia). If there is no mass lesion on CT scan of the head, a lumbar pucture (LP) can be performed, which may show an increased opening pressure, elevated protein, and decreased glucose. The CSF should be sent for cytology to look for metastatic cells. MRI shows diffuse enhancement of the involved subarachnoid spaces. Treatment includes radiation therapy and intrathecal chemotherapy given via a ventricular catheter or by LP. The prognosis is usually poor.

INFECTION

Infections in the CNS can be bacterial, viral, fungal, or parasitic. Bacterial infections can be subgaleal, osseous, epidural, subdural, leptomeningeal, intraventricular, or intraparenchymal. A *subgaleal abscess* is located between the galea and pericranium and is usually a complication of a traumatic or surgical wound. The skin overlying a subgaleal abscess is tender, warm, and swollen. Treatment consists of surgical drainage and antibiotics. *Osteomyelitis* is an infection of the bone. When the skull is infected, it is usually the result of the direct spread of an adjacent tissue infection such as a paranasal sinus infection, a subgaleal abscess, a penetrating wound infection, or a postoperative wound infection. Rarely, osteomyelitis of the skull is the result of hematogenous spread. Treatment includes systemic antibiotics, removal of the infected bone, debridement of the surrounding soft tissue, and addressing the underlying cause of the infection. Osteomyelitis also occurs in the spine, where it is usually the result of the hematogenous spread of bacteria. The infection can spread into the epidural space and create a spinal epidural abscess. An *epidural abscess* is more common in the spine than the head. A patient will usually present with a fever and spine tenderness, localized over the infected area of the spine. The workup should include blood cultures and an MRI of the spine. Epidural abscesses are treated with i.v. antibiotics and if the patient has a neurological deficit, emergent surgical drainage of the abscess and decompression of the spinal cord. A *subdural empyema* (subdural abscess) occurs around the brain. It is a purulent infection of the subdural space, which is widespread over the entire surface of the cerebral hemisphere. The source of a subdural empyema can be from an infection within the CNS, such as a meningitis, or from the spread of an infection from outside of the CNS, which has extended through the dura, such as a sinusitis, an infected traumatic or surgical wound, or a transcranial emissary vein thrombosis. On CT or MRI, an enhancing subdural mass is seen. Treatment includes emergent surgical evacuation of the subdural empyema. Unfortunately, a subdural empyema has a significant mortality rate.

Bacterial meningitis is an infection of the leptomeninges. Patients present with fever, lethargy, headache, nausea and vomiting, nuchal rigidity, seizures, and cranial nerve palsies. A patient suspected of having a bacterial meningitis should first undergo a CT of the head to rule out a mass lesion. With a negative CT scan of the head, an LP can be safely performed and CSF sent for a gram stain, culture, glucose level, protein level, and white blood cell count. CSF results consistent with a bacterial meningitis include a low glucose level (less than two thirds of the serum glucose level), a high protein level, and the presence of white cells with a predominance of polymorphonuclear lymphocytes. In addition, blood cultures should be sent, which may yield the causative organism. The treatment of bacterial meningitis is systemic i.v. antibiotics, and if a source of the meningitis is found such as a postoperative or traumatic CSF leak, treatment of any underlying cause should be done. The initiation of antibiotics should not be delayed until the completion of the CT scan of the head, the LP, and blood cultures in a sick patient because untreated cases are almost always fatal. Complications of bacterial meningitis include communicating hydrocephalus, subdural empyema, and cerebritis, leading to cerebral abscess formation

Cerebritis is a focal cerebral inflammation, which immediately precedes the development of an abscess. A cerebral abscess may arise from the direct spread of bacteria from an adjacent non-CNS infection or from the hematogenous spread of bacteria. The direct extension of an infection from the skull can occur with a mastoiditis, which leads to a temporal or cerebellar abscess, or a frontal sinusitis, which leads to a frontal abscess. Inoculation of bacteria through the meninges by an open skull fracture, gunshot wound, or surgical wound can also occur. Abscesses caused by direct extension are usually solitary. Abscesses caused by the hematogenous spread of bacteria occur with pneumonia, bacterial endocarditis, or diverticulitis. Cerebral abscesses are more common in patients with a right-to-left shunt, such as a cardiac septal defect or a pulmonary AVM, due to paradoxical emboli. Emboli usually lodge in a branch of the middle cerebral artery, because this vessel receives the largest proportion of cerebral blood flow. When cerebral abscesses are from the hematogenous spread of bacteria, they frequently are multiple. Patients without a preceding meningitis may not have systemic signs of infection. Focal signs, such as a hemiparesis or a focal seizure, can occur as the abscess grows and compresses the surrounding brain. Symptoms and signs of increased ICP, such as headache and decreased mental status, occur as the abscess enlarges and the surrounding brain becomes edematous. On CT or MRI, a thin-rimmed *ring-enhancing lesion* is seen. Treatment consists of sending blood cultures, administering i.v. antibiotics, and surgically draining the abscess. Corticosteroids may be given to treat the associated brain edema and an anticonvulsant may be used for seizure prophylaxis. Cerebral abscesses are more common in immunosuppressed patients.

Viral infections include meningitis and encephalitis. A *viral encephalitis* may present like a brain tumor or mass lesion. *Herpes simplex encephalitis* frequently presents as a temporal lobe mass causing an aphasia, upper-extremity weakness, seizure, or a combination of these. It may also present with generalized symptoms from increased ICP. MRI or CT frequently shows a hemorrhagic, necrotic, and sometimes cystic temporal lobe mass. Treatment includes a stereotactic biopsy to get a diagnosis or a craniotomy for biopsy and debulking of the mass.

Fungal infections are usually caused by opportunistic organisms in immunosuppressed patients. Commonly, they are associated with a pulmonary fungal infection. A meningitis or an abscess is possible. Complications include hydrocephalus.

Parasitic infections are uncommon in the United States. *Cysticercosis* is an infection of the pork tapeworm, *Taenia solium*. It can spread through the bloodstream to the meninges, the brain parenchyma, or the ventricular system. A patient may present with a seizure, focal deficit, or signs of increased ICP secondary to obstructive hydrocephalus. Cysticercosis also infects the spine and can be located intramedullary, which can cause a transverse myelitis, or extramedullary, which can cause a compressive myelopathy. *Echinococcosis*, also called *hydatidosis*, is an infection by

Echinococcus granulosus, the dog tapeworm. It spreads through the bloodstream to the white matter. These cysts are associated with little if any inflammation. It is possible for a cyst to act like a mass lesion and cause a neurological deficit. When this occurs, the cyst can be surgically excised.

DEGENERATIVE DISEASES OF THE SPINE

Degenerative changes affect both the cervical and lumbar spine. In the cervical spine, a disk or a fragment of a disk, degenerative changes in the ligaments, or bony grows called *osteophytes* can cause neurological symptoms. A cervical vertebral disk can herniate along the midline and compress the spinal cord or can herniate to one side of the spinal canal and compress a spinal root. In the cervical spine, the nerve root that is compressed is the one exiting at the level of the disk herniation. For example, a C6-7 disk compresses the C-7 root. A C7-T1 disk compresses the C-8 root. When a free fragment of disk is extruded into the canal or foramen, it is called a *soft disk* or a *herniation of nucleus pulposus,* which most commonly occurs in the lower cervical spine at C6-7 or C5-6, where most neck flexion and extension occurs. The usual history given by a patient with a herniated cervical disk is the symptoms began when he or she awoke in the morning and there is no history of trauma. Patients with herniated cervical disks complain of neck pain, which is increased with movement, particularly extension of the neck and lateral flexion of the neck toward the side of the herniated disk. Radicular symptoms and signs from a compressed nerve root include pain and hypoesthesia within the dermatome of that root (Fig. 1-17), weakness in the muscles innervated by that root, and loss of a deep tendon reflex mediated by that root. The pain experienced by the patient may be worsened by straining and coughing and improved with bed rest. With severe acute spinal cord compression, quadriparesis and bowel or bladder dysfunction occurs. On examination, the patient will have decreased range of motion of the neck, particularly in extension. MRI is the best study to look for free fragments of disk and cord abnormalities.

Any combination of the following pathological processes can cause stenosis of the cervical spinal canal (cervical stenosis) or stenosis of the intervertebral foramen: one or

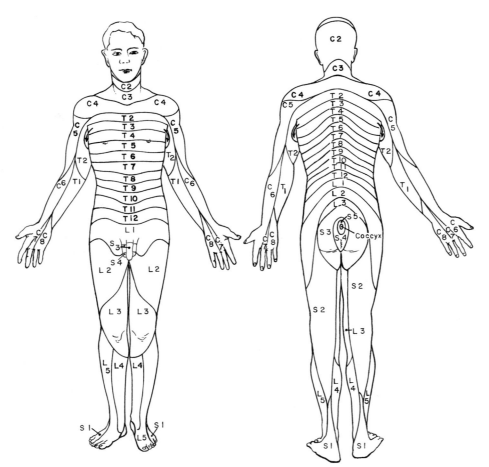

FIGURE 1-17. Dermatomes. The sensory innervation of the spinal roots. (From Barr, Kiernan. *The human nervous system.* JB Lippincott Co, 1993, with permission.)

more osteophytes (hard disks) located at the posterior edge of the vertebral bodies, hypertrophy or calcification of the posterior longitudinal ligament, hypertrophy of the ligamentum flavum, one or more medial disk bulges, hypertrophy of the dura, hypertrophy of the lamina of the vertebrae, and a congenitally narrow spinal canal. Osteophytes are formed at the superior and inferior end plates of the vertebral bodies. When cervical stenosis is caused by a long-standing degenerative process, it is called *cervical spondylosis*. The result is narrowing of the bony spinal canal causing chronic compression of the spinal cord, which results in myelopathic symptoms and narrowing of the intervertebral foramen causing chronic compression of exiting nerve roots, which results in radicular symptoms. *Myelopathy* is characterized by upper motor neuron dysfunction, which includes spasticity, hyperactive deep tendon reflexes, and the presence of a *Babinski sign*. A patient with spastic legs has difficulty ambulating and may suffer frequent falls. Bowel and bladder dysfunction, sexual dysfunction, and decreased sensation also occur. *Radicular symptoms* include lower motor neuron dysfunction, resulting in weakness of muscles innervated by the compressed root and hypoactive deep tendon reflexes of the same muscles. Radicular symptoms also include sensory loss in the dermatome innervated by the compressed root. Root compression can be worsened by osteoarthritis of zygapophyseal (facet) joints and joints of Luschka, which causes additional narrowing of the intervertebral foramina. On lateral cervical spine films, there is a loss of the normal cervical lordosis and straightening or even kyphosis of the cervical vertebral column, narrowed disk spaces, osteophytes, and the anteroposterior diameter of the spinal canal is narrowed. MRI is the best study to evaluate the spinal cord pathology, including the severity and location of the spinal cord compression and the presence of any signal change in the cord. CT is the best study for evaluation of the bony pathology.

The management for both an acute disk rupture and a chronic cervical stenosis is similar. If the patient presents with only radicular pain and sensory symptoms, but no motor, bowel, or bladder dysfunction, conservative management is initiated. This includes bed rest, pain medication, antiinflammatory medication, application of local heat, muscle relaxants, intermittent immobilization of the neck in a soft or hard collar (for comfort only, not for stability), and physical therapy. If a patient fails an adequate trial of conservative management, surgery is considered. If a patient has any motor weakness, bowel or bladder dysfunction, or myelopathic symptoms, surgery is usually necessary. Whether an anterior approach, such as an anterior cervical diskectomy, or a posterior approach, such as a laminectomy, is performed depends on the location of the pathological lesion.

Disk pathology occurs much less frequently in the *thoracic spine*, because there is less movement in this portion of the spine. The thoracic bony spinal canal is narrow, leaving little extra space around the spinal cord. Therefore, neurological deficits are common when a thoracic disk herniates into the spinal canal. Symptoms and signs include pain, sensory changes, and leg weakness. Thoracic disk herniations are seen in trauma and as chronic degenerative lesions and usually occur below T-8.

Disk herniations also occur in the *lumbosacral spine*. Herniated disks are pieces of the nucleus pulposus extruded into the spinal canal through a rent in the annulus fibrosis. If the disk fragment gets only partially through the annulus, it will create a bulge in the annulus. If the disk fragment gets through the annulus, a free fragment within the spinal canal results. Because the spinal cord usually ends around the L-1 vertebral body and most lumbar disk herniations occur at L5-S1 or L4-5, a patient will present with radicular symptoms. The compressed nerve root is the one exiting below the disk space with the herniation; e.g., L4-5 disk herniation will compress the L-5 root. With an L5-S1 disk herniation, the S-1 root is compressed. Less commonly, a far lateral herniation of a lumbar disk can compress the nerve root exiting in the intervertebral foramen of the same level; e.g., a far lateral L4-5 disk will compress the L-4 nerve root. Most lumbar disk herniations occur at L5-S1 or L4-5 because this is where most of the flexion and extension of the low back occurs. The patient may give a history of hearing or feeling a "pop" in the low back during exertion, after which the radicular symptoms began, or more commonly, the patient may give a history of slowly progressive symptoms. The radicular pain caused by a herniated lumber disk is increased with bending, sitting, standing, lifting, coughing, straining, or extension of the spine, and it is relieved with bed rest, particularly if the patient lies on his or her side with his hips and knees flexed. *Sciatica* is pain radiating down the posterior or lateral leg to the ankle or foot in the distribution of the sciatic nerve and commonly occurs on the same side as a herniated disk. Signs on examination include sensory loss in the dermatome (Fig. 1-17), weakness in muscles innervated by the compressed nerve root, low back tenderness, paravertebral muscle spasm, and loss of deep tendon reflexes effected by the compressed root. The *straight-leg raising test* is performed by having the patient lie flat on his or her back as the examiner slowly raises the fully extended legs of the patient one at a time. A positive result is when radicular symptoms are reproduced in the symptomatic leg. Back pain does not constitute a positive finding. Herniated lumbar disks are best imaged by MRI, which shows the fragment or disk bulge and the compressed nerve root. Treatment for a herniated lumbar disk can be conservative if the patient has only pain and sensory symptoms. Medical management includes strict bed rest, pain medications, local application of heat, antiinflammatory medications, and skeletal muscle relaxants. Physical therapy can be added later for low back strengthening. Surgery, usually a microdiskectomy, is indicated if a patient has weakness, progressive worsening of their exam, or chronic disabling pain. A herniated disc may recur after medical or surgical treatment.

Lumbar spinal stenosis—narrowing of the lumbar spinal canal, which compresses the cauda equina—is caused by one or more of the following: a congenitally narrow lumbar spinal canal, facet hypertrophy, hypertrophy of the ligamentum flavum, bulging of intervertebral discs, and spondylolisthesis. *Spondylolisthesis* is the anterior subluxation of a vertebral body on the vertebral body below it, most commonly L-5 on S-1. In addition to the canal being narrowed, the intervertebral foramina are narrowed, compressing the exiting nerve roots. Patients with lumbar spinal stenosis present with chronic radicular symptoms in the lower extremities. *Neurogenic claudication* (NC) occurs with lumbar spinal stenosis and can be differentiated from vascular claudication (VC) by history and physical examination. Both occur with walking, but a patient with VC can walk a predictable distance before he or she must stop due to pain while a patient with NC can walk variable distances before the onset of symptoms. The pain with NC is within one or several dermatomes, and the pain with VC is in a stocking distribution. The stenosis of the lumbar spinal canal is worsened by upright postures needed for standing and walking, because the lumbar spine is extended. Flexing the lumbar spine relieves the pain, which is accomplished by bending at the waist or sitting. Therefore, the NC patient must sit to get relief after walking, as opposed to a patient with VC who only needs to rest by standing still. In addition, relief with resting usually comes quicker to the patient with VC. On examination, decreased sensation in one or both legs is common, limitation of back movement, particularly forward flexion, is seen, and motor weakness and loss of deep tendon reflexes can occur. Signs of vascular insufficiency on examination, such as absent peripheral pulses and foot pallor with elevation, should not be present in a patient with NC. Plain x-rays may show spondylolisthesis, narrowing of the anteroposterior diameter of the canal, and disk space narrowing. Flexion and extension x-rays may be helpful. MRI is the best study to look at the cauda equina and the exiting nerve roots. CT is best for evaluating the bony pathology and a myelogram with a postmyelogram CT is helpful with complex cases. Initial treatment for a patient with lumbar stenosis and no weakness is medical. Surgery is indicated if a patient has weakness, progressive worsening of examination results, or chronic disabling pain.

The *cauda equina syndrome* is caused by a large compressive lesion usually located at L4-5. The signs and symptoms include bowel and bladder dysfunction, saddle anesthesia, motor weakness in multiple nerve root distributions, low back pain, sciatica, absence of both ankle reflexes, and sexual dysfunction. However, all of these symptoms and signs do not need to be present. *Saddle anesthesia* is numbness of the buttocks, the perineal region, and the posterior superior thighs. Sciatica, when present, may be bilateral. Emergent surgical decompression is needed.

SUGGESTED READING

American Association of Neurological Surgeons. *Guidelines for the management of severe head injury.* The Brain Trauma Foundation, New York, 1995.

Barr ML, Kiernan JA. *The human nervous system, an anatomical viewpoint.* Philadelphia: JB Lippincott Co, 1993.

Bracken MB, Shepard MJ, Collins WF, et al. A randomized controlled trial of methylprednisolone or naloxone in the treatment of acute spinal cord injury. *N Engl J Med* 1990;322:1405–1411.

Bracken MB, Shepard MJ, Holford TR, et al. Administration of methylprednisolone for 24 or 48 hours in the treatment of acute spinal cord injury. *JAMA* 1997;227:1597–1604.

Kaye A. *Essential neurosurgery.* Edinburgh: Churchill Livingstone, 1991.

2

IMMUNOLOGY AND TRANSPLANTATION

DANIEL KREISEL AND BRUCE R. ROSENGARD

BASIC SCIENCE

The function of the immune system is to protect the organism from pathogens.

Components of the Immune System

The immune system consists of primary and secondary lymphoid organs. *Primary lymphoid organs* (i.e., bone marrow and thymus) are defined as organs in which lymphocytes are produced. B lymphocytes originate and complete most of their maturation in the bone marrow. Subsequently, they migrate to the secondary lymphoid organs. T-lymphocyte progenitors originate in the bone marrow and then migrate to the thymus, where they undergo their positive and negative selection, a process in which highly autoreactive T-cell clones are eliminated, which is the basis for self-tolerance. This process of thymic "education" is also critical because T-cell activation requires that T cells see foreign proteins in association with self. After final maturation, T lymphocytes are exported to the periphery. Immune responses are induced in *secondary lymphoid organs* through interaction between antigen-presenting cells, T lymphocytes, and B lymphocytes. Secondary lymphoid tissues include encapsulated organs such as lymph nodes and spleen and unencapsulated tissue such as Peyer patches and bronchial-associated lymphatic tissue. Unencapsulated secondary lymphoid tissue lines the respiratory, gastrointestinal tract, and genitourinary tract and is also referred to as *mucosa-associated lymphoid tissue* (MALT). Components of secondary lymphoid organs include a framework of reticular tissue and bone marrow–derived cells that populate this framework. Lymphocytes enter lymph nodes by adhesion to and migration through specialized blood vessels. They leave secondary lymphoid organs via efferent lymphatic vessels. In contrast, antigen-presenting cells migrate from the periphery and enter lymph nodes via afferent lymphatic channels. Within lymphatic organs, B lymphocytes localize in primary foci, termed *germinal centers,* which are surrounded by the paracortical region, which is rich in T lymphocytes. Once antigen recognition takes place and an immune response is initiated, B lymphocytes proliferate and generate plasma cells, which subsequently migrate into the efferent lymphatics and exit into the circulation via the lymphatics. The MALT system is important for production of antibodies for mucosal secretion (Fig. 2-1).

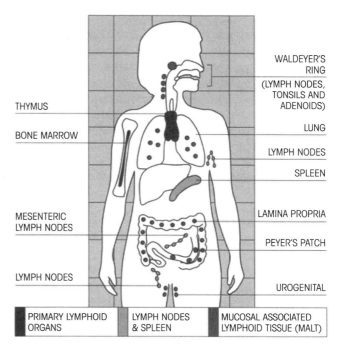

FIGURE 2-1. Primary and secondary lymphoid organs. (From Roitt I. *Essential immunology,* 8th ed. Oxford: Blackwell Science, 1994:148, with permission.)

CELLS OF THE IMMUNE SYSTEM

B Lymphocytes

B lymphocytes produce antibodies that mediate the *humoral immune response*. Structurally, antibodies are glycoproteins that are made up of four protein chains, two heavy chains, and two light chains, which are linked by interchain disulfide bonds (Fig. 2-2). Both heavy and light chains have constant regions at their carboxy terminals and variable regions at their amino terminals. In humans, immunoglobulins are separated into five classes or isotypes: IgA, IgG, IgD, IgM, and IgE. Both heavy and light chains have a constant region (Fc) that is identical for antibodies of a specific class. This constant region lacks the ability to bind antigen and is important for binding to complement and binding to Fc receptors on the surface of macrophages and natural killer (NK) cells. The variable antigen-binding region is referred to as *Fab*. Immunoglobulin classes differ in their ability to cross the placenta, cross mucosal barriers, activate complement, and bind to different cells of the immune system (Table 2-1).

The early stages of *B-cell development* are antigen-independent and are notable for genetic rearrangement of their heavy-chain and light-chain loci in order to generate their membrane-bound IgM immunoglobulin antigen receptor. The variable region of the antibody comprises both light and heavy chains and determines the specificity of surface receptors and secreted antibodies of B cells. B lymphocytes that encounter self-antigen are deleted at immature stages in the bone marrow. After completing most of their differentiation in the bone marrow, mature B lymphocytes exit into the periphery, where they can be found primarily in lymph nodes and spleen. If mature B cells recognize foreign antigen through their surface receptor, they are activated to undergo proliferation and differentiate into anti-

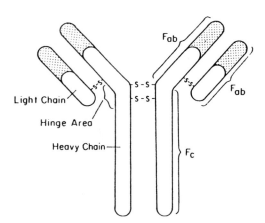

FIGURE 2-2. Two heavy and two light chains of IgG linked by disulfide bonds. (From O'Leary P. *The physiologic basis of surgery,* 2nd ed. Philadelphia: Lippincott-Raven, 1996:145, with permission.)

TABLE 2-1. MAJOR DIFFERENCES IN IMMUNOGLOBULIN ABILITIES ACCORDING TO IMMUNOGLOBULIN CLASS

	IgA	IgD	IgE	IgG	IgM
Cross placenta	−	−	−	+	−
Cross mucosal barriers	+	−	−	−	−
Complement activation	−	−	−	+	+
Binding to mast cells and basophils	−	−	+	−	−
Binding to macrophages	−	−	−	+	−

body-secreting plasma cells or alternatively into memory B cells. In addition to antigen recognition, B cells require help from T cells, particularly those bearing CD4 for their activation. This help is provided through cytokines such as IL-4, IL-5, and IL-6, as well as through direct cell-to-cell contact via CD40-CD40 ligand engagement. The first antibody produced during an immune response is IgM. CD40-CD40 ligand interaction between helper T cell and B lymphocyte is important for the subsequent isotype switch to IgG, IgA, or IgE. Both secreted antibodies and surface antigen receptors are composed of immunoglobulin proteins.

Antibodies can neutralize soluble foreign antigen. IgG and IgM can activate complement after binding to antigen. In addition, binding of antibodies to foreign antigen can lead to opsonization and clearance of the antigen-antibody complex through adherence to phagocytes. Antibody-dependent cell-mediated cytotoxicity can be exhibited by NK cells and macrophages and is dependent on their interaction with Fc receptors of antibodies after these bind to the target cells in a specific fashion.

T Lymphocytes

T lymphocytes mediate *cellular immune responses*. They arise in the bone marrow from pluripotent hematopoietic stem cells. T-cell differentiation in the thymus involves two distinct selection processes, which are triggered by different cellular components: Positive selection is triggered by epithelial cells in the thymic cortex and involves expansion of T cells specific for peptides bound to self–major histocompatibility (self-MHC) molecules. Cells that are not positively selected undergo programmed cell death, termed *apoptosis*, in the thymus. This process accounts for 95% of thymocyte death. Negative selection is triggered by bone marrow–derived dendritic cells in the thymic medulla and involves deletion of autoreactive T cells (Fig. 2-3). Thus, mature T lymphocytes that are exported to the periphery express T-cell receptors on their cell surface, which recognize foreign peptide in the context of self-MHC, but that are not reactive against self-peptides. The T-cell receptor is formed by two chains, α and β, which are embedded in the

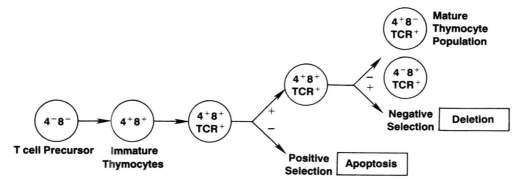

FIGURE 2-3. Intrathymic positive and negative selection of T-cell precursors. (From Fischer JE. *Surgical basic science.* St. Louis: Mosby, 1993:39, with permission.)

membrane. Similar to the B-cell receptor and secreted antibodies, it consists of constant and variable regions. All T lymphocytes express CD3, an accessory molecule, in close proximity to the T-cell receptor on their cell surface. The CD3 molecule is important for transduction of signals upon ligation of the T-cell receptor (Fig. 2-4). Two broad classes of T lymphocytes exist, which can be differentiated based on their phenotype and their function. T cells express either CD4 or CD8 accessory molecules, which bind to the constant region of MHC class II and class I, respectively. These accessory molecules stabilize the interaction between the T-cell receptor and the self-MHC/peptide complex. Functionally, CD4+ T cells synthesize variable soluble T-cell growth factors, which support the proliferation of both CD4+ and CD8+ T cells and are therefore termed *helper T cells.* CD8+ T cells have specific effector function and are termed *cytotoxic T cells.* CD4+ T-cell activation requires two signals: (a) engagement of the T-cell receptor by the MHC/peptide complex and (b) binding of specific receptors on the T cell with costimulatory molecules on the antigen-presenting cell. Engagement of the T-cell receptor in the absence of costimulatory signals can lead to anergy, an inactivation of T cells. Examples for costimulatory signals include interaction between CD28 on T cells with CD80 (B7-1) or CD86 (B7-2) on antigen-presenting cells and CD154 (CD40 ligand) on T cells and CD40 on antigen-presenting cells. T cells also express CTLA4, a molecule that is homologous to CD28 and shares the same ligands CD80 and CD86. Unlike CD28, which delivers a positive signal to helper T cells, CTLA4 delivers a strong negative signal, which inhibits expression of cytokines such as IL-2 and leads to cell-cycle arrest. Blockade of costimulatory signals has been shown to prolong allograft survival in experimental models and awaits trials in the clinical setting (Fig. 2-5).

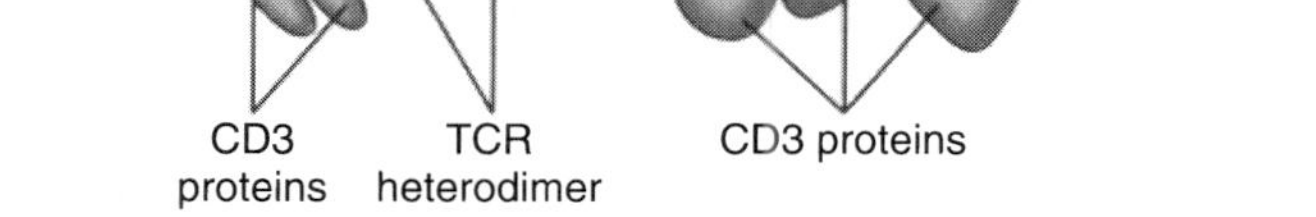

Activated CD4+ helper T cells produce several growth factors termed *cytokines.* CD4+ helper T cells can be divided into T_H1 and T_H2 cells based on their patterns of cytokine production and their corresponding regulatory effects. Cytokines produced by T_H1 cells, primarily IFN-γ and IL-2 help to generate CD8+ cytotoxic lymphocytes, mediate delayed-type hypersensitivity reactions, and induce activation of phagocytic cells. T_H2 cells produce cytokines, chiefly IL-4, IL-5, IL-10, and IL-13, which activate humoral immune responses by triggering IgM isotype switching with consequent production of IgG, IgA, and IgE. T_H2 cytokines also activate mast cells and eosinophils. Immature CD4+ T cells (T_H0 cells) differentiate into either T_H1 or T_H2 cells depending on the cytokine milieu in the microenvironment of activation. IL-12, which is secreted by mature dendritic cells and macrophages, deviates the immune response toward T_H1, whereas IL-4 polarizes helper T cells toward the T_H2 phenotype. Some investigators have speculated that deviation of the immune response toward T_H2 may diminish the immune response to transplanted organs (Fig. 2-6).

FIGURE 2-4. T-cell receptor. (From Contran RS, Kumar V, Collins T, eds. Robbins. *Pathologic basis of disease,* 6th ed. Philadelphia: WB Saunders, 1999:189, with permission.)

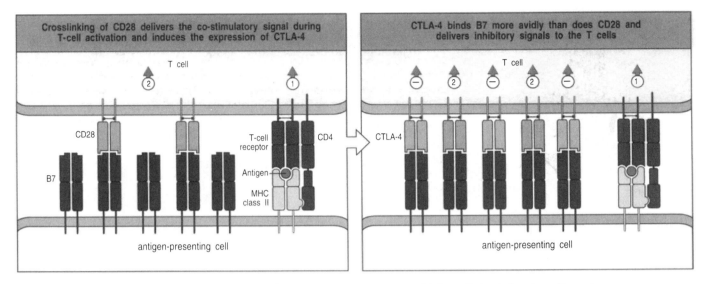

FIGURE 2-5. T-cell activation. (From Janeway CA. *Immunobiology*, 3rd ed. London: Current Biology, 1997:7.9, with permission.)

NK Cells

NK cells are derived from the lymphoid lineage of bone marrow–derived pluripotent stem cells. Unlike T cells, NK cells lack receptors for specific antigen on their surface. Phenotypically, they express CD2, CD16, and CD56. NK cells do not require prior sensitization to exert their cytotoxic effector function and do not acquire memory. Thus, like complement proteins, they are considered to be part of the innate immune system and play an important role before a specific immune response can be mounted. The activity of NK cells is inhibited by recognition of self class I MHC molecules on target cells. In addition, they are the effector arm of *antibody-dependent cell-mediated cytotoxicity* (ADCC). In ADCC, antibodies bind specifically to target cells, and then NK cells bind to the Fc portion of the antibody molecule via their CD16 molecule, which functions as a Fc receptor. This mechanism is important in eradicating virally infected cells (Fig. 2-7). NK cells are also thought to play an important role in the natural defense against cancer cells.

Complement

The complement system is a set of proteins that function nonspecifically to destroy invading pathogens. The system represents, in evolutionary terms, the most primitive system of innate immunity. The complement cascade can be activated through two different routes, termed the *classical* and *alternative pathways*. The classical pathway is triggered when antibodies of the IgG or IgM isotype specifically bind to foreign antigen. One of the complement proteins, C1q, binds to the Fc domains of the bound antibody, which is the initial event that activates the complement cascade. The alternative pathway can be triggered through infectious microorganisms in the blood, endotoxin, or extracorporeal circuits and also leads to attachment of C3b on the surface of the foreign antigen after spontaneous cleavage of C3 in the plasma. Classical and alternative pathways of complement activation therefore converge in the formation of C3 convertase (Fig. 2-8). The assembly of the membrane-attack complex is initiated by C5 binding to C5 convertase, which

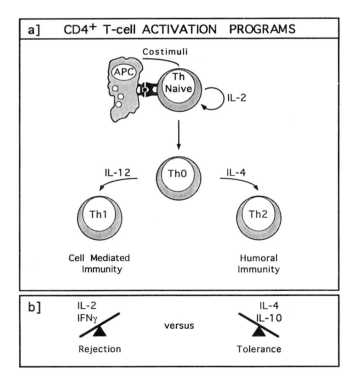

FIGURE 2-6. T_H1/T_H2 differentiation. (From Tilney NL, Strom TB, Paul LC. *Transplantation biology*. Philadelphia: Lippincott-Raven, 1996: 391, with permission.)

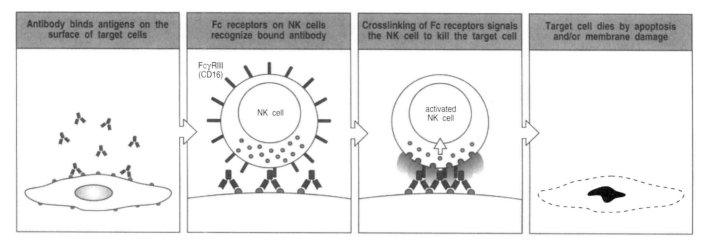

FIGURE 2-7. Antibody-dependent cell-mediated cytotoxicity. (From Janeway CA. *Immunobiology,* 3rd ed. London: Current Biology, 1997:8.29, with permission.)

is being formed after C3b binds to either the classical or alternative pathway C3 convertase. The C5b-9 membrane attack complex creates transmembrane channels and disrupts membrane integrity. These events can rapidly lead to thrombosis and interstitial hemorrhage. Small cleavage products of complement factors, such as C3a or C5a, are potent mediators of inflammation as well as chemotaxins, which can further augment damage to the graft. Neutrophil activation can also lead to formation of oxygen radicals, which is analogous to events of reperfusion injury.

Cytokines

Cytokines are soluble factors that are secreted by lymphocytes, dendritic cells, endothelial cells, macrophages, and other cells of the immune system. Cytokines that are

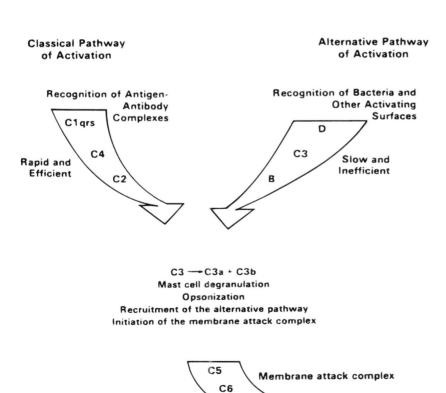

FIGURE 2-8. Pathways of complement activation. (From O'Leary P. *The physiologic basis of surgery,* 2nd ed. Philadelphia: Lippincott-Raven, 1996:146, with permission.)

TABLE 2-2. PRIMARY CELLULAR SOURCES, TARGET CELLS, AND BIOLOGICAL EFFECTS OF IMPORTANT CYTOKINES

Cytokine	Cellular sources	Target cells	Biological functions
IL-1	Macrophages	B lymphocytes T lymphocytes	Proliferation of activated B and T lymphocytes Fever response in hypothalamus
IL-2	T lymphocytes	T lymphocytes B lymphocytes NK cells	Proliferation of T lymphocytes Activation of NK cells
IL-3	T lymphocytes	Hematopoietic precursor cells	Growth and differentiation of hematopoietic precursor cells
IL-4	T lymphocytes natural killer (NK) T cells	T lymphocytes B lymphocytes Mast cells	Th_2 subset differentiation Isotype switch to IgG_1 and IgE Proliferation of hematopoietic precursor cells
IL-5	T lymphocytes	B lymphocytes	Proliferation of activated B lymphocytes Proliferation of eosinophils
IL-6	T lymphocytes Macrophages	T lymphocytes B lymphocytes	Differentiation of B lymphocytes Activation of T lymphocytes Primary signal for induction of hepatic acute phase proteins
IL-7	Bone marrow stromal cells	B lymphocytes T lymphocytes	Proliferation and activation of B lymphocyte and T lymphocyte precursors
IL-8	Monocytes	Neutrophils T lymphocytes	Chemotactic for neutrophils and T lymphocytes
IL-9	T lymphocytes	Th lymphocytes B lymphocytes Erythroid progenitors Mast cells	Growth of Th lymphocytes Growth and proliferation of B lymphocytes, erythroid precursors and mast cells
IL-10	T lymphocytes B lymphocytes Monocytes Macrophages Keratinocyte	T lymphocytes	Inhibits production of proinflammatory cytokines Interferes with macrophage-mediated antigen presentation Inhibits Th_1 function
IL-11	Bone marrow stromal cells	Cells of hematopoietic and nonhematopoietic lineage	Induction of acute phase proteins
IL-12	Macrophages Dendritic cells	T lymphocytes NK cells	Th_1 subset differentiation Activated NK cells
IL-13	T lymphocytes	T lymphocytes B lymphocytes	Decreases expression of proinflammatory cytokines Th_2 subset differentiation Induces IgE expression by B lymphocytes
IFN-τ	T lymphocytes	Macrophages T lymphocytes Endothelial cells NK cells	Activation of macrophages Induces and increases expression of major histocompatibility complex class I and II molecules Antiviral activity Activates NK cells
TNF-α	Monocytes Macrophages T lymphocytes B lymphocytes Endothelial cells NK cells	Activated T cells Most cells of hematopoietic and nonhematopoietic lineage	Activation of phagocytosis Induction of inflammatory reaction Tumor cell cytotoxicity Induction of acute phase proteins Antiviral activity
TGF-β	T lymphocytes B lymphocytes Macrophages Platelets Fibroblasts	Most lymphoid and hematopoietic cells	Antiproliferative effects on most cell types except fibroblasts Suppresses hematopoiesis and lymphopoiesis Inhibits activation of antigen presenting cells Suppresses NK cells and cytotoxic T cells

secreted by lymphocytes are also referred to as *lymphokines* and those secreted by mononuclear phagocytes are occasionally called *monokines*. However, these terms can be confusing because the same cytokines can be secreted by various cell types. Cytokines have both local and systemic effects. Locally they can act in either an autocrine or a paracrine fashion. They have a short half-life and interact with high-affinity cytokine-specific receptors on target cells. The expression of cytokine receptors is also regulated by cytokines in the microenvironment. In this way, cytokines can regulate each other's activity. Specific cytokines can have multiple effects and there is considerable redundancy among the function of different cytokines. IL-2 is critical for expansion of T lymphocytes following their initial activation. IL-2 receptors are not expressed on resting T lymphocytes. Inhibition of IL-2 production by the drugs cyclosporine or tacrolimus is the basis of clinical immunosuppression. The following table outlines primary cellular sources, target cells, and biological effects of important cytokines (Table 2-2).

Antigen-Presenting Cells

Antigen-presenting cells play an important role in the initiation of immune responses by taking up, processing, and presenting foreign antigen to T lymphocytes in the context of MHC molecules. Dendritic cells, macrophages, and B lymphocytes are the predominant cell types that have the capability to present antigen. An important characteristic of professional antigen-presenting cells is the ability to deliver a second *costimulatory signal*, in addition to presenting foreign peptides on their cell surface (signal one) (Fig. 2-9). Antigen-presenting cells vary in their means of antigen uptake and their surface expression of MHC and costimulatory molecules. B lymphocytes express class II MHC antigens on their surface but do not express costimulatory molecules constitutively. The expression of costimulatory molecules on B cells is inducible by several different inflammatory signals. B cells take up antigen in a specific manner utilizing their surface-bound immunoglobulin as receptors. In contrast, macrophages take up antigen efficiently through phagocytosis and do not express class II MHC antigens or costimulatory molecules constitutively. As with B cells, inflammatory signals induce these molecules. Dendritic cells are the most potent activators of naive T lymphocytes, because of their constitutive expression of class II MHC molecules and their high surface expression of costimulatory and adhesion molecules. In addition to delivery of signals through these accessory molecules, antigen-presenting cells secrete cytokines, which influence the response of T lymphocytes.

Histocompatibility

MHC antigens are cell-surface glycoproteins. These molecules, which encode the information necessary for antigen presentation and cellular recognition, are among the most polymorphic molecules within a species. Three classes of

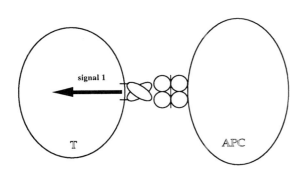

Signal 1 alone;

-Failure to activate
-T cell anergy (inability to respond on subsequent exposure to antigen)

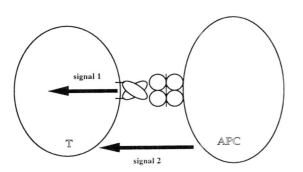

Signal 1 + second or costimulatory signals;

-Full activation
-Rescue from anergy

FIGURE 2-9. Two-signal model of T-cell activation. (From Tilney NL, Strom TB, Paul LC. *Transplantation biology*, Philadelphia: Lippincott-Raven, 1996:356, with permission.)

MHC antigens exist in humans. They have been mapped to chromosome 6 and are also termed *human leukocyte antigen* (HLA). Class I antigens (A, B, C in humans) are present on all nucleated cells and serve as the primary target for cytotoxic T lymphocytes (Fig. 2-10). They are composed of polymorphic heavy chains (α_1, α_2, α_3), which are noncovalently associated with a nonpolymorphic β_2-microglobulin light chain. NK cells eliminate cells that lack expression of MHC class I (e.g., tumor cells.) Class II antigens (DR, DQ, DP in humans) are composed of two polymorphic chains, referred to as the α and β chains (Fig. 2-11). They are expressed on the surface of bone marrow–derived antigen-presenting cells, such as mature dendritic cells, activated B lymphocytes, and activated macrophages. Under certain inflammatory conditions, expression of MHC class II can be induced on endothelial cells. Because solid organ grafts carry bone marrow–derived antigen-presenting cells within their interstitium, the recipient's immune system is exposed to intact MHC class I and class II of donor origin. The MHC class III loci encode for a miscellaneous group of proteins including complement components. Minor transplantation antigens are encoded outside the MHC loci. Minor transplantation antigens are difficult to characterize and are likely derived from various proteins serving general cellular housekeeping functions. Recognition of minor antigens occurs in a self-MHC-restricted fashion, in a manner identical to exogenous foreign peptides. Although minor antigen disparities can induce allograft rejection, the rigor of

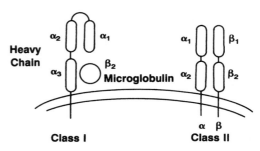

FIGURE 2-11. Major histocompatibility class I and class II antigen structure. (From Fischer JE. *Surgical basic science.* St. Louis: Mosby, :43, with permission.)

the rejection process is mostly determined by the degree of MHC disparity between donor and recipient. Multiple experiments have demonstrated that class II mismatches are of overwhelming importance in triggering rejection, presumably because disparities at class II loci drive $CD4^+$ helper T cells, which act *in vivo* to amplify immune responses. Therefore, MHC matching of donor and recipient is one strategy to minimize immune responses. While this approach is employed in the case of renal transplantation, MHC matching is not standard practice for heart and lung transplants because of time constraints related to permissible cold ischemic time and controversy over the significance of MHC matching. Tissue typing is performed to optimize matching for HLA-A, HLA-B, and HLA-DR, which have been identified as the most important histocompatibility loci. HLA-DQ is tightly linked to HLA-DR, and thus matching for HLA-DR is usually associated with matching for HLA-DQ. Considering inheritance of both maternal and paternal alleles at HLA-A, HLA-B, and HLA-DR loci, a six-antigen match is the best-case scenario in the case of transplantation of cadaveric organs. HLA genes are closely linked on chromosome 6. Each individual inherits a set of maternal and a set of paternal genes, which is also referred to as *haplotype*. In the case of living-related transplantation, MHC matches are referred to as *0, 1, or 2 haplotype matches*. Living-related 2 haplotype–matched renal transplants have been shown to have better long-term graft survival compared to 6 antigen-matched cadaveric renal transplantation. Although this may be related to the fact that 2 haplotype matches are also matched for HLA-C, HLA-DQ, and HLA-DP, it is more likely because the match is genotypically identical.

Rejection

Prevention and treatment of allograft rejection remain major challenges in the field of transplantation. The existence of different pathways of allorecognition is unique to the field of transplantation immunology. In conventional T-cell–mediated immune reactions, foreign antigen is taken up and processed by the host's antigen-presenting cells and

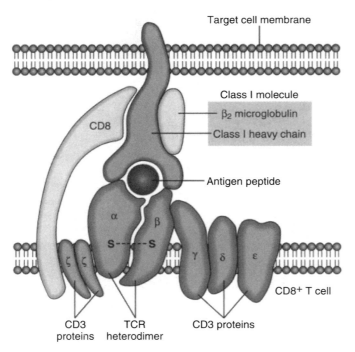

FIGURE 2-10. Antigen recognition by $CD8^+$ T lymphocyte. (From Contran RS, Kumar V, Collins T, eds. Robbins. *Pathologic basis of disease,* 6th ed. Philadelphia: WB Saunders, 1999:194, with permission.)

subsequently presented to T lymphocytes in a self-MHC-restricted fashion. After transplantation of an allograft, the recipient's antigen-presenting cells migrate to the graft, take up, process, and present allopeptide in a self-MHC-restricted fashion. This allorecognition pathway is referred to as *indirect allorecognition* (Fig. 2-12). However, the vigor of the immune response to an allograft is thought to be due to an alternate route of allosensitization. Donor bone marrow–derived antigen-presenting cells, which express donor MHC, are present in the interstitium of the allograft. At the time of transplantation, they rapidly migrate to the recipient's lymphoid organs and directly activate T lymphocytes. This process, unique to transplantation, is termed *direct allorecognition*. Activation of T lymphocytes leads to the release of proinflammatory cytokines, which promote the maturation of multiple immune effector mechanisms. Allorestricted T lymphocytes greatly outnumber T lymphocytes that react in a self-restricted manner.

Hyperacute rejection represents the most rapid form of allograft rejection, which generally manifests within minutes of graft revascularization. It occurs when the recipient has preformed cytotoxic antibodies directed against donor antigens. Preformed antibodies can be directed against several targets. Antibodies against foreign MHC molecules require prior sensitization via blood transfusion, pregnancy, or previous transplantation. Antibodies directed against blood groups or under rare circumstances against other tissue-specific antigens can also lead to hyperacute rejection. The injury is mediated by complement. Complement activation injures graft endothelium, which leads to fibrin and platelet deposition, vasoconstriction, and neutrophil adhesion. These result in rapid hemorrhagic necrosis of the graft. Fortunately, hyperacute rejection occurs very infrequently due to routine screening of recipients for lymphocytotoxic antibodies. If antibodies are detected by a panel of cells representing the common HLA antigens in a given region, then pretransplant cross-matching of the recipient's serum against donor lymphocytes (prospective cross-matching) is required. Hyperacute rejection affects the kidney more commonly than other solid organs.

The most frequent form of rejection seen clinically is *acute rejection*. It is mediated by T lymphocytes and generally occurs within a few weeks of transplantation. Recognition of foreign MHC leads to rapid clonal expansion of alloreactive T cells. CD4$^+$ T cells secrete cytokines, which are important for activation of effector CD8$^+$ cytotoxic T cells. CD8$^+$ cytotoxic T lymphocytes recognize donor MHC class I antigen and kill target cells through cell-to-cell contact. The elaboration of cytokines promotes nonspecific mechanisms such as activated macrophages, neutrophils, mast cells, and NK cells, which contribute to damage of the graft. Lastly, T-cell help is required for antibody class switching by B lymphocytes. Cytotoxic IgG antibodies participate in the pathogenesis of acute allograft rejection.

Although substantial progress has been made in the prevention and treatment of acute allograft rejection, *chronic rejection* remains the major cause of late graft failure. Likely examples of chronic rejection include obliterative bronchiolitis, cardiac allograft vasculopathy, and glomerulosclerosis. The liver is generally less susceptible to chronic rejection. Chronic rejection is typically seen months to years after transplantation. Both humoral and cell-mediated immunity have been suggested to participate in producing the damage leading to chronic graft rejection. In addition to histoincompatibility, nonimmune mechanisms such as ischemia-reperfusion injury, infections, and donor-recipient–size mismatching are thought to play an important role.

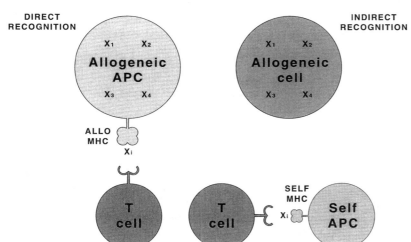

FIGURE 2-12. Direct and indirect allorecognition pathways.(From Bach FH, Auchincloss H. *Transplantation immunology.* New York: Wiley-Liss, 1995:98, with permission.)

Xenotransplantation

Xenotransplantation, the transplantation of tissue or organs between members of different species, represents one potential solution to the severe shortage of donor organs. Transplantation between closely related species such as between baboons and humans is also referred to as *concordant xenotransplantation*. Besides ethical considerations, one of the major risks associated with transplantation of organs from nonhuman primates to humans is zoonosis, the transmission of infectious agents such as herpesviruses and retroviruses. Discordant xenotransplantation is transplantation between widely phylogenetically disparate species, such as pigs and humans. The vigor of graft rejection increases with the degree of phylogenetic separation between the species. Although pigs offer significant advantages as organ donors for humans, one of the major biological challenges remains the prevention of hyperacute rejection. Hyperacute rejection is mediated through a combination of recipient natural antibodies, which cross-react against glycoproteins on the surface of endothelial cells of the donor organs, and complement. A promising approach to block hyperacute rejection has been the introduction of human genes into pigs encoding complement regulatory proteins. Examples of species restricted regulators of complement activation include decay-accelerating factor and CD59. Through transgenesis, these proteins have been expressed on the endothelium of the porcine donor organs and protect them from complement-mediated damage. Although this approach has successfully overcome immediate hyperacute rejection, other significant immunological barriers remain. Furthermore, additional concerns related to using porcine organs for humans are the risk of transmission of pathogens and the uncertainty about the long-term functional capabilities of pig organs in a xenogeneic environment.

Tolerance

Immune tolerance is defined as specific immunological nonresponsiveness and remains the holy grail of transplantation immunology. Operationally, tolerance refers to acceptance of the graft while maintaining the ability to mount immune responses against other environmental antigens. This would mean elimination or inactivation of alloreactive T lymphocytes. Four different mechanisms of T-cell tolerance have been postulated to explain specific inactivation of alloreactive T cells: deletion, anergy, suppression, and ignorance. *Deletion* means that reactive T lymphocytes are physically destroyed. *Central deletion,* the mechanism felt to be responsible for self-tolerance, refers to clonal deletion of new T lymphocytes in the thymus. T lymphocytes can also be physically eliminated in the periphery. *Anergy* defines a state of unresponsiveness to stimuli, which would normally be sufficient for T-cell activation. The anergic state is thought to result from an interaction of T lymphocytes with antigen-presenting cells delivering signal 1 foreign peptide in the context of an MHC molecule, without signal 2, costimulatory molecules. The anergic state can be reversed by exogenous administration of cytokines, particularly IL-2. Suppression is a mechanism of tolerance that remains highly controversial. Suppressor cells are felt to be a subset of cells capable of down-regulating immune responses. Their existence has been proposed based on experiments in which adoptive transfer of cells from long-term graft acceptors to naive syngeneic hosts has led to permanent acceptance of allografts in a donor-specific fashion. However, the inability to isolate, clone, and characterize suppressor cells has raised question about their nature and existence. *Immunological ignorance* is a state in which reactive T cells are present but are unable to respond normally to appropriate stimuli. However, they can be activated by environmental factors.

Immunosuppression

The success of organ transplantation over the last three decades is in large part due to refinements in immunosuppressive therapies. Because immunosuppressants impair the host's immune system in a nonspecific fashion, their administration carries the risk of significant side effects. In addition to tissue-specific adverse side effects that are associated with individual medications, general complications include opportunistic infections and malignancies. One approach to minimize the development of these complications includes titration of immunosuppressants to maintain therapeutic serum levels. Opportunistic infections are most frequent in the first 6 months after transplantation. Viral infections have a particularly high prevalence and have been associated with subsequent development of malignancy. Infections with cytomegalovirus (CMV), a member of the herpes family, are the most common. Although CMV is minimally symptomatic in healthy individuals, it frequently becomes symptomatic in immunosuppressed patients. Symptoms can include fever, malaise, gastrointestinal tract ulceration, renal insufficiency, pneumonia, and mental status changes. Another member of the herpes family that frequently affects transplant patients is Epstein-Barr virus (EBV), the pathogen responsible for mononucleosis. In healthy individuals, EBV infects B lymphocytes, which leads to lymphoproliferation. This is a self-limited process as infected B cells are killed by T cells. This control mechanism is impaired under the influence of T-cell immunosuppressants; hence, B cells proliferate in an unregulated fashion. Initially, the lymphoproliferation is polyclonal, but genetic alteration can lead to a true monoclonal B-cell lymphoma. In the polyclonal phase, EBV-related disease is referred to as *posttransplant lymphoproliferative disorder* and can be treated with reduction of immunosuppression and antiviral drugs such as valcyclovir. When a full-blown lymphoma develops, conventional chemotherapy is often required. In addition to viral infections, transplant recipients are prone to opportunistic infections with fungi such as nocardia and aspergillus and protozoa such as pneumocystis carinii and toxoplasmosis. Patients generally receive prophylaxis against pneumocystis with trimethoprim and sulfamethoxazole in the posttransplant period.

In the early days of transplantation, immunosuppression was achieved through whole-body or total-lymphoid irradiation. The biological effect was due to inhibition of DNA synthesis and cellular replication. Side effects included bone marrow suppression and direct toxicity to the lungs and gastrointestinal tract. Current immunosuppressive agents can be grouped into different categories based on their mechanisms of action. These include inhibition of initial activation of T lymphocytes, inhibition of cytokine synthesis, inhibition of cytokine signal transduction, antimetabolites, as well as polyclonal and monoclonal antibodies mainly targeting various lymphocyte receptors.

Corticosteroids intervene at many points in the immune system. They inhibit DNA and RNA production, and after forming complexes with intracellular receptors, they impair transcription of cytokines such as IL-1, IL-2, IL-6, IFN-γ, and TNF-α. In addition, they act in an antiinflammatory fashion by inhibiting margination of lymphocytes, decreasing chemotaxis and impairing function of macrophages and granulocytes. Long-term administration of corticosteroids is associated with multiple side effects including hypertension, hyperlipidemia, hyperglycemia, cataracts, osteoporosis, psychosis, pancreatitis, gastrointestinal tract bleeding, ulceration and perforation, poor wound healing, and growth retardation.

Cyclosporine A inhibits the transcription of IL-2 in activated T lymphocytes while sparing resting cells. It binds to a cytoplasmic protein cyclophilin, and the cyclosporine A cyclophilin complex inhibits calcineurin (Fig. 2-13). Calcineurin is a phosphatase responsible for activating a transcription factor for IL-2. Additionally, cyclosporine A also inhibits the transcription of IL-3, IL-6, IL-7, and IFN-γ. Clinically, plasma levels of cyclosporine A are closely monitored. Because cyclosporine is metabolized through cytochrome P-450, several medications can influence its plasma level. Phenobarbital and rifampin stimulate the cytochrome P-450 enzyme system and thereby induce metabolism of cyclosporine while ketoconazole and erythromycin have the opposite effect. The spectrum of cyclosporine's adverse effects includes nephrotoxicity, hypertension, hyperkalemia, hepatotoxicity, hyperlipidemia, and neurological symptoms such as tremors.

The macrolide antibiotic *tacrolimus* (FK 506), like cyclosporine A, interferes with intracellular calcium signaling. Instead of binding to cyclophilin, tacrolimus forms a

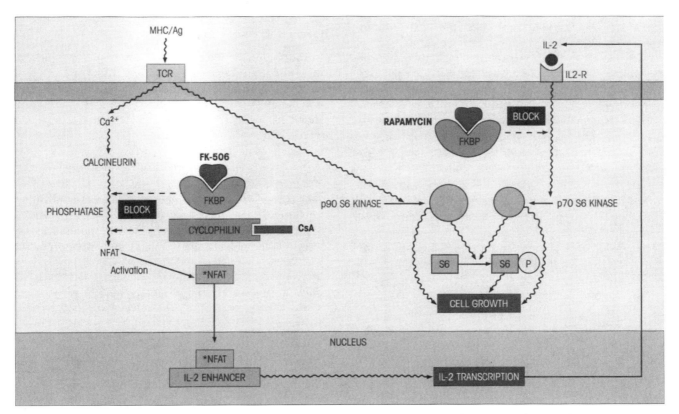

FIGURE 2-13. Mode of action of cyclosporine A, tacrolimus (FK 506) and rapamycin. (From Roitt I. *Essential immunology,* 8th ed. Oxford: Blackwell Science, 1994:351, with permission.)

complex with FK binding protein, and subsequently inactivates the phosphatase calcineurin which is an important activator of a transcription factor involved in production of IL-2 (Fig. 2-13). In addition, tacrolimus inhibits production of IL-3, IL-4, IFN-γ and the expression of the IL-2 receptor. It is far more potent on a per mg basis than cyclosporine A and is beneficial in rescuing grafts that are being rejected despite cyclosporine A maintenance therapy. Absorption of orally administered tacrolimus is less bile-dependent than cyclosporine A, which is important to consider in liver transplant recipients whose bile flow is diverted with a T tube. Similar to cyclosporine A, tacrolimus is nephrotoxic and is associated with hyperkalemia and hypertension. Additionally, it causes neurotoxicity and can lead to new onset diabetes mellitus.

Azathioprine is a purine analog, which is converted to its active metabolite in the liver and exerts its action through inhibition of DNA and RNA synthesis by blocking de novo purine synthesis and the salvage pathway (i.e., the interconversion among precursors of purine nucleotides) by incorporation into the genetic material as a fraudulent base. Azathioprine is commonly used in combination with corticosteroids and cyclosporine A as triple therapy. Its major side effects include hepatotoxicity and bone marrow suppression with severe neutropenia.

Mycophenolate mofetil inhibits inosinmonophosphate dehydogenase noncompetitively, an important enzyme of the *de novo* purine synthesis pathway. Because T and B lymphocytes lack significant activity of the purine salvage pathway, the *de novo* pathway is critical for these cells. Although mycophenolate mofetil is not associated with significant bone marrow suppression, it has some gastrointestinal toxicity.

Methotrexate inhibits DNA and RNA synthesis by blocking folic acid metabolism. It acts in an antiinflammatory fashion by inhibiting chemotaxis of macrophages. Adverse effects include myelosuppression, gastrointestinal toxicity, hepatic dysfunction, nephrotoxicity, and dermatitis.

Although *rapamycin*, a macrolide antibiotic, also binds to FK binding protein intracellularly, it does not interfere with production of cytokines but acts at later stages of the cell cycle by blocking cytokine-induced T-cell proliferation through inhibition of calcium-independent pathways (Fig. 2-13). Although rapamycin has been shown to be a potent immunosuppressant in experimental animal models and has been effective in clinical trials of renal transplantation, it has not been widely used in the clinical setting. Its major adverse effect is the induction of hyperlipidemia.

Both *polyclonal* and *monoclonal antibodies* are in clinical use as part of induction therapies or for rescue therapy and the treatment of acute rejection, occurring despite maintenance immunosuppression. Polyclonal antibodies include antilymphocyte sera and antilymphocyte globulin. These agents are antisera, produced by immunizing animals, most commonly horses or rabbits, with human lymphocytes. In *vivo*, these agents lead to profound depletion of T lymphocytes. Side effects include immune complex-mediated serum sickness, which commonly presents as a flu-like syndrome associated with lymphadenopathy and splenomegaly. In severe cases, patients can experience arthritis, vasculitis, glomerulonephritis, and neurological impairments. If severe side effects develop, administration of antibodies should be discontinued and plasmapheresis should be considered. Monoclonal antibodies target cell-surface epitopes that are important for activation of T lymphocytes. The most commonly used monoclonal antibody is OKT3. It binds to CD3, an epitope important for signaling through the T-cell receptor. OKT3 leads to prompt and complete T-cell depletion. As with polyclonal sera, OKT3 can be used as an induction agent or to treat episodes of acute rejection. Administration of OKT3 can be associated with fever and chills, diarrhea, arthralgias, hypotension, pulmonary edema, headache, aseptic meningitis, seizures, or coma. These symptoms are due to massive release of cytokines such as IFN-γ, TNF-α, or IL-1. In addition, OKT3 is associated with an increased risk for cytomegalovirus infection and the development of posttransplant lymphoproliferative disorders. Monoclonal antibodies directed against costimulatory or adhesion molecules have shown promise in experimental models and are being tested in clinical trials.

CLINICAL ASPECTS

Organ Preservation

In addition to advances in surgical techniques and immunosuppression, research efforts in organ preservation have led to improved outcomes in the field of transplantation. Optimal preservation during the period of ischemia allows for transport of organs, tissue typing, and maintenance of function, which is necessary for an uncomplicated postoperative course.

Before organs are removed from a cadaveric donor, they are cooled externally and by perfusion of the graft with cold preservation solution. Subsequently, they are stored at 4°C. One of the main principles of organ preservation is hypothermia in order to reduce metabolism and, therefore, oxygen demand. A decrease in temperature by 10°C leads to a twofold reduction in enzymatic activity and therefore decreases the rate at which intracellular enzymes degrade cellular components. Thus, storage at 4°C reduces enzymatic activity by a factor of 12 when compared to their activity at the body temperature of 37°C, which allows for an extended preservation period of cold ischemia. Refinement of preservation solutions has been an active area of investigation over the last few decades. These research efforts have been focused on defining components that minimize ischemic and reperfusion injury and hence reduce the incidence of primary graft dysfunction. Although hypothermia is essential to achieve a reduction in the metabolic rate, hypothermia has deleterious effects on cellular integrity and function. Cooling results in rapid reduction of energy stores with a drop in ATP. Decrease in cellular energy stores combined with hypothermia-induced inhibition of the Na^+/K^+ ATPase leads to an influx of water and cellular swelling. In addition, anaerobic glycolysis with accumulation of lactate leads to intracellular acidosis. Hypothermia also contributes to injury mediated through *radical oxygen intermediates*. This is due to degradation of ATP that leads to accumulation of hypoxanthine, which upon reperfusion with oxygen is broken down in a reaction that produces oxygen radicals. The most commonly used organ preservation solution is the *University of Wisconsin (UW) solution,* which was developed by Belzer and Southard in the 1980's. This solution includes ingredients that counterbalance the deleterious effects of hypothermia. Lactobionate has a large molecular mass and cannot permeate cell membranes rapidly. It provides osmotic support and suppresses hypothermic cell swelling. Raffinose, a trisaccharide with a large molecular mass, and hydroxyethyl starch are additional impermeants that counter intracellular osmotic forces and therefore reduce cellular edema. Adenosine and phosphate serve as precursors for ATP and help the cell to restore energy substrates upon reperfusion. Allopurinol, an inhibitor of xanthine oxidase and glutathione, a tripeptide that is important for maintaining enzymes in a nonoxidized form, have been added to UW solution to protect from damage induced by radical oxygen intermediates upon reperfusion. UW solution is rich in potassium, because it was thought that an intracellular milieu would be more protective for the cells. Magnesium serves as a cofactor for cation-dependent reactions. Glucose, an ingredient of other preservation solutions such as Euro-Collins, was not added to UW solution because its degradation to lactate through anaerobic glycolysis was thought to contribute to acidosis. In addition to glucose, Euro-Collins solution contains a high concentration of potassium, a low concentration of sodium, magnesium sulfate, and phosphate. UW solution has been shown to be superior to Euro-Collins solution with respect to graft function and extended periods of storage. Hypothermic storage in UW solution allows for preservation of kidneys up to 3 days, livers up to 2 days, and pancreas grafts over 24 hours. Although hearts have been successfully stored for up to 12 hours, most transplant centers are reluctant to exceed 4 to 6 hours of ischemia. The most common method to preserve lungs is by injection of the vasodilating agent prostaglandin E1 into the pulmonary artery, followed by a administration of a cold flush into fully inflated lungs, which ensures uniform perfusion, and subsequent storage in UW solution or Euro-Collins solution. An important aspect regarding preservation is the recognition that the lung graft can maintain a low level of aerobic metabolism by utilizing oxygen that diffuses from the alveoli to endothelial and parenchymal cells. Therefore, lungs are removed from the donor by clamping the trachea after a full ventilation, maintaining them in an inflated state. Another method, which was developed by Belzer and associates and has been used in clinical kidney transplantation, is continuous hypothermic perfusion. Although preservation of kidney grafts with continuous machine perfusion appears to be superior to simple hypothermic storage, particularly after extended periods of storage, this method is more cumbersome. Because most kidneys are transplanted within 24 hours of harvesting, a time span where cold storage offers excellent results, the majority of transplant centers preserve renal grafts by hypothermic storage.

Renal Transplantation

Joseph Murray successfully transplanted kidneys between identical twins in 1954 and was awarded the Nobel Prize in 1990 for his pioneering contributions to the field of transplantation. Over the last few decades, renal transplantation has become the treatment of choice for patients with end-stage renal disease secondary to a series of underlying conditions. It has evolved as a superior alternative to long-term dialysis, because it offers patients more independence, increases their quality of life, and is associated with better survival rates. These conditions include insulin-dependent diabetes mellitus, glomerulonephritis, polycystic kidney disease, hypertensive nephrosclerosis, systemic lupus erythematosus, and interstitial nephritis. Contraindications for renal transplantation include active malignancies, active infections, occult infections at hemodialysis and peritoneal dialysis sites, and end-stage vascular disease. Particular attention should be paid to the recipient's cardiovascular status, and if necessary, consideration should be given to pretransplant interventions, because these patients are at a high risk for suffering from myocardial infarctions postoperatively. Outcomes after renal transplantation are superior with grafts from living donors as compared to cadaveric organs. Advantages of living-related kidney transplantation include the potential for better HLA matching, decreased risk for acute tubular necrosis because cold ischemia time can be kept to a minimum, and optimal preparation of the recipient because it is an elective procedure. Moreover, brain death has deleterious effects on organ function. Exclusion criteria for cadaveric kidney donors include active infections, history of extracranial malignancy, viral infections such as human immunodeficiency virus (HIV) and hepatitis, a history of severe hypertension or diabetes mellitus. The living donor *nephrectomy* is performed either through an oblique flank incision or more recently with laparoscopic techniques in order to reduce postoperative discomfort and shorten hospital stays. In living donors, a longer renal vein and easier access to the renal artery make the left kidney the graft of choice. Exceptions to this strategy are donors who have multiple left renal arteries as demonstrated by preoperative angiogram. The ureter is divided in proximity to the bladder and the distal stump is ligated. Gonadal and adrenal veins are ligated, the renal vein is divided near its junction with the vena cava, and the renal artery is separated at its origin from the aorta. The *recipient operation* is performed through an extraperitoneal approach via an oblique incision in the left or right lower quadrant (Fig. 2-14A). Due to the ease of dissection, renal grafts are more commonly implanted on the right side. The incidence of lymphoceles can be reduced by dividing and tying lymphatics and minimizing dissection of the recipient iliac vessels. The arterial reconstruction of choice is an end-to-side anastomosis between the recipient's external iliac artery and the renal artery (Fig. 2-14B). Alternatively, an end-to-end anastomosis between the recipient's divided internal iliac artery and the renal artery can be performed. However, diabetic patients often have atherosclerotic disease in their internal iliac arteries, which may necessitate an endarterectomy before performing this type of arterial anastomosis. The venous anastomosis is performed in an end-to-side fashion between renal vein and external iliac vein. Of note, the external iliac vein tends to be more superficial on the right side. The method of choice for restoring continuity of the urinary tract is an ureteroneocystostomy. A 1-cm submucosal tunnel is created upon entry of the ureter into the bladder to minimize the incidence of vesicoureteral reflux during voiding. Before unclamping the vessels, most surgeons administer mannitol and furosemide to promote diuresis and sodium bicarbonate to counterbalance acidosis that develops from release of end products of anaerobic metabolism that have accumulated in the kidney during preservation. *Postoperative complications* after renal transplantation include acute tubular necrosis, which is usually due to an ischemic insult and is therefore more commonly observed in cadaveric grafts. The primary clinical manifestation of *acute tubular necrosis* is typically scant urine output immediately after the transplantation. This condition is generally self-limiting; important differential diagnoses include rejection, vascular or ureteral anastomotic complications, or nephrotoxicity secondary to immunosuppressants. Imaging studies such as renal scans, arteriography, and cystoscopy or renal biopsies may be necessary to exclude these conditions, which would mandate immediate interventions. *Vascular complications* such as thrombotic events or bleeding may necessitate emergent reexplorations to salvage the graft. Blood clots in the bladder, which may cause cessation of urinary output, can be treated with bladder irrigation. Lymphoceles can be treated with drainage into the peritoneum, which can be performed laparoscopically. Urine leaks, which can develop secondary to ischemia of the distal ureter, can be treated with external percutaneous drainage. Late development of renal artery stenosis, which can be secondary to technical or immunological causes, can be an important etiologic factor for the devel-

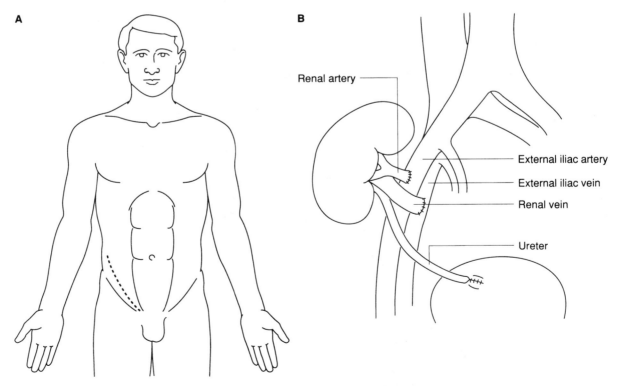

FIGURE 2-14. Renal transplantation **(A)** incision and **(B)** completed implantation. (From Greenfield LJ. *Surgery: Scientific principles and practice,* 1st ed. Philadelphia: JB Lippincott, 1993:517, with permission.)

opment of hypertension. A relatively rare complication of renal transplantation is *tertiary hyperparathyroidism*. Before renal transplantation, chronic renal failure with low serum calcium and elevated serum phosphorus leads to increased activity in the parathyroid gland, which is termed *secondary hyperparathyroidism*. Tertiary hyperparathyroidism defines a condition where parathyroid hyperfunction becomes autonomous after renal transplantation and is associated with hypercalcemia. Clinical manifestations include bone pain, renal calculi, gastrointestinal tract ulcers, and mental status changes. The treatment for tertiary hyperparathyroidism is total parathyroidectomy and autotransplantation of small portions of one parathyroid gland into the patient's forearm. *Rejection of the graft* remains the most frequent cause of graft failure. Hyperacute rejection becomes evident shortly after revascularization. It is caused by alloreactive antibodies, which fix and activate complement in the same manner as natural antibodies in discordant xenotransplants. Complement activates endothelium, making it a prothrombotic surface. Deposition of fibrin thrombi and platelet aggregates initiate an ischemic cascade. Rapid compromise of perfusion is associated with a bluish discoloration of the graft, which leads to cessation of graft function. This devastating complication necessitates removal of the graft. Cell-mediated acute rejection is the most common form of rejection and typically occurs within 3 months of transplantation. Clinical manifestations of acute renal-graft rejection include fever, graft tenderness, malaise, oliguria, and diastolic hypertension. Acute rejection is usually accompanied by an elevation in serum creatinine. Important differential diagnoses include fluid imbalances, infections, mechanical urinary tract obstructions, renal artery stenosis, and cyclosporine-induced nephrotoxicity. Because the diagnosis can be difficult to make on clinical grounds alone, imaging studies are usually obtained. Renal perfusion scans with radiolabeled tracers and ultrasound studies with color-flow Doppler can help exclude mechanical causes for graft dysfunction. Ultimately, a renal biopsy, usually obtained percutaneously, remains the gold standard to diagnose acute graft rejection. If acute rejection is diagnosed, prompt treatment with intravenous (i.v.) high-dose steroids or antilymphocyte preparations is initiated. Chronic rejection causes a gradual decline of renal-graft function over years and is an important factor for late graft loss. Clinical signs include proteinuria and microscopic hematuria, which are usually accompanied by a progressive rise in serum creatinine. The diagnosis of chronic rejection is made by renal biopsy, which shows thickening of the glomerular basement membranes, interstitial fibrosis, and proliferation of arterial smooth muscle cells. Currently, there is no definitive treatment for chronic kidney graft rejection. Consideration should be given to discontinuing potentially nephrotoxic medications, which further compromise graft function.

Clinical results after renal transplantation are excellent. In the case of HLA-identical living-related kidney transplants, 1-year graft survival exceeds 95%, and 1-year graft survival of 1-haplotype matched living-related kidneys is above 90%. For all cadaveric renal transplants, graft 1-year survival rates are in excess of 80%. Among cadaveric renal grafts, six antigen-matched grafts have a superior 1-year graft survival.

Liver Transplantation

The first successful human liver transplant was performed by Starzl in 1963. During the 1980's, liver transplantation evolved into effective treatment for end-stage liver disease. Significant improvements in the clinical results of liver transplantation were due to improvements in surgical and anesthetic technique, refinements in immunosuppressive regimens, the development of UW solution, which allowed for preservation of organ function after cold storage, and timing of the operation. Initially, hepatic transplantation was viewed as a life-saving intervention, which was performed on patients with very advanced liver disease. The procedure has evolved into a therapeutic intervention, which improves a patient's quality of life and therefore is performed at earlier time points of disease. *Hepatic cirrhosis* with consequent portal hypertension is the main indication for liver transplantation in the adult population. The most frequent etiologies of cirrhosis include alcoholic liver disease, viral hepatitis secondary to hepatitis B or C, Wilson disease, hemochromatosis, α_1-antitrypsin deficiency, primary sclerosing cholangitis, and primary biliary cirrhosis.

Other hepatic pathologies such as Budd-Chiari syndrome, portal vein thrombosis, and hepatocellular carcinoma can also be treated by transplantation. Up to 10% of all liver transplants are performed for patients with acute or fulminant liver failure. This devastating condition can be due to viral hepatitis, drug toxicity such as acetaminophen or carbon tetrachloride, or ingestion of various Amanita mushrooms. Rapid loss of hepatocellular function in these patients can lead to defective protein and clotting factor synthesis, hypoglycemia due to impaired gluconeogenesis, encephalopathy, and hepatorenal syndrome. Liver transplantation for acute liver failure is associated with a higher mortality than for chronic liver disease. Many transplant centers report favorable results in the treatment of small hepatocellular carcinomas with liver transplantation in combination with adjuvant chemotherapy. In light of the ongoing debate surrounding allocation of scarce donor organs, this topic remains an issue of great controversy. Liver transplantation is generally not offered to patients suffering from cholangiocarcinomas. *Pediatric patients* most commonly undergo hepatic transplantation for extrahepatic biliary atresia. Children suffering from biliary atresia often undergo a portoenterostomy (Kasai procedure) as the initial surgical procedure, which allows them to grow and increases the likelihood to obtain a suitable donor organ at a later time. The postoperative course after a Kasai procedure is occasionally complicated by recurrent episodes of cholangitis, which may be an indication for hepatic transplantation. *Contraindications* for liver transplantation include acute sepsis, extrahepatic malignancies, HIV seropositivity, hepatitis B surface antigen seropositivity, advanced cardiac or pulmonary disease, and inability to comply with an immunosuppressive regimen. The most frequent contraindication for liver transplantation for acute liver failure is uncontrolled infection. In addition, increasing requirements for vasopressors is a relative contraindication for hepatic transplantation in this setting. Donor livers are usually procured as part of multiple organ harvest procedures. Negative predictors of allograft function include prolonged ischemic time, donor hypotension, and poor nutritional status of the donor. The *recipient operation* is performed through bilateral subcostal incisions with midline extension. The major parts of the recipient procedure include hepatectomy, anhepatic phase, implantation of the donor liver, and postrevascularization period. Implantation includes anastomoses of suprahepatic inferior vena cava, infrahepatic inferior vena cava, portal vein, arterial reconstruction, which is commonly performed through an anastomosis of donor celiac axis to recipient common hepatic artery, and biliary reconstruction as an end-to-end anastomosis of donor and recipient common ducts over a T-tube stent or as a Roux-en-Y choledochojejunostomy between donor common bile duct and a defunctionalized limb of recipient jejunum (Fig. 2-15). Most liver transplants are performed with venovenous bypass. This bypass diverts blood from the recipient's portal vein and infrahepatic inferior vena cava to the central venous circulation and allows for more hemodynamic stability during the anhepatic phase.

The shortage of donor organs, particularly for the pediatric patient population, has led to the development of alternatives to the standard orthotopic liver transplant procedure. The intrahepatic segmental architecture allows for isolation of vascular pedicles that supply hepatic segments individually, thereby making partial liver transplantation a therapeutic option. Split-liver transplants provide two allografts from one donor liver, and reduced-size liver transplantation permits the surgical reduction of a liver to fit into the abdominal cavity of a child. Another approach to increase the donor pool for pediatric patients is living-related liver transplantation. Potential advantages of living-related liver transplantation are similar to those of living-related kidney transplantation: improved histocompatibility, shortened waiting times, shorter cold ischemic times, and use of an organ from a physiologically normal donor. The donor needs to be informed about the risks associated with a segmental hepatic resection. *Postoperative complications* of liver transplantation include primary nonfunction of the graft. This devastating complication has an incidence of less than 5% at most transplant centers and generally requires emer-

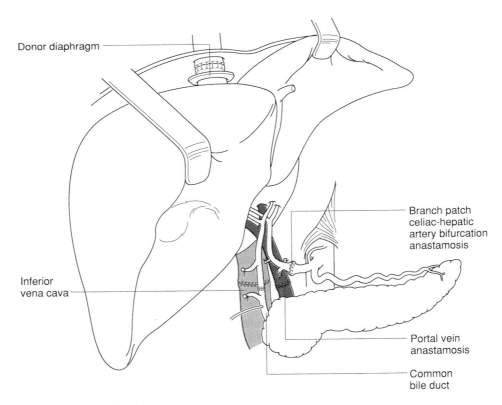

FIGURE 2-15. Completed liver transplantation. (From Greenfield LJ. *Surgery: Scientific principles and practice,* 1st ed. Philadelphia: JB Lippincott, 1993:534, with permission.)

gent retransplantation. Primary nonfunction has been attributed to ischemia-reperfusion injury and compromised nutritional status of the donor. *Hepatic allograft rejection* remains a major cause of morbidity after liver transplantation. Hyperacute rejection occurs very rarely in hepatic transplantation. Acute rejection occurs most commonly during the first 6 weeks after transplantation and is the most common form of rejection. This diagnosis can be suggested by clinical and laboratory parameters, including fever, lethargy, graft tenderness, leukocytosis, change in the color or quantity of bile, and elevations in serum bilirubin and hepatic enzymes. There exists no laboratory value or pattern of enzyme elevation that would be specific for hepatic allograft rejection. The gold standard for diagnosing acute hepatic rejection remains liver biopsy, which is usually obtained by percutaneous core needle biopsy. Histological findings include mononuclear portal or periportal inflammatory infiltrates with destructive cholangitis or endothelitis. Only minor inflammatory changes are seen in the hepatic lobules during acute rejection. Episodes of acute rejection are treated with steroid boluses, antilymphocyte therapy with OKT3, or tacrolimus. Chronic rejection has also been referred to as ductopenic rejection or vanishing bile duct syndrome. Patients usually experience an asymptomatic rise in alkaline phosphatase and γ-glutamyl transpeptidase and eventually the onset of jaundice. Histologically, they show arterial luminal narrowing and bile-duct loss. Because the bile duct is supplied by the arterial system, these two lesions tend to correlate. Chronic rejection can occur between 6 weeks and several years after liver transplantation. Severe cases of chronic rejection need to be treated with retransplantation. Other complications after hepatic transplantation usually relate to biliary *drainage of the graft*. During the early postoperative period, patients can experience biliary leaks or dislodgement of the T tube. Strictures of the bile duct, which develop secondary to ischemia, can complicate the later postoperative course. They can be generally managed with interventional radiologic or endoscopic techniques. One of the potentially most devastating complications of liver transplantation is *thrombosis of the hepatic artery*, which occurs more often in the pediatric population. This condition can lead to necrosis of hilar connective tissue, lymph nodes, and walls of the portal vein, as well as bile ducts with subsequent bile leaks. Diagnostic modalities are duplex ultrasound and arteriogram. Treatment options for hepatic artery thrombosis are emergent declotting and revascularization or retransplantation. Other vascular complications are portal vein thrombosis, which can present with increasing ascites and portal hypertension and has been successfully treated with surgical evacuation of the clot and reanastomosis and postoperative anticoagulation, and recurrent hepatic vein thrombosis after transplantation for Budd-Chiari syndrome. *Infectious complications* are related to the use of immunosuppressive medications and represent a major cause for morbidity and mortality after liver transplantation. Bacterial infections after liver transplantation include wound infections, pneumonias, liver abscesses, and biliary sepsis. Infectious processes of the hepatic allograft can develop secondary to vascular or biliary complications or can be the result of previous liver biopsies. A liver biopsy is often required to distinguish an infectious process from rejection, which can both present with fevers and worsening liver functions. Liver abscesses can usually be drained percutaneously. Infections with cytomegalovirus can affect several organ systems including lungs and gastrointestinal tract. It is also the most common cause of postoperative graft hepatitis and is most frequently encountered a few weeks after transplantation. CMV-negative recipients of CMV-positive grafts are particularly at risk for developing this serious complication. Patients usually have low-grade fevers and elevated liver enzyme levels. The treatment for this condition is reduction of the immunosuppression and administration of ganciclovir or valcyclovir. Outcomes after liver transplantation have improved significantly over the last 2 decades. Currently, the 1-year survival rate after liver transplantation is more than 85% at most institutions. Survival rates are dependent on the indication for the procedure; the best results are obtained in patients who undergo hepatic transplantation for cholestatic liver disease, and the worst results are reported for patients who suffer from hepatitis B or from malignancies. These patients often experience recurrences of their disease. In addition, outcomes are influenced by the severity of the recipient's disease before transplantation.

Pancreas Transplantation

The first pancreatic transplant was performed by Kelly at the University of Minnesota in 1966. Despite significant limitations, it was realized that a pancreas graft was able to provide an endogenous source for insulin and thus establish an euglycemic state in diabetic patients that was independent of exogenously administered insulin. Improvements in immunosuppression, organ preservation, and surgical technique have led to higher graft and patient survival rates. The *primary indication* for pancreas transplantation is the presence of type I diabetes mellitus. The effects of pancreas transplantation on progression and possible reversal of secondary diabetic complications, such as nephropathy, neuropathy and retinopathy, remain controversial. Pancreas transplantation can be performed either alone, after a kidney transplantation, or simultaneously with a kidney transplantation. *Simultaneous pancreas-kidney transplantation* is indicated for insulin-dependent diabetics, who suffer from advanced nephropathy. There are reports that the survival of the kidney graft is improved in this setting. Sequential pancreas transplants have been advocated because of the already existent immunosuppression. As outcomes for simultaneous pancreas-kidney transplants are more favorable, indications for pancreas transplantation alone are less well-defined. This procedure is generally reserved for highly selected patients with hyperlabile diabetes and early onset of secondary complications, who may benefit from metabolic control. However, the benefits of insulin independence need to be weighed carefully against the side effects of immunosuppressive drugs. Contraindications to pancreas donation include a history of type I or type II diabetes mellitus, history of pancreatic trauma, history of prior pancreatic surgery, pancreatitis, severe atherosclerosis, and intraabdominal contamination. The *donor pancreatectomy* is usually part of a multiorgan harvest and can be performed in combination with the hepatectomy (Fig. 2-16). The spleen can be used as a handle during the procurement to minimize damage to the pancreas. Cold preservation solution is perfused via abdominal aorta and portal vein. The portal vein is transected approximately 2 cm above the pancreas before its cannulation. This step prevents the development of pancreatic edema. The pancreatic graft can be separated from the liver on the back table. Before implantation, the pancreas graft needs to be prepared further. The portal vein may need to be elongated with a piece of donor iliac vein, and a donor common iliac artery bifurcation graft is sutured to splenic and superior mesenteric arteries to reconstruct the pancreatic arterial supply. The second portion of the duodenum remains attached to the head of the pancreas. Splenic vessels are ligated at the splenic hilum and the spleen remains in place to be used as a handle during the recipient operation. Although segmental pancreas grafts are being performed, most centers transplant whole pancreaticoduodenal grafts. Approaches to *manage the exocrine secretion* include ligation of the pancreatic duct, duct injection with synthetic polymers, as well as enteric or bladder drainage via the duodenal segment. The vast majority of pancreas grafts in the United States are performed with bladder drainage (Fig. 2-17). Advantages of this method include the ability to diagnose rejection by urinary amylase, cystoscopic access for transduodenal needle biopsies, lower rates of infection, and relative technical ease. Complications are mainly urologic and metabolic, such as hematuria, cystitis, and acidosis. The pancreas graft is transplanted ectopically to the iliac fossa with the arterial blood supply coming from the recipient iliac artery. Venous drainage is established through anastomosing the donor portal vein to the recipient iliac vein, which leads to nonphysiologic systemic drainage of insulin. Glucose levels are followed closely postoperatively, and patients are initially maintained on i.v. insulin infusions to keep serum glucose levels below 200 mg/dl. Duplex ultrasonography and radionuclide scanning can be used to assess the graft, if there is suspicion for compromised perfusion, fluid collections, or malfunction. Particular attention needs to be paid to fluid balance as well as bicarbonate and electrolyte losses in the initial postoperative period. Because *rejection* is the major etiology for graft loss, early diagnosis and treatment is critical to the outcome of pancreas transplantation. Rejection of the exocrine gland precedes rejection of the endocrine pancreas. Therefore, hyperglycemia may indicate advanced rejection and often irreversible damage to the graft. In combined kidney-pancreas transplants, rejection of the renal graft generally precedes pancreas graft rejection. Isolated

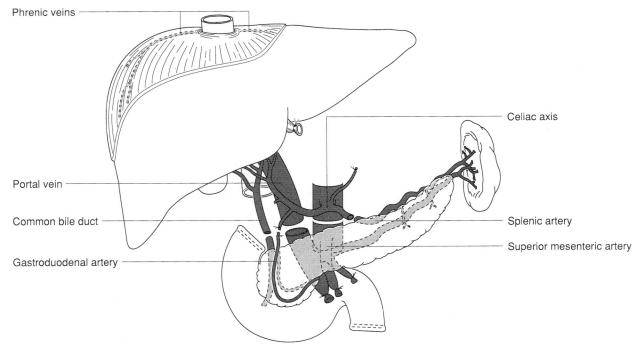

FIGURE 2-16. Donor pancreatectomy as part of multiorgan harvest. (From Greenfield LJ. *Surgery: Scientific principles and practice.* 1st ed. Philadelphia: JB Lippincott, 1993:514, with permission.)

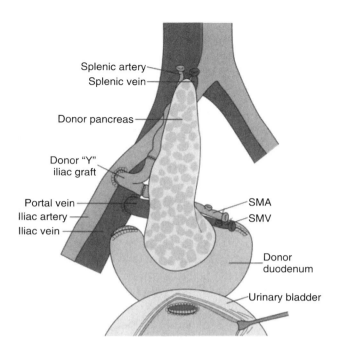

FIGURE 2-17. Bladder drainage of pancreas via duodenal segment. (From Miller TA. *Modern surgical care,* 2nd ed. St. Louis: Quality Medical Publishers, 1998:144, with permission.)

rejection of the pancreas graft alone is a rare occurrence. Thus, elevation of serum creatinine—usually combined with renal-graft biopsy—is a sensitive marker to guide therapy. Pancreatic graft rejection can be diagnosed by monitoring both exocrine and endocrine parameters in serum and urine, cytologic monitoring of pancreatic drainage or urine, noninvasive imaging studies such as ultrasonography or radionuclide scans, and finally allograft biopsies. Overall, pancreas transplantation—alone or in combination with kidney transplantation—has become an established treatment option for patients with insulin-dependent diabetes mellitus. One-year patient survival exceeds 90%, and 1-year pancreas graft survival, as defined by complete insulin independence, is greater than 70%. The effect of pancreas transplantation on secondary manifestations of diabetes is extremely important, because it would be desirable to halt or reverse conditions such as nephropathy, neuropathy, and retinopathy by establishing good metabolic control. There is evidence that recipients of successful combined kidney-pancreas transplants do not develop nephropathy in their transplanted kidneys. Although there are some encouraging reports with regard to improvements in neuropathy and retinopathy, the data here are controversial. Finally, studies have shown that successful pancreas transplantation is associated with improved quality of life.

Small Bowel Transplantation

In the 1980's, advances in immunosuppression combined with realization of shortcomings of long-term parenteral nutrition led to renewed efforts in clinical small bowel transplantation. Although there is a significant body of experimental work in small bowel transplantation dating back to the 1950's, the advent and success of total parenteral nutrition in the 1970's had temporarily limited interest in this procedure. Immunologic properties quite unique to the small intestine that represented significant immunologic barriers are high immunogenicity due to high expression of class II MHC on the surface of enterocytes and the propensity to develop graft-versus-host disease due to the large amount of lymphatic tissue in the gut. *Candidates for small bowel transplantation* include patients who suffer from short-gut syndrome and are dependent on total parenteral nutrition. Short-gut syndrome can be the result of massive surgical resection secondary to conditions such as embolic or thrombotic events, inflammatory bowel disease, necrotizing enterocolitis, malrotation, trauma, and certain neoplasms. Rarely, irreversible intestinal failure can be of functional origin with grave impairments of motility and absorptive capacities. The small bowel can be transplanted alone or in combination with a liver graft. There is convincing experimental evidence that liver grafts can act in an immunologically protective fashion and reduce rejection episodes of concomitantly transplanted organs. *Combined small bowel–liver transplants* are indicated for patients who suffer from irreversible liver disease secondary to total parenteral nutrition (Fig. 2-18). Loss of venous access is a potentially devastating problem in these patients, who are totally dependent on parenteral nutrition. In such circumstances, small bowel transplantation can become the only treatment option. Donor and recipient must be ABO blood group compatible and are usually matched for cytomegalovirus status. For isolated small bowel transplants, the entire small bowel and the right colon are removed with vascular pedicles including the superior mesenteric artery and origin of the portal vein. The donor superior mesenteric artery can be anastomosed directly to the recipient's superior mesenteric artery or an aortic segment of the donor containing the superior mesenteric artery can be connected to the recipient's infrarenal aorta. The venous drainage via the donor's superior mesenteric vein can be performed into the portal vein or systemically. Portal drainage may be the more physiologic option with first-pass of hepatotrophic substances through the liver. In combined small bowel–liver grafts, the donor portal vein is anastomosed to the recipient's portal vein so that the entire gastrointestinal tract drains into the transplanted liver. A donor aortic conduit containing both celiac arteries and superior mesenteric artery is anastomosed to the recipient's infrarenal aorta. Suprahepatic, infrahepatic caval as well as biliary anastomoses in this procedure are analogous to those employed in liver transplantation. Although the proximal portion of the intestinal graft is anastomosed to the recipient's small bowel, a stoma is created distally in order to be able to access the graft for mucosal biopsies in the postoperative period.

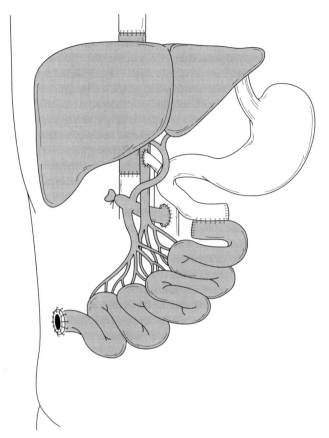

FIGURE 2-18. Combined small bowel–liver transplant. (From Asfar S, Zhong R, Grant D. *Surgical Clinics of North America. October 1994. Horizons in Organ Transplantation.* Philadelphia: WB Saunders, 1203, with permission.)

Heart Transplantation

The pioneering work that led to the establishment of clinical heart transplantation was conducted under the leadership of Shumway and Lower at Stanford University in the 1960's. The first successful human cardiac transplantation was preformed by Barnard in Cape Town in 1967. Introduction of cyclosporine into the immunosuppressive armamentarium in the 1980's led to improved patient survival and more widespread application of heart transplantation as a treatment modality for *end-stage heart disease.* Cardiac transplantation is indicated for patients who suffer from end-stage heart disease that is not amenable to medical therapy or other surgical interventions; the most common etiologies include idiopathic dilated cardiomyopathy, ischemic heart disease, and less commonly ventricular dysfunction secondary to valvular or congenital disease, malignant ventricular arrhythmia, or cardiac allograft vasculopathy. Congenital heart disease is the primary indication for heart transplantation in the pediatric population. Absolute contraindications to heart transplantation include fixed pulmonary resistance in excess of 6 Wood units that does not respond to vasodilators, severe hepatic or renal dysfunction, active malignancy, active systemic infection, and seropositivity for HIV. The major limiting factor to heart transplantation remains a shortage of suitable donor organs. This has led to attempts to expand the donor pool by considering donor parameters such as advanced age, high-dose inotropic support, seropositivity for hepatitis C, size mismatch, echocardiographic abnormality, and prolonged cold ischemic time. Absolute *contraindications to heart donation* include donor seropositivity for HIV, intractable ventricular dysrhythmias, extracranial malignancy, documented prior myocardial dysfunction, severe coronary artery or valvular disease, and death from carbon monoxide poisoning with a blood carboxyhemoglobin level greater than 20%. Donor and recipient operations need to be timed so that the ischemia time of the donor heart does not exceed 4 to 6 hours. The risk of postoperative myocardial dysfunction of the transplanted heart is minimized by proper donor management with invasive monitoring in an intensive care setting paying close attention to maintaining normothermia and regulating acid base, volume, and electrolyte status. Some transplant centers advocate hormonal resuscitation of the brain-dead donor with agents such as triiodothyronine, arginine, vasopressin, insulin, and methylprednisolone in an attempt to improve hemodynamics. The *donor cardiectomy,* which often is part of a multiorgan procurement, is performed through a median sternotomy. After dissection, the donor organ is arrested with a single dose of cardioplegic solution and rapidly cooled. Most hearts are transplanted orthotopically. *Heterotopic auxiliary heart transplantation* is a rarely performed procedure in which the donor heart is implanted in parallel to the native heart. Heterotopic implantation is considered when the donor heart is felt to be too small to support the recipient's circulation, when the native myocardium has the potential to recover, or when the recipient has elevated pulmonary resistance. *Orthotopic heart transplantation* can be performed using one of two different techniques. The biatrial technique—where the recipient heart is implanted using four anastomoses, the left and right atrial, the pulmonary artery, and the aorta— is considered the standard method (Fig. 2-19). The alternative method, which is termed *bicaval heart transplantation,* involves complete excision of the recipient heart except for a cuff of left atrial tissue around the ostia of the paired pulmonary veins and small cavoatrial cuffs and thus involves five anastomoses. Rarely, total orthotopic implantation is undertaken in which pulmonary venous cuffs are used, necessitating six anastomoses. Proponents of the more involved methods argue that they are associated with improved atrial function, a reduction of atrial arrhythmias, and improved tricuspid and mitral valve function. However, most surgeons feel that these advantages are only marginal and are outweighed by longer ischemic times and higher risk for anastomotic complications. Cornerstones of early *postoperative management* of orthotopic heart trans-

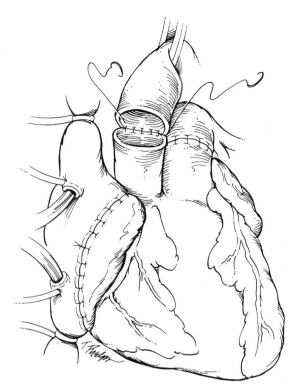

FIGURE 2-19. Aortic anastomosis at completion of orthotopic cardiac transplantation. (From Kaise LR, Kron IL, Spray TL. *Mastery of cardiothoracic surgery*. Philadelphia: Lippincott-Raven, 506, with permission.)

plant recipients are hemodynamic support and immunosuppression. Right ventricular dysfunction is a common occurrence in the early posttransplant period that requires the administration of inotropes and pulmonary vasodilators, including isoproterenol, phosphodiesterase inhibitors such as milrinone or amrinone, renal dose dopamine, and inhaled nitric oxide. Vagal denervation of the transplanted heart is associated with a resting heart rate of approximately 100 beats per minute. Donor sinoatrial and atrioventricular dysfunction caused by surgical trauma, ischemic injury, and the duration of cardiopulmonary bypass can often lead to early postoperative bradyarrhythmias. Most of these bradyarrhythmias respond well to pharmacological agents such as isopreterenol or to temporary epicardial pacing and usually resolve spontaneously. Therefore, permanent pacemakers should not be placed in the early postoperative period. On the other hand, early tachyarrhythmias are often associated with allograft rejection. Most heart transplant recipients receive triple-drug immunosuppression with cyclosporine or tacrolimus, azathioprine or mycophenolate mofetil, and steroids. Tacrolimus is felt to be equivalent to cyclosporine, and switching from cyclosporine to tacrolimus may be beneficial in circumstances of recurrent rejection. Increasingly, transplant centers believe that mycophenolate mofetil is superior to azathioprine as a maintenance immunosuppressant, as it appears to be associated with a reduced incidence of acute rejection. Induction therapy with cytolytic agents such as ATGAM, thymoglobulin, or OKT3 is generally used selectively in recipients with renal dysfunction or in presensitized patients. Induction therapy is associated with a higher risk for developing infectious complications and late lymphoproliferative disorders. Episodes of acute rejection are particularly common within the first few months after transplantation but account for fewer than 10% of early deaths after cardiac transplantation. Endomyocardial biopsy remains the gold standard for the diagnosis of acute rejection and it is generally believed that surveillance biopsies are important in the first year after transplantation. Acute allograft rejection is usually treated with pulse steroids. Cytolytic agents are reserved for episodes of severe rejection that are associated with hemodynamic compromise or steroid-resistant acute rejection. Infectious complications remain a serious complication of heart transplantation. Among heart transplant recipients, infections are responsible for 10% of early deaths and 30% of late deaths. Infections can be bacterial, fungal, parasitic, or viral in nature. Heart transplant recipients are particularly susceptible to infections with the herpesviruses, namely CMV, EBV, varicella-zoster virus, and herpes simplex viruses types 1, 2, and 6. Because CMV is a major cause of morbidity and mortality, some transplant centers have chosen approaches such as donor-recipient CMV matching or gancyclovir prophylaxis in high-risk recipients.

The major cause for late morbidity and mortality after heart transplantation is cardiac allograft vasculopathy. This pathological process involves the epicardial coronary arteries, intramyocardial arterioles, venous structures, and the great vessels of the allograft. Immunological mechanisms are thought to be primarily responsible for the development of cardiac allograft vasculopathy. Episodes of acute rejection are felt to portend the later development of this pathological condition. Nonimmunological mechanisms that contribute to the process include ischemia-reperfusion injury, drug toxicity, recipient hyperlipidemia, and recipient hypertension. The only definitive treatment for cardiac allograft vasculopathy is retransplantation. Overall, cardiac transplantation, with 1-year survival rates above 80% and 5-year survival rates well above 70%, is currently the best treatment option for end-stage heart disease.

Lung Transplantation

Hardy is credited with performing the first human single-lung transplantation in 1963. Several isolated attempts at lung transplantation were undertaken in the 1960's and 1970's. However, this early era of lung transplantation was highly unsuccessful and plagued by airway complications, rejection, and infection. The modern era of lung transplantation was ushered in by Reitz and his colleagues at Stanford University, who reported the first successful series of lung transplants by performing combined heart-lung transplants.

In subsequent years, long-term success with both single-lung and double-lung transplants was achieved by Cooper. In addition to changes in immunosuppressive regimens, refinements in surgical techniques of the bronchial anastomosis contributed to improved outcomes. Today, lung or combined heart-lung transplants are being performed for a wide spectrum of *end-stage pulmonary parenchymal* and *vascular disorders*. Patients suffering from end-stage lung disease generally have a life expectancy of less than 2 years. The main indications among obstructive lung diseases include idiopathic emphysema (at present, the most common indication), smoking-related emphysema, and emphysema secondary to alpha$_1$-antitrypsin deficiency. Septic diseases such as cystic fibrosis and bronchiectasis can be successfully treated with double-lung replacement. Restrictive lung diseases include idiopathic pulmonary fibrosis, sarcoidosis, and rare conditions, such as histicytosis X, bronchiolitis obliterans organizing pneumonia, asbestosis, or desquamative interstitial pneumonitis. Additionally, patients with primary pulmonary hypertension or Eisenmenger syndrome (pulmonary hypertension secondary to congenital heart disease) are candidates for lung or combined heart-lung transplants. *Combined heart-lung transplantation* is reserved for pulmonary hypertension with associated irreversible right heart dysfunction. *Double-lung transplants* are primarily performed for suppurative conditions, such as cystic fibrosis or bronchiectasis, in order to remove septic foci and avoid contamination of the donor allograft by the native lung, which would be the case with single-lung transplantation. Shortage of donor organs has expanded the indications for *single-lung transplantation* and, like hepatic transplantation, has led to development of novel approaches, such as living-related lobar transplantations. Contraindications for lung transplantation are comparable to those of other solid organ transplants, namely age, active infections, malignancies, and significant hepatic, renal, or cardiac diseases. Active cigarette smokers are not considered candidates for this procedure. Unlike heart and liver recipients, functional status, as assessed by treadmill testing, is a critical discriminant for those patients with sufficient reserve to recover from the surgery. When accepting donor lungs, it is important to rule out infectious processes. In addition, the PO_2 at 100% oxygen should exceed 350 mm Hg. Single-lung transplants have traditionally been performed through a posterolateral thoracotomy, although there is an increasing trend toward the use of muscle-sparing thoracotomies, anterior thoracotomies, and sternotomies to minimize postoperative discomfort. The lung receiving less blood perfusion is usually transplanted. Double-lung transplants have traditionally been performed through a clamshell incision (bilateral thoracosternotomy) with division of both internal mammary arteries. However, recently several groups have moved to bilateral anterior thoracotomy without sternal division to minimize wound complications. In the past, most centers attempted to avoid the use of cardiopulmonary bypass for this procedure, reserving its use for hemodynamic instability after implantation of the first lung or for inadequate ventilation or oxygenation after implantation of the first lung. However, a more liberal use of the pump seems to be gaining favor. *Complications* in the early postoperative period are mainly due to *surgical aspects* of the procedure, such as airway anastomotic stenoses or leaks, vascular anastomotic stenoses, ischemia-reperfusion injury, or cardiac decompensation. Anastomotic dehiscence is generally due to ischemia and necessitates prompt surgical intervention, stenoses may be amenable to noninvasive strategies, such as stent placement. Following this very early postoperative phase, *infectious complications* account for most morbidity and mortality. One has to remember that unlike other solid organ allografts, the lung has a direct exposure to airborne pathogens and therefore is more susceptible to various bacterial, viral, and fungal infections. Infections and episodes of *acute rejection* can have similar clinical manifestations. Bronchoscopy with transbronchial biopsies and bronchoalveolar lavage for microbiologic cultures are essential to differentiate these conditions. Both usually present with elevated temperature, leukocytosis, dyspnea, increased secretions, occasional rales on pulmonary auscultation, deterioration of pulmonary function, and infiltrates or pleural effusions on chest radiographs. Acute rejection episodes usually respond well to pulse treatment with steroids. Alternative regimens include OKT3, antithymocyte globulin, or ALG. Studies have indicated that the risk of developing posttransplantation lymphoproliferative disorders is particularly high in lung transplantation. EBV seronegativity of the recipient, CMV mismatch between donor and recipient, and treatment of rejection episodes with OKT3 have been associated with this complication. The primary cause of late mortality and morbidity after lung transplantation is *obliterative bronchiolitis*. More than one third of all lung transplant recipients develop this fibroproliferative process in the small airways. Obliterative bronchiolitis is generally believed to be a manifestation of chronic rejection. Infectious episodes, particularly due to cytomegalovirus, and ischemia-reperfusion injury are thought to increase allogenicity and antigenicity of the lung grafts and thereby may contribute to the development of obliterative bronchiolitis. One-year survival after lung transplantation is 70%, and 5-year survival is approximately 40%. Although these numbers are less favorable than survival figures for other solid organ transplants, lung transplant recipients have experienced significant improvements in their quality of life over the last decade.

SUGGESTED READING

Auchincloss H, Sykes M, Sachs DH. Transplantation immunology. In: Paul W, ed. *Fundamental immunology,* 4th ed. Philadelphia: Lippincott-Raven, 1998.

Cooper DKC, Miller LW, Patterson GA, eds. *The transplantation and replacement of thoracic organs,* 2nd ed., Boston: Kluwer Academic Publishers, 1996.

SURGICAL INFECTIONS AND ANTIMICROBIAL AGENTS

SARAH BOUCHARD AND HARRY L. ANDERSON III

Surgical infections are defined as infections that require operative treatment or those that may result from operative therapy. In surgical infections, pathogens are usually opportunistic and mixed, and they originate from the patient's endogenous flora. Because host barriers are by definition violated in patients who undergo surgery, these patients are particularly susceptible to the development of infection. The consequence of this violation can be delayed because more than 50% of postsurgical infections develop or are diagnosed after the patient is discharged from the hospital.

HOST DEFENSE MECHANISMS

Host defenses consist of a series of barriers, some of which may act synergistically to both prevent and contain infections. They can be classified as mechanical, microbial flora, humoral, cellular, and cytokine. The host may suffer serious deleterious consequences from an overresponse of host defense mechanisms. The skin, mucus membranes, and epithelial layers of the body serve to separate sterile body tissues from contact with the outer world. In addition to the mechanical barrier provided by these tissues, other mechanisms reinforce these protective effects. These include mucous and antibody secretion in the gut and the airway, which offers a physical, chemical, and biological barrier, the thicker skin of the soles and palms, chemical compounds secreted by the sebaceous glands, ciliary function of epithelial cells of the respiratory tract, and the low pH level of the alimentary tract.

Microbial Flora

The microbiologic flora of the gastrointestinal tract supports a type of *host defense.* This microflora is established in neonates after ingestion of microbes from the birth canal and from the first few feedings and remains fairly constant thereafter. Its presence seems critical for the development of the neonatal immune system. Endogenous microbes bind to gastrointestinal mucosal cells and to specific types of other bacteria. Thus, potential binding sites of pathogenic bacteria are occupied (colonization resistance) and a substantial physical microbacterial layer is present and maintained despite constant shedding of enterocysts.

The oropharynx contains both aerobic and anaerobic bacteria, consisting of Gram-positive aerobic and anaerobic microorganisms, lactobacilli, *Branhamella* sp, *Bacteroides melaninogenicus,* and *Bacteroides oralis.* Few oropharyngeal inhabitants will reach the intestine because of the low pH level in the stomach coupled with the rapid transit time. Passage of some microorganisms, however, may occur during meals due to buffering in the gastric pH. The upper small intestine contains few microorganisms, mostly Gram-positive aerobes and lactobacilli. On the other hand, the lower small intestine contains numerous aerobic and anaerobic organisms, particularly in the presence of an incompetent or absent ileocecal valve. In the colon, the aerobic bacteria (*Enterococcus faecalis, Escherichia coli, Enterobacteriaceae* sp) are outnumbered 300 to 1 by anaerobes (*Bacteroides fragilis, Fusobacterium,* and others). Microorganisms constitute up to 30% of fecal dry weight and up to 1,012 organisms are present per gram of feces.

Impaired Host Defenses in Surgical Patients

Patients with *cellular immunodeficiencies* are more susceptible to develop postoperative infections or infections requiring surgical interventions such as soft tissue infections. This category includes patients with diabetes mellitus, malnutrition, uremia, trauma, and burns. The absence of normal granulocyte oxidative activity in patients with chronic granulomatous disease renders them susceptible to infections by pathogens that require intracellular killing, such as *Staphylococcus aureus, E. coli, Pseudomonas, Serratia,* and *Salmonella*

The Children's Hospital of Philadelphia, Philadelphia, Pennsylvania; Hospital of the University of Pennsylvania, Philadelphia, Pennsylvania sp, and fungi. Asplenic patients, or those with disorders of opsonization, such as patients with sickle cell, are at increased risk of infections with encapsulated bacteria. Organisms such as *Streptococcus pneumonia*, *Haemophilus influenza*, and *Meningococcus* sp can then lead to fulminant meningitis and septicemia. Impaired cell–mediated immunity renders patients susceptible to infection by intracellular organisms, fungi, mycobacteria, viruses, and parasites. It is often seen in the very young and very old patients, with various congenital disorders such as DiGeorge syndrome (also called thymic aplasia), and in severe combined immunodeficiency disease. Acquired defects in cell-mediated immunity are also seen in viral infections, malignancy, steroids, chemotherapy, and radiation therapy.

Congenital and acquired deficiencies of the humoral defense system predispose patients to infections with encapsulated bacteria, toxin-producing bacteria, and viruses such as polio, hepatitis, and rubella. Exogenous administration of immunoglobulin offers some protection against some infections.

Surgical Breach of Host Defenses

Surgical operations may bring the sterile tissues or body cavities in contact with nonsterile regions, such as the gastrointestinal, genitourinary, and respiratory tracts and the oropharynx. General anesthesia itself depresses immune function by impairing lymphocyte response to foreign antigens and decreasing leukocyte capacity to lyse antibody-coated target cells. Malnutrition, the most common cause of acquired immunologic deficiency in surgical patients, and preoperative weight loss both adversely affect the body's resistance to infection.

The violation of sterile body tissues and cavities associated with the accumulation of blood, which is the best culture milieu that is seen in trauma patients, favors bacterial contamination and growth. Patients with severe injuries may also become anergic with decreased neutrophil chemotaxis. Burn patients are also particularly susceptible to infection. The decreased cellular response seen in these patients includes decreased chemotaxis, decreased lysosomal enzyme production, decreased immunoglobulin concentrations, and an absolute reduction in the number of T lymphocytes and the helper-T-cell/suppressor-cell ratio.

Patients with lymphedema and venous insufficiency are susceptible to infections because of the abnormal clearance of microorganisms through impaired vascular channels. Patients harboring foreign bodies are also at greater risk of infection because the host immune effectors often cannot reach the foreign object. Those with arterial insufficiency will have delayed wound healing, rendering them more prone to infections. In addition, the delivery of immune effectors is altered, compounding the problem.

Patients undergoing organ transplantation require long-term immunosuppression to prevent organ rejection. They are thus susceptible to an increased infection risk. Corticosteroids affect the host defense mechanisms at multiple levels. The atrophy of the skin and mucosa caused by steroids leads to breaks and increased susceptibility to infection and poor wound healing. Steroids also have a mild effect on humoral defenses, but their greatest effect is on cellular immunity.

Cyclosporin A affects the cytotoxic and proliferating capabilities of helper T cells through a decreased production of IL-2. Antithymocyte globulin and monoclonal antibodies suppress cell-mediated immunity through their effect on lymphocytes. Azathioprine causes lymphocytopenia and also mildly suppresses humoral and cellular immune responses.

Infections seen within 1 month of organ transplantation usually antedate the surgical procedure or may be due to the operation itself. Infections secondary to pharmacologic immunosuppression usually manifest themselves 6 weeks after transplantation.

Patients who have had a splenectomy are particularly vulnerable to infection with encapsulated bacteria. Their lifetime risk of developing overwhelming sepsis is 0.5%, with the greatest risk occurring within the first 2 years after splenectomy. The risk of overwhelming sepsis in these patients is 60 times greater than that for patients who have not had a splenectomy. Because of this risk, some recommend that pediatric patients who have had a splenectomy should receive penicillin prophylactically. The duration of prophylaxis remains controversial, because older recommendations were for lifelong treatment with oral antibiotics. Current recommendation for the pediatric patient (less than 5 years of age) is treatment for the first 3 years after splenectomy, because this represents the period of highest risk for developing overwhelming sepsis. All patients should receive immunization with meningococcal A and C, pneumococcal and *Haemophilus influenzae* type b vaccines. At least 50% of the mass of the spleen is necessary to maintain immune competence protection against encapsulated bacteria.

PATHOGENESIS OF SURGICAL INFECTIONS

It is difficult to predict the manifestation of a given pathogen in a given patient because of the variability of microbes' virulence and the strength of the host immune response. The development of surgical infections depends on four factors: microbial pathogenicity, host defenses, local environment, and surgical technique. Some characteristics that render specific bacteria virulent include the presence of capsules, pili, or flagella, and the production of toxins (endotoxins or exotoxins). Table 3-1 details some virulence factors with their given effect. Infection can also develop when nonvirulent pathogens are allowed to invade tissues because of compromised host immune defense mechanisms. Patients who have had surgery usually develop infec-

TABLE 3-1. VIRULENCE FACTORS[a]

Factor	Effect
Hemagglutinins	Adherence
Pili	Adherence
Capsule	Resist phagocytosis
Surface proteins	Resist phagocytosis
Enzymes	Impair intracellular killing
Inhibition of lysosomephagosome fusion	Impair intracellular killing
Toxins/enzymes	Cellular injury

[a]From DeGirolamo MP, Brennan PJ. Principles of surgical infectious disease. In: Svage EB, Fishman SJ, Miller LD, eds. *Essentials of basic science in surgery.* Philadelphia: JB Lippincott Co, 1993, with permission.

tion when resident or nosocomial skin and mucosal pathogens are inoculated in sufficient amounts into wounds at the time of trauma, surgical procedures, or other conditions subsequent to failure of the host immune response.

Bacteria

Bacteria are prokaryotic organisms because they lack a true nucleus, chromosomes, and a mitotic apparatus. Their DNA is contained in a single circular chromosome. Bacteria may also contain plasmids, which are autonomously replicating strands of DNA that may carry genes conferring resistance to antibiotics. These genes may be transferred between bacteria of the same or different species. Bacterial ribosomes are structurally and biochemically different from those of humans. Thus, antibiotics that act on bacterial ribosomes have little effect on those in human cells.

Bacteria possess a cell wall external to their cell membrane. This cell wall is much thicker in Gram-positive than in Gram-negative organisms and allows bacteria to resist large osmotic gradients without cell bursting. The *Gram-positive cell wall* is composed of peptidoglycan, a complex of polysaccharides and protein. Some Gram-positive bacteria can form spores in harsh living circumstances that are resistant to heat and freezing. The spore wall is composed of peptidoglycan. *Gram-negative* bacteria also possess an outer membrane containing lipopolysaccharide (LPS, which is also known as endotoxin). LPS has a lipid A core, but the LPS structure determines the antigen strain of the bacteria (e.g., the "O" antigen) (Fig. 3-1). Administration of antibodies directed against endotoxin would at first glance seem to improve survival in Gram-negative sepsis. Unfortunately, clinical studies have not demonstrated efficacy of the administration of monoclonal antibodies to endotoxin.

Some bacteria are surrounded by a thick gellike structure (capsule), which appears to protect against phagocytosis and therefore acts as a virulence factor. Bacteria may also possess pili and flagella. Pili are responsible for adherence to mucosal surfaces, an essential property for invasion, whereas flagella have a role in motility.

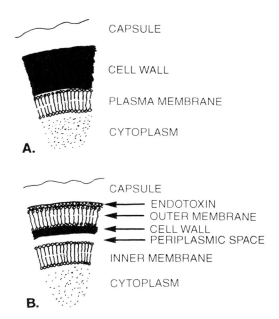

FIGURE 3-1. The wall of the Gram-positive organism **(A)** contains a much larger cell wall while the Gram-negative bacteria **(B)** has both an inner and outer membrane around the relatively thin cell wall. (From Fry DE. Surgical infections. In: O'Leary JP, ed. *The physiologic basis of surgery.* Philadelphia: Williams & Wilkins, 1996:185, with permission.)

Fungi

Fungi are eukaryotes, which implies that DNA separates into chromosomes during division. They possess mitochondria and an endoplasmic reticulum. The cell wall is external to the plasma membrane and is rigid, being composed of a polysaccharide called *chitin*. Some also possess a capsule that inhibits phagocytosis. Yeasts are unicellular fungi while molds are multicellular fungi. Systemic fungal infection results in granuloma formation and abscesses. Histoplasmosis, blastomycosis, coccidioidomycosis, and cryptococcosis are classified as endemic fungal infections, whereas infections with *Candida* and *Aspergillus* sp are classified as *opportunistic*.

Normal human hosts are usually not susceptible to severe fungal infections. Risk factors for the development of systemic fungal disease include intravenous (i.v.) cannulae, prolonged or broad-spectrum antibiotic administration, hyperalimentation, immunosuppression, burns, trauma, and malnutrition. Diagnosing a fungal infection may be challenging. Blood cultures may be negative in up to 50% of patients with severe fungal infection. Biopsies of tissue, ophthalmic examination for retinal involvement, and blood and urine culture may help the clinician make a decision regarding initiation of antifungal therapy.

Viruses

Viruses are the smallest pathogens and are obligate intracellular organisms. Each viral particle, or virion, consists of a central core of DNA or RNA surrounded by a protein coat (glycoprotein or lipoprotein), called a *capsid*, derived from the cellular or nuclear membrane of the host. The capsid serves to facilitate invasion of the host by cell penetration or fusion. Following viral entry into the host cell, the envelope is degraded by host enzymes, thereby exposing viral RNA or DNA to the cytoplasm. RNA (cytoplasmic) or DNA (nuclear) replication then takes place following RNA transcription and reassembly of the nucleocapsid. The newly formed viral particles are released following cell lysis. Viral diseases may occur secondary to cell lysis, inflammation, teratogenesis, and mutagenesis. Surgeons usually treat local manifestations of viral diseases, such as mucosal ulcers due to cytomegalovirus infection, rather than the overall systemic manifestation of the viral diseases.

The immunosuppressed transplant patient is one type of surgical patient predisposed to the development of viral illnesses. The herpesvirus family, including cytomegalovirus (CMV), are the most prominent pathogens encountered in this category. The Epstein-Barr virus is also seen and may lead to lymphoproliferative disease.

Toxins

Exotoxins are proteins and enzymes synthesized as virulence factors by bacteria that destroy host tissue and lead to loss of organ function. *Endotoxin* is the LPS derived from the outer layer of the cell wall of Gram-negative bacteria. As introduced above, the outer layer itself is composed of three parts: an O-specific polysaccharide that conveys serologic specificity, a core polysaccharide that shows cross-reactivity between Gram-negative organisms and allows the development of antibodies, and an innermost layer lipid A, which is the toxic component of LPS (Fig. 3-2). Endotoxins are released upon death of the bacterium. They induce fever by direct action on the hypothalamus and by stimulating the release of pyrogens such as IL-1, interferon, and tumor necrosis factor. Endotoxin can cause septic shock by inducing disseminated intravascular coagulation, activating the complement cascade, inducing the release of multiple vasoactive substances such as serotonin, collagenase, and prostaglandin, and by causing neutropenia, which may be followed by leukocytosis.

ANTIMICROBIAL AGENTS

Surgeons are faced on a daily basis with the prevention, diagnosis, and treatment of surgical infections. Antimicrobial agents are only an adjunct and not a replacement to the proper surgical therapy of infections. Such therapies might include the debridement of devitalized tissue, drainage of infected material (pus), the elimination of a continuous source of infection such as leaking viscera, and maximizing the blood supply to the infected area, which can facilitate the delivery of antibiotics to tissues. In the face of clinical improvement, there may be no need to alter the therapy administered to a patient despite return of negative cultures.

Classes of Antimicrobial Agents

The four most common classes of antimicrobial agents include the inhibitors of cell-wall synthesis, inhibitors of ribosomes activity, inhibitors of folic acid synthesis, and inhibitors of nucleic acid synthesis. Proper knowledge of the mechanisms of action of antimicrobial agents is essential to the selection and use of the most selective (specific) agent and combination of agents against the involved pathogens. Antibiotics from two different classes, when used together, can often have a synergistic antimicrobial effect on invading organisms rather than two agents of the same class, which compete and may use the same mechanism of action. The choice of antimicrobial agent will also depend on the suspected or proven pathogen (Table 3-2), the spectrum of the antibiotic, the ability to reach an appropriate drug level in affected tissues, allergies, cost, and underlying organ dysfunction such as renal failure, which might impair drug elimination. For hospital-acquired (nosocomial) infections, the local patterns of pathogen

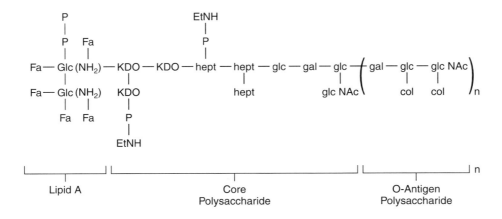

FIGURE 3-2. The chemical structure of lipopolysaccharide (endotoxin) includes lipid A, the O-antigen side chain and the core polysaccharide. Lipid A is the toxic moiety of endotoxin and interacts with various cells to induce the septic response.

TABLE 3-2. ANTIBIOTICS OF CHOICE BASED ON INFECTIOUS ORGANISM[a]

Organism	Drug of choice	Alternative agent
Aerobic gram-positive cocci		
Staphylococcus aureus	Nafcillin or oxacillin	Cefazolin or vancomycin
Methicillin resistant	Vancomycin ± gentamicin ± rifampin	Trimethoprim-sulfamethoxazole or ciprofloxacin
Staphylococcus epidermidis	Vancomycin	Rifampin
Streptococcus pneumonia	Penicillin G	Cefazolin, erythromycin, or vancomycin
Anaerobic organisms (gram-negative and gram-positive)		
Bacteroides		
Oral source	Penicillin G	Metrinidazole
Bowel source (*Bacteroides fragilis*)	Metronidazole	Clindamycin
Clostridium difficile	Metronidazole	Vancomycin
Clostridium tetani	Penicillin G	Tetracycline
Enterococcus faecalis	Ampicillin + gentamycin	Vancomycin + gentamycin
Aerobic gram-negative bacilli		
Escherichia coli	3rd-generation cephalosporin (ceftazidime or ceftriaxone)	Aminoglycasides, aztreonam
Klebsiella pneumonia	3rd-generation cephalosporin (ceftazidime or ceftriaxone)	Aminoglycasides, aztreonam
Pseudomonas aeruginosa	Antipseudomonal penicillin (ticarcillin, mezlocillin, piperacillin) + aminoglycoside	Aztreonam, ceftazidime, or imipenem
Fungi		
Aspergillus	Amphotericin B	Itraconazole
Candida		
Mucosal	Fluconazole	Ketoconazole, itraconazole
Systemic	Fluconazole	Amphotericin B
Cryptococcus	Amphotericin B	Fluconazole, itraconazole

[a]From Crawford GE, Emig M. An approach to the use of antimicrobial agents. In: Civetta JM, Taylor RW, Kirby RR, eds. *Critical care,* 3rd ed. Philadelphia: Lippincott–Raven 1997; and Marino PL. *The ICU book,* 2nd ed. Philadelphia: Lippincott Williams & Wilkins, 1997, with permission.

resistance to antimicrobial agents for the institution should be sought to allow proper initial selection of therapy.

Inhibitors of Cell-Wall Synthesis

Antimicrobials that possess a β-lactam ring (Fig. 3-3) bind to bacterial division-plate proteins, thus inhibiting cell-wall peptidoglycan synthesis and inducing autolytic bacteriolysis. The four-sided ring confers the bactericidal activity and is neutralized once the ring is disrupted. The β-lactams are distinguished from one another by their different side chains. Inhibitors of cell-wall synthesis include the penicillins (including those with extended spectrum, such as carboxypenicillins, ureidopenicillins, and the penicillins/β-lactamase–inhibitor combinations), cephalosporins, carbapenems, and monobactams. The different affinity of the β-lactams for Gram-negative and Gram-positive bacteria can be explained by the fact that these two types of microorganisms possess different division-plate proteins. For example, first-generation cephalosporins bind avidly to the division plates of Gram-positive organisms but poorly to those of Gram-negative organisms. The converse is true for the third-generation cephalosporins.

Penicillin is effective against Gram-positive aerobic and anaerobic streptococci, as well as some Gram-negative pathogens including *Neisseria meningitidis, Eikenella corrodens,* and *Pasteurella multocida.* It is the treatment of choice for clostridial infections as well as many other anaerobes (other than *B. fragilis*). Up to 90% of *S. aureus* infections, however, are resistant to penicillin. Extended-spectrum penicillins include ampicillin and amoxicillin. They are

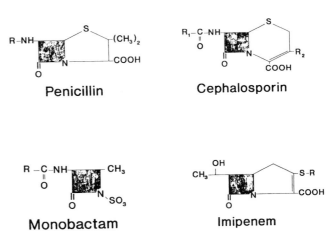

FIGURE 3-3. The four principle groups of β-lactam antibiotics include the penicillin, cephalosporin, monobactam, and imipenem families. The shaded area in each molecule reflects the common lactam ring. (From Fry DE. Surgical infections. In: O'Leary JP, ed. *The physiologic basis of surgery.* Philadelphia: Williams & Wilkins, 1996:192, with permission.)

effective against some Gram-negative pathogens including *H. influenzae*. Antipseudomonal penicillins include the ureidopenicillins (piperacillin, azlocillin, and mezlocillin) and the carboxypenicillins (carbenicillin and ticarcillin). Carbenicillin and ticarcillin can potentially cause hypernatremia because of their high sodium content, and they may also inhibit platelet aggregation. Cloxacillin, methicillin, nafcillin, and floxacillin are resistant to β-lactamases and are thus effective against *Staphylococcus* sp.

First-generation *cephalosporins* (cefazolin, cephapirin, cephalexin, cephradine, and cefadroxil) are very effective against streptococci and staphylococci but have little activity against Gram-negative bacteria. They also have little activity against enterococci and methicillin-resistant *S. aureus*. Second-generation cephalosporins include cefamandole, cefuroxime, cefaclor, loracarbef, cefprozil, and ceforanide and are effective against *H. influenzae*. The second-generation cephalosporins cefoxitin and cefotetan are highly effective against anaerobes, including *B. fragilis*. Cefotetan does have a potentially dangerous side effect of inducing thrombocytopenia. As a whole, the second-generation cephalosporins offer less coverage against Gram-positive organisms than the first-generation cephalosporins but offer greater efficacy against Gram-negative bacteria. The third-generation cephalosporins cefoperazone, ceftazidime, cefotaxime, ceftizoxime, ceftriaxone, and cefixime are most effective against Gram-negative enteric organisms and some anaerobes. Ceftriaxone has been associated with *pseudocholelithiasis* (ultrasonographic appearance of gallbladder sludge) and cholestatic jaundice. It does not effectively cover the *Pseudomonas* sp, but cefoperazone and ceftazidime both have greater activity against *Pseudomonas* infections. The fourth-generation cephalosporins (cefepime and cefpirome) have extended activity against *Pseudomonas* sp. None of the cephalosporin antibiotics are effective against *Enteroccocus* sp.

Imipenem, a carbapenem, provides the broadest coverage of all antibiotics. It covers *Pseudomonas* sp and *B. fragilis*. Some *Pseudomonas* sp (*Pseudomonas cepacia* and *Pseudomonas maltophilia*), methicillin-resistant *S. aureus*, *Enterococcus* sp, *Stenotrophomonas* (*Xanthomonas*) *maltophila*, and *S. epidermidis* organisms are resistant to imipenem. An important side effect of imipenem to remember is an increased incidence of seizures, particularly in patients with renal insufficiency.

The monobactam aztreonam offers broad coverage of Gram-negative bacilli including *Pseudomonas* sp. It does not cover Gram-positive bacteria nor anaerobes. It has a spectrum of activity similar to the aminoglycosides but is much less nephrotoxic and ototoxic. Clavulanic acid and sulbactam can be added to existing preparations of β-lactam antibiotics to offer protection against organisms producing β-lactamases.

Vancomycin inhibits bacterial cell-wall synthesis at a step earlier in the synthetic pathway than the β-lactams. It is effective against facultative and anaerobic Gram-positive organisms, including streptococci and staphylococci. It is the treatment of choice for methycillin-resistant *S. aureus* and *S. epidermidis* infections. Oral vancomycin is one treatment of choice for *Clostridium difficile* (so-called *antibiotic-associated*) colitis.

Inhibitors of Ribosomal Protein Synthesis

The *tetracyclines, chloramphenicol*, and the *macrolides* (erythromycin) inhibit bacterial ribosomal activity and therefore protein synthesis by various mechanisms. In addition to inhibiting protein synthesis, the *aminoglycosides* are thought to act on a second intracellular target because they exhibit bactericidal activity while the others are merely bacteriostatic.

The aminoglycosides are less effective under conditions of hypoxia and acidosis, and they are thus ineffective against anaerobic organisms. They work primarily against Gram-negative aerobic bacilli and have excellent activity against *Pseudomonas* sp. Two important side effects of all the aminoglycosides are nephrotoxicity and ototoxicity.

Chloramphenicol is more bacteriostatic than bactericidal. It is highly effective against Gram-negative bacilli and anaerobes (including *B. fragilis*). It does not cover *Pseudomonas aeruginosa* and nor *Staphylococcus* sp but has specific activity against vancomycin-resistant enterococci (VREC). More recently, quinupristin plus dalfopristin (Synercid) has been approved for use in the treatment of VREC and methycillin-resistant *S. aureus*. Major side effects of chloramphenicol include Gray syndrome (in premature infants), reversible bone marrow suppression, and aplastic anemia, as well as a disulfiram-like reaction with ingested alcohol. The erythromycins are also bacteriostatic and not bactericidal. They are mainly active against Gram-positive bacteria and are often used orally (in combination with neomycin) for bowel preparation before surgery.

The tetracyclines are bacteriostatic agents effective against *Streptococcus, Staphylococcus,* and *Neisseria* species. The tetracyclines are the treatment of choice for rickettsia, mycoplasma, chlamydia, lyme disease, and syphilis.

Inhibitors of Folic Acid Synthesis

Sulfonamides inhibit paraaminobenzoic acid incorporation into the dihydropteroic acid, reducing folic acid synthesis and thus purine synthesis. They offer broad coverage against Gram-positive and Gram-negative organisms but do not cover *Staphylococcus, Enterococcus, Serratia,* or *Pseudomonas* species. Trimethoprim acts to inhibit dihydrofolate reductase, an enzyme involved in purine synthesis. It offers broad activity against Gram-negative bacteria, except *P. aeruginosa*. Sulfonamides and trimethoprim act synergistically and are effective against *Staphylococcus, Streptococcus, Enterobacteriaceae, Shigella,* and *Salmonella* species. Major side effects of trimethoprim-sulfamethoxazole include allergic reactions, kernicterus (in newborns), renal damage, hemolysis in glucose-6-phosphatase-dehydrogenase deficiency, the Stevens-Johnson syndrome (erythema multiforme), and toxic epidermal necrolysis.

Inhibitors of DNA Synthesis

The fluoroquinolones act by binding to DNA helicase proteins and inhibit bacterial DNA synthesis. The fluoroquinolones have a very broad coverage, including Gram-negative and Gram-positive organisms, including methycillin-resistant *S. aureus* and *Pseudomonas* sp; they are not effective against anaerobes. The most commonly used fluoroquinolones include norfloxacin, ciprofloxacin, levofloxacin, and trovafloxacin.

Metronidazole acts by disrupting DNA transcription and microbial replication. It is the most effective antimicrobial against anaerobes including all *Bacteroides* species, protozoal infections (such as trichomoniasis), and amebiasis. Because of its low cost, it is also the treatment of choice for *C. difficile* enterocolitis. Side effects associated with the use of metronidazole include a disulfiram-like reaction with alcohol and peripheral neuropathy.

Antifungal Therapy

Amphotericin B is the most effective antifungal agent and is the drug of choice for systemic and severe localized fungal infections. It binds to fungal membrane sterols to cause cell lysis and is thus fungicidal. The acute side effects of amphotericin B administration are hypotension, nausea, vomiting, fever, and chills. A dose-dependent nephrotoxicity develops in up to 80% of patients. A progressive and reversible normochromic normocytic anemia may also develop. The nephrotoxicity can lead to renal tubular acidosis in patients receiving more than 500 to 1,000 mg accumulated dose. It is usually reversible. Patients should be kept well hydrated and their electrolytes monitored closely, particularly potassium, magnesium, and bicarbonate. If the creatinine level increases, the administration of amphotericin B should be stopped for 2 to 5 days and another agent selected. Dialysis may be necessary in cases of severe renal dysfunction.

KETOCONAZOLE AND FLUCONAZOLE

The azoles include ketoconazole and fluconazole, and both interfere with the formation of membrane sterols. Ketoconazole is effective for the treatment of mucocutaneous and mucosal *Candida* infections. Its variable absorption and poor tissue penetration prevent its use for more severe infections. Fluconazole is the most recent azole with good tissue penetration and less toxicity than amphotericin B. It achieves high levels in the cerebrospinal fluid and urine. Apart from nausea and vomiting, side effects associated with fluconazole administration are mild and may include impotence, increased cyclosporin and coumadin levels, and increased toxicity with Dilantin. It is indicated for esophageal and oropharyngeal *Candida* sp infections and for cryptococcal meningitis. It is well established as the first-line management of localized and systemic *Candida albicans* infections. Second-line therapy with a wider spectrum of action, such as iatroconazole, should be sought for infections that fail to respond to fluconazole.

SURGICAL PROPHYLAXIS

Antimicrobial prophylaxis is indicated for patients undergoing clean-contaminated surgical procedures, when debridement cannot be performed, when prosthesis are being inserted, in an emergency operation, and in the context of recent or active infection. Of the first-generation cephalosporins, cefazolin has the longest half-life and has been considered the prophylactic drug of choice for cardiac, orthopaedic, head/neck, and vascular surgical procedures. A second-generation cephalosporin with broader Gram-negative and anaerobic coverage such as cefoxitin is recommended by some for clean-contaminated and contaminated cases. The optimal timing of i.v. administration of antimicrobial prophylaxis in surgery is considered to be about 30 minutes before the incision, i.e., at about the time of induction of anesthesia. A single dose of the antimicrobial agent before the operation is sufficient prophylaxis for most surgical procedures. For colonic surgery, mechanical preparation of the bowel by intraluminal antiaerobic and antianaerobic decontamination (usually oral erythromycin and neomycin, because they are not systemically absorbed) has proven superior to either agent alone in preventing subsequent wound infection. The addition of i.v. antimicrobial coverage for skin flora has also been shown to decrease the occurrence of wound infection. Surgical prophylaxis of wound infection also entails the use of proper technique and the avoidance of tissue necrosis and ischemia.

The development of bacterial resistance is associated with unnecessary and overzealous antimicrobial use; therefore, prophylactic antibiotics should be used only when absolutely necessary. The spectrum of activity of the (those) drug(s) should be selected to be as *narrow* and *specific* as possible. The selection of broad-spectrum antibiotics for prophylaxis should be avoided. The prolonged continuation of prophylactic antibiotics in the postoperative period is similarly not justified. Prophylactic antibiotic use is not recommended for treatment of superficial burns, with central line insertion, urinary catheters, and tracheostomies.

Clostridium tetanii can be introduced into the body through soil contamination of a traumatic wound. The tetanus toxin is elaborated in the soft tissues of a nonimmune person, prevents neurotransmitter release by inhibitory neurons, and leads to spastic paralysis. A tetanus toxoid booster should be administered to vaccinated persons every 10 years. Upon identifying a potentially contaminated wound, a tetanus toxoid booster should be administered if the last booster dose was received more than 5 years prior to the current event. For patients never immunized or with an unclear immunization status, tetanus immunoglobulin should be administered immediately and the patients subsequently immunized with tetanus toxoid.

General Directed Therapy Guidelines of Common Surgical Infections

Directed therapy consists of targeting specific antimicrobial agents against identified pathogens once sensitivity reports are available. Therapy should be directed at both aerobic and anaerobic organisms because of the experimentally and clinically proven synergy between these microorganisms. The agent chosen should also have specific activity against various components of the infection. Single agent therapy with carbapenems or extended-spectrum penicillins or second-generation or third-generation cephalosporins can provide appropriate coverage for various surgical infections. In fact, single agent therapy is equivalent to an aminoglycoside plus anaerobic coverage for the treatment of peritoneal infections of numerous causes. Extended-spectrum agents should be reserved for patients infected with resistant organisms or several pathogenic organisms.

Wound Infections

Wounds are classified into three categories according to the likelihood and extent of bacterial contamination: (a) *clean* (bronchus or bowel not crossed), (b) *clean-contaminated* (minimal contamination, e.g., elective bowel resection in prepped bowels), and (c) *contaminated* (unprepped bowel, bowel obstruction with gross spillage, abscess, etc.). The accepted surgical infection rates for the above categories are 1.5%, 3%, and 5%, respectively. In addition to the degree of bacterial contamination, other important variables influence the development of wound infections, such as preoperative hair shaving (instead of the use of hair clippers), improper antiseptic skin preparation or breakage of aseptic technique, excessive use of electrocautery, forceps trauma to skin edges, use of braided sutures, the immunocompromised patient, and delayed administration of prophylactic antibiotics (i.e., after the creation of the surgical wound).

Experimental studies have shown that for many organisms, a bacterial load of 10^5 colony-forming units (CFU) per gram of tissue is the threshold for which contamination and subsequent wound infection are thought to occur. This number may be lower in the immunocompromised patient. The administration of antibacterial agents for prophylaxis of wound infections should be done 30 minutes prior to the skin incision and prophylaxis should be administered only for wounds in categories *b* and *c*. Patients with wounds classified as *clean* do not require prophylactic antimicrobial agent administration.

Proper surgical technique is first and foremost. Heavily contaminated wounds should not be closed primarily but should undergo delayed primary closure after 3 to 5 days. This period allows maximal accumulation of phagocytic cells within the wound bed and formation of a capillary-rich granulation tissue to facilitate wound healing. Contaminated wounds can also heal by secondary intention. Other local wound factors that increase the chance of developing an infection include the presence of foreign bodies (including sutures), sloppy approximation of tissues, strangulation of tissues by tying sutures too tightly, and the presence of dead tissue, hematoma, or seroma.

Intraabdominal Infections

Primary peritonitis occurs in patients on peritoneal dialysis or with ascites who do not have perforation of a viscus. *Secondary peritonitis* develops after spillage of microflora from a visceral perforation. Following antimicrobial treatment of secondary peritonitis, certain low-virulence pathogens may flourish and cause *tertiary* or *persistent microbial peritonitis*.

Several host defense mechanisms protect the peritoneal cavity from becoming infected, following a bacterial inoculation. *Local phagocytosis* of bacteria by resident macrophages constitutes the first line of local defense. Other phagocytic cells, such as polymorphonuclear cells, are recruited within hours of the initial stages of infection to engulf the offending microorganisms. *Trans-lymphatic absorption* occurs on the peritoneal surface of the diaphragm. Both fluid and particulate matter, including bacteria, are absorbed into lymphatic structures to drain in larger mediastinal lymphatic channels, and eventually in the bloodstream via the thoracic duct. Following intraabdominal inoculation, systemic bacteremia can occur within minutes due to the efficiency of this system. Organisms that escape both the clearance and phagocytic mechanisms will undergo *sequestration*. During this process, a fibrin-rich inflammatory exudate containing plasma opsonins forms and traps the bacteria. This fibrinous exudate acts in conjunction with the omentum and adjacent viscera to seal the leaking site from continued leak and contamination. This process is nonspecific, and once trapped in the fibrin peel, microorganisms are no longer accessible to phagocytes. When these host defense mechanisms are overwhelmed by the bacterial load, peritoneal contamination results in infection. Abscess formation probably results from the influx of fluid into the peritoneal cavity, which inhibits opsonization and phagocytosis.

Overall, an average of four to five microbial isolates occur in peritoneal infections, and both anaerobic and aerobic microorganisms are isolated in 80% to 90% of such patients. Common aerobic isolates include *E. coli* and other Gram-negative enteric bacilli, such as *Enterobacter* sp and *Klebsiella* sp. Gram-positive bacteria such as *Streptococcus*,

Staphylococcus, and *Enterococcus* species, and other Gram-negative pathogens (*Proteus* and *Pseudomonas* sp), as well as *Candida* species also occur. Frequently isolated anaerobes include *Bacteroides* sp, *Clostridium* sp, and anaerobic cocci.

The proper treatment of a perforated viscus is for the most part surgical. Concurrent antimicrobial therapy is an important component of this treatment and should provide both anaerobic and aerobic coverage. Single agent therapy can be adequate. Addition of antifungal or antienterococcal agents during the initial treatment is not recommended. A 3- to 5-day course of antimicrobial therapy is probably sufficient for cases with minimal peritoneal contamination and proper surgical care. Longer courses are indicated in the immunocompromised host and in cases of heavy bacterial contamination, and thus treatment must still be individualized. The presence of fever and persistently elevated white blood cell (WBC) count is associated with a high likelihood of ongoing or recurrent intraabdominal infection. Again, a thorough search should help identify the source of the persistent fever or leukocytosis. In this setting, *tertiary peritonitis* is often identified where certain pathogens were selected for, thereby thriving as a result of the initial antimicrobial therapy. Gram-positive cocci such as *S. epidermidis, E. faecalis,* and *Enterococcus faecium,* Gram-negative organisms such as *P. aeruginosa,* and other fungi will often be identified as the offending organisms of tertiary peritonitis. Therapy directed against these specific pathogens should be instituted.

Primary peritonitis associated with peritoneal dialysis should be treated with antibiotics, the addition of heparin to the dialysate, and an increase in the dwell time of the dialysate fluid. If these measures fail to control the infection, or in cases of fungal, fecal, or tuberculous peritonitis, the dialysis catheter should be removed.

Approach to the Necrotizing Soft Tissue Infection

The nomenclature and categorization of soft tissue infection is confusing because of its diversity. It involves an infectious process in the superficial muscular compartment, deep muscular fascia, superficial fascia, or a combination of the above. *Necrotizing fasciitis* ("flesh-eating bacteria") is probably the most serious soft tissue infection seen by surgeons. Although a rare occurrence, its mortality rate can be as high as 74%. Risk factors for the development of necrotizing fasciitis include peripheral vascular disease; i.v. drug use; immunosuppression from diabetes mellitus, malignancy, or alcoholism; obesity; or malnutrition. These infections are usually polymicrobial, involving Gram-positive bacteria such as *Staphylococcus, Clostridial,* and *Streptococcus* species, Gram-negative enteric bacteria, and Gram-negative anaerobes.

The severity of these infections and rapidity of their evolution often denotes a synergistic process among the microorganisms involved. However, some virulent organisms lead to a fulminant infection without the synergistic effect of other bacteria. These include *Clostridium* sp, *Pseudomonas,* and *Aeromonas* sp. Patients with necrotizing fasciitis initially present with nonspecific symptoms such as pain, high fever, and signs of local edema and erythema. The presence of systemic toxicity and severe pain out of proportion of the local findings also suggests the possibility of necrotizing fasciitis. The affected area is initially red, hot, shiny, swollen without sharp demarcation margins and is exceptionally tender. The skin will change to a grayish color, and within 3 to 6 days, cutaneous bullae and necrosis begin to appear. By this time, the area is no longer tender due to small vessels thrombosis and destruction of superficial nerves. The high mortality rate is probably due in part to the production of bacterial endotoxins. Tetanus and toxic shock syndrome with organ failure and death may also develop from toxins elaborated in the wound bed with minimal local classic signs of infection.

Once identified or highly suspected, soft tissue infections must be treated aggressively with surgical debridement of all the involved tissue until healthy margins are reached. This often results in destructive or disfiguring resection. Multiple debridement sessions are often required to remove any remaining necrotic tissue, and skin grafting may ultimately be necessary. One must look for skin discoloration; soft tissue necrosis; drainage of thin, watery, grayish, foul-smelling fluid; blebs; and crepitus. Performance of diagnostic studies or radiologic examinations should not delay immediate and definitive therapy in the operating room.

The hemodynamic status of the patient also requires careful evaluation and close monitoring. Hemodynamic instability may rapidly develop and may be the only obvious clinical sign of the underlying fulminant infectious process. Unlike other surgical infections, broad antimicrobial coverage against Gram-positive, Gram-negative, and anaerobes will usually require multiple agents to treat these infections appropriately. High doses of penicillin G are required to cover *Clostridium* species. Vancomycin or a semisynthetic penicillin will cover the Gram-positive organisms whereas Gram-negative coverage will be achieved with an aminoglycoside or a monobactam. Clindamycin or metronidazole will ensure anaerobic coverage.

Hyperbaric oxygen treatment in cases of clostridial gangrene has been advocated by some but remains controversial. Although the performance of a colostomy in patients with Fournier gangrene improves wound and patient care, it has not invariably improved outcome.

Septic Shock

Gram-negative bacterial sepsis is one of the most serious infectious processes occurring in the surgical population. It results in substantial morbidity, and up to 30% mortality. The mechanisms by which Gram-negative bacterial infection produces the detrimental physiologic host response is still a subject of active research. Increasing evidence implicates the bacterial LPS (endotoxin) as the portion of the Gram-negative cell membrane responsible for many of the toxic effects that occur during Gram-negative bacteremia. Immunologic responses to LPS include nonspecific polyclonal B-cell proliferation, macrophage activation and cytokine secretion, tolerance to a subsequent LPS or bacterial challenge, and production of antibody directed against various portions of the LPS molecule. The endotoxin from the cell wall of a Gram-negative bacteria triggers a chain of reactions involving the complement, clotting, fibrinolytic, and kinin pathways that lead to hemodynamic instability, increased vascular permeability, metabolic derangements, disorders of homeostasis, and ultimately organ failure. The physiologic responses to LPS administration are similar to those seen in Gram-negative sepsis and include hypotension, hypoxemia, acidosis, bacterial translocation across the gut, complement and coagulation cascade activation, WBC and platelet margination, and death.

The initiation of appropriate treatment early in the course of the disease has shown some beneficial effects. Empiric therapy against Gram-negative aerobes may have a salutary effect in febrile, neutropenic patients with hematologic malignancies.

Catheter and Prosthetic Device Infections

IV catheters can induce infectious complications such as cellulites, septic thrombophlebitis, abscesses, bacteremia, and endocarditis. Stiffer catheters are more thrombogenic and are associated with a higher infection rate, as are catheters with multiple lumina. Gram-positive organisms such as *S. epidermidis* and *S. aureus* are capable of adhering to synthetic polymers with great affinity and forming an exopolysaccharide slime layer that inhibits antimicrobial penetration. Removal of the catheter or prosthetic device and initiation of proper antimicrobial therapy should be done promptly upon the suspicion of a catheter infection. Recently, antibiotic impregnation of catheters with silver compounds, minocycline, rifampin, and other agents has been found to be effective in reducing catheter-borne bacteremia.

Urinary Tract Infections

In the patient without a urinary catheter, the presence of 10^5 CFU/mL is considered diagnostic of a urinary tract infection, whereas 10^2 to 10^3 CFU/mL is considered diagnostic in the presence of a urinary catheter. Because many antibiotics are excreted in the urine, infections are readily cleared after initiation of treatment. Urinary tract infections should not be underestimated, because they represent the most common cause of Gram-negative sepsis. A useful but somehow ignored adage to follow is "if the patient no longer needs the urinary catheter, remove it."

SUGGESTED READING

Chapnick EK, Abter EI. Necrotizing soft-tissue infections. *Inf Dis Clin North Am* 1996;10(4):835–855.

Gilbert DN, Moellering RC Jr, Sande MA. *The sanford* guide to antimicrobial therapy (*2000*), 30th ed. Hyde Park: Antimicrobial Therapy, 2000.

Gyssens IC. Preventing postoperative infections: current treatment recommendations. *Drugs* 1999;57(2):175–185.

4

TUMOR BIOLOGY

ISABELLE BEDROSIAN AND BRIAN J. CZERNIECKI

EPIDEMIOLOGY

Cancer remains the second most common cause of mortality in the United States, accounting for 22% of all deaths. Cancer affects all age groups, socioeconomic classes, and ethnic populations. Between 1973 and 1987, the incidence of cancer increased by 15% with melanoma showing the greatest rate of increase. The occurrence of a few types of tumors including cervical, endometrial, and gastric cancers decreased during this time. In men, lung and prostate cancers have the highest incidence, at about 20% each with the incidence of colorectal cancer presently at 15%. In women, breast cancer predominates with an incidence of 29%, followed by colorectal and uterine cancers at an incidence of 15% and 9%, respectively. Cancer *mortality rates* also increased between 1973 and 1987 with the greatest increase (13%) in patients older than 65 years. Overall, the 5-year survival rate for cancer patients is 40%. In women, the 5-year survival rate is closer to 50%, compared to 30% for men. Reasons for this discrepancy are not clear.

Striking geographic and ethnic patterns exist for many cancers highlighting the impact of environmental influences in the development of neoplasia. Although well-defined causative agents explain some geographic patterns, in other areas, causative factors remain unclear. In Japan, the high incidence of gastric carcinoma is linked to diets containing smoked and salted foods. However, other patterns such as the high rates of breast and colorectal carcinoma in North America compared to Africa and Asia and the high incidence of prostate carcinoma in African American men do not appear to be associated with clear causative factors.

In addition to geographic patterns, epidemiological studies have identified various dietary, chemical, viral, and physical agents important to the development of different cancers. These include tobacco smoking, which is the single most important causative agent for lung carcinoma, chronic hepatitis B, and hepatitis C infections that are linked to the development of hepatocellular carcinoma and sun exposure as a causative factor in melanoma. Other associations include human papillomavirus (serotypes 16 and 18) and cervical cancer, cryptorchidism and testicular cancer, aromatic amines and bladder cancer and tobacco smoking, blood group A, dietary salt, nitrosamines and more recently *Helicobacter* pylori in gastric cancer. Although epidemiological data have not been entirely consistent, a strong pattern has emerged linking high dietary intake of red meat, animal fat, and protein and low intake of fruit, vegetable, and fiber to increased risk for colorectal cancer. In prostate and pancreatic cancer, associations with environmental agents remain scant and although oral contraceptives and parity have been found to have an inverse correlation with ovarian cancer risk, the causative factors for this disease remain poorly understood. Further evidence for the importance of environmental factors in the development of carcinoma comes from studies of migrant populations such as Japanese immigrants to Hawaii. Within a few decades, and in marked contrast to cancer patterns in Japan, immigrants to Hawaii have increased risk for breast cancer but decreased risk for gastric carcinoma.

FAMILIAL INFLUENCES

Although compelling evidence supports the role of environmental factors in the development of cancer, familial cancer patterns have increased the awareness of the role of inherited factors. Inherited predisposition to cancer may be either in the form of direct causation of disease or more frequently, increased risk for specific cancers.

Familial (Hereditary) Breast Cancer

Familial aggregation is seen in 10% to 15% of breast cancers. Although first-degree relatives of patients with breast cancer have a threefold increased risk of developing the disease when compared to the general population, only about 5% of cases meet the criteria for familial breast cancer.

Hospital of the University of Pennsylvania, Philadelphia, Pennsylvania

These criteria include (i) early onset of breast cancer (average age of onset, 45 years), (ii) frequent bilateral disease, and (iii) an autosomal dominant inheritance pattern. In these families, there is also an increase in the incidence of ovarian, colorectal, esophageal, and gastric cancers and to a lesser extent sarcomas, lung, and adrenocortical cancers. Although genetic factors only account for 5% of all breast cancer cases, in women younger than 30 years, they may account for more than 25% of cases.

In 1990, a region on the long arm of chromosome 17 (17q21) was identified that contained a susceptibility gene in families with high-risk breast cancer. This gene was eventually identified as *BRCA 1* and appears to function as a tumor suppressor. Germ-line mutation of one allele is followed by a somatic event that inactivates the second allele in breast epithelial cells, thereby significantly increasing the risk for development of breast cancer. A second gene involved in susceptibility to breast cancer has also been identified, *BRCA 2,* and mapped to chromosome 13. Patients with either BRCA 1 or BRCA 2 have a lifetime risk of developing breast cancer of 85%. In those with BRCA 1, but not BRCA 2, the lifetime ovarian cancer risk is estimated to be 40% to 60%. BRCA 2 is more likely to be found in familial cases with male breast cancer. Together, BRCA 1 and BRCA 2 account for 75% of familial breast cancer cases.

Multiple Endocrine Neoplasia

Multiple endocrine neoplasia (MEN) syndromes are autosomal dominant disorders characterized by the development of synchronous or metachronous tumors in multiple endocrine glands. The tumors are characteristically multicentric and may be benign or malignant. *MEN 1* is characterized by anterior pituitary adenomas, parathyroid hyperplasia, and pancreatic islet cell tumors. Two glands are involved in over 50% of patients and approximately 20% have involvement of all three glands. A deletional mutation has been localized to the long arm of chromosome 11 although the gene involved remains unknown. In patients without affected kindred, the age at presentation ranges from the third decade in women to the fourth decade in men. In families with known affected members, evidence of this disorder can usually be found through screening in asymptomatic, affected individuals by age 18.

MEN 2A and MEN 2B are both characterized by the development of medullary thyroid carcinoma (MTC) and pheochromocytomas. In addition, patients with MEN 2A also are at risk for parathyroid hyperplasia, whereas patients with MEN 2B can display distinctive phenotypes such as marfanoid habitus, bony abnormalities, and mucosal neuromas. The *RET oncogene,* which codes for a tyrosine kinase receptor, located in the centromeric region of chromosome 10 is known to be involved. In MEN 2A, several missense mutations have been identified within the extracellular domain of this receptor. MEN 2A is also associated with deletional mutations in the short arm of chromosome 1. In MEN 2B, a single missense mutation has been characterized in the intracellular domain of the receptor, within the tyrosine kinase catalytic region. Although familial, these syndromes, particularly MEN 2B, can occur *de novo.*

Familial Medullary Thyroid Carcinoma

MTC is a malignancy of the parafollicular C cells in the thyroid gland. It accounts for only 5% to 10% of all thyroid malignancies. Eighty percent of MTC cases are sporadic. Among the familial cases, most are diagnosed as part of MEN 2 syndromes. Familial MTC, without other malignant endocrinopathies, is less common. Although sporadic and familial cases of MTC (including MEN 2A and MEN 2B) are histologically identical, familial cases are characterized by multifocal bilateral disease (Table 4-1). In addition, a premalignant, diffuse C-cell hyperplasia has been described in the familial cases. RET oncogene missense mutations on chromosome 10 have again been implicated.

Dysplastic Nevus Syndrome

Familial melanoma is uncommon; only 4% to 10% of patients with melanoma will have a positive family history in first-degree relatives. In most of these cases of familial melanoma, the genetic basis is unknown. The best characterized familial syndrome is the B-K mole syndrome or the dysplastic nevus syndrome. This syndrome is characterized clinically by the presence of multiple large (usually 6- to 15-mm) nevi, which are predominantly located on the back. In patients with dysplastic nevus syndrome and a family history of melanoma, the risk of developing melanoma approaches 100%, consistent with the autosomal dominant mode of inheritance of this syndrome.

Lynch Syndrome

Familial hereditary nonpolyposis colon cancer (HNPCC), or Lynch syndrome, accounts for approximately 5% to 10% of all colon cancers. The inherited mutation has been localized to chromosome 2. This gene product is believed to be important in DNA mismatch repair. There is an autosomal dominant mode of inheritance. HNPCC is defined by the Amsterdam criteria, which include (i) three or more relatives with colorectal cancer, (ii) one affected person is a first-degree relative to the other two, (iii) one or more cases diagnosed at less than 50 years of age, and (iv) colorectal cancer involving at least two generations. Patients with HNPCC characteristically present with multiple synchronous colonic tumors at earlier ages. Average age at diagnosis is 45 years. There is also a greater preponderance toward right-sided tumors. The syndrome is further characterized as Lynch I or site-specific colorectal cancer, with familial inheritance limited to colonic tumors, or Lynch II, or can-

TABLE 4-1. CLINICAL AND GENETIC ASPECTS OF MULTIPLE ENDOCRINE NEOPLASIA TYPES 1, 2A, AND 2B (MEN 1, MEN 2A, MEN 2B) AND FAMILIAL MEDULLARY THYROID CARCINOMA (FMTC)[a]

	MEN 1	MEN 2A	MEN 2B	FMTC
Chromosome	11q 12–13	Pericentromeric 10	Pericentromeric 10	Pericentromeric 10
Genetic defect	Unknown	RET mutation	RET mutation	RET mutation
Medullary thyroid carcinoma	No	Bilateral	Bilateral	Bilateral
Pheochromocytoma	No	70% bilateral	70% bilateral	70% bilateral
Parathyroid disease	Hyperplasia	Hyperplasia	No	No
Phenotype	No	No	Bony abnormalities, mucosal neuromas, marfanoid habitus, bumpy lips	No
Mode of inheritance	Autosomal dominant	Autosomal dominant	Autosomal dominant	Autosomal dominant
Course of medullary thyroid carcinoma	No medullary thyroid carcinoma	Variable, frequently indolent	More virulent	Most virulent
Pancreatic endocrine tumors	Yes	No	No	No

[a]From DeVita VT, Rosenberg SA, Hellman S, eds. *Cancer principles and Practice of Oncology* 5th ed. Philadelphia: Lippincott-Raven, 1997:1646, with permission.

cer family syndrome conferring also an increased risk for ovarian, endometrial, gastric, and urinary tract tumors.

Familial Adenomatous Polyposis

Familial adenomatous polyposis (FAP) is a rare syndrome accounting for less than 1% of all colorectal cancers. It is inherited in an autosomal dominant manner with high penetrance. The adenomatous polyposis coli (APC) locus, which is on chromosome 5, codes for a tumor suppressor gene. The mutation in the APC gene is presumed to be an early event in colorectal cancer carcinogenesis, allowing for the development of a hyperproliferative epithelium. Clinically it is characterized by the development of hundreds to thousands of colonic adenomatous polyps. These polyps are generally smaller than 5 mm. Average age at presentation of the polyps is 15 years and average age at diagnosis of cancer is 39 years. Left- versus right-sided cancer patterns generally mirror those seen in sporadic colorectal cancer. Many patients with FAP will also have polyps in the upper gastrointestinal tract. There are four variants of this syndrome. Patients with typical FAP have only gastrointestinal polyps and malignancies. In addition to the characteristic polyposis of FAP, patients with *Gardner syndrome* present with osteomas and desmoid tumors, and those with *Turcot syndrome* are at risk for development of brain tumors. Turcot, in contrast to the other variants, is inherited in an autosomal recessive pattern. Patients with APC have disease limited to the gastrointestinal tract but generally have fewer polyps and a later onset of cancer with an average age for diagnosis of 54 years. In addition, patients with APC have a higher tendency toward right-sided colon carcinomas.

HORMONAL FACTORS

Increasing evidence points to an important role of hormones in the etiology of several human cancers. Hormones probably act through increasing cell proliferation, thereby increasing the risk of a mutational event. The evidence is most convincing in *endometrial cancer*, where "unopposed estrogen" is a clear risk factor for the development of carcinoma and decreasing exposure to "unopposed estrogen" such as through use of oral contraception and pregnancy protects against development of endometrial cancer. Increased estrogen exposure, as determined by early menarche, late menopause, late age at first pregnancy and obesity, also appears to be an important risk factor in breast cancer development. Conversely, factors that diminish the estrogen exposure of the breast such as oophorectomy and more recently tamoxifen decrease breast cancer risk. Hormonal milieu may also be important in the etiology of *prostate cancer*; in various population studies, increased levels of testosterone, androstenedione, and estradiol have all been implicated. In *thyroid cancer*, a role for sex steroids is suggested by the preponderance of this disease in women and the decreased incidence after menopause. In addition, excess thyroid-stimulating hormone (TSH) may be important in tumor development because suppression of TSH can be effective treatment in thyroid carcinoma. Finally, the high incidence of osteosarcoma in adolescents correlates with a period of hormonally driven skeletal growth, suggesting again a possible etiology.

IMMUNODEFICIENCY AND AUTOIMMUNE DISORDERS

Clinical evidence from immunosuppressed and immunodeficient patients indicates that the immune system is important for prevention of malignancy, particularly malignancies of the lymphoreticular system. Solid organ *transplant recipients* have a 20% to 50% increase in relative risk compared to age-matched controls for developing secondary lymphoid malignancies. In addition, the incidence of squamous cell cancers of the skin, uterine cancer, and hepatobiliary cancers is also much higher in these patients. Replacement of azathioprine with cyclosporine for immunosuppression does not appear to decrease the overall incidence of malignancies in the transplant population but rather has altered the types of cancers seen.

Patients with *autoimmune disorders* such as Hashimoto disease, Sjögren disease, and nontropical sprue have higher rates of lymphoid malignancies and NHL. Kaposi sarcoma occurs with higher frequency in patients with acquired immunodeficiency syndrome (AIDS). Patients with AIDS also have an increased incidence of squamous cell cancers of the genitalia (women) and anorectum (men), frequently in conjunction with human papillomavirus infection.

Patients with cancer receiving chemotherapy, particularly alkylating agents, have higher rates of second malignancies. Acute leukemia is the most frequent second malignancy. Second malignancies typically occur 4 to 6 years after treatment of the primary cancer.

The exact role of the immune system in prevention of malignancy remains unclear. Natural killer (NK) cells, T cells, and B cells have all been suggested to play a role in eliminating aberrant cells. The increase in malignancies in immunocompromised states is believed to be due to both immune dysregulation and chronic antigenic stimulation.

Data from animal studies support a role for the cellular immune system in preventing viral carcinogenesis. Similarly, malignancies in immunocompromised individuals appear to be associated with viral infections and chronic antigenic stimulation. B-cell lymphomas are seen with increased frequency in such populations and often are associated with the Epstein-Barr virus. Kaposi sarcoma in patients with AIDS may be associated with herpes infections. The immune system does not seem to be important for prevention of chemical carcinogenesis.

CHARACTERISTICS OF MALIGNANT CELLS

Malignant transformation is often the result of *multiple mutations* of normal host genes. Most of these mutations

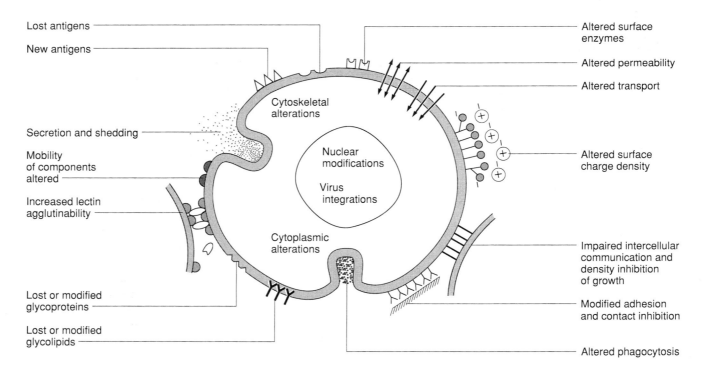

FIGURE 4-1. Alterations of transformed cells. (From Greenfield LJ, ed. *Surgery*, 1st ed. Philadelphia: JB Lippincott, 1993:417, with permission.)

occur spontaneously and may result from exposure to carcinogens, including physical and chemical carcinogens, foreign body irritations, and viruses. Most tumors arise from a single transformed cell or clone. Not all cells exposed to the same causative agent undergo transformation and importantly most transformations are lethal. Furthermore, from the small group of surviving transformed cells, some progress to terminal differentiation and others are recognized as nonself and eliminated by host immune cells. The two fundamental properties of neoplastic cells are "escape from normal growth regulation" and "the passage of the transformed genome to daughter cells."

Transformed cells exhibit many phenotypic, biochemical, and immunologic alterations (Fig. 4-1). These include changes in cellular morphology, loss of some antigens and acquisition of new surface antigens, altered transport, and impaired intercellular communication and modified adhesion and contact inhibition. In addition, karyotypic changes are often evident in transformed cells with an increase in aneuploid populations, frequent monosomy, trisomy, and other chromosomal aberrations. Although transformed cells demonstrate these alterations from normal host tissue, the definition of malignancy or neoplastic transformation requires the demonstration of "tumorigenesis on inoculation of transformed cells into a living host."

GROWTH AND PROLIFERATION OF TUMORS

To reach the smallest clinically detectable size of 1 g (1 cm^3), a solid tumor originating from a single cell will have undergone about 30 doublings. A 1-g tumor consists of approximately 10^9 cells. After an additional 10 doublings, the tumor mass reaches 1 kg or 10^{12} cells, at which point the tumor becomes lethal to the host. It is apparent therefore that most of a tumor's natural growth history occurs before it is clinically apparent (Fig. 4-2). Tumor growth is not however an exponential process; as the tumor reaches larger sizes, there is generally a deceleration of the growth rate presumably due to outgrowth of the blood supply and depletion of nutrients.

Tissue growth, including tumor growth, depends on three factors: growth fraction, cell-cycle time, and cell-loss fraction. Although many normal cells will exhibit high growth rates, overall tissue balance is maintained because of high turnover rates as well. In contrast, tumor cells exhibit a net growth because of an essential imbalance between cell proliferation and cell loss.

The *growth fraction* is the proportion of the tumor mass undergoing cell proliferation at a given point in time. The growth fraction of tumors (S phase) can be determined using flow cytometry or ^{3}H-thymidine labeling index. Clinically aggressive tumors have a growth fraction of around 10%. The maximum growth fraction of a tumor, 37%, occurs during the exponential linear segment of the tumor-growth curve that precedes clinical detection.

The *cell cycle* is the sequence of events that results in the formation of new daughter cells with a genetic makeup identical to that of the parent cell. Daughter cells may reenter the cell cycle with generation of new progeny, leave the cell cycle to enter a quiescent nonproliferative state, or leave the cell cycle to early cell death. Cells that are actively participating in the cell cycle are known as the *cycling* or *proliferating cells*. The duration of the cell cycle is similar for most tumors and ranges from 2 to 4.5 days.

The primary determinant of clinical growth of a tumor therefore is the balance between the growth fraction and the cell-loss fraction. In tumors, increases in the growth fraction are not balanced with increases in cell death and turnover. This discordance between cell proliferation and death, or

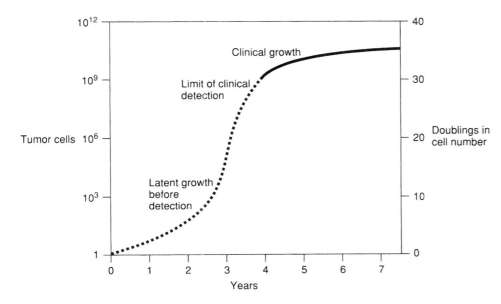

FIGURE 4-2. Tumor-growth characteristics. (From Greenfield LJ, ed. *Surgery*, 1st ed. Philadelphia: JB Lippincott, 1993:419, with permission.)

growth dysregulation, has been linked to alterations in cell growth regulatory genes or protooncogenes.

ONCOGENES

The identification of oncogenes has allowed a new understanding of the molecular basis of cancer. Oncogenes are altered forms of normal *protooncogenes,* which become activated by mutational changes. Protooncogenes are present at different stages of embryonic development and regulate cell proliferation and differentiation. They may be reactivated during periods of normal cellular proliferation such as wound healing or organ regeneration. However, mutational changes within protooncogenes give rise to oncogenes and a deregulated and dedifferentiated state of cell growth that is characteristic of neoplasms. Various mutations have been described that change a normal protooncogene into an oncogene. Point mutations of a single nucleotide change in the DNA, as seen in the *ras* gene family, can result in a protein with transforming activity. *Chromosomal translocations* involve the shifting of one segment of a chromosome onto another chromosome. One well-known example is the Philadelphia chromosome in CML, which results when the c-*abl* protooncogene is translocated from chromosome 9 to the *bcr* locus on chromosome 22, thereby generating the *bcr/abl* oncogene, which has enhanced tyrosine kinase activity. In Burkitt lymphoma, the c-*myc* protooncogene is translocated from chromosome 8 to either chromosome 2, 14, or 22, which results in the dysregulation of the c-*myc* oncogene.

Amplification of protooncogenes can also be found. In neuroblastoma, amplification of the N-*myc* gene correlates with poor outcomes. Deletional mutations, resulting in the loss of specific chromosome regions, usually with loss of tumor suppressor genes, likely play a permissive role in tumor development. Examples of deletional mutations include the deleted in colorectal cancer (DCC) gene in colon cancer, which results in loss of a cell-adhesion molecule and *p53* gene deletions commonly found in many tumors including lung cancer, colon cancer, and pancreatic cancer. Oncogenes can be classified into groups based on the function of the protein they encode.

Growth factor oncogenes: Growth factors are peptides that bind to cellular receptors to activate the intracellular second messenger systems that regulate growth and differentiation. Mutational changes in these oncogenes may result in constitutive expression of the gene product and therefore constant stimulation of the growth receptor. The *sis* oncogene, a variant of platelet-derived growth factor was the first such oncogene identified. Subsequently, *int-2, hst,* and *fgf-5* have been identified that code for proteins related to fibroblast growth factor.

Growth factor receptor oncogenes: Growth factor receptors have three domains (Fig. 4-3): (i) an extracellular ligand

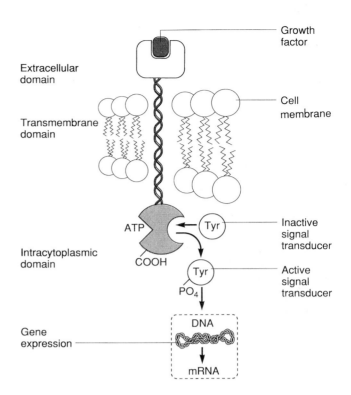

FIGURE 4-3. Growth factor receptor oncogenes. (From Greenfield LJ, ed. *Surgery,* 1st ed. Philadelphia: JB Lippincott, 1993:427, with permission.)

binding domain, (ii) a transmembrane domain, and (iii) the intracellular, cytoplasmic domain, which consists of a tyrosine kinase responsible for phosphorylation of tyrosine residues on intracellular proteins and subsequent activation of the second messenger system. Mutations at the genetic level can lead to alterations in any of these domains, resulting in constitutive expression of the receptor, increased affinity of the receptor for ligand, or a truncated receptor that lacks normal regulatory controls. Examples include the oncogenes her-2/*neu,* c-*kit,* and c-*fms.* Her-2/*neu,* which is overexpressed in 30% of breast cancers, belongs to the epidermal growth factor receptor family, whereas c-*kit* and c-*fms* share homology with platelet-derived growth factor family and the M-CSF receptor respectively.

Signal transduction oncogenes: The largest group of known oncogenes code for signal transduction proteins. These proteins are associated with the inner surface of the membrane and are responsible for the generation of intracellular signals in response to extracellular stimulation by ligand. Two major classes of oncogenes that belong to this group are the *ras* oncogenes that are characterized by binding to G proteins and the *src* family that has tyrosine kinase activity.

Nuclear oncogenes: These oncogenes encode for proteins that localize to the nucleus, where they regulate gene transcription. These oncogenes include c-*jun,* c-*fos,* c-*myb,* c-*myc*, and n-*myc*. The c-*fos* and c-*jun* oncogene products are components of the AP-1 transcriptional activator. These gene products form heterodimers that have enhanced affinity for the AP-1 target site on DNA, resulting in increased transcription of the AP-1 target genes. The *myc* family of oncogenes is found in a wide variety of tumors. Their potential for malignant transformation may be due to stimulation of cells out of the G1 phase and into the S phase.

Tumor suppressor genes: Tumor suppressor genes are negative regulators of cell proliferation. In contrast to the oncogenes listed above, it is the loss of tumor suppressor genes that leads to loss of normal growth inhibition signals and is therefore permissive for cell proliferation. Important tumor suppressor genes include *Rb, p53,* and *p21*. In retinoblastoma, loss of both alleles of the retinoblastoma suppressor gene (*Rb*) leads to malignant transformation of the retinal cell. The *Rb* gene is also lost in a number of adult tumors such as breast, small cell, lung, and ovarian cancers. Loss of the wild-type *p53* gene is implicated in the development of many tumors including cancers of the breast, lung, and colon. Both *p53* and *Rb* are nuclear phosphoproteins that may function as transcription regulators.

MULTISTEP CARCINOGENESIS

Carcinogenesis is a complex multistep process with three distinct stages: initiation, promotion, and progression. Each step is characterized by changes at the genetic level, resulting in alterations in the normal cell growth and differentiation process. When sufficient alterations in the normal growth and regulation of the cell have occurred, the cell may undergo malignant transformation. There is generally a prolonged latent time between initiation and promotion. Although promotion is a reversible step, progression into a fully mature tumor is not.

Multistep carcinogenesis has been best characterized in the formation of colonic tumors (Fig. 4-4). Colon cancer appears to arise as a result of mutations in at least 4 or 5 oncogenes. It appears that it is the cumulative acquisition of these mutations that is more important than the actual sequence. It is hypothesized that early events in colon carcinogenesis generally involve alterations of the FAP gene on chromosome 5. This mutation leads to a hyperproliferative epithelium and the development of an early adenoma. Subsequent mutations in the *ras* oncogene may lead to the development of an intermediate adenoma. In this state of accelerated mitoses, errors result that lead to deletions or loss of chromosomes 17 and 18 with the resultant loss of the *p53* and DCC genes, which allows progression to carcinoma. It is believed that further genetic alterations then predispose to the development of metastasis.

TUMOR METASTASIS

Metastasis of a tumor from its site of origin to distant sites is a complex process involving several stages that are not fully understood. Tumors can metastasize in one of four principal ways: direct extension across tissue fronts, spread through a cavity such as intraperitoneal or pleural seeding, lymphatic dissemination, and hematogenous metastasis. The route of dissemination is determined by the histologic characteristics and the location of the primary tumor. Steps in the formation of metastatic cancer include neovascularization at the primary site, invasion of tumor cells into blood or lymphatic vessels, transport and subsequent arrest in compatible organs, adherence of tumor cells to endothelial surfaces followed by extravasation at the site of metastasis, establishment of a new microenvironment and proliferation and establishment of metastases (Fig. 4-5). Importantly, less than 1% of tumors cells introduced into the circulation will survive to produce metastasis. Four principle groups of proteins are involved in this metastatic cascade.

First, tumor cells appear to have *lost contact inhibition.* Cell-adhesion molecules are important for maintaining cell-to-cell contact. In many tumors, these genes are down-regulated. E-cadherin is commonly lost in epithelial tumors. The DCC gene encodes for a cell-adhesion molecule that is typically lost in the development of colon cancer. Alternatively, embryonic forms of cell-adhesion molecules may be reexpressed, which may contribute toward altered cell motility and increased invasiveness. This is seen in colon cancer with loss of a differentiated form of carcinoembryonic antigen (CEA) and expression at high levels of the embryonic form of the molecule.

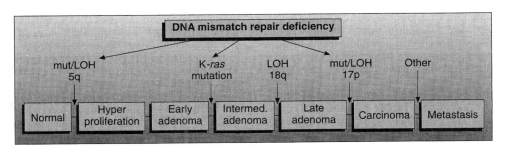

FIGURE 4-4. Multistep carcinogenesis. (From Kelley WN. *Textbook of internal medicine,* 3rd ed. Philadelphia: Lippincott-Raven, 1996:778, with permission.)

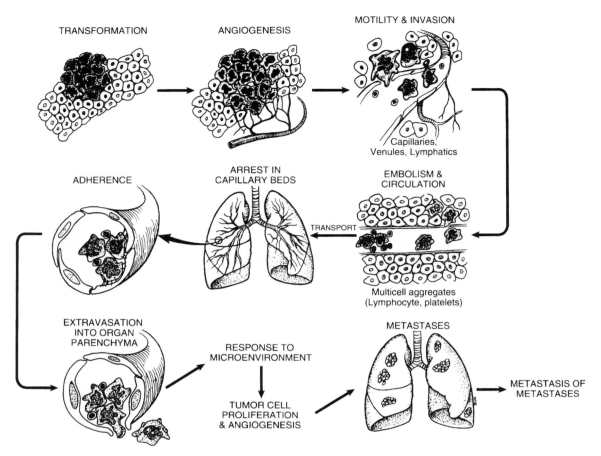

FIGURE 4-5. Steps in the formation of metastases. (From DeVita VT, Hellman S, Rosenberg SA, eds. *Cancer:* Principles and practice of oncology, 5th ed. Philadelphia: Lippincott-Raven, 1997:136, with permission.)

Second, there are *cytoskeletal changes,* which result in altered or increased cell mobility. This includes the product of the nm23 gene that results in phosphorylation of intermediate filaments with subsequent alteration of the cytoskeleton and cell shape. Other motility factors that have been identified include autocrine motility factor and hepatocyte growth factor.

Third, *angiogenesis* is essential for growth of the primary tumor as well as the development of metastasis. The greater the vascularization of the tumor, the greater the opportunity for metastasis. Clinically there is often a positive correlation between the tumor vessel density and the likelihood of metastasis. Angiogenesis is a balance between proangiogenic and antiangiogenic factors. Many proangiogenic factors have been identified including IL-8, transforming growth factor α (TGF-α), TGF-β, vascular endothelial growth factor (VEGF), and platelet-derived endothelial cell growth factor. Proangiogenic factors may be produced by tumor cells or by tissue mast cells and macrophages.

Lastly, malignant cells produce high levels of *tissue degradative enzymes.* These include lysosomal hydrolases, such as cathepsin B, collagenases such as collagenase IV, tissue inhibitors of metalloproteinases, and plasminogen activators.

TUMOR MARKERS

The potential clinical application of circulating tumor markers was first demonstrated in 1938 with the detection of elevated levels of acid phosphatase in the serum of patients with metastatic prostate cancer. Although the number of tumor markers entering clinical use continues to grow, no ideal marker has yet been identified. Nonetheless, tumor markers available today are important tools used in screening, diagnosis, and assessment of prognosis and therapeutic efficacy and as markers of recurrent disease.

Tumor markers can be classified as *tumor antigens, enzymes, hormones, oncogenes,* and *gene products.* Tumor antigens are further divided into *oncofetal antigens* and *tumor-associated antigens.* Oncofetal antigens, such as CEA and α-fetoprotein (AFP) are produced during normal fetal development, and although they do not disappear during

TABLE 4-2. CLASSIFICATION OF TUMOR MARKERS[a]

Tumor marker	Tumor antigen	Tumor histology
Tumor antigen		
	Carcinoembryonic antigen	Colorectal, pancreatic, breast, Hepatocellular, testicular
	Alpha-fetoprotein	
Tumor associated	Prostate-specific antigen	Prostate
	Tissue polypeptide antigen	Breast, gynecologic tumors
	CA 15-3	Breast
	CA 19-9	Colorectal, pancreatic, gastric
	CA 50	Colorectal, pancreatic, gastric
	CA 242	Ovarian, other gynecologic tumors
Enzymes	Neuron-specific enolase	Neuroendocrine
	Prostatic acid phosphatase	Prostate
Hormones	Beta-human chorionic	Testicular, trophoblastic
	Serotonin	Carcinoid
	Calcitonin	small cell lung cancer, medullary thyroid
	Cortisol	Adrenal cortical tumors
	Catecholamines	Pheochromocytoma
Oncogene	Erb B-2 (her-2/neu)	Breast, ovarian, prostate, stomach
	Ras	Colorectal, lung, prostate
	c-myc	Burkitt's lymphoma
	N-myc	Neuroblastoma
	Abl	Chronic myelogenous leukemia
	RET	Medullary thyroid carcinoma
	Rb	Retinoblastoma
	P53	Lung, colon
Other	M protein	Multiple myeloma
Cytoskeletal filaments	CYFRA 21-1	Non–small cell lung cancer

[a]From Sabiston DC, ed. *Textbook of surgery*, 15th ed. Philadelphia: WB Saunders, 1997:536, with permission.

adulthood, their reexpression at elevated levels is associated with disease states including malignancy. Tumor-associated antigens are distinctly different from those found on normal tissue and do not represent reexpression of fetal antigens. (Table 4-2).

TUMOR ANTIGENS

Oncofetal Proteins

CEA is a cell-surface glycoprotein consisting of a single polypeptide chain with a molecular weight of 180 kd. It is related to and shares antigenic determinants with biliary glycoprotein present in bile and nonspecific cross-reacting antigen found in normal lung, granulocytes, and epithelial cells. The CEA family is a subset of the immunoglobulin gene family. CEA modulates epithelial cell and collagen interactions. In states of high CEA expression, these interactions may be disrupted, allowing for greater cell movement and less ordered tissue architecture.

CEA is manufactured by fetal liver, pancreas, and gut and is present in normal adults at levels of less than 2.5 ng/mL. Levels of more than 5.0 ng/mL are elevated and those between 2.5 and 5.0 ng/mL are considered borderline. In addition to being elevated in various epithelial malignancies, CEA is elevated in a number of nonmalignant disease states including cirrhosis, pancreatitis, cholecystitis, ulcerative colitis, diverticulitis, and chronic obstructive pulmonary disease. CEA is cleared by hepatocytes and Kupffer cells and its half-life can vary from 1 to 7 days depending on hepatic function.

CEA is elevated in 60% of patients with colorectal cancer, 50% of patients with pancreatic and gastric cancer, and 20% of patients with breast cancer. CEA does not have sufficient sensitivity and specificity to be used as a screening or diagnostic marker. It does appear to have prognostic value though; CEA-positive patients with breast cancer have significantly worse outcome, as do patients with colorectal carcinoma with high preoperative CEA levels. Although patients with colorectal cancer with more advanced disease at presentation have higher CEA levels (Table 4-3), the

TABLE 4-3. CEA ELEVATION IN COLONIC CANCER[a,b]

Duke's stage	% patients with elevated CEA
A	3–5
B	25
C	33–45
D	65–90

[a]CEA, carcinoembryonic antigen.
[b]From Sabiston DC, ed. *Textbook of surgery*, 15th ed. Philadelphia: WB Saunders, 1997:538, with permission.

prognostic value of preoperative CEA levels in these patients seems to be independent of the stage of the disease. CEA appears to be of greatest value in detecting recurrence in patients with colorectal cancer. Postoperatively, elevated CEA levels are expected to return to normal in approximately 6 to 8 weeks after resection of a CEA-producing tumor. In approximately two thirds of patients, an elevated serum CEA level is the first manifestation of recurrent colorectal cancer and may precede clinically evident disease by 3 to 9 months. In patients with previous colorectal cancer, a CEA level greater than 10 ng/mL is consistent with a diagnosis of recurrence. Overall sensitivity and specificity of CEA for the detection of recurrence is 60% to 90%, respectively. The site of recurrent disease also appears to have impact on the sensitivity of this test. In patients with liver or retroperitoneal recurrence, the sensitivity is greater (75%), but the sensitivity is less (40% to 50%) in those with locoregional, pulmonary, or peritoneal recurrences. CEA levels may rise with recurrent disease even in patients with normal preoperative serum measurements. Finally, in metastatic colorectal cancer, CEA levels are useful for assessing response to chemotherapy. However, CEA determinations appear to be less reliable in assessing treatment response in other gastrointestinal malignancies.

AFP is an $\alpha 1$-globulin with a molecular weight of 70 kd produced by the fetal liver, gut, and yolk sac as well as hepatocytes and endodermally derived gastrointestinal tissues. AFP levels peak at 12 weeks of gestation and by 1 year of age decline to adult levels of less than 10 ng/mL. Half-life ranges from 4 to 6 days. AFP levels are elevated in 70% to 95% of patients with hepatoma, 60% to 75% of patients with nonseminomatous testicular cancers, and less frequently in patients with gastric, pancreatic, lung, and colorectal cancer. Abnormal levels are also seen in nonmalignant disease such as hepatitis, inflammatory bowel disease, and cirrhosis. AFP is not elevated during liver regeneration following hepatic resection.

AFP has been successfully used as a screening tool for patients at high risk for hepatocellular carcinoma (HCC). High-risk patients include those with cirrhosis or chronic hepatitis B infection. In this population, serum AFP is followed every 3 to 4 months with ultrasound examination every 4 to 6 months. Because only 40% of patients who have HCC in a noncirrhotic liver will have elevated AFP levels (compared to 85% of patients who have HCC within a cirrhotic liver), screening is not cost-effective in low-risk groups. False-positive screening results occur in about 20% of patients, particularly in those with cirrhosis and chronic active hepatitis, where 40% of patients may have baseline elevated AFP in the absence of HCC. However, AFP levels greater than 500 ng/mL are considered diagnostic of HCC in the presence of cirrhosis. False-negative screening results have been reported in 10% to 40% of cases. Measurement of AFP and β-HCG, is also important in the diagnostic workup of germ-cell neoplasms.

AFP is prognostically important in both HCC and testicular cancer. In testicular cancer, although higher AFP levels are associated with greater tumor burdens, patients with similar tumor burdens and elevated AFP, particularly if greater than 500 ng/mL, have poorer outcomes compared to patients with normal serum levels. In addition, testicular tumors with very high serum levels respond very poorly to chemotherapy. The better prognosis seen in HCC patients with normal AFP levels may be primarily due to the absence of cirrhosis.

Serial measurements of serum AFP are the best detector of recurrent HCC, with elevated AFP levels having greater sensitivity for recurrent disease than computed tomographic or ultrasound examination. A rise in serum levels is the first manifestation of disease in about one third of patients and elevated levels are eventually detected in most patients with recurrence. AFP levels also correlate well with treatment response in HCC. Spontaneous normalization of AFP has been reported in some patients despite the persistence of tumor, but this is an unusual event. Similarly, AFP is a useful marker to follow treatment response and recurrence in patients with testicular cancer. Elevated AFP may precede the development of radiologically evident recurrence by 2 to 14 months. In the 6% of patients whose tumor masses do not regress despite normalization of tumor markers conversion to a mature teratoma is seen.

TUMOR-ASSOCIATED ANTIGENS

Prostate-specific antigen (PSA) is a 30-kd glycoprotein found only in the cytoplasm of ductal and acinar cells of the prostate gland. It is therefore a prostate-specific marker and has replaced prostate acid phosphatase as a marker for prostatic diseases. Although specific for prostate in general, it is not specific to prostate cancer and elevations are also seen in patients with benign prostatic hyperplasia (BPH). Differentiating benign from malignant prostate enlargement is particularly difficult if PSA levels are in the intermediate range of 4 to 10 ng/mL. Therefore, use of PSA as a screening marker for early prostate cancer has been limited by this overlap. PSA levels greater than 10 ng/mL are generally considered suspicious for cancer.

A number of refinements in interpretation of PSA levels have been proposed to help discriminate between BPH and early prostate cancer and therefore refine the role of PSA as a screening marker. These include adjustments of normal limits for PSA based on age, PSA density, and PSA slope measurements. With increasing age and benign hypertrophy of the prostate, PSA levels increase, and thus, upper limits of normal have been age adjusted. Currently accepted uppernormal limits on PSA are 2.5 ng/mL for patients from 40 to 49 years of age, 3.5 ng/mL for ages 50 to 59, 4.5 ng/mL for 60 to 69 years, and 6.5 ng/mL for patients more than 70 years. PSA *density* measurements are determined as the amount of PSA per unit of prostate tissue. The volume of the prostate is estimated by ultrasound. The basis of this calculation is that prostate cancer has a higher PSA density than BPH. PSA *slope* is the rate of change of PSA density over time. PSA slope determinations of greater than 0.7 ng/mL per year in patients with PSA levels of less than 4.0 ng/mL or increase of more than 0.4 ng/mL per year in patients with PSA greater than 4 ng/mL would warrant evaluation for prostate cancer. PSA levels correlate with tumor burden; therefore, PSA is also used for monitoring the response to therapy and detecting recurrent disease. It is important to note that after radical prostatectomy, the PSA level is expected to fall to zero in the absence of metastasis.

CA 15-3 is a glycoprotein antigen elevated in breast, ovarian, and lung cancer. CA 15-3 is a differentiation antigen and is also present in breast milk. Elevated levels can be found in 20% of patients with benign breast disease. In breast cancer, the percentage of patients with elevated CA 15-3 increases with more advanced disease. Therefore, whereas only 50% of patients with nodal metastasis have a high CA 15-3 level, 80% of patients with systemic metastasis have an elevated CA 15-3 level. High CA 15-3 levels are also seen in 65% to 70% of patients with lung and ovarian cancer. Although CA 15-3 is not specific enough for use as a diagnostic marker; serum levels appear to correlate with response to therapy in patients with breast cancer, and CA 15-3 is monitored primarily in this patient group. It is also a helpful marker of breast cancer recurrence, with elevated levels often preceeding clinical and radiologic findings of recurrent disease by up to 18 months.

CA 19-9 is a carbohydrate antigen elevated in pancreatic, colon, and gastric cancers. It can also be elevated in pancreatitis, hepatitis, and sclerosing cholangitis; therefore, specificity of this tumor antigen for diagnostic purposes is limited. In patients with gastric and colon cancer, CA 19-9 measurements do not appear to offer any advantage over determinations of CEA; therefore, CA 19-9 remains most useful in the setting of pancreatic cancer. At presentation, over 80% of patients with pancreatic cancer have elevated levels of this antigen. Correlation between level of marker and extent of tumor has not been definitively established. CA 19-9 is not of use currently in monitoring response to therapy because no effective treatment exists for pancreatic carcinoma.

CA 125, also a glycoprotein antigen, is present in the fetal peritoneum, pleura, pericardium, and amnion. It has a half-life of 4.5 days. In adults, CA 125 can be detected in the epithelium of the fallopian tubes, endometrium, and endocervix by immunohistochemical staining. Although elevated levels are found in 80% of patients with nonmucinous ovarian carcinoma, CA 125 does not have specificity for ovarian cancer and can also be elevated in fallopian, endometrial, lung, and colon cancer as well as benign processes such as gynecomastia, pregnancy, menstruation, endometriosis, hepatitis, and cirrhosis. However, in patients with ovarian masses, an elevated CA 125 level may help in the diagnostic workup, with reports demonstrating 75% sensitivity and 90% specificity in this setting. CA 125 remains most useful in the management of patients with ovarian cancer. Elevated levels at diagnosis are consistent with larger tumor burdens and these patients have a poorer prognosis. CA 125 levels are used to follow response to therapy; persistently elevated CA 125 levels indicate failure of therapy. However, normalization of CA 125 levels is less useful as a measure of therapeutic efficacy because more than 50% of these patients will be found to have residual disease at the time of laparotomy. CA 125 levels in peritoneal washings may be more sensitive than serum levels for the detection of residual disease. Elevation of CA 125 is also an early finding in recurrent disease.

ENZYMES

Neuron-specific enolase (NSE) is an isoenzyme of enolase. It is found in high levels in neuroendocrine tissue and at such elevated serum levels can be detected in patients with pancreatic islet cell tumor, medullary thyroid carcinoma, adrenal tumors, gut carcinoids, and small cell lung cancer. In all cases except small cell lung cancer, other more sensitive and specific tumor markers exist and are preferred. In small cell lung cancer, over 80% of patients with extensive disease will have elevated serum NSE levels. In those with more limited disease, however, only 55% have a rise in serum NSE. NSE is particularly useful in patients with small cell cancer with CNS metastasis. NSE is found in the CSF of almost all patients with meningeal carcinomatosis and about one half of patients with CNS parenchymal metastasis. NSE levels also correlate with response to treatment in small cell lung cancer. However, this tumor marker is not sufficiently sensitive to detect minimal residual disease. Therefore, a normalized NSE level alone cannot be used for assessment of "cure."

HORMONES

β-HCG is a glycoprotein hormone consisting of two subunits. The α subunit is shared with the pituitary hormones LH, FSH, and TSH. The β subunit differs and determines the specificity of each hormone. β-HCG is a *placental hormone* that is useful as a tumor marker in gestational trophoblastic tumors and nonseminomatous testicular cancer. Three assays are available for determination of HCG levels; whole HCG, β-HCG, and an 83 amino acid fragment of β-HCG termed the β *core fragment*. Whereas the whole HCG molecule predominates in pregnancy, β-HCG and the β core fragment are the predominant forms in malignancies. β-HCG has a half-life of 36 to 48 hours and is therefore a useful early marker for assessment of efficacy of treatment.

β-HCG is a very sensitive marker in gestational trophoblastic neoplasms and nonseminomatous testicular cancers. Although β-HCG is also detected in 10% of seminomatous tumors, 20% of bladder cancers, 15% of epithelial ovarian tumors, and in a small percentage of other gynecologic cancers (cervical, vulvar, endometrial), its clinical utility in these circumstances is not well defined.

β-HCG is a very sensitive and specific tumor marker in gestational trophoblastic tumors. Elevated β-HCG levels after completion of normal pregnancy or after termination of a molar pregnancy is diagnostic of a malignant trophoblastic tumor. β-HCG is also of primary importance for assessing the response to therapy and determining recurrence. Absolute levels of β-HCG also have prognostic significance. Patients with gestational trophoblastic tumors and levels over 40,000 mIU/mL have a poor outcome. β-HCG is elevated in approximately two thirds of patients with nonseminomatous tumors and is combined with measurements of AFP for diagnosis, treatment response and detection of recurrence. Eighty-nine percent of patients with nonseminomatous testicular cancer will have either AFP or β-HCG elevated. Importantly, marker status is not used in planning initial surgical therapy; in the small minority of patients who become marker negative after initial orchiectomy, a retroperitoneal lymph node dissection is still required because a few patients will still be found to have nodal metastasis. As with AFP levels in patients with nonseminomatous testicular cancer, the absolute β-HCG levels also have prognostic significance. Patients with higher levels tend to respond poorly to treatment and have worse outcomes.

TREATMENT MODALITIES

Over the last several decades as understanding of tumor biology has grown, there has been a shift away from radical surgery and toward a *multimodal treatment* of cancer patients. With few exceptions (e.g., Wilms tumors), the overall survival of patients has not improved significantly with this new approach; however, morbidity has decreased and quality of life improved. Examples include improved cosmesis with lumpectomy and radiation therapy compared to mastectomy in breast cancer, improved limb salvage rates in patients with extremity sarcomas with marginal resection plus radiation compared to radical surgery. The surgeon maintains an important role in this new multidisciplinary approach and needs to be familiar with the prevention, diagnosis, definitive treatment, and palliation of cancer patients.

The principal role of the surgeon in the diagnosis of cancer lies in the acquisition of tissue for histologic evaluation. Although tissue confirmation of malignancy before definitive surgical treatment is ideal, occasionally this is omitted if the tumor is not easily accessible for biopsy or if biopsy would complicate or compromise the definitive operative intervention or if preliminary biopsy results would not alter the extent of the planned operation. A number of biopsy techniques are available for obtaining histologic tissue. *Aspiration* biopsy involves the aspiration of cells and fragments of tissue through a small gauge needle. Cytological assessment of this material provides a tentative diagnosis for the presence of malignant tissue. There is a small but definite error rate inherent in this biopsy technique. Therefore, large resections for cancer are generally not undertaken solely on the basis of aspiration biopsy results. *Needle* (core) *biopsy* requires the removal of a core of tissue using a specially designed needle. Although a core specimen provides enough tissue for definitive diagnosis of a neoplasm, in soft tissue tumors and bony sarcomas, differentiating between benign and malignant neoplasms using this technique remains difficult. *Incisional biopsy* refers to removal of a small segment of tissue from a larger mass through an open incision. This is the preferred method of diagnosis of soft tissue and bony sarcomas. *Excisional biopsy* involves removal of the entire suspect mass for histologic evaluation, usually taking little, if any, normal tissue at the margins. This is the preferred technique for diagnosis of tumors, provided they can be preformed without contaminating tissue planes and without compromising the definitive surgical procedure.

Several principles are important to consider when performing any type of surgical biopsy. *Needle tracks* and scars need to be placed such that they can be readily removed at the time of subsequent definitive surgery. Although reports of needle tract seeding with tumor are rare, these tracks must still be treated by excision or radiation. Incisions in the extremities should be placed longitudinally so as to make subsequent removal of underlying tissue compartments easier. Care should be taken not to contaminate new tissue planes. Large hematomas after biopsy risk further spread of tumor and care should therefore be taken to ensure hemostasis after completion of a biopsy. Instruments used to handle suspected sites of tumor should not be used again in potentially uncontaminated sites. The biopsy technique selected should provide adequate tissue for the pathologic evaluation. For the diagnosis of certain tumors, electron microscopy, tissue culture, or other techniques may be required and sufficient tissue should be obtained at the time of biopsy for all these studies. In addition, the handling of biopsy specimens is determined by the type of testing required. Biopsy tissue from breast cancer specimens, for example, should be saved in cold storage to allow for hormone receptor testing. Orientation of the biopsy specimen may be important for subsequent treatment, and the surgeon should mark distinctive areas of the tumor to assist in subsequent orientation by the pathologist.

Clinical, radiographic, and/or surgical staging need to be completed before definitive therapy. In order to perform adequate surgical staging, the surgeon must be familiar with the natural history of the cancer. In Hodgkin disease, for example, staging laparotomy remains appropriate in patients presenting with disease confined to the supradiaphragmatic sites. Patients with ovarian carcinoma are at risk for metastasis to the diaphragm; therefore, accurate staging requires an assessment of these areas. Extensive surgical staging may be required before undertaking major surgical procedures with curative intent. For example, involvement of the celiac and paraaortic lymph nodes in patients with esophageal cancer precludes resection for cure. However, in patients with tumors that are likely to spread to cervical, axillary, inguinal, or clinically suspicious lymph nodes, formal dissection of these lymph node basins is performed at the time of definitive surgical intervention. Preliminary biopsy of these nodes risks tumor spillage and compromise of the final surgical treatment of the tumor.

Surgery for Primary Cancer

Although surgery remains the most important aspect of treatment in most patients with cancer, it is important to realize that approximately 70% of patients will harbor micrometastasis at time of presentation. Therefore, accurate identification of patients who can be cured by local treatment alone is essential. The extent of local resection is influenced by several tumor-related factors. In areas where cosmesis or function may be compromised by extensive removal of tissue, narrower margins are taken, even though the risk of local recurrence may be slightly increased. The multifocal/multicentric nature of some tumors such as breast cancer or papillary thyroid cancer needs to be taken into consideration when the extent of operation is planned. An understanding of the growth pattern and local behavior of tumors is essential for the determination of the extent of local resection. Locally aggressive and invasive tumors with the capacity for diffuse infiltrative spread through contiguous tissue planes, such as gastric and esophageal carcinomas, require wide margins to clear areas of tumor infiltration. Finally, the extent of local surgery required has diminished with the availability of effective adjuvant treatment and the development of multimodal therapy for certain malignancies.

The decision to perform a *lymph node dissection* requires a risk versus benefit assessment. Removal of regional nodes interrupts lymphatic and venous flow and can lead to swelling of the extremity and an increased risk for development of infections after minor breaks in the skin. Although the benefit of determining nodal status is primarily to provide prognostic information and direct subsequent therapy, the role of routine regional lymphadenectomy as a therapeutic procedure remains controversial. Therefore, when considering a regional lymph node dissection, the likelihood that metastasis may be found in nodes that alter prognosis and impact therapy must be weighed against the potential morbidities of this intervention. Sarcomas, for example, even if high grade, rarely metastasize to regional nodes and therefore regional lymphadenectomy is not warranted, whereas invasive breast tumors, even if very small (less than 0.5 cm, T1a) carry a small but definite risk of nodal metastasis, justifying axillary dissections in this population. Even in patients with clinically suspicious nodes, the decision to perform a "therapeutic" lymph node dissection requires a risk versus benefit analysis. In certain circumstances, such as melanoma with regional nodal metastasis and no evidence of systemic disease, a lymphadenectomy for clinically suspicious nodes is justified because the morbidity is offset by the possibility of cure in a small percentage of such patients. However, extensive nodal dissections in pancreatic and gastric cancers to remove potentially involved nodes from multiple stations may not be warranted given the absence of consistent data that such an approach improves survival.

In general, the preferred approach to regional lymphadenectomy is to perform lymph node dissections en bloc with resection of the primary tumor, if at sufficient proximity, to prevent cutting across lymphatic channels. More recently, a more selective approach to standard lymphadenectomy has been advocated and tested in patients with clinically node negative melanoma and breast cancer. This approach involves removal of the *sentinel node,* the first node that drains the tumor mass, using blue dye and/or radioisotope. Sentinel node biopsy has been combined with serial sectioning and immunohistochemistry techniques to upgrade otherwise histologically negative nodes in 10% to 15% of breast cancer patients. Patients with tumor in the sentinel node are candidates for a full lymphadenectomy, and those with node-negative sentinel nodes are therefore spared a full lymph node dissection.

Resection of tumors that have invaded adjacent organs has generally been avoided on the assumption that such tumors have already metastasized to distant sites. However, on occasion this assumption is not justified, as some tumors can grow significantly without any evidence of systemic disease. The following considerations are important before undertaking en bloc multiorgan resections: (i) the distant metastatic potential of the tumor, (ii) the ability to reconstruct the resulting defects, and (iii) the risk of the operation to the patient. Resecting across tumors to avoid multiorgan resection is inappropriate because adjuvant therapies are unlikely to be effective in the setting of gross residual disease.

Surgery for Metastatic Disease

The decision to undertake resection of metastatic disease for cure requires assessment of (i) the likelihood that there is no additional occult metastasis, (ii) the morbidity of the operation, and (iii) the availability of effective medical therapies. As a general principle, patients with a limited number of metastases to a single site are most likely to be candidates for resection. This approach is particularly true for cancers in which there is no effective chemotherapy and in which there is metastasis to sites such as lung, liver, or brain. Metastasis to soft tissue sites, other visceral organs, and retroperitoneal nodes are generally associated with disseminated disease. The best outcomes have been seen with resection of *liver metastases* in patients with *colorectal cancer* and resection of *pulmonary metastasis* in patients with *sarcoma*. The interval between initial therapy and recurrence may reflect the biologic aggressiveness of the tumor but is not a contraindication to resection of metastasis.

Cytoreductive Surgery

In some instances of extensive locoregional disease, resection of all gross disease is not feasible. Debulking in these circumstances is practical only if there is effective systemic therapy for control and treatment of residual disease. This approach has been particularly effective in patients with ovarian tumors and Burkitt lymphoma. Except in the palliative setting, cytoreductive surgery is not appropriate treatment for patients with cancers that have no effective adjuvant therapies available. Additionally, the effectiveness of adjuvant therapies after debulking surgery generally requires that only microscopic residual disease be left behind.

Palliative Surgery

Palliative surgery is often required for relief of pain or to improve function and quality of life. The life expectancy of the patient, the availability of alternative, noninvasive interventions for palliation, the morbidity of the surgical procedure, and the likelihood that surgical intervention will be effective are important considerations in selecting patients for palliative surgery.

Surgery for Prevention of Cancer

With increased awareness about the hereditary nature of certain cancers and the identification of specific genetic defects, it has been possible to identify a high-risk population for prophylactic surgery to prevent the subsequent development of cancer. Examples include the identification of mutations in the *RET oncogene* in patients with *MEN 2* and in *familial MTC* and the *apc* gene mutations in *polyposis coli*. Polmerase chain reaction testing for the RET oncogene mutation has replaced measurement of calcitonin levels and has allowed early identification of patients that would benefit from prophylactic thyroidectomy. All patients with the polyposis coli gene mutation will eventually develop colon carcinoma, with 50% having been diagnosed by the age of 40. Patients carrying this mutation are therefore advised to undergo prophylactic colectomy by the age of 20. Patients with familial breast and ovarian cancers also represent high-risk populations; however, in these individuals, unlike patients with the RET oncogene and the apc gene mutations, the risk of developing cancer is not 100%. Therefore, extensive counseling is advised to determine the risks and benefits of prophylactic mastectomy or oophorectomy. Finally, certain *disease states* are known to *increase* the *incidence* of *subsequent carcinoma* (Table 4-4). In particular,

TABLE 4-4. DISEASE STATES ASSOCIATED WITH INCREASED RISK OF SUBSEQUENT MALIGNANCIES[a,b]

Underlying condition	Associated cancer	Prophylactic surgery
Cryptorchidism	Testicular	Orchiopexy
Polyposis coli	Colon	Colectomy
Familial colon cancer	Colon	Colectomy
Ulcerative colitis	Colon	Colectomy
MENII	MTC	Thyroidectomy
FMTC	MTC	Thyroidectomy
Familial breast cancer	Breast	Mastectomy
Familial ovarian cancer	Ovarian	Oopherectomy

[a]MTC, medullary thyroid cancer; FMTC, familial medullary thyroid cancer.
[b]From DeVita VT, Rosenberg SA, Hellman S, eds. *Cancer principles and practice of oncology.* Philadelphia: Lippincott-Raven, 1997:301, with permission.

about 40% of patients with *ulcerative colitis* will eventually die of colon cancer. Therefore, prophylactic colectomy should be considered in any patient with well-documented chronic ulcerative colitis. *Cryptorchidism* is associated with an increased risk of testicular cancer, which can probably be prevented by early prophylactic surgery.

PRINCIPLES OF RADIATION ONCOLOGY

Types of Radiation

Ionizing radiation is the energy absorbed by tissues that results in ejection of an orbital electron. Clinically this is measured as grays (Gy, 100rad = 1Gy) and is the amount of energy absorbed per unit mass. Ionizing radiation can be *particulate*, such as electrons, neutrons, or protons, or it can be *electromagnetic*, such as x-rays and γ-radiation. X-rays are produced extranuclearly using electrical machines, whereas γ-rays are produced intranuclearly through the decay of radioactive isotopes. The energy released by electromagnetic radiation is characterized as a wave or as a packet of energy (photon). The depth of penetration of tissue by ionizing radiation is related to the energy. Additionally, the absorption mechanisms differ at varying intensities. The range of electromagnetic energy used in clinical practice includes superficial radiation with energy ranging from 10 to 125 kV, orthovoltage radiation between 125 and 400 kV, and supervoltage or megavoltage radiation for energies over 400 kV. As the intensity of the electromagnetic radiation increases, the full energy of the radiation is not transferred to the tissue until some distance from the skin. This is called the *skin-sparing effect*.

Radiation Techniques

Brachytherapy describes placement of the source of radiation within the target tissue. This method uses isotopes such as gold-198, cesium-137, iridium-192, and iodine-125. Because the highest dose of energy is delivered to tissues immediately adjacent to the radiation source, precise placement of these radioisotopes is essential to maximize radiation delivery to tumor and minimize injury to adjacent normal tissues.

Teletherapy uses orthovoltage and megavoltage machines located at a distance from the patient. The dose absorbed by the target tissue depends on the tissue characteristics, radiation energy used, and distance from the source of radiation. This radiation can be modified by filters and collimators to minimize injury to adjacent normal tissue.

Radiation Biology

Ionizing radiation has both direct and indirect effects that ultimately render malignant cells incapable of cell division and proliferation. Data suggest that the critical target for radiation effect is DNA. Radiation effects, direct and indirect, are random. *Direct effects* of radiation result in chromosomal DNA breaks that then prevent replication. This is particularly true for high linear energy transfer radiation. Most of the biologic effects of radiotherapy, however, are probably due to *indirect effects* mediated via *free radicals*. Because the predominant molecule within mammalian cells is water, free radicals are generated by the interaction of radiation energy with water. These free radicals can interact with DNA and other important intracellular molecules to detrimental effect. Free radicals have short half-lives, but this can be altered and the effects of free radicals enhanced in the presence of molecular oxygen. Hypoxic tumors, therefore, are relatively radioresistant. A cell that has sustained radiation injury may undergo rapid apoptosis immediately following irradiation. However, most cells that are irradiated will not die until they undergo division. Additionally, some irradiated cells may divide, giving rise to one or more generations of daughter cells before some or all of the progeny become sterile. Alternatively, radiation injury may produce a cell that is unable to divide but is physiologically able to function for a prolonged period of time. Such cells do not appear histologically different from normal cells.

Cell Survival Curves

Cell survival after radiation injury is described in the form of radiation survival curves (Fig. 4-6). These curves have an initial shallow slope (shoulder) at low radiation doses, which becomes steeper as the dose is increased. The shoulder region is a measure of the ability of the cell to repair itself after irradiation (sublethal radiation). The slope of the steep portion of the curve reflects the radiosensitivity of the cells at the usual clinical doses delivered. Survival curves have been determined for normal and neoplastic cells in culture. There are no characteristic differences in survival

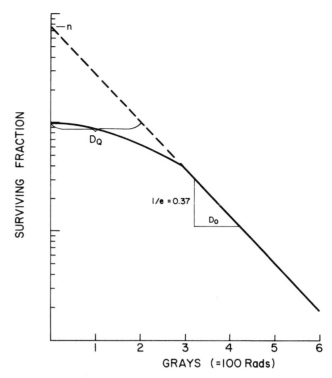

FIGURE 4-6. Radiation survival curve. (From DeVita VT, Hellman S, Rosenberg SA, eds. *Cancer:* Principles and practice of oncology, 5th ed. Philadelphia: Lippincott-Raven, 1997:315, with permission.)

curves between tumor cells and the normal tissues from which they are derived. In addition, the survival curves of radiosensitive and radioresistant tumors have been studied in culture conditions and also fail to demonstrate any differences. Therefore, the clinical responsiveness to radiation therapy appears to be more than simple acute differences in cell survival curves.

Radiation Response and Cell Cycling

The radiosensitivity of cells is also determined by their position within the cell cycle. Both tumor and normal cells are most sensitive to radiation damage in M phase and in G_2 phase and least sensitive during the G_1 and S phases. Following irradiation, *redistribution* refers to the progression of cells from the more resistant phases of the cell cycle to the more sensitive, and *repopulation* refers to the ability of tissue to reconstitute the volume of cells destroyed by radiation. Within tumors that are radiosensitive, the balance between cell killing and repopulation favors normal tissues over the tumor.

Effects of Oxygen

Molecular oxygen is the most important modifier of the biologic effects of ionizing radiation. The presence or absence of oxygen greatly affects availability and half-life of free radicals and therefore the number of cells killed by a given dose of radiation. For equivalent cell killing at every level along the cell survival curve, greater doses of radiation are required under hypoxic conditions. The oxygen enhancement ratio (OER) therefore is the ratio of dose required for equivalent cell killing in the absence of oxygen compared to the dose required in the presence of oxygen. The OER appears to be most relevant over the exponential part of the cell survival curve. Tumor cells grown in hypoxic conditions have less ability to repair damage from sublethal radiation; therefore, the differences in cell killing under hypoxic and normal conditions are not as significant over the "shoulder" region of the radiation survival curve.

Large tumors will have regions where tumors will escape the effects of radiation due to hypoxic conditions. Theoretically, with progressive cycles of cell death, conditions within the tumor are altered, rendering previously hypoxic sites now more oxygen-rich and more sensitive to radiation injury. This principle is called *reoxygenation*. However, this principle is not always clinically efficient, as evidenced by the relative radioresistance of larger tumors. The importance of oxygen in radiation killing has led to clinical experimentation to increase oxygen tensions with tumor sites using high-pressure oxygen and hypoxic cell sensitizers. Some studies have shown benefit in promoting cure rates when delivering radiotherapy in the setting of hyperbaric oxygen. However, the hyperbaric oxygen technique is cumbersome and limits the ability to modify the delivery of the ionizing radiation and is no longer clinically used in most centers. An alternative technique to increase oxygen tensions within tumors has been the use of hypoxic cell sensitizers. Some of the best studied agents are the nitromidazoles, which can substitute for oxygen and serve as hypoxic cell sensitizers.

Pharmacologic Modifiers

Halogenated pyrimidines such as bromodeoxyuridine and idoxuridine have been utilized to increase the effectiveness of a given dose of radiotherapy. When these are incorporated into DNA, the cells are more sensitive to radiation. Repair after sublethal damage is also limited by these agents. *Chemotherapeutic drugs* such as hydoxyurea can also augment the cell killing when combined with radiotherapy. Hydroxyurea preferentially destroys cells in the S phase, when they are most resistant to the effects of radiation.

Tumor Radiobiology

A sigmoid relationship is seen when plotting the probability of tumor control over increasing radiation dose. A similar relationship exists between the risk of complications and increasing radiation dose (Fig. 4-7). The difference in these two curves represents the desired *therapeutic range*. At progressively higher doses, there is little therapeutic gain but

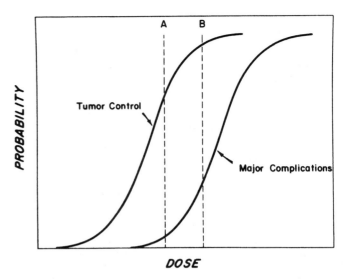

FIGURE 4-7. A: Relationship between radiation dose and tumor control. **B:** Relationship between radiation dose and risk of major complications. (From DeVita VT, Hellman S, Rosenberg SA, eds. *Cancer:* Principles and practice of oncology, 5th ed. Philadelphia: Lippincott-Raven, 1997:320, with permission.)

markedly increased probability of complications. These curves are determined by the characteristics of the tumor and of the transitioned normal tissue. The effects on organ function depend on the reproductive requirement of the irradiated cells. Many tissues have high cellular proliferation rates and are therefore particularly sensitive to acute radiation damage. These tissues include skin, bone marrow, the epithelial lining of the gastrointestinal tract, and germ-line cells. The sensitivity of the latter to radiation injury places patients at risk of mutagenesis and sterility. Tissues whose cells do not require frequent turnover are considered relatively radioresistant (e.g., bone, muscle, and liver). However, radiation damage to these slow proliferating tissues can be seen much later (late radiation complications) or may be seen if these tissues are subjected to injury that requires rapid cell proliferation. For instance, radiation to the liver has few consequences at moderate doses; however, if this is followed by hepatic resection, hepatic failure may result. Similarly, patients that have irradiation to the bone will have few consequences unless the bone is fractured. Under these circumstances, the fracture may fail to heal.

To minimize both acute and late injury to normal tissues during radiation treatments, several techniques have been developed. *Fractionation* is the process of delivering a given amount of radiation as a series of smaller fractions. This approach allows normal tissue time to repair some of the radiation damage. Fractionation allows tumor regression and subsequently reoxygenation to occur, thereby increasing the efficacy of subsequent fractions on tumor cell kill. In addition, the time between fractions allows cells to redistribute through the cell cycle to more radiosensitive phases. Hyperfractionation and accelerated fractionation are extensions of the fractionation principle. Hyperfractionation refers to even smaller fractions delivered several times per day. Accelerated fractionation uses standard fractionation doses and compresses them into a shorter overall treatment period by providing several doses per day.

Acute and Late Complications

Acute complications are seen as a consequence of radiation injury to the rapidly proliferating tissues of the gastrointestinal tract, skin, and lymphoid tissues. These rapidly dividing cells undergo repair and repopulation between radiation doses, but acute tissue reactions are a balance between loss and injury and time for repopulation and repair of injured sites. Acute reactions are also affected by fraction size. Therefore, if excessive acute complications are noted, a brief treatment break or a small decrease in fraction size may allow rapid resolution of the acute toxicities. Late complications of radiation include necrosis, fibrosis, fistula formation, nonhealing ulceration, and organ-specific damage such as spinal cord transection and blindness. These complications do not appear to be related to the rate of cellular proliferation. The primary determinants of late term complications are the total dose delivered and the size of each fraction. Treatment duration and interval between treatments do not appear to impact the risk of long term sequelae. Acute reactions also do not appear to predict the development of long-term complications.

Combining Radiation and Surgery

The rationale for combining radiation and surgery is that the mechanism of failure is different in these two modalities. Radiation tends to fail at adequately treating the central bulk of tumors under hypoxic conditions but can effectively treat small numbers of well-vascularized tumor cells at the periphery of tissue. Surgery, on the other hand, can effectively debulk the main tumor mass, but elimination of microscopic tumor at the periphery may be limited by the morbidity of a more radical surgical intervention. The combination of both modalities has resulted in the use of lower doses of radiation to eradicate microscopic tumor extensions left behind after a more limited surgical approach. Combining these two modalities has been most useful when preserving function and quality of life are important such as with *breast tumors* or with *extremity sarcomas*.

Radiation can be given either preoperatively or postoperatively. *Preoperative radiation therapy* has the advantage of sterilizing tumor at the edges of a planned resection. Preoperative therapy also aims to reduce the tumor volume, which may be important for otherwise large unresectable tumors or tumors close to important anatomic sites. Preoperative radiation may be administered to patients who suffer from low rectal carcinomas close to the sphincter. This may reduce the tumor sufficiently in size to allow for a sphincter preserving low anterior resection rather than an abdominoperineal resection. Preoperative radiation therapy does not appear to result in an increase in cure rates. Disadvantages to preoperative radiation treatment include downstaging of tumor, which precludes an accurate assessment of tumor stage at presentation. Surgical delay of 4 to 6 weeks is required if large (over 4,000 rad) doses are used to allow time for tissues to recover from injury.

Postoperative radiation treatment offers several advantages. Patients are more accurately staged and therefore more appropriately selected for adjuvant radiation therapy. Unnecessary radiation to patients who will not likely benefit is avoided and targets and volumes are more effectively selected based on intraoperative findings and pathologic review. Disadvantages to delaying radiation therapy to the postoperative period include reduction in tissue blood supply that may render tumor cells hypoxic, formation of adhesions, and fixation of small bowel loops with an increased risk of small bowel radiation injury.

Combining Radiation and Chemotherapy

In contrast to combination radiotherapy and surgery, combining radiation therapy with chemotherapeutic agents serves to *increase* the *therapeutic index* rather than diminish the dose of radiation delivered. Such chemotherapy agents include the hypoxic cell sensitizers, and actinomycin D, and hydroxyurea that modify the radiation survival curve. Local control also appears to be improved when radiation therapy is followed by or administered at the same time as chemotherapy.

Principles of Chemotherapy

The development of chemotherapy in the fifth and sixth decades of this century and its successful use in curing certain lymphoid tumors opened the doors to the widespread application of chemotherapy for solid tumors. However, the results with treatment of solid tumors were disappointing; in most cases, there was no substantial improvement of cure rates even when chemotherapy was used in the adjuvant setting rather than as a primary treatment modality.

The use of chemotherapeutic agents has been based on an understanding of tumor-growth kinetics, mechanisms of action, and mechanisms of drug resistance. The kinetics of tumor growth can be described in terms of Skipper's laws and gompertzian growth. Skipper's law states that the doubling time of tumor cells remains constant and that the percentage of cells that are killed with each dose of chemotherapy also remains constant. Skipper's law however applies only to cells that are proliferating and at any given time, only a fraction of tumor cells is in the proliferating compartment while most cells are in the G0 phase. Most human tumor growth approximates a sigmoid rather than an exponential curve (Fig. 4-2), which takes into account cells that are at rest (i.e., in the G0 phase) or dying. This growth pattern is referred to as *gompertzian growth*. The fraction of proliferating cells within a tumor population depends on the overall size of the tumor. In small tumors, this proliferating fraction is relatively high because of the efficient delivery of oxygen and nutrients. As tumors grow and outstrip their blood supply, their proliferating fraction decreases, resulting in a reduction in the growth rate of the tumor. The growth fraction is maximal when the tumor is about 37% of its maximum size. Gompertzian growth partially explains the refractory nature of many solid tumors to chemotherapy, because cells that are in the G0 phase are resistant to chemotherapy (intrinsic kinetic resistance). Tumors are most sensitive to chemotherapy when they are micrometastatic lesions, because the growth fraction and hence the chemoresponsive fraction is greatest in these small lesions. Conversely, large tumors have a smaller fraction of proliferating cells and therefore are less sensitive to chemotherapeutic agents. Elimination of all tumor cells is considered necessary for cure, because the immune system may not always recognize and eradicate microscopic residual disease.

Understanding the "mechanism of action" is important for appropriate selection of agents for combination therapy in order to minimize toxicity and drug interactions, as well as to prevent emergence of drug resistance. Chemotherapeutic agents have been placed into classes depending on the mode of action. *Alkylating agents* such as nitrosourea, cisplatin, carboplatin, melphalan, busulfan, and cyclophosphamide alkylate the DNA template causing single-strand and double-strand breaks and a misreading of the DNA code. *Antimetabolites* such as fluorouracil, methotrexate, 6-mercaptopurine, and cytarabine inhibit dihydrofolate reductase and reduce the cell folate pool, thereby inhibiting purine-nucleotide synthesis. This effect can be reversed by administering leucovorin, a reduced folate. *Antibiotics* such as adriamycin exert their antitumor effects through intercalation and disruption of the DNA template and the formation of free radicals. *Mitotic inhibitors* include the plant alkaloids vincristine and vinblastine, which inhibit spindle formation by binding to tubulin and etoposide (VP-16), which inhibits topoisomerase II. Paclitaxel (taxol), which is extracted from the bark of the Pacific yew tree, also disrupts mitosis. In addition, various *hormonal agents* are used in chemotherapy regimens such as luteinizing hormone-releasing hormone agonists in combination with the nonsteroidal antiandrogen flutamide in prostate cancer and tamoxifen in breast cancer.

In addition to kinetic resistance of cells in G0 phase, malignant cells often are either inherently resistant (intrinsic resistance) to chemotherapeutic agents or develop resistance after the start of therapy (acquired resistance). This resistance to chemotherapy ultimately results in treatment failure. Malignant human cells undergo spontaneous mutations even before a tumor is clinically evident. The likelihood of developing resistant clones continues to increase with tumor growth. An extensively studied mutation involves the *mdr* gene. This gene codes for a cell-surface P glycoprotein, which functions as a transmembrane efflux pump. The *mdr* gene is preserved through evolution and shares homology with several protein pumps in bacterial cell walls. This protein is normally found on the epithelial cells lining small bowel, colon, rectum, proximal tubules of the kidney as well as acinar and bile canalicular surfaces of the pancreatic and hepatic parenchymal cells and is also seen in tumors derived from these organs. P glycoprotein causes the extrusion of a wide variety of chemotherapeutic agents including vinca alkaloids, anthracyclines, and actinomycins before they reach their intracellular targets. The activity of P glycoprotein can be inhibited *in vitro* using calcium channel blockers, antiarrhythmic drugs, and monoclonal antibodies. However, these have not shown clinical efficacy in preventing the development of P glycoprotein–mediated resistance. Other mechanisms of resistance to chemotherapy include enhanced drug metabolism, reduced drug activation, development of alternative metabolic pathways, enhancement of target enzyme levels by gene overamplification, mutations in targets, or alteration in levels of intracellular targets.

Multiple-drug therapy, using agents from different classes, has become an important approach to ensure that there is broad coverage against the intrinsic resistance encountered within a heterogeneous tumor population. In addition, multidrug chemotherapy is important in slowing the development of acquired resistances and allows for maximal cell kill at doses usually below the dose-limiting toxicities of the individual agents used. Clinically, these theoretical considerations have been born out with increased responsiveness seen with most tumors when multiagent chemotherapy is used. However, this increase in response rates has not necessarily translated into improved survival. With some exceptions (choriocarcinoma, Burkitt lymphoma) single-agent chemotherapy does not produce durable remissions or cures. Table 4-5 lists current regimens of choice for several commonly seen tumors.

Dose response curves for chemotherapy agents generally are sigmoidal with a steep linear portion. Therefore, a small reduction in dose can have significant impact on efficacy. In some models, a 20% decrease in dose results in a 50% decrease in cure rate, although complete remission rates remain unchanged. These models have significant implications for clinical therapy in which suboptimal dosing can compromise long-term outcomes. Increasing dose intensity however is not useful in all settings. In particular, the administration of maximal or near maximal tolerated dosing is justified for those tumors where a cure is possible, such as Hodgkin disease and testicular cancer. In contrast, most solid tumors are not curable with chemotherapy even at extremely high doses used with autologous bone marrow transplantation. Increasing dose intensity is not justified in such patient groups. Other changes in chemotherapy such

TABLE 4-5. CURRENT CHEMOTHERAPEUTIC REGIMENS

Tumor	Regimen of choice
Squamous cell of the head and neck	Methotrexate, bleomycin, cisplatin
Transitional cell of the bladder	Cisplatin, mitomycin, vinblastine
Melanoma	Dacarbazine
Gastrointestinal adenocarcinomas	Fluorouracil
Breast cancer	CMF: cyclophosphamide, methotrexate, fluorouracil
	CAF: cyclophosphamide, adriamycin, fluorouracil
Testicular cancer	Bleomycin, vinblastine, cisplatin
Soft tissue sarcoma	Doxorubicin, dacarbazine
Lung cancer	Cisplatin, etopside or vinblastine, taxol
Insulinoma	Streptozocin
Carcinoid	Streptozocin, fluorouracil
Thyroid cancer	Radioiodine
Esophageal cancer	Cisplatin, fluorouracil

as continuous drug infusions, continuous drug infusions adjusted to circadian rhythms, and multiple daily dosing have resulted in reduced toxicities but have not affected survival.

The interval between doses is also important and is largely determined by the toxic effects on normal tissues and the time required for resolution of these toxicities. For most agents, the dose-limiting toxicity is myelosuppression with nadir counts at approximately 2 weeks and complete resolution by 3 to 4 weeks. Certain agents such as busulfan, nitrosourea, mitomycin C, and procarbazine cause delayed myelosuppression, which develops 4 weeks after initiation of therapy and can last several weeks. These agents are dosed every 6 to 8 weeks. Treatment with these agents also can lead to cumulative marrow toxicity and marrow failure.

The timing of chemotherapy within a treatment regimen depends on the particular clinical situation and the goals of therapy. *Patterns of chemotherapy administration* include induction, consolidation and maintenance chemotherapy, adjuvant chemotherapy, neoadjuvant chemotherapy, and palliative chemotherapy. *Induction chemotherapy* is the administration of high-dose chemotherapy given to induce a complete response in patients for whom chemotherapy is the only treatment modality. Although these are generally patients with hematologic malignancies, such regimens are also used in solid malignancies when patients have metastatic disease that precludes resection. If there is a complete response to induction chemotherapy, this is followed by a "consolidation phase" in which the same initial high dose of therapy is repeated to prolong remission or increase cure rate. After completion of consolidation therapy, a "maintenance phase" is given with lower doses of agents over longer terms designed to delay tumor-cell regrowth. In patients who do not have an adequate response to induction chemotherapy or who progress through induction chemotherapy, a salvage program is initiated typically using second-line agents that are less active. Responses to salvage therapy tend to be short-lived. *Neoadjuvant therapy*, or primary therapy, is given before surgical resection of the tumor. The benefits of this approach are to improve resectability and organ preservation. Neoadjuvant therapy also allows for an assessment of tumor response to the particular chemotherapy regimen, which can guide choice of therapy after resection. Theoretically, neoadjuvant regimens may treat micrometastatic disease and improve cure rates, but this has not been demonstrated clinically. The primary disadvantage is the risk that the tumor will not respond and then progress and become unresectable in the interim. Neoadjuvant treatments are usually offered to patients with locally advanced breast cancer, esophageal cancer, rectal carcinomas, and squamous cell cancers of the head and neck. *Adjuvant chemotherapy* is given after complete resection in cases where patients are at high risk for developing recurrent disease. The goal is to eradicate any micrometastatic disease and therefore increase the odds of cure. Therapy is usually high dose and given over a short interval. The agents used are generally the same as would be used in the palliative setting. The use of adjuvant therapy has been shown to have some survival benefit (8% to 10% improved chance of cure) in patients with breast, colon, and rectal cancers and for ovarian germ-cell tumors, osteosarcomas, and pediatric solid tumors. No benefit has been demonstrated in patients with pancreatic, gastric, cervical carcinomas, or melanomas. *Palliative chemotherapy* is designed to improve symptoms and possibly prolong life for patients with incurable disease. In these circumstances, quality of life is a significant consideration and dosing is adjusted to minimize toxicities.

Most chemotherapy is given *intravenously* and circulates systemically. However, cytotoxic concentrations may not be evenly distributed and sanctuary sites exist in the testis and central nervous system. When disease is limited to one organ, regional chemotherapy may be possible. These include *intraarterial chemotherapy* for treatment of metastasis to the liver or for disease limited to an extremity or to the head and neck. *Limb perfusion* requires vascular isolation of the limb and is usually combined with hyperthermia. This has most commonly been used in extremity melanoma, although limb perfusion for sarcoma has also been reported. *Intrathecal therapy* is used for treatment of meningeal carcinomatosis. *Intraabdominal chemotherapy* for peritoneal disease has been tested in gastric and ovarian cancers as well as in pseudomyxoma peritonei and peritoneal mesothelioma. One presumed advantage to these forms of regional therapy is the possibility of reduced systemic toxicity. However, many of these agents do not remain confined to the perfusion zone. In addition, regional therapy–specific toxicities have been reported such as the fluoropyrimidine-induced biliary sclerosis associated with hepatic intraarterial chemotherapy. Higher target-tissue concentrations are achieved with regional therapy and most studies show higher response rates compared to the administration of these same agents systemically. However, given the lack of controlled randomized trials, it is not clear that survival is improved with these regional approaches. In fact, many patients are not cured because of progression of disease both inside the treatment area and at distant sites.

Assessment of response to therapy is characterized as complete, partial, or minor. *Complete responses* are characterized as those that demonstrate regression of all clinically and radiographically evident disease that lasts for at least 4 weeks or one treatment cycle. *Partial response* is a reduction in the 2-dimensional measurements of the tumor by more than 50% but less than 100% that is durable for at least 4 weeks or through one treatment cycle. Tumors that respond with less than 50% decrease in size for at least 4 weeks or one treatment cycle or have a more than 50% reduction that lasts less than 4 weeks are considered to show a minor response to therapy. *Minor response* is not considered a significant response to treatment. In addition, it should be remembered that although partial and minor responses are characterized radiographically, such radiographically evident masses after treatment may not necessarily represent viable tissue but may instead be necrotic or fibrotic tissues.

Chemotherapy is invariably associated with *adverse side effects*. When chemotherapy is being administered with potential for cure, it is important to provide patients with symptom relief with antiemetics, blood products, antibiotics, growth factors, and other means to increase the likelihood that the planned course of treatment is completed. Patients receiving palliative chemotherapy who develop toxicities are best treated by adjustment of dose. Adverse reactions to some commonly used chemotherapeutic agents include nephrotoxicity associated with cisplatin, dose-dependent renal toxicity secondary to drug deposition within renal tubules with methotrexate, and hemorrhagic cystitis with cyclophosphamide and ifosfamide. In addition, some toxicities are observed only with prolonged therapy. These include doxorubicin-associated cardiotoxicity, bleomycin-induced and busulfan-induced pulmonary fibrosis, vincristine-induced neurotoxcity, and secondary leukemia associated with nitrogen mustard, nitrosourea, and etoposide. The adverse reactions seen with these agents are graded from 0 (no toxicity) to 4 (life threatening). Most regimens will reduce dosing if grade 3 toxicity is encountered.

Immunotherapy

Better understanding of cellular and humoral immune mechanisms have provided new strategies for manipulation of the host immune system, both *ex vivo* and *in vivo*, aiming to cause rejection of the tumor. These approaches include serotherapy (antibody-based therapy), nonspecific immunotherapy, adoptive immunotherapy, and active-specific immunotherapy with cancer vaccines.

Serotherapy

The use of *monoclonal antibodies* in cancer, for both diagnostic and therapeutic purposes, requires the presence of tumor-marker antigens on the surface of malignant cells, which distinguish them from normal host cells. Tumor markers that have been targeted by monoclonal antibodies include oncofetal antigens, oncogene products, and growth-factor receptors. Monoclonal antibodies have been coupled to gamma-emitting radioisotopes to detect occult foci of metastatic disease. Imaging can be accomplished either preoperatively using gamma cameras or intraoperatively using handheld gamma-detecting probes. Such radioimmunolocalization of tumor cells has been used in colon cancer using CEA or the tumor antigen TAG-72 as targets to determine the feasibility and direct the extent of curative resection. Therapeutic use of monoclonal antibodies was first studied using unconjugated antibodies. Antitumor responses using unconjugated antibodies rely on blocking the binding of tumor-growth factors to their cellular receptors or targeting the products of overexpressed oncogenes such as her-2/*neu* in breast cancer. However, tumor responses to unconjugated antibodies are few and if present, transient. To enhance the efficacy of serotherapy, antibodies have been conjugated to radioisotopes (iodine-125, iodine-131, yttrium-90) and toxins. One advantage of radioisotope labeling has been that radiolabeled antibodies need not be internalized to effect cell killing. Radiation from these isotopes can affect cells within a radius of 1 mm from the site of binding. This potentially overcomes the difficulties of heterogeneity in tumor-marker expression seen with tumors. One significant difficulty with the repeated use of mouse monoclonal antibodies in cancer therapy has been the development of a human antimouse antibody response. To limit this, recombinant DNA technology has been used to humanize these mouse monoclonal antibodies generating chimeric molecules that are mostly of human origin but retain the antigen recognition site from the mouse antibody.

Nonspecific Immunotherapy

To augment host antitumor responses, a number of nonspecific *immunomodulators* have been tested clinically. These include bacille Calmette-Guerin (BCG), *Corynebacterium parvum*, levamisole, and thymosin. In general, most of these efforts have been disappointing. BCG was first successfully used in 1969 for the treatment of acute lymphocytic leukemia. It has shown some efficacy with intralesional treatment of malignant melanoma, but this remains of limited clinical utility. Most effective has been the intravesical use of BCG in treatment of superficial bladder cancers, replacing cystectomy as the first line of treatment for this disease. *Levamisole,* in combination with 5-FU, has shown efficacy for adjuvant treatment of Dukes B2 and C *colon carcinomas.* BCG and the other nonspecific immunomodulators exert their effects by inducing the production of cytokines. Cytokines can have direct cytotoxicity against tumor cells (IFN-α, tumor necrosis factor α [TNF-α]) or can enhance cellular and humoral antitumor responses (IL-2, IL-4, IL-12). The ability to now produce pharmacological amounts of pure recombinant cytokines has made human testing with these compounds possible. INF-α has been most effective, with 75% to 80% response rates in patients with hairy cell leukemia and chronic myelogenous leukemia, although response rates in patients with solid malignancies has been significantly lower (10% to 20%). TNF-α exerts considerable antitumor cytotoxicity *in vitro.* However, in phase I and II trials severe side effects were encountered, which are likely due to the role of TNF-α in mediating shock. IL-2, a T-cell growth factor, has shown complete responses in 17% to 20% of patients with metastatic melanoma and metastatic renal-cell carcinoma. However, high-dose IL-2 therapy used to achieve these results is associated with significant toxicity. The wide-ranging effects of IL-2 including the induction of TNF-α and IL-1 have induced shocklike states.

Adoptive Immunotherapy

Adoptive immunotherapy involves the removal of circulating lymphocytes, with *ex vivo* expansion using IL-2 and then returning this expanded pool to the patient. These lymphokine-activated killer cells (LAK cells) appear to be distinct from natural killer cells (NK cells) and cytotoxic T lymphocytes. Despite promising animal studies, clinical protocols at the National Cancer Institute in patients with metastatic melanoma or renal-cell carcinoma demonstrated no difference in survival between IL-2 therapy alone and IL-2 plus LAK cells. To enhance the therapeutic specificity, tumor-infiltrating lymphocytes (TILs), rather than circulating lymphocytes, have also been studied in adoptive immunotherapy protocols. Response rates of up to 40% have been seen using TILs in combination with IL-2 in metastatic melanoma and renal-cell cancer patients.

Active-Specific Immunotherapy (Tumor Vaccines)

A number of approaches aimed at *active immunization* of patients against their tumors are currently under investigation. These active-specific immunotherapy protocols include the use of autologous tumor cells or a number of high-antigen-expressing allogeneic tumor-cell lines administered in conjunction with nonspecific immunomodulators such as BCG in melanoma patients. Immunization of patients with purified cellular components shared by many tumors, such as GM2, a ganglioside common to the plasma membrane of many melanomas, is also under study. The other area of active-specific immunotherapy in study in a number of clinical protocols is the use of dendritic cells. *Dendritic cells* are potent antigen-presenting cells. Dendritic cells pulsed with tumor antigens are able to elicit tumor-specific cellular immunity in both *in vitro* and animal studies. Dendritic cell studies are now under investigation in patients with lymphoma, metastatic melanoma, and prostate cancer. Some promising early results have been seen particularly in the melanoma trials.

Gene Therapy

Introduction of genes into malignant cells has been attempted both *in vivo* and *in vitro.* *In vitro* gene therapy involves the removal of cells from patients, *ex vivo* expansion of these cells with introduction of the normal gene and then return of the genetically modified cells back to the patient. A number of methods have been established for the successful transfer of genes into cells *in vitro* (Table 4-6). In contrast, the delivery of genes *in vivo* has proven to be more complex. The mainstay of *in vivo* gene therapy has been the use of replication-deficient viral vectors.

Cancer gene therapy falls in one of four areas. The genetic modification of tumor cells to secrete certain cytokines has shown efficacy in animal models. For human protocols, tumor cells removed from the patient are expanded *ex vivo,* cytokine gene transfer is performed *in vitro,* the cells are then irradiated to prevent further proliferation and then returned back to the patient. These tumor cells modified to secrete cytokines are used to up-regulate the host immune system. In contrast to systemic administration of cytokines, which is often associated with significant side effects, the secretion of cytokines by tumor cells theoretically attains maximal effects where most needed while minimizing side effects. Protocols using IL-2, IL-4, TNF-α, IFN-γ, GM-CSF, and IL-12 are all being tested. To

TABLE 4-6. GENE DELIVERY SYSTEMS[a]

Method	Ex vivo	In vivo	Expression
Direct injection of DNA	+	++	Transient
Electroporation	++	−	Stable after selection
Calcium phosphate precipitation	+	−	Stable after selection
Liposomes	+	++	Transient
Ligand DNA conjugates	−	++	Transient
Viral delivery			
Retrovirus	++	++	Stable
Adenovirus	+	++	Transient
Adeno-associated virus	++	?	Stable
Vaccinia virus	+	++	Transient
Herpesvirus	+	++	?

[a]From Greenfield LJ, ed. *Surgery,* 2nd ed. Philadelphia: Lippincott-Raven, 1997:504, with permission.

escape immune surveillance, many tumors down-regulate the expression of MHC class I and II molecules from the cell surface. Gene therapy with insertion of the genes coding the MHC molecules may up-regulate the expression of these immunomodulatory molecules in a tumor mass to allow recognition by the immune system. The development of cancer is believed to be the result of a series of genetic alterations resulting ultimately in a malignant cell. Correction of these genetic alterations may return the malignant cell to a normal state or may result in apoptosis. The targets of such gene therapy are *oncogenes* and *tumor suppressor genes*. Strategies for oncogene-directed therapy involve the use of antisense oligonucleotides. Instead of attempting replacement of the mutant gene with the normal allele, a piece of DNA is inserted that is complimentary to the mRNA of the oncogene. By subsequently blocking the translation of the mRNA, the oncogene product is not produced. For tumor suppressor therapy, one strategy is to introduce wild-type p53 into malignant cells, thereby inducing apoptosis. Other tumor suppressor genes under investigation include the DCC gene, which encodes for a cell-adhesion molecule, and nm23, which encodes for a nucleotide diphosphate kinase. Originally used in the treatment of brain tumors, the *suicide gene therapy* is based on the selective insertion of the herpes simplex thymidine kinase gene (HSVtk) into tumor cells. Addition of the drug ganciclovir leads to the formation of toxic nucleotides, which when inserted into newly synthesized DNA leads to autologous cell kill. Cytosine deaminase is another enzyme being used as a suicide gene. Cytosine deaminase converts 5-fluorocytosine into the antineoplastic agent 5-FU with resultant cell kill. Human trials using suicide gene therapy are underway or in development for treatment of mesothelioma, ovarian cancer, and hepatic metastasis. The reverse approach to suicide gene therapy has been to introduce the previously described multidrug resistance (mdr) gene into normal host cells. Host cells carrying the mdr gene should therefore be protected from the effects of high-dose chemotherapy. Bone marrow progenitor cells in particular have been targeted for mdr gene therapy. Because the P glycoprotein is not capable of exporting alkylating agents out of the cell, mdr gene therapy is of no benefit in chemotherapy regimens utilizing alkylating agents.

SUGGESTED READING

DeVita VT, Hellman S, Rosenberg SA, eds. *Cancer:* principles and practice of oncology, 5th ed. Philadelphia: Lippincott, 1997.

Tannock IF, Hill RP, eds. *The basic science of oncology,* 2nd ed. New York: McGraw-Hill, 1992.

5

MELANOMA, SARCOMA, LYMPHOMA, AND THE SPLEEN

MARC B. FARIES AND FRANCIS R. SPITZ

This chapter contains a diverse set of topics, each important in its own right to the general surgeon. The first three sections will deal with malignancies. Melanoma and sarcoma are diseases for which surgery is the primary treatment and the only potentially curative intervention. Surgery is also the best palliative modality for these diseases. Surgical treatment for lymphoma is unusual and is becoming even less common as medical treatments advance. However, surgeons are frequently involved in obtaining tissue for diagnosis and treating gastrointestinal lymphomas. The final section deals with the spleen. It is an organ frequently involved in lymphoma and other hematologic malignancies, and it will be considered here in that context as well as in the management of traumatic injury.

MELANOMA

The incidence of *melanoma* continues to increase worldwide, particularly in the United States. Since 1971 its incidence has increased by 83% (Fig. 5-1). The incidence is now 4 to 26 cases of melanoma per 100,000 population with the highest rates in the southern United States. By the year 2000, the lifetime risk of developing melanoma is estimated to be 1 in 90. Over the past 30 years, melanoma has also become more localized to the primary site, with 81% of melanomas localized in 1990 versus 73% in 1960. During the same period, the average thickness of melanomas has decreased from 3 mm to less than 1 mm, a trend that may reflect increased surveillance for primary lesions.

Differential Diagnosis of the Pigmented Lesion

The most common initial presentation of a patient is for evaluation of a *pigmented lesion*. The vast majority of such lesions are benign, but differentiation between benign and malignant is not always clear. The differential diagnosis of a pigmented lesion is extensive (Table 5-1).

Congenital nevi develop in approximately 1% of children before or shortly after birth. Risk of progression to melanoma correlates with size, with small lesions (0 to 1.5 cm) having little or no increased risk and lesions exceeding 20 cm in diameter having up to a 30% lifetime risk of developing into melanoma. *Acquired nevi* appear after the first few months of life and can be divided into junctional nevi, compound nevi, and intradermal nevi, among others. Differentiation of benign lesions from malignant can be

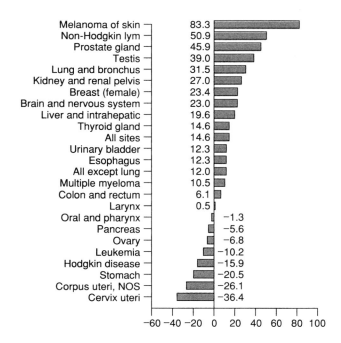

FIGURE 5-1. Change in incidence of cancer by type, 1973–1987. (From Chang AE, Johnson TM, Rees RS. Cutaneous neoplasms. In: Greenfield LJ, Mulholland MW, Oldham KT, et al., eds. *Surgery: scientific principles and practice*. Philadelphia: Lippincott-Raven, 1997:2232, with permission.)

Hospital of the University of Pennsylvania, Philadelphia, Pennsylvania

TABLE 5-1. PIGMENTED LESION, DIFFERENTIAL DIAGNOSIS

Melanocytic	Nonmelanocytic
Congenital nevus	Hemangioma
Acquired nevus	Kaposi's sarcoma
Atypical nevus	Pyogenic granuloma
Melanosis of the genitalia	Dernatofibroma
Blue nevus	Angiokeratoma
Solar lentigo	

difficult for even experienced clinicians. *Junctional nevi* are macular and generally have smooth, regular borders. They appear in childhood and adolescence and consist of a proliferation of melanocytes limited by the basement membrane. *Compound nevi* occur when melanocytes penetrate the basement membrane and are located in nests within the dermis. *Intradermal nevi* are entirely within the dermis and are clinically evident as dome-shaped or nodular and less pigmented.

History and Physical Examination

Patients undergoing evaluation of pigmented lesions should be evaluated for *risk factors* for melanoma. Elements of the history should include any family history of melanoma, as this is indicative of increased risk. Specific mutations have been identified in melanoma in four distinct genes. These mutations, located on chromosomes 1, 6, 7, and 9, are felt to play a role in developing melanoma. A genetic predisposition to melanoma is seen in families with familial atypical mole and melanoma syndrome. This disorder was formerly known as the *dysplastic nevus syndrome*.

An additional risk factor is a history of previous melanomas. Such patients have a ninefold increased risk for developing a second primary melanoma when compared to a population without a history of previous melanomas.

Another predisposing factor is previous exposure to environmental risk factors such as ultraviolet radiation. An increased risk of melanoma has been found with even one blistering sunburn. The increased exposure of the population to radiation from decreased ozone shielding of ultraviolet solar radiation and the increased use of tanning booths has been thought to contribute to the increasing rates of melanoma and other skin cancers.

In addition, compared to the black population, whites have an approximately 20-fold increased risk of developing melanoma. Finally, the history of the lesion itself should be elicited. Lesions that have recently developed or changed should arouse more suspicion than long-standing nevi that have not changed. Changes in size, shape, or color and any history of itching or bleeding may be indicators of malignant transformation.

Patients undergoing evaluation for a pigmented lesion should have all areas of their skin examined for evidence of other lesions. Patients with a large number of benign nevi are at increased risk of developing melanoma.

Individual lesions should be examined for several characteristics. These include the so-called *ABCDEs*: *a*symmetry, irregular *b*orders, variegated *c*olor, large *d*iameter, and *e*levated surface. When examining the color of a lesion, shades of red, pink, white, blue, black, or brown mixed together are suspicious. Lesions larger than 6 mm are also associated with malignancy. Although the presence of these characteristics may be suggestive of malignancy, their absence does not rule out melanoma.

Classification of Melanomas

Suspicious lesions should be *biopsied*. The incision should be oriented so that it can be incorporated into a subsequent wide local excision. Minimal margins of normal tissue should be obtained. Punch or incisional biopsies should be avoided, as an area of increased thickness or malignancy may be missed in the sampling. With large lesions in critical locations (such as above joints or near facial structures), an incisional biopsy may be the only practical option. Shave biopsies may also be used, but it may be difficult to accurately determine the thickness of a lesion that has been removed by shaving.

Melanomas can be classified into four main types based on their appearance and clinical behavior. *Superficial spreading melanoma* is the most common type. It is found in 70% of cases and often arises from preexisting nevi. Superficial spreading melanomas are initially characterized by the radial growth phase. Then, over variable periods of time, vertical growth develops within the lesion, often seen clinically as a raised papule.

Nodular melanoma is the second most common type and accounts for 15% to 30% of cases and lacks a radial growth phase. These tumors are characterized by a vertical growth phase without radial growth and are much more aggressive than superficial spreading. Clinically the lesions tend to be darker and more uniform and are more prevalent in men. Five percent of nodular melanomas lack pigment, which is associated with a higher rate of metastatic spread.

Lentigo maligna melanomas constitute 4% to 10% of cases and have a tendency to develop in older patients in sun exposed areas of the body such as the face. They are relatively more common in women and tend to be large, often greater than 3 cm in diameter. The lesions generally begin as tan but may become flesh-colored over time. They have a decreased propensity for metastatic spread.

Acral lentiginous melanomas are relatively uncommon. They make up only 2% to 8% of melanomas in white patients, but 35% to 60% of melanomas in patients with dark skin. Typically the lesions occur on the palms or soles. This class of melanoma is the most aggressive and has the highest risk of metastasis.

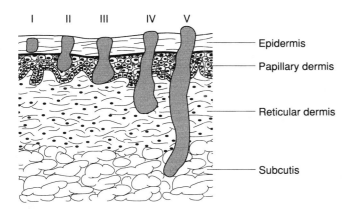

FIGURE 5-2. Clark's levels of invasion. (From Chang AE, Johnson TM, Rees RS. Cutaneous neoplasms. In: Greenfield LJ, Mulholland MW, Oldham KT, et al., eds. *Surgery:* scientific principles and practice. Philadelphia: Lippincott-Raven, 1997:2233, with permission.)

Other types of melanomas include mucosal and desmoplastic melanomas. Mucosal melanomas have a poor prognosis. Desmoplastic or neurotropic melanomas are a rare variant of melanoma. These tumors invade perineural tissues and the adventitia of blood vessels. Because of their tendency to recur locally, it is important to obtain microscopically clear margins at the time of resection.

Staging

The *staging system* for melanomas was developed by the American Joint Committee on Cancer (AJCC) and is based on the level or depth of invasion of the primary tumor (based on the systems of *Clark* and *Breslow*, respectively), involvement of regional lymph nodes, in-transit sites, and distant metastases. Fig. 5-2 outlines Clark's classification and Table 5-2 describes the staging system by the AJCC.

Revisions to the staging system are currently being made, which will eliminate Clark's levels from the evaluation of the primary tumor, modify thickness cutoffs to integer numbers of millimeters, consider in-transit metastases as equivalent to nodal disease, include the number of positive nodes rather than their size, and segregate different systemic metastases by site.

Surgical Treatment of Melanomas

Treatment of the primary tumor site consists of wide local excision. Width of margins is dictated by the thickness of the primary tumor, and several studies have led to decreasing margin requirements. One study done by the World Health Organization (WHO) randomized 612 patients with melanomas greater than 2 mm thick to undergo excision with 1- or 2-cm margins. There were four local recurrences, all of which occurred in patients with melanomas 1 to 2 mm thick in the 1-cm margin group. However, there were no statistically significant differences in disease-free or overall survival between the 1-cm and 2-cm margin groups. A subsequent study randomized 486 patients with intermediate thickness melanomas (1 to 4 mm) to either a 2-cm or a 4-cm margin. There were no statistically significant differences between the two groups in terms of local recurrence or overall survival. The wide margin group required skin grafting for closure more frequently than the narrow margin group. The results of this study were updated in 1996 to include 742 patients, and again no significant recurrence or survival differences were observed at that time. The Swedish Melanoma Study Group trial included 769 patients randomized to either 2-cm or 5-cm margins for melanomas 0.8 to 2.0 mm thick. No differences in local or regional recurrence or overall survival were seen during a median follow-up of 5.8 years. In 1998 the MD Anderson Cancer Center reported the results of a retrospective analysis of 278 patients with thick (greater than 4 mm) melanomas. Again no relation was found between margin width (greater than or less than 2 cm) and disease-free or overall survival.

Overall reasonable *guidelines for resection margin* are 1 cm for melanomas less than 1 mm thick and 2-cm margins for intermediate (1 to 4 mm) thickness melanomas. For thick melanomas, there are no significant data determining optimal margins, but higher local recurrence rates of 10% to 20% suggest wider margins should be attained where possible. Ensuring adequate resection margins in melanomas occurring on the digits generally requires amputation of the digit. The proximal phalanges can often be preserved, frequently with distal or subungual melanomas. An important goal with resection of melanomas of the hands and feet should be the preservation of a functional limb. For the

TABLE 5-2. AMERICAN JOINT COMMITTEE ON CANCER STAGING SYSTEM

Stage I	T1	Primary melanoma ≤0.75 mm thick and/or Clark level II, no nodal or systemic metastases
	T2	Primary melanoma 0.76 to 1.5 mm thick and/or Clark level III, no nodal or systemic metastases
Stage II	T3	Primary melanoma 1.51 to 4.00 mm thick and/or Clark level IV, no nodal or systemic metastases
	T4	Primary melanoma >4 mm thick and/or Clark level V, and/or satellites within 2 cm of the primary tumor, no nodal or systemic metastases
Stage III	Any T	Regional nodal and/or in-transit metastases. N1 ≤3-cm nodes, N2 >3-cm nodes
Stage IV	Any T	Systemic metastases
	Any N	

lower extremity, this entails weight bearing, which is dependent on the heel and ball of the plantar surface.

Most excision sites can be closed primarily, provided adequate skin flaps are raised on either side of the site. In the event that primary closure is not possible, a split-thickness skin graft should be applied in most areas. An important exception is the face, where for cosmetic and occasionally functional reasons, a full-thickness skin graft should be used.

Regional lymph nodes are often the first site of melanoma metastasis. If lymph nodes are the only site of tumor spread, their surgical resection may be curative. However, patients with metastatic spread to lymph nodes have markedly decreased survival and are therefore candidates for further, more aggressive treatment. Morbidity associated with lymph node dissections make elective removal of draining basins somewhat controversial, and a substantial effort has been made to determine which patients would benefit from *elective lymph node dissection* (ELND). In patients with thin (less than 1 mm) melanomas, primary wide local excision results in about a 95% cure rate, so elective lymph node dissection would appear unnecessary. Even if there is no clinical evidence of nodal disease, approximately 60% of patients with thick (greater than 4 mm) melanomas will have lymphatic spread diagnosed in a resected lymph node basin. However, 70% will already have distant disease and will not benefit from a lymph node dissection, except for control of clinically evident regional disease. Vigorous debate has persisted over the role of ELND for patients with intermediate (1 to 4 mm) melanomas. Early retrospective studies suggested some survival benefit in patients who underwent the procedure. However, more recently, the results of large randomized trials have become available. No survival benefit was seen in a prospective study by the WHO, in which 553 patients with extremity melanomas of all thicknesses were randomized to undergo ELND or observation. A subsequent WHO study examining patients with truncal melanomas of greater than 1.5-mm thickness also did not demonstrate an overall survival advantage for patients who had undergone ELND. However, survival was improved in a subgroup of patients retrospectively determined to have occult nodal metastases. Another trial, which was conducted at the Mayo Clinic and included 171 patients with all tumor thicknesses, also failed to show statistically significant differences. The Intergroup Melanoma Trial, which was designed in 1981 to examine this question, again failed to demonstrate a survival benefit for the entire group with melanoma. However, retrospective subgroup analysis demonstrated a significant benefit for patients less than 60 years old with intermediate thickness melanomas (1 to 4 mm). Subgroup analysis is vulnerable to false-positive results, and a subsequent prospective study was organized that included patients with intermediate thickness melanomas stratified by age and tumor characteristics. This study demonstrated a survival benefit for all patients with nonulcerated melanomas. Younger patients with trunk melanomas did particularly well, with about a 30% increased survival.

In patients who undergo lymph node dissection for clinically evident metastases or other indications, an effort should be made to perform a thorough lymphadenectomy. In the axilla, this includes level III nodes medial to the pectoralis minor. For groin dissection, this includes all superficial femoral nodes (Fig. 5-3.) These nodes fill the triangle between the sartorius laterally, the adductor muscles medially, and external oblique superiorly. The femoral vein is the deep margin of this group and removal of the group requires ligation of the saphenous vein. The inguinal ligament may need to be split to enable adequate exposure of the basin. Dissection of the deeper iliac and obturator nodes is indicated only if these appear clinically involved, there are three or more positive nodes in the superficial group, or a Cloquet node is involved, which is felt to be indicative of deeper lymphatic spread.

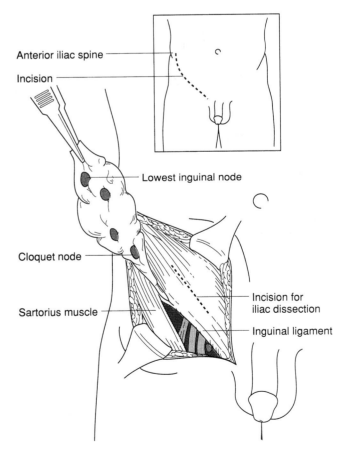

FIGURE 5-3. Technique of groin dissection. (From Chang AE, Johnson TM, Rees RS. Cutaneous neoplasms. In: Greenfield LJ, Mulholland MW, Oldham KT, et al., eds. *Surgery: scientific principles and practice.* Philadelphia: Lippincott-Raven, 1997:2240, with permission.)

For primary melanomas of the head and neck, lymphatic drainage patterns have been mapped and dictate appropriate areas for dissection. Parotid, submandibular, submental, jugular, and posterior triangle lymph nodes drain areas anterior to the ear and superior to the mouth. Anterior lesions inferior to the mouth drain to cervical nodes and posterior lesions drain to occipital, postauricular, posterior triangle, and jugular nodes. A radical neck dissection is generally performed for clinically apparent disease, and a less aggressive, modified dissection is done for an elective node dissection.

Complications of lymph node dissections include infection in 5% to 19%, seroma or lymphocele in 2% to 23%, and lymphedema in 2% to 27% of cases. Their incidence can be reduced by perioperative antibiotic therapy and limb elevation. Over the long-term, patients should be careful to protect the involved limb from insults such as trauma, burns, needle sticks (iatrogenic or accidental), and blood pressure measurements. Development of limb edema may be indicative of lymphatic recurrence. Lymphedema can be treated with limb elevation, application of compression stockings, or gentle diuresis. Severe cases of lymphedema may be treated surgically. Surgical treatment generally includes excision of subcutaneous tissues or microsurgical insertion of lymphatics into local veins using a needle and single securing suture.

Elective lymph node dissection must now be viewed in a considerably different light with the advent of *sentinel lymph node biopsy*. This technique, described by Morton in 1992, involves removal only of the specific lymph node or nodes that first receive drainage from the primary tumor site. Identification of the sentinel node is accomplished by injection of the primary tumor site with tracers shortly before the exploration, generally a vital blue dye and a radiocolloid.

This technique leads to identification of a sentinel node in 93% to 100% of cases. The accuracy of the procedure in evaluating the status of a lymphatic basin is excellent, with false-negative rates of 1% to 4%. The procedure allows identification of patients with subclinical spread to regional lymphatics, as defined by metastatic spread to the sentinel lymph node. These patients then have established staged III disease and should form the population most likely to benefit from complete regional node dissections. At the same time, unnecessary dissections are avoided in patients without lymphatic spread.

Adjuvant Therapy for Lymphatic Spread

Radiation therapy may be used as an adjunct to surgery for locoregional control. Patients with involvement of multiple regional lymph nodes or extracapsular spread should be considered for radiotherapy. When used alone in clinically node-negative patients or with surgery in node-positive patients, an 85% local control rate is achieved. It should be remembered, however, that the risk of complications after a combination of surgical resection of the lymphatic basin and radiation to the basin is severalfold greater than with either modality alone.

In-transit metastases are sites of tumor growth in subcutaneous tissues along the lymphatic drainage pathway between the primary tumor and the regional lymph node basin. There is a 2% to 3% incidence of these metastases. As they are an indication of tumor spread, in-transit metastases are associated with a poorer prognosis. In addition, the prognosis worsens with an increased number of in-transit metastases. In two out of three patients with in-transit metastases, regional lymph nodes are also involved.

Treatment includes excision and lymph node dissection. If the extent or location of disease renders them unresectable, radiation therapy may provide effective palliation. More recently, isolated limb perfusion has been used with good results in achieving local control. This technique involves vascular isolation of the limb and circulation of high doses of heated chemotherapeutic and biological agents. The most commonly used chemotherapeutic agent is melphalan. This has been combined with tumor necrosis factor alpha (TNF-α) and/or interferon-gamma (IFN-γ). Complete local response rates for melphalan alone are approximately 40%, and complete local responses as high as 90% have been reported for combinations of melphalan, TNF-α and IFN-γ. Intralesional injection of nonspecific immunostimulatory agents such as BCG has also been used with some response. Systemic chemotherapy is a poor option and should be used only as a last resort.

Distant Metastases

Initial evaluation of patients with melanoma should include a history and physical examination, chest x-ray, and liver function tests. If *distant disease* is suspected, a computed tomographic (CT) scan of the chest, abdomen, head, and pelvis should also be obtained, because melanoma spreads most commonly to lung, liver, brain, and bone in decreasing order of frequency. Cardiac, adrenal, pancreatic, visceral, and renal metastases are less commonly encountered. Brain metastases can lead to hemorrhage in 33% to 55% of cases, and strong consideration should be given to their resection. Indeed, a small percentage of patients with solitary brain metastases who undergo resection and radiation therapy survive longer than 5 years. As a rule, though, distant metastases portend a poor prognosis. Median survival after diagnosis is 11 months for lung metastases and 2 to 6 months for liver, brain, or bone metastases.

Treatment of systemic melanoma has not met with much success to date. In patients who are asymptomatic and in poor medical condition, observation alone is often warranted. Surgical resection of metastases can often provide effective palliation of symptoms and lead to a median survival of 16 to 23 months. Radiation therapy may also provide some benefit, particularly with hyperfractionated dosing. Although several chemotherapy regimens have achieved some response rates, success in improving survival has been more difficult to achieve. Combination regimens including DTIC, BCNU, and tamoxifen have resulted in response rates of up to 46% and complete responses in up to 11% of patients.

Biological therapies have also been tried with limited success. Cytokine therapy with IL-2 results in a 10% to 20% response rate, and some of these responses are dramatic. Numerous types of vaccines have also been used or are currently undergoing clinical trials. Infusion of monoclonal antibodies directed against melanoma-specific markers is also being evaluated, as are vaccines using dendritic cells pulsed with melanoma-associated tumor antigens.

Treatment of Local Recurrences

Overall there is approximately a 3% rate of local recurrences. *Recurrence* is defined as regrowth of tumor within 5 cm of the primary resection site. It occurs more frequently in patients with thick (greater than 4 mm) primary tumors (13%), ulcerated tumors (11.5%), and in lesions of the foot, hand, scalp, and face (5% to 12%). Initial local recurrences of low-risk tumors are treated with wide excision. On the other hand, multiple recurrences or recurrences from the high-risk tumor categories noted above should be treated with excision and consideration of isolated limb perfusion. Radiation therapy should be used when isolated limb perfusion is not possible. Local recurrence signals a worse prognosis, with a 3-year median survival and a 20% 10-year survival.

Prognosis

Multiple factors influence the prognosis of melanoma. These include location, gender, thickness, Clark level, ulceration, growth pattern, age, regression, and tumor-infiltrating lymphocytes. Melanomas of the trunk have a worse prognosis than those of the extremities. Primaries of the leg portend a worse prognosis than the arm, and scalp melanomas are worse than those in other head and neck locations are. Disease in women is associated with a better prognosis than in men, which may be due to the fact that they have a higher incidence of extremity melanomas and fewer ulcerated lesions. Matched for stage, however, survival is similar.

Thickness of the primary melanoma (Breslow scale) has been found to be one of the most reliable predictors of prognosis. Provided a representative biopsy is available, it is relatively simple for a pathologist to obtain this number, even with limited experience. The scale is divided into increments of thickness. Tumor thickness is inversely correlated with survival (Fig. 5-4).

The other common measure of depth of invasion, the Clark level, has also been shown to be highly predictive of prognosis. This measurement provides an indicator of biologic invasiveness, but it requires an experienced pathologist for optimal accuracy.

Ulceration is another powerful predictor of long-term survival. In stage I and stage II lesions with ulceration, there is a 50% 5-year survival, while survival for similar, nonulcerated lesions is 75%. In stage III lesions, ulceration decreases 3-year survival from 61% to 29%.

Growth pattern of melanoma is also predictive of survival. Acral lentiginous melanoma is associated with a poorer prognosis than superficial spreading and nodular melanoma. Superficial spreading melanomas are less aggressive than nodular melanomas. Lentigo maligna melanomas carry a slightly better prognosis than superficial spreading melanomas. Even lesions exceeding 3 mm in thickness have an 80% 10-year survival.

Presence of nodal or distant metastases is the strongest prognostic variable. Patients with clinically positive nodes have a 12% 10-year survival; those with occult positive nodes found during ELND have a 48% 10-year survival, while those who are node negative have a 64% 10-year survival.

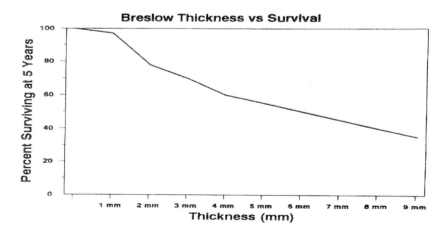

FIGURE 5-4. There is a linear relationship between increasing melanoma tumor thickness at diagnosis and decreasing survival.

There exists an inverse correlation between age and survival. Older patients generally present with thicker melanomas and do accordingly worse. Regression of lesions is a poor prognostic indicator, and tumor-infiltrating lymphocytes are associated with increased survival.

Multifactorial analysis reveals dominance of thickness, ulceration, and location as prognostic factors with lesser influence of initial surgical management, stage, and level of invasion.

SOFT TISSUE SARCOMA

Sarcomas are tumors derived from mesenchymal cells. The term *sarcoma* comes from the Greek *sar,* meaning flesh. For clinical purposes, a basic division exists between extremity and truncal sarcomas. Extremity sarcomas represent approximately half of adult sarcomas while truncal sarcomas represent 30%. About half of truncal sarcomas occur in the retroperitoneum.

Sarcomas have an age-adjusted incidence of 2 per 100,000 and represent about 1% of adult malignancies and 7% of pediatric malignancies. In the United States, there are approximately 6,000 cases per year, and cases are divided equally between men and women.

Etiology

Several genetic syndromes are associated with the development of sarcomas. Gardner syndrome is associated with the formation of multiple desmoid tumors. Li-Fraumeni syndrome, a familial cancer syndrome that is associated with an increased risk for soft tissue sarcomas, osteosarcomas, breast cancer, acute leukemia, brain tumors, adrenocortical carcinomas, and gonadal germ-cell tumors, is linked to a mutation in the p53 tumor suppressor gene. Neurofibromatosis I, or von Recklinghausen disease, is an autosomal dominant disorder characterized by multiple neurofibromas and café au lait spots. Sarcomas have also been associated with amplification of the MDM2 gene, whose product interacts with p53.

Environmental factors have also been linked to induction of sarcomas. It has been speculated that herbicides may play a role in some cases as well as previous radiation exposure. There is generally a considerable delay of 10 years or more between radiation exposure and onset of disease.

Stewart-Treves syndrome is defined as the development of an angiosarcoma associated with lymphedema, classically in breast cancer patients following removal of the tumor and axillary lymph node dissection.

Extremity Sarcomas

The clinical evaluation and treatment of sarcomas is dictated in part by their location. Extremity soft tissue sarcomas will be considered first followed by retroperitoneal sarcomas.

Diagnosis

Diagnosis begins with a complete history and a thorough physical examination. During the early course of disease, clinical manifestations are infrequent and a mass is the most common presenting complaint. Frequently a trivial traumatic event may have initially drawn attention to the area, although there is probably no causal relation between a history of trauma and the development of a sarcoma.

When a suspicious mass is discovered, a *biopsy* is indicated. In centers in which there is significant experience with sarcomas, a needle biopsy may be performed as a first step. Care should be taken to insert the needle through areas that would be incorporated into a definitive resection. However, in most centers, an open biopsy is the most reliable means of gaining a diagnosis. Lesions smaller than 3 cm can be completely excised while an incisional biopsy is often appropriate for lesions larger than 3 cm. It is critical that the dissection, including the skin incision, is planned so that the biopsy tract can be excised completely in the final resection. Incisional biopsies on extremities are performed through longitudinal skin incisions. Meticulous hemostasis is also important as hemorrhage dissecting down tissue planes can spread tumor cells and lead to the need for a much more extensive definitive resection.

Staging

Once a tissue specimen has been obtained, the pathologist can determine the histologic type of sarcoma. These include liposarcoma, fibrosarcoma, fibroxanthoma, leiomyosarcoma, rhabdomyosarcoma, lymphangiosarcoma, synovial sarcoma, and malignant neurilemoma. These categories are based on the appearance of the tumors and their presumed sites of origin. The most common soft tissue sarcomas in adults are malignant fibrous histiocytomas and liposarcomas while rhabdomyosarcomas and fibrosarcomas are the most prevalent types in the pediatric population. There is only a 65% concordance between different pathologists in assigning type. Pathologic grade is a much more significant prognostic parameter and is more reproducible between pathologists. It is based on differentiation of cells, cellularity of the specimen, amount of stroma, vascularity, degree of necrosis, and number of mitoses per high power field.

Radiologic imaging studies are invaluable prior to definitive resection of a sarcoma. The goal of these studies is to define the extent of the tumor so that a resection can be planned and patients can be informed of probable outcomes. The most commonly used imaging modalities for evaluation of soft tissue sarcomas are CT and magnetic resonance imaging (MRI) with or without magnetic resonance angiography (MRA). Although CT scanning is less expensive and easier to obtain, MRI provides better resolution of soft tissues. In addition, the relationship of tumors to blood vessels can be more accurately determined by MRA. Bone scanning is sensitive for bony involvement but is not specific enough to distinguish tumor extension from reactive inflammation. Angiography may be useful in selected cases of retroperitoneal or extremity sarcomas. Because sarcomas commonly spread to the lungs via the hematogenous route, a CT scan of the chest is also indicated to rule out metastatic disease.

The combination of histologic and radiographic information can then be used to stage the patient. Multiple staging systems have been used in the past. These systems are based on the histologic grade of the tumor, its size, and the presence of metastases in regional lymph nodes or distant sites. The AJCC produced a revised staging system in 1997. *Histopathologic grade* is divided into well differentiated (G1), moderately differentiated (G2), poorly differentiated (G3), and undifferentiated (G4). Tumors less than or equal to 5 cm in greatest dimension (T1) are separated from tumors greater than 5 cm (T2). The size classification is subdivided into superficial and deep tumors noted with the suffixes a and b, respectively. *Stage IV disease* is defined as the presence of regional lymph node metastases (N1) or distant metastases (M1) (Table 5-3).

This staging system has been found to correlate well with rates at 5 years of local recurrence, disease-free survival, and overall survival. Five-year survival is only 10% if metastatic disease is present (Fig. 5-5).

Surgical Treatment

Resection is the mainstay of treatment, though other modalities are useful as adjuvants. Sarcomas are characterized by a pseudocapsule. This cannot be used as a plane of dissection, as microscopic disease extends beyond the pseudocapsule and will inevitably lead to local recurrence. Local recurrence rates improved dramatically to 20% when this was recognized and radical resection was performed with excision of entire muscle groups. Significant morbidity was associated with this approach because it can lead to significant impairment of limb function or even amputation. In addition, in patients who went on to die from distant disease, the increased morbidity of radical resections

TABLE 5-3. AMERICAN JOINT COMMITTEE ON CANCER SARCOMA STAGING SYSTEM

Stage I
  A   Low grade, small, superficial/deep G1–2, T1a-b, N0, M0
  B   Low grade, large, superficial G1–2, T2a, N0, M0
Stage II
  A   Low grade, large, deep G1–2, T2b, N0, M0
  B   High grade, small, superficial/deep G3–4, T1a-b, N0, M0
  C   High grade, large, superficial G3–4, T2a, N0, M0
Stage III
       High grade, large, deep G3–4, T2b, N0, M0
Stage IV
       Any metastasis any G, any T, N1, or M1

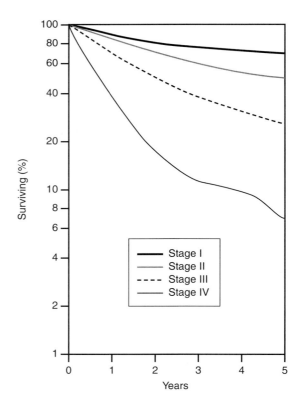

FIGURE 5-5. Sarcoma survival by stage of disease. (From Sondak VK. Sarcomas of bone and soft tissue. In: Greenfield LJ, Mulholland MW, Oldham KT, et al., eds. *Surgery:* scientific principles and practice. Philadelphia: Lippincott-Raven, 1997:2250, with permission.)

was unnecessary. Recent focus has therefore been placed on preservation of limbs and limb function by limiting resection.

Limb preservation has been increased by acceptance of a 2-cm resection margin in the setting of low-grade sarcomas less than 5 cm in diameter (Fig. 5-6). In the case of high-grade sarcomas, limb function can be preserved through a combination of limited resection and adjuvant radiotherapy. Equivalent disease-free and overall survival rates have been reported with limb-sparing procedures in conjunction with radiotherapy, compared to amputation.

Adjuvant Therapy

Radiotherapy can be administered before, after, or during surgery and is indicated in patients with tumors greater than 5 cm or close resection margins. It may be given as beam radiation or in the form of brachytherapy. There have been no studies directly comparing these methods of administration and no marked difference in local control has been noted with each method measured separately. Each technique offers some advantages and disadvantages, which may guide the physician's choice of modality. Preoperative radiotherapy has the advantages of requiring a smaller field of radiation exposure as well as a lower dose

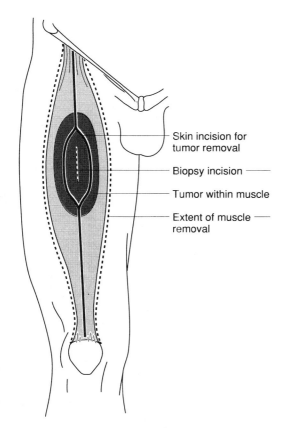

FIGURE 5-6. Plan for sarcoma resection showing longitudinal biopsy incision and wide excision border, sparing limb function. (From Sondak VK. Sarcomas of bone and soft tissue. In: Greenfield LJ, Mulholland MW, Oldham KT, et al., eds. *Surgery:* scientific principles and practice. Philadelphia: Lippincott-Raven, 1997:2257, with permission.)

than postoperative radiation due to relative hypoxia at the resection site. However, preoperative radiation has been demonstrated to have a significantly higher wound complication rate than postoperative radiation without a significant benefit in terms of local recurrence or survival. Therefore, preoperative radiotherapy is generally reserved for patients whose tumors are initially considered too large to resect with acceptable morbidity.

Brachytherapy is a relatively new technique in which radioactive isotopes are placed in close proximity to the tumor for a period of 5 to 6 days. Although this technique is associated with similar rates of wound complications as postoperative external beam radiotherapy (provided therapy is delayed at least 5 days after surgery), it has the advantages of less radiation scatter and a much shorter duration of therapy. Brachytherapy is only indicated in the setting of high-grade lesions while external beam radiation is indicated for low-grade lesions.

Adjuvant systemic *chemotherapy* has also been used in patients with sarcoma. Trials of postoperative chemotherapy have generally demonstrated no survival benefit. A recent metaanalysis of individual data from previous trials revealed statistically significant improvements in local recurrence-free and disease-free survival rates in patients who received doxorubicin-containing postoperative chemotherapy. However, the same analysis did not show any improvement in overall survival, and postoperative chemotherapy cannot be considered standard therapy.

Preoperative or neoadjuvant chemotherapy has also had fairly poor results with doxorubicin-based regimens, resulting in 3% to 27% response rates. Preliminary studies using combinations of doxorubicin and ifosfamide have shown some improvement in response rates. Approaches using only chemotherapy as adjuvant treatment have been largely abandoned in favor of protocols that combine multiple modalities.

Sequential or concurrent use of chemotherapy and radiation therapy has demonstrated promising short-term results, with improvements in local control, disease-free survival, and overall survival. However, these results will require longer follow-up and confirmation before the combined modality therapy moves beyond the investigational stage.

Finally, localized therapy in the form of *isolated limb perfusion* (ILP) with chemotherapeutic agents such as melphalan in combination with TNF-α and/or IFN-γ can be used in cases where local control or limb salvage is particularly challenging. Toxicity in the perfused limb is generally not severe and is often related to necrosis of the tumor. Systemic toxicity can be severe if there is a leak of perfusate into the systemic circulation.

This technique provides only regional therapy, so its application is limited to certain specific situations. These include locally advanced disease that would otherwise require amputation for local control. ILP has demonstrated limb salvage rates of greater than 80%. In addition, ILP may be used in patients with stage IV disease that is advanced at the site of origin. ILP may preserve the function of the affected limb and quality of life over the anticipated short period of survival of these patients.

Sarcomas spread via the hematogenous route. Therefore, regional lymph node involvement is unusual and elective lymph node dissection is generally not indicated. One possible exception is in the case of epithelioid sarcomas in which metastases to regional lymph nodes are found in approximately 20% of cases. Nodal metastases are also seen in 10% of rhabdomyosarcomas and 5% of malignant fibrous histiocytomas.

Local recurrence of sarcoma is associated with a poor prognosis. However, it has not been determined if there exists a causal relationship to decreased survival. The site of recurrence may be a source for further metastasis. However, the fact that even amputation of the recurrent site does not improve survival suggests that distant disease may have already been present at the time of the local recurrence. Local recurrences should be treated by excision. Considerations for preservation of limb function are analogous to those in primary resections, and radiotherapy should also be considered. Even if the site has been previously irradiated, brachytherapy or intraoperative radiotherapy may be options for additional treatment. Finally, chemotherapy should be considered for patients with local recurrences of high-grade tumors. Approximately two thirds of patients who undergo resections for local recurrences will experience long-term survival.

Patients who die from their disease generally succumb to distant metastases. The tumors with higher histologic grades and those exceeding 5 cm in size have a higher propensity to metastasize. Longer intervals from the treatment of the primary tumor to occurrence of metastatic disease are associated with a better prognosis. The lungs are the most common site of metastasis. Pulmonary lesions should be resected, provided the patient can tolerate the operation and has adequate pulmonary reserve. Survival at 5 years in patients with completely resected pulmonary metastases is 15% to 30%.

Retroperitoneal Sarcoma

Retroperitoneal sarcomas are considerably less common than extremity sarcomas, making up only 15% to 25% of all cases. However, these tumors carry a much worse prognosis, as 80% are high grade, and due to a relative lack of clinical signs during early stages of disease, they are frequently not diagnosed until they have reached a relatively advanced stage. The progress in patient outcomes and quality of life, which has been evident in the treatment of extremity sarcoma, has not been mirrored in retroperitoneal sarcomas.

Diagnosis

Most patients present with an abdominal mass (80%) and many have lower extremity neurological symptoms (42%) or pain (37%). Most tumors are greater than 10 cm in diameter at the time of presentation and the most common histologic types are liposarcoma (41%), leiomyosarcoma (27%), and malignant fibrous histiocytoma (7%).

Evaluation of a suspected retroperitoneal sarcoma should include CT scanning to evaluate the local extent of disease and the presence of hepatic metastases. It is important in this anatomic region to distinguish sarcoma from lymphoma and germ-cell tumors, which are amenable to chemotherapy. This can be accomplished with a CT or ultrasound-guided fine-needle aspirate, or if that is inadequate, a guided core biopsy. If lymphoma or germ-cell tumor is not part of the differential diagnosis, biopsy is only performed if neoadjuvant therapy is considered. An abdominal/pelvic MRI and/or MRA may be necessary to delineate involvement of adjacent vasculature. Metastatic workup should include a CT scan of the chest.

Treatment

Chemotherapy has not been shown to be effective for these tumors and radiation is limited by toxicity to adjacent structures. As a result, surgery offers the only effective treatment. Complete gross resection is possible in over three fourths of initial presentations and frequently requires resection of neighboring organs. Patients who have unresectable tumors on the basis of radiologic studies may be candidates for neoadjuvant chemotherapy and radiation in an attempt to decrease tumor size to the point where it is resectable. Resection should be attempted only if a complete resection is anticipated, because incomplete resection has not been shown to offer any benefit in survival (Fig. 5-7).

Approximately one fourth of patients with complete gross resections will have positive microscopic margins. Patients who have high-grade sarcomas do significantly worse than those with low-grade tumors (median survival 33 months versus 149 months). Approximately half of the patients who suffer local recurrences will have disease that is grossly resectable. Resection is the only effective treatment for such a recurrence. Trials of tumor debulking or cytoreduction combined with other intraoperative modalities such as photodynamic therapy, hyperthermic intraperitoneal chemotherapy, and intraoperative radiotherapy have shown some promise but are currently only investigational. Distant disease most frequently occurs in the liver (44%), lung (38%), or both (18%). If the distant disease is isolated, it should be considered for resection. Patients with metastatic disease have only a 10-month median survival.

Because early recognition of metastases—while resection is still possible—offers patients the only hope of cure, patients with no evidence of disease should be followed closely for signs of recurrence. This follow-up should include history and physical examination every 3 months for the first 2 years with a chest radiograph every 6 months. Any radiographic abnormalities should be further evaluated with a CT scan of the chest. The site of the primary tumor should be evaluated with MRI scanning every 6 months for the first 2 years, particularly if the primary tumor was in a deep location. After the first 2 years, patients should

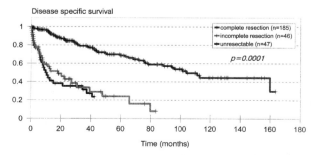

FIGURE 5-7. Incomplete resection provides no survival benefit. (From Lewis JJ, Leung D, Woodruff JM, et al. Retroperitoneal soft tissue sarcoma. *Ann Surg* 228(3):355–365, with permission.)

undergo a history and physical examination every 6 months for the following 3 years.

LYMPHOMA

Surgeons are often asked to participate in the care of lymphoma patients for specific reasons: diagnosis, intravenous access, or to treat complications of the disease. Hematologic malignancies are the most common malignancies of children younger than 15 years and constitute 6% to 8% of adult cancers.

Lymph Node Biopsy

One of the most common reasons for surgical consultation for patients with lymphoma is for obtaining tissue for diagnosis. The importance of tissue architecture in pathologic classification and the need for a significant amount of tissue for special studies leads to the need for surgical biopsy rather than fine-needle aspirate or core biopsy. One exception to this is for evaluation of recurrence when a needle biopsy may be sufficient.

Generally the largest node is removed because this provides the greatest chance for a positive result and the greatest amount of tissue for study. Though ease of removal is a consideration for choosing the biopsy site, cervical or axillary nodes are generally preferred over inguinal nodes, as nodal enlargement due to reactive inflammation is less likely.

Hodgkin Lymphoma

These patients typically present in young adulthood with nontender lymphadenopathy. Cervical lymph node basins are the most commonly involved sites at presentation, with axillary, inguinal, mediastinal, and retroperitoneal basins involved less frequently. Patients may report the presence of other symptoms such as fever (greater than 38°C), night sweats, or weight loss of more than 10% of body weight over a 6-month period. These are the so-called *B symptoms* in Hodgkin disease and are used in staging, as discussed below.

In addition to a complete history including duration of the enlargement or recent injury to sites drained by that lymphatic basin, the evaluation of patients referred for lymph node biopsy should include a physical examination, with complete evaluation of all accessible lymphatic tissue. This includes palpation of all superficial lymph node basins, oropharyngeal examination with evaluation of tonsils, and abdominal palpation for hepatic or splenic enlargement. Laboratory studies should include a complete blood count with differential and peripheral blood smear examination.

Staging in Hodgkin disease is based on the extent of disease and the presence or absence of the symptoms. Stage I disease is limited to a single lymph node region or single extralymphatic site. Stage II is characterized by involvement of two or more lymph node regions on the same side of the diaphragm or one extralymphatic site with only adjacent lymph nodes involved. In stage III disease, lymph nodes on both sides of the diaphragm or the spleen (denoted with an *S*) are involved, and stage IV consists of diffuse or disseminated involvement of one or more extralymphatic sites with or without associated lymph node involvement. The absence of symptoms is denoted with an *A* in staging and their presence is denoted with a *B*.

Staging workup includes liver function tests and chest radiographs. CT scans are frequently used to evaluate the presence of mediastinal or retroperitoneal lymphadenopathy. Bone marrow biopsies provide additional information regarding the extent of disease.

The cornerstones of treatment of Hodgkin lymphoma are radiation therapy for stage I and IIA disease, and chemotherapy in combination with radiation for patients with stage III disease and above.

The *staging laparotomy* has historically played an important role in the complete evaluation of patients with Hodgkin disease. The goal of this procedure is to provide a thorough evaluation of the abdomen and retroperitoneum for the presence of disease and thereby distinguish between low-stage and advanced lymphoma. The procedure entails a midline laparotomy and palpation of the liver, small bowel, colon, and mesentery. Intraoperative ultrasound may be used as an adjunct to palpation for evaluation of deeper areas within solid organs. Splenectomy and wedge biopsies of the liver are also performed with additional Tru-cut biopsies of deeper hepatic tissue. Each major nodal group is then dissected. Nodes associated with the hepatic artery and celiac axis are removed via an incision in the gastrohepatic ligament. Nodes from the porta hepatis are also removed with particular attention to the so-called *sentinel node* at the junction of the portal vein and duodenum. Finally, the aorta is exposed inferior to the transverse mesocolon and nodes removed down to the inferior mesenteric artery. If there are any nodes that are suspicious based on evaluation at laparotomy or preoperative lymphangiography, these should also be removed with concomitant oophoropexy in anticipation of radiation to the pelvis (Fig. 5-8).

Improved radiographic imaging has led to a reduced need for staging laparotomies to choose a therapeutic approach (Fig. 5-9). Patients with early stage disease and favorable histology almost always have disease limited to supradiaphragmatic nodal tissue and can be safely treated with mantle radiation therapy only. In addition, improved efficacy and safety of chemotherapy have led to its more liberal administration in more advanced Hodgkin disease without laparotomy. However, staging laparotomy is still useful in cases where negative results would obviate the need for chemotherapy.

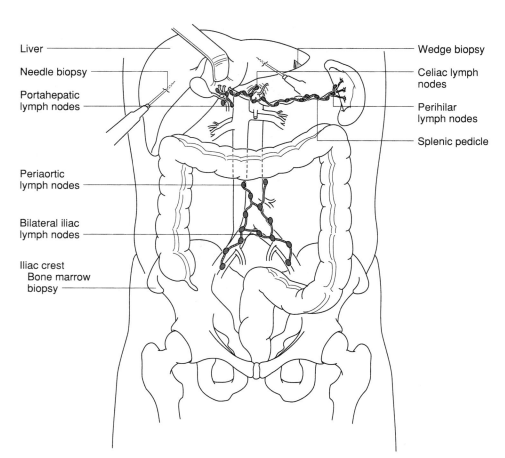

FIGURE 5-8. Biopsy sites during staging laparotomy. (From Meyer AA. Spleen. In: Greenfield LJ, Mulholland MW, Oldham KT, et al., eds. *Surgery: scientific principles and practice.* Philadelphia: Lippincott-Raven, 1997:1275, with permission.)

Non-Hodgkin Lymphoma

Non-Hodgkin lymphoma is increasing in incidence in the United States and now represents approximately 7% of malignancies. Some of this increase can be attributed to increasing numbers and life expectancies of patients with acquired immunodeficiency syndrome (AIDS). Patients typically present with lymphadenopathy. Histologically the tumors are classified as diffuse versus follicular, small cell versus large cell, and cleaved versus noncleaved nuclear morphology. Most cases are of B-cell origin (80%). Using pathologic information, non-Hodgkin lymphomas are classified as low, intermediate, or high grade based on their prognosis.

Surgeons are typically called on to obtain tissue for diagnosis. The use of a staging laparotomy is extremely limited in patients with non-Hodgkin lymphoma, because this disease generally does not progress in the orderly manner that Hodgkin lymphoma does and patients therefore typically present with advanced disease.

Gastrointestinal Lymphomas

The *stomach* is the most common site of extranodal non-Hodgkin lymphoma in the United States. Gastric lymphoma

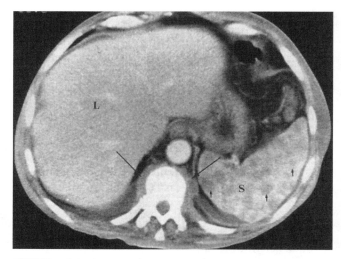

FIGURE 5-9. Computed tomography scan demonstrating involvement of both the spleen and paraaortic lymph nodes. (From Brant WE. Pancreas and spleen. In: Brant WE, Helms CA, eds. *Fundamentals of diagnostic radiology,* 2nd ed. Philadelphia: Lippincott Williams & Wilkins, 1998:710, with permission.)

is the second most common tumor of the stomach, representing 2% to 7% of primary gastric malignancies. Patients typically present with abdominal pain (71% to 85%), weight loss (11% to 68%), nausea or vomiting (14% to 28%), bleeding (7% to 23%), or rarely, perforation (0% to 6%).

Patients will usually undergo endoscopic evaluation, which has recently become increasingly effective in diagnosing lymphoma, with reports of 92% to 100% sensitivity. The technique is not completely accurate though, as 25% of cases of gastric lymphoma are diagnosed only as cancer, and not lymphoma, before operation.

There are several systems for staging GI lymphomas. The Ann Arbor system uses the suffix E to identify lymphomas that originate in extranodal tissue. The TNM staging system is also used. Tumor stage is based on level of invasion, nodal stage is based on the presence and location of lymph nodes positive for tumor, and metastasis stage is based on the presence of distant metastasis (Table 5-4).

This system correlates well with patient survival but does not take tumor grade into account. A third system proposed as the result of a workshop in 1994 presents a system for pathologic classification that incorporates tumor grade. Prognosis correlates with both stage and grade and correlates more closely when both variables are considered.

Treatment for gastric lymphomas is highly variable. Numerous studies have demonstrated that surgery alone is an effective therapy for early (stage I_E or II_E) stage disease. However, other studies have demonstrated no additional benefit to surgery in patients treated with chemotherapy and radiation therapy. One difficulty in evaluating these results is that there are no prospective randomized trials of surgical versus nonsurgical treatment. Single-modality treatment with surgery, radiation, or chemotherapy is appropriate for early stage disease, and multimodality treatment including chemotherapy is indicated for more advanced (stage II_E or stage I, high grade) disease. Most centers employ surgical treatment in patients with early stage disease as well as in patients with advanced stages of disease who present with bleeding or obstruction.

Gastric Mucosa Associated Lymphoid Tissue Lymphoma

Gastric mucosa-associated lymphoid tissue (MALT) lymphoma is a collection of lymphoid tissue in the stomach that resembles the mucosa-associated lymphoid tissue rather than nodal lymphoid tissue. It is felt to be a precursor of gastric lymphoma and is associated with *Helicobacter pylori* infection. Proliferation of malignant, monoclonal B cells is stimulated by IL-2 released by nonneoplastic T cells in response to the infection. Treatment with antibiotics to eliminate the infection is highly effective in cases of low-grade MALT lymphoma. Patients who fail to respond completely to antibiotic therapy should undergo surgical resection and possibly chemotherapy based on the pathology of the surgical specimen.

Other Gastrointestinal Lymphomas

Lymphomas of the small bowel are less common in the United States but are the most common extranodal lymphoma in the Middle East. These tumors have a higher incidence in patients who suffer from celiac disease and are typically located in the proximal jejunum. These tumors can present with obstruction, intussusception, or bleeding. They are multiple in 20% of cases, and treatment is limited resection with chemotherapy. Radiation therapy can be considered as an additional modality. However, its usefulness is limited by radiation enteritis. Survival at 5 years is about 40%.

Colonic lymphomas are quite rare, although they are the most common noncarcinomatous tumors of the large bowel. Occasionally systemic non-Hodgkin lymphoma can lead to diffuse lymphomatous polyposis. Treatment of these tumors also consists of local resection of involved bowel with adjuvant therapy dictated by the stage and grade of the disease. Overall survival at 5 years after complete resection is 50%.

SPLEEN

Surgical intervention is frequently required in the care of patients with splenic complications of hematologic disorders or trauma. This section will consider the normal

TABLE 5-4. PRIMARY GASTRIC LYMPHOMA STAGING: TNM

Tumor stage (depth of invasion)
T1: lamina propria or submucosa
T2: muscularis propria
T3: subserosa
T4: serosa (adjacent structures free)
T5: adjacent structures

Metastasis stage
M0: no metastases
M1: distant metastases

Nodal stage
N0: node negative
N1: perigastric nodes
N2: perigastric nodes >3 cm from stomach or along hepatic, left gastric, splenic or celiac arteries
N3: hepatoduodenal, paraaortic, or distant abdominal nodes
N4: nodes beyond N3

Stage	Tumor	Nodes	Metastasis	5-yr survival
I	T1	N0,N1	M0	100%
II	T1	N2	M0	88.9%
	T2,T3	N0,N1,N2	M0	
III	T4,T5	Any N	M0	52.1%
	Any T	N3,N4	M0	
IV	Any T	Any N	M1	25%

anatomy and function of the spleen and discuss surgical care of patients with abnormalities manifested in the spleen due to disease or trauma.

Anatomy and Normal Function

The spleen arises from embryologic mesoderm along the left side of the dorsal mesogastrium and attains a weight of 100 to 150 g in the normal adult. It is a solid, purplish organ located in the left upper quadrant that measures approximately 12 × 7 × 4 cm and stretches from the eighth to the eleventh rib. Its blood supply arises from the splenic artery off the celiac trunk and from the short gastric arteries, arising from the left gastroepiploic artery. It is surrounded by a fibroelastic capsule 1 to 2 mm in thickness. In humans there is no significant smooth muscle in the capsule to affect autotransfusion in response to circulating catecholamines, as is the case in dogs and cats. The spleen is attached by so-called *ligaments* of connective tissue to surrounding structures. These include the gastrosplenic ligament containing the short gastric arteries as well as the avascular splenorenal, splenophrenic, and splenocolic ligaments.

The parenchyma of the spleen is divided into the red and white pulps, which are the sites of filtration of senescent or abnormal red blood cells and other unwanted elements from the blood and generation of effective lymphoid immune responses, respectively. Blood is carried into the spleen from the hilum via trabecular arteries, which branch further and form the central arterioles. The central arteriole is surrounded by white pulp over much of its course and empties either into the red pulp from open-ended penicillary arterioles or into venules through a closed circulation without being directly exposed to the red pulp. After entering venous sinusoids, it proceeds to trabecular veins and exits via the splenic vein (Fig. 5-10).

The red pulp is composed of spongelike areas of tissue known as the *cords of Billroth*. They contain a large number of macrophages that function to remove aged or defective red blood cells. They also remove inclusions from cells such as Heinz or Howell-Jolly bodies. In autoimmune hemolytic anemia, these macrophages recognize and destroy red blood cells coated with autoantibodies. Bacteria, cellular debris, and other abnormal debris are also filtered in the red pulp.

The spleen is one of the secondary lymphoid organs. The majority of splenic lymphoid activity occurs in the white pulp. One particularly important lymphoid function performed by the spleen is the generation of primary antibody responses. It is well suited to this function, as serum and any foreign antigens contained within it are skimmed from trabecular and central arteries and percolate through the white pulp and sinusoids where they may be taken up, processed, and presented by macrophages or dendritic cells. This generally takes place in the T-cell dominated periarterial sheaths. Lymphocyte responses are generated in lymphoid nodules that are primarily composed of B cells and follicular dendritic cells and are spaced out along the artery. If an antigen is properly presented by antigen-presenting cells and recognized by lymphocytes, a germinal

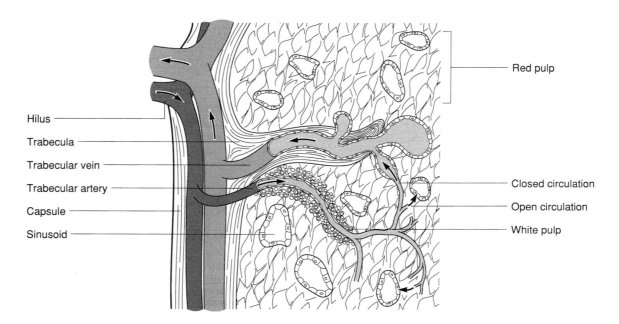

FIGURE 5-10. The splenic microcirculation is shown with depictions of both open and closed circulation. (From Meyer AA. Spleen. In: Greenfield LJ, Mulholland MW, Oldham KT, et al., eds. *Surgery:* scientific principles and practice. Philadelphia: Lippincott-Raven, 1997:1265, with permission.)

center containing proliferating lymphocytes forms within the follicle. The spleen is central to the development of new antibody responses characterized by the production of IgM.

The spleen has other functions including production of monocytes and lymphocytes and storage of 30% to 40% of the body's platelets. It serves as a site of hematopoiesis during early development and in some pathologic conditions.

Splenomegaly

Surgical consultation is frequently sought for splenomegaly. The differential diagnosis includes infectious, hematologic, neoplastic (both hematologic and nonhematologic), congestive, inflammatory, and infiltrative processes.

Malaria is the most common *infectious* cause for splenic enlargement in tropical regions of the world, while splenomegaly due to mononucleosis is more prevalent in the developed world. In addition, AIDS, viral hepatitis, cytomegalovirus, tuberculosis, hepatic echinococcosis, and congenital syphilis may lead to splenomegaly.

Hematologic disorders are among the most common causes of splenic enlargement. These include disorders of red blood cells such as spherocytosis, early sickle-cell disease, thalassemia major, paroxysmal nocturnal hemoglobinuria, hemoglobinopathies, and autoimmune hemolytic anemia. Generally, in these disorders the spleen is congested due to an attempt to clear abnormal erythrocytes from the circulation. In advanced stages of sickle-cell disease, the spleen eventually undergoes autoinfarction due to occlusion of its vasculature by distorted red blood cells.

Myeloproliferative disorders are characterized by overproduction of one or more hematologic cell lines. These syndromes include polycythemia vera, myelogenous leukemia, and idiopathic thrombocytosis. Myeloproliferative disorders are often accompanied by replacement of bone marrow with fibrous tissue, or myelofibrosis, leading to extramedullary hematopoiesis. This combined with infiltration of the spleen with abnormal blood components can result in massive splenomegaly.

Hematologic neoplasms such as lymphomas and leukemias are also responsible for a significant proportion of enlarged spleens. Hairy cell leukemia is commonly associated with pancytopenia and splenomegaly and select cases respond well to splenectomy as primary treatment.

Extrasplenic tumors such as melanomas and lung and breast malignancies may also metastasize to the spleen. Generally, involvement of the spleen occurs when the primary tumor becomes widely metastatic. In addition, nonhematologic primary tumors such as sarcomas, hemangiomas, and hamartomas may arise in the spleen.

Congestion within the portal venous system, which may be due to primary hepatic disease, thrombosis of the hepatic, portal, or splenic veins, or failure of the right side of the heart, can also result in splenomegaly. Pancreatitis is the most common cause of *splenic vein thrombosis*. This condition frequently results in gastric varices and can be treated with splenectomy. The likelihood of functional hypersplenism increases with the duration of congestion and splenomegaly.

Inflammatory or *autoimmune conditions* may result in reactive hyperplasia of the spleen and splenomegaly. This is seen in a variety of disorders including infectious mononucleosis, autoimmune hemolytic anemia, and systemic lupus erythematosus. Rheumatoid arthritis, when accompanied by splenomegaly and neutropenia, is known as *Felty syndrome*. This condition is associated with antibodies against granulocytes and responds well to splenectomy.

Splenomegaly may also result from *infiltration with extracellular or intracellular material*. Sarcoidosis and amyloidosis are examples of disorders in which extracellular accumulation occurs. Several enzymatic defects that result in abnormal storage or degradation products such as gangliosides and mucopolysaccharides can lead to their accumulation in the reticuloendothelial system and consequently enlargement of the liver, spleen, and lymph nodes. Gaucher disease (β-glucocerebrosidase deficiency) and Niemann-Pick disease (sphingomyelinase deficiency) are examples of such disorders.

Splenectomy

Splenectomy is indicated as treatment for severe symptoms of splenomegaly and hypersplenism, as a diagnostic procedure, and in some cases of splenic trauma.

Splenectomy may be indicated in some cases to relieve the effects of increased splenic size alone. In such cases, the massive size of the spleen causes symptoms such as shortness of breath, early satiety, and weight loss secondary to displacement of neighboring structures such as the stomach or diaphragm.

In other cases, the spleen may need to be removed due to clinical consequences of its function, as in the case of *hypersplenism*. Though hypersplenism may be associated with splenomegaly, the syndrome is currently defined based on its functional consequences rather than organ size. The clinical picture is one of deficiency and increased turnover in one or more hematologic cell lines with increased or normal cellularity of the bone marrow. Hypersplenism may in rare cases be a primary disorder, but it is generally secondary to another systemic abnormality. In such cases of secondary hypersplenism, the spleen functions normally, but abnormalities in blood components lead to excessive destruction or sequestration in the spleen.

Some *hematologic diseases* are responsive to splenectomy. *Hereditary spherocytosis*, the most common symptomatic familial hemolytic anemia, is characterized by defective erythrocyte membranes due to a deficiency in spectrin. The red blood cells are relatively fragile and are therefore destroyed after only a few passes through the splenic cords, resulting in anemia, jaundice, intractable leg ulcers, and an increased incidence of gallstones. Splenectomy should be delayed until after the age of 3 in order to reduce the incidence of infectious complications. Though the red blood cell defect persists after splenectomy, symptoms are generally relieved completely. Cholecystectomy should be performed at the time of splenectomy in patients who have developed pigment gallstones before the procedure. *Hereditary elliptocytosis* is a similar, though less severe, disorder of red blood cell membranes. Splenectomy may be indicated in these patients depending on the severity of associated symptoms. *Thalassemia major* and *sickle-cell disease* are red blood cell disorders characterized by abnormal hemoglobin and increased red blood cell destruction. Splenectomy is not generally indicated in either disorder, but it may decrease transfusion requirements in some cases of thalassemia and may be useful in some episodes of splenic sequestration in sickle-cell disease. *Autoimmune hemolytic anemia* is characterized by autoantibodies to red blood cells, which develop after exposure to certain drugs, during the course of a collagen vascular disease or infection, or in up to 50% of cases, without an identifiable cause. Penicillin, quinidine, hydralazine, and methyldopa are the drugs most commonly implicated in inducing autoimmune hemolysis. Antibodies are classified as *warm* or *cold,* depending on the temperature at which they optimally bind to red blood cells. Cold antibodies are typically of the IgM isotype, and warm antibodies are usually IgG. Some patients suffer only a self-limited acute episode of the disease. Corticosteroids induce a remission in about 75% of cases and are the first-line treatment for patients who suffer from more severe forms of the disease. Approximately two thirds of these patients will suffer a relapse after steroid withdrawal. Splenectomy is indicated only for patients with warm antibodies in whom steroids have failed or are contraindicated. Removal of the spleen is therapeutic in about 80% of these patients. Other medical therapies such as azathioprine or cyclophosphamide have been used in patients for whom steroids and splenectomy have failed.

Hematologic disorders may also result in increased *platelet destruction,* and splenectomy is an effective treatment in some of these cases. *Idiopathic thrombocytopenic purpura* (ITP) is characterized by IgG antibodies directed at platelets. The spleen contributes both to the production of these antibodies and to the sequestration of antibody-bound platelets. Though as indicated by the name, a specific etiology is not known, the disease may be associated with a lymphoproliferative disorder, drug reaction, bacterial or viral infection, or other autoimmune disorders such as systemic lupus erythematosus. Clinical manifestations of the disease include thrombocytopenia with platelet counts generally below 50,000, prolonged bleeding times with fairly normal clotting times, and normal to hyperplastic megakaryocytes. The spleen is generally not enlarged. Bleeding from the gums or gastrointestinal tract may occur, and women, who make up 75% of patients, often suffer excessive menstrual bleeding. Though acute ITP frequently is self-limited, patients may require active treatments. Steroids are the first-line treatment in this disorder. Patients who do not respond within the first 6 to 8 weeks of treatment, or who relapse after withdrawal of steroids, should undergo splenectomy. Approximately 75% to 85% of these patients will attain a permanent response with increased platelet counts or normalization of bleeding diathesis even if the platelet count does not fully return to normal. Persistence of symptoms may indicate the presence of an accessory spleen. Technetium scanning is a sensitive method of detecting accessory spleens, which should be removed if they are found. Intracranial hemorrhage due to ITP is an indication for emergent splenectomy.

Thrombotic thrombocytopenic purpura (TTP) is defined by a pentad of clinical features: fever, thrombocytopenic purpura, hemolytic anemia, neurological manifestations, and renal dysfunction. Arteriolar damage results in activation or destruction of multiple blood components, resulting in anemia, thrombocytopenia, and thrombosis. Cerebral hemorrhage and renal failure are the most frequent causes of death in these patients. Plasmapheresis and replacement with fresh-frozen plasma replacement has proven to be the most effective treatment. Splenectomy is indicated in cases refractory to plasmapheresis. Steroids and dextran may also provide some benefit. Most patients can achieve remission with one or more of these therapies.

Splenectomy has been used to stage *Hodgkin disease* for several decades, but this practice has become less frequent in recent years. Laparotomy often leads to changes in staging with 25% to 35% of patients having higher stage disease and 5% to 15% having lower stage disease than clinically suspected. However, it is controversial whether this improved accuracy of staging translates into improved clinical outcomes. In addition, there is evidence that splenectomized patients are more likely to develop acute myeloid leukemias and myelodysplasia. It is generally believed that staging laparotomy still has a role for patients who do not have B symptoms, who have no hilar disease, and whose mediastinal disease occupies less than one third of the chest diameter. Hodgkin disease may also be staged laparoscopically. Use of this technique decreases postoperative ileus and length of hospitalization, which may increase the use of operative staging.

Splenic rupture is defined as disruption of the spleen's parenchyma, capsule or vasculature, and is the most common indication for splenectomy. The spleen is the most common site of major abdominal injury after blunt trauma, but it may also be injured in penetrating trauma and by abdominal retractors during surgery. Rupture may also occur spontaneously or after minimal trauma, in cases of splenomegaly.

The possibility of splenic injury may be suggested by information obtained in the history and physical examination of the trauma patient. History of blunt or penetrating trauma to the left upper quadrant should raise suspicion of splenic injury, as should left upper abdominal tenderness or evidence of diaphragmatic irritation such as left scapular pain (*Kehr sign*).

Diagnostic procedures to further evaluate the possibility of splenic injury include diagnostic peritoneal lavage (DPL), focused ultrasound examination for trauma, and CT scanning. The choice of examination is dictated by the clinical setting. DPL is a simple, rapid procedure that may be done in the emergency room or trauma bay. Its sensitivity in cases of splenic injury is close to 100%, though it lacks specificity and the ability to grade splenic injuries. Focused ultrasound examinations for trauma are increasingly common in the United States. The examination consists of four ultrasonic views: the pericardium, the left and right flanks, and the bladder. The goal of each view is to detect abnormal fluid. A dark stripe imaged between the spleen and left kidney on the left flank view is indicative of free fluid in that region, consistent with splenic rupture. In experienced hands, this technique is very sensitive in detecting fluid, but similar to DPL, it lacks specificity. CT scanning is the test of choice in hemodynamically stable patients. The technique is very sensitive and specific for injuries of the spleen and other solid organs of the abdomen, including retroperitoneal injuries. It provides information regarding the severity of splenic disruption and can demonstrate the presence of ongoing hemorrhage.

The paradigm for management of splenic injuries has changed over the last 20 years. Throughout most of this century, splenic injuries were routinely managed with splenectomy, but recognition of postsplenectomy sepsis in the pediatric population led to increased splenic salvage procedures and nonoperative management in that population during the 1960s. This change was mirrored in adult patients in the late 1980s. At New York University from 1978 to 1989 only 13% of cases of splenic injury were managed nonoperatively. At the same institution, 54% of splenic injuries were treated nonoperatively from 1990 to 1996. Nonoperative management is now favored for patients who are hemodynamically stable, have blunt injuries or stab wounds, and injuries isolated to the spleen. Unstable patients, those with shattered spleens and those requiring ongoing transfusion for splenic bleeding or other abdominal injuries, should undergo laparotomy. Nonoperative treatment of splenic injury may also include angiographic embolization of bleeding vessels. Patients who are stable but who demonstrate a blush of contrast from the spleen during CT scanning should proceed to the angiography suite. The role of nonoperative management continues to expand, and even patients with relatively high-grade splenic injuries, elderly or neurologically injured patients, and patients with abnormal spleens are considered for nonoperative management.

Splenic trauma patients who are managed conservatively are initially observed in the intensive care unit for 2 or more days, followed by bed rest on a general care floor for several additional days. Stable patients after this period who are tolerating a regular diet may be discharged but are permitted only very limited activity for approximately 3 weeks. Thereafter, a more normal activity level may be resumed, but contact sports and other vigorous activity remain prohibited for 8 weeks to 6 months after the injury. Follow-up CT scanning remains controversial. Several centers still perform CT scanning on a routine basis 2 to 4 days after the injury and have reported discovering vascular blushes in two thirds of patients who eventually failed nonoperative management. Other groups have not found routine follow-up CT scans useful and will scan only for clinical indications.

Splenic salvage, rather than splenectomy, should be considered for patients who undergo laparotomy for splenic injury. Minor injuries may be addressed through application of packing or topical hemostatic agents. More extensive injuries may require debridement of devitalized tissue, ligation of bleeding vessels, suture repair of the splenic capsule, or a partial splenectomy (Fig. 5-11). Patients with splenic avulsion, major hilar trauma, or instability due to associated injuries should not be considered for splenic salvage.

The overall prognosis for splenic injury is largely based on the severity of associated injuries. For isolated splenic trauma, mortality is generally 1% or less.

Technical Considerations of Splenectomy

The spleen is generally approached through a midline or left subcostal incision. The former is used in trauma cases. The ligamentous attachments of the spleen are taken down to mobilize the spleen. These normally avascular attachments may develop collateral vessels in myeloid metaplasia and secondary hypersplenism. The short gastric vessels are doubly ligated, but care must be taken to preserve gastric circulation. The hilar vessels are then dissected and ligated. During elective splenectomies, the hilar dissection may be completed before mobilization of ligamentous attachments. Initial ligation of the splenic artery serves to decrease the size of the spleen and facilitate complete mobilization. The pancreatic tail is in very close proximity to the splenic hilum, so careful dissection is required to avoid damaging the pancreas during the hilar dissection. In patients undergoing splenectomy for hematologic disease, a careful search should be made for accessory spleens in the peritoneal cavity, as their presence frequently causes postoperative recurrent hypersplenism.

There is controversy regarding preoperative embolization as a method of reducing splenic size and intraoperative blood loss. Data supporting the use of this technique have failed to clearly demonstrate a benefit to date, and it is not utilized at our institution.

Many patients undergoing splenectomy in the context of hematologic disorders have had numerous previous blood transfusions and may therefore have developed antibodies

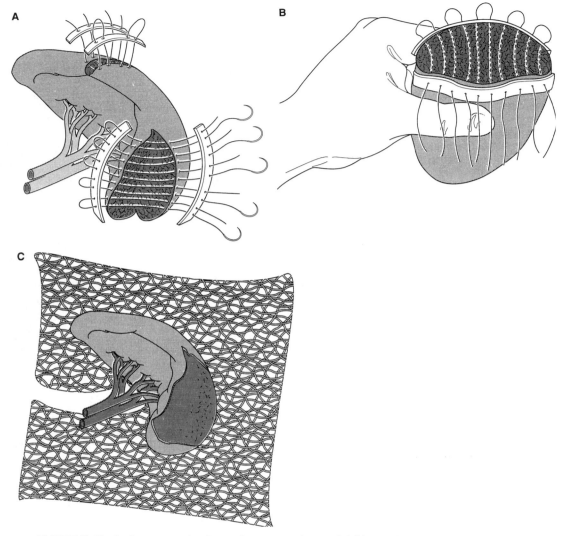

FIGURE 5-11. **A:** Suture repair of capsular tears and superficial lacerations. **B:** Suture compression after partial splenectomy. **C:** Wrapping of spleen with poly(glycolic) acid mesh after the capsule had been traumatically stripped away. (From Meyer AA. Spleen. In: Greenfield LJ, Mulholland MW, Oldham KT, et al., eds. *Surgery: scientific principles and practice.* Philadelphia: Lippincott-Raven, 1997:1279, with permission.)

to blood products. This makes cross-matching of banked blood difficult, and ample time must be allowed to complete the task before surgery.

Gastric decompression should be accomplished both intraoperatively and postoperatively until bowel function has returned. This prevents gastric distention, which may hinder intraoperative exposure and place strain on short gastric ligatures.

Laparoscopic Splenectomy

Improvements in video technology and laparoscopic instruments as well as increased surgical experience with laparoscopic techniques have resulted in many more splenectomies being performed laparoscopically. The procedure is typically performed with the patient in either lithotomy or right lateral decubitus position. Port placement is variable but typically includes a 10-mm umbilical camera port and 3 to 5 other ports for placement of instruments and retractors. Initially the short gastric vessels are exposed, clipped, and divided. The hilum is then dissected, and the splenic artery and vein are isolated and divided individually using an endoscopic stapling device. The spleen can then be removed either by enlarging one of the port site incisions to allow for removal or by morcellation within a plastic retrieval bag placed into the peritoneal cavity.

The indications for laparoscopic splenectomy are the same as those for open splenectomy, although several relative contraindications for using the laparoscopic approach exist. Trauma patients are not appropriate candidates, because unstable patients cannot tolerate the operative time required to perform the technique, and stable patients are generally treated with nonoperative therapy or splenorrhaphy. Massive splenomegaly is a relative but not absolute contraindication, as similar results to cases involving smaller spleens have been reported.

In general the operative times have been found to be longer with the laparoscopic approach and the operative costs higher. The blood loss, transfusion requirements, and complication rates are generally similar. The postoperative ileus and length of hospital stay are significantly decreased, leading to an overall cost comparable to that of the open technique.

Complications of Splenectomy

Splenectomy, both when it is elective and when it is performed for isolated trauma, is generally well tolerated. Mean operative blood loss is between 250 and 400 mL in most series, and transfusions are required in about 10% to 15% of patients. An incidence of subphrenic abscess as high as 3.4% has been reported in some trauma series. However, when patients with isolated splenic injuries, or patients undergoing elective splenectomy, are considered alone, the rate is well below 1%. Leukocytosis and thrombocytosis are frequently observed in the postsplenectomy patient. These elevations generally occur 1 to 2 days after surgery and may persist for several weeks. These laboratory abnormalities generally are not clinically significant, but antiplatelet agents such as aspirin should be considered if the platelet count increases to over 1×10^6 cells per mm^3. Delayed complications may also arise from splenectomy. These include pseudoaneurysm formation of the splenic artery and pancreatic fistula or pseudocyst formation due to iatrogenic pancreas injury.

Patients who have undergone a splenectomy are more susceptible to infections than the general population. Although this increase has been reported as up to 200 to 600 times the normal risk, this translates into an estimated incidence of less than 0.2%. The risk is somewhat higher in the pediatric population, with an estimated incidence of 0.6%. The disease process leading to splenectomy appears to affect risk, with posttraumatic splenectomy engendering the least risk. The first 2 years after splenectomy are most dangerous in both the adult and pediatric populations, but some increased risk continues throughout the patient's life.

Encapsulated bacteria are the most frequent infectious agents in *overwhelming postsplenectomy infection* (OPSI). *Pneumococcus* is the most common organism, accounting for between 50% and 90% of cases. *Haemophilus influenzae,* another significant agent, accounts for 32% of OPSI deaths. *Neisseria meningitidis* is a third important encapsulated organism. The clinical course of OPSI is frequently fulminant. Patients may develop fever and mild symptoms of infection, followed rapidly by severe sepsis and death. Progression from good health to death may occur in less than 24 hours. Treatment of patients who may be developing OPSI must be early and aggressive. Empiric antibiotic therapy is instituted with drugs tailored to treat resistance patterns of pneumococci prevalent in the respective area.

Vaccines exist for the three encapsulated organisms noted above. Because the spleen plays an important role in the development of new immune responses, the vaccine should be given at least 2 weeks before splenectomy. In emergent cases, such as trauma, in which preoperative administration of vaccines is not feasible, the vaccines must be given postoperatively. The optimal timing for postsplenectomy vaccination is discussed controversially. Some authors advocate early vaccination while others feel a delay until the patient is in positive nitrogen balance would optimize the immune response.

Pediatric patients are frequently treated with prophylactic antibiotics because they are at a higher risk of developing OPSI. Prophylactic antibiotics have traditionally consisted of penicillin or amoxicillin, but changing bacterial resistance patterns has made this recommendation less uniform. Patients located in areas of high resistance to penicillin should receive trimethoprim/sulfamethoxazole or possibly amoxicillin/clavulanic acid. There is also no uniform recommendation with regard to the duration of prophylactic antibiotic therapy. Some authors suggest that treatment may be stopped at the age of 6 while others advocate the continuation of therapy until the age of 18. Some authors also recommend treating even adult patients with prophylactic antibiotics for the relatively high-risk 2-year postsplenectomy period.

SUGGESTED READING

Lewis JJ, Brennan MF. Soft tissue sarcomas. *Current problems in surgery.* Chicago: Yearbook Medical Publishers, October, 1996.

McClelland RN. *The spleen. Selected readings in general surgery,* Vol 24, No 8. University of Texas, Southwestern Medical Center at Dallas, Texas, 1997.

6

WOUND HEALING

ALEXANDER S. KRUPNICK AND N. SCOTT ADZICK

Wound healing is the tissue's response to injury. Although usually taken for granted, this process has been the subject of intense research over the last several decades. As more details unfold, one can see the resemblance of wound healing to embryogenesis, tissue and limb regeneration, and neoplasia. Similarity of growth factors to products of oncogenes is more than a coincidence. Transformation by the *sis* oncogene of the simian sarcoma virus involves autocrine stimulation by a platelet-derived growth factor–like (PDGF) molecule, and the *erb* B oncogene shares homology with the epidermal growth factor receptor, both of which are instrumental in normal wound healing. The fact that numerous "medically treated" diseases such as rheumatoid arthritis, cirrhosis, and pulmonary fibrosis are due to excessive scarring further emphasizes the importance of these mechanisms to the physician in general. To the surgeon, who approximates tissue while relying on the normal healing process to join it together, the understanding of wound healing is a must.

DESCRIPTION OF HEALING

All wound healing reflects the body's attempt to restore tissue to its structural and functional preinjury state. This response to injury involves either regeneration or repair. Regeneration necessitates the dedifferentiation of cells, migration to the site of injury, and redifferentiation into lost or injured tissue. Although amphibians can grow back limbs and appendages, regeneration does not truly occur in people. Although liver and bone both have the ability to regenerate, healing of other adult tissues involves repair by scar formation.

Most of the work in tissue injury and repair has been performed in the skin, but similar principles and processes are involved in the healing of other tissues as well. Because skin is the main focus of the body's interaction with the external milieu, a rapid and efficient restoration of its integrity is vital to the organism's survival. The classification of healing is determined by the method of injury. Repair can be classified into healing by first, second, and third intention.

Healing by *primary*, or first, intention results after a focused, small area of injury occurs due to a surgeon's scalpel or a small cut. Little injury to the surrounding tissue is incurred and the wound edges are easily approximated with minimal distortion. Rapid reepithelialization occurs on the surface with dermal and soft tissue integrity restored through new matrix formation and scarring.

The large tissue defect resulting from an animal bite or a shotgun blast can present a formidable challenge to the healing process. The epithelial edges cannot simply come together, and a large, often infected, tissue defect needs to be tackled. Healing by *secondary intention* involves the interplay of granulation, wound contraction, and reepithelialization to fill in the defect and restore tissue integrity. A large scar often remains at the site of injury. *Tertiary*, or third intention, healing occurs when a large or contaminated wound is closed in a delayed fashion, several days after the injury. This allows for local decontamination of necrotic tissue by both surgical debridement and the action of leukocytes. The base of the wound has had time for the accumulation of the neovascular ground substance and white blood cells known as *granulation tissue*. Increased local concentration of white blood cells make the wound more resistant to infection or abscess formation, and delayed closure can be achieved with improved cosmetic results and a smaller scar. Burn experience dictates that closure of a wound with bacterial counts less than 10^5 organisms per gram of tissue can lead to successful delayed closure.

STAGES OF WOUND HEALING

Wound healing has been described as a series of stages, each one dominated by a certain cell, cytokine, and wound

Hospital of the University of Pennsylvania, Philadelphia, Pennsylvania; The Children's Hospital of Philadelphia, Philadelphia, Pennsylvania

TABLE 6-1. VARIATION IN THE CONTENT OF THE WOUND DURING THE HEALING PROCESS[a]

	Coagulation stage (injury–1 hr)	Inflammatory stage (1 hr–day 4)	Proliferative stage (day 3–day 21)	Remodeling stage (day 21–6 months)
Matrix	Fibrin	Fibrin, proteoglycans	Collagen, proteoglycans	Collagen
Dominant cell	Platelet, vascular endothelium	Neutrophil, macrophage	Fibroblast	Fibroblast, myofibroblast
Cytokines	PDGF, TGF-β	TGF-β, PDGF, aFGF, bFGF	TGF-β, lactate	TGF-β

[a]Each step in the healing of a wound is a coordinated interaction between a background matrix, a cell or group of cells, and cytokines. The constituents of the wound vary during different stages of maturation (PDGF, platelet–derived growth factor; TGF-β, transforming growth factor-β; aFGF, acidic fibroblast growth factor; bFGF, basic fibroblast growth factor).

matrix. Although this model is a gross oversimplification full of inaccuracies, it can make the process easier, and in fact possible, to understand. As each phase of the process is completed, the cellular signals elaborated during that phase set the background for the next stage of development. The gradual transformation of a blood clot formed at the site of injury to the relative avascular collagen matrix organized along lines of tension occurs through four identifiable stages. The initial insult of tissue injury is followed by (i) the coagulation phase, (ii) the inflammatory phase, (iii) the proliferative phase, and (iv) the remodeling phase.

Just as the temporal component of the healing process is organized into four stages, the physical architecture of the wound consists of three separate elements that vary in content during the healing process. These elements include (i) the background matrix, (ii) the cells localized to the wound, and (iii) the cytokines elaborated in the healing tissue. The background matrix forms the scaffolding and organizes the structure of the wound. Cells migrating into the wound modify the background matrix while cytokines aid in cell-to-cell communication and help to orchestrate the process of wound healing. Each step is actually a dynamic and organized interaction between the cellular cytokine and matrix component (Table 6-1).

Coagulation Stage (Injury to 1 Hour)

The traumatic disruption of vascular endothelium results in the outpouring of blood at the site of injury. Exposure of tissue phospholipids and glycoproteins (known as *tissue thromboplastin*) to procoagulant factors initiates the formation of a localized clot. The extrinsic pathway can form a large amount of clot within seconds and is limited only by the amount of tissue thromboplastin, factor VII and X, at the site. The intrinsic pathway is much more controlled, relying on the platelet surface for activation and control (Fig. 18-2, Chapter 18).

Fibrin, the final common pathway of clot formation serves as the first, *provisional matrix* for the healing wound. Fibrinogen is a 340,000 dalton hexamer composed of three fibrinogen chains encoded on three different genes. It is synthesized in the liver and circulates in the blood at a concentration of 3 g/L in the healthy state. Thrombin cleavage of the amino terminus promotes self-polymerization into staggered overlapping protofibers. Lateral protofibril polymerization results in a thick fibrin network that forms a clot. The preliminary fibrin clot, however, is unstable and friable. Stability is conferred by covalent cross-linking of adjacent fibrin strands. Plasma transglutaminase (factor XIII) produces these intermolecular bonds by covalently linking the lysine and glutamine residues between adjacent chains (Fig. 6-1). The final product is an extensive fibrin network that can bind cytokines and lymphocytes as well as act as scaffolding for cell migration during the repair process (Fig. 6-2).

Cells interact with constituents of the extracellular matrix through *fibronectin*, a protein that reversibly binds to the cell's plasma membrane. It consists of two 250-kd polypeptide chains linked by a disulfide bond (Fig. 6-3). The molecule has numerous domains of repeating amino acid sequences that can simultaneously bind fibrin, heparin, and collagen to facilitate cell adhesion. This makes it the perfect intermediary between the numerous macromolecules and cells. It is the "glue" that holds the provisional matrix together. Cellular adhesion is mediated through cellular receptors that interact with the arginine-glycene-asparagine (RGD) sequence found on fibronectin. Plasma fibronectin is initially synthesized by the liver and incorporated into the growing clot. Eventually most of the fibronectin in the wound is synthesized locally by endothelial cells, fibroblasts, and macrophages. Interestingly, malignant cells are often deficient in fibronectin, and unlike untransformed cells, they can undergo anchorage-independent proliferation and invasion.

The *platelet* is the *first cell* at the scene of tissue injury. Aside from its role in the coagulation cascade, it is one of the key players in initiating the healing of a wound. Platelets are anuclaete cells of myeloid lineage derived from bone marrow megakaryocytes. Their multifaceted involvement in inflammation, coagulation, and even host defense (coating of bacteria and tumor cells) may reflect the residual function of a primitive inflammatory cell. Platelets possess IgE receptors on their surface and can to some extent participate in the allergic response.

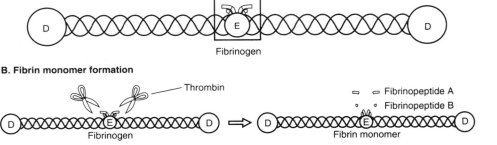

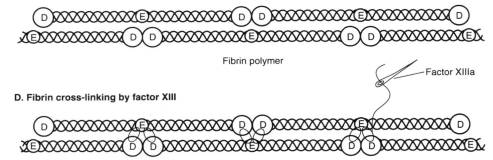

FIGURE 6-1. Conversion of fibrinogen to fibrin. Final cross-linking by factor XIII forms a highly stable structure. (From Besa EC, Catalano PM, Kant JA, et al. *Hematology.* Baltimore: Williams & Wilkins, 1992: 226, with permission.)

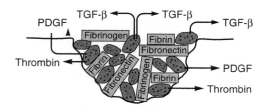

FIGURE 6-2. The fibrin clot forms a preliminary matrix that binds and releases cytokines and fibronectin and functions as scaffolding for cell migration. (From Colletti LM, Kunkel SL, Strieter RM. Cytokines. In: Greenfield LJ, Mulholand MW, Oldham KT, et al., eds. *Surgery: scientific principles and practice,* 2nd ed. Philadelphia: Lippincott-Raven, 1997:118, with permission.)

Activation of platelets occurs initially by exposure to collagen and later by thrombin generated during the clotting cascade. The cytokine products, which are released and synthesized by activated platelets at the site of injury, orchestrate the transition to the inflammatory phase and help to coordinate the wound-healing process (Table 6-2). The alpha granules contain platelet-specific proteins such as *PDGF* and *transforming growth factor* β (TGF-β). Synthesis of thromboxane from arachidonic acid and release of epinephrine and serotonin from platelet-dense bodies act to further enhance vasoconstriction and prevent exsanguination at the scene. C5a is a powerful chemotactic agent that is derived from complement cleavage by neutral proteinases and released from the activated platelet. Exposure of platelet glycoprotein IIb/IIIa results in the binding of fibrin and fibrinogen cross-linked to other platelets in order to form a platelet/fibrin clot. This further aids in hemostasis.

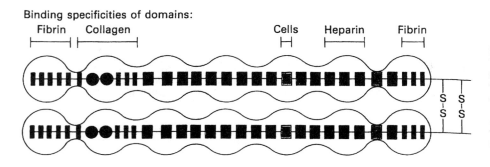

FIGURE 6-3. Structure of fibronectin. The two polypeptide chains consist of several domains simultaneously binding various macromolecules. This molecule is a key intermediary for cell binding and migration along a fibrin or collagen matrix. (From Connnective tissue proteins. In: Stryer L. *Biochemistry,* 3rd ed. New York: WH Freeman and Company, 1988: 1278, with permission.)

TABLE 6-2. PLATELET PRODUCTS

Location	Product
Platelet alpha granules: growth factors	Transforming growth factor β, platelet derived growth factor
Platelet dense granules	Epinephrine, serotonin, calcium
Platelet surface receptor	Platelet glycoprotein IIIa, platelet glycoprotein IIb
Products synthesized by platelets	Thromboxane A_2, 12-HETE

The *vascular endothelium,* once thought to be a passive participant, is now known to be an active player in wound healing. The immediate vascular response to tissue injury is vasoconstriction, which is mediated by action potentials directly generated in the blood vessel by injury. After this initial response, vasoconstriction is maintained on the order of minutes through the action of epinephrine, serotonin and thromboxane A2 generated by activated platelets. Thromboxane A2 also reciprocally activates platelets, causing further aggregation. Low-dose aspirin works during this phase of platelet activation by irreversibly inhibiting cyclooxygenase and resultant thromboxane synthesis. Unlike the endothelial cell, the platelet is anucleate and cannot synthesize further cyclooxygenase. It is inactivated for the rest of its lifespan.

The initial phase of vasoconstriction is followed by vasodilation, which allows blood-borne factors to enter the wound. Vasodilation is mediated by histamine derived from platelet decarboxylation of L histidine. Further dilation is produced by endothelial-derived products of cyclooxygenase (PGE1 and PGE2), bradykinin and endothelium-derived relaxing factor or nitric oxide. Vasodilation results in local tissue hyperemia and edema associated with the "tumor" and "rubor" of inflammation. More important than the generation of edema, local activation of endothelium at the site of injury allows cellular homing to the site of injury.

Adhesion molecules are expressed on the surface of activated endothelial cells and leukocytes. Initial contact in the area of recruitment is mediated by the constitutively expressed leukocyte L selectin and E selectin of the activated endothelial cell. This induces a loose adhesion or "rolling" of the cell along the vascular surface. The neutrophil slows down enough to be activated in the proinflammatory milieu of the wound. Firm adherence or "trapping" of the cell at the site of injury is mediated by the leukocyte integrins and the endothelial cell ICAM (intercellular adhesion molecule). The leukocyte is guided by chemotactic gradients and uses loose spaces between endothelial cells to gain access to the area of inflammation. This process is known as *diapedesis.* High endothelial venules are areas of specialized postcapillary veins with enlarged cuboidal endothelial cells. Loss of kinetic energy to the capillary bed facilitates prolonged contact of blood-borne elements with the endothelial surface. In these structures, the highest density inflammatory endothelial receptors are expressed, and they serve as the main portal of cellular entry into the inflammatory tissue (Fig. 6-4).

Cytokines are proteins used for cellular communication. Confusion in the nomenclature can exist because the molecule is initially named for the first cell from which it is isolated but significant overlap in function and cell of origin exists for each cytokine. Secreted from one cell in minute quantities and binding to a receptor in a recipient cell to induce a response, cytokines can be autocrine, produced by a cell to act on itself, or paracrine, acting on nearby cells.

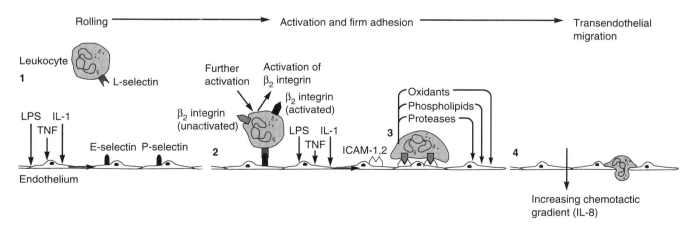

FIGURE 6-4. The process of leukocyte recruitment into areas of inflammation. At first, the cell exhibits a rolling type of motion due to loose adhesion between L selectin and E selectin. Progressive activation results in the expression of more adhesion molecules, firmer connections between the leukocyte and endothelial cell surface, and finally transendothelial leukocyte migration. (From Colletti LM, Kunkel SL, Strieter RM. Cytokines. In: Greenfield LJ, Mulholand MW, Oldham KT, et al., eds. *Surgery: scientific principles and practice,* 2nd ed. Philadelphia: Lippincott-Raven, 1997:117, with permission.)

Systemic action and overproduction of cytokines can lead to multisystem organ dysfunction seen with uncontrolled injury or inflammation. *Growth factors* are cytokines that specifically stimulate the proliferation of cells. They are important to wound healing not only because of their mitogenic properties but also because of their propensity to attract inflammatory cells into the wound, activate cells, and stimulate production and degradation of extracellular matrix. Of the many growth factors secreted in the provisional wound, two, PDGF and TGF-β, dominate.

PDGF is one of the earliest cytokines to appear in the healing wound. It is a hetero-dimer protein consisting of an A and a B chain, which are also potent growth factors and are independently synthesized on two separate genes. PDGF is synthesized by the megakaryocyte and packaged in platelet alpha granules. Platelet activation immediately releases PDGF, but its activity is soon supplemented due to synthesis at the scene of injury by macrophages, endothelial cells, and fibroblasts. Aside from its chemotactic activity for neutrophils, fibroblasts, and smooth muscle cells, PDGF stimulates a series of autocrine and paracrine activities. Acting through a surface tyrosine kinase receptor, PDGF stimulates production of fibronectin and hyaluronic acid by fibroblasts, but most importantly it facilitates the activation of macrophages. The activation and stimulation of macrophages allows production of other cytokines necessary for the inflammatory process. PDGF-stimulated accumulation, activation, and proliferation of fibroblasts increases noncollagenous extracellular matrix deposition and the synthesis of fibronectin and glycosaminoglycans (GAGs), which are important for the following inflammatory phase.

TGF-β is one of the key cytokines in controlling tissue repair. Although many of its functions overlap those of PDGF, TGF-β predominates in the wound and controls key steps throughout all phases of wound healing. It also makes its initial appearance in the wound after degranulation of the platelet alpha granules, but local synthesis maintains its concentration in the wound throughout the healing process. TGF-β is strongly chemotactic for neutrophils, T cells, monocytes, and fibroblasts. Increasing concentration of TGF-β activates monocytes as they approach the wound, further supplementing its own synthesis as well as synthesis of other factors necessary for healing. More important than its role in cellular activation and proliferation, TGF-β is a potent inducer of extracellular matrix production. Unlike PDGF, it stimulates the production of not only fibronectin and GAGs but also collagen types I, II, and V. TGF-β inhibits matrix degradation by inhibiting gene expression and synthesis of proteases and increasing synthesis of protease inhibitors.

Overproduction of TGF-β is a key step in excessive fibrosis. Limited or topical injection of TGF-β in rats can reverse wound healing impaired by corticosteroids and diabetes while systemic injection can induce pulmonary fibrosis, cirrhosis, and scleroderma. TGF-β has also been shown to increase keratinocyte migration across the wound surface and accelerate reepithelialization by increasing production of keratinocyte cell-surface integrins. Clearly TGF-β is an important promoter of all phases of tissue repair; its role in diseases of excessive scarring will be outlined later.

By the completion of this phase, the blood clot formed at the site of injury has undergone the first step in its transformation toward the healing wound. Bound to the provisional fibrin matrix are activated and degranulated platelets bathed in a chemotactic gradient of TGF-β and PDGF. Selective migration of proinflammatory cells into the wound signals the next step in the repair process.

Inflammatory Stage (1 Hour to 4 Days)

The *neutrophil* marginates, extravasates, and accumulates within 30 to 60 minutes at the scene of injury, initiating the inflammatory phase of the healing response. The neutrophil is a fully differentiated granulocyte derived from the myeloid lineage in the bone marrow. It is a migratory, phagocytic cell that circulates in the blood for 7 to 10 hours before extravasation into tissue. Although it may exist in the tissues for 1 to 2 days, it cannot replicate and once spent is rapidly cleared. Highly responsive to chemotactic gradients set up by components of complement such as C5a and C3a, fibrin degradation products, and bacterial *N*-formylpeptides, and "trapped" by activated endothelium, the neutrophil is the first leukocyte at the site of injury.

Unlike that of other inflammatory cells, the neutrophil's role is limited to phagocytosis and debridement of the wound. It engulfs foreign material, removes necrotic debris, and destroys infiltrating bacteria. Contents of primary, secondary, and tertiary granules (Table 6-3) are released

TABLE 6-3. NEUTROPHIL PRODUCTS

Granule	Content	Primary function
Primary (azurophilic) granules	Bacteriocidal (cationic proteins, myeloperoxidase) Proteinases (elastase, proteinase 3, cathepsin)	Bacterial killing, digestion of organic molecules
Secondary (specific) granules	Cell surface receptors (FMLP receptors, C3b receptors) Bacteriocidal (lysozyme, lactoferrin)	Contains reserves of cell surface receptors and bacteriocidal proteins to bind free iron
Tertiary granules	Gelatinase, C3b receptors	

including proteinases, collagenases, and bactericidal proteins. The nicotinamide adenine dinucleotide phosphate (NADPH) oxidase enzyme system produces the toxic oxygen species superoxide anion ($O_2^{\cdot-}$) to facilitate phagosomal killing of ingested microbes. Patients with chronic granulomatous disease have a defective NADPH oxidase system that is unable to generate O_2 radicals. Neutrophils can phagocytose bacteria but are unable to kill, leading to chronic unresolved infections. Although neutrophils help to expedite repair, they are not essential to the process of wound healing. Healing continues in the absence of neutrophils, but with a higher rate of infection.

Macrophages appear in the wound within 4 to 5 hours of injury and peak around 72 hours, replacing the neutrophil as the dominant cell. Even though macrophages are present in all tissues, most wound macrophages are derived from the circulatory monocyte. Originally a bone marrow granulocyte, the monocyte circulates in the blood stream until it is induced to accumulate by chemotactic stimuli. Once it has left the circulatory system, the tissue monocyte, now known as the macrophage, establishes itself in the wound. Unlike the neutrophil, which is essential only to wound debridement, the macrophage is the central cell in organizing the inflammatory stage of wound healing. Although it continues the initial debridement started by the neutrophil (engulfing most of the spent neutrophils in the process), it is a virtual chemical factory, elaborating growth factors and cytokines necessary for the maturation of the wound. Animals depleted of monocytes and macrophages heal poorly with minimal scar formation and form chronic nonhealing wounds.

Numerous cytokines are elaborated by the activated macrophage. TGF-β is elaborated by the macrophage as well as the platelet and lymphocytes. Other products such as tumor necrosis factor (TNF) act locally to activate the endothelium and increase the synthesis of tissue thromboplastin. Systemically TNF can induce the fever, hypotension, and hypermetabolism associated with septic shock. Although not yet clinically applicable, pretreatment with antibodies to TNF has been shown to prevent the systemic effects of septic shock despite exposure to TNF or LPS endotoxin. Tumor cachexia and the negative nitrogen balance associated with the presence of malignancy are due to the suppression of lipoprotein lipase and stimulation of glycogen breakdown by TNF. Cachexia is associated with both chronic infection and malignancy.

IL-1 is another early response cytokine secreted by the macrophage. The effects of IL-1 and TNF overlap. IL-1 also produces the sepsis syndrome in concert with TNF. Local endothelial activation is increased by expression of E selectin and ICAM. A prothrombotic state is induced by synthesis of tissue thromboplastin. IL-6, also know as *hepatocyte-stimulating factor,* regulates the hepatic acute-phase response. Alterations in the physiologic set point for a variety of parameters induce a catabolic state. Synthesis of hepatic acute-phase-response proteins such as fibrinogen, C-reactive protein, haptoglobin, and serum amyloid A signifies a proinflammatory state. The increased erythrocyte sedimentation rate seen during acute and chronic infection is due to the increased levels of acute-phase reactants in serum.

Angiogenesis

A local decrease in the oxygen tension and an increase in lactic acid concentration is due to the anaerobic metabolism of neutrophils and the disruption of vascular channels by injury. These factors stimulate the macrophage to synthesize angiogenic growth factors. *Acidic* and *basic fibroblast growth factors* (aFGF, bFGF) stimulate angiogenesis. Both cytokines bind the same cellular receptor on endothelial cells, but bFGF is about 10 times more potent than aFGF. Other than the macrophage, endothelial cells themselves secrete aFGF and bFGF, as do local fibroblasts and smooth muscle cells. Endothelial basement membrane binds and serves as a reservoir of FGF. The release of this cytokine is facilitated by degradation and breakdown of the basement membrane during debridement of the wound, further emphasizing the role of meticulous surgical debridement in the formation of a healthy well-vascularized granulation bed.

Migration begins as the microvascular endothelial cells release collagenases that partially digest their own basement membranes. Migration down the chemotactic gradient set up by bFGF and TGF-β is accomplished by adhesion of surface receptors to fibrin-bound fibronectin. An initially amorphic mass of endothelial cells is organized into a capillary bed through synthesis of type IV collagen and a basement membrane. The wound now takes on a pink granular appearance due to the invasion of numerous capillaries into the neodermis. This new connective tissue is known as *granulation tissue.*

Granulation tissue is also rich in proteoglycans, which form another important component of the wound matrix. Proteoglycans consist of a repeating polysaccharide based around a protein core (Fig. 6-5). These very large polyanions bind water and cations, forming a hydrated gellike extracellular medium known as the *ground substance* of connective tissue. This effect frees space between the fibrin matrix to open the wound for incoming cellular migration and further matrix deposition. GAGs make up the polysaccharide chain in the proteoglycan. A negative charge is created by either a carboxyl or a sulfate group and results in a hydration shell of H_2O around the molecule. Initial deposition of nonsulfated GAG such as hyaluronic acid is replaced by sulfated GAGs such as heparin sulfate, chondroitin sulfate, and keratin sulfate as the wound matures.

High levels of hyaluronic acid (HA) dominate the early wound matrix. Although not a true proteoglycan due to the absence of a protein core, this massive GAG is detected in the wound as early as day 1 and peaks around day 3. By 1

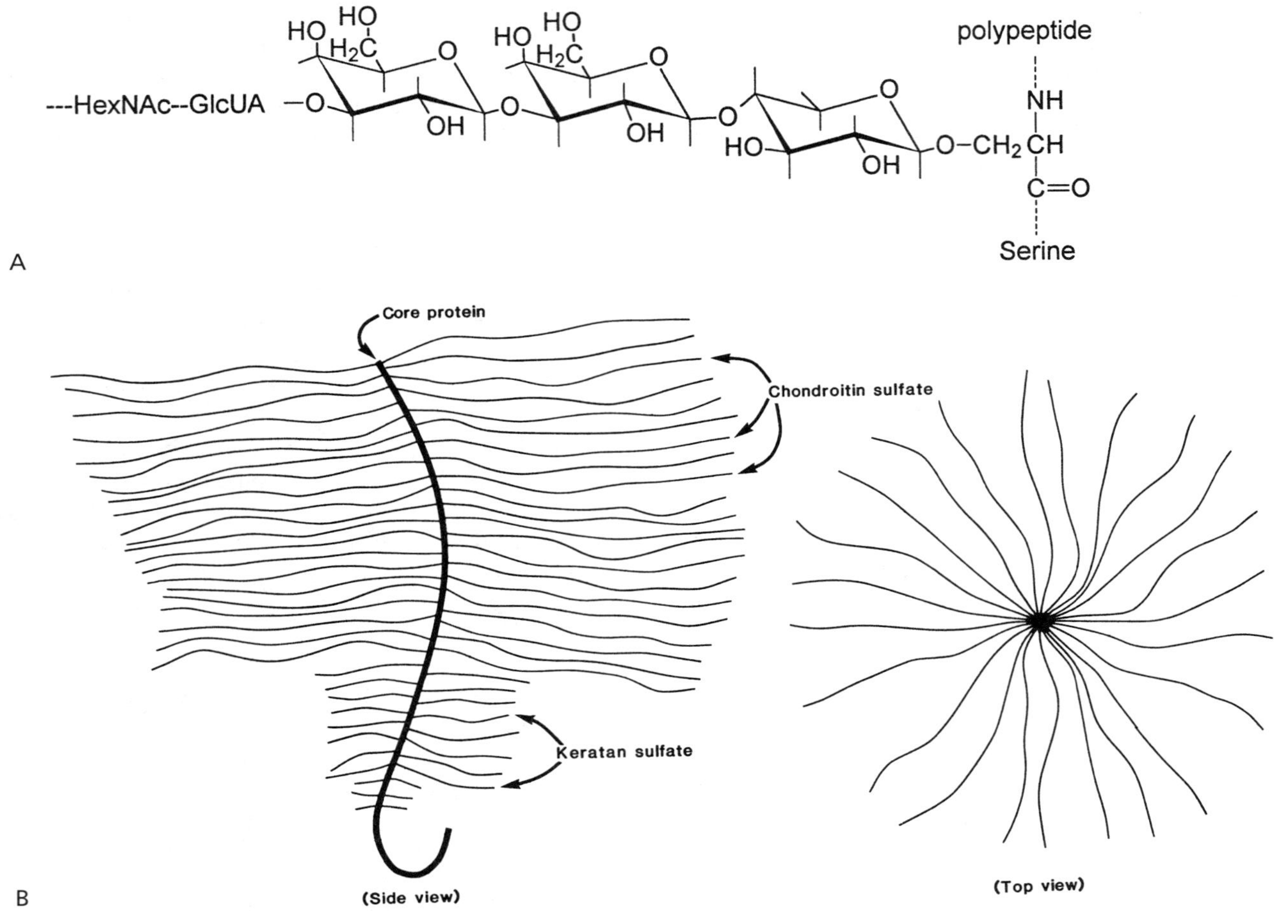

FIGURE 6-5. The structure of a proteoglycan (chondroitin sulfate). A polysaccharide chain is covalently linked to a polypeptide chain to form a large bottle-brush–like molecule. These large polyanions bind water and cations, forming a hydrated gellike extracellular medium. (From Cohen RM, Roth KS, eds. *Biochemistry and disease:* bridging basic science and clinical practice. Baltimore: Williams & Wilkins, 1996:433. Champe PC, Harvey RA, eds. *Biochemistry.* Philadelphia: JB Lippincott Co, 1987:84, with permission.)

week, HA levels drop back to baseline as sulfated GAGs replace the ground substance. Fetal wounds, which heal with minimal or no scarring, are rich in GAGs. HA is the principal GAG present in the fetal wound and remains in the wound matrix much longer than in the adult. Experimental evidence shows that an environment high in HA tends to promote cellular migration and proliferation while sulfated GAGs facilitate differentiation and collagen deposition. It is possible that an HA-rich matrix decreases scar formation and permits healing by regeneration characteristic of the fetal wound.

The highly vascular granulation tissue, debrided by the action of neutrophils and macrophages and bathed in proinflammatory cytokines, is now primed for the pivotal step in the formation of a scar. *Fibroplasia* is defined as the deposition of collagen by fibroblasts while forming the definitive wound matrix. The provisional fibrin matrix is used by the fibroblast for migration into the wound. By day 3, the migration of fibroblasts signifies the transition to the proliferative stage of wound healing.

Proliferative Stage (Day 3 to Day 21)

Fibroplasia is the production of fibrous collagenous tissue. It is the key event of the proliferative phase. Smooth transition toward this phase relies on turning down the inflammatory response and initiating fibroblast migration and collagen synthesis. Debridement and decontamination of the wound by neutrophils removes the proinflammatory stimulus. Production of local cytokines stops once the inflammatory stimulus is removed and the short half-life of most cytokines decreases their concentration. The decrease in wound neutrophils is due to their short lifespan and lack of stimuli for extravasation. Decreased surface expression of endothelial ICAM prevents neutrophil diapedesis and further decreases their concentration.

Fibroblast migration into tissue begins by day 3, and by day 5, it is the dominant cell in the wound. Mediators of fibroblast migration include numerous growth factors released during the inflammatory phase. PDGF and TGF-β are both highly chemotactic for fibroblasts. Fibroblasts will orient along gradients established by these cytokines, and the initial migration is soon supplemented by local expansion.

Interaction of the fibroblast with the extracellular matrix is facilitated by tissue fibronectin. Fibroblast fibronectin receptors are large transmembrane proteins referred to as *fibronexi*. They interact with both the extracellular fibronectin RGD sequence and the intracellular cytoskeleton, allowing transmembrane signal transduction and the coordinated migration of fibroblasts along fibronectin-fibrin strands. *Traction morphogenesis* refers to this uniform orientation of fibroblast migration by the fibronectin-fibrin strands. Fibroblast-to-matrix coupling is facilitated by fibronectin, which plays a similar role in most cellular migration including reepithelialization, angiogenesis, and wound contraction. Without it, cell migration within the tissue matrix is impossible.

The early wound matrix is rich in nonsulfated GAG such as HA. The negatively charged hydrophilic molecules act as a binding site for cytokines, allowing the formation of chemotactic gradients governing fibroblast migration. Aside from their role in the hydration of extracellular matrix and as a repository for cytokines, proteoglycans are increasingly recognized as regulators of cell behavior. High concentrations of HA have been associated with rapid and organized migration of fibroblasts into a wound. Although a cause-and-effect relationship has not been established, this efficient and orderly migration, as seen in the fetal wound, might contribute to more organized collagen deposition with little or no scar formation. Deposition of sulfated GAGs, seen in the later phases of adult wound healing, stimulates fibroblast differentiation and disorganized collagen synthesis typical of adult wounds.

Collagen Synthesis

By definition, a *scar* is a disordered collection of collagen that replaces native tissue at the site of injury. Collagen forms insoluble fibers with high tensile strength. It is the dominant structural component of the final scar and succeeds fibrin as the definitive matrix. Several types of collagen are found in human tissue and each has a different structural and functional component (Table 6-4). Type I collagen predominates throughout the body and is the principle collagen of a mature scar. Type III collagen is found in association with type I, and its concentration is increased during the initial phases of wound healing and in the developing fetus. Type II collagen makes up cartilage, and type IV collagen, unlike types I and III, tends to aggregate in sheets rather than fibrils and forms the background structure of basement membranes. Type V collagen is found in the cornea, and

TABLE 6-4. COLLAGEN DISTRIBUTION

Type I	All connective tissue, 90% of body collagen
Type II	Cartilage, vitreous humor
Type III	Fetal tissues, healing wound, blood vessels, cornea
Type IV	Basement membranes
Type V	Cornea

along with Type III collagen, type V maintains its transparency. Up to 14 types of collagen have been identified to date and some types have as yet unknown functions.

As a molecule, collagen is unique for several reasons. It contains two amino acids that are not found in any other protein: 4-hydroxyproline and 5-hydroxylysine. Proline and lysine are incorporated into the growing collagen chain in the usual manner, but after incorporation, 40% of the proline residues in the collagen molecule are converted into hydroxyproline by *prolyl hydroxylase*. Fourteen percent of the lysine residues become hydroxylated at C-5 by *lysyl hydroxylase* during posttranslational modification. Both enzymes depend on ascorbate (vitamin C) to maintain the iron atom in the active site of the molecule reduced. Because molecular oxygen acts as the donor of the oxygen atom, lack of ascorbic acid or hypoxia results in deficient function of both enzymes, failure of hydroxylation, and weaker collagen.

Another unique aspect of the collagen molecule is its unusually high content of the amino acid *glycine* (Fig. 6-6). Molecular analysis reveals that one third of all amino acids consist of glycine. Only by understanding the 3-dimensional

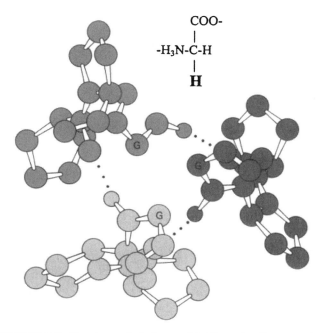

FIGURE 6-6. Structure of glycine and folding of collagen molecule with each glycine (G) directed toward the center of the chain. (From Connective tissue proteins. In: Stryer L. *Biochemistry*, 3rd ed. New York: WH Freeman and Company, 1988:265, with permission.)

conformation of the collagen molecule triple helix can the significance of this relationship be understood. Because it is the smallest amino acid, containing only a hydrogen atom as its side chain, glycine occupies very little space. It is precisely this small structure that allows the glycine molecule to fit inside the triple helix, forming the intermolecular hydrogen bonds that hold the triple helix together.

Fibroblasts begin the process of collagen formation by intracellular synthesis of the baseline protein. Posttranslational modification consists of proline and lysine oxidation and triple helix formation between the three alpha chains. Additional peptides, called *propeptides,* exist at both the amino-terminal and carboxyl-terminal ends (Fig. 6-7). Propeptides have a very different structure from the rest of the chain, are not rich in proline, hydroxyproline, or glycine, and do not aggregate into a triple helix. They prevent early intracellular aggregation of collagen and require removal before progression of synthesis.

The molecule, now known as *procollagen,* is secreted into the extracellular matrix. Orientation of the secreted procollagen molecules is maintained by the orientation of fibroblasts along the direction of fibrin-fibronectin strands known as *traction morphogenesis.* Cleavage of the terminal propeptides is performed by the extracellular *procollagen peptidases.* With the ends trimmed, the triple helix, now known as *tropocollagen,* undergoes spontaneous terminal and lateral elongation by the formation of cross-links with other tropocollagen bundles. Sequential assembly eventually leads to the mature collagen fiber oriented along the direction of fibroblasts (Fig. 6-8).

Extensive intramolecular and intermolecular bonds form the basis for the innate strength of collagen. The three alpha chains are hydrogen bonded to each other. Hydrogen bonds between these molecules are a direct result of the physical proximity afforded by the glycine residue. More stability is conferred by ionic bonds due to the hydroxylation of proline. Covalent joining of two hydroxylysine residues and

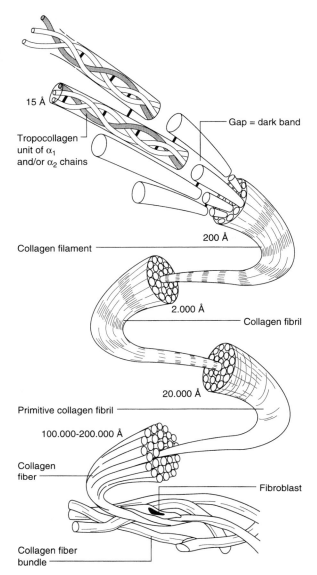

FIGURE 6-8. Sequential assembly of tropocollagen leads to the production of filaments, fibrils, and fibers. (From Fine NA, Mustoe TA. Wound healing. In: Greenfield LJ, Mulholand MW, Oldham KT, et al., eds. *Surgery: scientific principles and practice*, 2nd ed. Philadelphia: Lippincott-Raven, 1997:71, with permission.)

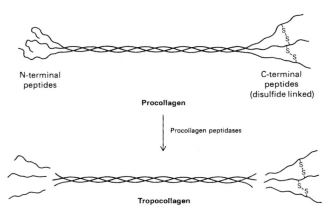

FIGURE 6-7. Cleavage of propeptides results in the progression of procollagen synthesis to tropocollagen. (From Connective tissue proteins. In: Stryer L. *Biochemistry,* 3rd ed. New York: WH Freeman and Company, 1988:269, with permission.)

one lysine residue (Table 6-5) forms further intermolecular cross-links. *Lysine oxidase* (separate from lysine hydroxylase) is a copper-containing enzyme that forms these intramolecular cross-links via aldol condensation between two lysine residues. Overall strength of the final molecule is due to the cooperative interaction of numerous relatively weak bonds.

The similarity between the final collagen matrix and the preliminary fibrin matrix is striking. Both appear extracellularly in an inactive form (fibrinogen and procollagen) and require enzymatic cleavage before assembly (by thrombin and propeptidase). Extensive intermolecular and intramolecular cross-links are required for strength and assembly of

TABLE 6-5. ENZYMES INVOLVED IN COLLAGEN PRODUCTION

Prolyl hydroxylase	Hydroxylation of prolene residues
Lysyl hydroxylase	Hydroxylation of lysine residues
N- and C-terminal propeptidases	Cleavage of terminal propeptides
Lysine oxidase	Linkage of lysine residues

the final macromolecule (factor XIII and lysine oxidase), and formation of both occurs near the cell surface (platelet and fibroblast). Defects in the synthesis of collagen can lead to structural disorders, just as a deficiency in a procoagulant leads to a bleeding diathesis. Vitamin C deficiency (ascorbic acid) leads to the inefficient function of prolyl and lysyl hydroxylase. Collagen synthesized in the absence of ascorbic acid is insufficiently hydroxylated and less stable. This leads to the disease known as *scurvy*, causing skin lesions, gum fragility, and poorly healing wounds. The clinical condition and the benefits of citrus fruits in alleviating this ailment has been recognized for centuries as extensively described by James Lind in his 1753 Treatise on the Scurvy:

> They all in general had putrid gums, the spots and lassitude, with weakness of their knees. ... The consequence was that the most sudden and visible good effects were perceived from the use of oranges and lemons; one of those who had taken them, being at the end of six days fit for duty.

Regulation of Collagen Synthesis

Collagen accumulation begins by day 3 to day 5 and reaches a maximum level by 2 to 3 weeks. Although collagen synthesis and breakdown continues at a supernormal rate, there is no further change in the overall content of collagen after 21 days. The exact signals that initiate and terminate the synthesis of collagen are still being investigated. TGF-β has been found to increase the transcription of alpha chain ribonucleic acid, and the extracellular matrix itself has been found to regulate aspects of collagen synthesis and serve as a repository for cytokines. High lactic acid concentration and hypoxia increase the rate of collagen accumulation once the oxygen levels are raised. Experimental evidence indicates that collagen synthesis is not a constitutive property of the fibroblast but is normally inhibited at the transcription level by NAD+, and its metabolite ADP-ribose. Lactate accumulation reduces the NAD+ and consequentially ADP-ribose pool by reducing it to NADH. This results in a disinhibition of collagen synthesis by fibroblasts. Although absolute hypoxia prohibits the creation of mature collagen due to the lack of O_2 as a substrate for lysine and proline hydroxylase, these enzymes require a much lower P_{O_2} level than that needed for cellular respiration. Collagen synthesis can go on with a tissue P_{O_2} level as low as 20 mm Hg. Lactate also elicits secretion of TGF-β by macrophages further up-regulating collagen synthesis. As angiogenesis

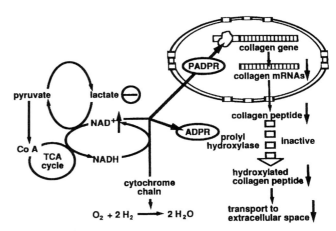

FIGURE 6-9. Lactate accumulation reduces the NAD+ and ADP-ribose pool by reducing it to NADH. Collagen synthesis is consequentially uninhibited until the NAD+ pool is restored. (From Jennings RW, Hunt TK. Overview of postnatal healing. In: Adzick NS, Longaker MT, eds. *Fetal wound healing.* New York: Chapman & Hall, 1992:40, with permission.)

proceeds, more substrate, O_2, and ascorbic acid becomes available to the fibroblast, increasing its rate of synthesis. Once the vascular system develops to the point of removing the majority of lactic acid, NAD+ and ADP-ribose reaccumulate and down-regulate collagen synthesis (Fig. 6-9).

Lactate accumulates during the inflammatory phase of tissue remodeling due to the traumatic disruption of vascular endothelium and the anaerobic metabolism of the macrophage and neutrophil. In a way, it acts as the predominant cytokine during the proliferative phase by signaling the fibroblast to begin synthesis of the collagenous background matrix. Transition to the remodeling phase occurs about 3 weeks after wounding.

Remodeling Stage (21 Days to 6 Months)

The transition to this phase is defined by reaching collagen equilibrium. Although both synthesis and breakdown of collagen continue, the total amount does not increase after 3 weeks. By 6 weeks, the wound is generally at 50% of its original strength. The strength of the wound increases for 6 months or longer, reaching up to 70% of the strength of native tissue. The tensile strength increases due to the gradual replacement of the disorganized collagen array with a more organized structure directed along the lines of tension. More intramolecular bonds form and the relative change in the type of collagen also increases wound strength. The adult skin consists of 80% type I and 20% type III collagen. Fetal skin and the healing wound have a higher type III content, which is gradually replaced with type I collagen during the remodeling phase. Capillary density in the tissue decreases as the metabolic requirements dwindle. The wound loses its pink beefy appearance and starts to reflect the pale color of collagen. New collagen is formed as old collagen is broken down. Although the metabolic requirements of the wound are significantly less, an ongoing supply of substrate is still required. This is illustrated by the fact that in scurvy not only do new wounds fail to heal, but old scars open up as well once the rate of collagen breakdown outstrips that of synthesis.

Wound Contraction

Wound contraction is instrumental in the healing of open wounds. Although a collagenous scar replaces the area of damage, contraction of normal tissue around the wound decreases the cross-sectional area of the scar from that of the original wound. Because human skin is loosely connected to fascia and muscle underlying it, wound contraction can decrease the area of scar by as much as 30% to 90%. The *myofibroblast* is instrumental in the process of wound contraction. It is derived from the fibroblast and develops intermediate characteristics of a smooth muscle cell. Actin fibers span the long axis of the myofibroblast and gap junctions connect the cells to each other. Coupling and orientation of the myofibroblast cytoskeleton with the extracellular collagen is facilitated by transmembrane fibronexi. The force for wound contraction is generated by the actin bundles and transmitted to the cell-matrix connections. Granulation tissue rich in myofibroblasts responds to pharmacological agents similar to smooth muscle and contracts upon surface application of epinephrine.

In contrast to wound contraction, which occurs early in the healing process, *scar contracture* refers to the pathologic contractile process following complete wound closure. It is the end result of wound contraction and may be caused by the contraction itself, fibrosis, adhesions, or surrounding damage. Prolonged pathological persistence of the myofibroblast within the remodeled scar also correlates with scar contracture. This can be detrimental in certain locations due to the distortion of neighboring tissue and the decrease in the range of motion of a joint or digit. Scar contracture over the elbow or hand after a burn injury can severely limit motion and use of the extremity.

Reepithelialization

Reepithelialization is made easier by wound contraction, which brings the margins closer together. Within hours of injury, the epithelial cells at the basal layer of the wound edge undergo a morphologic change by loosening cell-to-cell and cell-matrix contacts, increasing mitotic activity and proliferating. Loss of contact inhibition initiates the signal to repopulate the wound, and the fixed basal cells near the edge of the wound divide as their daughter cells begin the process of migration toward the center of the wound. Epithelial cell migration exhibits a rolling type of motion as each cell sends out pseudopods, attaching to the underlying extracellular matrix by integrins receptors. Once the cell starts to migrate, it does not replicate until epithelial continuity is restored and replication occurs only by basal cells at the edge of the wound. Migration under fibrinous exudate, or the dry "scab" of the wound, gradually separates it from the underlying matrix. An infected wound with ongoing inflammation or copious amounts of necrotic debris will undergo delayed epithelialization, resulting in unsightly hypertrophic scarring.

Once the denuded wound surface is covered by a monolayer of keratinocytes, epithelial integrity is reestablished and contact inhibition restored. The keratinocytes lay down type IV collagen as part of their basement membrane and restore hemidesmosome attachments to the underlying matrix. Hemidesmosomes connect by a series of intermediate proteins to the dermal collagen network and provide stability for the neoepithelium. Replication of the basal cells and their vertical migration restores the layers of the epidermis. Cell differentiation occurs as the cells progress upward and increased amounts of keratin are produced at the epidermal surface.

Migration occurs not only from the margins of the wound but also from hair follicles and dermal appendages. Epithelialization occurs at a maximum rate of 1 to 2 mm per day and restoration of epithelial integrity depends on the number of dermal appendages remaining and the health and vascularity of the underlying neodermis. Although chronic wounds are characterized by lack of reepithelialization, the problem usually lies in the underlying bed. Epithelial coverage of most surgical wounds is complete by 48 hours. The operative dressing can then be removed and the patient may shower with the incision protected by a layer of epithelium. If the wound edges are not approximated and healing by secondary intention must occur, reepithelialization generally takes longer but is complete in most healthy wounds by 7 to 10 days.

Fetal Wound Healing

Whenever dermal integrity is violated, a scar (unorganized collection of collagen) results. Although some amphibians and phylogenetically lower animals can heal by regeneration, the human adult undergoes the process of wound healing in order to form a scar. A fetus manifests the ability for scarless healing. A major difference lies in the degree of inflammation exhibited by fetal skin. Fetal wounds support a sparse inflammatory response with few neutrophils and monocytes present at the site of injury. The relative lack of monocytes and the immature state of these cells lead to a deficiency of TGF-β in the fetal wound. TGF-β is known to stimulate fibrosis and promote scar formation. Experimental introduction of TGF-β into the fetal wound increases scar formation even early in gestation. The fetal wound matrix is also rich in GAGs, particularly HA. An HA-rich environment promotes cell migration and proliferation, which is necessary for regeneration. The fetal fibroblast lays down an organized reticular pattern of extracellular matrix rich in type III collagen. These fibers are indistinguishable from adjacent normal tissue, reminiscent of regeneration rather than scar formation. Because pathological scarring and fibrosis plagues all aspects of medicine, contributing to problems caused by laparotomy-induced adhesions, surgical strictures, and post–hepatitis cirrhosis, finding ways to control scarring is the goal of ongoing research.

CLINICAL IMPLICATIONS

Excessive Scar Formation

Excessive fibrosis results from an aberration of the healing response. *Hypertrophic scars* are characterized by an abundance of disorganized dermal collagen. They occur mostly in individuals with darker skin, frequently of Asian, African, and Middle Eastern background. Deep dermal burns that take longer than 3 weeks to heal frequently manifest hypertrophic scarring. Although they can reach significant size, hypertrophic scars respect the boundaries of the original injury and do not extend into surrounding tissue. *Keloids,* on the other hand, behave in a malignant manner, invading surrounding tissues and extending beyond the original boundaries of injury. True keloids are uncommon, occur in dark-skinned people and are probably transmitted in an autosomal dominant manner. Histologically, keloids are characterized by an overabundance of large active fibroblasts, synthesizing broad hyaline bands of collagen. Unlike hypertrophic scars, whose cellularity grows less with time, keloids retain their population of fibroblasts, which often become triangular in shape. Treatment for both disorders is unsatisfying. Although hypertrophic scars can be reexcised, and improved cosmetic appearance achieved with pressure garments and silicone sheeting, keloids usually reoccur after such treatment. Although some improvement has been achieved with steroid injections into the lesion, no therapeutic magic bullet yet exists for this disease.

The development of hypertrophic scars and keloids has been attributed to relative "cytokine poisoning" by TGF-β. It is chemotactic for macrophages, induces and up-regulates its own production, participates in angiogenesis, and stimulates collagen production by the fibroblast. Scarless fetal healing occurs in the relative absence of TGF-β from the wound and addition of exogenous TGF-β induces scar formation. Systemic administration of TGF-β can result in fibroproliferative disorders such as cirrhosis, pulmonary fibrosis, and scleroderma. Persistence of this cytokine is the link between prolonged inflammation (e.g., due to bacterial contamination of the wound) and scarring. Future therapies for keloid and hypertrophic scars will focus on modulating the amount of TGF-β in the wound through neutralizing antibodies, soluble TGF-β receptors, and control of TGF-β gene transcription and translation.

Chronic Wounds

A *chronic wound* is defined as one that persists for longer than 3 months. Leg ulcers represent the most common type of chronic nonhealing wound, and 90% of all leg ulcers in the United States are due to venous stasis and valvular insufficiency. The venous stasis ulcer exemplifies several changes; the most prominent of which is "brawny edema" of the surrounding tissue or limb. Although initially extremity edema is a result of high hydrostatic pressure and transudation of plasma, eventually the local capillary bed distends with widening of the space between endothelial cells. This allows larger molecules such as fibrinogen to escape from the capillary bed into the extravascular space. Polymerization of fibrin occurs outside the vessel wall, forming a "perivascular cuff" that acts as a barrier to oxygen and nutrient diffusion. Extensive extravascular fibrin polymerization results in brawny edema. The fibrin cuff also acts as a nonspecific binder of growth factors limiting their availability to the healing wound. When fluid from a chronic wound is compared to fluid from an acute wound, there is indeed a decreased level of growth factors and cytokines. Decreased tissue oxygenation leads to the formation of a necrotic center with superinfected debris. This limits keratinocyte migration from the periphery, providing less wound coverage and further increasing bacterial colonization.

Meticulous debridement of the wound down to healthy well-vascularized tissue is the first step in stimulating the healing of a chronic wound. This removes unnecessary necrotic tissue, decreases bacterial proteases, and allows keratinocyte migration. Control of extremity edema through elevation and pressure garments can decrease protein exudation into the surrounding tissue. Once extravascular fibrin polymerization occurs, however, the process is rarely reversible. Pain control at the site of injury, once thought to be important for patient comfort only, is now understood to be vital in the healing process. Activation of the sympathetic nervous system and a high catecholamine concentration causes peripheral vasoconstriction, limiting the availability of oxygen and nutrients to the healing wound. Alleviation of pain not only increases patient comfort and allows more meticulous debridement but also facilitates increased oxygenation of the wound.

Diabetes and Wound Healing

Diabetic patients are particularly vulnerable to impaired healing and chronic wounds. The most common wound in the diabetic patient is a lower extremity pressure ulcer. Peripheral neuropathy allows the placement of prolonged and unequally distributed pressure on insensate toes and feet. Elevation of tissue tension above the capillary filling pressure of 25 mm Hg produces ischemia by occlusion of the microcirculation. Because the skin is more resistant to pressure necrosis than the underlying soft tissue, it is not uncommon to find a small ulcer overlying a large area of subcutaneous necrosis. Poor function of neutrophils in a hyperglycemic environment leads to a higher degree of infection. Peripheral vascular disease is prevalent in the diabetic population and contributes to delayed wound healing. Small vessel disease also accompanies diabetes and is manifested by endothelial proliferation in small arterioles and basement membrane capillary thickening. Both processes compromise the oxygen available for hydroxylation and synthesis of collagen. Rigid nondeforming erythrocytes form due to nonenzymatic glycosylation of cell-membrane proteins and accentuate microvascular disease by plugging capillary beds. Glycosylated hemoglobin also has a higher affinity for oxygen, making less of it available to tissues. Insulin is essential for fibroblastic activity, and when it is suppressed, collagen deposition is limited. Despite all the mitigating factors, healing is not impaired in a well-perfused area of a controlled diabetic patient.

Immunosuppression and Wound Healing

The success of solid organ transplantation and the prolonged survival of organ recipients have brought the issue of wound healing in the immunosuppressed patient to the forefront. Patients receiving corticosteroids as part of the immunosuppression regimen may respond poorly to conventional therapy. Corticosteroids interfere with numerous steps in the initial inflammatory response, including prostaglandin synthesis, leukocyte migration, and production of cytokines by the macrophage. Reduction of the initial inflammatory response can attenuate successive steps in the healing process. Steroids may also impair wound repair by inhibiting other factors in the repair process such as fibroblast function and collagen synthesis. Skin of patients taking chronic steroids often becomes thin and fragile due to the imbalance of collagen synthesis and breakdown.

Vitamin A, in oral doses of 25,000 U per day, tends to overcome the inhibitory effects of steroids, at least temporarily. The effect may be mediated by TGF-β, which is decreased by steroids and returned to normal by vitamin A therapy for about 7 days after injury. Once inflammation has developed, steroids affect healing less, but the negative affect on collagen synthesis still persists. Other drugs used for immunosuppression such as antimetabolites and cyclosporine have variable effects on the healing process.

The precise mechanism by which human immunodeficiency virus (HIV) affects the healing process is unknown. Wound healing is a significant problem after anorectal surgery in patients affected with HIV and is directly related to the stage of the disease. Patients with CD4+ T-lymphocyte counts less than 50 cells per μL were four times more likely to have unhealed wounds at 3 months than those with CD4 counts of greater than 50 per μL. The decreased ability to fight infection can also result in bacterial overgrowth in wounds, further retarding the healing process.

SUGGESTED READING

Adzick NS. Wound healing. In: Sabiston DC Jr, ed. *Textbook of surgery*, 15th ed. Philadelphia: WB Saunders, 1997:207–220.
Adzick NS, Longaker MT, eds. *Fetal wound healing*. New York: Chapman & Hall, 1992.
Clark RAF, ed. *The molecular and cellular biology of wound repair*, 2nd ed. New York: Plenum Publishing, 1996.

7

BURN INJURY AND MANAGEMENT

ALEXANDER S. KRUPNICK AND N. SCOTT ADZICK

A burn can present as the ultimate wound. Over 2 million burn injuries occur annually in the United States. Most of these injuries (about 80%) are relatively small and can be well cared for in the outpatient setting. Around 20% of patients, however, require admission to the hospital due to the extent of the burn, extremes of age, the presence of associated injuries, comorbid conditions, or the possibility of child abuse. As many as 7,000 patients die each year as a result of or due to complications from burn injuries. Characteristics that influence the occurrence and course of a burn injury include the extremes of age, with young children and the elderly less likely to escape injury in a house fire, smoking patterns, alcohol abuse, and socioeconomic class.

Advances in the treatment of burns have had a tremendous impact on patient survival and recovery. There are now close to 140 designated burn centers in the United States. The success of the combined team approach to burn resuscitation and management piloted by these centers is evidenced by increased patient survival. Before 1950, a pediatric patient with a 50% body surface burn had a 50% chance of survival. Similar mortality is rarely seen today, even with burns over 90% of total body surface area (TBSA). Burn shock resulted in 20% to 40% of burn-related deaths prior to 1950 but has been virtually eliminated today due to the meticulous study and improvement of fluid resuscitation. Early burn wound excision and advances in nutritional support have decreased the mortality from wound sepsis and postburn hypermetabolic response. Pulmonary sepsis, which often follows inhalation injury, is now the primary cause of death in the burn victim. Increased survival has shifted attention toward long-term functional and cosmetic outcome, with physical and psychological rehabilitation playing more of a key role in patient survival and quality of life.

BURN INJURY PATHOPHYSIOLOGY

Survival depends on the moisture and bacterial barriers provided by the normal skin. The skin envelope is made up of two principal layers: the epidermis and the dermis. The epidermis consists of a keratinized squamous epithelium that extends into underlying dermal appendages. The basal cells in the innermost layer, next to the dermis, undergo mitosis and exhibit an upward maturation program associated with the production of keratin. Although the keratinocyte progresses through five separate morphological layers, its final destination before sloughing is in the stratum corneum or the cornified layer. This layer consists of flattened fused cell remnants composed of the fibrous protein keratin. The dermis supports the basal layer of the epidermis and provides support, flexibility, and strength through its attachment to the subcutaneous tissues and fat (Fig. 7-1).

Classification of the burn injury is based on the degree of damage and penetration of the skin and subcutaneous tissues (Table 7-1). A *first-degree burn* results in only superficial damage to the epidermis. This type of insult frequently results from a sunburn or a hot water scald and is exquisitely painful and red due to the inflammation at the site. Despite its clinical appearance, the wound will usually heal within 5 days without scarring by epidermal regeneration. A *second-degree*, or *partial-thickness*, *burn* involves both the epidermis and the dermis. Blister formation occurs as the dermal–epidermal junction separates and serous interstitial fluid accumulates in this space. Intact nerve endings transmit both tactile and pain sensations while hair follicles as well as other dermal appendages remain intact. Because the dermis is affected, healing proceeds through scar formation, unlike simple regeneration of the epidermis. Superficial partial-thickness burns will usually heal within 21 days, going through the classic stages of scar formation and wound contraction. Epithelialization from the surrounding edges as well as dermal appendages provides coverage for the wound. Deep-dermal partial-thickness burns can take a significantly longer time to heal. Minimal remaining dermal appendages and a large

---

Hospital of the University of Pennsylvania, Philadelphia, Pennsylvania; The Children's Hospital of Philadelphia, Philadelphia, Pennsylvania

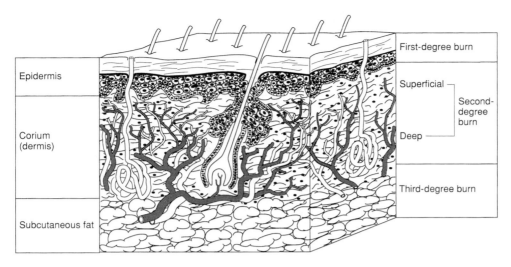

FIGURE 7-1. Depiction of skin. Degree of burn injury is classified based on depth of penetration. (From Sheridan RL, Tompkins RG. Burns. In: Greenfield LJ, Mulholand MW, Oldham KT, et al., eds. *Surgery: scientific principles and practice*, 2nd ed. Philadelphia: Lippincott-Raven, 1997:423, with permission.)

wound often result in delayed reepithelialization and hypertrophic scar formation. Excision and grafting of this extensive damage must often be performed, similar to a full-thickness burn.

Full-thickness, or *third-degree, burns* result from prolonged contact with flame, hot steam, or high-voltage electrical injury. Damaged tissue extends through the epidermis, and all of the dermis is destroyed. Extensive third-degree burns are classified further as *fourth-degree* if subcutaneous fat, muscle, connective tissue, and bone are involved. The damaged tissue has a dry leathery appearance due to dehydration and denaturation of proteins. The area is insensate due to complete destruction of sensory nerve endings. The extensive damage can not heal on its own and always requires surgical repair and grafting.

Estimating the degree of the burn immediately after the accident often leads to errors in judgment. Although a completely charred limb after a high-voltage electrical injury is difficult to miss, distinguishing a deep second-degree burn from a third-degree burn can be difficult. To make the process easier to understand, the injury should be conceptualized as consisting of three zones. A central zone of cellular death with complete coagulation and precipitation of proteins is surrounded by a zone of viable tissue, but with compromised perfusion due to thrombosis of some of the feeding vessels. Depending on the adequacy of the resuscitation, this zone can return to normal and maintain cell viability or progress to ischemia and necrosis. The third and outermost zone of hyperemia represents minimal vascular and cellular damage with viable tissue and early healing. Due to the progression of cellular damage in the partially compromised zone of the burn, the degree of the burn should never be estimated in the field or even early in the emergency department; rather efforts should initially focus on other potentially life-threatening injuries according to standard advanced trauma life support (ATLS) protocol. Only after other injuries have been excluded and fluid resuscitation has begun should the burn be fully assessed.

TABLE 7-1. CLASSIFICATION OF BURNS BASED ON DEPTH

Burn	Structures involved	Clinical characteristics	Healing characteristics
First degree	Epidermis	Red, painful, no blisters	Will heal without a scar in 5 days
Superficial second degree (partial thickness)	Epidermis and superficial (reticular) dermis	Bright red, very painful, blistering, blanches with pressure	Will heal within 21 days, reepithelialization from dermal appendages and wound margin
Deep second degree (partial thickness)	Epidermis and deep (papillary) dermis	Pale waxy, decreased blanching, painful but decreased pain sensation	Delayed healing and reepithelialization with hypertrophic scar formation
Third degree (full thickness)[a]	Epidermis and all of dermis and subcutaneous tissue	Dry, leathery, insensate, charred	Requires surgical excision and grafting

[a]Fourth degree sometimes applied when subcutaneous tissue involved.

BURN-SHOCK RESUSCITATION AND SYSTEMIC EFFECTS OF THE BURN

Burn shock is characterized by a combination of systemic hemodynamic and local tissue alterations. Originally classified into two separate phases of ebb (hypofunction) and flow (hyperfunction), burn shock affects nearly every organ system. Progression to the hyperdynamic stage depends on successful fluid resuscitation and support during the hypofunctional stage. Before the advent of modern fluid resuscitation, most deaths were encountered during this early stage of burn recovery.

Hemodynamic Changes and Fluid Resuscitation

Immediately following injury, the hemodynamic changes in the cardiovascular system predominate all other organ-specific alterations. These changes mandate treatment priority to limit volume deficits and the progression toward full-blown shock. The damaging effects of heat and cellular necrosis alter capillary permeability at the site of injury. The magnitude of the extravascular volume shift is proportional to the size and extent of the burn. Clinically evident edema occurs within the burned tissue in 15 to 30 minutes and peaks in 8 to 12 hours. Extravasation and precipitation of protein at the site of cellular damage increases the local osmotic load, leading to more tissue edema.

The loss of fluid from the vascular tree also proceeds systemically in areas unaffected by the burn. A generalized diffuse capillary leak develops with increased microvascular permeability. Various humoral factors liberated from damaged tissue as well as cytokines produced by the activated leukocytes within the tissue are responsible for this phenomenon. The most frequently mentioned cytokine is *histamine*. Its major effect is in the postcapillary venules, resulting in widening of the intracellular junction space. The concentration of histamine increases within 1 minute of thermal injury and blood levels are proportional to burn size. Systemic capillary leak rises precipitously in the first 6 hours and slowly over the next 18 hours. By 24 hours after injury, equilibrium is reached, and even though *trans*-capillary albumin flux rates remain mildly elevated, edema formation ceases.

Cardiac output decreases within minutes after burning in proportion to burn size. Originally, a circulating myocardial depressant factor was hypothesized to be responsible for this change, but animal studies have largely discounted this theory. Despite the decreased cardiac output, the heart is typically hyperdynamic during this period, as evidenced by an increased ejection fraction and elevated velocity of myocardial fiber shortening. Hypovolemia and hemoconcentration resulting in elevated hematocrit and depressed left ventricular end diastolic volume are now known to be responsible for the decreased cardiac output and low flow state. Administration of fluid is necessary immediately after a burn injury to ameliorate these hemodynamic changes and stop the progression of shock.

Fluid resuscitation is aimed at supporting the patient through the first 24 hours of hypovolemia by replacing the volume sequestered due to thermal injury. Although the myriad clinical and experimental data fail to support one formula as superior to another, the most commonly used equation (and one usually questioned on surgical examinations) is the Parkland formula for resuscitation. A balanced salt solution in the form of Ringer lactate is administered intravenously (i.v.) for a total volume of 2 to 4 mL/kg per each percent of TBSA burned. This estimates the amount of fluid sequestered due to the effects of the burn. Only areas of second- and third-degree burn should be included in the calculation because first-degree superficial burns rarely lead to fluid shifts. One half of the Ringer lactate is administered over the first 8 hours while the second half is given over the following 16 hours. This schedule coincides with the progressive correction of total body and wound capillary permeability seen after injury. It should be noted that the fluid needs are calculated from the actual time of injury and not the patient's arrival in the emergency department or the establishment of i.v. access. A delay in resuscitation mandates making up for lost time in the field with more vigorous fluid administration until deficits are corrected.

Successful fluid resuscitation will lead to systemic edema due to the diffuse capillary leak. Efforts at limiting the progression of edema by decreasing the volume of crystalloid administered will always lead to underresuscitation and should be avoided. Investigational use of different fluid regiments during the initial resuscitation period has shown little superiority to crystalloid. Colloid administration in the form of albumin has been advocated due to the potential effect of increasing the intravascular osmotic gradient and preventing extravasation of fluid. Because the microvascular system is permeable to even large proteins such as albumin immediately after the burn, little reduction in edema is seen within the first 24 hours. Colloid administration is used during the postresuscitative phase after the first 24 hours and the correction of the capillary leak. Hypertonic saline containing 250 mEq of sodium per liter has also been advocated to reduce the total volume of fluid administered. Its use, however, has been plagued with a higher incidence of renal failure and organ dysfunction due to hypernatremia.

No formula or fluid can replace frequent evaluation of the patient's intravascular volume and physiologic response. Blind adherence to the formulas without monitoring the patient can lead to tragedy. A urinary output of 0.5 to 1.0 mL/kg per hour in the adult and 1 to 2 mL/kg per hour in children generally indicates adequate intravascular volume. Signs of hypoperfusion such as mental status change, decreasing urine output, or ongoing hypotension indicate a failing resuscitation. Administration of more than 6 mL/kg per percentage of TBSA burn over the first 24 hours is also indicative of a failing resuscitation. Patients whose resuscitation has been delayed, who have extensive and deep burns underestimated in size, or those who have suffered inhalation injury frequently need larger volumes. Inhalation injury increases fluid requirements due to the release of vasoactive mediators from injured pulmonary parenchyma. These patients will frequently benefit from low dose dopamine for hemodynamic support or placement of a pulmonary artery catheter to guide further fluid administration. A successful resuscitation can result in the administration of huge amounts of fluid. An average 70 kg man with a 50% TBSA burn will require a staggering 7 to 14 L of fluid within the first 24 hours to replace deficits. In the 1940s and 1950s, inadequate fluid administration during the first day of injury resulted in a 20% to 40% death rate. With the advent of modern, vigorous fluid resuscitation, that figure has been reduced to only a few percentage points. Despite the vast improvement in the resuscitation methods, some patients, unfortunately, cannot be resuscitated.

Successful support through the initial resuscitation and the early hypodynamic phase is followed by a prolonged hyperdynamic phase. Cardiac output and metabolic rate can double over resting values (Table 7-2). Supranormal levels of catecholamines and glucagon, combined with decreased levels of insulin and thyroid hormone, result in protein catabolism, lipolysis, muscle wasting, and hepatic fat deposition. Elevated oxygen consumption and increased body temperature to as high as 38.5°C is often seen. Cardiomyopathy and heart failure due to the prolonged elevation of catecholamines is not a rare occurrence in those with predisposing coronary artery disease. Attempts had been made in the past to ameliorate the hypermetabolic response and the deleterious side effects with selective β blockade, but this has had no impact on survival. Although nursing the patient in a heated environment closer to his or her ambient temperature can ameliorate some metabolic needs, most of the hypermetabolic response is driven by the needs of the wound. Blood flow to the wound is significantly and disproportionately increased compared to that of healthy unburned tissue. Studies of burns to the lower extremity have shown that blood flow to the injured limb increases in proportion to the burn while flow to the contralateral, unburned limb is not affected. Glucose consumption and lactate production are significantly higher in the area of the burn and remain unchanged in unaffected tissue. Because pharmacological manipulation to diminish the hypermetabolic state can negatively affect the delivery of nutrients for wound healing in the burned tissue, modern therapy focuses on metabolic and nutritional support during this phase rather than amelioration of the response. Early excision of the burn with wound closure and coverage has come to the forefront as the most successful method to alleviate the increased metabolic needs and improve patient outcome.

Postresuscitation fluid management centers mainly around excretion of the salt load infused during the resuscitative period. A daily loss of 10% of the weight gained during the initial resuscitation should allow the patient to return to preburn weight by 8 to 10 days after injury. Although mild hyponatremia may be present immediately after resuscitation (lactated Ringer solution is hyponatremic), hypernatremia is the most common electrolyte disturbance. This is mainly due to the loss of the water vapor barrier in the skin and insensible free water loss. Fluid management after the first 24 hours relies on calculating and properly replacing this free water loss while monitoring the postresuscitation diuresis.

Gastrointestinal Changes

The gastrointestinal system behaves in a stereotypical manner after thermal injury. Decreased mucosal blood flow during the ebb phase is almost universal. Although blood flow is restored to normal with vigorous fluid resuscitation, focal ischemia in the gastric and duodenal mucosa can be observed as early as 3 to 5 hours postburn. Diminished blood flow weakens mucosal defenses, and if left unprotected, transmural changes can lead to ulceration, scarring, or perforation. Acute ulceration of the stomach and duodenum, known as a *Curling ulcer,* is not due to acid hypersecretion but lack of mucosal defense. Perforation and bleeding from these ulcers were formerly the most life-threatening gastrointestinal complications, but the early institution of gastric acid control has virtually eliminated them. The goal of therapy is to maintain gastric pH level of more than 5 with i.v. or preferably enteral histamine antagonists. Although past concerns regarding the increased incidence of pneumonia due to the neutralization of gastric acidity have been brought up, recent studies show that sucralfate, while also providing adequate stress ulcer control, was associated with a similar incidence of bronchopneumonia. The frequency and time of Gram-negative colonization of the airway was similar in both groups.

Decreased blood flow to the colon can also result in mucosal alteration. Although acute perforation of the colon

TABLE 7-2. INCREASE IN METABOLIC ENERGY EXPENDITURE AFTER BURN[a,b]

% TBSA	V_{O2} (mL/min/m^2)	kcal/24 h	REE (fraction of calculated BEE)
0–20	156	2,232	1.35
20–40	174	2,404	1.43
40–60	209	2,782	1.67
>60	247	3,155	1.97

[a]Metabolic expenditure increases proportionally with burn size. REE was measured while BEE calculated using Harris-Benedict equation.
[b]From Saffle JR, et al. Use of indirect calorimetry in the nutritional management of burned patients. *J Trauma* 1985;25(1):32–39.

has been identified in the burn patient, this condition is relatively rare and is more likely to be seen in individuals with persistent hypotension due to inadequate fluid resuscitation or supervening sepsis. Gastrointestinal permeability, however, is increased and bacterial translocation is frequent in the burn patient. Animal studies of the murine model with a 30% full thickness burn have identified the presence of radiolabeled *Escherichia coli* in the mesenteric lymph nodes as early as 1 hour after a burn injury. Early data suggest a possible beneficial effect of selective decontamination of the gastrointestinal tract in decreasing the incidence of Gram-negative sepsis. Future studies will determine the clinical utility of this therapy.

Ileus is almost universal in patients with TBSA burns of over 25%, and a nasogastric tube should be placed in the emergency department to prevent aspiration and pneumonitis. Gastrointestinal mobility returns by the third to fifth postburn day. Enteral nutritional support should be started immediately upon return of gastrointestinal function (patients who are not obtunded and have suffered minor burns can even benefit from enteral fluid during the initial resuscitation phase). Early enteral nutrition not only helps support the increased metabolic needs of the burn (Table 7-2) but also preserves gastrointestinal integrity, decreases bacterial translocation and wasting of visceral protein, and prevents acalculous cholecystitis. Because infectious complications are the most common cause of morbidity in the burn patient, complete enteral nutritional support can prevent the need for long-term central access and associated infectious complications. Oral intake of sufficient caloric and protein requirements can be maintained in an awake individual or a postpyloric feeding tube can be positioned under fluoroscopic guidance in the intubated patient. Sudden onset of ileus, feeding intolerance, or hyperglycemia in one previously tolerating enteral feeds should prompt a search for a source of infection, as this is most likely the reason for deterioration.

Glutamine may have a uniquely beneficial effect on total body nitrogen balance. In times of stress, the gut mucosa will exclusively utilize glutamine for energy requirements. This results in a systemic glucose sparing effect, allowing it to be utilized by tissues with an obligate glucose requirement. In the absence of glutamine, the gut mucosa becomes atrophic, and the addition of glutamine to feedings will increase mucosal cellularity and barriers. Addition of glutamine to total parenteral nutrition also spares the fall in skeletal muscle protein synthesis and improves systemic nitrogen balance, reinforcing glutamine's role in the overall protein economy.

Pulmonary System

Various changes in the pulmonary system are seen after a burn injury while circumferential burns of the thorax or inhalation injury produce their own pattern of dysfunction. In patients without chest wall burns or inhalation injury, the initial hypovolemia may result in a rapid, shallow breathing pattern. The ventilatory pattern 3 days after a burn is reflective of the overall hypermetabolic state. Hyperventilation with minute ventilation two to three times normal is common during this period. As a consequence, a respiratory alkalosis is the most common acid-base disturbance in the recovering patient. Mild hypoxemia may be present concurrently due to some pulmonary edema and shunting after vigorous fluid resuscitation. Burn-related hyperventilation typically recedes as the wound heals, but any supervening pulmonary or systemic complications can deplete the already stressed pulmonary reserve and require mechanical ventilation.

Pneumonia is currently the most common infectious complication in the burn patient and is considered the primary cause of death in 50% of fatal burn cases. Improvement in burn wound care and the use of topical antimicrobials has decreased the incidence of burn wound sepsis. This has consequentially decreased the incidence of hematogenously spread pneumonia. The sudden appearance of a solitary, round infiltrate on a routine chest x-ray (CXR) can be the first indication of a hematogenous pneumonia. An infected wound or vein harboring an area of septic thrombophlebitis is frequently the source of infection. The area of thrombophlebitis must be completely excised or drained and cannot be treated with antibiotics alone. Today pneumonia in the burn patient, as in any other sick patient in the intensive care unit (ICU), is acquired by the tracheobronchial rather than hematogenous route and is caused by *Staphylococcus aureus* or Gram-negative opportunistic bacteria. Atelectasis frequently precedes this complication and can be seen gradually developing on the CXR as an ill-defined pneumonic process. Antibiotic choice and duration is based on obtained tracheobronchial cultures and the patient's response.

Inhalation Injury

Inhalation injury presents as a clinical condition complicating the burn injury. It is evident in almost 20% of patients with a 50% TBSA burn and increases mortality from 18% to 50%. The pattern of airway injury can be divided into three distinct entities: (i) injury to the upper airway, (ii) injury to the lower airway, and (iii) carbon monoxide poisoning. Upper airway injury is limited to structures above and including the vocal cords. The pathophysiology relates to direct thermal injury by flame, heat, or steam. The patient may present with singed eyebrows, facial hair, or evidence of burns in and around the mouth and nose. Upper airway stridor secondary to difficulty in moving air is often present, and upper airway edema, erythema, or a carbonaceous coating can be seen during endoscopy or laryngoscopy. Because the disease process involves progressive edema, increasing over the first 24 to 36 hours and then subsiding, elective intubation during this time can support the patient and stent the supraglottic structures from collapse and obstruction. Although corticosteroids could shorten this period, their use should be avoided due to immunosuppressive effects and the already high incidence of infectious complications in the burn patient. Individuals with minor upper airway injuries can be managed expectantly without intubation, provided they are monitored closely during the period of progressive edema and intubated at any sign of respiratory distress.

Lower airway injury is rarely caused by direct thermal damage. The very successful evolution of the nasopharynx as a dissipater of heat—warming cold winter air and cooling down dry summer heat—does not allow transmission of thermal energy to the lower airways (except in isolated cases of severe steam inhalation). Damage is caused by the direct products of thermal combustion. Smoke contains over 200 chemicals that are damaging to the bronchial mucosa. Destruction of type I pneumocytes leads to difficulties in gas exchange and destruction of type II pneumocytes leads to inefficient surfactant secretion and small airway collapse. This results in airway obstruction, intrapulmonary shunting, and progressive hypoxia with respiratory failure. Casts of dead cells are sloughed into the small airways causing inefficient ventilation and further ventilation/perfusion mismatch. Clearance of the endobronchial debris is also compromised by the loss of the ciliary clearance mechanism.

Clinically, the patient does not manifest evidence of respiratory distress for 24 to 48 hours until the sloughing of cells lining the tracheobronchial tree is seen. History of confinement in a closed space should raise the physician's suspicion for inhalation injury, but routine diagnostic studies, CXR, and initial blood work are notoriously insensitive for lower airway injury. The workup of the patient with suspicion for inhalation injury should begin with bronchoscopy. An appropriately sized endotracheal tube is fitted over the bronchoscope before the start of the procedure, and if the patient requires intubation during bronchoscopy, the tube can be simply slipped over the scope into the trachea without additional manipulation or removal of the bronchoscope. Upper airway injury is excluded as the supraglottic passages are examined for signs of injury or the presence of edema. Evidence of mucosal inflammation, ulceration, deposition of carbon particles, or loss of definition of the septa dividing the bronchial orifices is indicative of lower airway injury. A false-negative examination can result from insufficient resuscitation and failure of inflammatory changes to develop in the underperfused mucosa. Inability to fully visualize the smallest airways can also lead to false-negative results. If the patient is suspected of having an inhalation injury, but the diagnosis cannot be confirmed by bronchoscopy, a ^{133}Xe ventilation/perfusion lung scan should be performed. A ^{133}Xe ventilation scan is frequently positive early after airway injury, showing patchy areas of ventilation/perfusion mismatch corresponding to areas of inhalation injury. Delaying this diagnostic maneuver by 72 hours can lead to a false-negative result once the hypermetabolism-induced hyperventilation sets in. Together the ventilation/perfusion scan and diagnostic bronchoscopy have an over 93% accuracy rate in detecting inhalation injury and are the diagnostic tests of choice for this disease process.

Treatment of the patient with inhalation injury relies mostly on supportive care during the recovery period. In those with mild disease, the use of frequent pulmonary toilet and warm humidified oxygen might be enough. Progressive hypoxia or respiratory distress necessitates endotracheal intubation and mechanical ventilation. Frequent therapeutic bronchoscopy is needed in those unable to clear the copious secretions due to mucosal sloughing. High fraction of inspired oxygen (FIO_2) requirements may be decreased with the judicial use of positive end-expiratory pressure, allowing recruitment of available airways. High frequency jet ventilation has been shown to decrease the incidence of barotrauma and facilitate the clearance of secretions. Steroids are again contraindicated because their antiinflammatory effects render the patient immunocompromised, exposing him or her to further infectious complications.

Pulmonary infections are the most common cause of morbidity and mortality in the burn patient, and their frequency is exaggerated by inhalation injury. Between 20% and 50% of those with an inhalation injury will develop pneumonia. Susceptibility to pulmonary infection by Gram-negative organisms, which colonize the burn patient, is accentuated with decreased mucosal defenses of the injured airway. Serial sputum cultures and gram stains should be obtained at the first sign of clinical deterioration and guide antimicrobial therapy.

Carbon Monoxide Poisoning

Carbon monoxide (CO) poisoning is frequently encountered in burns within an enclosed space. CO is an odorless product of hypoxic combustion and has an affinity for hemoglobin 200 times that of oxygen. By displacing O_2 from its binding site, it leads to cerebral hypoxia, anoxia, and tissue death. The classic picture of an obtunded patient with plethora and cherry red lips is rarely seen, except in premorbid cases of CO poisoning. CO exposure should be suspected based on neurological complaints such as confusion, light-headedness, and headache. Because the pulse oximeter does not detect carboxyhemoglobin, a normal transcutaneous saturation does not preclude CO poisoning. Only by measuring the level of carboxyhemoglobin on a blood gas CO oximeter can the level be determined. Normal levels range from 3% to 5% in nonsmokers and 7% to 10% in smokers. A higher blood concentration is pathologic and a 50% carboxyhemoglobin level is considered lethal.

CO poisoning should always be suspected in an individual burned within an enclosed space with the above neurological findings. Because determination of blood carboxyhemoglobin value is impossible in the field, treatment should be empiric. Because CO competes with O_2 for hemoglobin binding sites, its half-life of 4 hours at room air can be decreased to 60 minutes by the administration of 100% oxygen. Hyperbaric oxygen treatment at 2 atmospheric pressures can reduce the half-life further to 30 minutes and possibly minimize neurological sequelae. The cumbersome resuscitation of the burned patient in an enclosed hyperbaric chamber, however, precludes its general use. Immediate treatment with 100% face mask or endotracheal tube O_2 in the field usually reduces CO levels to normal by the time the patient arrives in the emergency department. Even though this treatment may prevent prolonged tissue hypoxia, neurological evidence of CO poisoning can persist. Postexposure neurological problems include parkinsonism, cortical blindness, deafness, memory deficits, and frank psychosis in 0.2% to 11% of individuals with CO exposure. Most victims either die or recover from their symptoms, but few develop permanent impairment. The cause of central nervous system damage is probably due to cellular hypoxia, but the exact mechanism is unknown.

Hydrogen cyanide (CN) is a combustion product of nitrogen-containing plastic polymers and is often present in industrial fires. Because both must occur in a closed space, cyanide poisoning without CO poisoning is rare. When CN inhibits oxidative phosphorylation by combining with the cytochrome complex and halting mitochondrial aerobic activity, lactic acidosis and tissue anoxia are seen despite normal blood oxygen content. Symptoms including an altered level of consciousness, dizziness, headache, tachycardia, and tachypnea are indistinguishable from those of CO poisoning. Because the standard blood CN level testing can take hours to perform, treatment is again based on clinical suspicion. The patient is given i.v. sodium thiosulfate that detoxifies cyanide to the harmless compound thiocyanate and hydroxycobalamin (vitamin B12) to produce inactive cyanocobalamin.

Renal System

Most of the changes in renal function are a direct result of the fluid and electrolyte imbalance. Immediately after the burn, the intravascular depletion and hypovolemia contribute to decreased renal perfusion and low urinary output levels. Although early oliguric renal failure and tubular necrosis are possible from prolonged hypovolemia, adequate fluid resuscitation will inevitably restore renal flow and function. Renal blood flow and the elimination of renally excreted drugs are augmented during the hyperdynamic phase of burn recovery. Late renal failure is usually caused by inappropriate doses of nephrotoxic drugs or multisystem organ failure due to septic complications.

Victims of high-voltage electrical injury and those with deep thermal burns or associated soft tissue injury can incur a high myoglobin load. Patients with heavy loads of hemochromogens in their urine are prone to develop acute renal failure unless a brisk diuresis is achieved. On top of resuscitation protocols, fluid should be administered in such quantities to achieve a urinary output level of 75 to 100 mL per hour. Failure to achieve this output despite sufficient fluid administration is one of the only indications for giving a diuretic within the initial resuscitation period. The patient is either given lasix or mannitol until the desired level of urine output is achieved and the pigment clears from urine. Because myoglobin is more soluble in an alkaline solution, some clinicians advocate alkalinizing the urine by the addition of bicarbonate to the resuscitation fluid. Although this maneuver may effectively clear pigment from the blood stream, its superiority over a simple brisk diuresis has not been proven. Once a diuretic has been administered, the urine output can no longer remain a safe indicator of intravascular volume status and a Swan-Ganz catheter should be placed to guide further fluid resuscitation.

Hematologic and Immunologic Changes

Biphasic changes are also seen in the coagulation system. At first, there is a marked depression of coagulation parameters characterized by a relative thrombocytopenia, a drop in fibrinogen level, and an increase in fibrin split products indicative of low-grade disseminated intravascular coagulation. Animal studies have shown that platelet microthrombi and local activation of the coagulation cascade in the area around the burn are responsible for this consumptive coagulopathy. Thromboxane and other arachidonic acid metabolites are produced locally in the burn wound and released from platelets. Local thrombosis in the zone of stasis can contribute to further ischemia and progressive tissue damage, leading to the conversion of a partial-thickness to a full-thickness burn. Some experimental data indicate that local and systemic administration of prostaglandin inhibitors can attenuate these responses and increase tissue salvage.

Immediately following resuscitation, there is a prompt return to a normal and even supranormal level of platelets, fibrinogen, and other procoagulant proteins such as factor V and factor VIII. This change is accompanied by a parallel decrease in protein C and antithrombin III. Despite this apparent prothrombotic state, thromboembolic phenomenon is surprisingly low in the burn population. Several large series have noted a deep venous thrombosis rate of less than 1% with only a 0.5% rate of pulmonary emboli, a rate much lower than in the trauma or ICU population as a whole. Due to the numerous potential complications associated with subcutaneous heparin such as prolonged bleeding during surgical debridement, hematoma formation under newly placed skin grafts, heparin-induced thrombocytopenia, and paradoxical arterial thrombosis, some centers have abandoned the routine use of subcutaneous heparin in the burned patient and favor other methods of prophylaxis.

Unlike other organ systems, the immunologic response to a burn injury is characterized by a global and persistent decrease in function. Immunosuppression is evident in all burned patients and directly proportional to the burn size. A global alteration is seen with decreased IL-2 production and T-cell activation, decreased polymorphonuclear leukocyte activity, and a deficiency of immunoglobulin and complement components. The exact etiology of the decrease in both specific and nonspecific immune function is unknown and could be due to the consumption of factors during early activation of the immune system or the presence of suppressor mechanisms. A minor beneficial effect of the relative immunosuppression is delayed rejection of allogeneic skin grafts, but because the burned patient is already susceptible to infection from loss of the skin barrier, most of the effects are deleterious. A temporal relationship between the onset of infectious complications and the degree of cellular immune dysfunction has been documented, reinforcing the correlation between the two conditions. With careful postburn management and prevention of setbacks from infectious complications, immune function generally returns to normal 2 to 3 weeks after the burn. Current research is focused on boosting the immune response with colony-stimulating factors and administration of IL-2. Among the numerous therapies investigated, early wound debridement and closure has been shown to restore neutrophil migration, further stressing the importance of early excision and grafting for patient survival.

CLINICAL MANAGEMENT AND TRIAGE OF THE BURNED PATIENT

Prehospital Care

Unlike other trauma victims, the burned patient is still undergoing injury when rescuers initially arrive. Ongoing heat and combustion of clothes can extend the area of the burn. Exposure to corrosive chemicals will lead to progressive tissue damage and contact with electrical wiring will result in ongoing electrocution. The first responder should separate the patient from the source of heat or electricity, remove all clothing, and dilute with copious lavage any chemical agents causing injury. Neutralization of acid or alkali solution should be avoided because the exothermic reaction will elaborate more heat and result in further injury. Irrigation with water should be carried out to remove as much of the offending agent as possible. Cold application to burned tissue may reduce the heat contact and arrest propagation of tissue destruction if applied within 10 minutes of injury but will only contribute to hypothermia beyond that time. Following the cooling or irrigation, a clean sheet and blanket should be placed over the patient to conserve body heat and prevent hypothermia.

A primary survey according to ATLS protocol should be carried out and any patient with obvious respiratory distress or inhalation injury needs to be intubated in the field. One hundred percent FIO_2 by face mask or endotracheal tube is administered during transport to assist in oxygen delivery and facilitate the disassociation of CO. Intravascular fluid status is estimated in the field. Because hemodynamic instability within 30 minutes of injury is rare in an isolated burn injury, establishing i.v. access in the field is not always necessary due to the high rate of infectious complications experienced by the burned patient. If delayed transport to a care facility is anticipated or the patient requires fluid or pressors due to another injury, i.v. access should be established. The preferable route of access is a peripheral i.v. through unburned tissue, but if no site is available, burned tissue or a central vein can be used for fluid administration.

Emergency Department Evaluation

Upon arrival to the emergency department, the primary survey is again repeated, airway patency is reaffirmed, permanent i.v. access is established using sterile technique, and fluid resuscitation is begun. Impairment of ventilation and respiratory excursion can be seen with circumferential burns to the thorax. An *eschar* is defined as the nonviable mass of dead cells and denatured protein covering a full-thickness burn. This tissue has lost the elastic properties of unburned skin and is insensate and avascular. Developing edema in an eschar covering the thoracic cavity can interfere with free chest wall movement and ventilation. Burn escharotomy is performed as an emergency department or bedside procedure using a scalpel or elecrocautery. The purpose is to allow the edges of the eschar to separate, not to remove the eschar. Chest escharotomies should be placed in the anterior axillary line bilaterally, extending from the clavicle to the costal margin. If the eschar still restricts free chest wall and abdominal motion, the anterior axillary escharotomies can be connected by a similar subcostal incision (Fig. 7-2). The incision should be performed through charred and destroyed tissue without incising unburned subcutaneous tissue. Performed in this manner, the procedure is painless and bleeding is minimal.

A brief history surrounding the accident should be obtained from the conscious patient. Comorbid illnesses or medical conditions such as cardiopulmonary or renal dysfunction can complicate the postburn course. The use of medications, allergies, and tetanus status must be determined. If the patient is within 10 years of his last tetanus immunization, 0.5 mL of tetanus toxoid should be administered. If the patient is improperly immunized, tetanus toxin antibody should be given concurrently in the contralateral arm. Loss of consciousness or an explosion could signal other bodily and closed head injuries. An electrocardiogram should be obtained and continuous cardiac moni-

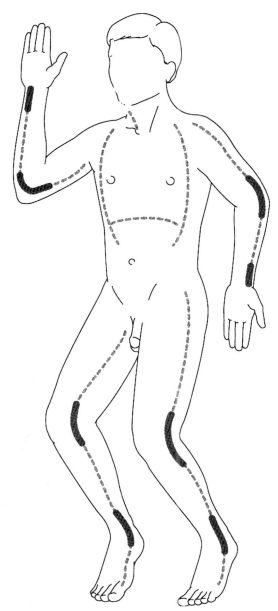

FIGURE 7-2. Preferred sites for escharotomy incisions. (From Moylan JA, Wellford WJ, Pruitt BA. Circulatory changes following circumferential extremity burns evaluated by the ultrasonic flowmeter: an analysis of 60 thermally injured limbs. *J Trauma* 1971;11(9):767, with permission.)

toring for arrhythmias should be instituted during the 72 hours after a high-voltage injury.

A secondary survey is used to evaluate other immediate life-threatening injuries and only then is the extent of the burn fully assessed. Focusing on the surface manifestation of the burn, no matter how horrific, can cause the care provider to overlook other life-threatening injuries. A head-to-toe examination is needed to evaluate possible mechanical injury to the neck or skull. Examination of the eyes and staining with fluorescein can disclose even subtle burns or abrasions to the cornea. Treatment with irrigation and ophthalmic antibiotics can manage all but the most extreme ophthalmic burns or chemical injuries. Stability evaluation of the neck is performed and appropriate radiographic studies ordered. Cardiac and pulmonary status is reassessed, as progressive edema or respiratory distress in those with inhalation injury may require delayed intubation. Serious intraabdominal injury in the hypovolemic patient can be frequently overlooked at the scene of the accident and should be reassessed at this time. All burned patients receive immediate stress ulcer prophylaxis with histamine blockers or antacids.

Assessment of peripheral extremity perfusion is critical in the emergency department and during the first few days after the burn. Edema of constricting circumferential eschar tissue can compromise blood flow to the arms and legs. Deep muscle or tissue swelling after an electrical injury can cause a true compartment syndrome, necessitating fascial release. Both are detected by the progressive swelling and change in the consistency of an extremity. Paresthesia and decreased range of motion with progressive fluid administration are both clues to impending extremity compromise. The five *P*'s of a compartment syndrome (pain, paresthesia, pallor, pulselessness, and poikilothermy) can be difficult to detect in a charred extremity and a simple clinical suspicion is sufficient reason for an escharotomy. Doppler pulse signal of the distal vasculature such as the palmar and digital vessels can be used to assess the distal circulation, but arterial changes may be a late sign in the developing compartment syndrome. Extremity escharotomies are performed in a similar fashion to those on the chest. Incisions through the dead tissue are made along planes designed to avoid major sensory and cutaneous nerves, and care is taken not to incise viable subcutaneous tissue (Fig. 7-2). Fasciotomy is an additional procedure performed only on patients with deep thermal or electrical burns if surface escharotomies fail to decompress the burned limb.

After the presence of other life-threatening injury is eliminated, the extent of the burn is assessed. The surface area burned is calculated using the rule of nines (Fig. 7-3). This method divides the body into 11 parts, each making up 9% of the TBSA (head, arms, anterior chest, posterior chest, anterior abdomen, lower back, upper legs, lower legs). The perineum makes up 1% of the TBSA. The sum adds up to 100%. A diagram of the patient's burns can help avoid serious miscalculations. Only second- and third-degree burns are used to calculate resuscitation requirements, and fluid administration is adjusted immediately upon calculating needs. Another useful technique assumes the patient's hand, without the fingers extended, is equal to 1% of the TBSA. Smaller and less extensive burns can be calculated using this method. In young children, a higher proportion of TBSA is occupied by the head, and more precise charts and calculations are used to guide pediatric fluid administration.

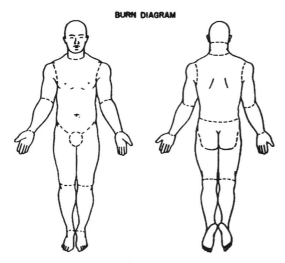

FIGURE 7-3. Burn estimate based on body surface area.

In contrast to the assessment of the burn size, initial evaluation of burn depth is notoriously inaccurate. Although the appearance of very superficial first-degree and deep third-degree burns is classic, differentiating a superficial second-degree burn from a deep second-degree or a third-degree burn during the early stages of resuscitation is next to impossible. Numerous technical aids such as laser Doppler flowmeter, vital dyes, and staining have been devised to aid in this determination, but they are full of inaccuracies and limitations. Fortunately, accurate estimation of burn depth is not necessary during resuscitation and fluid administration because second- and third-degree burns are treated the same. The matter becomes important several days after the burn when management decisions need to be made on which wounds will heal by themselves with minimal hypertrophic scarring and cosmetic complications and which wounds will need excision and skin grafting. Better surgical technique and improved function and cosmetic appearance of grafted wounds have shifted the clinical bias to early excision and grafting of most deep second-degree burns and even some superficial second-degree burns.

Triage

Minor wounds comprise 95% of all burns. Initial burn wound management can be carried out in the emergency department for those patients who will not require hospitalization. The burned area is gently cleaned with a mild disinfectant and only loose nonviable skin is removed. Blisters over 2 cm should be excised because they commonly rupture, but smaller ones can be left intact to act as a protective covering for the underlying tissue. After the wound is dressed, the patient is discharged home and seen in follow-up every 3 days. If the area remains free of infection, the patient is monitored as an outpatient until the wound heals. Any sign of wound infection mandates immediate hospitalization and initiation of topical antibiotics.

Despite the success of outpatient therapy, over 100,000 patients require hospitalization due to burn injury each year. Indications for inpatient care vary from person to person and are modified based on the circumstances surrounding the injury. Patients with second- and third-degree burns involving more than 20% TBSA generally need to be admitted for fluid resuscitation and surgical management of the wound. Lesser burn injuries with associated inhalation, concurrent trauma, or preexisting medical conditions are also better managed in a hospital setting. Significant electrical injury including lightening injury carries the added risk of ventricular and atrial arrhythmias. Cases of suspected child abuse and neglect should be admitted no matter what the extent of the actual burn (Table 7-3).

A high level of awareness is required by the physician caring for burned children in order to pinpoint and identify child abuse. The physician's suspicions should be aroused when the magnitude of injury is inconsistent with the history offered. Certain patterns of burn injury are incompatible with accidental exposure and point to more serious and intentional injuries of abuse. Characteristic forced immersion or "doughnut" burns are seen in infants and children who are intentionally placed in a hot or scalding bath. An area of second- or third-degree burn is sharply demarcated from surrounding uninjured tissue. Central sparing on the back or buttocks results when the area is forcefully compressed against the bottom of the container, avoiding exposure to the hot liquid (Fig. 7-4). This pattern is difficult to replicate with an accidental immersion when damage is equally distributed over the exposed area. Forced contact burns are caused by deliberate contact with a rigid hot object. The configuration and shape of the burn conforms to that of the object, such as a hot grate, and is uniform in all directions due to prolonged contact. Accidental burns always manifest an unequal pattern of injury as the child moves away from the heat. Burned children with a suspicion of intentional abuse should always be hospitalized and injuries reported to the appropriate local agency. Radiographic evidence of several long bone fractures at different stages of healing also points to possible child abuse.

TABLE 7-3. INDICATIONS FOR HOSPITAL ADMISSION AFTER BURN INJURY

Second and third degree burns over 20% TBSA
Second and third degree burns over 10% TBSA in children and elderly
Fourth degree burns over 5% TBSA
Any size burn with concurrent multisystem trauma
High voltage electrical injury
Suspicion of child abuse

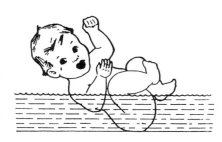
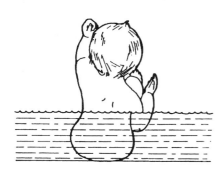
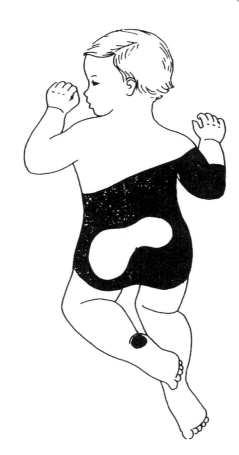

FIGURE 7-4. Typical pattern of submersion injury result in central buttock sparing. (From Lenoski EF, Hunter KA. Specific patterns of inflicted burn injuries. *J Trauma* 1997; 17(11):843–844, with permission.)

MANAGEMENT OF THE BURN WOUND

Excisional Management

For many years, burns were treated by daily washings, removal of loose and dead tissue, and application of topical ointments. The wound eventually healed by reepithelialization from the surrounding tissue or the burn eschar spontaneously separated. The underlying granulation tissue could then be covered by a split-thickness skin graft. Because full-thickness burns usually lose their protective eschar due to collagenase production from bacterial overgrowth, underlying granulation tissue was often heavily colonized. A 50% graft taken over this bed was considered acceptable and prolonged healing with hypertrophic scar formation and contracture was the norm in burn recovery. Nutritional support through the hypermetabolic phase and the frequent need for systemic antibiotics to treat burn infections and sepsis prolonged hospitalization. Patients remained in the hospital for several weeks to months.

The understanding of the deleterious systemic effects of burned tissue has changed this expectant management to one of early wound excision and coverage. The typical hospital course can now be divided into stages of burn evaluation and resuscitation, burn wound excision, temporary closure, and finally definitive closure of the wound. The advantages of early excision include a shortened duration of hypermetabolism, earlier reversal of immunologic impairment, decreased incidence of burn wound infection, and hypertrophic scarring, leading to shorter hospitalization and an earlier return to work.

Wounds that benefit from early excision and grafting include all full-thickness and deep partial-thickness burns. Due to the increased fibrosis and hypertrophic scarring associated with any wound that has not fully healed by 3 weeks, excision and grafting of even superficial second-degree burns can be of benefit to the patient. This is the time when estimation of burn depth is critical to optimize management. Differentiating a superficial partial-thickness burn that will spontaneously heal from a deeper injury necessitating excision requires clinical judgment and will change the course of management.

In the 1950s, scalpel excision down to investing fascia was used to remove full-thickness burns. For treatment of partial-thickness burns, the technique of tangential excision was later introduced. This technique is now used almost universally for deep and even full-thickness burns. Similar to harvesting a full-thickness skin graft, a dermatome or Humby guarded knife (Fig. 7-5) is used to remove the dead tissue and eschar. Rather than immediate removal of a large quantity of tissue, the burn is removed in successive thin layers until all nonviable tissue is excised. The presence of

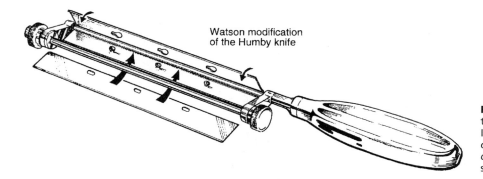

FIGURE 7-5. Humby guarded knife for tangential burn excision. (From McGregor IA, McGregor AD. *Fundamental techniques of plastic surgery and their surgical applications,* 9th ed. New York: Churchill Livingstone, 1995:43, with permission.)

dense bleeding from the capillary bed indicates healthy viable tissue. Maximum effects of this technique are realized if excision is carried out after resuscitation and as soon as the patient is cardiovascularly stable (generally within 72 hours of burn injury). Waiting longer decreases the benefits of early excision and allows for burn wound colonization and infection.

Although tangential excision adds a level of precision to determining the viable/nonviable tissue interface and allows maximal sparing of healthy tissue, this technique is not without limitation. Blood loss during excision can be formidable, and although tourniquet use can decrease bleeding in the extremities, it can also obscure healthy tissue. Topical thrombin and epinephrine is used for hemostasis, although systemic absorption limits epinephrine use only to small areas. Prolonged operating time can also contribute to systemic hypothermia and stress. Tangential excision is limited to 1 to 2 hours of operating time and 10% to 20% TBSA. The patient returns to the operating room within the next several days for further excision until all nonviable tissue is removed.

Expectant Management

Although early excision and grafting is now widely practiced, not all wounds can be treated in this manner. Patients with additional trauma and multiorgan injury or an inhalation injury might not be stable enough for a trip to the operating room. Small burns of an indeterminate depth covering cosmetically important areas such as the face, palms, soles, and genitals need to be monitored for signs of early healing and exact determination of burn depth. Patients with a large body surface burn cannot be debrided in one sitting and eschar will still remain between operations.

The burn wound is initially sterile but quickly colonized by endogenous bacteria. At first, Gram-positive bacteria predominate, but by the fifth postburn day, Gram-negative organisms colonize the burn. Bacteria proliferate and penetrate the avascular, protein-rich media of the eschar until they reach the nonviable/viable tissue interface. If host defenses are adequate, bacteria simply promote early eschar sloughing via local production of proteases. If host defense is compromised, as is commonly seen, systemic invasion can occur. Management of the unexcised burn wound was revolutionized in the 1960s with the widespread use of *topical antimicrobial agents.* Three topical agents are currently used in routine burn wound care. Each has specific limitations and side effects. Chemotherapy should be tailored to fit each individual's needs (Table 7-4). These agents must be differentiated from *topical antibiotics,* which are widely available but whose use should be discouraged due to the develop-

TABLE 7-4. TOPICAL ANTIMICROBIAL AGENTS

Agent	Spectrum of activity	Advantages	Side effects
Silvadene (silver sulfadiazine)	Gram-positive, yeast, most gram-negative except pseudominas and E. cloacae	Ease of application, painless	Poor eschar penetration, limited **neutropenia,** cannot use with sulfa allergy
Sulfamylon (mafenide acetate)	Most gram-positive and gram-negative	Good eschar penetration, broadest spectrum of activity	Pain upon application, **carbonic anhydrase inhibitor,** cannot use with sulfa allergy
Silver nitrate soaks	Most gram-positive and gram-negative, yeast	Can be used in those with sulfa allergy	Staining of tissue and material, poor eschar penetration, bulky dressings, **leaches electrolytes from tissue**

ment of resistant organisms and sensitization of the patient to the antibiotic. Topical bacitracin is an exception to this rule and is often used for outpatient burn management.

Silver sulfadiazine (Silvadene) burn cream is a 1% suspension and probably the most commonly used agent on the market. Its bacteriostatic activity comes from both the Ag+ ion and the polymerized sulfa compound. It is well tolerated by patients, does not cause pain upon application, and does not stain sheets or cloth. Its disadvantages include poor eschar penetration and limited activity against certain Gram-negative organisms such as some strains of *Pseudomonas* and *Enterobacter cloacae*. Many patients also develop neutropenia after exposure to this agent. This is usually a self-limited process and the leukocyte counts quickly return to normal upon discontinuation. They remain at normal levels even if the drug is reinstated.

Mafenide acetate (Sulfamylon) is available as an 11% suspension. This agent is also bacteriostatic, but unlike Silvadene, it penetrates freely the full thickness of the eschar down to the subeschar space. This compound also offers the broadest spectrum of activity against most Gram-negative and *Pseudomonas* organisms. The agent is best for patients with heavy eschar colonization or those who have failed other methods of topical therapy. Two disadvantages that limit its use are pain upon application and activity as a carbonic anhydrase inhibitor. Systemic absorption leads to bicarbonate wasting by the kidney and results in acidosis. Patients treated with this agent often develop compensatory hyperventilation to correct for the acid-base imbalance. Both mafenide acetate and Silvadene contain a sulfa compound as an active ingredient and should not be used on patients with a sulfa allergy or glucose-6-phosphate dehydrogenase deficiency.

Topical silver nitrate soaks (0.5%) are now less commonly used than in the past. Although it also has a broad spectrum of activity, this agent is difficult to use because it must be applied in the form of multilayered soaks. It does not penetrate the eschar, and the silver ion precipitates immediately upon contact with any proteinaceous substance. Although part of its bacteriostatic effect, this reaction tends to discolor unaffected skin of both the patient and the nursing staff. Clothes, bedsheets, and everything else in the ward is similarly affected. The bulky dressings limit full range of motion of joints and its use predisposes to major electrolyte disturbances. This agent leaches sodium, potassium, chloride, and calcium from both the wound and the patient. Symptomatic hyponatremia, hypochloremia, and hypokalemia, necessitating frequent electrolyte checks and repletion, are common.

Topical agents can control the bacterial population but do not sterilize the burn. Wound sepsis caused by *Pseudomonas aeruginosa*, formerly very common, has become rare due to wound surveillance and care. *S aureus*, from pulmonary and i.v. catheter sources, is now the most common organism isolated from the blood of the burned patient. To prevent systemic complications, one must identify burn wound infections at the earliest possible time. Conversion of a partial-thickness to a full-thickness burn, early eschar separation, and dark brown or black discoloration of the wound all point to burn wound infection (Table 7-5). Histologic examination of a burn wound biopsy is the most sensitive way to diagnose invasive infections. A tissue sample of the eschar and underlying unburned tissue is obtained using a scalpel. Part of the sample is sent to the microbiology laboratory for identification of the organisms and part is sent to pathology for frozen section analysis. Quantitative colony counts of less than 1×10^5 organisms per gram of burned tissue indicate absence of wound infection and another source of sepsis must be identified. Colony counts of more than 10^5 per gram of tissue usually indicate the presence of invasive infection, particularly if microorganisms are seen extending into viable uninjured tissue. Vascular or lymphatic invasion is also indicative of systemic infection. If one of the nondiffusible antimicrobial agents is being used, it should be stopped and therapy switched to mafenide acetate to increase eschar penetration. Systemic antibiotics are administered based on microbial sensitivity and the patient is scheduled for prompt wound excision.

Viral infections of a burn wound are uncommon and when they do occur are mostly herpetic. *Herpes simplex virus I* infection usually occurs in healing partial-thickness burns of the nasolabial area. Diagnosis is best made by biopsy of a cutaneous lesion and healing is expedited by the topical application of acyclovir ointment. Systemic herpesvirus infection is rare and the diagnosis should be suspected in the burned patient with signs of systemic sepsis and rapidly spreading cutaneous herpetic lesions. Treatment is changed to i.v. acyclovir, but the disease is usually fatal.

TABLE 7-5. SIGNS OF BURN WOUND INFECTION

Gross characteristics	Microscopic characteristics
Conversion of partial thickness to full thickness burn	Colony count over 10^5/g tissue
Rapid eschar separation	Microorganisms in subeschar space
Areas of dark brown or black discoloration	Microorganisms in viable tissue
Hemorrhage in underlying fat	Invasion of blood vessels (perivascular cuffing)
Ecthyma gangrenosum (metastatic septic lesions in unburned tissue—sign of *Pseudomonas* sepsis)	Invasion of lymphatics

TABLE 7-6. BURN WOUND COVERAGE OPTIONS

	Permanent	Temporary
Biologic	Autograft, cultured epithelial autograft	Allograft, Xenograft, Amnion
Synthetic	Integra	Biobrane

WOUND COVERAGE

The benefits of early excision are realized only if the wound is properly covered. Both biological and synthetic dressing have been developed for this purpose and can be grouped as *permanent* and *temporary agents* (Table 7-6).

Permanent Coverage

A split-thickness *autograft* consisting of epidermis and a variable proportion of dermis provides the best coverage for a freshly excised wound. Autografts 0.010 to 0.015 inches thick are harvested from unburned skin. Almost any site can be used to harvest a split-thickness skin graft. Preferable sites include the thigh, upper arm, and flat portions of the torso. The scalp presents as a favorable site in those with extensive burns with rapid reepithelialization and freedom from hypertrophic scar formation. Because the harvest of a split-thickness skin graft leaves intact dermal adnexal remnants, reepithelialization of the donor site is complete within 14 to 21 days. The same site can be used for multiple harvests, but the grafts are thinner and of poorer quality with each successive harvest.

If a graft is placed on a suitable bed of tissue it initially adheres by a fibrin clot. Revascularization is achieved by the growth of capillary buds from the recipient area to the undersurface of the graft. Revascularization is well advanced by day 3 and fibroblasts invade the fibrin clot to form the definitive connection within 1 week. Failure of graft take is usually a result of heavy granulation bed colonization or the formation of subgraft hematoma. To prevent this complication and expand the surface area covered by the split-thickness skin graft, the graft is usually meshed in a ratio of 1.5:1 up to 9:1 (Fig. 7-6). Reepithelialization occurs from the small bridges of skin centrally to cover all of the wound. Because the meshed pattern never fully disappears, areas of the great cosmetic concern such as the face and dorsum of the hand should be covered with unmeshed graft. Burns involving the joints should also be covered with unmeshed autograft to prevent formation of contractures.

Harvesting of adequate split-thickness skin grafts is impossible in those with massive burns. Elderly individuals also present with thin friable dermis and the wounds created by autograft harvest can be as difficult to heal as the original burn. Commercially grown sheets of cultured autologous keratinocytes (*cultured epithelial autograft*) have

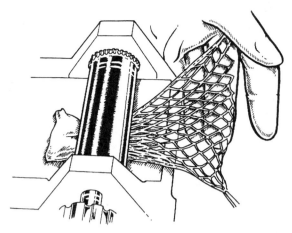

FIGURE 7-6. The mesher was originally designed to create slits (or pie crust) in a split-thickness skin graft to prevent the formation of a subgraft hematoma. Now it is used more often to expand the surface area of the autograft. (From McGregor IA, McGregor AD. *Fundamental techniques of plastic surgery and their surgical applications,* 9th ed. New York: Churchill Livingstone, 1995:57, with permission.)

been used to close excised burns in such patients. Three to four weeks are required to grow keratinocytes in sufficient quantity to cover the wound. Because this layer lacks a supporting dermis or epithelial appendages, it will remain dry and nonpliable. Low resistance to mechanical trauma, late wound contracture, and cracking of this layer also limit its clinical usefulness. The staggering cost to cover a large body surface can be prohibitive.

A synthetic bilaminate skin substitute has been developed in order to take advantage of dermal support. Integra consists of a dermal analog composed of chondroitin 6-sulfate enriched collagen fibrils covered by a thin silicone epidermal analog. Ingrowth of fibroblasts and granulation tissue into the collagen fibrils is complete by 3 to 4 weeks. The silicone upper layer is then peeled off and the neodermis covered by an ultrathin skin graft. Absorption of the collagen fibrils and replacement by native fibroblasts restore autologous tissue and forms a structure similar to native dermis. The use of an extrathin split-thickness skin graft allows earlier healing and reharvesting of donor sites. This product, however, is extremely expensive and is not yet universally available.

Temporary Coverage

Temporary overage of the freshly excised burn wound must be provided while waiting for permanent coverage in the form of regenerating autograft sites or cultured autologous keratinocytes. *Cutaneous allograft* (homograft) is the temporary biological dressing of choice against which all other dressings must be compared. It is harvested from cadavers free of disease and cutaneous malignancy. Shelf life can be extended and supply can be increased with refrigeration and cryprotective techniques. The allograft is placed over the wound in a similar manner as an autologous graft. The initial process of "take" is also similar to the autograft, and adherence is promoted by a fibrin layer with capillary ingrowth into the graft. Immune recognition and rejection of the graft as foreign occurs within several weeks as the graft sloughs. In the meanwhile, the allograft prevents wound desiccation, limits bacterial proliferation, and conditions the wound bed by promoting granulation tissue (presumably due to the elaboration of growth factors and cytokines). Limitations of cutaneous allograft such as its finite shelf life and the potential transmission of disease, hepatitis, and HIV have led to the development of other methods for temporary wound coverage.

Cutaneous xenograft, usually harvested from pigs, offers some advantages of human allograft and has no shortage of supply. Xenografts, however, never support true tissue ingrowth and allow the survival of a greater number of subgraft bacteria. Amniotic tissue can be used to cover the wound but has the same risk of disease transmission as allograft and requires frequent replacement due to desiccation. Biobrane is a synthetic, bilaminate wound dressing composed of a nylon mesh enclosed in a silicone outer membrane. It can be used as a temporary dressing to prevent desiccation or can cover a partial-thickness burn during reepithelialization. Because true union does not occur with the synthetic membrane, suppuration can occur in the subgraft space.

ELECTRICAL BURNS

Electricity damages tissue through conversion of electrical energy to heat. Because this is a function of both current density and tissue conduction, it is not uncommon for an area of small cutaneous damage to overlie a large amount of dead and devitalized tissue. *Myoglobinuria* is common with muscle destruction and the small cutaneous injury can often lead the inexperienced observer to underestimate the degree of damage. High-voltage and lightening injury often result in cardiopulmonary arrest, requiring resuscitation at the scene. *Hyperkalemia* from extensive tissue necrosis can also cause cardiovascular compromise and must be treated. Even minor electrical injuries can predispose to future arrhythmias and cardiac monitoring must be instituted for at least 72 hours.

Patients develop a compartment syndrome as the damaged muscle swells beneath investing fascia. Classic signs of a compartment syndrome are often difficult to discern in a charred extremity and the earliest symptoms of pain and swelling mandate fascial release. Operative debridement of devitalized tissue should be performed as soon as the patient is stable. Even if fasciotomies are not required, the degree of subcutaneous damage can not be estimated solely from the surface burn. The presence of viable superficial muscle does not guarantee that the underlying periosteal muscle is not necrotic.

Neurological changes can be seen after an electrical injury. Immediate neuropathy occurs directly from electrical injury and usually resolves with time. Late manifestations are more permanent and follow the thrombosis of the nutrient vessels to the spinal cord or large nerve trunks. Localized deficits, ascending paralysis, or even quadriplegia is not uncommon after an electrical injury. Compression fractures of the vertebrae can occur due to tetanic contractions at the time of electrocution and the delayed formation of cataracts can result from electrical contact in the head or neck.

A special form of electrical injury occurs in children who suffer burns from chewing on a live electric cord. A deep second- or third-degree burn forms on the lip and commissure of the mouth. Significant early or delayed bleeding can occur from the labial artery, justifying observation in the hospital. Even horrendous injuries to the lip or mouth can heal with good cosmetic results and further elective reconstruction can proceed after healing.

CHEMICAL BURNS

A strong acid or base destroys tissue by the denaturation and precipitation of protein and liberation of thermal energy. Tissue injury is ongoing as long as the offending agent remains in contact with skin. The first responder at the scene must remove all contaminated clothes and irrigate the area with copious amounts of water. Neutralization of the agent is discouraged because the exothermic reaction will elaborate more heat and lead to further tissue destruction. Wound irrigation needs to be carried out for at least 30 minutes after acid exposure and even longer with strong alkali due to deeper tissue penetration. Skin is tanned as it is destroyed by strong acid. This can often have the benign appearance of a suntan rather than the true full-thickness burn. Fluid requirements can be underestimated and excision delayed based on this misdiagnosis.

Hydrofluoric acid burn is a specific hazard to those working in the refinery industry or chemical manufacturing. Besides destroying tissue by changing its pH, hydrofluoric acid also causes injury by complexing with calcium. An initial painless period is followed by severe pain and necrosis. Topical application or subcutaneous injection of calcium gluconate into affected tissue limits damage and controls pain. *Systemic hypocalcemia* can occur after massive exposure and is treated by i.v. infusion of calcium.

FROSTBITE

Cold injury resembles a burn in many ways, but unique pathophysiologic alterations make treatment unique. For freezing to occur, ambient tissue temperature must fall to −2°C or −3°C. Tissue destruction occurs by the intracellular formation of ice crystals, and distortion of cellular architecture. Unlike the burn, damage is unevenly distributed throughout the extremity due to changing tissue tolerance to cold. The skin is relatively resistant to freezing, but other tissues, particularly nerves and blood vessels, are quite sensitive. As tissue temperature drops below 10°C, the cutaneous microvasculature displays alternating periods of vasoconstriction and vasodilation. This protective response, known as the *hunting reaction,* protects extremities from cooling while sacrificing core temperature. This mechanism is abolished in cases of systemic hypothermia.

The vascular system is particularly susceptible to cold and appears to be the primary target of freezing injury. Endothelial damage is apparent during thawing as platelet aggregates form and occlude the microvasculature. This obstruction results in opening of arteriovenous shunts, and although flow to the frozen extremity rises upon rewarming, flow to the damaged tissue is decreased.

Treatment of frostbite should focus on immediate rewarming of the injured extremity in an attempt to retard further damage. The frozen extremity should be placed in a circulating water bath at 40°C. Temperatures higher than 40°C can lead to independent tissue damage and lower temperatures rarely accomplish rapid thawing. Rewarming should be accomplished in 30 minutes and slow rewarming results in more extensive microvascular damage. Edema of the extremity is usually evident upon thawing but is rarely extensive enough to require fluid resuscitation. The depth of frostbite is classified into three levels similar to those of burn injury (Fig. 7-1), but accurate assessment of depth and tissue viability is impossible upon rewarming. Unlike in the burn, the mummified tissue over a frostbitten extremity does not result in physiological alterations and serves as a protective covering for underlying tissue. Demarcation can take weeks to months and premature debridement can sacrifice viable tissue. Local care focuses on prevention of infection while the tissue demarcates with avoidance of early eschar excision.

SUGGESTED READING

Greenfield E, Jordan B. Advances in burn wound care. *Critical care nursing clinics of North America.* Vol 8:2. Philadelphia: WB Saunders, 1996.

Pruitt BA Jr, Goodwin CA Jr, Pruitt SK. Burns, including cold, chemical, and electric injuries. In: Sabiston DC Jr, ed. *Textbook of Surgery,* 15th ed. Philadelphia: WB Saunders, 1997.

8

ANESTHESIA

MICHAEL B. RODRICKS AND C. WILLIAM HANSON III

Anesthesia, perhaps more so than any other specialty, has its roots in the United States. William T.G. Morton, on October 16, 1846, gave the first public demonstration of general anesthesia at the Massachusetts General Hospital. From this initial display, the discipline of anesthesiology was born.

It is imperative that the surgeon be familiar with the basic concepts of operative anesthesia. To function most effectively in the operating room, the surgeon and the anesthesiologist must work together as a team. Information pertaining to sudden or large amounts of blood loss, adequacy of relaxation, and forewarning before clamping or unclamping of hemodynamically significant vessels should be conveyed to the anesthesiologist. The anesthesiologist, in turn, has a responsibility to inform the surgeon of important information (such as hemodynamic stability, adequacy of urine output, etc.) as it arises.

The principles of operative anesthesia include the five A's. Amnesia, analgesia, anxiolysis, akinesia, and areflexia are generally desired qualities of an anesthetic. *Akinesia* ensures a quiet surgical field, allows the surgeon to function efficiently, and prevents mishaps associated with patient movement. *Areflexia* implies attenuation or abolishment of the hemodynamic responses associated with surgery.

PREOPERATIVE ASSESSMENT

An anesthetic begins with the preoperative assessment. This evaluation may take place on the day of surgery, in the patient's hospital room the night before surgery, or in a physician's office or preoperative evaluation center days to weeks before a scheduled surgery. The obvious advantage of an evaluation 1 or more days before surgery is that it allows further studies to be performed if indicated and interventions to take place so that the patient may be "optimized."

The preoperative evaluation begins with a thorough history. Particular attention to previous anesthetics is important: The type of anesthesia given, the nature of the surgery, and the patient's level of satisfaction with the anesthetic should be noted. A personal or family history of adverse reactions to anesthesia is elicited. Assessment of cardiac and pulmonary function is crucial because most major perioperative complications involve these organ systems. A history of congestive heart failure, angina, hypertension, arrhythmias, or myocardial infarction warrants further investigation. The ability of a patient to walk at least two blocks or up two flights of stairs without dyspnea or angina is indicative of adequate cardiac reserve. The evaluation of the pulmonary system includes an inquiry for reactive airway disease, chronic obstructive pulmonary disease, tobacco use, and recent upper respiratory tract infections. Patients should be strongly encouraged to refrain from tobacco use before surgery. Twenty-four hours of smoking abstinence will reduce carboxyhemoglobin levels, although an improvement in mucociliary transport takes several weeks of no smoking. Based on the patient's state of health, a physical status is assigned (Table 8-1). Physical status is a means of classifying patients based on their overall condition and does not take the planned procedure into account.

The patient's *current medications* need to be reviewed during the preoperative assessment. A number of common drugs have potential interactions with anesthetic agents. Chronic alcohol abuse will cause tolerance to anesthetic agents while acute alcohol intoxication will result in decreased anesthetic requirements. Diuretics tend to cause hypovolemia and hypokalemia. Beta-blockers may blunt sympathetic nervous system (SNS) responses as well as induce bronchospasm and bradycardia.

A *physical examination* with special emphasis on the vital signs, airway, heart, lungs, and central nervous system (CNS) is performed. Particular attention should be placed on the airway evaluation. Dental injury is the leading cause of malpractice cases against anesthesiologists. *Laboratory data* should be ordered on the basis of findings on history and physical examination, keeping in mind the planned procedure. With the new emphasis on cost containment, gone are the days of ordering a full set of studies on all patients. The haphazard ordering of laboratory tests is not only

---

Hospital of the University of Pennsylvania, Philadelphia, Pennsylvania

TABLE 8-1. THE PHYSICAL STATUS CLASSIFICATION OF THE AMERICAN SOCIETY OF ANESTHESIOLOGISTS

Physical status	Definition
PS-1	A healthy patient (free of systemic disease)
PS-2	A patient with mild systemic disease that results in no functional limitations
PS-3	A patient with moderate to severe systemic disease that results in some functional limitation
PS-4	A patient with severe systemic disease that is a constant threat to life and incapacitating
PS-5	A moribund patient who is not expected to live 24 hours with or without surgery
PS-6	A brain-dead patient for organ harvest
E (emergency)	Any patient in whom an emergency operation is required; e.g., a healthy patient undergoing an emergency procedure is classified as PS-IE

expensive, but also rarely of any utility. A general guideline for ordering laboratory studies is provided in Table 8-2.

Anesthetic Technique

Based on the proposed surgery, the patient's condition and preference, the surgeon's needs, and the anesthesiologist's opinion, an anesthetic technique is chosen. General anesthesia, regional anesthesia, peripheral nerve block, and monitored anesthesia care represent the various options. *General anesthesia* implies a loss of consciousness, either by inhaled or intravenous (i.v.) agent. *Regional anesthesia* is specific for a given region of the body; it typically does not alter consciousness. *Epidural, spinal,* and *caudal anesthesia* (collectively known as *neuraxial blockade*), though acting at the spinal cord and it's spinal nerves, all represent regional modalities. The hemodynamic alterations and respiratory consequences of neuraxial blockade can be significant. A *peripheral nerve block* is achieved by infiltration of a nerve or nerves to anesthetize a given distribution. Peripheral nerve blocks are an attractive option for patients with poor cardiac or pulmonary reserve, as hemodynamic and respiratory perturbations are minimized. Monitored anesthesia care is the administration of sedation and analgesics for patient comfort. The surgeon often infiltrates the operative site with a local anesthetic to provide additional analgesia.

MONITORING

Certain tools have become standard intraoperative monitors for virtually all anesthetics in modern operating rooms. They include the pulse oximeter, noninvasive blood pressure monitor, electrocardiogram, temperature monitor, and a means of assessing adequacy of ventilation (i.e., an end-tidal carbon dioxide monitor).

Patients undergoing general anesthesia may breathe spontaneously or if paralyzed, be placed on a ventilator. There are various ventilator monitors and alarms built into most modern anesthesia machines. Respiratory rate, tidal volume, oxygen concentration being delivered, and a low oxygen concentration alarm are universal. Airway pressure monitoring allows the detection of low circuit pressure (in the event of a disconnection from the ventilator) and high circuit pressure (which may alert one to a kink in the circuit, main stem bronchus intubation, patient respiratory effort, etc.).

Most operating rooms employ end-tidal capnometry or mass spectrometry as routine monitors during general anesthesia. Capnometry measures the level of carbon dioxide (CO_2) in the circuit and serves as a reliable indicator of a tracheal intubation. The presence of CO_2 in exhaled gas is the gold standard of a successful endotracheal intubation, although the endotracheal tube may be mispositioned in a main stem bronchus. With normal lungs, end-tidal CO_2 is approximately 5 mm HG below arterial CO_2 and capnometry serves as a reliable noninvasive measure of systemic partial pressure of CO_2. End-tidal capnometry and the interpretation of the waveform of exhaled CO_2 can give a great deal of information about the patient's cardiopulmonary status; for example, bronchospasm can be diagnosed from a delayed upstroke in the end-tidal capnogram, while cardiac arrest is heralded by a sudden loss of end-tidal CO_2.

Mass spectrometry is used to measure the end-tidal concentration of oxygen, nitrogen, carbon dioxide, nitrous

TABLE 8-2. GENERAL GUIDELINES FOR PREOPERATIVE TESTING

Test	Indication
Hemoglobin concentration	Surgery with potential for significant blood loss, women of child-bearing age, patients over the age of 60, as indicated by H & P
Coagulation profiles	Current treatment with anticoagulants, as indicated by H & P
Blood chemistries	Current diuretic treatment, patients over the age of 60, as indicated by H & P
Electrocardiogram	Patients over the age of 40, history of hypertension, as indicated by H & P
CXR	Thoracic surgery, evidence of pulmonary disease
PFTs	Thoracic surgery in a patient with evidence of pulmonary disease

oxide, and inhalational anesthetics, permitting real-time correlation between exhaled concentration of gases and anesthetic level.

An *intraarterial catheter* may be inserted for frequent blood gas and electrolyte monitoring or "beat to beat" blood pressure monitoring where a narrow blood pressure range must be maintained (Table 8-3). The radial artery is the preferred site of placement of an arterial line, in the absence of contraindications.

A *central venous line* may be used to monitor intravascular volume for patients in whom left ventricular filling pressures can be presumed to correlate with central venous pressures (CVPs). In an emergency situation (such as exsanguination), it may be impossible to cannulate a peripheral vein, leaving central venous access as the only option. A central venous catheter may also be used to infuse vasoactive medications or aspirate air from or infuse volume into the central circulation (Table 8-4). In addition, central access provides a means for total parenteral nutrition administration in patients unable to receive enteral feeds.

The internal jugular, subclavian, or femoral vein may be chosen for cannulation. The internal jugular vein is easier to access and more reliable for pulmonary artery catheter placement than the subclavian vein. The right subclavian vein is a notoriously difficult site from which to perform right heart catheterization. One to two percent of subclavian line placements are complicated by the development of a pneumothorax. Despite having a higher complication rate and being more difficult to place, subclavian lines are better tolerated by the patient and less work from a nursing standpoint than neck vein catheters. In an emergency situation, the femoral vein is the preferred site of central line placement. Femoral lines, however, are prone to the development of line sepsis and thrombosis. They should be removed as soon as possible.

The *pulmonary artery catheter* is preferred to the central venous line when there are abnormalities of the tricuspid valve, right ventricle, pulmonary vasculature, mitral valve, or pericardium—i.e., conditions under which the pulmonary artery occlusion pressure (PAOP) is a more accurate measure of left ventricular end-diastolic volume (LVEDV) than the CVP (Table 8-5). It is also felt by some to be a reliable early indicator of left ventricular ischemia. This presupposes that ischemia is the cause of sudden increases in PAOP due to a precipitous decrease in left ventricular compliance. The use of PAOP as an indicator of left ventricular preload relies on the assumption that there is a predictable proportional relationship between pulmonary artery diastolic pressure, PAOP left ventricular end-diastolic pressure, and LVEDV. Mitral valve disease, high levels of positive end-expiratory pressure, catheter position in the lung, and alterations in left ventricular compliance can all confound the relationship between PAOP and LVEDV.

A *urinary catheter* permits indirect evaluation of renal and splanchnic blood flow in patients with normal kidneys.

TABLE 8-3. INDICATIONS FOR PLACEMENT OF ARTERIAL LINES

	Risk of procedure
Cardiac surgery	Infection
Major vascular surgery	Thrombosis
Pulmonary resections	Vasospasm
Intracranial operations	Hematoma
Major trauma procedures	Air embolization
Major organ transplant (liver)	—
Deliberate hypotension	—
Deliberate hypothermia	—
Patients having surgery with significant pulmonary disease, significant cardiovascular disease, obesity	—

TABLE 8-4. INDICATIONS FOR PLACEMENT OF CENTRAL VENOUS LINES

	Risks
Cardiac surgery	Bleeding
Surgery with large volume shifts	Infection
Potentially hypovolemic patients, i.e., bowel obstruction	Carotid puncture
Shock	Pneumothorax
Massive trauma	Nerve damage
Need for total parenteral nutrition	Thoracic duct trauma (with left-side placement)
Vasopressor requirement	Venous thrombosis
	Air embolization
	Venous or cardiac perforation

TABLE 8-5. INDICATIONS FOR PLACEMENT OF A PULMONARY ARTERY CATHETER

	Risks
General surgery:	
Major surgery in patients with heart disease	Those of central venous cannulation plus:
Patients with significant coronary artery disease	
Septic surgical patients	Arrhythmias
Massive trauma	Pulmonary arterial rupture
Shock	Knotting
Planned aortic clamping	Endocardial or valvular damage
Severe preexisting respiratory failure	—
Preexistent pulmonary emboli	—
Cirrhosis	—
Liver transplant	—
Cardiac Surgery:	
Poor left ventricular function	—
Recent infarction	—
Valve replacement (on left side)	—
Pulmonary hypertension	—

Urine output of greater than 0.5 mL/kg per hour is consistent with adequate renal blood flow in an adult. A catheter is typically used in any lengthy operative procedure, in the event of ongoing resuscitation, or when impaired renal blood flow is a concern.

Cutaneous application of a *peripheral nerve stimulator* allows an objective assessment of the level of neuromuscular blockade when paralytic agents are used. A train of four electrical stimuli (40 to 50 mA) is applied over 2 seconds (2 Hz), typically to the ulnar nerve where the adductor pollicis muscle (thumb opposition) is monitored for effect. When non-depolarizing drugs (pancuronium, *cis*-atracurium) are used, the train demonstrates "fade," with the last twitch smaller than the first. This is analogous to the "fatigue" seen with myasthenic patients.

A number of specialized monitors may be employed during procedures where there exists the potential to compromise the integrity of the CNS. Electroencephalographic (EEG) monitoring is used for carotid endarterectomies and by some centers for coronary artery or cardiac valvular surgery. Somatosensory evoked potentials are useful for monitoring the spinal cord and its vascular supply (i.e., thoracic aneurysmectomy). Monitoring may be done by the anesthesiologist or more typically by a dedicated technician.

Transesophageal echocardiography (TEE) has become a mainstay for the intraoperative monitoring of select patients. It is currently employed primarily in the cardiac surgical suites. TEE permits real-time evaluation of left ventricular wall-motion and end-diastolic volume. It is used to detect air embolism, aortic dissection, valve malfunction, and myocardial ischemia as manifested by regional wall-motion abnormalities.

Bispectral analysis of the EEG can be used to judge anesthetic depth. Intraoperative recall, a very undesirable event, has been shown to be minimized with the use of bispectral analysis. Intraoperative use of bispectral analysis allows the use of lower doses of anesthetic agents, which in turn provides for a shorter "wake-up time" following completion of surgery. Bispectral analysis is, however, a poor predictor of patient movement, which is often reflexive in nature.

INHALATIONAL AGENTS

General endotracheal anesthesia typically implies some combination of oxygen with or without nitrous oxide and a volatile agent (such as halothane or isoflurane). Ether and chloroform are no longer used in the United States because of their toxicity and flammability. It is not commonly recognized that under appropriate conditions (such as hyperbaric pressures), a wide variety of gases, including inert gases, can act as anesthetics. Nitrogen narcosis, or "rapture of the deep," demonstrates nitrogen's ability to act as an anesthetic at high pressures.

The primary effector site of anesthetic gases is the CNS, with the lungs providing a conduit for delivery of the gas to the CNS. The standard measure of potency for inhaled anesthetics is arbitrarily defined as the minimum alveolar concentration (MAC) of a given gas at 1 atm that produces immobility in 50% of subjects exposed to a noxious stimulus. MAC is expressed in terms of percentage of 1 atm, so that the MAC of nitrous oxide, which is 105%, is unachievable at sea level but becomes reachable with more atmospheric pressure.

The inhalational agents in common use today include nitrous oxide, halothane, isoflurane, enflurane, sevoflurane, and desflurane (Table 8-6). Each has its own unique set of properties. It is an inhalational anesthetic's partial pressure in the brain that results in anesthesia. Therefore, more soluble agents are slower in onset and offset but are more potent (lower MAC) than less soluble agents. Other important characteristics include cardiovascular respiratory depression, airway irritation, amount of agent metabolized as well as effects on blood flow to vital organs.

Nitrous oxide is a colorless, odorless gas. It is the least soluble of the agents currently in use; therefore, it is not very potent (MAC of 105%). Its lack of potency results in its use as an adjuvant gas at relatively high partial pressures. Its major shortcoming is the tendency to diffuse into closed air-containing spaces. It is, therefore, contraindicated in the presence of a pneumothorax, small bowel obstruction, air embolism, middle ear surgery, etc. A second potential problem with nitrous oxide is its predilection

TABLE 8-6. CHARACTERISTICS OF INHALATION ANESTHETICS

Agent	MAC[a]	Adverse effects
Nitrous Oxide	105	Bone marrow depression, pernicious anemia, diffused into air containing cavities (contraindicated in presence of pneumothorax, small bowel obstruction, etc.)
Halothane	0.7	High solubility (slow onset and offset), sensitized heart to dysrhythmogenic effects of epinephrine, potential cause of hepatitis
Enflurane	1.7	May cause seizures at high doses
Isoflurane	1.2	Potential to cause coronary steal
Desflurane	6.0	Pungent odor, may cause airway irritation
Sevoflurane	2.0	Metabolism produces free fluoride ions with potential to cause impaired renal function

[a]MAC, minimum alveolar concentration.

to oxidize vitamin B12 into an inactive state. Prolonged exposure may thus result in peripheral neuropathies and megaloblastic anemia.

Halothane is a potent agent with a pleasant odor. It is not irritating to the airways, acts as a potent bronchodilator, and is often used for masked induction of children. Because of its high solubility, halothane is slow in onset and offset. It is known to cause a variety of cardiac arrhythmias (atrial and ventricular), particularly in the presence of increased epinephrine levels. Its use has been limited in recent years because of concerns about *halothane hepatitis*, which is likely immune mediated, potentially fatal, and most often afflicts middle-age obese women. A family predisposition to halothane hepatitis has also been noted.

Because of the development of newer agents with more favorable characteristics, *enflurane* is not commonly used today. A shortcoming of enflurane is its metabolism, which produces a potentially nephrotoxic fluoride ion. Seizure activity may be seen with the use of high doses of enflurane. Isoflurane causes the least myocardial depression of the inhalational agents. It does, however, cause vasodilation, which will lower blood pressure. Vasodilation of coronary arteries has the potential to divert blood from fixed lesions, the so-called *coronary steal syndrome*. This syndrome seems primarily theoretical, as isoflurane does not tend to cause ischemia in the clinical setting.

Desflurane is a very insoluble agent, with a composition similar to that of isoflurane. Because of its low solubility, desflurane has a very fast onset with a quick recovery profile. It is therefore associated with shorter times to extubation after completion of surgery. A pungent odor makes desflurane unsuitable for masked induction, and it may precipitate coughing. Catecholamine surges may cause a transient tachycardia, which appears to be self-limited.

Sevoflurane is a nonpungent agent, which is particularly suited for masked induction. It falls between isoflurane and desflurane in terms of solubility. Sevoflurane, like enflurane, is metabolized with the production of fluoride ion; therefore, it should not be used in patients with renal failure.

INTRAVENOUS ANESTHESIA

Traditionally, operative anesthesia has consisted of an inhalational anesthetic combined with i.v. use of agents such as opiates and paralytics in a balanced technique. With the development of new drugs, total i.v. anesthesia has become a more common technique. Propofol, in particular, has proven to be a very reliable agent; combined with an opiate and a muscle relaxant, total i.v. anesthesia is an attractive alternative to a balanced technique.

Barbiturates

The traditional agents for the i.v. induction of anesthesia include thiopental and methohexital. They undergo hepatic metabolism and urinary excretion. *Sodium thiopental* (Pentothal) is the most commonly encountered barbiturate. It is highly lipophilic, quick in onset, and short acting because of rapid redistribution after a single dose. With repeated doses, peripheral fat stores become saturated with sodium thiopental and recovery is much slower.

Barbiturates (Table 8-7) depress medullary and pontine respiratory centers and may cause profound respiratory depression when administered as a bolus. They also act as cardiovascular depressants and cause peripheral vasodilation and myocardial depression when given with typical induction doses. The reduced doses of barbiturates administered should be decreased in the presence of hypovolemia or hypotension. Acute intermittent porphyria may be precipitated by administration of barbiturates to predisposed individuals. A beneficial effect of these agents is the reduction in cerebral metabolism and oxygen consumption. They provide cerebral protection in the face of focal ischemia but not in the event of global ischemia (such as cardiac arrest).

Benzodiazepines

Benodiazepines are primarily used as anxiolytics; however, they may also be used for induction and in combination with other agents for total i.v. anesthesia. *Midazolam*,

TABLE 8-7. INTRAVENOUS AGENTS

Drug	Induction dose[a]	Duration[b]	Unique properties[c]
Barbiturates:			
Thiopental	3.0–5.0 mg/Kg	Minutes	↓ ICP
Benzodiazepines:			
Midazolam	0.2–0.4 mg/Kg	30–90 min	Profound amnestic
Opioids:			
Fentanyl	5.0–100 mg/Kg	6–24 h	Stable BP and CO
Miscellaneous:			
Propofol	1.5–2.5 mg/Kg	Minutes	↑HR ↓SVR
Ketamine	1.0–2.0 mg/Kg	15–60 min	Bronchodilator; ↑HR, ↑SVR

[a]To induce anesthesia as a sole agent in a healthy adult.
[b]Will vary considerably from patient to patient. Range represents usually clinically important duration of action.
[c]BP, blood pressure; HR, heart rate; ICP, intracranial pressures; SVR, systemic vascular resistance.

because of its short duration of action (30 to 90 minutes), is the predominant benzodiazepine encountered in anesthetic practice. Midazolam is a sedative-hypnotic with profound amnestic properties. It has minimal depressant effects on the cardiovascular and respiratory system when used alone; however, as an adjuvant agent, it has more significant depressive effects on these systems. Benzodiazepines have no analgesic properties and are therefore often combined with opiates. Flumazenil is a specific benzodiazepine reversal agent. Bolus administration of flumazenil may cause seizure activity in patients on chronic benzodiazepine therapy.

Opioids

Opioids are not sedative-hypnotics and have minimal amnestic properties. They interact with opioid receptors in the CNS and mediate effects on pain, mood, respiration, circulation, and bowel and bladder function. The liver is the site of opioid metabolism.

In general, opioids are not associated with decreased cardiac contractility. Blood pressure may, however, fall as a result of vagally mediated bradycardia and blunting of the SNS. There is a direct dose-dependent depression of ventilation with opioid administration. Peristalsis is slowed and gastric emptying is delayed by opioids. Opioids have a prominent effect on the gastrointestinal tract. Peristalsis is slowed and gastric emptying is delayed. Nausea and vomiting, as well as constipation and urinary retention, are common side effects to using opioids.

Morphine and *meperidine* have been associated with histamine release. Both are known to have active renally excreted metabolites, which will accumulate in patents with renal failure. The combination of meperidine and monoamine oxidase inhibitors has been linked with untoward reactions, including sudden death. Fentanyl, a synthetic agent, has minimal cardiovascular effects and a short half-life. It has thus become the opioid of choice for most anesthesiologists. Fentanyl does, however, have a high potential for abuse. It is the most widely abused drug by anesthesiologists.

All opioids are utilized as components of a particular anesthetic technique: anesthesia with sedation; balanced inhalational and i.v. anesthesia; and for postoperative pain management (e.g., epidural opioids). They are unable to provide total i.v. anesthesia both because of respiratory depression and the potential for intraoperative awareness that exists even in the face of massive doses.

Propofol

Propofol is a lipid soluble agent with a very short (4- to 8-minute) half-life. It has excellent amnestic and sedative properties; however, it has no analgesic effects. Cardiovascular depression results in a drop in blood pressure, which may be profound in cases of hypovolemia or depressed left ventricular function. Because of its short half-life and antiemetic properties, propofol is now the most commonly used induction agent. Continuous infusions of propofol (100 to 200 mg/kg per minute) can be used in combination with other agents (such as opioids) for total i.v. anesthesia.

Ketamine

Ketamine is a phencyclidine derivative that induces a dissociative state of anesthesia. Unlike other agents, ketamine stimulates the SNS, causing an increase in heart rate, blood pressure, and cardiac output. Ketamine has negligible effects on ventilatory drive and is associated with bronchodilatation. Cerebral blood flow and oxygen consumption are increased with the administration of ketamine. Because of this, it is undesirable in patients with head injury and/or elevations in intracranial pressure. Its stimulation of the SNS makes ketamine contraindicated in the presence of coronary artery disease or uncontrolled hypertension. Emergence dysphoria and hallucinations are commonplace following ketamine-based anesthesia.

Muscle Relaxants

There are a number of rational reasons for the use of neuromuscular blocking agents (Table 8-8). They are known to facilitate intubation as well as surgical exposure, to ensure immobility, and to enable a patient to be anesthetized with

TABLE 8-8. MUSCLE RELAXANTS

Agent	Intubating dose (mg/Kg)	Duration	Clearance	Autonomic effects	Of note
Depolarizing:					
Succinylcholine	1.5–2.0	3–5 min	Enzymatic	+ vagatonic	↑K, arrhythmias
Nondepolarizing:					
Pancuronium	0.08–0.10	90 min	Renal	Vagolytic	Tachycardia
Cisatracurium	0.20	60 min	Enzymatic	—	Organ-independent elimination
Vecuronium	0.10	60 min	Renal, hepatic	—	Cardiovascularly inert
Rocuronium	0.6–1.0	60 min	Hepatic	—	Rapid onset of intubating conditions
Rapacuronium	1.0–1.5	20 min	Hepatic	—	Histamine release; renally excreted active metabolite

TABLE 8-9. ADVERSE EFFECTS OF SUCCINYLCHOLINE

1. It is a known trigger for malignant hyperthermia.
2. A prolonged duration of action is seen in patients with atypical pseudocholinesterase or severe liver disease.
3. Increases in intragastric, intraocular, and intracranial pressures follow its administration.
4. Arrhythmias including bradycardia, junctional arrhythmias, and ventricular dysrhythmias may occur because of vagotonic effects.
5. While usually mild (a rise of 0.5–1.0 mEq/dl is typical) and transient, hyperkalemia follows succinylcholine administration. This effect can be profound in patients with burns, upper and lower motor neuron injuries or disease, and after significant trauma. The hyperkalemic response is most pronounced beginning 24 hours after a burn or injury and lasts 6 months. In predisposed patients, the precipitous rise in potassium may cause cardiac arrest.
6. Because of the potential for undiagnosed muscular dystrophy, succinylcholine is relatively contraindicated in children.

lower concentrations of inhalational agents. Degree of paralysis can be objectively assessed with a peripheral nerve stimulator.

There are two major types of neuromuscular blocking agents: depolarizing and nondepolarizing. There are numerous nondepolarizing agents commonly used today, though the only depolarizer used is *succinylcholine*. Succinylcholine binds to the acetylcholine receptor, causing an initial depolarization that is heralded by fasciculations and subsequent flaccid paralysis. It eventually dissociates from the receptor and is metabolized by plasma pseudocholinesterase to succinic acid and choline. The major advantage of succinylcholine is its rapid onset, provision of reliable intubating conditions in 60 seconds, and ultrashort duration of action (3 to 5 minutes). Succinylcholine, however, is associated with various adverse side effects (Table 8-9).

Nondepolarizing agents do not act at the acetylcholine binding site, but at another part of the receptor. Their mechanism of action is a competitive inhibition of acetylcholine binding. Pharmaceutical companies have long been searching for a nondepolarizing agent that will match succinylcholine in speed of onset and have an ultrashort duration of action. Such an agent has not yet been produced.

Nondepolarizing agents can be reversed with acetylcholinesterase inhibitors such as neostigmine and edrophonium. Their mechanism of action is via inhibition of acetylcholine breakdown. Intrasynaptic levels of acetylcholine rise, allowing for displacement of the neuromuscular blocker.

LOCAL ANESTHETICS

Local anesthetics can be classified as either *amides* or *esters* on the basis of their intermediate linkage structure (Table 8-10). An easy way to differentiate amides from esters is on the basis of their name. Agents in the amide family have two *i*'s in their name (lidocaine, ropivacaine), and esters have a single *i* (procaine, cocaine). Certain generalizations can be made about the two groups based on the nature of their linkage. Plasma cholinesterase is responsible for the metabolism of the ester family of agents while local anesthetics with an amide linkage undergo hepatic metabolism. In general, the ester agents are shorter acting than the amides, tend to be less toxic on a milligram-per-milligram basis. However, they have a higher incidence of "true" allergic reactions based on cross-sensitivity to paraaminobenzoic acid.

Local anesthetics act on the sodium channels of nerve membranes. Binding to specific receptors within the inner portion of sodium channels, these agents stabilize the channel in the inactivated state. The initiation and conduction of action potentials is thus terminated, causing a loss in sensory and motor function as well as autonomic nervous system blockade.

Local anesthetics may be used topically or subcutaneously and in a wide variety of perineural locations for major nerve block. The choice of agents is based on the location, desired duration of action, and toxicity. Addition of epinephrine to a local anesthetic causes vasoconstriction of that region. This will prolong an agent's duration of action, limit systemic absorption and toxicity, and may serve as a marker for intravascular injection (tachycardia occurs). Alkalinization of a local solution (with bicarbonate) will speed onset, as it is the nonionized form that diffuses down and inactivates sodium channels.

Lidocaine is perhaps the most commonly used local anesthetic, having a wide margin of safety, a moderate duration of action, and intrinsic sedative and antiarrhythmic properties when given i.v. It is an amide, it diffuses well, and it is used in various concentrations for virtually all blocks. The maximum dose of lidocaine for infiltration is 5 mg/kg (7 mg/kg if epinephrine is added).

TABLE 8-10. LOCAL ANESTHETICS

Local	Duration	Use[a]
Esters:		
Procaine	Short	l, m, s
Cocaine	Short	t
Tetracaine	Intermediate	t, s
Amides:		
Lidocaine	Intermediate	t, l, m, e, s
Bupivacaine	Long	l, m, e, s
Ropivacaine	Long	l, m, e, s
Mepivacaine	Intermediate	l, m, e

[a] t, topical; l, local; m, major nerve block; e, epidural; s, spinal.

Bupivacaine is an amide agent that provides a good sensory and motor block, lasting approximately twice as long as lidocaine. It is, however, more toxic than lidocaine because its ability to bind avidly and durably to cardiac sodium channels, resulting in conduction abnormalities, arrhythmias, myocardial depression, and even cardiac arrest. The maximum dose for infiltration is 3 mg/kg. *Ropivacaine* is a relatively new amide agent. It shares a similar pharmacokinetic profile with bupivacaine. The major advantage of ropivacaine over bupivacaine is a decreased toxicity, which provides an enhanced therapeutic index.

Mepivacaine has a similar margin of safety and dose range to those of lidocaine, but with a slightly longer duration of action. It is an amide, it diffuses well, and it is used primarily for major nerve blocks. *Procaine* is a very short-acting ester that has a very wide margin of safety, is rapidly metabolized by serum pseudocholinesterase, and is used primarily for local infiltration.

Because of its abuse potential, *cocaine* has fallen into disfavor as a local anesthetic, although it is the prototypical drug for this purpose. It has potent vasoconstrictive properties and spreads well. Its licit use is largely confined to topical mucosal application. It is a short-acting ester, with potent cerebral excitatory effects. *Tetracaine* is the longest acting ester and has a duration of action comparable to that of the amides. It is used topically and in spinal anesthesia where its narrow hemodynamic margin of safety is of less consequence.

A major concern about the use of local anesthetics is their cardiovascular and CNS toxicity. Toxicity is mediated by changes in sodium conductance in the affected organs. Toxicity is frequently said to occur at a given dose for a given weight; yet, there are several fallacies to this statement. First, toxicity is primarily related to the blood level seen in an affected organ, so only 10 mg of lidocaine in a cerebral artery may be toxic. Systemic blood levels can also vary as a function of the rate of absorption from a site (Fig. 8-1). Drugs given for intercostal nerve blocks are absorbed much more rapidly than drugs given subcutaneously; therefore, although the two blocks may result in the same ultimate blood level for the same dose, the intercostal nerve block will result in a higher peak concentration. Weight can also be a confusing variable and a patient in congestive heart failure weighing 80 kg will have a very different volume of distribution for lidocaine than a lean 80-kg athlete—thus, quite different blood levels for the same dose of drug.

Given these caveats, some generalizations can be made about cardiovascular and CNS toxicity. Toxicity is dose related, with higher doses predictably causing more symptoms. CNS symptoms tend to precede cardiovascular symptoms. Five to ten times the convulsive dose of any local anesthetic is required to cause cardiovascular collapse. The first signs of CNS toxicity are light-headedness, dizziness, a metallic taste in the mouth, circumoral tingling, and tinnitus. These symptoms may progress and culminate in tonic-clonic seizures. Local anesthetically induced seizures may be terminated with barbiturates or benzodiazepines. Sufficiently high levels of local anesthetics, particularly bupivacaine, may cause cardiac arrest. In a patient under general anesthesia, the initial presenting sign of an overdose may be cardiovascular collapse. Treatment of such an event is with cardiopulmonary resuscitation and institution of cardiac bypass.

Care must be taken when utilizing local anesthetics. Measures to limit the total dose or the rate of uptake will tend to lessen toxicity—i.e., use of lower concentrations or the addition of a vasoconstrictor. The use of benzodiazepines, barbiturates, or inhalational anesthetics decrease CNS toxicity by raising the seizure threshold.

MALIGNANT HYPERTHERMIA

Malignant hyperthermia is a much feared, although uncommon, complication of anesthesia. It has an incidence of 1 in 15,000 anesthetics in children and 1 in 50,000 anesthetics in adults. Known triggers of malignant hyperthermia include all inhalational agents as well as succinylcholine. The pathophysiology of malignant hyperthermia is an abnormal calcium release in skeletal muscle, which causes sustained muscle contractions.

The usual first sign of malignant hyperthermia is an elevation in the end-tidal carbon dioxide level. Other findings include tachycardia, dysrhythmias, skeletal muscle rigidity, and eventually, an elevated body temperature. Laboratory abnormalities include a combined metabolic and respiratory acidosis, hyperkalemia, and extremely high levels of creatine kinase.

Treatment includes immediate discontinuation of surgery and inhaled anesthetics, hyperventilation with 100% oxygen, diuresis to protect the kidneys, and active cooling measures. Dantrolene is the drug of choice for treatment of malignant hyperthermia. It acts by interfering with calcium release from the sarcoplasmic reticulum.

REGIONAL ANESTHESIA

Regional anesthesia implies sensory and or motor blockade of some regions of the body with local anesthetic. The major regional modalities include epidural and spinal anesthesia as well as peripheral nerve blocks. Regional blockade may be used as the sole form of anesthesia or as an adjunct to general anesthesia. The advantages of regional anesthesia include postoperative pain relief; the ability to avoid general anesthetics and their resultant myocardial depressant

Intravenous>tracheal>intercostal>caudal>paracervical>epidural>brachial plexus>sciatic>subcutaneous

FIGURE 8-1. Systemic absorption of local anesthetic.

effects; the opportunity to monitor CNS function during the surgery; higher rates of graft viability following peripheral revascularization procedures; and particularly with hip surgery, decreased intraoperative blood loss and lower rates of deep venous thrombosis.

Epidural anesthesia results from the administration of local anesthetic into the epidural space. Using one of a variety of methods, a needle is used to traverse (in order) the skin, subcutaneous tissue, supraspinous ligament, interspinous ligament, and ligamentum flavum. The epidural space is reached after penetration of the ligamentum flavum. Most typically, a catheter is threaded into the epidural space for subsequent use. Placement of a spinal is similar to that of an epidural; however, the epidural space is traversed and the subarachnoid space entered, which is heralded by return of cerebrospinal fluid. A much finer needle is typically employed for spinal anesthesia and it is less common to place an indwelling catheter. As the spinal cord terminates at the L1-2 level in adults, at least one interspace below this is chosen for spinal anesthesia.

The systemic implications of major conduction anesthesia (epidural or spinal) may be significant. In addition to their sensory and motor effects, local anesthetics effect a chemical sympathectomy in the affected body region. This results in vasodilation and when the block is proximal to the high thoracic cardiac accelerator fibers, bradycardia. The combination of bradycardia and peripheral pooling of blood can cause profound hypotension. The hypotension may result in nausea (from parasympathetic predominance) as well as mental status changes (from impaired cerebral blood flow). As the sympathetic ganglia are predominantly in proximity to the thoracic spinal cord, thoracic epidurals are notorious for causing hypotension. Treatment of hypotension includes the head-down position, fluid administration, and inotropic agents. Small (5 to 10 mg) doses of ephedrine can correct the bradycardia and the hypotension. With restoration of a normal blood pressure measurement, the nausea and mental status changes are usually reversed. A high spinal implies levels of local anesthetic sufficiently high enough to impair breathing. This condition is very distressing to the patient and requires positive pressure ventilation (possibly intubation) as well as circulatory support, as hypotension and bradycardia are common.

A spinal headache may occur following spinal anesthesia or after inadvertent dural puncture during an attempted epidural placement. Spinal headaches are the result of cerebrospinal fluid leaks resulting in a decreased cerebrospinal fluid pressure. These headaches are exacerbated by the erect position and ameliorated by assumption of a supine position. Spinal headaches can occur anywhere but are usually frontal in location. Associated features may include visual changes and tinnitus. Treatment of a spinal headache includes bed rest, i.v. hydration, caffeine, and if these "conservative" measures fail, an epidural blood patch. An epidural blood patch involves the sterile placement of 10 to 20 mL of blood into the epidural space. It affords almost immediate relief in 95% of patients suffering from a spinal headache.

Neurological sequelae, although much feared, are very rare following spinal or epidural anesthesia. The formation of an epidural hematoma or an epidural abscess with compression of the spinal cord is the most likely scenario. Such a situation mandates immediate surgical decompression.

Commonly used *peripheral nerve blocks* include those of the brachial plexus, the sciatic and femoral nerves, the intercostal nerves, the ilioinguinal nerve, and the nerves of the ankle. The anesthesiologist may with skillful placement of local anesthetic, anesthetize only the region of surgical interest. Advantages of peripheral nerve blocks over neuraxial blockade include greater hemodynamic stability, less risk of respiratory embarrassment, avoidance of the possibility of a spinal headache, and a decreased incidence of nausea.

Complications of peripheral nerve block include hematoma, block failure, intravascular injection, and rarely infection or nerve damage. An intercostal nerve block may cause a pneumothorax and respiratory decompensation. This fact must be kept in mind as intercostal nerve blocks are often used for pain relief in trauma patients with rib fractures.

Patient selection and preparation is crucial prior to the administration of a regional anesthetic. Certain patients, due to altered mental status, high anxiety levels or psychiatric disorders, are not suitable candidates for a regional technique. By thoroughly explaining to the patient what to expect, the anesthesiologist can ease a patient's anxiety level. Patients are particularly afraid that they will be awake or feel pain during the procedure. Through the skillful use of sedation, a patient under the regional modality may have no recall of any intraoperative events. A contingency plan, however, must exist before beginning any case under regional anesthesia. In the event that the patient begins to feel pain (the block wears off, surgery is more extensive than anticipated, etc.), can no longer hold still, or desires to "go to sleep," general anesthesia will be induced. The contraindications to regional anesthesia, although few in number, must be kept in mind when considering one of these techniques. They include lack of patient consent, coagulopathy, sepsis, skin infection in the area of proposed needle placement, and preexistent neurological deficit/neuropathy.

SUGGESTED READING

Barash PG, Cullen BF, Stoelting RK, eds. *Clinical anesthesia,* 2nd ed. Philadelphia: Lippincott, 1996.
Miller RD, ed. *Anesthesia,* 5th ed. Philadelphia: Churchill Livingstone, 2000.
Morgan GE, Mikhail MS, eds. *Clinical anesthesiology,* 2nd ed. Stamford: Appleton & Lange, 1996.
Stoelting RK, Miller RD, eds. *Basics of anesthesia,* 3rd ed. New York: Churchill Livingstone, 1994.

9

FLUIDS, ELECTROLYTES, SHOCK, TRAUMA RESUSCITATION

VICENTE H. GRACIAS, BRIAN S. KING, and PATRICK M. REILLY

Care of the surgical patient extends far beyond the operating room. The recognition that both trauma resuscitation and postoperative patient care are primarily the responsibility of the surgeon demands that the training resident becomes familiar with the treatment of shock. Appropriate surgical care also demands a firm understanding of the fluid and electrolyte balances, which govern normal and abnormal human physiology.

BODY FLUID COMPARTMENTS

The total volume of water within the human body is defined as *total body water* (TBW). TBW in men is 60% of body weight, whereas in women, the average TBW is 50% of body weight. As one ages, a decrease in TBW content occurs because the amount of fat within the body usually increases and fat has less water than other tissues. TBW is contained in three interconnected compartments. The intracellular compartment contains 67% of TBW and the extracellular compartment 33%. The extracellular compartment is made up of an intravascular space (8% TBW) and an interstitial space (25% TBW). Changes in one compartment ultimately lead to changes in all compartments (Table 9-1).

The principal cations in the body are sodium and potassium. Sodium is primarily found in the extracellular fluid (ECF) and potassium in the intracellular (ICF). The principal anions in the extracellular space are Cl^- and HCO_3^- while phosphates and negatively charged proteins are in the intracellular space. Sodium is the principal regulator of the ECF volume and indirectly regulates TBW because the addition or loss of water in the ECF causes a reciprocal redistribution of water in the ICF (Fig. 9-1). The renin-angiotensin system is the key mechanism in controlling the ECF volume by regulating sodium excretion. Renin is secreted by the juxtaglomerular apparatus and cleaves angiotensinogen to angiotensin. Angiotensin I is further cleaved to angiotensin II by angiotensin-converting enzyme, primarily found in the vascular endothelium of the lung. Angiotensin II modulates both peripheral vascular resistance and aldosterone release from the adrenal cortex. Aldosterone increases sodium reabsorption in the distal renal tubules and collecting system. The result is an increased sodium reabsorption and increased potassium excretion (Fig. 9-2). Aldosterone release is also stimulated by increased potassium levels, corticotropin, and prostaglandins. Atrial wall distension causes the release of atrial natriuretic peptide, which has an inhibitory effect on renal sodium reabsorption.

OSMOLALITY

Osmolality is defined as the number of osmoles of solute particles per liter of water. The osmotic forces generated across a semipermeable membrane are determined by the concentration of the solutes on each side of the membrane. The movement of water across a semipermeable membrane is primarily influenced by the number of particles on either side of the membrane, not the molar concentration. One mol of sodium chloride (NaCl) dissociates in water to Na^+

TABLE 9-1. BODY FLUID COMPARTMENTS[a]

Total body water	Body weight (%)	Total body water (%)
Total	60	100
Intracellular	40	67
Extracellular:	20	33
Intravascular	5	8
Interstitial	15	25

[a]From Wait RB, Kahng KU, Dresner LS. *Fluids and electrolytes and acid-base balance in surgery: scientific principles and practice,* 2nd ed. Greenfield LJ, Mulholand MW, Oldham KT, Zelenock GB, Lillemore KD, eds. Philadelphia: Lippincott–Raven, 1997:242, with permission.

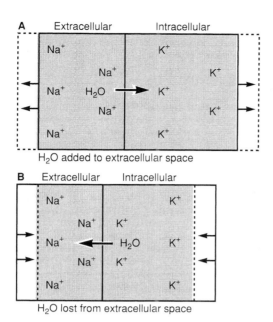

FIGURE 9-1. A: When free water is added to the extracellular space, the osmolality transiently decreases, causing water to move intracellularly until a new equilibrium is reached. **B:** A similar situation occurs due to water loss from the extracellular space. (From Wait RB, Kahng KU, Dresner LS. Fluids and electrolytes and acid-base balance. In: Greenfield LJ, Mulholand MW, Oldham KT, et al., eds. *Surgery: scientific principles and practice*, 2nd ed. Philadelphia: Lippincott-Raven, 1997:244, with permission.)

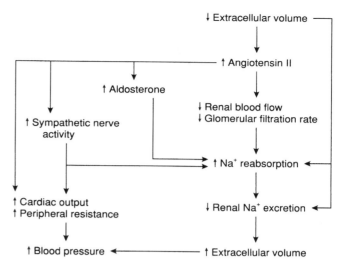

FIGURE 9-2. Effects of angiotensin II release due to a decrease in extracellular volume. (From Wait RB, Kahng KU, Dresner LS. Fluids and electrolytes and acid-base balance. In: Greenfield LJ, Mulholand MW, Oldham KT, et al., eds. *Surgery: scientific principles and practice*, 2nd ed. Philadelphia: Lippincott-Raven, 1997:247, with permission.)

and Cl^- produces 2 osmol, whereas 1 mol of a larger but nondissociating molecule, such as glucose or urea, produces only 1 osmol. The osmolar force created by dissociated NaCl is greater than that of a larger molecule that does not freely dissociate. Therefore, more water is influenced to cross the semipermeable membrane by NaCl, which is said to have a higher effective osmolality. The effective osmolality is synonymous with tonicity. The unit of measurement for these particles is the osmole (osm) or milliosmole (mOsmol). During normal physiologic states, osmolality remains fairly constant at an average of 289 mOsmol/L. The main effector of osmolality and therefore tonicity is antidiuretic hormone (ADH). As osmolality falls below 289 mOsmol/L, ADH levels decline. Without the ADH effect, renal tubular permeability to water falls and urine becomes maximally dilute. As the plasma osmolality rises above 289 during dehydration, ADH levels rise, the renal tubules become more permeable to water, and the urine becomes concentrated.

Water and Electrolyte Balance

Water loss can be characterized as sensible (able to be measured such as urine and stool) and insensible (evaporation through skin and respiratory effort). A person normally consumes about 2,000 mL of water per day. About one third of this comes from water bound to food and the remainder originates from free water intake. Daily salt intake averages 50 to 90 mEq per day Na^+, or 3 to 5 g/dL NaCl. The normal sodium requirement is in the range of 1 to 2 mEq/kg per day. The kidney provides fine control over the sodium balance within our bodies. Renal conservation during hyponatremia can result in urinary losses of less than 1 mEq per day. Potassium balance is maintained by two mechanisms. First, intracellular and extracellular shifts of potassium in exchange for protons can occur in response to imbalances. Second, renal excretion and intestinal losses help maintain potassium levels within acceptable boundaries. Normal daily potassium requirements are about 0.5 to 1 mEq/kg.

Parenteral Fluid and Electrolyte Therapy

Basic water and electrolyte requirements are determined by the imbalance created by ingestion and sensible losses (feces, urine). Insensible losses play a role when fever is present at temperatures of above 37.2°C (99°F).

Fluid replacement in surgical patients who may have drains, fistulas, ileostomies, etc., have unique needs that must be considered. A firm understanding of the electrolyte composition of the differing effluents is critical to providing adequate fluid replacement therapy. During intraoperative resuscitation, unique factors come into play. Evaporative loss during abdominal surgery is estimated to be about 1,000 mL per hour. Replacement with isotonic solutions should take not only blood loss but this evaporative loss into consideration.

Common Electrolyte Imbalances

Sodium

Sodium concentration is largely responsible for determining plasma osmolality. In general, free water volume excess or loss causes hyponatremia and hypernatremia, respectively. Therefore, the most common cause of hyponatremia is volume excess, rather than a deficit, in the sodium content. However, hyponatremia can occur in the presence of volume excess or euvolia as well. Hypotonic hyponatremia is associated with a low P_{osm}. Postsurgical or postinjury hormonal reactions cause an increased release of ADH, which in turn may exacerbate hyponatremia particularly in the face of a patient receiving a hypoosmolar solution for fluid replacement postoperatively. Hypertonic hyponatremia may result from transient shifts of fluid from the intracellular space to the extracellular space. Hyponatremia can, therefore, occur from an overabundance of solutes. The presence of large molecules such as glucose or mannitol creates an osmolar gradient that drives water from the intracellular space into the extracellular space and creates a hypertonic hyponatremia. Isotonic hyponatremia is caused by an isotonic expansion of the extracellular space. This can be seen among patients receiving isotonic sodium-free solutions during surgery such as the irrigation solution during a transurethral prostatectomy (TURP). Laboratory measurement of sodium from the serum of patients with hyperproteinemia or hyperlipidemia can relate low sodium values termed *pseudohyponatremia*.

The differential diagnosis for hyponatremia begins by excluding hypertonic hyponatremia (caused by hyperglycemia) and pseudohyponatremia. If circulating volume is low, the diagnosis of dehydration is obvious and the kidney or an extrarenal source is losing sodium. Hyponatremic dehydration may be due to renal sodium losses usually due to the result of diuretic use or chronic renal failure. A urine sodium level of above 20 mEq/L in the face of hyponatremia can diagnose renal sodium loss. Extrarenal sodium loss is likely due to loss of enteric effluent through a nasogastric tube, fistula, diarrhea, etc. This leads to an increased renal sodium reabsorption, and therefore, urine sodium levels of below 20 mEq/L. Hyponatremia in the face of normal circulating volumes is generally due to the syndrome of inappropriate antidiuretic hormone secretion (SIADH). Certain drug interactions (sulfonylureas, antidepressants) can also lead to electrolyte imbalances. Patients with hyponatremia generally present with lethargy, confusion, nausea, and vomiting. This may progress to seizures and coma. Symptoms relate to the acuteness of the electrolyte imbalance.

Hypovolemic patients benefit primarily from rehydration. Isotonic saline or lactated Ringer are the crystalloids of choice to restore the circulating intravascular volume. Hypervolemic hyponatremia can generally be corrected with water restriction. SIADH should initially be treated with water restriction. Hypertonic saline should be used only in the presence of severe symptoms or if the sodium level is less than 110 mmol/L. Rapid correction of hyponatremia can lead to central pontine myelinolysis.

Hypernatremia in the surgical population is generally caused by the loss of free water in excess of sodium. Hypovolemic hypernatremia is caused by the loss of hypotonic fluid from the body. Common etiologies include gastrointestinal (GI) losses from diarrhea, and cutaneous losses from massive burns. Hypervolemic hypernatremia is commonly due to iatrogenic manipulation such as the exogenous administration of too much sodium in resuscitation fluid or sodium bicarbonate infusion. Isovolemic hypernatremia is generally due to the replacement of hypotonic losses with isotonic solutions during total parenteral nutrition (TPN) administration. Physiologic isovolemic hypernatremia can result as a normal response to inflammation from high fever with sweating or from trauma such as head injury causing *diabetes insipidus*.

Symptoms are generally neurological in nature and include lethargy, weakness, and at times irritability. Progression leads to seizures and coma. Correction of hypernatremia should always be instituted slowly. Rapid normalization of sodium levels can lead to cerebral edema. A simple method of correction involves calculating the free water deficit and replacing only one half of that amount during the first 24 hours. Diabetes insipidus can be treated with desmopressin replacement intranasal or parenteral.

Potassium

Potassium is the main intracellular cation and the major contributor to intracellular osmolality. Only 2% of total body potassium is found in the extracellular space and normal extracellular serum concentration is 3.3 to 4.9 mmol/L. Normal intake is approximately 50 to 100 mmol per day. Potassium balance, like sodium balance, is mainly controlled by renal excretion although there is some minor extrarenal excretion through the GI tract as well. High plasma concentrations, alkalosis, ADH, aldosterone, and increased sodium delivery to the distal tubules stimulate potassium secretion. Extracellular potassium levels are influenced by intracellular and extracellular fluxes of potassium ion that occur through various mechanisms. Increasing insulin levels causes potassium to move into the cell with glucose influx. Alkalosis causes potassium to shift into cells in exchange for intracellular protons (H^+). Conversely, acidemia induces cellular influx of H^+ in exchange for the efflux of K^+.

Hypokalemia is generally the result of excessive renal loss. This is often the result of patients treated with excessive diuretics, although extrarenal loss and decreased oral intake can also lead to hypokalemia. Decreased intake is generally iatrogenic and caused by the administration of IV fluids with inappropriate low amounts of potassium. Intracellular shifts of potassium into cells in an alkalotic environment can also cause an effective hypokalemic state, as can the administration of insulin to hyperglycemic patients. Colonic pathology such as diarrhea or increased secretion through a villous adenoma can also result in excessive potassium loss. Amphotericin B can also produce potassium depletion.

Mild hypokalemia is generally asymptomatic. More pronounced hypokalemia (K^+ of less than 3 mmol/L) is manifest by muscle weakness and ileus. Patients are also predisposed to cardiac arrhythmias and electrocardiogram (ECG) abnormalities classically involve T-wave depression, prominent U waves, and prolongation of the QT interval. The primary treatment of hypokalemia is obviously potassium repletion. A measured decrease in potassium of 1 mEq/L represents a total body potassium deficit of about 100 to 200 mEq. The rate and therefore the route of potassium replacement depend on the presence and severity of symptoms, namely cardiac rhythm disturbances. Oral preparations are appropriate for mild hypokalemia. Potassium should be administered intravenously (i.v.) if the symptoms are severe, if serum concentration is below 2 mmol/L, or if the patient is unable to take oral potassium. Potassium can safely be administered at a rate of 10 to 20 mEq per hour, and if more rapid repletion is required, cardiac monitoring must be instituted. Resistant hypokalemia is generally associated with patients who are also hypomagnesemic, and generally these patients respond well to repletion of magnesium before correction of their potassium deficit. If at all possible, the safest and easiest method of potassium repletion remains an oral preparation.

Diminished renal function is perhaps the most common problem leading to *hyperkalemia*. Other etiologies include crush injuries with release of potassium from injured tissues, reperfusion injury, cell lysis (chemotherapy), and succinylcholine administration.

Mild hyperkalemia is generally asymptomatic. More severe hyperkalemia (K^+ of more than 6.5 mmol/L) results in cardiac rhythm disturbances and symmetric peaked T waves on an ECG. More serious forms of hyperkalemia can prolong the QRS interval and deepen the S wave, causing a characteristic sinusoidal pattern on the ECG. Mild hyperkalemia can be treated with restriction of potassium intake and administration of a loop diuretic. Severe hyperkalemia with EGG abnormalities must be treated urgently. Calcium gluconate infusion will help stabilize myocardial membrane potentials. Intracellular shift of potassium in exchange for H^+ can be induced by the alkalization of blood with the infusion of sodium bicarbonate. This intracellular shift can also be produced with the infusion of insulin and glucose. Definitive therapy of hyperkalemia must still be instituted. Potassium resin binders (kayexalate) can generally institute potassium excretion at an appropriate rate within 2 to 4 hours of administration. Appropriate hydration should always be maintained. Hemodialysis can be used in patients with severe life-threatening hyperkalemia and in those patients with renal failure.

Calcium

Calcium is a crucial cation whose homeostasis is tightly controlled. About 99% of calcium within the body is located within bone. Calcium balance depends on bone exchange, intestinal absorption, and renal excretion, all of which are controlled primarily by parathyroid hormone (PTH) and vitamin D. PTH regulates bone resorption and renal excretion, and vitamin D regulates intestinal absorption. Most physiologic mechanisms and effects of calcium are due to its ionized form that makes up approximately 45% of the calcium in the body. Normal serum-ionized calcium ranges between 4.1 to 5.1 mg/dL. Because laboratory measurement of the ionized form is more difficult than measurement of total calcium, many laboratories report only total calcium values. The remainder of calcium is mostly bound to albumin and other serum proteins. Because of this, any change in serum protein level can also affect the ionized calcium level. For example, a decrease in albumin concentration of 1 g/dL decreases measured calcium levels by 0.8 mg/dL; this should be remembered when a patient presents with hypocalcemia in the laboratory profile. Normal calcium intake is approximately 500 to 1,000 mg per day.

Calcium is well known for its intracellular signaling properties. Calcium influx occurs through calcium channels, and specific intracellular binding molecules such as calmodulin can interact with calcium to generate intracellular signals. The majority of intracellular calcium is stored within the endoplasmic reticulum and release is tightly controlled.

Calcium regulation is affected primarily by PTH. Calcium homeostasis, as mentioned earlier, is dependent on a balance between bone turnover, intestinal absorption, and renal excretion. Decreasing levels of calcium cause a rise in PTH level. This rising PTH level in turn causes an increase in activation of vitamin D to 1,25-dihydroxyvitamin D_3, both of which stimulate bone absorption by increasing osteoclastic activity. Intestinal absorption of calcium is controlled primarily by 1,25-dihydroxyvitamin D_3, which stimulates calcium absorption from the small intestine. In addition, elevated ionized calcium levels result in an increase in calcitonin, which increases osteoblastic activity. Distal tubular reabsorption of calcium is increased by PTH and vitamin D and decreased by calcitonin. Calcium homeostasis is depicted in Fig. 9-3.

In the surgical population, *hypocalcemia* is generally seen after parathyroidectomy or thyroid surgery when the parathyroids have been devascularized or parathyroid gland resection has been too aggressive. After resection of a parathyroid adenoma, hypocalcemia can occur because of atrophy of the remaining glands and a precipitous drop in PTH levels. Hypocalcemia is still seen due to vitamin D

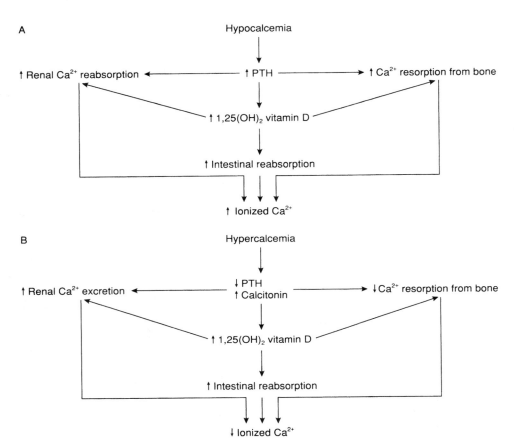

FIGURE 9-3. Physiologic compensatory effects of **(A)** hypocalcemia and **(B)** hypercalcemia. (From Wait RB, Kahng KU, Dresner LS. Fluids and electrolytes and acid-base balance. In: Greenfield LJ, Mulholand MW, Oldham KT, et al., eds. *Surgery: scientific principles and practice*, 2nd ed. Philadelphia: Lippincott-Raven, 1997:258, with permission.)

deficiency, secondary to malnutrition or malabsorption. Calcium sequestration can occur with pancreatitis. Hypomagnesemia can impair PTH release and function, causing a decrease in serum calcium. Chronic renal failure leads to deficiency in 1,25-dihydroxyvitamin D_3 and subsequently a diminished intestinal absorption of calcium.

Hypocalcemia is manifest by *hyperactivity* of muscles and reflexes. Muscle cramps and perioral tingling are early signs of low calcium. Classic signs include Chvostek sign (facial muscle spasm elicited by tapping over the facial nerve) and Trousseau sign (carpal-pedal spasm elicited by blood pressure cuff placed on an arm). ECG changes show prolonged QT interval and prolongation of the ST segment. Ventricular arrhythmias can also occur.

Severe forms are manifest by muscular tetany. Laboratory hypocalcemia without symptoms may be a manifestation of low serum albumin and not a true decrease in the levels of ionized calcium. A patient with symptoms can best be treated with an infusion of calcium gluconate. Long-term treatment involves oral replacement of calcium generally in combination with an oral form of vitamin D.

Hypercalcemia also has a long list of etiologies. The most common cause overall is primary hyperparathyroidism. The most common cause of elevated calcium in the hospital environment is a malignancy with either metastatic disease or parathormone activity causing hypercalcemia. In addition to these conditions, thiazide diuretics, multiple myeloma, Paget disease, hyperthyroidism, TPN, immobility, sarcoid, and milk alkali syndrome can all cause hypercalcemia. Parathormone activity is generally due to tumors involving lung, breast, thyroid, kidney, and parathyroid.

Mild hypercalcemia is generally asymptomatic. Hyperparathyroidism may present with bone disease and nephrolithiasis. Neuromuscular effects are seen with levels of more than 12 mg/dL. These include fatigue, weakness followed by personality changes, psychoses, and possibly coma. ECG changes classically involve a shortened QT interval and arrhythmias. GI complaints such as abdominal pain, nausea, and vomiting are described. Nephrocalcinosis can ultimately lead to renal failure.

Elevation of serum calcium concentrations to above 12 mg/dL requires urgent treatment. Maximizing renal excretion of calcium is the first step in therapy. NaCl and loop diuretics can rapidly correct calcium levels. Calcitonin has proven effective in hypercalcemia associated with malignancy. Phosphate binders (Pamidronate disodium) have also been used with success in treating hypercalcemia. Long-term treatment involves diagnosing the underlying etiology such as hyperparathyroidism or tumor and providing adequate treatment. Primary hyperparathyroidism is readily treated by resection. Hypercalcemia secondary to parathormone activity responds to tumor resection in many cases. Metastatic disease may necessitate the use of mithramycin or calcitonin on a long-term basis to inhibit bone resorption. Steroid therapy has also been used to treat hypercalcemia related to metastatic disease.

Magnesium

Half of the total body content of magnesium is bound to bone. The remaining magnesium is mostly intracellular, and less than 1% of total magnesium is located in the extracellular space. Magnesium is absorbed by the small intestine and primarily excreted by the kidneys. Bony reserves constitute the major store of available magnesium. Magnesium currently has no proven hormonal control.

Common causes of hypomagnesemia include excessive renal or GI loss as well as malabsorptive states (steatorrhea) and nutritional deficiency. Other causes include protracted i.v. or TPN therapy, loop diuretics, chronic alcoholism, renal dysfunction, and primary hyperaldosteronism. Hypomagnesemia is often accompanied by hypokalemia.

Magnesium deficiency presents similar to hypocalcemia. Neuromuscular and cardiovascular abnormalities predominate. Weakness and fatigue are followed by deep tendon hyperreflexia and muscular spasm. ECG results may show QRS widening and prolongation of the QT interval. Electrolyte disturbances may also be caused by hypomagnesemia. Hypocalcemia and hypokalemia may result from an extended period of hypomagnesemia.

Mild deficiencies can be treated with oral replacement. More severe deficits (Mg^{+2} less than 1.0 mEq/L) need to be corrected by IV replacement and possibly cardiac monitoring if the deficit is pronounced. Magnesium sulfate ($MgSO_4$) infusion of 1 to 2 g per hour for several hours (3 to 6 hours) can be started and subsequently reduced as deficits correct. Magnesium oxide is the preferred oral preparation. In patients with renal failure, magnesium dosages should be reduced appropriately according to creatinine clearance.

Hypermagnesemia is rare. The primary cause of hypermagnesemia is renal failure. Hypermagnesemia may also be caused by severe tissue injury, as occurs with crush injury or rhabdomyolysis. Severe metabolic acidosis and dehydration can also lead to elevated magnesium levels. Mild hypermagnesemia is generally asymptomatic. More severe hypermagnesemia leads to depressed deep tendon reflexes and neuromuscular activity. With extremely high levels, paralysis and coma can develop. Eventual cardiac arrest can occur. ECG may show sinus bradycardia and prolonged PR, QRS, and QT intervals.

Treatment involves volume expansion with a crystalloid infusion, generally combined with diuresis and correction of the acid-base disorders. In severe cases, calcium gluconate may aid in antagonizing the effects of magnesium. In life-threatening elevation levels, hemodialysis may be the only alternative to decrease levels quickly.

ACID-BASE BALANCE

An acid is a chemical that donates hydrogen ion (H^+), and a base is a chemical that accepts H^+. The acidity of a solution is determined by the concentration of H^+ ($[H^+]$). The pH is defined as the negative log of $[H^+]$: $pH = -\log [H^+]$ (mol/L).

Main intracellular buffers include organic phosphates, bicarbonate, and peptides. Extracellular buffers include hemoglobin and the most important bicarbonate. This buffer system is efficient because the body possesses large amounts of bicarbonate and CO_2. The product of this acid neutralization, or CO_2, is easily removed via the lungs.

All acid-base evaluations start with a simple laboratory test, an arterial blood gas (ABG). This provides information as to arterial pH, $PaCO_2$ (normal 35 to 45 mm Hg), and HCO_3^- levels (normal 22 to 31 mmol/L). There is a narrow range of pH in which enzymes and other chemical reactions within the body can function. This narrow range is maintained by the buffering systems present within our bodies. Normal pH level is 7.35 to 7.45. Acid-base equilibrium is dependent on the serum concentration of H^+, $P_{CO}2$, and HCO_3^-.

Metabolic acidosis is generally the result of overproduction of acid that causes a decrease in the amount of bicarbonate available as a buffer. As acid production overwhelms buffering capacity, a pronounced acidosis is seen on pH monitoring. Renal acid secretion and the reabsorption of bicarbonate help maintain physiologic pH in equilibrium, and metabolic acidosis can result from too much acid production or from the renal loss of bicarbonate. As the capability for renal acid excretion is surpassed by production (lactic acidosis/ketoacidosis), acidosis worsens. In the face of renal failure, acidosis can also be manifest from the decreased ability of the kidneys to reabsorb bicarbonate.

The anion gap is a quick method of determining the balance between cations and anions in our bodies. The anion gap equals $[Na^+] - ([Cl^-] + [HCO_3^-])$ and is usually 12 ± 2 mEq/L. Calculation of the anion gap is useful when clinically investigating an acidosis that is present on pH monitoring. A high anion gap of above 12 ± 2 mEq/L generally involves the production or addition of organic acid into the extracellular space, namely lactic acid associated with anaerobic metabolism or ketoacidosis. Increased gap metabolic acidosis can also be caused by the ingestion of drugs or toxins. The most common etiologies include the ingestion of salicylates, ethylene glycol, or methanol. Decreased excretion due to renal failure should also not be overlooked. Renal tubular acidosis or the loss of alkali from the GI tract most commonly causes nongap (normal anion gap) acidosis. Diarrhea and intestinal or pancreatic fistulas can lead to pronounced acidosis from the large amount of bicarbonate that can be lost. The amount of bicarbonate within the effluent determines how severe the buffering system decompensates.

The major effects of metabolic acidosis involve the *cardiovascular system*. Profound vasodilation occurs. Coupled with decreased cardiac contractility, metabolic acidosis can greatly impair the overall delivery of oxygen to tissue and further increases lactic acid production. Renal excretion of ammonia, hence acid, increases, as does the resorption of bicarbonate to help maintain equilibrium and remove more acid. Renal compensation, however, is a slow process and takes days to occur. Respiratory compensation occurs through hyperventilation and the removal of carbon dioxide, but complete compensation through hyperventilation can not be achieved without the addition of renal compensation.

The major treatment for acute metabolic acidosis is treatment of the underlying cause. Volume resuscitation must be ensured, as should the treatment of any infection. Support of the respiratory compensatory mechanisms with intubation may be in order until resuscitation and definitive treatment of sepsis or hemorrhage can be instituted. Bicarbonate infusion is generally not beneficial with mild to moderate acidosis and should be reserved for severe cases, only those when pH level falls below 7.2 to 7.0. Remember acidosis causes a right shift in the oxyhemoglobin dissociation curve and decreases Hg affinity for oxygen. This effect may actually be beneficial at the tissue level where oxygen off-loading is increased under these conditions. More chronic forms of acidosis, such as those associated with renal failure and renal tubular acidosis, require chronic replacement of alkali. Diabetic ketoacidosis should be treated with volume resuscitation and insulin infusion while monitoring glucose and acidosis.

The most common causes of *metabolic alkalosis* in the surgical patient include diuretic therapy (contraction alkalosis) and the loss of hydrogen chloride (HCl). Contraction alkalosis due to volume depletion can often be seen in postoperative patients who have not been fully resuscitated. Decreased renal blood flow due to volume depletion reduces the amount of bicarbonate that can be filtered and excreted. Nasogastric suctioning is the most common method of creating a loss of HCl and subsequent alkalosis. The removal of HCl from the stomach causes a net loss of acid and allows for excess buildup of bicarbonate within the serum. Nasogastric suctioning also causes a volume loss that inhibits the kidney from fully compensating for the extra bicarbonate. Metabolic alkalosis can also occur due to exogenous infusion of bicarbonate. These types of metabolic alkalosis are termed *chloride responsive* because repletion of Cl⁻ corrects the imbalance. Chloride unresponsive metabolic alkalosis is uncommon and may be caused by hyperaldosteronism, a rare syndrome of renin hypersecretion known as Bartter syndrome, or marked hypokalemia. Hypokalemia and intracellular shift of protons, as mentioned earlier, can result in a metabolic alkalosis. Marked hypokalemia also results in net renal acid secretion (as potassium is scavenged) and bicarbonate resorption aggravating metabolic alkalosis.

Signs of metabolic alkalosis are generally rare due to the insidious nature of the imbalance. In acute alkalotic states, patients may exhibit confusion, stupor, or even coma. Measurement of urinary chloride can aid in the differentiation of these disorders. Urinary chloride level of less than 15 mmol/L is seen with nasogastric tube (NGT) suctioning, emesis, and diuretic therapy. Urinary chloride level of more than 20 mmol/L implies mineralocorticoid excess, severe hypokalemia, alkali loading, or simultaneous diuretic use.

Compensation often occurs through hypoventilation. Correction of the underlying cause is the treatment of choice. Volume repletion and the correction of hypokalemia can be easily performed. Rarely is it necessary to administer acid i.v. to correct a severe metabolic alkalosis. If necessary, ammonium chloride or HCl can both be used to correct severe symptomatic alkalosis.

Respiratory acidosis is caused by hypoventilation that leads to an increase in PCO_2 and a decrease in blood pH level. The most common etiologies include impaired respiratory drive, secondary to medication and chronic pulmonary disease such as emphysema. Another quite common cause is inappropriate ventilator settings that result in respiratory acidosis secondary to inappropriate reduction of minute ventilation.

Chronic respiratory acidosis among patients with pulmonary disease generally presents with the classic signs and symptoms of chronic pulmonary disease. Acute changes present with restlessness, headache, tremor, and in more severe cases stupor or coma. As with metabolic acidosis, respiratory acidosis, if severe, can lead to vasodilation, depressed cardiac function, and catecholamine resistance. Therapy should involve the diagnosis and treatment of the underlying cause. If the respiratory acidosis is severe, securing an adequate airway with endotracheal intubation may need to be the first step in supporting the patient. Chronic hypercapnia may result from primary alveolar hypoventilation in the face of chronic pulmonary disease. These patients have generally remained well compensated until an overlying pneumonia or bronchitis tips the balance. Oxygen should be supplemented. Because the patient with chronic obstructive airway disease may depend on mild hypoxemia to support the respiratory drive, loss of this respiratory drive can occur, but this concept is controversial. Adequate saturation in these patients must be maintained although at lower levels than normal. There is no role for exogenous bicarbonate infusion in this clinical setting.

Respiratory alkalosis is caused by hyperventilation, which in turn causes a decrease in blood PCO_2 and an increase in the pH level. The hyperventilation may be due to pain, hypoxia, pneumothorax, pulmonary disease, mechanical ventilation, or drugs. Findings in this condition are generally nonspecific. Chronic respiratory alkalosis associated with pulmonary disease is generally well tolerated and asymptomatic. Patients with acute respiratory alkalosis may exhibit anxiety, shortness of breath, dizziness, and nervousness. Left untreated, this proceeds to paresthesia and obtundation. As with most acid-base disorders, one must treat the underlying cause. The underlying stimulus for the hyperventilation should be addressed. Pulmonary disease may require bronchodilator therapy and supplemental oxygen, and pneumonia should be treated with antibiotics. Pain should also be controlled. Hypoxia due to pneumothorax requires chest tube insertion. Pulmonary edema may involve diuretic therapy and an appropriate cardiac workup. If the respiratory alkalosis is caused by mechanical ventilation, steps to decrease minute ventilation should be instituted.

Mixed Acid-Base Disorders

Normal acid-base derangement follows a predictable pattern of buffering that can easily be calculated using simple formulas. When buffering of acid-base disorders does not follow orderly acid-base physiology, a mixed disorder should be sought. When pH level approaches normal value and the PCO_2 and HCO_3^- are abnormal, some form of mixed acid-base disorder is generally present and functioning to compensate for an underlying physiologic acidosis or alkalosis. Generally, mixed acid-base disturbances are the combination of two or more underlying primary acid-base disturbances. All combinations are possible with one exception, respiratory alkalosis and respiratory acidosis can not occur at the same time. The most common surgical patterns seen are when either a respiratory alkalosis is compensating for a metabolic acidosis as in sepsis or a metabolic alkalosis is compensating for a chronic respiratory acidosis and the patient presents with vomiting or overzealous diuretic therapy. When a patient is on a ventilator, any mixed acid-base disturbance is possible depending a how appropriate the minute ventilation setting is to the underlying clinical acid-base scenario.

SHOCK

Shock is the clinical syndrome that arises from the inadequate perfusion of tissues. When tissue perfusion diminishes to the point that oxygen delivery is inadequate to meet the demands of cellular metabolism, shock ensues. Alterations in cellular metabolism lead to cellular dysfunction, expression of inflammatory mediators, and cellular injury. If perfusion is quickly restored, cellular injury is limited and the progression of shock can be halted. However, if oxygen delivery remains inadequate, irreversible cellular injury occurs and end-organ damage can result. Shock should therefore be viewed as a continuum ranging from subclinical cellular perfusion injury to the multiple-organ dysfunction syndrome (MODS).

Recognizing that shock may present with varying degrees of severity is paramount to initiating treatment. Timely restoration of perfusion is the core concept when treating shock regardless of the etiology. Even when the cause of shock is not immediately apparent, treatment, to include volume resuscitation, is initiated immediately to halt the progression of the syndrome leading to MODS while elucidating the underlying pathology.

Despite the fact that there is a trend to avoid subdividing the shock syndrome into a traditional classification scheme and instead to concentrate on correcting the common underlying defect of tissue hypoperfusion, a classification system is sometimes useful. It can provide the clinician with direction as to the etiology of the underlying disorder that is causing shock. Treatment of shock may vary depending on the etiology, but the categories listed in Table 9-2 are not mutually exclusive. Several etiologies may contribute to the clinical picture of shock, making diagnosis and treatment challenging. For example, traumatic shock may be complicated by sepsis or by a neurogenic component in the case of spinal cord injuries. The classification scheme outlined in Table 9-2, however, serves better to define the various etiologies of shock and to provide some guidance as to the initial clinical management.

Hypovolemic shock is the most common type of shock and results from intravascular volume depletion. The most frequent cause of hypovolemic shock is hemorrhage. However, hypovolemic shock may also ensue from excessive third-space plasma losses, as might occur in pancreatitis, severe burns, or bowel obstruction. Additionally, it may arise from excessive renal, GI, or insensible losses.

As the name implies, *cardiogenic shock* is the result of pump failure. Both extrinsic and intrinsic mechanisms of diminished cardiac output are incorporated into this classification of shock. Extrinsic cardiogenic shock is sometimes referred to as *compressive* (or obstructive) cardiogenic shock and occurs due to increased extracardiac forces, which limit blood return to the heart. Tension pneumothorax, pericardial tamponade, and extreme levels of positive end expiratory pressure (PEEP) are examples of forces that may limit blood return to the heart and result in shock. Clinically,

TABLE 9-2. CLASSIFICATION OF SHOCK

Hypovolemic	Cardiogenic	Neurogenic	Vasogenic
Hemorrhage	Intrinsic		Septic
Third space volume loss	Extrinsic		Anaphylactic, traumatic, hypoadrenal

these patients may present with symptoms of hypovolemic shock, but they generally have distended neck veins, which should direct the clinician to look for cardiac compression. Intrinsic cardiogenic shock results from myocardial dysfunction. Right-sided heart failure may ensue after a large pulmonary embolus that causes an acute increase in right ventricular pressure. This normally low-pressure system cannot compensate for sudden large increases in pressure. Left-sided heart failure may be due to myocardial infarction, cardiomyopathy, valvular heart disease, and rhythm disturbances.

Sympathetic denervation from spinal cord injury, spinal anesthesia, or severe head injury produces generalized arteriolar vasodilation and venodilation resulting in neurogenic shock. Traumatic spinal cord injuries generally must occur above the level of T-6 to cause disruption of the sympathetic outflow tract, resulting in *neurogenic shock*. Relative hypovolemia results when the normal blood volume is suddenly insufficient to fill the acutely increased intravascular space. These patients present with the characteristic findings of warm extremities and normal to decreased heart rate despite profound hypotension.

Vasogenic shock is similar to neurogenic shock in that it results from a sudden decrease in vascular tone, resulting in relative hypovolemia; however, the mechanisms are quite different. Vasoactive mediators are responsible for this type of shock, and causative mechanisms include systemic inflammatory response syndrome (SIRS) or sepsis, anaphylaxis, and acute hypoadrenal states. *Vasoactive shock* is differentiated from neurogenic shock in that sympathetic outflow is intact, and these patients are generally quite tachycardic and tend to be more refractory to volume resuscitation.

Pathophysiology of Shock and Organ Responses

Tissue hypoperfusion is the common feature of all shock syndromes, regardless of the etiology. This hypoperfusion leads to cellular injury and the elaboration of inflammatory mediators. Restoration of perfusion at the cellular level is the common goal of resuscitation of all forms of shock. Steps taken to restore perfusion while investigating the pathology causing the shock syndrome may mean the difference between reversible cellular dysfunction and progression to MODS. In general, when the oxygen demands of the cell are not met, there is an uncoupling of oxidative phosphorylation and the cell begins to metabolize glucose anaerobically, which leads to a buildup of lactate. Cellular efficiency is impaired and the cell membrane loses the ability to maintain its sodium gradient via the active ionic pump, leading to cellular swelling. As the process continues, cellular inflammatory mediators are released, which sets up a vicious cycle of further cellular injury and the shock syndrome progresses.

Cardiovascular Response

The cardiovascular system undergoes significant compensatory adaptations in an attempt to maintain perfusion to vital organs. The principal determinants of cardiac function in the normal heart are preload and contractility. In accordance with the Frank-Starling mechanism, stroke volume (SV) is dependent on ventricular end-diastolic volume. As intravascular volume decreases, the amount of blood returning to the heart is diminished. This causes a decrease in the SV. The normal cardiovascular response to this situation is twofold: Heart rate (HR) increases to maintain cardiac output (HR × SV), and at the same time, compensatory venous mechanisms are activated to maintain cardiac filling.

The venous system contains two thirds of the total circulating blood volume, including 20% to 30% within the splanchnic venous system. Most of this blood volume resides within the small venous capacitance vessels, which tend to collapse in the fall of hypotension, passively shunting blood toward the heart. Additionally, active venoconstriction (via α-adrenergic activity) further augments venous return.

Selective vasoconstriction also occurs via α-adrenergic stimulation in response to shock. Based on the distribution of sympathetic fibers innervating arterioles and precapillary sphincters, blood flow to the skin is sacrificed early, followed by renal and splanchnic viscera. The resultant increase in systemic vascular resistance helps to maintain the arterial pressure despite decreasing cardiac output. As long as the systolic arterial pressure remains above 70 mm Hg, autoregulatory mechanisms maintain blood flow to the cerebral and coronary vessels.

Pulmonary Response

The acute pulmonary vascular response to shock parallels that of the systemic system. Angiotensin II mediates an increase in pulmonary vascular resistance to maintain pressure. Tachypnea occurs largely in response to the increased sympathetic tone as well as the increased metabolic acidosis. The increased respiratory rate causes a decreased tidal volume but increased dead space and minute ventilation.

Acute respiratory distress syndrome (ARDS) is a continuum of progressive lung injury and may be a direct consequence of shock. The pulmonary endothelium has a higher ratio of large to small pores compared to other tissue beds. This makes the lung particularly susceptible to injury from the inflammatory mediators of shock. The hallmark of ARDS is that the pulmonary edema occurs despite normal or even decreased left heart pressures (pulminary capillary wedge pressure [PCWP] of less than 18). Intrapulmonary shunting results in hypoxemia as underventilated or even collapsed lung segments are perfused. Surfactant levels are decreased, and combined with pulmonary edema, this leads to a decrease in lung compliance.

The earliest clinical findings of acute lung injury include moderate tachypnea and anxiety. Blood gas findings include respiratory alkalosis and mild hypoxemia. Chest x-ray findings may lag behind the clinical picture by as much as 24 hours and are of little value early in the course of ARDS.

Renal Response

When subjected to shock, the physiologic response of the kidney is to preserve salt and water. A drop in blood flow to the kidney causes a reflex constriction of the renal afferent arteriole, which results in a drop in the glomerular filtration rate (GFR). As GFR decreases, circulating ADH and aldosterone levels rise, producing oliguria. With a drop in filtration, there is back-diffusion of filtered urea, causing a rise in the serum urea nitrogen level out of proportion to the creatinine level, which is known as *prerenal azotemia*. At this point, the process is reversible if adequate volume resuscitation is initiated.

Prolonged decreases in renal blood flow may result in ischemia and acute tubular necrosis (ATN). Restoration of renal blood flow at this point results in a reperfusion injury. This may present as a loss of renal concentrating ability such that urine output is no longer an accurate measure of adequate perfusion (high-output ATN). Conversely, if the ischemic injury was profound, the renal tubules may be clogged with cellular debris (oliguric or anuric ATN) so that urine output remains low despite adequate resuscitation. This injury may resolve over time or may progress to renal failure.

General Approach to Diagnosis and Management of Shock

The goal in the management of shock is to restore perfusion and subsequent oxygen delivery to tissues; this goal is the same regardless of the cause of shock.

Early assessment of volume status is critical in the approach to the patient in shock. Patients in mild shock who respond appropriately to volume may not need invasive monitoring. However, if the cause of shock is not immediately apparent (as is the case with hemorrhage), a pulmonary artery catheter will assist in discerning the cause of shock as well as help direct and optimize the resuscitation. Volume expansion to a PCWP of between 15 and 18 mm Hg is the goal. Patients in shock with a PCWP of more than 18 mm Hg should be suspected of having cardiogenic causes. Frequent reassessment is vital to treating shock and the goals of resuscitation include (i) PCWP of 15 to 18 mm Hg, (ii) MAP of 60 to 80 mm Hg, (iii) SVo_2 of 65% to 75%, (iv) O_2 saturation level of more than 92%, and (v) urine output of more than 0.5 mL/kg per hour.

Treatment of Specific Shock Syndromes

It is not always easy to discern the specific type of shock causing hypoperfusion. There may also be an overlap between the shock syndromes complicating the clinical picture, particularly in the trauma patient. However, understanding the physiologic characteristics of the various shock syndromes and management techniques specific to each allows the clinician to direct therapy more effectively. Table 9-3 outlines some of the physiologic variables found in the various shock syndromes.

Hypovolemia is the most frequently encountered shock syndrome in surgical patients. The clinical signs and symptoms of hypovolemic shock depend on the severity of the intravascular volume deficit. The first sign of hypovolemic shock generally does not occur until the patient has lost 15% to 30% of circulating blood volume. Even then, the signs may be subtle, including a mild tachycardia and slight narrowing of the pulse pressure. After greater than 30% blood loss, there is a more profound tachycardia and a mild drop in blood pressure. A thorough examination also reveals a loss of normal skin turgor, decreased urine output, and progressive mental status changes as blood loss progresses. It may not be until the patient has lost over 2 L of blood (more than 40% of total circulating volume) that shock becomes obvious, as compensatory mechanisms begin to fail.

The initial management of hypovolemic shock includes assessing the patient's airway and breathing. Direct pressure on obvious external bleeding is the best way to control obvious hemorrhage. Two large-bore i.v. lines should be placed and 1 to 2 L of balanced crystalloid solution should be rapidly administered. If the patient does not have a rapid response to this initial bolus, blood transfusion must be considered. Cross-matched blood is preferable, but type-specific or type O Rh-negative can be used in emergent situations. In situations in which the patient has no response to initial volume resuscitation, emergent operative intervention may be necessary to control life-threatening hemorrhage. The use of colloid other than blood or the use of hypertonic saline in acute hypovolemic shock is controversial. Currently, there is no data to suggest that these

TABLE 9-3. PHYSIOLOGIC CHARACTERISTICS OF THE VARIOUS FORMS OF SHOCK[a,b]

Type of shock	CVP and PCWP	Cardiac output	Systemic vascular resistance	Venous O_2 saturation
Hypovolemic	↓	↓	↑	↓
Cardiogenic	↑	↓	↑	↓
Septic:				
Hyperdynamic	↓↑	↑	↓	↑
Hypodynamic	↓↑	↓	↑	↑↓
Traumatic	↓	↓↑	↑↓	↑↓
Neurogenic	↓	↓	↓	↓
Hypoadrenal	↓↑	↓	↑↓	↓

[a]CVP, central venous pressure; PCWP, pulmonary capillary wedge pressure.
[b]From Maier RV. *Shock in surgery: scientific principles and practice*, 2nd ed. Greenfield LJ, Mulholand MW, Oldham KT, Zelenock GB, Lillemoe KD, eds. Philadelphia: Lippincott–Raven, 1997:197, with permission.

solutions improve outcome in the acute setting, so their routine use is not recommended.

The placement of a central venous catheter to monitor central venous pressure or a pulmonary artery catheter may also be necessary if the patient is not responding to resuscitation as expected. Endpoints of resuscitation in the absence of invasive monitoring include normalization of heart rate and blood pressure, urine output of 0.5 to 1.0 mL/kg per hour, normal capillary refill, and normal sensorium.

Traumatic shock is currently considered separately from hypovolemic shock. The reason for this is that traumatic shock generally has an additional component of vasogenic shock that is absent with pure hypovolemic shock. The direct tissue injury that occurs in the setting of trauma causes an additional release of inflammatory cellular mediators that adds a component of vasogenic shock to the picture of hypovolemia. Patients with traumatic shock frequently require a more aggressive resuscitation than one might expect based solely on their intravascular losses. In addition to being more refractory to resuscitation, patients with traumatic shock are more likely to progress to SIRS and MODS as a result of the additional inflammatory process initiated by the extra injury.

Therapy after cardiogenic shock is directed toward correcting the pump failure. Invasive monitoring is essential to guide resuscitation. Initial therapy includes administration of supplemental oxygen, optimization of hemoglobin level to 10 to 12 g/dL, optimization of preload (PCWP of 15 to 18 mm Hg), and control of tachycardia. An aggressive search must be undertaken to quickly rule out extrinsic causes of cardiogenic shock (pneumothorax, tamponade, excessive PEEP). Once extrinsic compression has been ruled out or treated, one is left with treating intrinsic cardiogenic shock. This usually requires inotropes. Dobutamine is generally the inotrope of choice because it improves contractility and reduces afterload. Milrinone is also gaining favor in some centers. This phosphodiesterase inhibitor is a vasodilating agent and improves contractility by increasing the intracellular availability of cyclic adenosine monophosphate. The net effect of milrinone is similar to that of dobutamine, but it tends to cause less cardiac irritability (dysrthymias) and produces less tachycardia than dobutamine.

If efforts to improve preload, augment contractility, and decrease afterload with fluid and drugs fail, then one must consider the use of an intraaortic balloon pump (IABP). This device is positioned in the descending thoracic aorta, inflates during diastole, and deflates just before systole to augment diastolic flow and coronary perfusion while decreasing ventricular afterload and myocardial O_2 consumption.

Neurogenic shock results from the interruption of sympathetic vasomotor input and may occur following spinal cord injury, spinal anesthesia, or severe head injury. Hypotension is the rule and may be accompanied by a mild tachycardia from a systemic catecholamine surge, but it can often be seen with bradycardia due to unopposed vagal parasympathetic tone. In stark contrast to hypovolemic or cardiogenic shock patients, neurogenic shock patients present with extremities that appear warm and well perfused. Gastric dilation and ileus are also common and may aid in the diagnosis, but most often the diagnosis is obvious due to the associated neurological deficit.

After a patent airway and a breathing patient is ensured, the mainstay of treatment is volume administration. The patient has a relative hypovolemia because of the sudden relative increase in intravascular space. It may be necessary to augment the patient's blood pressure with the use of an α-agonist such as phenylephrine during the volume resuscitation, but this can generally be weaned off as intravascular volume replacement is accomplished.

Septic shock is a form of *vasogenic shock* that develops as a consequence of the metabolic and circulatory derangements that accompany systemic infection. It is considered separately here because two distinct presentations are associated with septic shock. *Hyperdynamic* septic shock (warm sepsis) generally occurs first. In the early stages of sepsis, a hyperdynamic profile exists, with tachycardia, elevated cardiac output, peripheral vasodilation, and a marked increase in oxygen consumption. As sepsis progresses, the syndrome becomes *hypodynamic* (cold sepsis). The cellular mitochondria are no longer able to utilize oxygen and the O_2 consumption amount drops, marked by an increase in SVo_2 despite a falling cardiac output. This is an ominous prognostic sign and generally heralds cardiovascular collapse.

Treatment of septic shock is aimed at treating the causative organism while supporting perfusion with volume and pressors. Undrained collections must be aggressively sought to remove the nidus of infection. If operative intervention is required for control of the septic process, it is best undertaken when the hemodynamic status has been optimized. Waiting until the patient progresses to cold septic shock lessens the chance of recovery.

Shock due to *relative adrenocortical insufficiency* is a rare form of vasogenic shock and is rarely seen in an initial patient encounter. This etiology of shock must be considered in any patient who has a history of glucocorticoid use (within previous 6 months) or in severely ill patients who suddenly become refractory to volume and pressor resuscitation. Patients with significant metabolic stress due to trauma, operation, or serious medical illness may appear septic but do not respond to resuscitation. A high index of suspicion is necessary to make the diagnosis of addisonian crisis, but this diagnosis is rewarded with prompt stabilization with the administration of corticosteroids. Clues that may aid the clinician include hypoglycemia in a hypotensive patient or hyponatremia with hypokalemia. Eosinophilia has also been reported in association with relative adrenal insufficiency in the intensive care unit setting.

10

HERNIAS

ROBERT A. LARSON AND JO BUYSKE

The study and treatment of hernias has been an important part of surgery since ancient times. A large part of any general surgical practice is devoted to the diagnosis and treatment of hernias and their complications. Consequently, it is important for the surgeon to fully understand the types of hernias that can occur, their natural history, the pertinent regional anatomy, and the treatment options available.

In the broadest sense, a *hernia* is the protrusion of an organ through a confining wall. The most common type is the inguinal hernia, in which the properitoneal fat or abdominal viscus protrudes through a defect in the abdominal wall; when one says "hernia," this is what usually comes to mind. Other clinical entities, however, are also hernias by definition. These include umbilical hernias, congenital diaphragmatic hernias, incisional hernias, omphaloceles, gastroschisis, and even hiatal hernias. The etiology, presentation, treatment, and potential complications of these conditions are all different; the aim of surgical treatment is to restore the herniated organ to its normal position and to repair the anatomic barriers.

Several terms are used to describe hernias and the status of the herniated organs. A *reducible* hernia is one in which the herniated contents can be returned to their anatomic position manually; they may, however, spontaneously herniate again after the manual control is removed. A hernia is called *incarcerated* if its contents cannot be returned to their normal position in a nonsurgical manner. This type of hernia is often associated with complications and may require urgent or emergent treatment. An incarcerated hollow viscus may become obstructed while any incarcerated organ may have its blood supply compromised, resulting in a dangerous strangulated hernia. When less than the full circumference of the bowel wall becomes entrapped in a hernia defect, that segment of bowel wall may become ischemic (strangulated) without the bowel becoming obstructed. This is called a Richter hernia and most commonly involves a loop of small bowel (Fig. 10-1).

Hospital of the University of Pennsylvania, Philadelphia, Pennsylvania

ABDOMINAL WALL HERNIAS

The lower abdominal wall is made up of three musculoaponeurotic layers covered by subcutaneous fat and skin (Fig. 10-2 and Table 10-1). The external oblique muscle arises from the 5th through 12th ribs with its fibers running in an inferomedial direction. As the fibers pass medially, they become aponeurotic near the midclavicular line at the linea semilunaris. The aponeurosis contributes to the anterior rectus sheath before inserting into the linea alba in the midline. The inferior aspect of the aponeurosis inserts onto the iliac crest laterally and the pubic tubercle medially. The portion of the external oblique aponeurosis that stretches between the anterior superior iliac spine and the pubic tubercle is somewhat thickened and folds back onto itself, forming the *inguinal* (Poupart) *ligament*. Medially, the inguinal ligament reflects back onto the pectin pubis as the *lacunar ligament*. Just superior to the medial part of the inguinal ligament, there is a triangular opening in the external oblique aponeurosis. This is the *superficial inguinal ring*, through which the spermatic cord in men, or the round ligament in women, exits the inguinal canal. The superficial

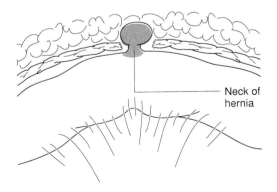

FIGURE 10-1. Richter hernia of the small bowel. (From Knol JA, Eckhauser FE. Inguinal anatomy and abdominal wall hernias. In: Greenfield LJ, Mulholland M, Oldham KT, et al., eds. *Surgery: scientific principles and practice*, 2nd ed. Philadelphia: Lippincott-Raven, 1997:1218, with permission.)

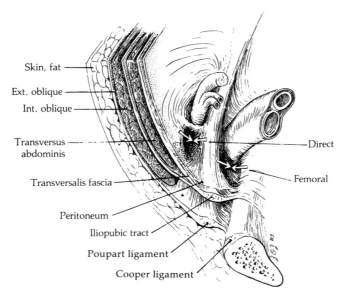

FIGURE 10-2. Muscular support of the abdominal wall in relation to the formation of direct, indirect, and femoral hernia. (From Nyhus LM. Iliopubic tract repair of inguinal and femoral hernia: the posterior (preperitoneal) approach. In: Nyhus LM, Baker RJ, eds. *Mastery of surgery,* 2nd ed. Boston: Little, Brown and Company, 1992:1853, with permission.)

inguinal ring plays no role in the development, diagnosis, or treatment of inguinal hernias.

The *internal oblique muscle* is the middle layer of the abdominal wall musculature. It arises from the lumbar fascia, the iliac crest, and the lateral half of the inguinal ligament and inserts, via its aponeurosis, onto the linea alba. The aponeurosis of the internal oblique contributes to both the anterior and posterior rectus sheathes above the arcuate line and solely to the anterior rectus sheath below the arcuate line. The fibers of the internal oblique are directed in a superomedial direction, at approximately right angles to the fibers of the external oblique. The often-cited *conjoined tendon,* a fusion of the internal oblique and transversus abdominis aponeuroses in the medial aspect of the inguinal canal, is present in only 5% of individuals. More commonly, the internal oblique arcs cranially around the inguinal canal and contributes little to the strength and integrity of the region.

TABLE 10-1. LAYERS OF THE ANTERIOR ABDOMINAL WALL

Skin
Subcutaneous fat
Scarpa's fascia
External oblique muscle
Internal oblique muscle
Transversus abdominus muscle
Transversalis (endoabdominal) fascia
Properitoneal fat
Peritoneum

The *transversus abdominis* is the innermost muscular layer of the abdominal wall. It arises from the lower six ribs, lumbar fascia, iliac crest, and the iliopubic tract. The fibers of the transversus abdominis course transversely, the medial aspect being an aponeurosis that contributes to the rectus sheath. Above the arcuate line, the aponeurosis contributes to the posterior rectus sheath along with the internal oblique; below the arcuate line, it joins the internal and external oblique to form the anterior rectus sheath. The inferior edge of the transversus abdominis aponeurosis inserts onto Cooper ligament's.

Every muscle is encased in a fascial sheath that gives it tensile strength and binds the fascicles together. The deep fascia of the transversus abdominis muscle is important in the stability of the inguinal region and is called the *transversalis fascia.* This fascia is continuous with the inner facial layers of all muscles encasing the abdominal cavity and is often called the *endoabdominal fascia.* The transversalis fascia plays a central role in the development of inguinal hernias. The *deep inguinal ring* is a defect in the transversalis fascia located about halfway between the anterior superior iliac spine and the pubic tubercle. It is through the deep ring that the spermatic cord or round ligament exits the abdominal cavity and enters the inguinal canal.

The *inguinal canal* begins at the deep inguinal ring and ends at the superficial inguinal ring. The floor of the canal is formed by the transversalis fascia, which is reinforced medially to variable degrees by the aponeuroses of the internal oblique and transversus abdominis. The roof of the canal is made up of the external oblique aponeurosis and, laterally, fibers of the internal oblique muscle. The superior wall of the canal is formed by the arching fibers of the internal oblique and transversus abdominis muscles, and the inferior wall is made up of the inguinal and lacunar ligaments.

Hesselbach triangle defines a region of the abdominal wall through which a direct inguinal hernia protrudes. The triangle, located in the medial inguinal region, is bounded by the inferior epigastric artery laterally, the inguinal ligament inferiorly, and the rectus sheath medially (Fig. 10-2).

The anatomy of the *spermatic cord* is intimately related to that of the abdominal wall and inguinal canal (Table 10-2). At the center of the spermatic cord are the vas deferens, testicular vessels, and the obliterated (usually) processus vaginalis. As the cord passes through the deep ring, the transversalis fascia extends onto the cord, forming the inter-

TABLE 10-2. RELATION OF ABDOMINAL WALL LAYERS TO SPERMATIC CORD LAYERS

Abdominal wall	Spermatic cord
External oblique	External spermatic fascia
Internal oblique	Cremaster muscle
Transversalis fascia	Internal spermatic fascia
Peritoneum	Processus vaginalis

nal spermatic fascia. The internal oblique muscle extends onto the cord as the cremaster muscle while the external oblique muscle fascia adds the external spermatic fascia at the superficial inguinal ring.

The *iliopubic tract* is a thickening of the endoabdominal fascia at the juncture of the transversalis fascia and the iliopsoas fascia. It stretches from the anterior superior iliac spine to the superior pubic ramus and pubic tubercle. It is located deep to and slightly superior to the inguinal ligament and forms the inferior margin of the deep inguinal ring. As it passes medially, it makes up the anterior and medial walls of the femoral canal.

Cooper ligament's is a prominence of periosteum at the insertion of the transversalis fascia, iliopubic tract, and lacunar ligament onto the superior pubic ramus. It follows the iliopectineal line of the pubic ramus in a posterolateral direction. This is a stout structure that is important in the McVay technique and in some properitoneal hernia repairs (see below).

Knowledge of the location of nerves that course through the inguinal region is important in order to avoid injuring these structures and for the administration of regional anesthesia. The *iliohypogastric nerve* and *ilioinguinal nerves* originate from the L-1 nerve root and penetrate the transversus abdominis muscle at about the middle of the iliac crest. They pierce the internal oblique muscle at the level of the anterior superior iliac spine, traveling obliquely downward underneath the external oblique aponeurosis. The ilioinguinal nerve runs just superior to the spermatic cord and passes through the superficial inguinal ring to innervate the scrotum or labium majus. The genital branch of the *genitofemoral* nerve arises from the L-1 and L-2 nerve roots. It enters the inguinal canal inferior to the deep inguinal ring and remains in close apposition to the spermatic cord, providing motor innervation for the cremaster muscle and sensory innervation to the scrotum and medial thigh.

The *femoral canal* is a potential space deep to the inguinal ligament through which abdominal viscera can herniate. It is bounded laterally by the external iliac vein, superiorly by the inguinal ligament, posteriorly by Cooper ligament's. Medially, the canal is bounded by, and usually closed by, the reflected fibers of the iliopubic tract as it inserts onto Cooper ligament's. The canal enters the thigh deep to the inguinal ligament and enters the femoral triangle through the fossa ovalis, a defect in the fascia lata where the greater saphenous vein joins with the femoral vein.

GROIN HERNIAS

The vast majority (75%) of abdominal wall hernias occur in the inguinal region. Men are more than five times more likely to develop a hernia than women, and it has been estimated that up to 5% of the male population develop symptomatic hernias.

Inguinal hernias are divided into two categories, indirect and direct. *Indirect inguinal hernias* arise, by definition, lateral to the inferior epigastric artery and vein, i.e, outside of Hesselbach triangle. They traverse the deep inguinal ring via a patent processus vaginalis. The indirect sac is present within the cremaster muscle and is located on the anteromedial aspect of the cord. The hernia travels through the inguinal canal for a variable distance, depending on the patency of the processus vaginalis, and may reach the scrotum. Because these hernias exit the abdominal cavity through a relatively narrow opening, they are termed *funicular*. Because of the well-defined neck of the hernia sac, these hernias are more prone to incarcerate and strangulate bowel than broad-based, or diffuse, hernias, such as direct inguinal hernias. Indirect inguinal hernias are the most common abdominal wall hernias in both men and women, making up 50% of all hernias.

Direct inguinal hernias arise medial to the inferior epigastric vessels and are produced by a weakness in the floor of the inguinal canal, i.e., the transversalis fascia and transversus abdominis aponeurosis. Direct inguinal hernias are the second most common type of hernia, making up 25% of hernias. They tend to occur in older age groups and in active persons; both groups tend to develop weakness of the tissues of the inguinal floor from chronic stress and injury. These hernias are broad-based (diffuse) and generally do not have a tight neck. Because they lack a preformed sac extending to the testicle (like indirect hernias), direct hernias rarely reach the scrotum. Additionally, most recurrent inguinal hernias are direct. This results from failure to correct a weakness in the inguinal floor at the time of indirect inguinal hernia repair or breakdown of an inadequate repair of the inguinal floor.

A *sliding hernia* is an advanced indirect inguinal hernia in which the peritoneal hernia sac has progressed so far through the internal ring that a retroperitoneal organ is drawn into the hernia defect (Fig. 10-3). Consequently, a portion of the posterior wall of the hernia sac is actually the wall of the sliding viscus. The organs usually associated with this condition include the cecum on the right, sigmoid colon on the left, and occasionally the bladder or ovary. It is important to recognize the presence of a sliding hernia at the time of repair to avoid injury to the herniated organ.

When a patient has ipsilateral direct and indirect hernias, i.e., defects on either side of the inferior epigastric vessels, they are said to have a *pantaloon hernia*. This condition usually occurs in long-standing indirect hernias in which the internal ring is severely dilated and the inguinal floor is displaced medially. The repair of pantaloon hernias is the same as for any large indirect hernia.

A *Littré hernia* is one that contains a Meckel diverticulum. The original case described was that of a femoral hernia, but the true distribution has been found to be 50% inguinal, 20% femoral, 20% umbilical, and 10% miscellaneous. Littré hernias are more common in men and on the

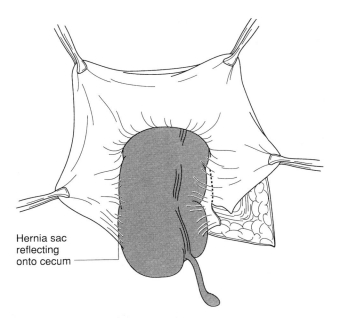

FIGURE 10-3. Right-side sliding inguinal hernia containing the cecum. (From Knol JA, Eckhauser FE. Inguinal anatomy and abdominal wall hernias. In: Greenfield LJ, Mulholland M, Oldham KT, et al., eds. *Surgery: scientific principles and practice*, 2nd ed. Philadelphia: Lippincott-Raven, 1997:1219, with permission.)

right side. They often present with symptoms of intestinal strangulation without obstruction, as seen in a Richter hernia. The repair of the hernia defect is the same as that of a common hernia; however, a Meckel diverticulectomy should be done concurrently.

The *etiology of inguinal hernias* is related to congenital variations in the inguinal anatomy and the fatigue of the abdominal wall supporting structures over time. There are two mechanisms by which the inguinal region is supported during periods of abdominal straining. When the transversus abdominis muscle contracts, the transversalis fascia and internal ring are retracted superolaterally. This pinches the internal ring closed and moves the ring under the internal oblique, thus providing additional anterior support. Contraction of the transversus abdominis also provides a buttress for the medial aspect of the inguinal canal. In the relaxed state, the transversus abdominis muscle frequently arches over the medial inguinal canal, leaving only the transversalis fascia to make up the inguinal floor. During contraction, however, the transversus abdominis arch stretches transversely and moves into apposition with the inguinal ligament. This provides additional support to the medial canal during periods of abdominal straining. Congenital variations in the distance of the transversus abdominis muscular arch from the inguinal ligament may preclude its apposition to the inguinal ligament. This lack of support may contribute to the fatigue of the tissues of the inguinal floor and thus to the development of direct inguinal hernias.

The presence of a patent processus vaginalis has been considered the sine qua non of indirect inguinal hernias. Autopsies on children, however, have shown that up to 25% continue to have a patent processus vaginalis, despite a much lower incidence of indirect herniation. Other factors, such as the size of the internal ring and the physiologic buttressing mechanisms described above, play important roles. Although a patent processus vaginalis provides a potential hernia sac, it may take years of stress and trauma to the internal ring before abdominal contents are able to herniate.

There is evidence that defects in collagen metabolism can contribute to the development of hernias. Patients who developed inguinal hernias were found to have decreased collagen content and decreased collagen formation in rectus sheath biopsies compared to controls without hernias. More research is needed in this area before definite conclusions can be drawn.

Any condition that chronically increases intraabdominal pressure can contribute to the development and progression of abdominal wall hernias. Frequently associated conditions include morbid obesity, chronic pulmonary disease with frequent coughing, urinary obstruction, chronic constipation, pregnancy, and poorly controlled ascites. Indeed, any elderly person with the recent development of a hernia should be screened for the possibility of colonic or urinary obstruction.

The history and physical examination are the primary tools used to diagnose hernias. Most inguinal hernias are asymptomatic until the patient notices a lump in the groin, the appearance of which may be associated with a pulling or tearing sensation that can radiate into the scrotum. The symptoms are often worse with activity and improve with recumbency. An inciting event, such has heavy lifting or straining, can frequently be elicited. The patient should be questioned about the presence of bowel symptoms, such as distention, vomiting, intermittent diarrhea, and constipation. The details of any previous hernia repairs is important. Additionally, any condition causing increased intraabdominal pressure should be ruled out, as mentioned above. If the situation permits, these problems should generally be dealt with before herniorrhaphy because the increased intraabdominal pressure may contribute to failure of the repair.

The examination of the patient is best initiated with the patient standing. The inguinal region is inspected for the presence of a lump with and without the patient performing a Valsalva maneuver. In men, the examining finger is then invaginated into the scrotum up to the superficial inguinal ring. A Valsalva maneuver should bring the herniated contents into contact with the examining finger. In women, the inguinal region is palpated directly over the superficial inguinal ring. It is often not possible to distinguish between an indirect and direct inguinal hernia by examination alone. This does not pose a problem, however, because the operative approach is likely to be the same for both.

If the patient presents with a hernia but without signs of strangulation (fever, intestinal obstruction, persistent pain in the hernia) an attempt at reduction can be made. Sedation is often useful to help the patient relax the abdominal muscles, improving the chance for a successful reduction. The technique of gentle, continuous pressure applied directly over the hernia is the safest option. If an aggressive attempt for reduction is made, there is a risk of reducing unsuspected dead bowel that could progress to perforation and sepsis. Alternatively, the hernia may be reduced en masse, a situation in which the viscera and hernia sac are reduced into the abdomen together. This converts an inguinal hernia into an internal hernia with the continued risk of strangulation. Patients who present with symptomatic incarcerated hernias are best served with prompt operative herniorrhaphy.

Although the diagnosis of an inguinal hernia is often straightforward, several conditions must be considered when evaluating a patient with a lump in the groin. Other possible diagnoses include inguinal adenopathy, undescended testis, spermatocele, varicocele, hydrocele, lipoma, metastatic testicular cancer, and femoral hernia. If the diagnosis is uncertain, ultrasound or computed tomography (CT) can be helpful.

Treatment

Over the past century, many different herniorrhaphy techniques have been described, most of which are now only of historical interest. Of the remaining techniques still in use, several general principles are shared by all. The choice of technique is very much a function of one's training; however, the use of a tension-free repair using prosthetic mesh has become very common.

As mentioned above, if the patient presents with a painful incarcerated hernia or signs of bowel ischemia, urgent repair is indicated. If ischemic bowel is found, it can often be resected through the same incision, but a standard laparotomy is indicated if control of the bowel is lost or a complete exploration of the abdomen is indicated.

Anesthesia for most inguinal herniorrhaphies can be provided by local field block. Providing a combination of iliohypogastric and ilioinguinal nerve block with a regional field block is generally adequate. The exceptions include large and complex hernias that may require more than 90 minutes to repair, recurrent hernias, or when deep intraperitoneal manipulation is anticipated. Epidural or spinal anesthesia is also an option for procedures on the lower abdominal wall, particularly when the operative time is anticipated to be too long for local blockade. General anesthesia is required for intraabdominal operations and for patients with strangulated hernias.

For the anterior repairs described below, the groin is explored through an oblique incision parallel to the inguinal ligament and following Langer line's. The incision is carried down through Scarpa fascia to the external oblique aponeurosis, which is incised parallel to its fibers from the deep inguinal ring through the superficial ring. Great care must be taken to avoid injuring the underlying ilioinguinal and iliohypogastric nerves. The spermatic cord is carefully encircled at the level of the pubic tubercle and mobilized to the deep ring. Careful dissection through the cremaster muscle reveals the indirect hernia sac on the anteromedial aspect of the cord. The sac should be carefully dissected free from the spermatic cord, opened to ensure the reduction of all contents, ligated at the deep ring, and excised. If the sac extends into the scrotum, no attempt should be made to retrieve the sac distal to the pubic tubercle because of the risk of damaging collateral blood supply to the testis. In this situation, the sac should be divided at the pubic tubercle and the distal segment left open to prevent a hydrocele. During the repair of a direct inguinal hernia, one should make a careful search for the presence of a small indirect sac, which if present should be ligated.

Reconstruction of the floor of the inguinal canal is commonly required in adult inguinal herniorrhaphy, and the creation of a tension-free repair is one of the important aspects in preventing recurrence. It is also crucial to use only strong musculoaponeurotic structures in the repair; the attenuated tissues at the site of a hernia will usually not hold a reconstruction. An important technique used in many procedures to help reduce the tension in a repair is the *relaxing incision*. In general, an incision is made in the aponeurosis overlying a muscle, parallel to the repair but several centimeters away. This allows the aponeurosis to slide over the underlying muscle and reach the area of the repair with less tension. The muscle prevents herniation through the newly created defect.

Surgical Procedures

For an indirect hernia in which there is no attenuation of the floor of the inguinal canal, simple high ligation and excision of the hernia sac is adequate. This is often only possible in young people and is the standard procedure in the pediatric population. In children, the recurrence rate for simple sac ligation is about 0.1%.

In adults, the deep inguinal ring is often dilated to some degree. In the Marcy repair, after the sac has been ligated, the deep ring is tightened by placing several interrupted sutures medial to the spermatic cord. In women, the deep ring can be closed completely after dividing the round ligament.

One of the most common inguinal hernia repairs is the *Bassini repair*. In this technique, after the indirect hernia sac has been ligated, the inguinal floor is buttressed by approximating the transversalis fascia and transversus abdominis aponeurosis to the shelving edge of the inguinal ligament. This may require a relaxing incision in the anterior rectus sheath to minimize tension. Recurrence rates vary from 5% to 20%, with small hernias faring better.

The *Shouldice,* or Canadian, repair (Fig. 10-4) reconstructs the floor of the inguinal canal by dividing the transversalis fascia from the deep ring to the pubis and then imbricating it to itself and the inguinal ligament with two suture lines. The transversus abdominis aponeurotic arch is then approximated to the inguinal ligament, also with two suture lines. This technique has had excellent results in large series, with 0.6% recurrence rates. As with the Bassini repair, relaxing incisions may be required to minimize tension.

In the *McVay* or *Cooper ligament's repair* (Fig. 10-5), the attenuated floor of the inguinal canal is excised and the underlying iliopectineal line exposed. The floor is then reconstructed by approximating the transversus abdominis aponeurosis and transversalis fascia to Cooper ligament's from the pubis to the medial aspect of the femoral vein. At the femoral vein, a transition stitch moves the suture line to the more superficial iliopubic tract for the lateral extent of the repair. A relaxing incision is frequently required in this procedure. Because this technique effectively closes off the femoral canal medial to the femoral vein, it is often used in femoral hernia repairs.

The presence of tension in a hernia repair has long been known to increase the risk of recurrence. Tension may also increase the discomfort that patients experience postopera-

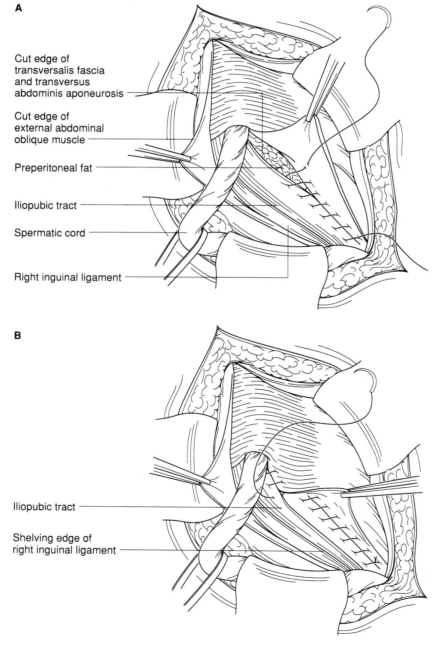

FIGURE 10-4. The Shouldice inguinal hernia repair involves **(A)** the approximation of the lateral cut edge of the transversus abdominis aponeurosis and transversalis fascia to the undersurface of these same structures near the edge of the rectus abdominis muscle. The second suture line **(B)** joins the medial cut edge of the inguinal floor to the iliopubic tract and shelving edge of the inguinal ligament. (From Knol JA, Eckhauser FE. Inguinal anatomy and abdominal wall hernias. In: Greenfield LJ, Mulholland M, Oldham KT, et al., eds. *Surgery: scientific principles and practice*, 2nd ed. Philadelphia: Lippincott-Raven, 1997:1223, with permission.)

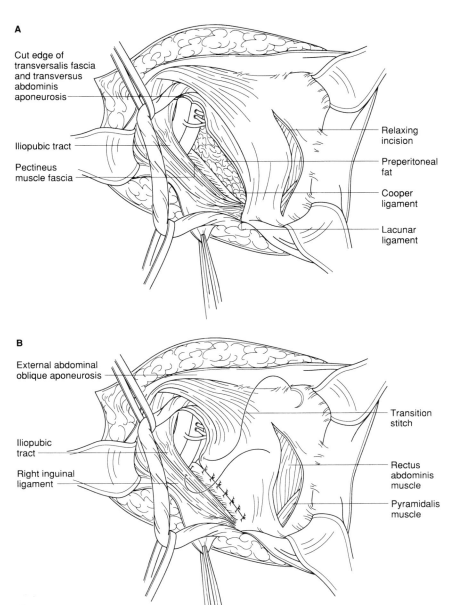

FIGURE 10-5. The Cooper ligament's of McVay repair can involve a relaxing incision (A) and approximation of the conjoined structures medially to the Cooper ligament's laterally (B) with placement of the transition stitch through the conjoined structures, Cooper ligament's, pectineus muscle fascia, and iliopubic tract. The internal ring is approximated by bringing the transversalis fascia and transversus abdominis muscle medially to the iliopubic tract laterally. (From Knol JA, Eckhauser FE. Inguinal anatomy and abdominal wall hernias. In: Greenfield LJ, Mulholland M, Oldham KT, et al., eds. *Surgery: scientific principles and practice*, 2nd ed. Philadelphia: Lippincott-Raven, 1997:1224, with permission.)

tively, delaying their return to normal activities. To minimize the tension in the repair and thus reduce recurrences and improve patient recovery, the use of prosthetic mesh, or the *Lichtenstein repair*, to repair the inguinal floor with very little tension has become a widely used technique (Fig. 10-6).

The mesh, usually an inert material such as polypropylene (Marlex) or ePTFE (Gortex), is placed over the inguinal floor, posterior to the spermatic cord, and is sutured to the inguinal ligament inferiorly and the transversus abdominis aponeurosis or internal oblique aponeurosis superiorly. The mesh is split laterally to allow space for the cord to exit the deep ring. In addition to the patch, a mesh plug is often placed within the deep ring beside the spermatic cord to help reinforce the laxity in the ring that can occur in large hernias.

The mesh incites a fibrotic reaction in the wound that adds to the strength of the repair, and recurrence rates are quite low with this technique, usually less than 0.5%. The slight (0.6%) risk of the mesh becoming infected must be considered, however, and the placement of mesh in an obviously infected wound is generally contraindicated.

In addition to the anterior approaches to hernia repair, it is possible to use a *posterior*, or properitoneal, approach. This technique is applicable to the treatment of recurrent inguinal hernias, incarcerated or strangulated inguinal hernias, and femoral hernias. For recurrent inguinal hernias, the properi-

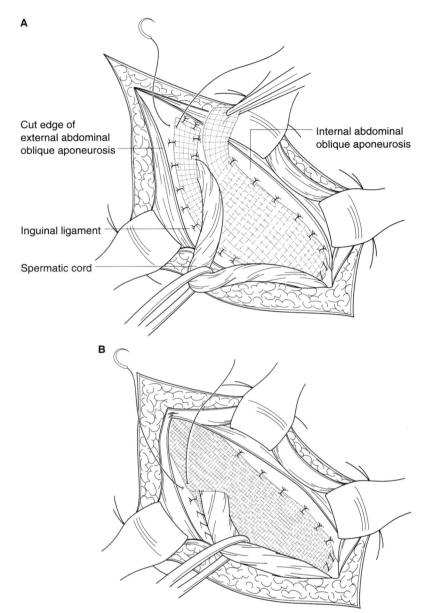

FIGURE 10-6. The placement of mesh to create a tension-free repair of an inguinal hernia was initially popularized by Lichtenstein. (From Knol JA, Eckhauser FE. Inguinal anatomy and abdominal wall hernias. In: Greenfield LJ, Mulholland M, Oldham KT, et al., eds. *Surgery: scientific principles and practice*, 2nd ed. Philadelphia: Lippincott-Raven, 1997:1225, with permission.)

toneal approach allows one to avoid the densely scarred tissues of the reoperative groin and thus reduce the risk of nerve or spermatic cord injury. In cases of incarcerated or strangulated hernias, the properitoneal approach allows the bowel to be isolated before it is reduced, thereby preventing the premature reduction of dead bowel or contamination of the operative field. The use of a properitoneal approach allows for the repair of femoral hernias without disturbing the inguinal floor, in contrast to the McVay technique.

The incision is made somewhat superior to that used for a conventional anterior approach, keeping the incision superior to the deep inguinal ring. The abdominal wall layers are divided down to the properitoneal fat plane that lies immediately deep to the transversalis fascia. The peritoneum is then bluntly pushed away from the abdominal wall inferiorly, thus exposing the internal surface of the inguinal region. After reduction of the hernia by gentle traction and amputation of the sac, the hernia defect is repaired by approximating the transversus abdominis aponeurosis to Cooper ligament's medially and then starting at the medial edge of the femoral vein, to the iliopubic tract laterally. The hernia defect can also be repaired by suturing prosthetic mesh to the inner abdominal wall. This is similar to the technique used in the laparoscopic approaches to hernia repair.

The disability experienced after an anterior herniorrhaphy imposes a significant expense on both the patient and society. *Laparoscopic approaches* to hernia repair propose to offer improved recovery time without significantly increased recurrence rates; the drawbacks include increased cost, increased technical skill required, and the possibility of serious complications. These procedures are usually done under general anesthesia and are contraindicated in high-risk patients. The most widely accepted indications for a laparoscopic approach are the presence of bilateral or recurrent hernias. With bilateral hernias, both sides can be repaired at the same operation without added disability. In recurrent hernias, the laparoscopic approach allows one to avoid the scarred tissue planes of the previous repair, thus reducing the risk for spermatic cord or nerve injury.

There are currently two techniques for laparoscopic inguinal herniorrhaphy, the transabdominal properitoneal (TAPP) repair and the totally extraperitoneal (TEP) repair. Both of these techniques place a mesh patch over the deep inguinal ring and the floor of the inguinal canal in the properitoneal position, similar to the open properitoneal procedure.

In the TAPP herniorrhaphy technique, a pneumoperitoneum is established and the inguinal regions are examined with the laparoscope. Femoral and indirect hernias are identified as protruding defects in the peritoneum, whereas direct hernias are generally broad-based defects filled with peritoneal fat. It is important to have a thorough understanding of the anatomy of this region to identify the landmarks for this procedure: the spermatic vessels, the obliterated umbilical artery, the inferior epigastric vessels, and the external iliac vessels. The peritoneum is divided transversely, just superior to the deep inguinal ring, and upper and lower flaps are created using blunt dissection. A sheet of prosthetic mesh, large enough to cover the entire inguinal and femoral region, is placed in the properitoneal space (Fig. 10-7). Because staples are used to secure the mesh, great care must be taken to avoid injury to the neurovascular structures in the region. After the mesh is in place, the peritoneum is reapproximated to prevent it from coming in contact with bowel.

In the TEP procedure, the properitoneal space is entered via an infraumbilical cutdown. A pneumatic balloon can be placed in the space to facilitate the dissection, which is carried down to include the space of Retzius. The entire inguinal floor is exposed, along with the femoral region and the obturator canal. A sheet of prosthetic mesh, large enough to cover the entire region, is then placed into the properitoneal space. Most surgeons do not use staples to secure the mesh, thus reducing the risk of neurovascular injury. As the properitoneal space is deflated, the peritoneum covers the mesh and holds it in place. There is approximately a 5% to 10% conversion rate from a TEP repair to a TAPP repair due to difficulty with the dissection or tearing of the peritoneum.

Little data are currently available on the long-term recurrence rate for laparoscopic hernia repairs, but in general, the recurrence rate for the TAPP technique is about 0.7%, and about 0.4% for the TEP technique. Patients generally tolerate the procedure well and are able to return to unrestricted activity within 3 or 4 days. Complication rates are related to the expertise of the surgeon, but average around 7% to 10% and include epigastric vessel injury, enterotomy, cys-

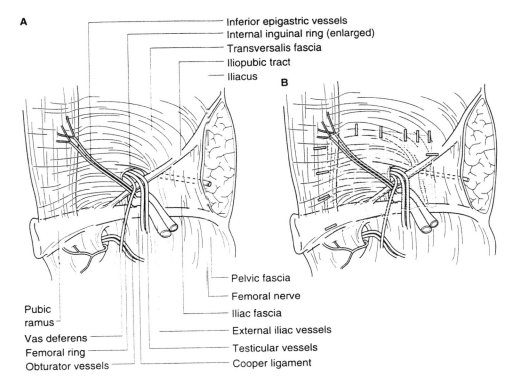

FIGURE 10-7. Internal anatomy of a right groin hernia **(A)** and placement of mesh during a laparoscopic repair **(B)**. (From Knol JA, Eckhauser FE. Inguinal anatomy and abdominal wall hernias. In: Greenfield LJ, Mulholland M, Oldham KT, et al., eds. *Surgery: scientific principles and practice*, 2nd ed. Philadelphia: Lippincott-Raven, 1997:1226, with permission.)

totomy, urinary retention, trocar site hematoma, bowel obstruction, and infection.

The treatment of *recurrent inguinal* or *femoral hernias* can be a difficult surgical problem. Recurrences can be due to the failure to recognize the presence of an indirect hernia sac during the repair of a direct inguinal hernia. Other causes include progressive tissue fatigue and the use of weak tissues in the initial repair. The creation of a repair under tension can also contribute to the development of a recurrence.

Most recurrences occur in the medial aspect of the repair, near the pubic tubercle. These can be dangerous because the defect is generally small and nondistensible, thus increasing the risk for incarceration and strangulation. The repair of recurrent hernias poses a greater risk for spermatic cord and neurovascular injury than a primary repair. The dissection through the scarred tissue planes is often difficult. If adequate tissues are present, or if a previously untreated indirect hernia is found, a standard repair can be performed. This is often not the case, however, and many surgeons prefer to repair recurrent hernias with prosthetic mesh. The use of properitoneal approaches, either open or laparoscopic, is another option particularly well suited for the treatment of multiple recurrent hernias. These techniques allow the surgeon to avoid the previous operative field entirely, thus reducing the risk to inguinal canal structures and avoiding the use of attenuated or scarred tissues in the repair.

Femoral hernias pass through the femoral canal (Fig. 10-2) beneath the inguinal ligament and into the femoral triangle of the upper thigh. They are more common in women (33% of groin hernias) than in men (2% of groin hernias), but are less common than inguinal hernias in both sexes.

Femoral hernias are often difficult to diagnose and often remain asymptomatic until incarceration or strangulation occurs. The history of a bulge in the lower groin or upper medial thigh can often be elicited. The presence of a reducible mass in the lower inguinal region supports the diagnosis, but it can be difficult to distinguish a femoral from an inguinal hernia in some patients. Other conditions that can cause a tender mass in the infrainguinal region include lymphadenopathy (infectious, metastatic, etc.) and saphenous varicies. If the diagnosis is not clear after a thorough history and physical examination, ultrasound or CT studies may be helpful.

The aim of treatment for femoral hernias is to close the femoral canal, which lies medial to the femoral vein. This is generally done using Cooper ligament's as the deep margin of the musculoaponeurotic repair. When an anterior approach is performed, the transversus abdominis aponeurosis is sutured to Cooper ligament's, i.e., the McVay repair. This is the most common approach used to treat femoral hernias. Recurrence rates for the McVay repair vary from 5% to 10%.

Properitoneal approaches, both open and laparoscopic, are also appropriate for the treatment of femoral hernias using the techniques described above for inguinal hernias. In the open technique, either a mesh or a direct repair can be performed. Laparoscopic techniques can be more challenging due to the difficulty often encountered in reducing a femoral hernia. The laparoscopic approach is contraindicated in cases of incarcerated or strangulated hernias.

Regardless of the approach, femoral hernias are difficult to reduce. Occasionally, it becomes necessary to make a counter incision in the upper thigh over the hernia bulge to help free the sac. It may also be necessary to divide the inguinal ligament to reduce the hernia. The inguinal ligament is then repaired with nonabsorbable sutures, producing no significant deficit.

ANTERIOR ABDOMINAL WALL HERNIAS

The anterior abdominal wall is the site of several types of hernias. They are, in general, less common than groin hernias. Due to the risk of bowel strangulation, however, it is important to be able to diagnose these hernias accurately and to treat them properly.

The *umbilicus* is a site of potential weakness in the anterior abdominal wall. The round ligament, urachus, and obliterated umbilical arteries converge at the inferior rim of the umbilicus, a site of fascial attenuation.

In children, an umbilical hernia is a congenital defect found in approximately 10% of white infants and in 40% to 90% of black infants. There is also a higher incidence in premature infants. In most children, the hernia will spontaneously close within 2 years. There is a very low incidence of complications of umbilical hernias in children, leading many surgeons to withhold surgical treatment until the child is at least 4 years old, by which time the majority have resolved. Early treatment is indicated in cases of incarceration, symptomatic hernias, or defects larger than 5 cm, which are unlikely to close spontaneously.

In adults, umbilical hernias do not spontaneously regress as in children. Abdominal straining and conditions leading to increased intraabdominal pressure tend to expand the hernia defects over time. Because of the risk of incarceration or strangulation of bowel, surgical treatment is indicated if the patient's overall condition permits.

The *treatment* of umbilical hernias is generally performed on an outpatient basis using epidural or general anesthesia. Small hernias that are unlikely to require intraabdominal manipulations can be repaired under local anesthesia. A curvilinear infraumbilical incision is used, and the hernia sac can usually be isolated by blunt dissection. The hernia contents, usually omentum, are reduced, and the fascial edges of the hernia defect are identified. The defect is closed transversely; if the defect is large, prosthetic mesh may be required. The traditional "pants over vest" imbricated closure does not provide added strength but does increase the tension in the repair. All attempts are made to preserve the umbilicus for cosmetic reasons in all but multiple recurrent cases.

Hernias occurring above the umbilicus, through the linea alba, are referred to as *epigastric hernias*. Congenital variations in the decussation patterns of the linea alba can lead to weak areas in the epigastrium. In the setting of repetitive stresses or persistent elevations in intraabdominal pressure, defects can develop in these areas of weakness. The resulting epigastric hernias occur in about 3% to 5% of the population, more commonly in men and usually from 20 to 50 years of age. About 20% of epigastric hernias are multiple and 80% are located slightly off the midline.

Epigastric hernias are generally small and contain properitoneal fat but can become quite large and contain a peritoneal sac. Small hernias are generally the most symptomatic; as the hernia enlarges, the sharp pains give way to dull aches. The presence of a painful midline epigastric mass is often enough to make the diagnosis.

The treatment of epigastric hernias must take into account the frequency of multiple defects. Small defects can be closed primarily, but a thorough palpation of the linea alba should be made at the time of surgery to determine whether additional asymptomatic defects are present. Some surgeons have advocated the use of diagnostic laparoscopy to examine the abdominal wall at the time of hernia repair. Infrequently, large defects may require prosthetic mesh for tension-free closure. Recurrence of epigastric hernias occurs in about 5% to 10% of patients.

A *spigelian hernia* is a rare spontaneous hernia of the anterior abdominal wall. The hernia protrudes through a weakness in the spigelian fascia (Fig. 10-8), which is defined as the segment of the transversus abdominis aponeurosis between its origin (at the semilunar line) to the edge of the rectus sheath. The weakest site along the spigelian fascia is at the point where it crosses the arcuate line in the lower abdomen; this is where most of the hernias occur.

Spigelian hernias can be difficult to diagnose. They are often small and can dissect between the aponeurotic layers of the abdominal wall, making it more difficult to palpate a distinct mass. A point of tenderness can usually be found at the site of the hernia defect. Having the patient perform a Valsalva maneuver can help make a hernia palpable and usually causes increased pain at the site of the hernia defect. If the diagnosis is in question, an ultrasound or CT examination of the anterior abdominal wall is often useful.

The fascial defects in spigelian hernias are often small, making them prone to incarcerate or strangulate. Consequently, these hernias should be repaired when identified. Generally, a simple reduction of the hernia sac and primary repair of the fascial defect is sufficient treatment.

Incisional hernias continue to be a difficult problem with which every general surgeon must contend. The incidence of incisional hernias has been estimated to be about 10%, most becoming apparent within the first postoperative year, although one third develop after 5 years.

Several risk factors have been identified, which predispose patients to develop incisional hernias. In addition to

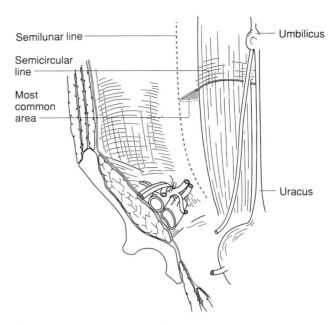

FIGURE 10-8. A spigelian hernia occurs through the linea semilunaris and inferior to the linea semicircularis. (From Knol JA, Eckhauser FE. Inguinal anatomy and abdominal wall hernias. In: Greenfield LJ, Mulholland M, Oldham KT, et al., eds. *Surgery: scientific principles and practice*, 2nd ed. Philadelphia: Lippincott-Raven, 1997:1228, with permission.)

the risk factors for the development of other abdominal wall hernias, such as increased intraabdominal pressure, factors such as increased age, nutritional depletion, male gender, and jaundice also increase the risk for incisional hernias. Poor surgical technique at the original operation often sets the stage for the development of an incisional hernia. The use of weak tissues in the repair, inadequate fascial bites, and too much tension in the closure are the most common causes of technical failures. The development of a postoperative wound infection also greatly increases the risk that the closure will break down, up to a fivefold increase in some studies.

Small incisional hernias with tight necks are prone to strangulate herniated abdominal contents. Larger hernias are less likely to strangulate but will frequently be incarcerated due to the development of adhesions between the intraabdominal contents and the hernia sac. All hernias should be repaired if the patient's physical condition will allow. The success of the repair depends on several important factors, including the use of healthy fascial tissues in the repair, closure with minimal tension, and prophylaxis for wound infection. Small defects can often be closed primarily, but large hernias present a difficult problem. In massive hernias, a substantial portion of the abdominal viscera may be present within the hernia. If this condition is long-standing, the viscera may lose their "abdominal domain" and respiratory embarrassment may follow reduction and repair of the hernia. Several surgeons advocate the use of progressive pneumoperitoneum to increase the intraabdominal volume prior to repair.

The repair of incisional hernias must be performed using healthy tissues and without tension. General anesthesia is preferred to allow for abdominal wall relaxation and because intraabdominal dissections are often required to free adherent viscera from the hernia sac. The closure itself may be made primarily or with the use of prosthetic mesh.

Primary closures are usually successful only for defects less than 3 to 4 cm in size. Relaxing incisions placed in the lateral aspects of the anterior rectus sheath, the Keel procedure, often will allow the medial aspect of the anterior sheath to be closed in the midline. For larger hernias, the use of prosthetic mesh, most commonly Marlex, has become invaluable. Several methods for the placement of the mesh have been described, including extrafascial, subfascial, and intraperitoneal techniques. For any procedure, however, it is important to have the mesh overlap the fascia for 4 to 8 cm and to secure the mesh to the fascia with nonabsorbable sutures. Placement of the mesh directly in contact with the bowel presents the risk for future erosion of the mesh into the bowel and the formation of a fistula. Most surgeons prefer to place tissue (peritoneum, omentum) between the mesh and bowel if possible. Care should be taken to prevent fluid collections under the subcutaneous flaps made during these procedures. Fluid collections

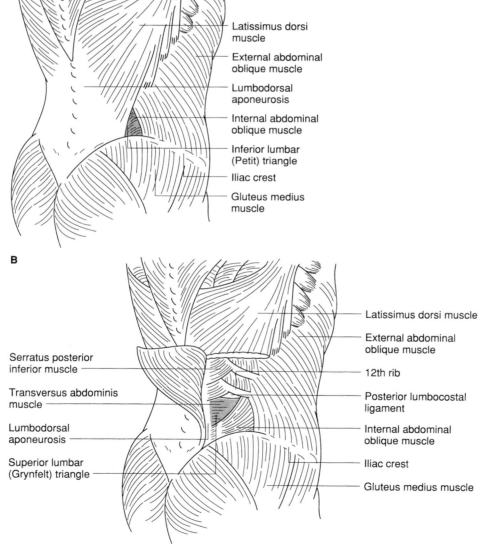

FIGURE 10-9. A hernia in the lumbar region can occur through the **(A)** inferior lumbar triangle and the **(B)** superior lumbar triangle. (From Knol JA, Eckhauser FE. Inguinal anatomy and abdominal wall hernias. In: Greenfield LJ, Mulholland M, Oldham KT, et al., eds. *Surgery: scientific principles and practice*, 2nd ed. Philadelphia: Lippincott-Raven, 1997:1210, with permission.)

are prone to infection, and the use of closed suction drains is advisable with large flaps.

The recurrence rate for incisional hernias is 30% to 50% overall. The use of mesh to provide a tension-free repair, however, has been associated with recurrence rates as low as 10%. Multiple recurrent hernias present even greater challenges and are even more prone to recur, so prevention, by adherence to the principle of wound closure, is the best treatment.

Hernia defects can develop through the musculoaponeurotic structures of the posterolateral abdominal wall in the *lumbar region*. These hernias, although rare, have a significant incidence of incarceration and are often difficult to diagnose.

The posterolateral abdominal wall, like the anterior abdomen, is made up of several layers. The deep layer is made up of the quadratus lumborum and psoas major posteriorly and the transversus abdominis laterally. The next layer is formed by the internal oblique and the serratus posterior inferior, and the superficial layer is made up by the external oblique and the latissimus dorsi muscles (Fig. 10-9).

Spontaneous hernias in the lumbar region usually occur at two locations, known as the superior and inferior lumbar triangles. The superior lumbar triangle of *Grynfeltt* is bounded by the 12th rib, the superior margin of the internal oblique muscle, and the sacrospinalis muscle. The floor of the superior triangle is formed by the transversus abdominis muscle, and the roof is the latissimus dorsi. The bounds of the inferior lumbar triangle of *Petit* are formed by the iliac crest, the latissimus dorsi, and the external oblique.

The majority of lumbar hernias occur spontaneously, but up to 25% are posttraumatic, including postoperative. The superior lumbar triangle is the most common site of spontaneous lumbar hernias. The latissimus dorsi muscle plays an important role in maintaining the integrity of the lumbar region. Operative procedures that weaken or reposition the latissimus dorsi, such as latissimus dorsi flaps or flank exposures of the retroperitoneum, can predispose the development of a hernia. The presentations of a lumbar hernia can vary from a localized dull ache to symptoms of strangulation. Most often, the complaint is of a lump in the flank associated with dull pain.

Lumbar hernias progress in size over time, and as they enlarge, they become more difficult to repair. They also have a 10% incidence of incarceration and strangulation; thus, the general recommendation is to repair lumbar hernias when they are found, as long as the patient can withstand an operation. There are many different approaches to repair, but there are not sufficient numbers to proclaim one technique as the best. In general, the patient is placed in the lateral decubitus position and the hernia is approached directly. Native musculoaponeurotic tissues can be used for the repair if they are adequate and tension can be avoided, otherwise a prosthetic mesh technique can be done. Recurrences are rare after lumbar herniorrhaphy.

PELVIC HERNIAS

Pelvic hernias are a form of internal hernia, occurring through the muscles that make up the pelvic floor. They generally occur in older patients and can be difficult to diagnose due to the lack of a palpable bulge on physical examination. They bear the same risks as hernias of the abdominal wall, however, and patients often present with symptoms of intestinal obstruction or strangulation.

The pelvis is lined by several muscles that serve as diaphragms, allowing the passage of structures from the abdominal cavity into the lower extremities and perineum while containing the abdominal viscera. The anterior pelvic wall is composed of the pubic bones and the origins of the obturator internus muscle. The lateral pelvic walls are covered primarily by the obturator internus muscle and the enveloping endopelvic fascia, which cover the underlying obturator foramen. The obturator canal is located in the superior part of the obturator foramen and is surrounded by the fibers of the obturator internus muscle. Through this canal pass the obturator nerve, artery, and vein into the deep medial thigh. The pelvic floor is formed by the levator ani and coccygeus muscles, together known as the *pelvic diaphragm*. The urogenital diaphragm is located in the anterior aspect of the pelvic floor, between the anterior edges of the levator ani muscles.

Obturator hernias are acquired defects through the obturator canal, along the tract taken by the obturator neurovascular bundle as it exits the pelvis. These hernias occur primarily in elderly women and have a predisposition for the right side. The diagnosis of these hernias is difficult because of the lack of specific findings on physical examination. The hernia is rarely palpable in the groin; however, a mass may be felt on vaginal or rectal examination. The classic sign is a radicular pain extending down the medial thigh with abduction or internal rotation of the knee. This Howship-Romberg sign, although useful, is present in less that half of patients with an obturator hernia. The most common presentation is crampy abdominal pain and small bowel obstruction. Because of the difficulty in making the diagnosis, treatment is often delayed and the mortality for this type of hernia can be as high as 40%.

The treatment for obturator hernias is operative, most commonly via a transabdominal approach. Any nonviable bowel should be resected and the hernia sac is removed, as with other hernias. It is often not possible to close the defect primarily, requiring the placement of a prosthetic mesh patch. Recurrences are rare with obturator hernias.

Perineal hernias occur through the pelvic diaphragm. Almost all of these are the result of multiple pregnancies or surgery of the pelvic floor. These hernias are frequently asymptomatic and easily reducible; strangulation and incarceration are rare. The diagnosis can often be made by a careful history and physical examination, most importantly the vaginal and rectal examinations.

The treatment for perineal hernias is direct repair, preferably via a transabdominal approach. Small defects can often be closed directly, but larger hernias with patulous musculoaponeurotic tissues require prosthetic mesh patch repair.

Sciatic hernias are extremely rare defects that occur through the greater or lesser sciatic foramina. Patients often present with a gradually enlarging mass in the infragluteal region. Symptoms of sciatic nerve compression may also be present, as can symptoms of bowel obstruction or ischemia. The diagnosis is often difficult to make, and ultrasound or CT scanning can be helpful.

Sciatic hernias can be repaired via both the transabdominal and transgluteal approach, but the transabdominal approach is recommended if signs of bowel obstruction or strangulation are present. The repair usually requires the use of a prosthetic mesh, but great care must be taken not to injure the neurovascular structures in the area.

PEDIATRIC DEVELOPMENTAL HERNIAS

The diaphragm develops between the fourth and eighth weeks of gestation as the transverse septum and pleuroperitoneal folds fuse. Failure of these structures to fuse in the posterolateral region results in a patent foramen of Bochdalek through which abdominal contents can herniate (Fig. 10-10). Foramen of Bochdalek hernias make up the majority of congenital diaphragmatic hernias (CDHs), occurring in 1 out of every 4,000 to 5,000 live births. Because the left hemidiaphragm closes later in gestation than the right, most (about 90%) CDHs occur on the left. Left-side hernias generally contain small bowel, spleen, colon, and stomach, while right-side hernias contain the right lobe of the liver and small bowel. Because the intestines are displaced into the thorax before they are fixed to the retroperitoneum, all foramen of Bochdalek hernias are associated with intestinal malrotation.

The foramen of Morgagni hernia is a defect in the anterior aspect of the diaphragm where it inserts onto the sternum. They can be located on either the right or left. Most commonly, they are asymptomatic and found incidentally on a chest x-ray.

The major problem associated with CDHs is pulmonary hypoplasia. The presence of abdominal viscera in the chest early in gestation prevents the normal development of the bronchoalveolar tree on the ipsilateral side. The development of the pulmonary vasculature is also affected, resulting in significant pulmonary hypertension, which can contribute to the persistence of fetal circulation and right to left shunting of blood through the patent foramen ovale and ductus arteriosus. These factors produce profound hypoxia, hypercarbia, and acidosis early after birth.

With today's close prenatal monitoring, most cases of CDH are found on routine maternal ultrasound examinations. At birth, infants with significant pulmonary hypopla-

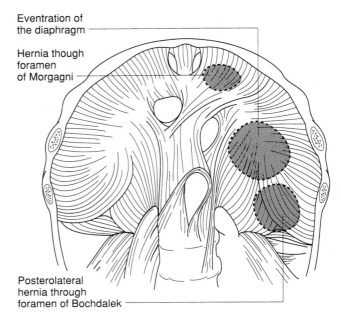

FIGURE 10-10. Congenital diaphragmatic defects include the posteriorly located Bochdalek hernia or an anterior hernia through the foramen of Morgagni. Congenital eventration of the diaphragm is usually caused by a defect in the muscularization with the majority of the diaphragm being principally membranous rather than muscular. (From Coran AG, Oldham KT. Pediatric thorax. In: Greenfield LJ, Mulholland M, Oldham KT, et al., eds. *Surgery: scientific principles and practice*, 2nd ed. Philadelphia: Lippincott-Raven, 1997:2020, with permission.)

sia develop severe respiratory distress, often requiring mechanical ventilation. The infants abdomen is usually scaphoid, and breath sounds are absent on the side of the hernia. The diagnosis is often confirmed with a chest x-ray showing the intestines in the thorax. In some cases, it is difficult to differentiate a CDH from cystic adenomatoid malformations or intralobar sequestrations. An upper gastrointestinal (GI) barium study is diagnostic in this situation.

The initial aim of treatment for infants with CDH is management of their respiratory distress. Immediate surgery to repair the hernia has been found detrimental and a period of stabilization is warranted. Most centers wait up to 24 hours after stabilization before operating. Ventilatory support consists of mechanical ventilation and pharmacologic support to reduce the pulmonary hypertension. The prevention of barotrauma is critical, and patients are often placed on high-frequency jet ventilation to avoid high peak inspiratory pressures. In extreme cases, when hypoxia and hypercarbia cannot be reversed by conventional ventilation, infants can be placed on extracorporeal membrane oxygenation (ECMO) until their pulmonary function recovers.

The hernia is repaired through an upper abdominal transverse incision. The abdominal viscera are reduced and the hernia sac, if present, should be removed. There is often a rim of diaphragm along the posterior wall of the defect that can be used in the repair. It is frequently possible to close the defects primarily with interrupted nonabsorbable sutures. If the defect is too large, abdominal wall muscle flaps can be created to provide closure. Occasionally, a prosthetic patch, usually Gortex, is required to close the defect, but they are associated with a small incidence of hernia recurrence.

The overall survival rate for infants who become symptomatic with a CDH early after birth is about 50%; however, the availability of ECMO for postoperative respiratory support has increased the survival to 60% to 80%. There is a growing experience with fetal surgery at a few large centers utilizing prenatal tracheal occlusion to stimulate in utero pulmonary development and ameliorate the consequences of pulmonary hypoplasia.

Gastroschisis is a defect in the anterior abdominal wall that is usually to the right of an intact umbilical cord. It is probably due to the intrauterine rupture of the umbilical sac. Unlike omphalocele, there is no peritoneal sac with gastroschisis. The bowel is thus in direct contact with the amniotic fluid, which is an irritant, causing the development of a thick, exudative serosal reaction.

Gastroschisis is about twice as common as omphalocele. It is usually diagnosed on prenatal ultrasound examination. About 40% of these patients are either premature or small for gestational age. In contrast to infants with omphalocele, the incidence of associated congenital anomalies is small. There is a 10% to 15% incidence of intestinal atresia associated with gastroschisis, but chromosomal syndromes are rare.

The treatment of gastroschisis begins with adequate fluid resuscitation and prevention of sepsis. Significant third space fluid losses occur due to the exposed bowel. Once adequate hydration has been achieved and parenteral antibiotics initiated, operative repair of the defect is indicated. The bowel must be carefully inspected for sites of atresia or perforation. Usually, it is necessary to extend the defect vertically to allow for reduction of the viscera. In 80% of infants with gastroschisis, it is possible to reduce the bowel and close the defect primarily. However, in 20% of cases, the abdominal cavity is not large enough to accommodate all of the herniated viscera without producing excessively high intraabdominal pressures. This situation can impair ventilation, reduce venous return to the heart, and compress the bowel mesentery, resulting in ischemia. In these cases, a Silastic silo is sutured to the fascial edge of the defect to provide a temporary covering for the viscera. The silo is kept sterile, and on the second or third postoperative day, a gradual reduction in size of the silo is started in the intensive care unit. The viscera can be gradually reduced into the abdominal cavity over the course of several days. Once all of the viscera have been returned to the abdomen, the infant is returned to the operating room to remove the silo and close the defect.

These patients often have a profound adynamic ileus that can last for several weeks. Consequently, the early initiation of total parenteral nutrition (TPN) is important. The overall survival of infants with gastroschisis is about 90%, with most deaths being due to sepsis or complications of atresias.

An *omphalocele* is an abdominal wall defect occurring through the umbilical ring that occurs in 1 out of 5,000 live births. Unlike gastroschisis, omphaloceles are covered by a sac made up of an outer layer of amnion and an inner layer of peritoneum; the umbilical cord inserts into the sac. These infants have a 30% to 70% incidence of associated anomalies, including cardiovascular, genitourinary, GI, and central nervous system defects. They also have an increased incidence of malignant tumors, such as Wilms tumor and neuroblastoma.

The diagnosis of omphalocele is usually made by prenatal ultrasound examination. At birth, about 90% of infants with an omphalocele will have an intact sac. Care should be taken to keep the sac clean and moist, because it provides a natural barrier to fluid loss and abdominal sepsis. In cases where the sac has ruptured, there are increased fluid requirements, as with gastroschisis.

Small defects can often be repaired primarily or by the creation of a ventral hernia. Larger defects, however, may require a staged reduction of the abdominal viscera by the placement of a Silastic silo (see gastroschisis above). Alternatively, when the defect is very large or when the infant is unable to withstand an operation due to concurrent illness, nonoperative treatment using the topical application of an escharotic agent is acceptable. Typically, merbromin (Mercurochrome), mafenide (Sulfamylon), or silver nitrate solution are applied to the sac twice a day. This stimulates the epithelialization and contraction of the sac over time. As long as the sac remains intact, definitive repair can be delayed until the infant is able to withstand an operation.

Unlike in infants with gastroschisis, the intestines in an infant with omphalocele have not been irritated by the amniotic fluid and are not thick and edematous. Consequently, the incidence and duration of adynamic ileus is less and enteral feedings can be initiated earlier. The survival of infants with omphalocele is related to the severity of the additional anomalies and chromosomal defects. The overall mortality rate varies widely from 30% to 60%.

11

STATISTICS AND EPIDEMIOLOGY

ALPHONSO BROWN AND RUDOLF N. STAROSCIK

A sound background in basic epidemiology and biostatistics is a necessary prerequisite in order for a surgeon to make informed decisions when reviewing the literature or study data. This chapter will focus on the fundamental skills needed to evaluate the rapidly growing and often conflicting medical literature.

FUNDAMENTALS OF STUDY DESIGN

This section will review the basic types of study design and provide an overview of when and why each particular design should be used in order to better interpret the medical literature. Epidemiological studies may be classified into two categories: *descriptive studies* and *explanatory studies*. Descriptive studies serve principally to chronicle clinical and scientific observations, which may then serve as a basis for subsequent investigative studies. Case reports and case series are examples of descriptive studies.

A *case report* provides a clinical description of a single patient, and case reports are used to document a rare or uncommon presentation of a disease. A case report can provide information about the diagnosis and management of rare cases and may also be used for future hypothesis generation. A major limitation of case reports is that they cannot be generalized to other subjects and cannot prove causation of disease. In addition, because the sample size is one, statistical analysis can not be performed.

A *case series* is a clinical description of a group of patients with a specific disease or condition. It provides descriptions of clinical symptomatology as well as interventions and outcomes. Most case series allow characterization regarding several aspects of an illness, which is usually a rare disease, or an atypical presentation of a common illness. Case series can not prove causation but may provide information, which can then be used to generate hypotheses for further investigation. Due to the lack of a control group, statistical analyses also can not be performed in a case series.

Unlike descriptive studies, *explanatory studies* can be used to make inferences about causality. Explanatory studies can be further subdivided into experimental studies, such as a randomized clinical trial, and observational studies, such as case-control and cohort studies.

Observational Studies

A *case-control study* may be defined as a study in which patients with a given disease of interest are paired with control subjects (Fig. 11-1). All study participants are then queried about one or several exposures of interest with the principle goal of demonstrating an association between a prior exposure of interest and the development of disease. The case-control study design allows the study of a number of risk factors or potential etiologies for a given disease. This design should be used when the disease to be studied is very rare or takes a long time to develop. It is often thought of as an efficient study design because the study can usually be completed in a short time and on a smaller budget than a cohort study. An example of a simple case-control design is a study in which the last 50 cases of gastric lymphoma seen at one institution are pooled and matched with 50 normal controls. If one wants determine whether prior ulcer disease is a risk factor for gastric lymphoma, all the subjects could be asked about their past history of peptic ulcer disease or gastritis.

Because patients and subjects in case-control studies must recall in detail past exposure, these studies are particularly susceptible to the introduction of bias. *Recall bias* occurs when subjects selectively recall past events, and *interviewer bias* occurs when an interviewer, who is aware of the exposure of clinical interest, interviews some subjects more selectively than others. Usually the patients interviewed more intensely are those who the interviewer suspects have the exposure of interest. *Information bias* can occur during retrospective review of data. Researchers who review the data and are aware of the study hypothesis as well as the patients history may be influenced in the way they select cases and controls for the study.

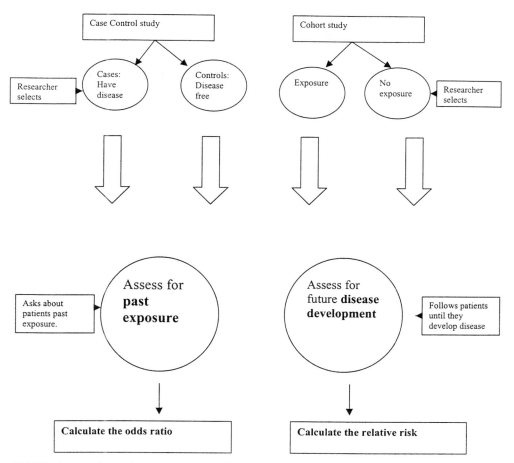

FIGURE 11-1. Schematic representation of the difference between a case-control and a cohort study.

The strength of association between exposure and disease in a case-control study is often reported as the exposure odds ratio. The *exposure odds ratio* may be defined as the likelihood of the development of disease in the exposed group relative to that of those who were are not exposed. If you constructed a standard 2 × 2 table (Fig. 11-2A) and defined the odds of exposure among those with disease as a/c and the odds of exposure among the controls as b/d, the exposure odds ratio would become $(a/c)/(b/d)$.

A *cohort study* may be defined as a study design in which patients who share a common exposure thought to be a precursor to the development of a specific disease are followed for a given period in order to see whether they actually develop disease (e.g., following a group of smokers for 30 years to determine who will develop lung cancer). Cohort studies are excellent for defining the development of new cases of disease (incidence) and investigating the potential causes of a condition. A cohort study design should be used (i) to study rare exposures and their ability to cause disease, (ii) to determine the temporal relationship between exposure and disease, and (iii) to minimize the types of bias described for case-control studies. In addition, a major advantage of the cohort study over the previously mentioned study designs is the ability to prove causality. Although explanatory studies such as randomized trials are the most valid study designs for establishing causality, the resources may not be available or it might not be feasible to conduct such a study. Some problems with cohort studies include their expense, the very long time needed to conduct the study, and the potentially high rate of patient attrition and loss to follow-up. Unlike the case-control design, the cohort study design can assess the incidence of a disease secondary to a given exposure in a population at risk. The *relative risk* may be defined as the risk of disease in the exposed population divided by the risk of disease in the unexposed population. The 2 × 2 table method may also represent this relationship (Fig. 11-2B).

	Disease +	Disease −
Exposure +	a	b
Exposure −	c	d

A

	Disease +	Disease −
Exposure +	a	b
Exposure −	c	d

B

FIGURE 11-2. A: An example of a 2 × 2 table used to calculate the odds ratio from a case-control study. (*a*, the subjects who have disease and the exposure of interest; *b*, the subjects who have the exposure of interest and no disease; *c*, the subjects who have not been exposed but have disease; *d*, the subjects who do not have the exposure of interest or disease). Note that *a* + *c* equals all the patients with disease (the cases); *b* + *d* equals the total number of patients without disease (the controls). **B:** Calculation of the relative risk of a cohort study by the 2 × 2 table. Given *a*, *b*, *c*, and *d* as previously defined in the example for case-control studies, the relative risk of disease development given exposure may be represented as follows: $RR = a/(a + c)/b/(b + d)$.

Experimental Studies

The *randomized clinical trial* is the most powerful type of study design and can provide definitive evidence of causality by means of an intervention. The major difference between this study design and the observational study design is that the researcher administers the intervention under control. This design should be employed whenever ethically possible and affordable. If done well, the randomized clinical trial eliminates the effect of the various types of confounding variables and biases, which may invalidate case-control and cohort studies. As with the cohort study, the randomized trial may be expensive and large losses to follow-up may also be an issue.

STATISTICAL METHODS AND DATA INTERPRETATION

Statistical methods can be classified as either descriptive or inferential. *Descriptive statistics* refer to the utilization of statistics to describe or summarize actual data. This type of statistic may be used, e.g., to characterize the eye color traits of the population of African American females in the United States. *Inferential statistics* use a small sample of patients to make assumptions about the population as a whole. Gallup polls and surveys use inferential statistics to make general comments about the population based on a small sample of opinions.

A *population* refers to the total set of individuals or objects about which the researcher wants to draw a conclusion. A *sample* is a smaller set taken from the population of interest, which contains characteristics felt to be representative of the total population. Each object within a given population is called an *element*. The total number of elements is equal to the number of objects in the population and is usually denoted by *N*. The way in which a sample is selected is called the *sample selection process*. The investigator's primary goal when selecting a sample is to select one that will be representative of the entire source population. *Randomization* refers to the process of selecting a sample from the population such that each individual has an equal chance of being selected. A sampling method that yields a random sampling of the source population has the greatest chance of truly being representative of the population from which it was drawn. Bias occurs when an error in the sampling method distorts our sampling method such that the final sample is not representative of the source population.

Data for both descriptive and inferential statistics can be organized into one of the following four categories: interval, ratio, ordinal, or nominal. These classifications for all data can be remembered using the mnemonic *IRON*. *Interval data* can be placed in a meaningful order based on an accepted convention with similar intervals between data points. The readings on a thermometer are an example of interval data. *Ratio data* is similar to interval data except it has an absolute zero frame of reference (e.g., 0 lb on a scale and 0 mm Hg on a blood pressure cuff). *Ordinal data* can be placed in a meaningful order, but no information is available on the intervals between data points. Data ordered by conventions such as first, second, and third represent ordinal data. Groups based on descriptive qualities such as white/black, male/female, and fat/skinny categorize *nominal data*. Unlike the other data types, nominal data can not be ordered and there is no meaning to intervals between the data points. Nominal data is often referred to as *categorical* because it groups data into categories.

Data can also be described as *discrete* or *continuous*. Discrete data can only take on certain values within a given range, such as the ordinal counting of numbers 1, 2, 3, 4.... Continuous data can take on any value within a given range. All real numbers between 1 and 2 would be an example of continuous data. Classifying data in this manner is important because the statistical analysis is dependent on the type of data being analyzed. Investigators characterize the distribution of a data set by descriptors, which provide information about the points in the data set. The measures most commonly used are the mean, median, and mode. The *mean* of a data set is the sum of all the elements divided by the number of elements in the distribution. The mean of a distribution is sensitive to extreme values; therefore, you must be careful to take extreme values into account when interpreting the mean. The *mode* of a distribution is the observed value that occurs with the greatest frequency. If there is more than one value that occurs multiple times within a distribution, then the distribution is said to be *multimodal*. Unlike the mean, the mode is insensitive to values that lie at the extremes of the distribution. The *median* of a distribution is the figure that exactly divides the data in half. When the number of elements is odd, the median is the middle one. When the number of elements is even, the median is the value that lies halfway between the two middle scores. The median is relatively insensitive to extreme values within the distribution (Fig. 11-3A).

Despite having the same mean, certain distributions may still look different (Fig. 11-3B). Though the median, mode, and mean are the same, the variability of the data can be significantly different. To accurately describe a data set, there must also be commentary on the measures of variability. The three measures of variability are the *standard deviation*, the *range*, and the *variance*. The variance of a distribution is the mean of the squares of all the deviation scores in the distribution. The variance of a population is symbolized by θ^2. The variance of a sample is given by the square of the sample's standard deviation. The range is simply the difference between the lowest and highest scores in the distribution. The population standard deviation is the square root of the variance. These three variables define the degree of splay of a distribution, and when taken together with mean, median, and mode, they uniquely describe the shape of the distribution. A normal distribution, also called a *Gaussian distribution*, is a bell-shaped curve, which is uniquely defined by a mean and a standard deviation. The mean and standard deviation are called the *parameters* of the curve, and taken together, they uniquely define a given normal distribution.

INFERENTIAL STATISTICS

When performing data analyses, you often can not survey the entire population and will instead analyze a small sample that you feel is representative of the population as a whole. The method of using a sample population to draw inferences about the population is called *inferential statistics*. As can be expected when you draw a sample, there may be an error in the way the sample is collected. In fact, several samples from the same population may not be similar to each other at all, each having a different mean and standard deviation. This sampling error is overcome by considering the overall distribution of the means of the samples drawn. The distribution of sample means is

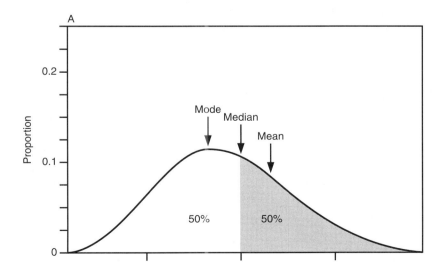

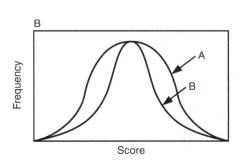

FIGURE 11-3. A: Representation of the mode, median, and mean of a normal distribution. **B:** Example of two normal distributions in which the mode, median, and mean are similar but the variances differ.

described by one of the most powerful theorems in statistics: the central limit theorem. The central limit theorem states that the random sampling distribution of means will always tend to be normally distributed irrespective of the distribution of the source population of the samples. The z score allows for calculation of the probability of a given element within a population lying a given number of standard deviations from the mean. Unfortunately, when performing studies, you often do not know the mean of the source population and instead the only available data are the sample data. In this situation, the sample standard deviation and mean become the known parameters, which you will use to approximate the unknown true population mean. The *estimated standard error of the mean* is a statistic used as approximation to the population standard deviation. The formula for the standard error of the mean may be expressed as $s_x = S/\sqrt{n}$, where n is the number of patients in the sample and S is the sample standard deviation. Because you are using the sample to make inferences about the population mean, you can not use the z statistic. In this situation, a new statistic called the t statistic is used. The t test is an inferential statistic, which is used to try to make inferences about how many standard deviations the sample means lies from the true population mean.

The paired t test is similar to the t test except it is utilized when the study subjects serve as their own control. For example, if you wanted to test a new sunscreen in a group of patients and decided to let each subject play in the sun for 6 hours and then to have the burned areas graded by a trained researcher, two weeks later, you can repeat this experiment after application of sunscreen. The researchers can then compare the new sunburn with the prior results. The data in this example are paired because each subject serves as his or her own control.

Analysis of variance (ANOVA) statistic is the statistical test used when comparisons are being made between the means of three or more variables. The calculation of the ANOVA statistic is somewhat complicated; however, the major point to remember is to utilize this statistic when drawing conclusions about the means of three or more groups. For example, to determine which three blood pressure medicines provide the best antihypertensive effect, you could randomly select from a group of similar subjects with moderate hypertension. These subjects can be separated into three groups and each group given one of the three antihypertensive agents. The mean blood pressure for each group before and after the treatments could then be calculated and compared using ANOVA.

A *correlation* is said to occur between two variables if it can be shown that there is a relationship between two variables such that one variable can be utilized to predict the value of the other. A dependent variable is a variable whose outcome is predicted by another variable, the independent variable. Correlations between variables may be thought of as positive or negative and are usually signified by a correlation coefficient r. The correlation coefficient r varies from −1 to 1. A perfect-positive correlation is represented by a value of 1; similarly, a perfect-negative correlation is represented by a value of $r = -1$. If two variables are highly correlated, it then becomes possible to predict the value of the dependent variable by the independent variable. *Linear regression* is a statistical technique in which the value of one variable, x, is used to predict the value of the other variable, Y, by means of a simple linear mathematical function. The simple linear regression equation is usually of the form $Y = a + bx$, where a is the Y intercept, b is the slope of the best-fit line, and x is the dependent variable. Linear regression should be used to make predictions of one variable on the basis of the other. For example, a linear regression model can be used to predict blood pressure in individuals who have body mass indices of greater than 30.

Nonparametric statistical tests are performed on data that are not normally distributed or can not be defined by certain parameters such as the mean and standard deviation. When dealing with data represented by categories (such as male, female, race, marital status, currently employed), rather than a normal distribution, you can categorize a proportion of individuals who fall into a given category versus the proportion of individuals who fall into an alternative category. The statistical test used to test for differences between the observed and expected proportion of individuals with a given outcome is referred to as the *chi-square statistic*. If you wanted to determine whether living near a radio transmitter increases the risk of developing leukemia, a simple study design would select two groups of individuals. The exposure group consists of individuals who lived near a radio transmitter for 10 years, and the second group could be a similar family that had never lived near a radio transmitter. You could then follow the groups for 10 years and assess the development of leukemia. The entire study could be represented by a 2 × 2 table (Fig. 11-4A).

If living near a radio transmitter has no effect on the risk of developing leukemia, then you would expect the proportion of cases of those developing leukemia to be similar in both groups. Thus, the percentage of expected cases is 110 (total number of cases in both groups) divided by 300 (the total number of subjects). The 36.7% or 0.367 represents the proportion of leukemia you would expect in either group based on the natural history of this disease, assuming that living near a radio transmitter does not increase one's risk. Using this expected disease percentage, you can then generate a new 2 × 2 table of expected frequencies as follows:

Expected number of exposed among those with leukemia = 0.367 × 100 = 36.7

Expected number of exposed among those without leukemia = 0.367 × 200 = 73.3

Expected number of unexposed among those without leukemia = (150 + 40)/300 = 0.6333 × 100 = 63.3

Exposure	Leukemia	No leukemia
Yes	60	50
No	40	150

Observed cases of disease

Exposure	Leukemia	No leukemia
Yes	36.7	73.3
No	63.3	126.7

Expected cases of disease

FIGURE 11-4. A: Observed incidence of leukemia in the two groups. **B:** Expected incidence of leukemia in the two groups assuming that living near power lines or a radio transmitter does not change the frequency of the disease.

Expected number of exposed among those without leukemia = 0.633 × 200 = 126.7

This gives us a new table of expected frequencies (Fig. 11-4B).

The chi-square statistic tests whether the difference between the actual observed frequencies and the expected frequencies are due to chance or represent a real difference. In this example, a real difference would occur if living near a radio transmitter truly caused cancer. The chi-square statistic is calculated by summing the square of the difference between the observed and expected result in each cell and then dividing that by the expected frequency in each cell. For example, the results would be as follows:

Chi-square = $(60 - 36.7)^2/36.7 + (40 - 73.3)^2/73.3$
$+ (40 - 63.3)^2/63.3 + (160 - 126.7)^2/126.7$
$= 35.17$

The larger the chi-square value the more likely the difference between the observed and expected frequencies are real and not due to chance. To determine whether the results are significant, you would then have to look at an available table of chi-square values.

The *Fisher exact test* is very similar to the chi-square test except it is used for small sample sizes and when any one of the expected frequencies from the chi-square analysis is less than 5. The *McNemar* test is also a special variant of the chi-square test used only when the study subjects are used as both the case and the control. This is similar to the paired *t* test.

Putting It All Together: Which Statistical Test to Use When?

The key questions to ask when trying to determine which statistical test to use are (i) what is/are the outcome(s) being measured or compared and (ii) is the data continuous or categorical?

HYPOTHESIS TESTING AND THE EFFECT OF CHANCE

The Null and Alternative Hypothesis

Researchers are concerned whether the results of a study occur by chance or are due to a true difference. The likelihood that a study result has occurred by chance and is not really true is called the *alpha error* of the study. By convention, alpha is usually set at 0.05, but alpha may be anything the researcher chooses. An alpha error is committed when you accept the results of a study as being real but really they occurred by chance or dumb luck. *Beta error* refers to the probability of rejecting a study result as false when it actually is true. In other words, the results of the study were real and not due to chance, but you chose to reject the results. By convention, beta is usually set at 0.20.

The *power* of a study is defined as the ability of a study to detect an outcome of interest. The power of a study is an important variable to consider because if a study does not have enough power, it may not be able to detect the outcome of interest even if the study results are positive. For this reason, it is important that a power determination is performed before any study begins. The formula for calculation of the power of a study is dependent on the type of study and varies according to the type of variables being studied (IRON) and the distribution of the data set (parametric or nonparametric). A derivation of the various power calculations is beyond the scope of this text; the usual convention is that the power to detect a given outcome is set at 80%. A formula is then used to calculate the number of subjects needed to perform the study and detect the expected outcome with power 0.80. Choosing a smaller sample might invalidate the results even if differences are detected. Alpha equals the significance level you hope to achieve. By convention, alpha is usually set at 95%. The value for beta is usually set at 20%. The power of the study to detect the difference is (1 − beta) by convention the power is usually set at 0.80.

The following example provides the utility of consulting a statistician and calculating a sample size needed to fulfill the power requirement of at least 0.80. Suppose you wanted to determine whether open cholecystectomy carries an increased risk of biliary leak compared to laparoscopic cholecystectomy and you would like to detect a difference of at least 5% between the mean rate of complications between each group because you feel this would be a clinically significant difference in complications; so you decide to perform a randomized controlled trial by randomizing patients to open versus laparoscopic cholecystectomy. After undergoing the operation, the patients will be followed for 3 months to see what percentage develop biliary leaks. Assuming the standard deviation for the sample is 6, you enroll 50 patients in each arm and follow them for 3 months. Is this study significantly powered to detect a difference in complication rates of at least 5% with 80% certainty? After performing the calculations, you discover that $N = 6,659$. Thus, you would need 6,659 patients per group to detect a clinical difference of 5%. A researcher might not realize that such a large number of patients is needed to detect a 5% difference. Realizing this before the start of the study can save a lot of time, effort, and frustration. This example illustrates the importance of performing a power calculation before embarking on an expensive clinical trial.

The Meaning of Statistical Significance and Confidence Intervals

Statistical significance, or the p value, is very similar to alpha, as it is the probability that the observed scientific result occurred by chance. For example, a p value of 0.05 means that there is a 95% chance that the observed outcome was real and a 5% likelihood that it occurred by chance alone. By convention, a p value of 0.05 is chosen to demonstrate statistical significance. Unfortunately, knowing whether a result is due to chance or represents the true value does not provide any information on whether the result is clinically meaningful and what the size of the actual observed outcome is. For example, suppose you demonstrate that wearing tight underwear results in infertility in one in a billion cases and the results are statistically significant with a p value of less than 0.05. Although the result may unlikely be due to chance based on the observed p value, the clinical utility of knowing that wearing tight underwear has a one in a billion chance of causing infertility might not be considered clinically significant. Therefore, when interpreting p values, you must be sure to consider clinical significance as well as statistical significance. This point is extremely important considering that any outcome can be made statistically significant by increasing the size of the sample used in the experiment. In other words, if a large enough sample is used, you will be able to calculate a statistically significant p value because p is a function of the size of the sample.

A supplement to the p value that is often cited in scientific studies is the 95% confidence interval. The 95% confidence interval is the range over which the true study outcome would lie 95% of the time. In other words, if you were to repeat the study an infinite number of times, the result would lie between the extremes of the 95% confidence interval 95% of the time. Unlike with the p value, testing for the 95% confidence interval can tell you just how clinically significant the result may be because you can look at the upper limit of the confidence interval. If a study is performed to determine whether sleep deprivation increases motor vehicle accidents and the results indicated that sleeping 2 hours a night increases the chance of an accident 20 times over the individual who sleeps 8 hours a night, the 95% confidence interval on your estimate of risk might be from 8 to 32. This confidence interval indicates that at a minimum, sleep-deprived individuals may be at 8 times the risk of an accident or as high as 32 times the risk. If the confidence interval crosses 1, however, you must also take into account the possibility that no difference between the two groups exists. Finally, the width of the confidence interval tells something about the accuracy of the study result: The more narrow the confidence interval, the more accurate the result, and the wider the confidence interval, the less accurate the result. An easy way to narrow the width of a 95% confidence interval is to increase the sample size N.

STATISTICS IN EPIDEMIOLOGY

Epidemiology is the study of determinants, descriptors, and distribution of biological disease. The epidemiologist is principally concerned with the determinants of disease risk. The *prevalence* of disease is the number of existing cases of a given disease among all the individuals at risk at one time. The *incidence* of disease is the number of new cases of disease occurring over a given time among all those at risk for the disease. Prevalence and incidence are used throughout epidemiology to assess characteristics of given study populations. The prevalence and incidence are used in the calculation of outcome measures such as odds ratios and relative risks. In addition, prevalence is useful in the evaluation of diagnostic testing.

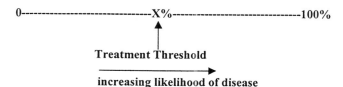

FIGURE 11-5. Decision to treat based on the results of a test.

Diagnostic Tests

In clinical practice, physicians are required to interpret the results of diagnostic tests. The results of these tests are then translated into probabilities that the physician uses to make decisions about the likelihood of a given disease in a patient. All diagnostic tests may be thought of as consisting of two fundamental parts: the test result and the test's ability to predict the occurrence of the disease. The data from a test result may be in any form: dichotomous, interval, nominal, or continuous. The ability of the test to predict the presence or absence of a given patient with a given disease is described by a set of parameters called the *operating characteristics of the diagnostic test.*

To define how well a test predicts the disease state, you must compare it to a standard, which always correctly predicts the disease state. A test that always accurately predicts the disease state is called the *gold standard*. The decision by a physician to perform a given medical intervention is usually based on the physician's determination that the benefit of the intervention significantly outweighs the risk of not providing therapy. This decision-making process can be represented schematically (Fig. 11-5). The treatment threshold X represents the probability of disease below which a physician will not provide a treatment intervention. Beyond the treatment threshold, the probability of disease is so high that the physician feels comfortable providing a recommendation for intervention. Diagnostic testing serves the purpose of moving a physician further to the right on Fig. 11-5, thereby enabling him or her to make treatment decisions with greater confidence. The treatment threshold is entirely physician dependent, and its location will vary depending on several factors such as physician experience, disease severity, and availability of diagnostic testing.

Definition of Terms

All diagnostic tests yield results, which can be summarized in the 2 × 2 table (Fig. 11-6). The test operating characteristics include the *sensitivity* of a test, which is the probability of having a positive test given that the patient truly has disease: $TP/(TP + FN)$. The sensitivity is sometimes

	Disease +	Disease −
Test +	TP	FP
Test −	FN	TN

FIGURE 11-6. A 2 × 2 table used in the calculation of the test operating characteristics of a hypothetical diagnostic test. (*TP*, the percentage of patients with a positive test result who truly have disease; *FP*, the percentage of patients with a positive test result who do not have disease; *FN*, the percentage of patients with a negative test result who truly have disease; *TN*, the percentage of patients with a negative test result who do not have disease.)

referred to as the *true-positive rate*. *Specificity* of a test is the probability of having a negative test given that the patient does not have disease: $TN/(TN + FP)$. The specificity is often referred to as the *true-negative rate*. The *prevalence* of disease is the percentage of subjects in the study population who truly have disease: $(TP + FN)/(TP + FN + TN + FP)$.

The sensitivity, specificity, and prevalence of disease uniquely identify the test operating characteristics of a given diagnostic test. The sensitivity and specificity of a given diagnostic test will vary according to the severity of disease; therefore, when you apply a diagnostic test to patients with varying degrees of disease severity, the test operating characteristics will change. The sensitivity and specificity of diagnostic tests enable the clinician to answer the question "What is the probability of having the disease given the results of a positive test?" Because most patients do not present to the physician with a diagnosis, the more useful question is What is the likelihood that a patient has disease if his or her test result is positive? The probability of this outcome is known as the *positive predictive value* of a diagnostic test. The likelihood that a patient does not have disease if his or her test is negative is referred to as the *negative predictive value* of a diagnostic test. The positive and negative predictive values of a diagnostic test can also be determined using the 2 × 2 table (Fig. 11-7).

	Disease +	Disease -
Test +	TP	FP
Test-	FN	TN

FIGURE 11-7. A 2 × 2 table used to calculate the positive and negative predictive values of a diagnostic test. (*PPV,* those with true disease and a positive test result/all those with a positive test result (*PPV = TP/[TP + FP]*); *NPV,* those without disease who have a negative test result/all subjects with a negative test result (*NPV = TN/[FN + TN]*).

CLINICAL ECONOMICS
Outcome Measures

The analyses performed by decision models can assess outcomes such as death or morbidity. Due to the current focus on quality of health care and cost of health care, many studies have focused on outcomes that not only reflect lives saved but also reflect issues related to cost and quality of life. These types of economic studies reflect four fundamental types of studies.

The types of studies are (i) cost-effectiveness analysis, (ii) cost-utility analysis, (iii) cost-benefit analysis, and (iv) cost-minimization analysis.

Cost-effectiveness Analysis

A *cost-effectiveness analysis* is an analysis in which costs are related to a single common effect (e.g., management of pancreatic cancer), which may differ in magnitude between the alternative options. Results are often expressed in units of cost per life-years gained. This type of study is often used to compare clinical interventions and when you have a fixed budgetary constraint usually referred to as the acceptable upper limit (AUL). The AUL is usually reflective of what society is willing to pay for a service. Thus, a clinical intervention may save many more lives but at an unacceptably high monetary cost.

Cost-utility Analysis

A *cost-utility analysis* is an economic analysis in which an assessment is first made of the preferences that an individual or society may have for a particular set of health outcomes. This assessment is called the *utility of the outcome.* Because utilities incorporate the preferences of the target population, they are usually measured in terms of quality-adjusted life-years (QALYs). A cost-utility analysis assesses cost as a function of QALYs gained when you select one intervention. The calculation of specific utilities is beyond the scope of this text (refer to the selected readings at the end of this chapter for further study).

Cost-benefit Analysis

A *cost-benefit analysis* compares the costs and consequences of alternatives in dollars. It is often used when the outcomes to be compared do not have a similar common effect. The overall goal of these types of analyses is to provide an estimate of the resources used by each analysis compared to the resources served or created by implementation of that strategy. Usually the baseline strategy of comparison is a do-nothing strategy.

Cost-minimization Analysis

A *cost-minimization analysis* compares two clinical interventions and specifically looks at which intervention is the least costly. It is primarily used to evaluate two very similar regimens for their overall costs. These various economic analyses can be incorporated into decision models or in separate analyses. Parameters such as costs are usually estimated by using Medicare claims data and are thought to represent the most accurate reflection of costs. If Medicare claims data are not available, you can use hospital-specific claims data. The major difference here is that claims data are institution-specific and may not represent the actual reimbursement to the institution.

SUGGESTED READING

Bernard Rosner. *Fundamentals of biostatistics,* 4th ed. Belmont, California: Duxbury Press, 1995.

Fletcher R, Fletcher S, Wagner EH. *Clinical epidemiology: the essentials,* 3rd ed. Philadelphia: Williams & Wilkins, 1996.

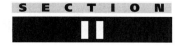

GASTROINTESTINAL SYSTEM

12

THE ESOPHAGUS

MICHAEL LANUTI AND JOSEPH S. FRIEDBERG

ANATOMY

The esophagus proper is a 25-cm mucosal-lined hollow tube of circular and longitudinal muscle with no serosa. The esophagus begins as a continuation of the pharynx and terminates at the cardiac part of the stomach. The transition from pharynx to cervical esophagus occurs at the lower border of the sixth cervical vertebra. The cervical esophagus (estimated 5-cm length) begins below the cricopharyngeus muscle, which is a continuation of the inferior constrictor of the pharynx. The space posteriorly within the inferior constrictor between fibers of the thyropharyngeus and the cricopharyngeus muscles is an area of potential weakness commonly referred to as the *Killian triangle* and is the site where a Zenker diverticulum develops. Both parasympathetic and sympathetic systems contribute to the *innervation* of the esophagus. The vagus nerve and its recurrent laryngeal branches innervate the striated muscle of the cervical esophagus and the upper esophageal sphincter and therefore play a critical role in coordination of pharyngoesophageal peristalsis. The lower two thirds of the esophagus is composed of smooth muscle and is supplied by the vagus nerve and by intrinsic autonomic nerve plexus that are located in the esophageal wall. The adult position of the vagus nerve is the result of the unequal growth of the greater curve of the stomach relative to the lesser curve, resulting in rotation of the left vagus anteriorly and the right vagus posteriorly at the level of the diaphragmatic hiatus.

Measurements obtained during endoscopic examination reveal an average distance of 38 to 40 cm (men) from incisor teeth to the cardiac part of the stomach. Along its course, the esophagus maintains three regions of anatomic narrowing, which include the upper esophageal sphincter, the bronchoaortic constriction at the level of T-4, and the diaphragmatic hiatus at the level of T-10. Topographically, the cervical esophagus lies slightly to the left of midline, allowing adequate access via a left neck incision. The midthoracic esophagus deviates to the right of the descending aorta (Fig. 12-1) and can be accessed readily via a right thoracotomy incision, as described in the Ivor-Lewis approach to total esophagectomy. The distal esophagus courses anteriorly and to the left of midline at the level of the lower esophageal sphincter and in general is most easily approached via a left thoracotomy or thoracoabdominal incision. Only the lower 5 to 7 cm of the esophagus are below the diaphragm. Throughout its length, the attachments of the esophagus to adjacent structures other than the posterior trachea are weak. This accounts for the relative ease by which the esophagus can be bluntly mobilized out the mediastinum during *trans*hiatal esophagectomy. The thoracic duct ascends posterior and to the right of the distal esophagus, but at the level of T-5, it passes posterior to the aorta and ascends on the left side of the esophagus emptying into the left subclavian vein.

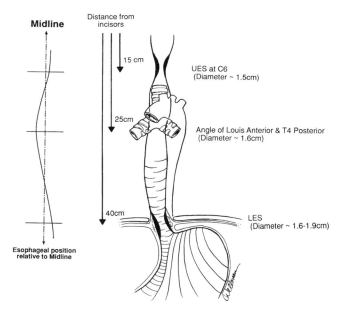

FIGURE 12-1. Topography of the esophagus with pertinent clinical endoscopic measurements in adults. (From Nyhus LM, Baker RJ, Fischer JE, eds. *Mastery of surgery*, 3rd ed. Boston: Little, Brown and Company, 1996:722, with permission.)

Hospital of the University of Pennsylvania, Philadelphia, Pennsylvania

Generally, the *arterial blood supply* to the esophagus originates in a segmental fashion (Fig. 12-2). The cervical esophagus receives its main arterial inflow from the inferior thyroid artery. The thoracic portion of the esophagus receives its blood supply from bronchial arteries and directly from the aorta. The intraabdominal esophagus receives its blood supply from both the left gastric artery and the inferior phrenic artery. Blood vessels run longitudinally in the submucosa and terminate in fine capillary networks before penetrating the muscle layer of the esophagus. *Venous drainage* from the esophagus also occurs segmentally. The cervical esophagus drains into the inferior thyroid vein, whereas the thoracic esophagus drains into the azygos/hemiazygos system as well as into intercostal veins. Distal esophageal venous drainage occurs mainly through the left gastric vein (coronary vein). The left gastric vein provides the collateral conduit to permit the formation of esophageal varices in portal hypertension.

Lymphatic drainage of the upper two thirds of the esophagus is usually cephalad. Cervical esophageal tumors drain to internal jugular, paratracheal, and deep cervical lymph nodes. Efferent lymphatics in the midthoracic esophagus drain into subcarinal nodes and into nodes at the inferior pulmonary ligament. Lower one-third esophageal tumors tend to drain caudad to paraesophageal and celiac nodes. Lymph node metastases in the thoracic and lower esophagus can be found centimeters away from the primary lesion as a consequence of the rich submucosal network of lymphatics, which allow *trans*mural extension of tumor. Conversely, the cervical esophagus has more direct segmental lymphatic drainage into regional nodes.

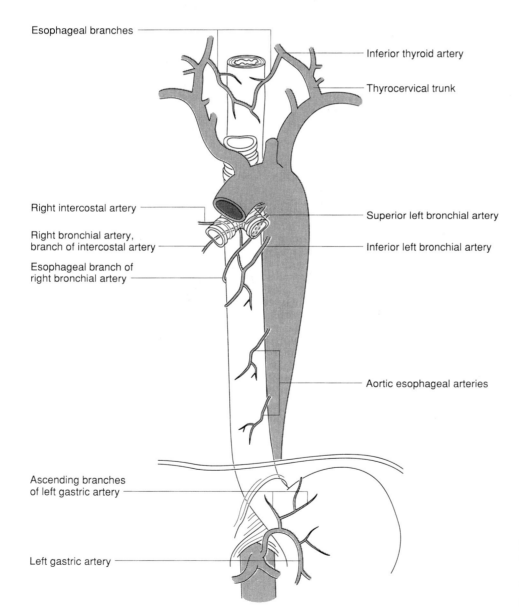

FIGURE 12-2. Arterial blood supply of the esophagus. (From Greenfield LJ. *Surgery: scientific principle and practice*, 1st ed. Lippincott-Raven Publishers, 1996:597, with permission.)

EMBRYOLOGY

During the fourth to fifth week of gestation, the developing esophagus is partitioned from the trachea by the tracheoesophageal septum. Anomalous partitioning occurs with an incidence of 1 in 3,000 to 4,500 livebirths. Esophageal atresia results from posterior deviation of the tracheoesophageal septum, and tracheoesophageal fistula occurs due to the incomplete separation of the two structures. These conditions are usually seen together and esophageal atresia is associated with a tracheoesophageal fistula 85% of the time. Polyhydramnios, or the accumulation of excessive amniotic fluid in utero, suggests esophageal atresia due to the failure of normal swallowing and resorption of amniotic fluid by the fetus and placenta. Infants with esophageal atresia tend to drool excessively shortly after birth and at the first feeding present with choking, coughing, and cyanosis. Failure of the nasogastric tube to pass into the stomach with the tip of the tube caught up in the proximal esophagus is the telltale sign of atresia. If intraabdominal air is concurrently seen on a plain radiograph, the presence of distal tracheoesophageal fistula can be inferred because air can enter the distal gastrointestinal (GI) tract only through this anomalous connection (Fig. 12-3). Immediate management includes prevention of further aspiration by decompressing the blind ending pouch with a sump drain. Operative therapy is aimed at correcting both anomalies by dividing the tracheoesophageal fistula and restoring esophageal continuity.

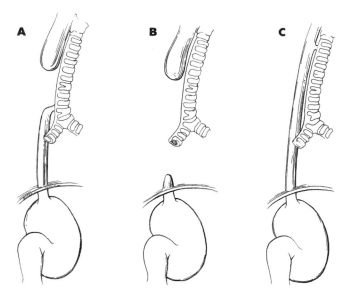

FIGURE 12-3. The three most common types of esophageal atresia/tracheoesophageal fistula include **(A)** proximal atresia with distal tracheoesophageal fistula, **(B)** esophageal atresia without fistula, and **(C)** tracheoesophageal fistula without atresia. (From Coran AG, Behrendt DM, Weintraub WH, et al. *Surgery of the neonate.* Boston: Little, Brown and Company, 1978, with permission.)

ESOPHAGEAL PHYSIOLOGY

The tongue, soft palate, and cricopharyngeus muscle, namely, the *upper esophageal sphincter* (UES), provide the propulsion necessary to move a food bolus into the body of the esophagus. The body of the esophagus acts as a propulsive pump with its valve. The terminal valve of the esophageal pump is the *lower esophageal sphincter* (LES). The LES is not an anatomic muscular sphincter, but a functional sphincter more appropriately termed the "distal esophageal high-pressure zone" (HPZ). The fundus of the stomach simulates a pressure reservoir constantly filling the antral pump. The pylorus in concert with the antrum restricts the size of food particles passing distally, forcing them to return to the fundic reservoir for further digestion. Failure of any of these components individually or in combination leads to abnormalities.

During *swallowing,* the larynx is elevated and pulled forward, opening the retrolaryngeal space and bringing the epiglottis under the tongue. The backward tilt of the epiglottis covers the opening of the larynx to prevent aspiration. The entire pharyngeal phase of swallowing occurs within 1.5 seconds. As a food bolus enters the body of the esophagus, cricopharyngeal pressure reaches twice the resting level of 30 mm Hg. When the maximal cricopharyngeal pressure is reached, a peristaltic wave begins in the upper esophagus.

The swallowing center in the medulla coordinates the complete act of swallowing by discharging impulses through the 5th, 7th, 11th, and 12th cranial nerves as well as through the motor neurons of cervical nerves C1-3. The afferent nerves of the esophagus are the glossopharyngeal and superior laryngeal branch of the vagus nerve. Once triggered, the swallowing response is always the same highly organized pattern of outflow. Motor disorders of the pharyngeal phase of swallowing are characterized by abnormalities of incomplete, premature, or delayed relaxation of the UES.

Once the swallowed bolus of food reaches the esophagus, orderly primary peristalsis propels the material into the stomach over a pressure gradient from −6 mm Hg intrathoracic to +6 mm Hg intraabdominal. The smooth muscle action in the lower one third of the esophagus facilitates the propulsion of food across this barrier. Consecutive swallows produce similar primary peristaltic waves. If the smooth muscle portion of the esophagus is distended at any point, it initiates relaxation of the LES and propagation of a contractile wave that sweeps down the esophagus. The secondary peristaltic wave may be helpful in clearing the esophagus of a large bolus that failed to be propagated by the primary wave. Despite the rather powerful occlusion pressure, the propulsive force of the esophagus is relatively weak.

Disruption of the normal peristaltic pattern results in esophageal motor disorders. Loss of peristalsis throughout the body of the esophagus and failure of the LES to relax on swallowing are characteristic of achalasia. In contrast, scleroderma results in the loss of contraction of the smooth muscle portion of the esophagus and is primarily myogenic in etiology. The absence of distal esophageal contractions and LES tone is diagnostic of this condition. Absence of esophageal contractions in the proximal striated portion of the esophagus generally occurs with inflammatory conditions that affect skeletal muscles, such as dermatomyositis.

ESOPHAGEAL FUNCTION TESTS

Structural and physiologic abnormalities of the esophagus can be analyzed via many different modalities, all of which can be grouped as *esophageal function tests* (EFTs). These modalities include endoscopy, barium esophagram, 24-hour pH monitoring, manometry, the Bernstein test, and computed tomographic (CT) scanning.

Endoscopy is generally the first evaluation for esophageal disease. It allows visualization of a wide range of disease processes and permits both diagnostic and therapeutic measures. The main risks are aspiration and esophageal perforation. The locations of esophageal landmarks are measured endoscopically from the incisor teeth. The cricopharyngeus is normally at 15 cm in adults and is the first area of physiologic narrowing encountered in the esophagus. Moreover, this region is the most common site of *endoscopic perforation*. The tracheal bifurcation and indentation of the aortic arch is between 24 and 26 cm from the incisors. The position of the gastroesophageal (GE) junction (identified as the place where the stomach, with vertically running rugae, becomes the tubular esophagus, with smooth muscle mucosa) occurs normally at approximately 38 to 40 cm in adults.

Barium esophagram is a powerful radiologic tool used in the evaluation of dysphagia and complements endoscopy in providing both structural and functional information. The esophagus is relatively fixed at its upper and lower ends; however, these points of fixation move cephalad 1 to 2 cm during swallowing. The pharyngoesophageal region is evaluated in the upright position. Aspiration can be readily identified on video esophagram by documenting residual barium in the larynx after a swallow. Esophageal body peristalsis is studied with the patient in the prone position. A swallowed bolus normally generates a stripping wave, which clears the bolus completely. Motility disorders characterized by disorganized activity with simultaneous contractions give rise to tertiary waves, often with a segmented appearance to the barium column resembling a "corkscrew." A hiatal hernia can best be visualized with the patient in the horizontal position.

Esophageal manometry provides a measurement of the contractility of the esophageal body and sphincters. It is a modality that is used to investigate nonobstructive dysphagia, noncardiac chest pain, and gastroesophageal reflux disease (GERD). Manometry is also known as the most accurate way of locating the distal HPZ (LES) before placement of a pH electrode for 24-hour pH monitoring in patients suspected of having GERD. Esophageal manometry defines the amplitude and length of the distal HPZ. It does not determine whether the LES is competent. A manometric study consists of four components: (i) assessment of the LES, (ii) measurement of LES relaxation, (iii) esophageal body manometry, and (iv) assessment of the UES. These assessments become integral in the diagnosis of esophageal dysmotility disorders.

The *Bernstein test* is a provocative maneuver in an attempt to reproduce reflux symptoms by administering 0.1 N-HCl into the esophagus via a catheter positioned 15 cm above the LES. The test basically measures esophageal mucosal sensitivity. A positive test result is scored when the patient spontaneously reports symptoms during infusion of acid and relief during infusion of saline. It has been largely replaced by the use of 24-hour pH monitoring. The Bernstein test identifies the patient with an acid-sensitive esophagus but does not indicate the presence or absence of GERD or esophagitis.

The *24-hour pH monitoring* has made it possible to quantify the degree of esophageal acid exposure in normal subjects and to categorize different patterns of reflux in patients with GERD. It is usually performed after the LES has been located by manometry. In adults, the probe is placed 5 cm above the manometrically determined upper border of the LES or HPZ. Reflux episodes are defined as periods when esophageal pH level is less than 4.0. It is indicated in any patient with symptoms suggestive of GERD having failed a 12-week course of acid-suppression therapy and more importantly in patients who are being considered for antireflux repair. In addition to measurement of acid exposure, pH monitoring can be used to detect excessive alkaline exposure in the esophagus. This concept becomes important in the workup of a Barrett esophagus and its association with bile and duodenal juice. An esophageal bile probe has been developed to detect the presence of bilirubin during a 24-hour period in an ambulatory setting.

CT scanning of the esophagus is important in localizing esophageal lesions in reference to other structures, particularly the trachea, left main bronchus, and aorta. Furthermore, esophageal lesions can be clinically staged based on involvement of adjacent structures and the presence of lymphadenopathy.

DYSMOTILITY DISORDERS

There are four identifiable categories of *primary motor disorders*: achalasia, diffuse esophageal spasm, nutcracker esophagus, and hypertensive LES. An additional category termed "nonspecific motor disorder" includes all patients whose motor function is clearly abnormal but does not fall into any of the defined categories. The most common causes of pharyngoesophageal dysphagia are neuromuscular diseases such as cerebrovascular disease, myasthenia gravis,

Parkinson disease, motor neuron disease, multiple sclerosis, and polymyositis.

Achalasia is characterized by incomplete relaxation of the LES along with a peristalsis of the esophageal body. Neuronal degeneration in the myenteric plexus has been implicated in the pathophysiology of esophageal dysmotility. There is some evidence that previous viral (varicella-zoster virus) or parasitic infection (*Trypanosoma cruzi,* Chagas disease) may be responsible. The loss of inhibitory neurons to the LES results in incomplete relaxation. Patients with achalasia classically present with dysphagia, regurgitation, and weight loss. Generally, regurgitation occurs during or at the end of a meal. Respiratory symptoms are common and are due to aspiration. Chest pain is also common in patients with achalasia. Esophageal dilation occurs later in the disease course, rendering an air fluid level on plain film and a classic *bird's beak* appearance on barium esophagram (Fig. 12-4). Achalasia is a *premalignant* esophageal lesion with carcinoma developing as a late complication in 1% to 10% of patients who have this condition for an average time of 15 to 25 years. Histologically, these tumors are usually squamous cell carcinomas and likely the result of mucosal irritation. Other sequelae of achalasia include pneumonitis, bronchiectasis, hemoptysis, and retention esophagitis.

Conservative treatment for achalasia consists of calcium channel blockers; however, the effect is short-lived. The mainstay of treatment is either balloon dilatation or surgery. Repetitive pneumatic dilatations can potentially achieve relief of dysphagia in about 70% of patients with achalasia. Surgical intervention should include a variant of the Heller myotomy, either *trans*thoracic or *trans*abdominal, with division of the circular muscle of the lower esophagus. Most esophageal surgeons advocate a complete esophagocardiomyotomy for achalasia with some type of fundoplication to prevent the subsequent development of GERD.

Diffuse esophageal spasm (DES) is a benign primary disease of the esophageal body and is clinically characterized by substernal chest pain or dysphagia. Manometric abnormalities in DES can be classically characterized by the frequent occurrence of simultaneous and repetitive esophageal contractions with abnormally high amplitude and duration. Its radiographic appearance resembles that of a *corkscrew esophagus* (Fig. 12-5). The LES in patients with DES usu-

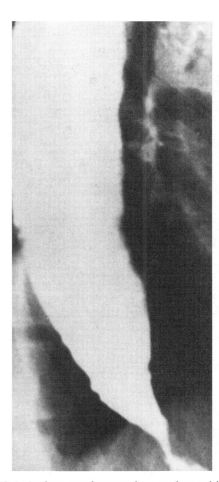

FIGURE 12-4. Barium esophagram in a patient with achalasia demonstrating a persistent "bird's beak" taper at the gastroesophageal junction. (From Bell RH, Rikkers LF, Mulholland MW. *Digestive tract surgery: a text and atlas.* Philadelphia: Lippincott-Raven Publishers, 1996:34, with permission.)

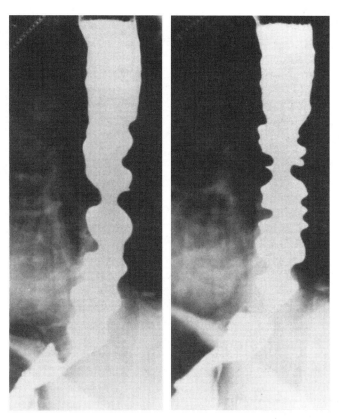

FIGURE 12-5. Barium esophagram demonstrating tertiary contractions of the circular muscle "corkscrew" characteristic of diffuse esophageal spasm. (From Bell RH, Rikkers LF, Mulholland MW. *Digestive tract surgery: a text and atlas.* Philadelphia: Lippincott-Raven Publishers, 1996:38, with permission.)

ally shows normal resting pressure and relaxation. Most patients with DES do not have associated GERD. DES is associated with stress and irritable bowel syndrome. The chest pain of DES is often indistinguishable from that of angina pectoris of cardiac origin. Many patients undergo coronary artery evaluation before the diagnosis can be made. Medical treatment of DES employs the use of calcium channel blockers or long-acting nitrates to abolish the strong simultaneous contractions. Surgery for DES is generally not as successful as it is for achalasia and is considered only when symptoms are refractory to medical management.

Nutcracker esophagus is the most common primary motility disorder of the esophagus. It is used to describe a manometric phenomenon in which the amplitude of esophageal body peristalsis is greater than 2 standard deviations above normal (peaks of more than 180 mm Hg). The dominant symptom of the condition is central crushing chest pain that occurs more frequently at rest. Patients are normally referred from cardiologists with normal coronary angiograms. Myotomy for isolated nutcracker esophagus with symptoms of chest pain has a low success rate. The mainstay for treatment is muscle relaxants such as calcium channel blockers and nitrates.

An elevated basal pressure of the LES characterizes *hypertensive* LES. Patients commonly present with chest pain and dysphagia. LES relaxation and esophageal body peristalsis are normal in these patients. Symptoms in these patients may be caused by a prolonged postrelaxation contraction of the LES. Myotomy of the LES may be indicated for dysphagia in patients who do not respond to medical therapy or dilatations.

Scleroderma, or systemic sclerosis, is a collagen vascular disease, which is characterized by skin induration, fibrous replacement of visceral smooth muscle, and progressive loss of visceral and cutaneous function. Progressive fibrosis of the distal two thirds of the esophagus results in loss of normal peristalsis. Heartburn and GERD are often severe. A standard antireflux medical regimen including proton pump inhibitors generally controls the reflux symptoms and esophagitis associated with scleroderma. In selected patients with advanced esophageal scleroderma, *trans*hiatal esophagectomy with a cervical esophagogastroanastomosis may effectively eliminate reflux esophagitis and restore the ability to swallow comfortably.

ESOPHAGEAL DIVERTICULA

Esophageal diverticula can be divided into two functional categories: pulsion and traction. This is an old classification proposed before the realization that all esophageal diverticula are associated with abnormalities of esophageal motility. *Pulsion diverticula* arise from elevated intraluminal pressure forcing mucosa and submucosa through the esophageal wall creating a "false" diverticulum. Both pharyngoesophageal (Zenker) and epiphrenic diverticula are considered pulsion diverticula. *Traction diverticula* are the result of an adjacent inflammatory process (i.e., mediastinal lymph nodes) that adhere to the esophagus and pull the entire wall "true diverticulum" toward them as they heal and contract (Fig. 12-6). *Parabronchial diverticula* are characterized as traction diverticula at the level of the midesophagus and are usually associated with mediastinal granulomatous disease (e.g., histoplasmosis, tuberculosis). They are characteristically small and asymptomatic.

A *Zenker diverticulum* normally arises at a point of potential weakness within the inferior pharyngeal constrictor (Fig. 12-7), between the oblique fibers of the thyropharyngeus muscle and the more horizontal fibers of the UES (cricopharyngeus muscle). These diverticula are associated with cervical dysphagia, regurgitation of undigested particles, recurrent aspiration, and halitosis. Accepted surgical treatment includes cervical esophagomyotomy and resection of the diverticulum. Alternative surgical approaches

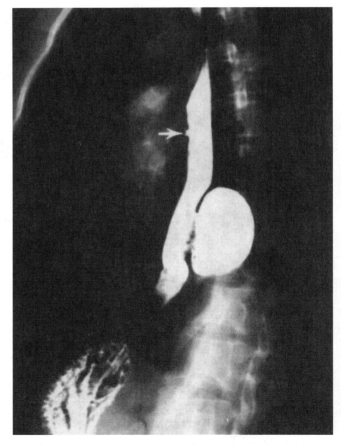

FIGURE 12-6. Esophagram of a patient with a large epiphrenic pulsion diverticulum and a small midesophageal traction diverticulum (*arrow*). (From Sabiston DC Jr. *Textbook of surgery: The biological basis of modern surgical practice*, 15th ed. Philadelphia: WB Saunders, 1997:731, with permission.)

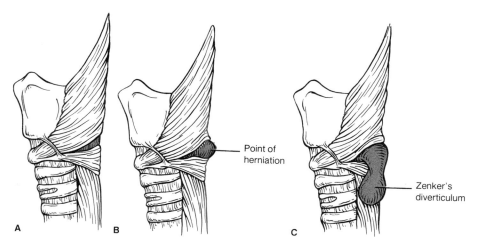

FIGURE 12-7. Formation of a Zenker diverticulum. **(left)** Herniation of the pharyngeal mucosa and submucosa occurs at the point of transition (*arrow*) between the oblique fibers of the thyropharyngeus muscle and the more horizontal fibers of the cricopharyngeus muscle. **(center and right)** As the diverticulum enlarges, it dissects toward the left side and downward into the superior mediastinum in the prevertebral space, forming a false diverticulum. (From Bell RH, Rikkers LF, Mulholland MW. *Digestive tract surgery: a text and atlas.* Philadelphia: Lippincott-Raven Publishers, 1996:33, with permission.)

include diverticulopexy with cricopharyngeal myotomy. Recently, *trans*oral endoscopic division of the common wall between the diverticulum and the esophagus has been reported as an alternative strategy.

Epiphrenic, or subdiaphragmatic, diverticula generally occur within the distal 10 cm of the esophagus and are pulsion diverticula that arise secondary to motor dysfunction or mechanical obstruction. Mildly symptomatic patients with diverticula smaller than 3 cm often require no treatment. Those patients with moderate to severe symptoms, such as dysphagia or chest pain and an enlarging pouch, are candidates for surgery. Preoperative assessment of esophageal function including evaluation of the LES should be performed. Surgical intervention via a left thoracotomy involves resection of the diverticulum accompanied by a long extramucosal thoracic esophagomyotomy down to the GE junction. Additionally, some authors advocate an antireflux procedure if the LES is divided during the myotomy.

GASTROESOPHAGEAL REFLUX DISEASE

Gastroesophageal reflux disease (GERD) occurs when esophageal acid exposure exceeds that of a normal population. This can be measured only by 24-hour pH monitoring. The pathophysiology of GERD may be from a defect in the LES, the esophageal body, or the stomach (Fig. 12-8). Although the etiology of GERD is clearly multifactorial, the greatest emphasis has been placed on the LES or the so-called *distal esophageal HPZ*. Resting pressure of the LES provides one of the primary components of the antireflux mechanism. Patients with a mean HPZ level of less than 6 mm Hg or a sphincter length of less than 2 cm are likely to have an incompetent LES and reflux gastric fluid into the esophagus. Esophageal clearance also plays a critical role in the prevention of esophageal injury. In a normal esophagus, reflux of gastric contents is cleared by a combination of gravity and reactive peristalsis. This minimizes the time of mucosal exposure to the reflux gastric contents. Patients with primary motor disorders are therefore predisposed to more severe esophagitis. Of note, the presence of a hiatal hernia has also been associated with more complications of GERD; however, not every patient with a hiatal hernia suf-

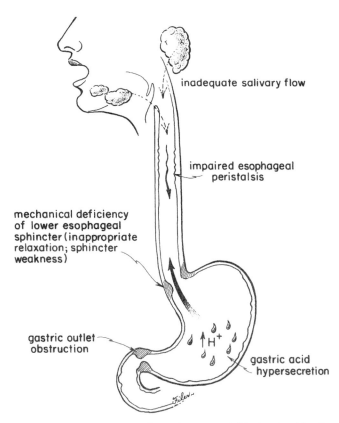

FIGURE 12-8. Pathophysiologic factors variably involved in the genesis of esophageal injury from gastroesophageal reflux disease. (From Cameron JL. *Current surgical therapy*, 5th ed. St. Louis: Mosley;1995:25, with permission.)

fers from esophagitis, and vice versa. Although alkaline bilious reflux has been identified to cause severe esophagitis, a more severe erosive esophagitis can be observed when acid, pepsin, and bile are combined—much more so than any of the three components alone. Additionally, delayed gastric emptying has been suggested to play an important role in as many as 40% of patients with reflux esophagitis.

Symptoms are classified as *typical* (heartburn and regurgitation) or *atypical* (noncardiac chest pain, asthma, recurrent pneumonia, and loss of dental enamel). Symptoms are often worse after meals and aggravated by postural changes. In some patients, symptoms occur only at night, waking the patient from sleep. Potential complications of GERD include esophagitis, aspiration pneumonia, esophageal strictures, Barrett metaplasia, and esophageal shortening. The GE mucosal junction may become thickened or fibrotic, producing an annular weblike constriction called a *Schatzki ring*. Intermittent dysphagia may occur when the ring size is 20 mm or less, but dysphagia is almost always present when the ring measures 13 mm or less. A Schatzki ring occurs precisely at the epithelial squamocolumnar junction and signifies the presence of a hiatal hernia if seen radiographically on barium esophagram. However, it does not necessarily indicate GE reflux or esophagitis and does not require therapy if it is asymptomatic. On the other hand, a Schatzki ring presenting with severe dysphagia can be managed with endoscopic dilatation.

Surgical intervention for GERD is reserved for those patients with refractory symptoms on maximal medical therapy. Evaluation for an antireflux procedure includes objective evidence for the presence of GERD by 24-hour pH monitoring, and esophageal manometry to rule out any primary motor disorder of the esophagus. Moreover, the disease should be caused by a defect amenable to surgical therapy, such as a mechanically defective LES. Long-term relief of symptoms can be achieved in 90% of patients undergoing an antireflux procedure (e.g., Nissen fundoplication). Laparoscopic Nissen fundoplication has been thoroughly evaluated in the surgical literature and has been accepted as the standard of care for antireflux surgery.

A *Barrett esophagus* is a histologic diagnosis and describes a condition whereby the normal esophageal squamous mucosa is replaced with columnar epithelium. Barrett-like changes are found in 10% to 20% of patients with GERD. Columnar mucosa can normally extend proximally over the entire length of the LES and can commonly occupy 2 cm of distal esophagus. A Barrett esophagus is defined as the condition in which the esophagus is lined with columnar mucosa more than 3 cm proximal to the distal end of the muscular esophageal tube. Patients with Barrett metaplasia have a 40 to 75–fold increase in the development of esophageal adenocarcinoma. Endoscopy with biopsy is the primary diagnostic technique for a Barrett esophagus. Biopsies should be performed at 1-cm intervals along any suspicious segment of mucosa. Once a Barrett esophagus is diagnosed, medical acid-suppressive therapy should be instituted. If biopsies show low-grade dysplasia, then biannual endoscopic surveillance with biopsy is recommended to detect high-grade dysplasia and early carcinoma. Some authors advocate laparoscopic Nissen fundoplication for early Barrett esophagus with low-grade dysplasia. Antireflux operations are effective in relieving esophagitis and preventing further metaplasia but are not effective in causing regression of the columnar mucosa nor in eliminating the risk of esophageal cancer. Patients who have been labeled negative for any dysplasia on endoscopic biopsy should have surveillance on a yearly basis. The aims of therapy are to prevent evolution of Barrett esophagus by improving esophageal clearance, to optimize LES function, and to minimize the contributions of abnormal gastric function. A number of substances reduce LES pressure including caffeine, nicotine, fats, chocolate, alcohol, peppermint, theophylline, anticholinergic agents, Valium, opiates, and calcium channel blockers. LES tone and gastric emptying may be improved with the use of prokinetic agents such as metoclopramide or cisapride. The treatment of biopsy-proven high-grade dysplasia "carcinoma *in situ*" remains controversial, yet most authors would recommend surgical resection via either a *trans*hiatal or *trans*thoracic approach. In patients who are at high risk or elderly with the potential for high morbidity or mortality, an argument can be made for endoscopic therapy such as photodynamic therapy. Evidence now exists that high-grade dysplasia is not merely a marker for carcinoma, but that 33% to 50% of patients with this complication of a Barrett esophagus already have invasive esophageal adenocarcinoma.

ESOPHAGEAL PERFORATION

Esophageal perforation can be classified into three main categories: spontaneous (15%), traumatic (20%), or iatrogenic (58%). The mortality rate associated with this condition is from 10% to 15% in patients treated less than 24 hours following injury, whereas the mortality increases to more than 50% if intervention is delayed. The absence of serosa in the esophagus predisposes to rupture at lower pressures compared to the rest of the alimentary canal. Ruptures of the lower esophagus usually perforate into the left thoracic cavity, and ruptures of the midesophagus usually perforate into the right thoracic cavity. Instrumental perforations of the esophagus may occur during esophagoscopy, endotracheal intubation, or passage of oral-gastric tubes. Instrumental perforation is most common in the cervical esophagus at the level of the cricopharyngeal constrictor and just above the cardia.

Common manifestations of esophageal rupture include pleural effusion, pneumothorax, pneumomediastinum, atelectasis, and subcutaneous emphysema. A patient who reports chest pain or manifests fever after instrumentation of the esophagus should be considered to have perforation until proven otherwise. Barogenic esophageal rupture (increased pressure against a closed glottis), namely Boerhaave syndrome, classically shows a Mackler triad: vomiting, lower thoracic pain, and subcutaneous emphysema. The perforation commonly occurs at the level of the left lateral wall of the esophagus just above the diaphragm. When a strain-induced tear occurs below the cardia, bleeding rather than perforation is the dominant feature. This is the case with the Mallory-Weiss syndrome in which the mucosal laceration is on the gastric side of the GE junction. Diagnosis can be frequently determined with history and physical examination alone. Esophageal perforation can be associated with a Hamman sign, which is defined as a mediastinal crunch secondary to mediastinal emphysema. However, confirmatory radiographic studies are usually obtained: (i) chest radiograph to identify pneumomediastinum or (ii) a dilute barium esophagram to identify location of the leak. Of note, mediastinal emphysema takes at least 1 hour to be demonstrated and is present in only 40% of patients. Chest radiograph results are normal in 10% of patients with esophageal perforation.

Treatment options for esophageal perforation consist of operative and nonoperative management. Absolute indications for operative repair include pneumothorax, mediastinal emphysema, sepsis, shock, or respiratory failure. Surgical options include reinforced primary closure, drainage alone, exclusion and diversion, and placement of an intraluminal stent. Primary repair, if possible, should be the procedure of choice. Resection is reserved for massive necrosis or malignant obstruction, and some authors advocate resection even if surgical intervention is beyond 48 to 72 hours from the time of injury. Perforated carcinoma necessitates resection or placement of an intraluminal stent if the tumor is unresectable.

CAUSTIC INJURY

The incidence of *caustic injury* to the esophagus is bimodal in age distribution, encountered most frequently in children less than 5 years of age and having a much lower secondary peak in late adolescence. The most common chemicals implicated in corrosive burns are alkali (65%), acid (16%), and occasionally bleach. The degree of injury depends on the character, concentration, and pH of the material, as well as the duration of contact with the mucosa. Liquid alkali is odorless and tasteless, thus making accidental or suicidal ingestion of a large amount feasible. *Alkali* causes liquefaction necrosis and penetrates deeply into the surrounding tissues. In contrast, *acid* has an unpleasant taste commonly causing choking and gagging. This leads to epiglottic burns, threatening airway patency. Acid produces coagulation necrosis and less penetration. Intraesophageal acid has a short transit time and tends to spare the esophageal mucosa but produce coagulation necrosis of the stomach. *Bleaches* are esophageal irritants and pose no serious complications or mortality.

Mucosal injury requires 20 to 30 days to heal. Deep injury is associated with edema and local infection with concomitant fibrosis. Strictures develop in 20% of patients and are usually extensive. Assessment begins with flexible esophagoduodenoscopy within the first 24 hours where staging can be performed. Therapy consists of broad-spectrum antibiotics and corticosteroids, but these measures do not significantly decrease early complications or late stricture formation. Surgical exploration is indicated for hemorrhage, endoscopic burns extending beyond the pylorus, and peritonitis. If partial or total gastric necrosis exists, *trans*hiatal esophagogastrectomy with end-cervical esophagostomy, mediastinal drainage, and feeding jejunostomy should be performed. GI continuity is restored with colonic interposition approximately 2 to 3 months after resection.

It is well-recognized that caustic strictures have a propensity to undergo malignant degeneration. The latent period between lye ingestion and the development of carcinoma can be as long as 40 years. All patients with lye strictures should undergo endoscopic or cytologic surveillance to detect early tumors.

FOREIGN BODIES

Ingested foreign bodies usually present at areas of anatomic narrowing within the GI tract. As previously mentioned, esophageal anatomic narrowings include the UES, crossing of the aortic arch, the left main bronchus, and the LES. If a foreign body becomes impacted, esophageal damage can occur because of direct penetration, which leads to perforation or submucosal tearing and bleeding. Foreign body ingestion occurs predominantly in the pediatric population. The most common esophageal foreign body seen on radiographs is a coin. Symptoms of foreign body ingestion in children include coughing or wheezing because of airway compromise. In adults, symptoms include odynophagia, dysphagia, and drooling with obstruction. Diagnosis should begin with routine radiographs and dilute barium if the foreign body is radiolucent. In the absence of an identifiable foreign body, flexible endoscopy is indicated in patients with persistent symptoms. Blunt objects can be removed with esophagoscopy. Sharp foreign bodies should always be removed because perforation can occur in 15% to 30% of patients, usually at the ileocecal valve. Surgical removal is indicated if a sharp object can not be removed endoscopically or a blunt object has not advanced for 3 days. Drug-filled condoms should be removed surgically to avoid the risk of rupture and potential chemical overdose.

BENIGN ESOPHAGEAL NEOPLASMS

Benign tumors of the esophagus are rare and constitute only 0.5% of esophageal neoplasms. They are classified into two major groups: mucosal and intramural. *Leiomyomas* represent 60% of all benign esophageal neoplasms and are by far the most common benign intramural tumors. They are usually found in patients between 20 to 50 years of age. Sixty percent of all benign esophageal neoplasms are leiomyomas. More than 80% of esophageal leiomyomas occur in the distal two thirds of the esophagus and are multiple in up to 10% of patients. Symptoms include dysphagia, pain, and digestive symptoms including anorexia, regurgitation, belching, and nausea. These tumors produce a characteristic smooth concave defect with sharp borders on barium esophagram. Endoscopy is mandatory to rule out a malignant epithelial process. Treatment is usually surgical because of the uncertainty of diagnosis. Although small tumors can be removed by enucleation, large tumors may require esophageal resection. Thoracoscopic techniques have also been successfully applied in the resection of some of these tumors.

Benign polyps of the esophagus are rare and typically arise in the cervical esophagus. Peristaltic contractions result in progressive lengthening of their pedicles. Most occur in older men and are frequently attached to the cricoid cartilage. These polyps tend to be solitary and are sometimes amenable to endoscopic electrocoagulation of the pedicle. The recommended approach, however, is resection through a lateral cervical esophagostomy, delivering the polyp from the esophagus, resecting its mucosal base, and repairing the defect under direct vision.

Esophageal hemangiomas are rare, constituting 2% to 3% of benign tumors. Although predominantly asymptomatic, they could be a source of upper GI bleeding. If found incidentally, esophageal hemangiomas should be followed by periodic endoscopy. Laser endoscopy provides effective control of little bleeding; however, surgical resection is required for recurrent bleeding.

The *esophageal duplication cyst* is a variation of the foregut cyst. It extends along the length of the thoracic esophagus and is lined by squamous epithelium. Seventy-five percent of esophageal duplication cysts present in childhood, and more than 60% are located on the right side of the esophagus. Similar to other foregut cysts, esophageal duplication cysts are frequently associated with vertebral and spinal cord anomalies. Diagnosis can be made by their characteristic radiographic appearance. Because esophageal cysts have a tendency to bleed, ulcerate, or become infected, excision is generally recommended. This can generally be performed via an extramucosal resection with a relatively low morbidity rate.

MALIGNANT ESOPHAGEAL NEOPLASMS

Esophageal malignant disease is among the most dismal of visceral tumors, with an overall 5-year survival rate of 8% to 24%. Esophageal carcinoma has remarkable variability in prevalence worldwide. In the United States, the annual incidence of esophageal carcinoma is 6 out of 100,000 men with approximately 12,000 new cases annually. In the Peoples Republic of China, the annual national mortality for esophageal carcinoma is 19.6 out of 100,000 men. In Iran, the annual incidence is 180 out of 100,000 men, perhaps linked to the use of opium and the ingestion of very hot tea. The influence of local dietary habits and environmental factors on the widely disparate incidences has been the subject of extensive epidemiologic studies. From a demographic standpoint, esophageal carcinoma can be divided by its histopathology into squamous cell carcinoma (SCCA) and adenocarcinoma. There is a predilection toward men in both groups. Of note, the incidence of SCCA is at least four times higher in black men than in white men. When studied on an age basis, esophageal carcinoma is a disease of advancing age, with the condition rarely being diagnosed before the age of 40 years.

The etiology of the different pathological types of esophageal cancer varies significantly. The most consistently implicated etiological factors for SCCA are alcohol and tobacco. Carcinogens (e.g., *N*-nitrosamines) in the environment have also been associated with SCCA. Certain acquired diseases of the esophagus, including achalasia, chronic esophagitis, radiation esophagitis, caustic injury, and human papillomavirus, have been implicated in the development of SCCA. The disease occurs more often in the upper and midthoracic esophagus (55%) compared to the distal esophagus (37%).

Recently, there appears to be a significant increase in the incidence of adenocarcinoma in Western countries. The most important predisposing factor is Barrett columnar-cell metaplasia, which is present in over 80% of patients with adenocarcinoma of the distal esophagus. In contradistinction to esophageal SCCA, alcohol and tobacco do not play a major role in the pathogenesis of adenocarcinoma. Epidemiological evaluation of nutritional risk factors have suggested a decreased incidence of adenocarcinoma of the esophagus with the intake of raw fruits and vegetables, but an overall increased risk with obesity. Adenocarcinoma usually occurs in the distal one third of the esophagus.

Patients with esophageal carcinoma often present with dysphagia and weight loss and are often malnourished at the time of presentation. Surgical resection in the form of esophagogastrectomy or total esophagectomy remains the optimal palliative treatment for patients with cancer of the esophagus without evidence of distant disease. Depending on the location of the tumor, a number of different surgical approaches can be utilized. These include the *trans*thoracic or thoracoabdominal approach (via a left thoracotomy [Fig. 12-9]), the Ivor-Lewis operation (right chest and abdominal incision [Fig. 12-10]), and *trans*hiatal esophagectomy (left cervical and abdominal incision).

Once a diagnosis of invasive carcinoma has been made, evaluation of systemic disease begins with a simple chest radiograph. Barium esophagram aids in tumor localization

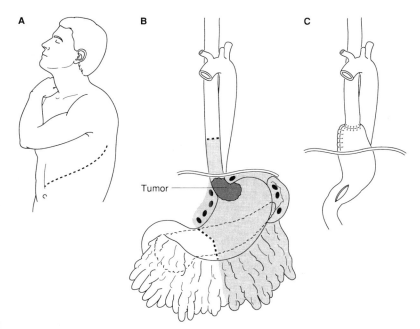

FIGURE 12-9. Standard thoracoabdominal esophagogastrectomy for lesions of the distal esophagus and cardia. **A:** Incision. **B:** Margins of resection (*shaded area*). **C:** Completed reconstruction with intrathoracic esophagogastroanastomosis and either pyloromyotomy or pyloroplasty to prevent postvagotomy pylorospasm. (From Ellis FH, Jr. Treatment of carcinoma of the esophagus and cardia. *Mayo Clin Proc* 1960;35:653, with permission.)

and extent of intraluminal extension. CT and magnetic resonance imaging (MRI) can be used to evaluate visceral extension of tumor. Endoscopic ultrasound (EUS) has demonstrated superiority (90% overall staging accuracy) in determining T stage and N stage but is limited in assessing the M stage of disease. In summary, the most effective and precise way to stage patients with esophageal carcinoma is to combine CT or MRI (to rule out distant metastases) with EUS to assess depth of tumor penetration and the presence or absence of regional lymph nodes. Finally, bronchoscopy should be employed in the upper third of lesions to rule out direct invasion of the trachea.

Surgical resection for carcinoma located in the upper and middle thirds of the esophagus are best approached via a right thoracotomy combined with an abdominal incision (Ivor-Lewis procedure) to mobilize the necessary conduit (e.g., stomach or colon). Tumors arising in the lower third of the esophagus or at the GE junction are usually approached by a left thoracoabdominal approach or by a *trans*hiatal approach. The left thoracoabdominal approach requires taking down the left hemidiaphragm and ultimately performing a midthoracic esophagogastoanastomosis. Because of the complexity of the procedure, complications occur in 10% to 15% of cases. Advantages of the thoracoabdominal approach as well

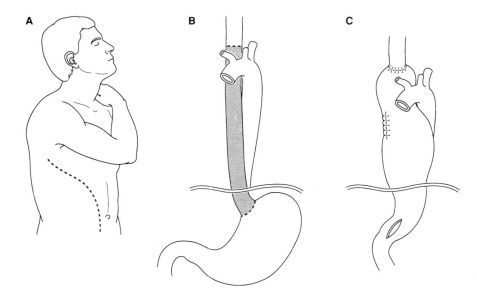

FIGURE 12-10. Standard Ivor-Lewis esophagogastrectomy for lesions of the lower and middle third of the thoracic esophagus. **A:** The continuous thoracoabdominal incision and the separate thoracic and abdominal incisions that may be used. **B:** Portion of the esophagus to be resected (*shaded area*). **C:** Completed reconstruction with high intrathoracic esophagogastroanastomosis and gastric drainage procedure. (From Ellis FH, Jr. Treatment of carcinoma of the esophagus and cardia. *Mayo Clin Proc* 1960;35:653, with permission.)

as the Ivor-Lewis approach include excellent exposure and the ability to perform an extensive lymphadenectomy. In contrast, *trans*hiatal esophagectomy does not permit a formal lymph node dissection and provides limited exposure.

The *trans*hiatal approach is most applicable for patients with Barrett dysplasia where extensive mediastinal lymph node dissection is not needed. Regardless, the approach can be utilized for carcinoma of any portion of the thoracic esophagus and is indicated for all types of esophageal cancer. The operation consists of an abdominal and left cervical incision to allow for a proximal cervical esophagogastrostomy. *Trans*hiatal esophagectomy avoids the morbidity of an intrathoracic anastomosis, with an overall mortality rate of less than 5%. Moreover, cervical anastomotic leaks are much better tolerated than intrathoracic anastomotic leaks. Comparable survival figures have been reported with *trans*thoracic approaches with formal lymph node dissection and *trans*hiatal approaches without lymph node dissection for tumors in the middle and distal thirds of the esophagus (Table 12-1). Stomach reconstruction for any of the above-mentioned procedures requires division of the short gastrics, left gastric, left gastroepiploic, and right gastric arteries while preserving the right gastroepiploic artery as the sole vascular pedicle for conduit viability.

In the United States and many other Western countries, most (80%) patients with esophageal carcinoma present with advanced disease with involvement of regional lymph nodes, and hence the overall 5-year survival rate is between 10% and 15%. Treatment options include endoscopic palliative techniques (e.g., self-expanding stents) versus single-modality measures (e.g., chemotherapy, radiation, and surgery) versus multimodality measures (neoadjuvant chemotherapy/radiation therapy and surgery). Chemotherapy alone or radiation alone does not impact significantly on median survival. Chemotherapy given with concurrent radiotherapy has been shown to be superior to chemotherapy alone in esophageal cancer. A recent randomized, prospective trial examining the role of neoadjuvant chemotherapy in both SCCA and adenocarcinomas failed to demonstrate any impact on resection rate, relapse-free survival, or overall survival compared to surgery alone.

Recently, there have been several studies investigating the potential of combined therapy with radiation, chemotherapy, and surgery. These studies generally used a combination of 5-fluorouracil (5-FU) and cisplatin or mitomycin. There have been two large randomized trials to evaluate this regimen in patients with resectable SCCA and adenocarcinomas. Bosset studied 282 patients with SCCA treated with cisplatin and 37 Gy radiation followed by surgery compared to surgery alone and found no improvement in survival. In contrast, Walsh studied 113 patients with adenocarcinoma and used cisplatin with a 96-hour infusion of 5-FU and 40 Gy radiation and observed a significant increase in the 3-year survival rate.

The role for the palliative treatment of unresectable or recurrent esophageal tumor is rapidly expanding. Patients who are candidates for these techniques are those who have metastatic disease at presentation, recurrence of disease, or refuse primary curative therapy. Some specialized centers provide these alternative techniques including the use of endoprostheses to restore patency and function, as well as tumor ablative techniques. The most serious complication of deployment of endoprostheses or endoscopic thermal ablative therapy is perforation. Another new technique with numerous possible applications in the treatment and palliation of esophageal neoplasia is photodynamic therapy (PDT). PDT involves the administration of exogenous photosensitizers, which are then preferentially localized to neoplastic tissue. Light at a specific wavelength is delivered by laser fiber through the endoscope, activating oxygen-free radicals to induce cellular damage. Currently, this modality is being evaluated in clinical trials at multiple centers.

TABLE 12-1. EFFECT OF EXTENT OF RESECTION (THREE-YEAR SURVIVAL)

Esophageal tumor site	Transthoracic esophagectomy with en bloc lymph node dissection	Transhiatal esophagectomy without formal lymph node dissection
Middle third	14% (29)[a]	17% (40)[b]
Distal third	33% (37)	31% (47)

[a]From Skinner, DB. En bloc resection for neoplasms of the esophagus and cardia. *J Thorac Cardiovasc Surg* 1983;85(1):59–71, with permission.
[b]From Orringer, MB. Transhiatal esophagectomy without thoracotomy for carcinoma of the thoracic esophagus *Ann Surg* 1984;200:282–288, with permission.

SUGGESTED READING

Baue AE, Geha AS, Hammond GL. *Glenn's thoracic and cardiovascular surgery.* Stamford: Appleton & Lange, 1996:691–950.

Bosset JF, Gignoux M, Triboulet JP, et al. Chemoradiotherapy followed by surgery compared with surgery alone in squamous cell cancer of the esophagus. *N Engl J Med* 1997;337:161–167.

Walsh TN, Noonan N, Hollywood D, et al. A comparison of multimodal therapy and surgery for esophageal adenocarcinoma. *N Engl J Med* 1996;335(7):462–467.

13

THE STOMACH AND DUODENUM

JAGAJAN J. KARMACHARYA AND JON B. MORRIS

ANATOMY

The stomach and duodenum are derived from the caudal portion of the embryonic foregut, as a dilation during the fifth week of gestation. The typical morphology is completed by the sixth to seventh week of gestation. The primitive stomach is invested within the ventral mesentery and the dorsal mesenteries. In postnatal life, the ventral mesentery is represented as the lesser omentum, consisting of the falciform ligament and the gastrohepatic and hepatoduodenal mesenteries. The greater omentum is the former dorsal mesentery and it forms the gastrosplenic and the gastrophrenic ligament. The rate of growth of the left gastric wall outpaces that of the right wall, thus establishing a lesser and greater curvature. Rotation of the gut causes the left vagal trunk to lie in its anterior portion and the right trunk lies posterior. The stomach lies most commonly between the tenth thoracic and the third lumbar vertebral segments, fixed at these points by the gastroesophageal junction proximally and the retroperitoneal junction distally.

The stomach is divided into four parts, serving as guidelines in planning surgical resection (Fig. 13-1). The cardia is located immediately distal to the gastroesophageal junction while the fundus is the portion above the gastroesophageal junction. The body (corpus) is the central part marked distally by the angularis incisura, a crease on the lesser curvature, just proximal to the terminal nerves of Latarget. The distal segment of the stomach is the pylorus, which upon palpation feels relatively thickened.

Anteriorly, the stomach comes in contact with the left hemidiaphragm, the left lobe of the liver, the anterior portion of the right lobe of the liver, and the parietal surface of the abdominal wall. On its posterior surface, its topographic relations are as follows: the left diaphragm, the left kidney, the left adrenal gland, neck, tail, and body of the pancreas, the aorta, the coceliac trunk, and the periaortic nerve plexus. Nestled in the concavity of the spleen is the left lateral portion of the stomach. The transverse colon and its mesentry lies below and close to the greater curvature.

An abundant network of extramural and intramural collaterals connects the blood supply to the stomach. Most of its blood supply is derived from the celiac trunk. The left gastric artery, the first branch of the celiac trunk, and the right gastric artery, a branch of the hepatic artery, supply the lesser curvature. Branches of the splenic artery, the short gastric arteries, and the left gastroepiploic supply the greater curvature. It is also supplied by the right gastroepiploic artery, a branch of the gastroduodenal artery. The venous drainage parallels the arterial supply (Fig. 13-2).

Lymphatic drainage from the proximal portion of the lesser curve drains into the superior gastric lymph nodes surrounding the left gastric artery and from the distal portion to the suprapyloric lymph nodes. Pancreaticosplenic nodes and subpyloric and omental nodes drain the proximal and the antral portions of the greater curve, respectively. Ultimately, all of the lymph nodes drain via the base of the celiac axis. Disease processes can bypass and present beyond the primary nodes due to extensive intramural and extramural communications.

Two vagal trunks emerge through the esophageal hiatus of the diaphragm. The left trunk is on the anterior surface of the esophagus and the right is posterior, between the esophagus and the aorta. The anterior vagus nerve gives off the hepatic branch and follows the lesser curvature giving off branches to the anterior gastric wall (Fig. 13-3). The posterior vagus branches into the celiac division and the posterior division, the later supplies the posterior gastric wall. Mostly afferent, the vagal trunks transmit information to the central nervous system. Ten percent of the vagal fibers are motor or secretory efferents. Parasympathetic fibers originate in the dorsal nucleus of the medulla. They synapse in the myenteric and submucosal plexus and secondary neurons then directly innervate the gastric smooth and epithelial cells.

Pain from the stomach and the duodenum are sensed through the afferent fibers of the sympathetic system. These

---

The Children's Hospital of Philadelphia, Philadelphia, Pennsylvania; Hospital of the University of Pennsylvania, Philadelphia, Pennsylvania

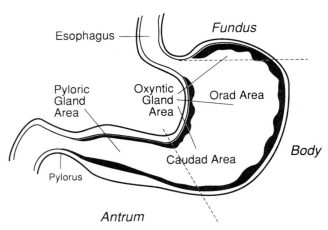

FIGURE 13-1. The stomach is anatomically divided into four parts with different anatomic functions. (From Johnson LR. Secretion. In: Johnson LR, ed. *Essential medical physiology.* New York: Raven Press, 1992:482, with permission.).

The gastric mucosa is lined by simple columnar cells with three types of gastric glands: cardiac, oxyntic, and antral. The *cardiac glands* occupy the narrow transition zone between the stratified squamous epithelium of the esophagus and the simple columnar cells of the stomach. The cardiac glands are branched structures, containing mucus glands, undifferentiated glands, and endocrine glands. The functional importance of the cardiac gland, other than the secretion of mucus, is not completely understood. The fundus and the body of the stomach contain the tubular *oxyntic gland* in which the acid-secreting parietal cells are prominent (Fig. 13-4). The oxyntic gland also contains the chief cells that synthesize pepsinogen. The gland is divided into three regions: (i) the isthmus, containing surface mucosal cells and a few parietal cells; (ii) the neck, containing a high concentration of parietal cells and few mucosal cells; and (iii) the base, containing chief cells, few parietal cells, scattered mucosal cells, and undifferentiated cells.

fibers are derived from T-5 through T-10 spinal segments, entering *gray rami* communicantes to the prevertebral ganglia. Presynaptic nerves then pass through the greater splanchnic to the celiac plexus. Postsynaptic fibers from the celiac plexus innervate the stomach.

The parietal cell has a unique canalicular structure that extends from the basal cytoplasm to the gastric lumen. This canalicular system becomes very prominent and conspicuous on stimulation. The surface area of the canaliculi is increased by the presence of microvilli. The parietal cells have high oxidative rates, as reflected by the

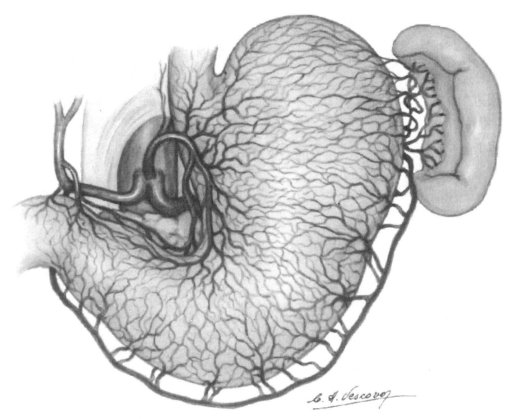

FIGURE 13-2. The stomach is an extremely vascular organ with blood supply from the left and right gastroepiploic arteries, left and right gastric arteries, and the short splenic vessels. (From Etala E. *Atlas of gastrointestinal surgery.* Philadelphia: Williams & Wilkins, 1997:879, with permission.)

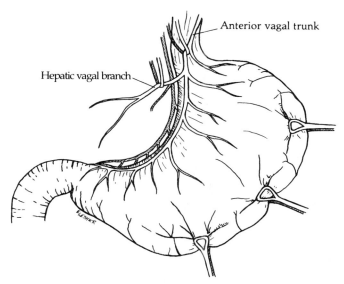

FIGURE 13-3. The vagus nerve forms two vagal trunks on the anterior and posterior surface of the stomach. The anterior vagal trunk gives off the hepatic vagal branch. (From Sawers JL. Selective vagotomy and pyloroplasty. In: Nyhus LM, Baker RJ, eds. *Mastery of surgery,* 2nd ed. Philadelphia: Little, Brown and Company, 1992:674, with permission.)

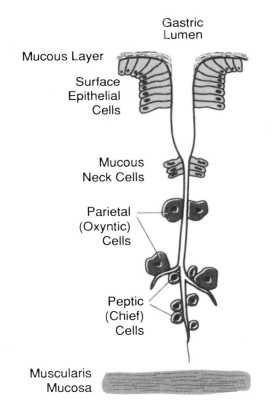

FIGURE 13-4. The oxyntic gland is divided into three regions: (i) the surface, containing mucosal cells; (ii) the neck, containing mainly parietal cells and a few mucosal cells; (iii) and the base, containing mainly chief cells. (From Johnson LR. Secretion. In: Johnson LR, ed. *Essential medical physiology.* New York: Raven Press, 1992:482, with permission.).

increased number of mitochondria, particularly during stimulation.

The *antral gland* is located in the distal stomach, or antrum, as well as the pyloric channel (Fig. 13-1). Gastrin-secreting cells are a distinctive feature of this gland and can be identified morphologically by numerous dense granules containing this hormone. Upon stimulation, gastrin diffuses through the basal membrane and into the bloodstream. Endocrine cells are generally found in all three regions.

PHYSIOLOGY

The stimulation of acid secretion occurs in three phases: cephalic, gastric, and intestinal. The basal acid secretion is 2 to 5 mEq per hour in a fasting state and is determined by the ambient histamine secretion plus the vagal tone. The *cephalic phase* begins with thought, sight, and smell of food, mediated by the vagus nerve, and is abolished by vagotomy. Cholinergic stimulation is by direct action on gastrin cells. Binding of acetylcholine and related cholinergic agonists to muscarinic receptors results in mobilization of intracellular calcium via protein phosphorylation, resulting in hydrogen ion secretion. The maximal output in a normal person is 10 mEq per hour during the cephalic phase.

Entry of food marks the beginning of the *gastric phase*. The most important stimulative factors are the presence of partially hydrolyzed food and gastric distention. Small peptide fragments and amino acids, particularly tryptophan and phenylalanine, stimulate the release of gastrin. This acid regulatory peptide is derived from its prehormone (preprogastrin). Increased intracellular levels of amines stimulate the release of gastrin. Local cholinergic intramural reflexes also increase the sensitization of the parietal cells to the effects of gastrin. The acid secretion is the effect of activation of gastrin receptors situated in the basolateral membrane. Gastrin, like histamine and acetylcholine, acts via the membrane-bound parietal-cell proton pump or the hydrogen ion pump. The hydrolysis of adenosine 5'-triphosphate drives the transport of H^+ to the lumen of the canaliculi. This requires the cotransport of K^+ to the cytosolic membrane. The diffusion of K^+ along with Cl^- ions to the canaliculi allows for the maintenance of this electrochemical gradient. H^+/K^+–adenosine triphosphatase (ATPase) pump activation results in increased OH^- generation. The enzyme carbonic anhydrase converts this toxic product to HCO_3^-, which is exchanged for the canalicular Cl^- ions, thus maintaining the cytoplasmic supply of Cl^- ions on a one-to-one basis for each H^+ secreted and the maximal acid output is between 15 to 25 mEq per hour for an average meal (Fig. 13-5).

The entry of gastric contents into the intestine marks the *intestinal phase*. The hormones entero-oxyntin, secretin, somatostatin, peptide YY, gastric inhibitory peptide, and neurotensin have been proposed as the mediators during

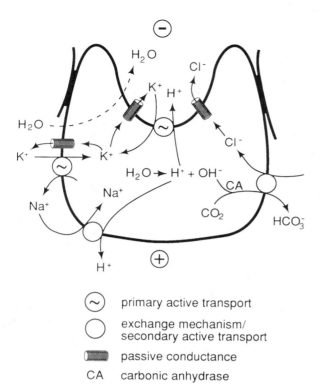

FIGURE 13-5. The gastric parietal cell produces hydrochloric acid and creates and acidic intraluminal gastric environment. (From Johnson LR. Secretion. In: Johnson LR, ed. *Essential medical physiology.* New York: Raven Press, 1992:485, with permission.)

this phase of gastric-acid secretion that is at present incompletely understood.

The stomach also serves to store, mix, and regulate the release of the ingested contents. Peristaltic waves pass from the body of the stomach toward the pylorus. The gastric pacemaker is located in the proximal one third of the greater curvature of the fundus with a basic electrical rhythm of 3 cycles per minute. These intrinsic pacemaker activities of gastric smooth muscle cells reflect partial depolarization. The distal spread of electrical activity does not result in smooth muscle contraction unless there is further depolarization. Stimulation and the opening of Ca^{2+} channels result in depolarization and a generation of an action potential that determines the contraction and the maximal peristaltic wave.

Postprandial gastric distention, texture, volume, and osmolality of meals also influence the peristaltic wave. The most important factor is vagally controlled distention known as "receptive relaxation," which allows the accommodation of food in the proximal stomach. This function is lost in patients who have undergone truncal vagotomy. The distal propagation of food occurs once the food is ingested due to increased contractile activity of the proximal stomach. As the antral wave of contraction arrives, the pylorus closes and opens every 2 to 3 seconds. Small amounts (5 to 15 mL) of liquid and floating particles (chyme) are passed into the duodenum while the rest of the ingested food particles are propelled in a retrograde manner, churning the material, mixing it with gastric juices plus pepsin, thus allowing for digestion and trituration (reduction of size) to occur as the large food particles are squeezed within the stomach's distal muscular walls.

After every meal, about 1,000 mL of gastric juice is secreted by the stomach. The most important components are mucus, HCO_3, pepsinogen, and intrinsic factor. Mucus consists of high-molecular-weight glycoproteins and 95% water produced by the parietal and oxyntic glands. Mucus is important in lubrication and protection of the gastric mucosa. This mucoid gel forms the layer on the gastric mucosal surface known as the "unstirred layer." Bicarbonate ions formed as a byproduct of acid secretion (Fig. 13-5) are trapped in this layer, maintaining neutrality over the gastric mucosa despite the low luminal pH. The combination of HCO_3^- and the unstirred layer of the mucoid gel act as mechanical barriers to the effects of acid. Although numerous factors modulate the secretion of HCO_3^-, prostaglandin (PGE_2) production is paramount (Table 13-1). The loss of protective effects of the mucus and the HCO_3^- layer due to use of nonsteroidal antiinflammatory medications (NSAIDs) can result in ulceration.

Pepsinogen is synthesized by the chief cells and is stored as visible granules. The precursor zymogen is activated by a falling pH level, resulting in the cleavage of a polypeptide fragment to the active enzyme pepsin. Pepsin catalyzes the hydrolysis of peptide bonds containing phenylalanine, tyrosine, and leucine. The most important stimuli for pepsin secretion is stimulation of muscarinic receptors of the M1 type (cholinergic). The major function of pepsin is to initiate protein digestion. It functions optimally at a pH level of 2.0 and is irreversibly denatured at a pH level of 7.0 or greater.

A mucoprotein, *intrinsic factor,* is also secreted by the parietal cells of the gastric mucosa. This factor is necessary for the absorption of cobalamin (vitamin B_{12}) from the terminal ileum. Histamine, acetylcholine, and gastrin stimulate intrinsic factor secretion. Atrophy of the parietal cells, characteristic of pernicious anemia, results in a deficiency of intrinsic factor and anemia. This deficiency can be cor-

TABLE 13-1. FACTORS MODULATING GASTRIC MUCOSAL PROTECTION[a]

Stimulation	Inhibition
cAMP	NSAID
Prostaglandins	α-adrenergic agonists
Cholinomimetics	Bile acids
CCK	Acetazolamide
Glucagon	Ethanol

[a]cAMP, cyclic adenosine monophosphate; CCK, cholecystokinin; NSAID, nonsteroidal antiinflammatory drug.

rected by parenteral administration of vitamin B_{12}. Total gastrectomy results in the permanent dependency of parenteral vitamin B_{12} administration.

PEDIATRIC AND NEWBORN CONSIDERATIONS

Intestinal atresia is estimated to occur at an incidence of 1 per 2,700 livebirths. Jejunoileal atresia and stenosis make up most of these cases and result from a late intrauterine mesenteric vascular compromise. *Duodenal atresia and stenosis,* on the other hand, occurs due to early failure of recanalization of the duodenal lumen. Aside from etiology, another important difference between duodenal and the more distal jejunoileal atresia is the higher incidence of associated systemic malformation. Although less than 10% of those with distal atresia have a concurrent major anomaly, trisomy 21 syndrome is detected in 30% of infants with duodenal atresia, and a large portion of these patients suffer malformation of the cardiac, musculoskeletal, or central nervous system. Annular pancreas is also found in 20% to 30% of patients with duodenal obstruction but most likely represents an associated embryologic defect rather than the primary cause of obstruction.

The presentation of congenital duodenal anomalies can vary from mild partial obstruction caused by a mucosal web to complete atresia, resulting in total obstruction. Maternal polyhydramnios can be detected *in utero* with complete atresia, but stenosis rarely results in excess amniotic fluid. Clinical presentation of complete obstruction is typically characterized by vomiting within hours of birth or after the attempted first feeding. Because most cases of obstruction occur distal to the ampulla of Vater, the vomitus is usually bilious in nature and abdominal distention is rarely observed due to the high level of obstruction. Passage of an orogastric tube yields a large amount of bilious gastric fluid and an upright abdominal radiograph reveals the characteristic "double bubble" sign of a dilated, air-filled stomach separated from the dilated first portion of the duodenum by the pylorus. Lack of air in the distal small bowel or colon confirms complete atresia while scattered small amounts of air point to a partial obstruction or stenosis.

Treatment involves immediate orogastric decompression and intravenous (i.v.) rehydration. Careful search for other congenital anomalies and correction of electrolyte imbalances typically precedes operative intervention, which is accomplished by bypassing the obstruction via a duodenostomy.

Hypertrophic pyloric stenosis is the most common surgically correctable cause of emesis during infancy, with an incidence rate as high as 1 in 300 livebirths. Although the exact etiology has not been defined, evidence exists for genetic predisposition and possible sex-linked inheritance due to a preponderance of this condition in firstborn males. The classic presentation is one of a previously healthy firstborn males between the fourth and sixth week of life with new onset of emesis. The emesis is typically nonbilious and forceful or "projectile" in nature due to the high pressure generated by the hypertrophic gastric muscles. Visible peristaltic waves can often be observed in the epigastrium preceding the vomiting episode. Immediately after vomiting, the infant will usually crave further feeding with recurrent emesis after every meal.

Diagnosis can be confirmed by careful palpation of the epigastrium, revealing a firm, mobile, olive-size mass to the right of the midline corresponding to the hypertrophic pylorus. Abdominal ultrasonography or an upper gastrointestinal (GI) contrast study can confirm the diagnosis if the mass is not palpable. Treatment involves rehydration, correction of electrolyte imbalances, and relief of obstruction by a pyloromyotomy. Oral feedings can resume within several hours of surgery and most patients are discharged within the next 24 to 48 hours.

PEPTIC ULCER DISEASE

Duodenal Ulcer

Peptic ulcers are defined as ulcers caused by the action of gastric acid upon decreased epithelial defenses. These ulcers can occur in the stomach or duodenum.

There has been an overall decrease in ulcer mortality and hospitalization rates in the United States and other Western countries over the past two decades. This has been attributed to treatment of peptic ulcer disease with powerful antisecretory drugs, an integrated approach to this disease with medical, surgical, and endoscopic intervention, and the treatment of *Helicobacter pylori* infection. About 300,000 new cases are diagnosed every year with 4 million people receiving some type of medical or surgical therapy. A racial predilection for duodenal ulcers does not exist. Rarely, genetic factors are important such as the autosomal dominant condition hyperpepsinogenemia I (Table 13-2).

TABLE 13-2. POSTULATED PATHOGENETIC FACTORS IN PATIENTS WITH DUODENAL ULCER[a]

Acid secretion
Increased acid secretory capacity
Increased basal secretion
Increased pentagastrin-stimulated output
Increased meal response
Abnormal gastric emptying
Environment
Cigarette smoking
Nonsteroidal antiinflammatory drug
Helicobacter infection
Mucosal defense
Decreased duodenal bicarbonate production
Decreased gastric mucosal prostaglandin production

[a]From Mulholland MW. Duodenal ulcer. In: Greenfield LJ, Mulholland MW, Oldham KT, et al., eds. *Surgery: scientific principles and practice,* 2nd ed. Philadelphia: Lippincott-Raven Publishers, 1997:759, with permission.

Pathogenesis

The current theory underlying the pathogenesis of peptic ulcer disease involves the disequilibrium of acid secretion and mucosal defense. Environmental factors such as smoking and use of alcohol and NSAID's have all been implicated in ulcerogenesis. Cigarette smoking is a major risk factor. Smoking has been shown to impair ulcer healing, increase the rate of recurrence, and decrease effective medical therapy, resulting in the need for surgical intervention. The suggested mechanisms include altered mucosal blood flow, increased bile reflux, decreased mucosal PGE_2 production, and increased acid stimulation. All these are key factors that affect patients who continue to smoke. Clearly, counseling regarding cessation of smoking is mandatory. Widespread belief that dietary factors cause ulcers is not generally supported by adequate scientific evidence. Alcohol in moderation is not harmful, but there is evidence to indicate that alcohol consumption in excess impairs ulcer healing.

NSAID use can result in a variety of duodenal and gastric lesions, leading to hemorrhage, superficial erosions, and deep ulcerations. The Food and Drug Administration estimates the rate of NSAID-induced ulcers to be 2% to 4% per patient year. The mechanism involves the systemic suppression of PGE_2 production and withdrawal of NSAIDs results in rapid healing. All NSAIDs pose the risk of peptic ulceration, and elderly patents should used NSAIDs with caution. Concurrent use of NSAIDs with alcohol and tobacco increases the rate of ulceration.

In 1982, Warren and Marshall demonstrated a spiral urease-producing, Gram-negative organism that caused antral gastritis and peptic ulceration. They also showed that eradication of the organism resulted in healing of the ulcer. Since then there has been an accumulation of data to support the role of *H. pylori* as the causal bacterial organism in ulceration. Evidence supporting the pathogenesis of *H. pylori* in duodenal ulcer disease is summarized in Table 13-3.

TABLE 13-3. SUPPORT FOR THE ROLE OF *HELICOBACTER PYLORI* IN ULCER DISEASE[a]

1. *H. pylori* positive patients almost always demonstrate antral gastritis, characterized by nonerosive mucosal inflammation.
2. *H. pylori* binds only to gastric epithelium.
3. Eradication of *H. pylori* results in resolution of gastritis with antimicrobials, and recurrence is associated with reinfection.
4. Intragastric administration of isolated organism in animal models and in two humans resulted in lesions of chronic superficial gastritis.

[a]From Mulholland MW. Duodenal ulcer. In: Greenfield LJ, Mulholland MW, Oldham KT, et al., eds. *Surgery: scientific principles and practice,* 2nd ed. Philadelphia: Lippincott-Raven Publishers, 1997:768, with permission.

Unlike patients suffering from gastric ulceration, some patients with duodenal ulcers present with *increased acid secretion* due to an increase in parietal-cell mass in the gastric mucosa or an increase in sensitivity to circulating gastrin. Exaggerated gastrin secretion could also be due to mediators of inflammation such as IL-2. Patients with duodenal ulcers demonstrate a prolonged postprandial acid-secretory response, and in contrast to normal individuals, duodenal acidification fails to slow gastric emptying. Increased basal secretion can be demonstrated by nocturnal collection of gastric acid, which is probably mediated by exaggerated vagal stimulation. Local duodenal defenses might also be compromised in patients with duodenal ulcers and mucosal HCO_3^- secretion is lower than in normal subjects. Decreased PGE_2 production may also result in loss of cytoprotective effects.

Clinical Features and Treatment

Many patients report epigastric pain that is worse in the morning. The pain is frequently described as burning, stabbing, or gnawing and is commonly relieved by eating or taking antacids. Pain referred to the back signals perforation or penetration into the head of the pancreas. Physical examination is typically nonspecific in uncomplicated cases. Differential diagnosis can include nonspecific dyspepsia, gastric neoplasia, cholelithiasis, pancreatitis, and pancreatic neoplasia. The diagnostic evaluation typically involves either a barium contrast study or an endoscopy. Acid secretory studies are no longer used routinely. Endoscopy generally is preferred to barium examination due to a higher sensitivity and specificity in experienced hands. Endoscopy also provides a means for tissue diagnosis in the same setting. Of all the dyspeptic patients referred for endoscopy, 13% have duodenal ulcers, 10% have gastric ulcers, 2% have gastric cancer, and up to 15% have esophagitis. Duodenal ulcers have a typical appearance with sharp edges and a clean smooth base. Recent hemorrhage is characterized by an eschar or exudate. The ulcers are usually surrounded by a local inflammatory response. The most common site for occurrence is the first part of the duodenum. Histologically, duodenal ulcers demonstrate gastric metaplasia in the surrounding tissue, infiltration with chronic and acute inflammatory cells, and fibrosis. Radiographic signs of an acute ulcer usually are seen in profile or enface, and erosion of the normal smooth outline is seen. Changes associated with chronicity and scarring can be evident with distortion of the duodenal bulb or psuedodiverticulum formation. Despite the predilection for higher acid secretion in those with duodenal ulcer, circulating serum gastrin levels are typically normal and measuring gastrin levels is only helpful if you suspect Zollinger-Ellison syndrome (normal basal gastrin levels vary from 50 to 100 pg/mL).

Since the discovery of the *H. pylori* contribution to the pathophysiology of peptic ulcer disease, the diagnosis of infection and posttreatment eradication of infection has become paramount to successful therapy. The presence of the organism can be diagnosed by endoscopic or nonendoscopic methods. *Serology* is a reliable marker of initial infection because most people harboring the organism will develop circulating antibodies. Serology results, however, will remain positive for a prolonged time, even after the eradication of the bacteria, so serology is unreliable in documenting clearance. The urea breath test is a more reliable, nonendoscopic measure of infection. It relies on the principle that labeled urea is converted into ammonia and labeled carbon dioxide by the *H. pylori* urease in the stomach. The carbon dioxide is then absorbed through the stomach wall and can be detected upon expiration. *Endoscopic diagnosis* relies on the ability to see the characteristic organism within endoscopic biopsies of the gastric mucosa.

Medical therapy is directed toward both the healing of the ulcer and the definitive cure. The former is achieved by reduction of acid secretion and the later by the eradication of *H. pylori*. Powerful antisecretory drugs include *histamine antagonists* (cimetidine, ranitidine) and proton pump inhibitors (omeprazole). Histamine receptor antagonists bind competitively to parietal-cell histamine receptors, producing reversible inhibition of acid secretion. Peak plasma concentrations are generally reached within 1 to 3 hours after oral administration. They are secreted in the urine; thus, renal failure significantly alters plasma clearance. Under this regimen, a duodenal ulcer can heal in 80% of patients within 6 weeks. If the medication is stopped, however, half the patients may present with recurrent ulceration within the year. This can be avoided by long-term, single-dose bedtime administration of a histamine antagonist.

Proton pump inhibitors should be reserved for patients refractory to this first line of therapy. *Omeprazole* in therapeutic doses causes near-complete inhibition of acid secretion. This drug acts specifically in the gastric mucosa, binding to the parietal-cell-membrane–associated $H^+/K^+/ATPase$. Several studies demonstrate the efficiency and superiority of proton pump inhibitors with higher healing rates (80% within 2 weeks), reduction in associated epigastric pain but a similar recurrence rate after cessation of this drug as with histamine antagonists. Long-term maintenance on omeprazole is not recommended, as the effects of sustained hypergastrinemia are not known and continuous anacidity is not necessary for ulcer healing.

If long-term maintenance is necessary, an attractive option is *sucralfate*, an aluminum salt of sulfated sucrose. This polymer acts by providing a protective coat over the gastric and duodenal mucosa, which binds bile acids, inhibits pepsin while stimulating mucus, prostaglandin and bicarbonate secretion. The side effects are minimal and there is virtually negligible systemic absorption. It is also the drug of choice for ulcer therapy during pregnancy. When administered at a dose of 1 g four times a day, ulcer healing is achieved within 4 weeks in 80% of patients. *Misoprostol*, a prostaglandin analog, should be avoided during pregnancy because of its abortifacient properties. Three fourths of patients treated with misoprostal achieve healing in 4 weeks. The major setback with doses required for antisecretory effects is diarrhea. Antacids should be used as supplements to antisecretory drugs mentioned above.

Eradication of *H. pylori* infection eliminates recurrent ulceration, unless recurrent ulceration is due to reinfection (10% of cases). Various therapeutic combinations exist and treatment with bismuth subsalicylate, metronidazole, tetracycline, and omeprazole has the highest cure rate (94% to 98%), but compliance is difficult to achieve. Less expensive alternatives consist of clarithromycin and metronidazole or amoxicillin with omeprazole for 1 week. An equally effective regimen involves the combination of antibiotics with a histamine receptor antagonist for 2 weeks. It is generally accepted that acid-suppressive therapy continue for 6 weeks after eradication of *H. pylori*.

Surgical treatment for duodenal ulcer disease is indicated if optimal medical treatment fails or if the patient presents with the classical complications of peptic ulcer disease such as hemorrhage, perforation, or obstruction. Widely used procedures include truncal vagotomy with drainage, truncal vagotomy and antrectomy, and proximal gastric vagotomy. Truncal vagotomy must be combined with a drainage procedure, as denervation will result in impaired pyloric coordination and gastric emptying. The method of drainage usually selected is a pyloroplasty. Heineke-Mikulicz pyloroplasty is most commonly performed, as it offers the advantage of preserving continuity of the duodenal loop, hence the integrity of the hormonal milieu (Fig. 13-6). If the duodenum is scarred, then another option involving the creation of a posterior gastrojejunostomy should be considered.

The most complete acid reduction is achieved by *truncal vagotomy* combined with resection of the gastric antrum. This entails a 50% resection of the distal stomach and the remnant is anastomosed to the duodenum (*Billroth I resection*) or to the proximal jejunum (*Billroth II resection*) (Fig. 13-7). The morbidity rate of this operation is higher due to the combination of partial gastric resection with vagotomy and complications are higher then with vagotomy alone.

Proximal vagotomy involves resection of the nerve fibers to the acid-secreting fundic mucosa while preserving the fibers to the antrum and the pylorus, thus preserving gastric emptying. The denervation of the nerve fibers begins at about the distal 5 to 7 cm of the esophagus and extends along the lesser curvature to 5 cm of the proximal pylorus (Fig. 13-8).

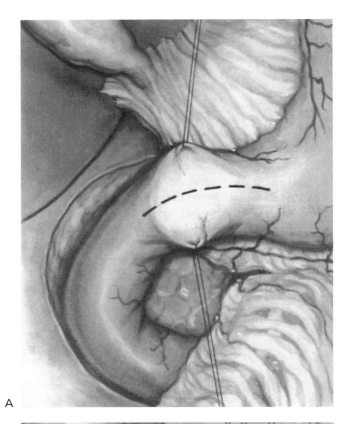
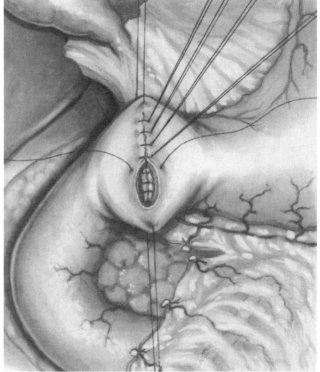

FIGURE 13-6. The Heineke-Mikulicz pyloroplasty enlarges the gastric outlet by closing a longitudinal pyloric incision **(A)** in a transverse fashion **(B)**. (From Etala E. *Atlas of gastrointestinal surgery.* Philadelphia: Williams & Wilkins, 1997:1085, with permission.)

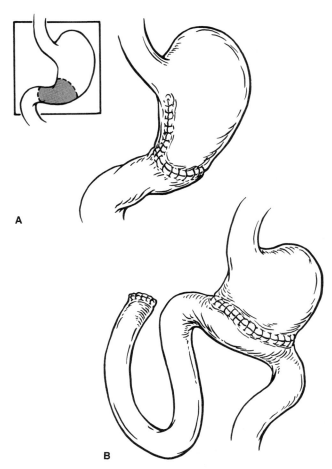

FIGURE 13-7. The anatomic differences between an antrectomy with a **(A)** Billroth I reconstruction and a **(B)** Billroth II resection. (From Mulholland MW. Peptic ulcer disease. In: Bell RH, Rikkers LF, Mulholland MW, eds. *Digestive tract surgery: a text and atlas.* Philadelphia: Lippincott-Raven Publishers, 1996: 180, with permission.)

Complications of Ulcer Surgery

The physiologic consequences of truncal vagotomy are listed in Table 13-4. All forms of vagotomy cause postoperative hypergastrinemia due to decreased luminal acid, loss of inhibitory feedback, and loss of vagal inhibition. In most cases, the result is chronic hypergastrinemia due to gastrin-cell hyperplasia. Antrectomy combined with truncal vagotomy causes greater reduction in acid secretion then vagotomy alone. This operation also decreases gastrin levels due to the removal of gastrin secretion from the antrum.

Any form of vagotomy alters gastric emptying, as vagus-mediated receptive relaxation is lost. Liquids are emptied at a faster rate due to the alteration in gastroduodenal gastric pressure gradient, as for any given volume, the gastric pressure rises sharply. Truncal vagotomy affects the motor activ-

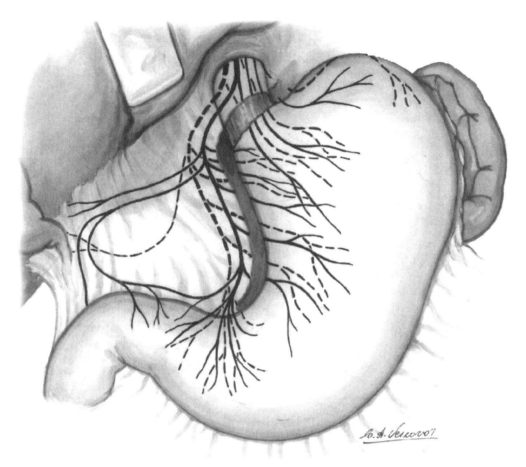

FIGURE 13-8. Unlike the truncal vagotomy, the proximal gastric vagotomy selectively denervates the lesser curvature of the stomach but spares the nerves to the pylorus and antrum. (From Etala E. *Atlas of gastrointestinal surgery.* Philadelphia: Williams & Wilkins, 1997:1047, with permission.)

TABLE 13-4. PHYSIOLOGIC ALTERATIONS CAUSED BY TRUNCAL VAGOTOMY[a]

Gastric effects
Decreased basal acid output
    Reduced cholinergic input to parietal cells
Decreased stimulated maximal acid output
    Diminished sensitivity to histamine gastrin
    Decreased meal-induced acid secretion
Increased fasting and postprandial gastrin
Gastrin cell hyperplasia
Accelerated liquid emptying
Altered emptying of solids
Nongastric effects
Decreased pancreatic exocrine secretion
    Decreased pancreatic enzymes and bicarbonate
Decreased postprandial bile flow
Increased gallbladder volumes
Diminished release of vagally mediated peptide hormones

[a]From Mulholland MW. Duodenal ulcer. In: Greenfield LJ, Mulholland MW, Oldham KT, et al., eds. *Surgery: scientific principles and practice,* 2nd ed. Philadelphia: Lippincott-Raven Publishers, 1997:768, with permission.

ity of both the proximal and the distal stomach. This decreases gastric emptying but can be improved when combined with some form of pyloroplasty. Proximal vagotomy on the other hand preserves the mixing and triturating capacity of solid food and emptying of solids is near normal.

Early complications of peptic ulcer surgery include duodenal stump leakage after a Billroth II resection, gastric retention, and hemorrhage. Later complications are recurrent ulcer, gastrojejunocolic and gastrocolic fistula, dumping syndrome, alkaline gastritis, anemia, postvagotomy diarrhea, chronic gastroparesis, and afferent loop syndrome. Recurrent rate of ulceration after a proximal vagotomy is 10% but is slightly lower when a truncal vagotomy is combined with pyloroplasty. There is a significant decrease in ulceration when truncal vagotomy is combined with antrectomy. The ulcers almost always develop in the intestinal side of the anastomosis. Patients classically complain of pain that is improved by eating or by antacids. In some patients, the pain is referred to the shoulder.

Complications such as hemorrhage or perforation can also occur. The treatment for these complications is similar to that of the original ulcer. Patients presenting with severe diarrhea, weight loss, and a history of abdominal pain preceding the onset of diarrhea define the classic characteristics of a gastrocolic fistula. Low protein level and fluid electrolyte imbalance are typical. Barium enema is the investigation of choice. Fluid and electrolytes should be restored in the initial management of these patients with plans for excision of gastrojejunal segment and restoration of colonic continuity.

Dumping syndrome is characterized by GI and vasomotor symptoms. It occurs to some extent in most patients with impaired gastric emptying but becomes a problem in about 2% when truncal vagotomy is combined with antrectomy. The exact cause is not known but is believed to result from the sudden osmotic load of ingested food in the small bowel. Symptoms include palpitations, sweating, weakness, dyspnea, flushing, nausea, abdominal cramps, belching, vomiting, diarrhea, and occasionally syncope. These symptoms classically occur shortly after a meal. In severe cases, patients may lie down for 30 to 40 minutes to achieve relief. A dietary regimen of low carbohydrates with meals high in fat and protein content, as well as restriction of fluid intake with meals, is met with some success. Most patients' symptoms improve with time. A somatostatin analog, octreotide, at 50 to 100 µL subcutaneously before a meal, may reduce symptoms of dumping in some patients. Although its mechanism of action is uncertain, it may act by reducing splanchnic blood flow, inhibiting release of vasoactive peptides, decreasing peak plasma insulin, and slowing intestinal transit time.

The clinical triad of postprandial epigastric pain, evidence of bile reflux, and histological evidence of gastritis constitute *alkaline reflux gastritis*. The epigastric pain must be differentiated from recurrent ulceration, biliary and pancreatic conditions, afferent loop obstruction, and esophagitis. Endoscopic examination results may show bile reflux and a patchy nonulcerative edematous mucosa. A more quantitative study may be obtained by i.v. ^{99m}Tc dimethyl iminodiacetic acid administration. As the radionuclide is excreted in the bile, an external scintigraphy can measure the reflux of bile into the stomach. Dietary and drug therapies improve the symptoms, but the definitive treatment involves the prevention of reflux by creating a Roux-en-Y gastrojejunostomy with a 50- to 60-cm efferent jejunal limb.

Iron deficiency anemia develops in one third of the patients after partial gastric resection due to the failure of organic iron absorption. Ferrous sulfate or ferrous gluconate, the inorganic form of iron, is normally absorbed and can be used to overcome this form of iron deficiency.

Gastric Ulcer

The peak incidence of gastric ulceration occurs in patients 40 to 60 years of age. Ninety-five percent of the ulcers are located along the lesser curvature. The signs and symptoms are similar to those of duodenal ulcer. Gastric ulcers are divided into four different types. *Type I ulcers* are usually found along the lesser curvature. Antral gastritis is always present, and in most cases, *H. pylori* infection is present. *Type II ulcers* are usually prepyloric and occur in association with duodenal ulcers.

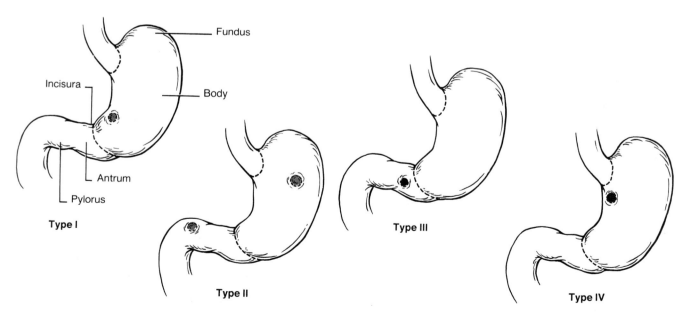

FIGURE 13-9. Gastric ulcers can be classified into four types based on location and pathogenesis. (From Mulholland MW. Peptic ulcer disease. In: Bell RH, Rikkers LF, Mulholland MW, eds. *Digestive tract surgery: a text and atlas.* Philadelphia: Lippincott-Raven Publishers, 1996:190, with permission.)

Type III ulcers occur in the antrum as a result of NSAID use. *Type IV ulcers* occur high on the lesser curvature and are similar in pathophysiology to type I ulcers (Fig. 13-9).

Patients present with a history of epigastric pain that is relieved by food or antacids. The pain of gastric ulcers appears soon after eating and other times is aggravated by eating. Endoscopy should be performed to rule out a malignant gastric ulcer. Benign ulcers are characterized by flat edges, as opposed to malignant ulcers that classically have rolled-up edges. At least six biopsies from the margins should be obtained at the time of initial endoscopic examination to differentiate benign from malignant ulcers. An upper GI series can also demonstrate a gastric ulcer. Radiographic characteristics of a malignant ulcer include a prominent rim of radiolucency around the ulcer (meniscus sign) and a large ulcer size (more than 2 cm), which is associated with an increased incidence of malignancy. The principal complications of gastric ulcer disease include bleeding, obstruction, and perforation.

The etiology of gastric ulceration is often similar to that of duodenal ulcers, but patients with gastric ulcerations are rarely acid hypersecretors and the pathogenesis lies mostly in the loss of the mucosal defense. Factors such as cigarette smoking, NSAID abuse, and *H. pylori* infection are involved. The medical treatment is the same as that for duodenal ulcers. A repeated endoscopic evaluation is recommended at 2 to 3 months, particularly if the ulcer was greater than 2 cm, and *H. pylori* eradication should be confirmed after a course of medical management. Currently, surgical treatment for a primary, nonmalignant gastric ulcer is rarely indicated, but in the past, the best surgical procedure was a distal hemigastrectomy. Today, most surgical procedures are reserved for treatment of nonhealing gastric ulcers as well as complications of ulcer disease such as bleeding, perforation, or obstruction.

Upper GI Hemorrhage

The most common causes of upper GI bleeding requiring hospital admission include peptic ulceration, esophageal or gastric bleeding from portal hypertension, and gastritis, with peptic ulcer disease being the most common. An *upper GI bleed* is defined as originating proximal to the Treitz ligament and is usually bright red or dark depending on etiology. The presence of coffee-colored vomitus denotes that blood has been in the stomach long enough for hemoglobin conversion to methemoglobin to occur. Melena (i.e., the passage of black tarry stools) is a nonspecific sign that in general is a poor guide for the rate of bleeding and represents that the blood has been in the intestine for some time. Melena can be produced by a total blood-volume loss of 50 to 100 mL. The black color is due to hematin, the product of heme oxidation by bacterial and intestinal enzymes. Hematochezia, or the passage of bright-red blood per rectum, due to upper GI bleeding is very unusual.

Patients presenting with a history of hematemesis or melena of less than 12 hours require hospital admission. After assessment of the patient's circulatory status, a physical examination should be preformed. Patients should be questioned about predisposing factors for upper GI bleeding including NSAID use and other bleeding tendencies. A large nasogastric tube should be placed to check for the presence of intragastric blood, and a positive lavage result can confirm an upper GI source of bleeding. A negative lavage, consisting of bile but no blood, generally indicates a source distal to the Treitz ligament but can create some diagnostic confusion because as many as 20% of bleeding duodenal ulcers may result in a negative lavage. During the initial evaluation, a blood sample should be drawn for crossmatch, hematocrit, hemoglobin, and liver function tests. A very low hematocrit level without signs of shock indicates gradual blood loss because the hematocrit is usually at normal levels or only slightly lowered during acute bleeding prior to volume equilibration.

After the patient is stabilized and the blood volume is restored, endoscopy should be performed (within 24 hours). Improved outcome is associated with endoscopic therapy for both esophageal sources of variceal bleeding and ulcers. Rarely, it is necessary to use angiographic techniques to demonstrate or embolize a bleeding vessel. In 80% of the cases, the source of bleeding can be identified and treated endoscopically. Monitoring the patient by blood pressure level, pulse rate, central venous pressure measurement, hematocrit level, hourly urinary volume, and gastric aspirates is essential to avoid underestimation of blood loss and to determine the need for blood transfusion. A persistently hypotensive patient that requires more then 4 units of blood or 1 unit every 8 hours usually has a poor prognosis for medical management and must be considered for surgical therapy.

Rebleeding from peptic ulcer disease occurs in about 25% of patients treated medically and is more common in patients with gastric rather than duodenal ulcers. Rebleeding has been associated with up to a 30% death rate; these patients should be treated by early surgical intervention to reduce that number. Those at a higher risk of rebleeding include patients older than 60 years, those that initially presented with hematemesis, those with a visible vessel actively bleeding during endoscopy, and those with a hemoglobin level below 8 g/dL upon admission. These patients usually rebleed within the first 48 hours of hospital admission and will generally benefit from surgical intervention. The use of histamine blockers or proton pump inhibitors reduces the risk of rebleeding in the long run but does not affect active bleeding.

Perforated Peptic Ulcer

The most common site of perforation for peptic ulcer is the anterior gastric or duodenal wall. Erosions of ulcers through the anterior wall tend to present as perforation rather than bleeding due to the absence of major blood vessels on this surface. So-called "kissing ulcers" or posterior bleeding ulcers complicating an anterior perforation are rare and carry a high mortality rate. Initially, patients present with a chemical peritonitis from the gastroduodenal contents, which over a 12- to 24-hour period evolves into a bacterial peritonitis. It is uncertain how many perforations are sealed by the undersurface of the liver, but if this is the case, a subphrenic abscess is a likely complication.

Following a gastric perforation, the patient will present with a sudden onset of severe upper abdominal pain, typically several hours after a meal. Pain may be referred to the shoulder or to the back. A history of peptic ulcer disease is not a consistent finding. Classically, patients are severely distressed, lie still with knees drawn up, and take shallow breaths. There may be a temporary improvement of symptoms with the onset of bacterial peritonitis, as the initial chemical peritonitis is diluted by the peritoneal fluid. Patients are usually afebrile upon presentation, and on physical examination, there is boardlike rigidity of the abdomen. The continual loss of air from the perforation can result in tympany and abdominal distention. Peristaltic sounds are usually reduced or absent.

However, there are patients who present with abdominal pain but without the classic physical findings. The incidence of this masked presentation is higher in hospitalized patients who are being treated for other unrelated causes. The significance of the pain often goes unnoticed, resulting in a delay of appropriate treatment. A reasonable initial approach is to obtain an abdominal radiograph or upright chest film, which will demonstrate free intraperitoneal air. Duodenal leaks can track down the paracolic gutter and cause signs and symptoms that may be confused with appendicitis or colonic diverticulitis. Subclinical perforations can also be sealed off by the omentum or liver and present as a subdiaphragmatic or subphrenic abscess.

Laboratory findings usually will show a mild leukocytosis (12,000/µL) in the early stages, which can rise during the course of illness. Serum amylase levels are usually mildly elevated. Free subdiaphragmatic air on an upright chest x-ray is the most definitive diagnostic finding and is present in about 85% of the patients.

If the patient is uncomfortable sitting up, a left lateral decubitus film can be obtained to look for free air. If the diagnosis remains unclear, an abdominal CT scan, which is very sensitive to free intraperitoneal air, can be obtained or 400 mL of air may be insufflated into the stomach via a nasogastric tube to demonstrate the perforation. A contrast study can also be a reliable tool when free air is not visible.

Treatment is dictated by the overall condition of the patient. Fluid resuscitation and i.v. antibiotics should be started. A nasogastric tube should be passed and abdominal films acquired. The surgical method of repair involves sealing the perforation with an omental patch (Graham Steell patch). With the availability of powerful antiacid secretory agents and successful treatment of *H. pylori* medical management generally can prevent recurrence, and surgical treatment of ulcer disease with a truncal vagotomy or pyloroplasty is rarely necessary today. However, perforation in the presence of pyloric obstruction is best treated by pyloroplasty or a gastroenterostomy.

Nonoperative treatment with fluids and antibiotics is occasionally chosen but is associated with a high rate of peritoneal and subphrenic abscess. This conservative approach does not necessarily carry a higher mortality rate and has been shown to be effective if the risk of operative intervention is prohibitive. An increased mortality rate is associated with a delay in treatment, in the elderly, or in the presence of other systemic illnesses.

Pyloric obstruction

Pyloric obstruction from peptic ulcer disease is a less common condition compared to perforation. Duodenal ulcers cause obstruction more frequently than gastric ulcers. Malignant ulcers causing obstruction are becoming more common due to the decreasing complications of nonmalignant ulcer disease. Most patients have a long history of peptic ulcer disease and up to one third have had some treatment for a previous obstruction or perforation. Anorexia and vomiting of undigested food with no biliary staining is the usual presentation. Weight loss is seen only if the patient has delayed seeking medical attention, and malnutrition and dehydration are not always present. A succussion splash can be elicited in some patients from gastric dilation and retained gastric contents, but a visible peristaltic wave in the abdominal wall is rare in adults. The usual laboratory studies reveal a metabolic alkalosis with hypochloremia, hypokalemia, hyponatremia, and increased bicarbonate. Tetany has been reported in severe cases of alkalosis due to prolonged vomiting. Prerenal azotemia may result as GFR is reduced.

A large nasogastric tube should be passed into the stomach and gastric contents lavaged. Medical therapy consists of decompression of the stomach, allowing resolution of pyloric edema and amelioration of pyloric muscular spasm. In most circumstances, improvement is seen after 72 hours of this conservative management and a liquid diet is tolerated. Gradually, solid food is introduced. Saline load test (infusion of 700 mL of saline and its aspiration after 30 minutes) is indicative of ongoing pyloric obstruction if more than 350 mL is aspirated. The test is diagnostic, but it is not predictive of how the patient will handle solid food.

Endoscopic evaluation is extremely important in this condition. Endoscopy is favored over an upper GI series because biopsies can be taken to exclude malignancy. If medical therapy and decompression for 1 week do not relieve the obstruction or the patient is able to take liquids only, intervention is indicated. Endoscopic-guided balloon dilation can relieve symptoms in most patients, but long-term relief of obstruction is obtained in only 40% of patients. The surgical treatment of choice in cases of chronic or recurrent obstruction is usually a truncal vagotomy and drainage procedure.

Stress Ulcers

Stress gastritis is defined by ulcers occurring after major shock. The causes include shock, sepsis, burn over more than 35% of body surface area (Curling ulcer), or trauma. Stress gastritis can also occur due to central nervous system disease (Cushing disease). The pathogenesis is mainly due to decreased mucosal resistance as an effect of ischemia, decreased production of prostanoids, and thinning of the mucous layer; and the mucosa becomes vulnerable to acid pepsin and lysosomal enzymes. Ulcers associated with central nervous system pathology (Cushing disease) are generally associated with increased gastrin levels and increased gastric acid secretion.

Most of the ulcers occur in the acid-secreting portion of the stomach and bleeding ulcers are more common than perforation. Perforation is more common, however, in a Cushing ulcer. The ulcers are shallow and discrete with little inflammation and edema. The condition becomes clinically prominent 4 to 5 days after the onset of the initial illness. Prophylaxis with a histamine receptor antagonist can decrease the incidence and avert bleeding. Antacids given hourly by a nasogastric tube can also be effective as long as the gastric pH level remains above 3.5. Sucralfate can also be used as a prophylactic drug and is as effective as antacids or histamine receptor antagonists.

Initial therapy involves resuscitation and treatment of the underlying condition. Hemorrhagic shock should be corrected with whole blood replacement and antimicrobial therapy should be started to combat sepsis while any abscess or undrained collection is drained. Medical management of gastric bleeding can be achieved by gastric lavage. This can control bleeding 80% of the time, but infusion of a vasoconstricting agent by selective angiographic catheterization may sometimes be needed. *Trans*catheter embolization with Gelfoam, metal coils, or autologous blood clots are possible alternatives but rarely necessary.

Despite aggressive medical therapy a definitive surgical procedure is unavoidable in some patients. The possible choices include vagotomy and pyloroplasty, vagotomy and antrectomy, vagotomy and subtotal gastrectomy, and total gastrectomy. There is no evidence supporting the superiority of one procedure over the other. There is a trend toward vagotomy and pyloroplasty with suture ligation to control bleeding points. The mortality rate is high (30% to 60%) in patients with acute hemorrhagic stress ulcers requiring surgical intervention.

GASTRIC CANCER

The incidence of gastric cancer in the United States is decreasing, but the reason for this decline is not known. The factors that play a key role in the pathogenesis of gastric carcinogenesis include diet, exogenous chemicals, intragastric synthesis of carcinogens, genetic factors, infectious agents, and antral gastritis. Dietary factors probably play an important role in countries such as Japan and other countries where the incidence is high. Studies of individuals emigrating from endemic areas to Western countries show a lower incidence of gastric cancer after migration. Dietary nitrites and their derivatives such as nitrosamines have been shown to induce gastric cancer under experimental conditions, but specific dietary factors have yet to be identified in humans. As recent information has become available, *H. pylori* was recently classified as a carcinogen by the World Health Organization. *H. Pylori* infection also causes atrophic gastritis, which is a recognized precursor of gastric adenocarcinoma. However, it is not known if eradication of *H. pylori* infection will prevent gastric cancer.

Patients with long-standing pernicious anemia characterized by fundic mucosal atrophy, hypochlorhydria, hypergastrinemia, and loss of parietal and chief cells are at increased risk (twice that of age-matched controls) of developing gastric cancer. The other premalignant lesion that has a distinct risk of leading to gastric malignancy is an adenomatous polyp. Ten to twenty percent of patients with polyps greater then 2 cm in diameter develop gastric cancer. The amount of dysplasia and carcinoma *in situ*, as well as the number of polyps increase the risk of cancer.

Gastric cancers usually are adenocarcinomas. The morphologic types include *ulcerating carcinoma* where a deeply penetrating malignant ulcer involves the entire gastric wall. *Polypoid carcinoma* is defined as a large intraluminal tumor with late metastasis. *Superficial spreading carcinoma* is an early gastric cancer that is often confined to the superficial layers of the gastric wall. Unlike other subtypes, only one third of these present with metastatic disease. Screening programs in countries with a high prevalence of this disease have improved survival rates (5-year survival rate of 90%) if this type of tumor is detected early, compared to deep and penetrating lesions. *Linitis plastica* is a spreading tumor involving all the layers of the gastric wall. The stomach loses its pliability early due to malignant infiltration and metastasis occurs early. Most commonly, patients present with *advanced disease* where there is evidence of spread outside of the stomach.

An alternative method classifies gastric cancer by the degree of differentiation. Inflammatory, glandular (intestinal), and diffuse (stromal) are the common histological features used in the classification. Tumors eliciting an inflammatory response are generally found to have a better prognosis. Gastric cancer is predominately found in the antrum along the lesser curvature. This is also a common location for benign gastric ulcers. Ulcers along the greater curvature and the cardia are likely to be malignant.

Patients with gastric cancer frequently present with new onset of discomfort on top of a history of chronic dyspeptic symptoms. Anorexia develops early with concurrent weight loss. Vomiting is associated with pyloric obstruction while involvement of the cardia is associated with dysphagia. A mass can be palpated in some patients, and the liver is enlarged in about 10% of patients. Occult blood can be detected in the stool of 50% of patients, but frank anemia is present in fewer individuals. Physical signs of dissemination include a palpable Virchow node in the left supraclavicular space, indicating metastasis along the thoracic duct, and intraperitoneal spread may cause enlarged ovaries (Krukenberg tumors) or palpable peritoneal deposits on rectal examination known as a *Blumer shelf*. Distant metastasis can involve the liver, lungs, brain, or bone. Carcinoembryonic antigen level is usually elevated in disseminated tumors.

The initial diagnostic procedure of choice is an upper endoscopy. Polyps or ulcers that are suspicious for malignancy should be sampled. An upper GI series can be diagnostic in most instances, but the false-negative rate can be as high as 20%, so patients with gastric ulcers seen on an upper GI series should undergo endoscopic ulcer biopsy.

Surgical resection is the only curative treatment, but only half of the resectable tumors are potentially curable due to micrometastasis. The location of the tumor dictates the extent of resection necessary. Antral tumors necessitate a distal gastrectomy with a proximal resection margin of approximately 6 cm from the tumor and 3 to 4 cm from the duodenum, along with an en bloc resection of the omentum, the subpyloric lymph nodes, and the left gastric artery and lymph nodes. Bowel continuity is established, preferably using a Billroth II procedure. Proximal tumors usually require a total gastrectomy while tumors of the cardia require an esophagogastrectomy, splenectomy, and intrathoracic esophagogastrostomy. Frozen sections of the margins, particularly the proximal margin, is recommended before an anastomosis.

Antral tumors with extragastric spread or pyloric obstruction require a palliative gastrectomy. If a gastrectomy is impossible, then a palliative gastrojejunostomy for bypass is the procedure of choice. Adjuvant chemotherapy and/or radiation therapy have not proven efficacious. The overall 5-year survival rate for gastric cancer in the United States is 12%.

14

THE SMALL BOWEL

SAMANTHA K. HENDREN AND NOEL N. WILLIAMS

ANATOMY AND PHYSIOLOGY OF THE SMALL BOWEL

Anatomy

The anatomy of the small bowel makes it highly specialized for digestion, absorption, endocrine function, and immunologic defense. It is characterized by a massive surface area and the presence of digestive enzymes, immune cells, multiple hormones, paracrine and neurocrine substances, and a complex nervous system.

As a whole, the small bowel is a tubular organ about 13 feet long. The mucosa and submucosa form circular folds called "valvulae conniventes," which decrease in number and prominence distally. Blood supply, nerves, and lymphatics travel via the mesentery to the bowel wall. Arterial supply is from the superior mesenteric artery (SMA), and venous drainage via the superior mesenteric vein into the portal vein. Lymphatic channels run with the vessels and drain into the cisterna chyli, which empties into the thoracic duct. Parasympathetic innervation comes from the celiac division of the posterior trunk of the vagus nerve, and sympathetic supply comes from celiac and superior mesenteric ganglia. Sympathetic afferents mediate the perceived periumbilical pain resulting from bowel distention.

The *duodenum* (Fig. 14-1) is the first 20 to 30 cm of the small bowel. The first portion of the duodenum is the duodenal bulb, where 90% of duodenal ulcers occur. This portion overlies the pancreatic head and gastroduodenal artery. The blood supply comes from the supraduodenal branch of the hepatic artery and the gastroduodenal artery. The second portion of the duodenum is retroperitoneal; it displays characteristic mucosal folds known as "Kerckring folds." It is attached to the head of the pancreas. The major ampullae of Vater and minor ampulla of Santorini (present in 50% to 60% of the population) enter the second portion of the duodenum posteriorly. The third, or transverse, portion is attached to the uncinate process of the pancreas in the retroperitoneum. It is wedged between the SMA and the aorta. The arterial supply of the second and third portions is from the anterosuperior and posterosuperior pancreaticoduodenal arteries, arising from the gastroduodenal artery, as well as from the anteroinferior and posteroinferior pancreaticoduodenal arteries, arising from the SMA. The forth, or ascending, portion of the duodenum derives its blood supply from the first jejunal branch of the SMA.

The *ligament of Treitz* is a striated muscle band extending from the right crus of the diaphragm and a fibromuscular band connecting the duodenum to the celiac axis. The jejunum is the small intestinal portion extending from the ligament of Treitz to two fifths of the distance to the ileocecal valve. The arterial supply of the jejunum is from the first jejunal branch of the SMA.

The distal three fifths of the small bowel (after the ligament of Treitz) is known as the "ileum." The jejunoileal mesentery contains the SMA branches, lymphatics, and fat. This mesentery is fixed to the posterior abdominal wall in a line extending from near the ligament of Treitz to the right lower quadrant. Along the length of the small bowel, the luminal diameter decreases gradually and the folds become much less pronounced.

Histologically, the bowel is composed of four concentric layers: mucosa, submucosa, muscularis, and serosa (peritoneal). The mucosa is made up of villi and crypts and is responsible for secretion and absorption (Figs. 14-2 and 14-3). The submucosa contains blood vessels, lymphatics, and nerves. There are two muscle layers: an inner circular layer and an outer longitudinal layer. The myenteric plexus of Auerbach and a plexus of ganglia for nonmyelinated nerve fibers are located within the muscular layers.

The *mucosal villi* and *crypts* are covered by columnar epithelial cells specialized with apical *microvilli* for absorption. Peptidases and disaccharidases are located on the apical surface of the epithelial cells, and a significant proportion of protein and carbohydrate breakdown takes place at the luminal surface. The enterocyte cytoplasm contains lysosomes with hydrolytic enzymes to aid in digestion. *Goblet cells* are interspersed between the columnar cells.

Hospital of the University of Pennsylvania, Philadelphia, Pennsylvania

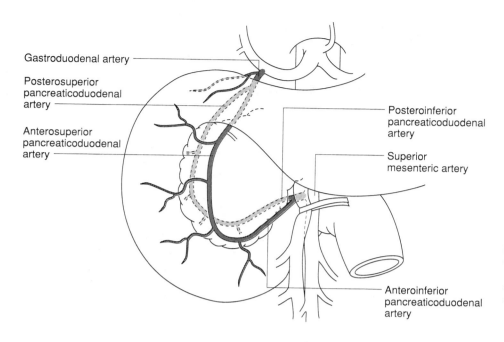

FIGURE 14-1. Gross anatomy of the duodenum. (From Greenfield LJ, Mulholland MW, Oldham KT, et al., eds. *Surgery: scientific principles and practice,* 2nd ed. Philadelphia: Lippincott-Raven Publishers, 1997, with permission.)

These exocrine cells have a narrow base and a head filled with mucinogen droplets that are secreted to lubricate and protect the gut epithelium. *Paneth cells* are located at the bases of the villi in the crypts of Lieberkühn; these cells contain granules with lysosomal enzymes. The submucosa of the duodenum and upper jejunum contains Brunner glands, which produce a viscous alkaline solution that protects the mucosa.

The gut immune system includes the leiolymphocytes (enteric T cells) that are distributed throughout the mucosa and submucosa, with suppressor and cytolytic activity. Peyer patches are specialized collections of lymphatic tissue primarily located in the submucosa of the ileum.

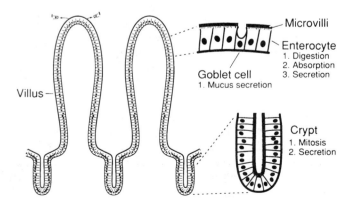

FIGURE 14-2. Two sectioned villi and a crypt from the small intestinal mucosa. (From Johnson LR. *Essential medical physiology.* New York: Raven Press, 1992:508, with permission.)

Physiology

Digestion and absorption are covered in Chapter 17, but a few points will be mentioned here. Digestion begins with mastication and salivary enzymes. Chyme in the stomach is mixed and hydrolyzed, delivering a liquid product to the duodenum, where cholecystokinin (CCK) and secretin mediate the release of bile and pancreatic secretions. Most absorption occurs in the jejunum through active and passive mechanisms. The ileum is specialized for absorption of vitamin B_{12} and bile salts, and resection of the terminal ileum, as in Crohn's disease, results in deficiencies of both. The liquid that passes through the gut consists of about 1.5 L of ingested liquid and 5 to 10 L of gut secretions (1 to 2 L salivary, 2 to 3 L gastric, 0.5 L bile, 1 to 2 L pancreatic, and 1 or more L intestinal). Eighty percent of this fluid is reabsorbed by active and passive mechanisms, primarily in the small bowel and right colon. Surgery and disease of the small bowel can disrupt this complex process.

The *bacterial population* of the gut contributes to both normal function and pathology of the gut. At birth, the gut is sterile, but immediately after birth, colonization begins. In the adult, relatively high bacterial counts exist in the oropharynx and esophagus, particularly of Gram-positive and anaerobic species. These high bacterial counts result in severe infections when perforations occur. In the stomach and small bowel, the bacterial flora also resembles the oropharynx, but smaller numbers of bacteria are present. Bacteria here are often sensitive to penicillin and first-generation cephalosporins. In the colon, there are large numbers of mainly Gram-negative and anaerobic species.

The gut bacteria function to metabolize fecal sterols, producing the short-chain fatty acids that feed colonocytes.

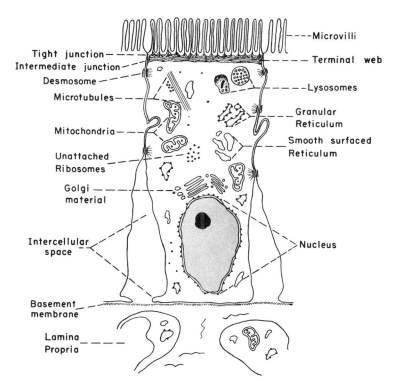

FIGURE 14-3. An intestinal epithelial cell. (From Trier JS, Rubin CE. Electron microscopy of the small intestine: a review. *Gastroenterology* 1965;49:574, with permission.)

The bacteria also metabolize bile acids, fat-soluble vitamins, vitamin B_{12}, and complex carbohydrates. In addition, the normal flora appears to be necessary for normal motility and secretions of the intestines. Obstruction, dysmotility, and antibiotics disrupt the ecology of gut flora and lead to overgrowth, which can result in malabsorption, infectious enteritis/colitis, and increased bacterial translocation. The phenomenon of bacterial translocation, particularly in the critically ill patient, is a topic of active investigation. Bacterial translocation from the gut probably contributes to the systemic inflammatory response syndrome and to infectious complications in this patient population.

Bowel Immunity

The small bowel is the largest immune organ in the body. Its major mechanisms of defense include enteric proteolytic enzymes, mucin, peristalsis, rapid epithelial turnover, and the normal flora, in addition to immune cells and antibodies. The gut-associated lymphoid tissue (GALT) is composed of aggregated tissue (Peyer patches, lymph nodes, and lymphoid follicles) and nonaggregated cells (free leukocytes).

The nonaggregated lymphoid tissue consists of intraluminal, intraepithelial, and lamina propria leukocytes. Fifteen percent to twenty-five percent of gut epithelial cells are immune cells, including lymphocytes, macrophages, mast cells, eosinophils, and neutrophils. Intraluminal antigens can induce an increase in the number of immune cells, by *trans*epithelial migration of cells after antigen presentation. The gut's B lymphocytes are specialized to produce IgA. IgA exists primarily as a dimer, connected by a J chain and connected to a molecule that aids in *trans*epithelial delivery of the antibody (Fig. 14-4). The entire complex is called "secretory IgA." The complex provides protection by binding

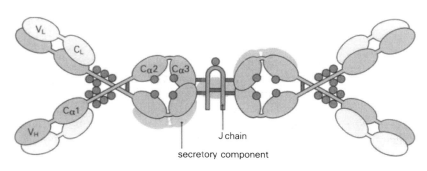

FIGURE 14-4. Structure of human secretory IgA. (From Roitt IM, Brostoff J, Male DK. *Immunology*. Philadelphia: JB Lippincott Co, 1989, with permission.)

threatening intraluminal antigens and preventing uptake of or inactivating the bound molecules or organisms.

The most specialized aggregated gut lymphoid tissues are the Peyer patches, found in the ileum. These are collections of lymphoid follicles involved in antigen presentation and processing, leading to production of mature antigen-specific B-cell populations. Specialized epithelium overlying the Peyer patch contains M cells, which phagocytose luminal contents for presentation to underlying follicles. The patches are located on the antimesenteric ileal mucosa.

Motility of the Small Bowel

Gut motility is essential for the normal functions of digestion, absorption, immune surveillance, and elimination, as well as for the prevention of pathologic overgrowth of endogenous microorganisms.

The intestinal wall contains inner circular and outer longitudinal smooth muscle layers. The smooth muscle cells have a resting membrane potential of 40 to 50 and a basal electrical activity, consisting of slow arboral waves that occur at a rate of 11 to 12 per minute. Myoelectric impulses can travel prograde through longitudinal smooth muscle via intercellular tight junctions. The control of muscular contractions is due to intrinsic and extrinsic neural stimuli, as well as hormonal influences. The *myenteric nerve plexus* exists between the circular and longitudinal muscle layers. Excitatory neurons utilize acetylcholine as their neurotransmitter while inhibitory impulses use adenosine 5'-triphospate, vasoactive intestinal polypeptide (VIP), somatostatin, serotonin, or substance P as neurotransmitters.

Interdigestive motility is characterized by the *migrating motor complex* (MMC), periodic arboral peristaltic contractions that travel from stomach to terminal ileum every 90 to 120 minutes. This is the basic motility pattern that results in arboral propagation of cellular debris, bacteria, and chyme. Interdigestive motility is divided into four phases of myoelectric activity. Phase I is quiescent; phase II contains irregular accelerating spike activity; phase III is an activity front with rapid spikes and muscular contraction (phase III is the MMC); and phase IV is the slowing of activity. In the postprandial period, this pattern is replaced for 3 to 4 hours by rapid spiking activity, similar to phase II of the interdigestive cycle. This results in a random pattern of muscular contractions, probably designed to mechanically mix the chyme and allow for absorption. Overall, the postprandial pattern does propel chyme forward somewhat, but not in the coordinated fashion of the MMC.

The MMC is initiated by the intrinsic gut nervous system, but its activity is influenced by extrinsic central nervous system (CNS) and hormonal actions, as well as by medications. Motilin, pancreatic polypeptide, somatostatin, histamine, metoclopramide, and morphine appear to initiate the MMC. Neurotensin, gastrin, CCK, insulin, and the sight or smell of food interrupt the MMC. The importance of parasympathetic regulation of gut motility is seen after vagotomy, which often results in postprandial diarrhea. This may be due to persistence of the interdigestive motility pattern after meals. Nonetheless, the denervated bowel will adapt and function relatively normally over time, highlighting the importance of hormonal and intrinsic factors in motility.

Disorders of motility usually consist of hypomotility or ileus. This is usually a temporary phenomenon due to systemic disease, medication, or surgery. Postoperative ileus is thought to result from the high catecholamine state after surgery. The MMC is disturbed for about 24 hours after laparotomy. Anesthetic agents disrupt gastric more than small bowel motility, resulting in postanesthesia nausea and vomiting. Generally, small bowel function returns first, then stomach, then colon. Bowel resection temporarily blocks peristaltic waves and the MMC at the site of resection; however, motility usually quickly returns to normal. Although most motility disturbances are temporary, occasionally a patient will present with pseudoobstruction due to a rare familial or primary hypomotility syndrome.

Gut Hormones

The gut is the largest endocrine organ in the body. Gastrointestinal (GI) organs produce and respond to myriad peptide hormones via endocrine, paracrine, and neurocrine mechanisms. Developmental and functional links between the CNS and the endocrine system in the gut are suggested by the great degree of overlap between endocrine and CNS mediators. The idea that these systems function together is referred to as the "brain-gut axis." Substance P was the first neuro/endocrine transmitter/hormone to be identified, but many others have followed, including serotonin, somatostatin, CCK, gastrin, and VIP.

Some of the gut peptides serve as neurotransmitters in the enteric nervous system or in the CNS. However, when performing paracrine or endocrine signaling, they generally act through cell-surface receptors. At least two second-messenger systems (cyclic adenosine monophosphate [cAMP] and calcium cyclic guanosine 3',5'-monophosphate [Ca/cGMP]) function in this system. Glucagon, secretin, VIP, and gastric inhibitory polypeptide are known to work via cAMP second-messenger systems. Insulin, somatostatin, and several other hormones do not have clear second-messenger systems but nonetheless have diffuse cellular effects on glucose, ion transport, enzyme activation, and DNA, RNA, and protein synthesis.

Early researchers noted the unique staining properties of the hormone-producing cells within the gut and referred to these cells by names that reflect their staining properties, such as "chromaffin" or "argentaffin." Later, the amine precursor uptake and decarboxylase (APUD) concept was developed to describe the perceived common metabolic functions of these cells. Most but not all gut endocrine cells process endogenous amines in this way, and other common cellular features are important, such as the presence of specific cytoplasmic granules, high esterase or cholinesterase content, and high glycerol-3-phosphate dehydrogenase content. Our understanding of the *in vivo* actions, interactions, and significance of the gut hormones is imperfect but improving (Fig. 14-5).

Gastrin is a peptide hormone produced by the G cell in the gastric antrum and duodenum. Gastrin release is induced by the presence of protein or calcium in the gastric lumen, or gastric antral distension. The primary action of gastrin is stimulation of gastric acid secretion by the parietal cell. A gastrin-secreting tumor, or gastrinoma, causes the Zollinger-Ellison syndrome (ZES). Gastrinomas occur most commonly in the pancreas and duodenum and are often multiple. ZES has clinical features of severe, intractable peptic ulcer disease, diarrhea, and hypokalemia.

CCK is a peptide hormone produced by I cells in the duodenum and jejunum, and less commonly in the ileum. Fat and protein in the small intestinal lumen stimulate CCK release. The best-known effects of CCK involve its regulation of biliary smooth muscle. CCK causes gallbladder contraction and relaxation of the sphincter of Oddi. CCK is also a potent stimulant of pancreatic enzyme, insulin, and glucagon secretion, and it potentiates the pancreatic exocrine stimulatory effects of secretin. It also causes relaxation of the lower esophageal sphincter, slowing of gastric emptying, and possible slowing of intestinal transit. These effects may be caused by CCK-mediated interruption of the MMC. It also seems to function as an enterogastrone, inhibiting the stimulated release of gastric acid in certain settings, such as fat intake. No CCK-secreting tumors are known, but impaired CCK release can complicate celiac disease and corrects with treatment of the disease. CCK is also found as a neurotransmitter in the CNS, where it appears to mediate anxiety and panic states.

Secretin is a helical peptide that shares structural similarities with pancreatic glucagon and VIP. It is produced by S cells, which are located throughout the small bowel. The most potent stimulant for secretin secretion is intraluminal acid, particularly with a pH level of less than 4.5. Secretin has been called "nature's antacid," as most of its effects result in decreased acidity of the duodenal contents. Secretin's actions include stimulation of the exocrine pancreas to secrete large volumes of alkaline pancreatic juice. It has synergy with CCK in pancreatic stimulation. Its biliary effects include promoting biliary bicarbonate, chloride, and water secretion and decreasing bile-salt concentration. Gastric effects include the stimulation of pepsin release and antagonism of gastrin.

Somatostatin is secreted from D cells throughout the GI tract as prosomatostatin, a prohormone that is processed into two physiologically active peptides. Somatostatin-secreting cells are densely localized around the pylorus, duodenum, and pancreatic islets. D cells have the unique feature of dendritic processes that lie in close contact with blood vessels. Somatostatin has also been found within nerves of the peripheral nervous system. Somatostatin release is stimulated by intraluminal fat, protein, acid, and sucrose. Highest secretion appears to occur during the interdigestive period.

Somatostatin has various effects on the GI tract. It inhibits several other peptide hormones and affects gut motility and absorption. In the stomach, it is released in response to duodenal acidification and inhibits gastric acid secretion. It also reduces serum gastrin levels in patients with gastrinomas. In the intestine, it inhibits amino acid absorption and blocks glucagon-induced jejunal water and electrolyte secretion. These effects may account for its therapeutic usefulness in diarrhea. In the pancreas, it inhibits release of insulin, glucagon, and pancreatic polypeptide. Somatostatin appears to cause direct feedback inhibition of insulin release. Pancreatic somatostatin release is also stimulated by glucose and amino acids, the same stimuli that cause insulin secretion. In the brain, somatostatin inhibits growth hormone and thyroid-stimulating hormone release

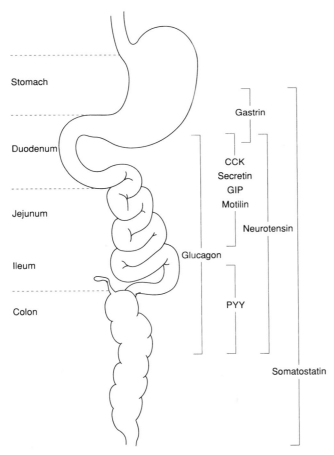

FIGURE 14-5. Distribution of gut hormones. (From Greenfield LJ, Mulholland MW, Oldham KT, et al., eds. *Surgery: scientific principles and practice,* 2nd ed. Philadelphia: Lippincott-Raven Publishers, 1997, with permission.)

from the pituitary gland. Somatostatin-secreting tumors of the pancreatic D cells cause diabetes, malabsorption, cholelithiasis, and hypochlorhydria. These rare tumors are slow growing but highly malignant. Somatostatin analog has multiple clinical uses, as discussed below.

Motilin is secreted by M cells in the upper small intestine. Motilin is released primarily in the fasting state and seems to stimulate the onset of the MMC. Fat ingestion and acid in the duodenum produce increased plasma levels. Motilin acts on smooth muscle in the upper GI tract to stimulate motility, and motilin-stimulated myoelectric complexes start in the small intestine and propagate distally. Erythromycin is a motilin agonist that is clinically useful in treating gastroparesis. Motilin causes contraction of the LES in the fasting state, probably through a neural mechanism. Motilin is also a neurotransmitter in the CNS.

VIP is a gut neurotransmitter with a similar structure to secretin and glucagon. This peptide is localized to the neural systems of the gut, CNS, peripheral nervous system, and urogenital tract. Although it is found in nerves throughout the small bowel, colon, gallbladder, and pancreas, it is particularly localized to the nerves that innervate the GI and genitourinary sphincters. VIP causes relaxation of smooth muscle in blood vessels and sphincters. It has multiple GI effects, but most prominently, it increases intestinal secretion through stimulation of adenylate cyclase. *VIPoma* is a VIP-secreting islet cell tumor that produces a clinical syndrome of watery diarrhea, hypokalemia, and achlorhydria (WDHA or Verner-Morrison syndrome). Nonpancreatic tumors of nerve, endocrine, or bronchogenic origin may also produce VIP.

Substance P is a neuropeptide found in gut nerves, gut endocrine cells, brain, and spinal cord. In the gut, substance P is released in response to increased intraluminal pressure and distension, and it stimulates contraction of GI smooth muscle.

Serotonin, or 5-hydroxytryptamine, is secreted by enterochromaffin or argentaffin cells throughout the GI tract. It is also found in mast cells, thyroid, pancreas, and lung. Serotonin acts on nerve cells and smooth muscle cells to cause smooth muscle contraction. It may be an important mediator in gut motility and may mediate some chronic diarrheal states. *Carcinoid tumors* are malignancies of the serotonin-producing cells of the appendix, small bowel, and rectum. These tumors are discussed in detail later in this chapter.

There are multiple other gut peptide hormones of minor importance, which will not be discussed here.

Clinical applications of gut peptides are becoming increasingly common, including uses in diagnostic studies and treatment of disease. Other than insulin, *somatostatin* currently has the greatest clinical application of the gut peptides. It successfully treats the symptoms of islet cell and other neuroendocrine tumors, including carcinoid, Zollinger-Ellison syndrome, VIPoma, and acromegaly. Somatostatin receptors are found on many tumor cell surfaces, and studies are underway in using somatostatin to localize and perhaps treat various cancers. Somatostatin is effective in the treatment of variceal upper GI tract bleeding. It is effective in ameliorating the symptoms of dumping syndrome, and it can convert high-output enterocutaneous fistulae to low output. Its usefulness in pancreatitis has not yet been proven.

The stimulatory effect of *secretin* on pancreatic secretions and pancreatic duct dilation has been used with ultrasound and endoscopic retrograde cholangiopancreatography (ERCP) to evaluate duct anatomy and functioning. Intravenous (i.v.) secretin stimulates gastrin release in patients with ZES and has revolutionized the diagnosis and monitoring of this disorder. At the time of this writing, however, secretin was not available in the United States. The active C-terminus sequence of gastrin, pentagastrin, has been used for evaluation of gastric acid secretory functioning and can rule out achlorhydria in patients with hypergastrinemia. Because gastrin (and CCK) appears to stimulate the growth of GI tumors, proglumide, a gastrin antagonist, is undergoing trials in the treatment of metastatic colon cancer. CCK is used with ultrasound or dimethyl iminodiacetic acid scanning to evaluate suspected acalculous gallbladder disease. Therapeutic CCK administration may prevent acalculous cholecystitis and gut mucosal atrophy in patients on total parenteral nutrition (TPN). The GI tumor stimulatory and appetite-modulating effects of CCK are likely to be harnessed in new pharmacologic agents. CCK antagonists are also being studied as antianxiety agents, due to CCK's brain activity mediating panic attacks.

Glucagon is used in emergency treatment of accidental insulin overdose, and it is used to relax the GI smooth muscle during some radiologic and endoscopic tests. It relieves spasm of the sphincter of Oddi during ERCP. Pancreatic polypeptide (PP) may be useful in treating diabetes after pancreatitis, which is characterized by glucose intolerance of the liver. PP also is used to test for vagal integrity. Macrolide antibiotics such as erythromycin are motilin agonists. They are commonly used to promote gastric emptying and GI motility.

EMBRYOLOGY

The small bowel is the anatomic segment of the gut extending from the duodenal bulb to the ileocecal valve. The portion of the duodenum proximal to and including the ampulla of Vater is derived from the *primitive* foregut, and the remainder of the small bowel is derived from the *midgut*. *Endoderm* of the primitive gut gives rise to the epithelium and glands, and the muscular and connective tissue components are derived from *splanchnic mesenchyme*.

The midgut starts as a simple tube that elongates to form a loop suspended from the dorsal abdominal wall by elongated mesentery containing the SMA. The midgut loop physiologically herniates into the proximal umbilical cord between 6 and 10 weeks of gestation, and it communicates with the yolk sac via the yolk stalk or vitelline duct during this time. While inside the umbilical cord, the midgut rotates 90 degrees counterclockwise around the SMA. It rotates a further 180 degrees during its return into the abdomen at 10 weeks. The small bowel mesentery then shortens, and the intestines are fixed to the posterior abdominal wall by peritoneal fusions, resulting in the retroperitoneal position of the ascending and descending colon and duodenum (Fig. 14-6).

The common congenital anomalies of the gut result from failure of normal rotation and fixation as described above. Failure of rotation of the midgut results in malrotation anomalies, and the small intestine resides in the right side of the abdomen while the entire colon is on the left. Failure of peritoneal fixation of intestinal segments or failure of the mesentery to shorten can lead to volvulus with bowel ischemia *in utero* or during life. Congenital atresia or stenoses of the small bowel are thought to result from just such *in utero* segmental volvulus, with scarring of the infarcted bowel segment. A Meckel diverticulum represents the remnant of the proximal yolk stalk or vitelline duct.

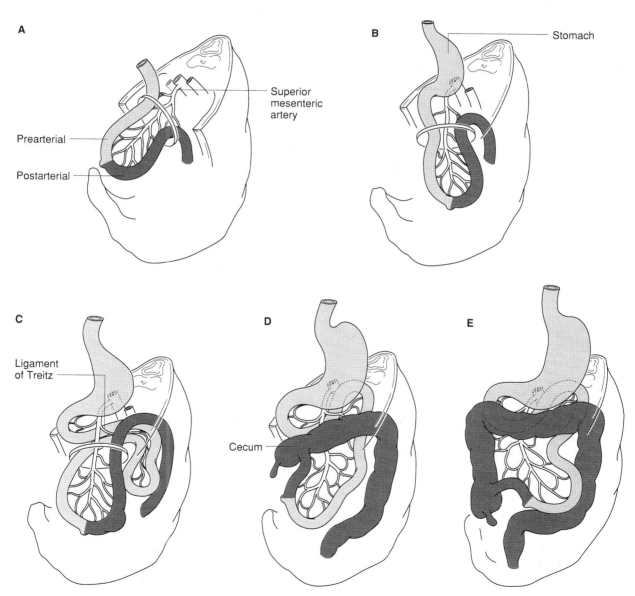

FIGURE 14-6. Normal midgut rotation **(A)** starting during the 5th week of gestation and **(E)** completing during the 12th week. (From Greenfield LJ, Mulholland MW, Oldham KT, et al., eds. *Surgery: scientific principles and practice,* 2nd ed. Philadelphia: Lippincott-Raven Publishers, 1997, with permission.)

PEDIATRIC SMALL BOWEL DISEASES

Malrotation

Malrotation refers to a spectrum of diseases in which the normal 270-degree counterclockwise rotation of the midgut around the SMA fails to occur. This leads to abnormal positioning and/or fixation of the gut. Instead of a broad mesenteric base extending from the left upper quadrant (LUQ) to the right lower quadrant (RLQ), the small bowel mesentery may be an excessively mobile, long, narrow stalk containing the SMA, with the risk of volvulus and ischemic gut. Most cases of volvulus occur in infancy, with 50% in the first month of life.

Malrotation can be asymptomatic, but when volvulus occurs, bilious vomiting occurs in two thirds of patients. Bilious vomiting in the newborn or infant is always an emergency, and 95% of patients with midgut volvulus will present with vomiting. Abdominal distention, pain, and blood per rectum (30%) or hematemesis may also be present. Radiographic examination shows a dilated stomach and duodenum proximal to the volvulus, the *double bubble sign,* with a relatively airless abdomen distally. If there is complete absence of distal air, it is impossible to differentiate malrotation from atresia, although these diseases may occur together with some frequency. In the patient who is stable, an upper GI tract contrast study is performed to further characterize the disease. The study reveals the characteristic pattern of abnormal duodenal and jejunal positioning to the right of the spine. The cecum and jejunum often lie parallel in the right upper quadrant (RUQ), connected together by Ladd bands.

Emergency laparotomy is performed after nasogastric tube decompression, administration of antibiotics, and rapid replacement of fluid and electrolytes. At surgery, a right transverse or midline laparotomy incision is made. The Ladd procedure consists of the following steps: counterclockwise rotation of the bowel (one to two complete turns) to reduce the volvulus, division of Ladd bands, resection of nonviable portions of gut with primary anastomosis, and examination for intrinsic duodenal obstruction; and appendectomy. The cecum must be mobilized from the RUQ into the LUQ by dividing the Ladd bands, which are folds of peritoneum connecting the duodenum and cecum. The bands are divided until the superior mesenteric vessels are seen, with separation of the cecum into the LUQ, leaving the duodenum in the RUQ. This maneuver broadens the mesenteric base, and postoperative adhesions fix the bowel in roughly this position, making repeat volvulus unlikely. Although this should also relieve any extrinsic duodenal obstruction, an associated intrinsic duodenal obstruction should also be ruled out. If any evidence of duodenal obstruction is present, a Foley catheter may be placed through the duodenum from above and withdrawn with the balloon inflated. An appendectomy is always performed, because the RUQ position of the appendix at the end of the case will create a diagnostic difficulty if appendicitis occurs.

If the entire midgut appears gangrenous, the surgeon must consider reduction of the volvulus, followed by a second-look operation 12 to 24 hours later. If the entire gut is still nonviable, support has traditionally been withdrawn without resection. In the modern era of TPN, however, some surgeons may opt for resection and continued support of these infants.

Other syndromes associated with malrotation of the gut are duodenal obstruction due to Ladd bands and mesocolic internal hernias. Malrotation should generally be corrected when it is discovered at any age because of the potentially devastating consequences of midgut volvulus.

Intestinal Atresia or Stenosis

Intestinal atresias or stenoses occur in about 1 in 2,700 livebirths. *Atresia* refers to a complete congenital bowel obstruction while *stenosis* refers to an incomplete obstruction. With modern care and TPN, the survival rate is greater than 90%. The pathophysiology of atresia and stenoses is felt to be *in utero* volvulus and ischemia, with scarring of the affected segment. The volvulus may result from a failure of normal rotation and fixation of the bowel, with abnormally long or mobile mesentery.

Atresias are classified into four types. Type 1 (20%) is characterized by an obstructing intraluminal diaphragm, with continuity of the muscular layer of the gut. Type 2 atresias (35%) have a fibrous cord between the two noncommunicating segments. Type 3 atresias have total separation of the two segments, with a mesenteric defect. Type 3B is an "apple peel" deformity, where the atrophic distal segment is coiled around a retrograde ileocolic artery blood supply. Type 4 (6%) refers to the presence of multiple atresias (Fig. 14-7).

Unlike other small bowel atresias and stenoses, *duodenal atresias* are due to failure of recanalization of the gut during the first trimester. The duodenal lumen is normally transiently obliterated by epithelial overgrowth early in gestation. Vacuolization of the solid cord stage normally begins at 8 to 10 weeks of gestation, and failure of this process results in duodenal obstruction. Many of these infants have associated malrotation. Duodenal obstruction may also be associated with anomalous biliary ducts or an annular pancreas. These associated anomalies may actually contribute to the obstruction, such as extrinsic obstruction of the second portion of the duodenum by annular pancreas or a preduodenal portal vein. One third of babies with duodenal atresias have other major anomalies while only 10% of babies with jejunoileal atresias have other major anomalies. Thirty percent of babies with duodenal atresia have Down syndrome. In contrast to the duodenal atresias, jejunoileal atresias are thought to be due to ischemic injury to the gut during gestation. Ten percent to twelve percent of babies with jejunoileal atresias have cystic fibrosis; a sweat test and evaluation for associated meconium ileus are indicated in all these infants.

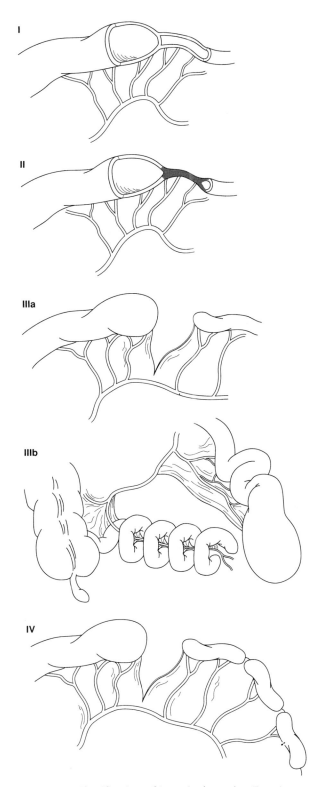

FIGURE 14-7. Classification of intestinal atresias. Type I, muscular continuity with a complete web; type II, fibrous cord with intact mesentery; type IIIa, discontinuous muscle and mesentery; type IIIb, apple-peel deformity; and type IV, multiple atresias. (From Greenfield LJ, Mulholland MW, Oldham KT, et al., eds. *Surgery: scientific principles and practice,* 2nd ed. Philadelphia: Lippincott-Raven Publishers, 1997, with permission.)

Proximal to the stenosis, the gut is extremely dilated while the distal gut is tiny. The total length of the distal segment may be decreased. One might expect maternal polyhydramnios to be a universal sign, due to lack of fetal ingestion of amniotic fluid, but polyhydramnios is present in less than 50% of cases. Most babies present with a failure to pass meconium, vomiting—often bilious—or jaundice. Twenty percent to thirty percent do pass meconium, highlighting the fact that the segment was once open *in utero*. A double bubble sign on x-ray is typical of proximal obstruction, which must be differentiated from malrotation by contrast study of the upper GI tract. More distal atresias have x-ray findings of small bowel obstruction (SBO). Upper GI tract contrast study defines the site of obstruction. Barium enema may show microcolon distal to the obstruction.

Treatment of an intestinal atresia consists of nasogastric tube decompression and fluid and electrolyte resuscitation, followed by surgery. At operation, side-to-side anastomosis is used for the duodenum, and end-to-oblique anastomosis is used for jejunoileal atresias. TPN is used postoperatively. Short-gut syndrome may occur if the gut resected is excessive, but most outcomes are good.

Intussusception

Ninety-five percent of intussusceptions occur in children and are primarily the entity called "ideopathic intussusception of infancy." Two to four cases per 1,000 births occur, and there is a 3:2 male to female preponderance. Two thirds of babies with intussusception present before 1 year of age. There are more cases in the spring and winter, when viral gastroenteritis is more frequent. Viral gastroenteritis may lead to hypertrophy of Peyer patches in the terminal ileum, which act as a lead point. Only 2% to 8% of patients have an identifiable lead point, such as a Meckel diverticulum, polyp, enteric cyst, or hematoma in Henoch-Schönlein purpura. Figure 14-8 depicts the anatomy of intussusception.

Characteristic clinical findings consist of colicky abdominal pain, vomiting, and passage of bloody mucus with a currant-jelly appearance. A sausage-shaped mass in the RUQ of the abdomen is frequently palpable. Fever is also common. After administration of a broad-spectrum antibiotic, a barium enema is the principle diagnostic and therapeutic maneuver for intussusception. Neither sedation nor anesthesia is used. A Foley catheter is inserted into the rectum, and barium is allowed to run into the colon from a height of about 3.5 feet above the table. The barium is followed using intermittent fluoroscopy. Several attempts are made until the intussusception reduces. Glucagon can be administered i.v. as a last-ditch effort to promote success of the barium reduction before surgery is undertaken.

When barium enema is unsuccessful, surgery is performed through a RLQ, muscle-splitting incision. The intussusception is reduced by pushing the lead point, never by pulling. If reduction can not be performed without

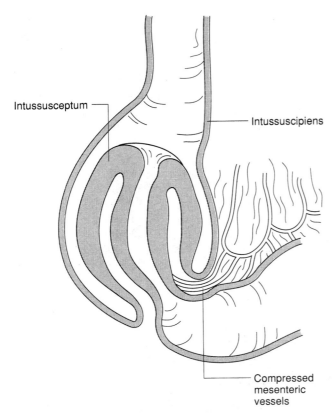

FIGURE 14-8. Intussusception. (From Greenfield LJ, Mulholland MW, Oldham KT, et al., eds. *Surgery: scientific principles and practice*, 2nd ed. Philadelphia: Lippincott-Raven Publishers, 1997, with permission.)

serosal tears, a resection is performed with primary anastomosis. If reduction is successful by operation or barium enema, 1 day of antibiotics and observation follows. New methods of air enema reduction or saline enema reduction using ultrasound are in development. Recurrence rates vary between 5% and 7%, regardless of whether barium or operative reduction is performed.

In the rare cases of adult intussusception, tumors form the lead point in 65%. Postoperative cases may involve suture lines, adhesions, or long intestinal tubes. As in pediatric cases, contrast studies, particularly barium enema, are the mainstay of diagnosis. However, reduction by hydrostatic pressure of barium should not be performed in adults; laparotomy is instead indicated.

Meckel Diverticulum

A Meckel diverticulum results from failure of the vitelline or omphalomesenteric duct to obliterate *in utero*. The vitelline duct is the primitive connection between the yolk sac and the midgut. A Meckel diverticulum is a true diverticulum, with all layers of bowel wall present. It is found arising from the antimesenteric border of the distal ileum. The "rule of twos" is a useful mnemonic for characterizing a Meckel diverticulum: It is present in 2% of people, it is about 2 inches long, it is usually located within 2 feet of the ileocecal valve, and if symptomatic, it usually presents before the age of 2. The diverticulum may contain ectopic mucosa from the stomach (25%), pancreas, duodenum, jejunum, colon, or biliary duct. Frequently, there are associated congenital anomalies such as cardiac anomalies, omphalocele, atresias, malrotation, Hirschsprung disease, and Down syndrome. A Meckel diverticulum is the most common vitelline duct anomaly, but others are depicted in Fig. 14-9.

The signs and symptoms of a Meckel diverticulum result from either (a) local effects of the ectopic mucosa, such as bleeding; (b) obstruction, which may involve intussusception with the diverticulum as a lead point; or (c) diverticulitis and its complications. In newborns, obstruction is the most common presentation, and in older infants and children, bleeding is the most common presentation. Acid produced by ectopic gastric mucosa may produce ulceration of the unprotected nearby bowel, presenting with bleeding, pain, or perforation. An unusual presentation is an incarcerated inguinal or umbilical hernia containing a Meckel diverticulum, called a Littré hernia.

The diagnostic study of choice when a Meckel diverticulum is suspected is a Meckel scan, which is a $^{99m}Tc^{99m}Tc_4$ pertechnetate radionuclide scan localizing gastric mucosa, including ectopic gastric mucosa. Sensitivity is increased if pretreatment with pentagastrin, H_2 blocker, and glucagon is administered.

Complications of a Meckel diverticulum are treated with wedge or segmental resection of the diverticulum. If ulcerations are present, a segmental resection is performed, because the ulcerations involve the normal bowel wall around the diverticulum. The diverticulum may have a separate blood supply from the primitive vitelline artery, arising separately from the small bowel mesentery. Asymptomatic Meckel diverticula are usually resected in children, but not in adults, who are unlikely to develop complications.

Necrotizing Enterocolitis

Necrotizing enterocolitis (NEC) is primarily a syndrome of low-birth-weight infants. It occurs in approximately 2.4 of 1,000 livebirths. The onset occurs during the first 2 weeks of life. Some cases of NEC can be treated medically, but 62% of babies with NEC need operations and 30% die. The pathophysiology of NEC has been quite controversial. Initially, researchers felt it was related to hypoxic or other physiologic stress during delivery or the newborn period. Umbilical artery catheters, exchange transfusions, certain drugs, and birth asphyxia were cited as etiologic factors. However, the perinatal hypoxic stresses felt to be etiologic were found to be just as common in infants without NEC. More recently, evidence has begun to accumulate that NEC

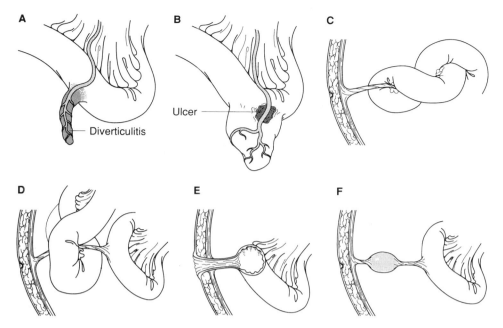

FIGURE 14-9. Yolk stalk malformations. A Meckel diverticulum can result in symptoms from **(A)** diverticulitis or **(B)** acid-induced ulceration with hemorrhage. A Meckel diverticulum may be associated with an abdominal wall band that predisposes to **(C)** volvulus and **(D)** intestinal obstruction. **E:** Patent omphalomesenteric duct. **F:** Omphalomesenteric sinus and cyst. (From Greenfield LJ, Mulholland MW, Oldham KT, et al., eds. *Surgery: scientific principles and practice,* 2nd ed. Philadelphia: Lippincott-Raven Publishers, 1997, with permission.)

is primarily an infectious disease in a compromised host with immature immune and gut barrier defenses.

Clinical findings that support the infection hypothesis include the following: (a) NEC occurs in epidemic waves, (b) these epidemics can be stopped with strict infection control measures, (c) common microorganisms are identified in these epidemics, (d) NEC develops at least 10 days postnatally when a perinatal hypoxic insult should have resolved, (e) an NEC-like disease occurs in vulnerable hosts after ingestion of clostridium, and (f) breast-feeding and enteral immunoglobulins are protective against NEC.

Grossly, the disease is characterized by mucosal necrosis and ulceration with pseudomembrane formation. Marked bowel distension, pneumatosis, skip areas, and antimesenteric perforations are other clinical features. Commonly affected sites are in the ileum and proximal colon. Babies who develop sepsis from bacterial translocation have a worse outcome, particularly when the sepsis is polymicrobial. Commonly isolated organisms include *Escherichia coli, Klebsiella,* coagulase-negative strep, and *Clostridia.* Nineteen percent of babies with NEC develop pannecrosis in which 75% of the gut dies, or more. This is almost universally fatal.

The diagnosis of NEC is usually made when an appropriate clinical scenario is combined with symptoms of abdominal distension, vomiting, heme-positive stools, temperature instability, and lethargy. Abdominal radiographs reveal *pneumatosis* in most cases (up to 98%). Other findings that support the diagnosis include the presence of reducing substances in the stool, portal vein gas, pneumoperitoneum, intraperitoneal fluid, and a fixed persistently dilated loop on abdominal x-ray. A negative breath hydrogen test result is sometimes used for ruling out NEC. In babies with a questionable diagnosis, upper GI contrast study or ultrasound may be helpful.

Unless perforation or necrosis has occurred, initial management of NEC is nonoperative. A nasogastric tube, TPN, and antibiotics based on stool, peritoneal, and blood cultures are given. Vancomycin/gentamycin and vancomycin/cefotaxime are typical regimens. These choices reflect the common presence of coagulase-negative staphylococci, whose delta toxins may contribute to the pathogenesis of NEC. Patients are closely monitored for evidence of intestinal necrosis, and if this does not occur, feedings are slowly resumed. Stools are tested for reducing substances or blood, and if either is present, the feedings are stopped. Indications for operation include perforation, unrelenting sepsis, erythema of the abdominal wall, abdominal mass, a fixed dilated loop on x-ray, positive paracentesis, portal vein gas, and clinical deterioration. Paracentesis is performed in patients failing to improve with medical management, and if yellow-brown fluid with bacteria on a Gram stain is found, an operation is immediately undertaken.

Operative management usually involves a right transverse supraumbilical incision. Peritoneal cultures for aerobic and anaerobic organisms are collected. The entire gut is examined, and all unquestionably necrotic or perforated segments are resected. The guiding principle is bowel conservation. Also, every effort is made to preserve the ileocecal valve. The most proximal site of resection is brought out as a diverting ostomy. When pannecrosis is found, a proximal diverting jejunostomy may improve the viability of apparently necrotic gut, although some surgeons will simply close the abdomen and forgo further treatment.

The long-term consequences of NEC include strictures at the sites of healed ischemic segments. As many as 25% of patients may develop clinically significant strictures, particularly in the colon and terminal ileum.

Meconium Ileus

Meconium ileus is usually an early manifestation of cystic fibrosis (CF), a common autosomal-recessive genetic disease caused by a defective chloride channel. Ten percent to twenty percent of newborns with CF present with meconium ileus. Meconium ileus is responsible for about 30% of neonatal bowel obstructions. The obstruction begins *in utero*. It is caused by impaction with abnormal meconium concentration, containing decreased water and increased albumin.

Babies present with constipation, distension, and bilious vomiting in the first days of life. The rectum and anus are small. Abdominal x-ray reveals obstruction and a "ground-glass" appearance of the abdomen. No contrast should be given from above, but a gastrograffin enema is both diagnostic and therapeutic. Microcolon and pellets of meconium in the terminal ileum are found. Often, the infant will pass the meconium after the enema is administered. Enemas may be repeated multiple times in uncomplicated meconium ileus. A sweat test showing increased chloride and sodium makes the diagnosis of CF. About 50% of cases are complicated by perforation of the ileum. Other complications include volvulus, intestinal atresia, gangrene, meconium pseudocyst at the site of perforation, or meconium peritonitis. *Meconium peritonitis* is a chemical (aseptic) peritonitis secondary to prenatal bowel perforation. These babies may be very ill with massive distension and erythema and induration of the abdominal wall. The massive distension sometimes leads to respiratory compromise.

Complicated meconium ileus requires surgery. Before surgery, antibiotics are given and hydration is performed. At surgery, the ileum is found to be packed with tarlike meconium, which is inspissated into a solid gray mass more distally. There may be microcolon, due to obstruction and disuse. In the absence of perforation or peritonitis, treatment may consist only of T-tube ileostomy for irrigation. In complicated cases, all compromised bowel is resected, with an endileostomy and mucus fistula for irrigation. The ileostomy may be closed in 3 weeks.

Meconium plug syndrome is a variant of meconium ileus found in patients without CF, but with colonic dysmotility due to immaturity, Hirschsprung disease, neonatal small-left-colon syndrome, or left-sided megacolon. These infants present with little to no meconium and distension. Gastrograffin enema reveals a meconium plug, usually at the splenic flexure. The enema often stimulates passage of the plug.

Duplications

A *duplication* is an anomaly in which any portion of the GI tract has an adjacent hollow viscus sharing a common wall with the true structure. The embryologic etiology of duplications is not well understood, and theories of abnormal splitting of the notochord and abnormal recanalization of the bowel have been proposed. Duplications take two forms: Most (75%) are enteric cysts that do not communicate with the bowel lumen, and the remaining (25%) are true tubular duplications that may or may not communicate. All duplications contain some sort of GI mucosa. Ectopic gastric mucosa is common, and ulcerations complicate those duplications that communicate with normal bowel.

Two thirds of patients present within the first 2 years of life. Symptoms include the following: partial intestinal obstruction, abdominal pain due to large quantities of fluid accumulating within a noncommunicating cyst, bleeding from severe peptic ulceration, and compression of vascular or other adjacent structures. Duplications in the chest can cause respiratory compromise. The diagnosis is often made by ultrasound in infants. Computed tomography (CT) scans are also helpful. Ten percent of patients have more than one duplication. Treatment consists of complete excision or enterotomy and partial excision with mucosal stripping. Internal drainage with stripping of ectopic mucosa is also an accepted form of treatment.

Omphalocele and Gastroschisis

Omphalocele describes the herniation of bowel through a defect at the base of the umbilical cord into a sac composed of peritoneum and amnion. *Gastroschisis* is an abdominal wall defect lateral to the umbilical cord with bowel protruding, but no peritoneal sac. The combined incidence is probably about 1 in 4,000 livebirths. The etiology of these conditions is controversial, but the cause of omphalocele is probably failure of advancement of the lateral mesoderm around the umbilical cord or persistence of the body stalk. Gastroschisis is more poorly understood, but one theory states that it is actually an *in utero* rupture of an omphalocele, and another theory postulates that it is due to dissolution of one of the umbilical veins, with underdevelopment of a hypoperfused portion of the abdominal wall.

Infants with omphalocele frequently have associated trisomy 13, 18, or 21 syndrome. Malrotation is common in both conditions. Other associated anomalies include the prune belly syndrome and the Beckwith-Wiedemann syndrome. Gastroschisis is associated with fewer anomalies, except for undescended testes and intestinal atresias due to ischemia of the herniated gut *in utero*. Twenty percent of patients with gastroschisis develop NEC.

Both of these anomalies are now frequently diagnosed by fetal ultrasound, which can show them as early as 13 weeks of gestation, when the midgut has normally returned to the abdominal cavity. *Maternal α-fetoprotein* levels are elevated in both conditions. Elective delivery, often by cesarean section, results in improved outcomes. Once the infant is delivered, the repair of a gastroschisis is a relative emergency while omphalocele repair is only urgent, not emergent, because a sac protects the herniated bowel. One major difference between these two conditions is the presence of the herniated bowel. In gastroschisis, the herniated bowel has been in contact with the urea-rich amniotic fluid and may be severely thickened, cracked, and friable as a result. The bowel in omphalocele is normal; however, omphalocele cases are often complicated by the high rate of associated anomalies.

TPN and nasogastric decompression are instituted immediately for infants with both defects. Conservation of body heat can be a major problem in these infants, and warm saline gauze or occlusive plastic wraps are instituted. Hydration is performed and antibiotics are given.

Surgical repair options include primary repair for small defects or delayed primary closure with skin flaps or Silastic sheeting (silo). Construction of an abdomen-enlarging pouch or silo allows for gradual reduction of the pouch contents into the abdomen at the bedside, with gradual stretching of the abdominal wall. The limitations on abdominal wall closure are usually respiratory compromise and impaired venous return to the heart due to inferior vena cava compression when abdominal pressures are excessive. Closure of skin results only in a large hernia that can be repaired in a staged fashion during childhood.

BENIGN DISEASES OF THE SMALL BOWEL

Small Bowel Obstruction

SBO is defined as a failure of aboral passage of bowel contents due to mechanical blockage. Mechanical SBO is a common surgical emergency; however, with modern management, mortality rate has been reduced to 5%. There are numerous etiologies that lead to mechanical SBO (Table 14-1). External hernias were previously the most common cause, but now 75% of SBO cases are due to adhesions from previous surgery. Five percent of patients who undergo abdominal surgery will eventually develop an SBO, and 15% of those who do will develop recurrent SBOs.

Investigations into the mechanisms of adhesion formation have revealed foreign-body reactions to sutures, intestinal contents, and talc within adhesions. Serosal irritation or injury appears to result in fibroblast and inflammatory cell infiltration. Tissue plasminogen activator appears to prevent adhesions.

Malignancies are responsible for about 10% of obstructions, and abdominal wall hernias for 5% to 10%. Other etiologies include internal hernia, volvulus, Crohn's disease, intraabdominal abscess or mass, intussusception, radiation stricture, foreign body, gallstone ileus, Meckel diverticulum, intramural hematoma, and mesenteric ischemia. Mechanical obstruction must be differentiated from paralytic ileus, because the two diseases are managed differently.

Symptoms of SBO include crampy intermittent abdominal pain, nausea and vomiting, distension, and obstipation. The site of the obstruction will influence the constellation of symptoms, with profuse bilious vomiting, minimal distention, and late obstipation in proximal obstruction versus scant increasingly feculent vomiting, obstipation, and prominent distension in distal obstruction. In early obstruction, bowel sounds are hyperactive but become hypoactive as the obstruction progresses. Mild diffuse tenderness is expected in uncomplicated SBO, but focal tenderness and signs of peritonitis develop if transmural necrosis complicates the obstruction. Other signs of bowel compromise that require urgent exploration include fever, leukocytosis, and hemodynamic instability. An indolent presentation is more likely due to malignancy or radiation

TABLE 14-1. CLASSIFICATION OF ADULT MECHANICAL INTESTINAL OBSTRUCTIONS[a]

Intraluminal	Extrinsic
Foreign bodies	Adhesions
Barium inspissation (colon)	Congenital
Bezoar	Ladd or Meckel bands
Inspissated feces	Postoperative
Gallstone	Postinflammatory
Meconium (cystic fibrosis)	Hernias
Parasites	External
Other (e.g., swallowed objects, enteroliths)	Internal
	Volvulus
Intussusception	External mass effect
Polypoid, exophytic lesions	Abscess
	Annular pancreas
Intramural	Carcinomatosis
Congenital	Endometriosis
Atresia, stricture, or stenosis	Pregnancy
Web	Pancreatic pseudocyst
Intestinal duplication	
Meckel diverticulum	
Inflammatory process	
Crohn's disease	
Diverticulitis	
Chronic intestinal ischemia or postischemic stricture	
Radiation enteritis	
Medication induced (nonsteroidal antiinflammatories, potassium chloride tablets)	
Neoplasms	
Primary bowel (malignant or benign)	
Secondary (metastases, especially melanoma)	
Traumatic	
Intramural hematoma of duodenum	

[a]From Greenfield LJ, Mulholland MW, Oldham KT, et al., eds. *Surgery: scientific principles and practice* 2nd ed. Philadelphia Lippincott-Raven Publishers, 1997:819, with permission.

enteritis. Severe hypovolemia and hypochloremic, as well as hypokalemic metabolic alkalosis are frequently present in simple SBO, due to intravascular volume depletion by vomiting and fluid losses into the intestinal lumen. Leukocytosis is a late finding.

An abdominal x-ray or an obstruction series will usually make the diagnosis of SBO. These plain films should always include supine and decubitus or upright films. The obstruction series in SBO usually shows distended small bowel (more than 3 cm) with air-fluid levels and a paucity of colonic air. Paralytic ileus may be differentiated from SBO by the lack of a distally decompressed, or "airless," colon on plain films. However, this distinction is blurred by the fact that colonic air can be consistent with early or partial obstruction. *Closed loop obstruction* due to volvulus or multiple adhesions may be noted on plain film, and exploration should be carried out urgently. Upper GI series (UGIS) with small bowel follow-through or enteroclysis can be helpful in differentiating partial from complete SBO. Thin barium (not gastrograffin) is used unless perforation or strangulation is suspected. *Enteroclysis,* or small bowel enema, is a GI contrast study in which a tube is advanced into the small bowel and thin barium is instilled with serial images taken. It has increased sensitivity in identifying a site of obstruction or a mucosal abnormality, compared to UGIS with small bowel follow-through. Finally, barium enema may be helpful if colonic obstruction is suspected.

The use of CT scan in SBO is controversial, but this modality is increasingly utilized as a part of the conservative management of SBO. A CT scan with oral and i.v. contrast is helpful when the diagnosis of inflammatory bowel disease (IBD) or malignancy is suspected. Other potential benefits of CT scanning include increased sensitivity for the identification of free air, increased accuracy in identifying the anatomic site of obstruction, and a somewhat improved ability to see signs of bowel ischemic necrosis, termed *strangulation obstruction* (although frank bowel necrosis can be missed on CT). Again, it is important to stress that clinical signs of strangulation (tachycardia, focal abdominal tenderness, fever, and leukocytosis) in the obstructed patient warrant exploration. The pursuit of imaging studies in this setting constitutes an unjustified delay.

Prompt diagnosis and treatment of SBO is important because simple SBO can progress to strangulation and bowel necrosis. The pathophysiology of strangulation obstruction includes the following steps: progressive distension of the bowel with gas and fluid; bacterial overgrowth; progressive blockage of lymphatic, then venous, then arterial gut circulation; and finally ischemic necrosis with bacterial translocation, sepsis, and death. Because accumulation of gas and fluid in the bowel lumen is the first step toward strangulation, early decompression with a nasogastric tube is mandatory.

Multiple factors contribute to intraluminal fluid accumulation in SBO patients. Inhibition of absorption and stimulation of secretion are caused by the following factors: increased intraluminal pressure (particularly the high pressures reached in closed loop obstruction), release of paracrine and hormone substances (VIP, prostaglandins), changes in blood flow, and bacterial toxins. Static intestinal contents are digested, leading to increasing intraluminal osmolarity and further secretion of fluid into the gut. In response to increased pressure, blood flow initially increases, but eventually the intraluminal pressure exceeds intramural capillary and venous pressure, with edema, bacterial invasion, inflammation, and further blood-flow compromise. The source of gaseous distension in SBO is swallowed air (80%); however, methane and hydrogen disulfide are present in small quantities.

The bacterial population of the gut contributes to the pathophysiology of obstruction. Obstruction, dysmotility, and antibiotics disrupt the ecology of gut flora and lead to overgrowth. In obstruction, bacterial endotoxins likely stimulate secretion, possibly through prostaglandin, neuroendocrine mediators, or nitric oxide. In addition, the myoelectric function of the gut is altered during obstruction, with initial increased contraction against the obstruction followed by receptive relaxation of the gut proximal to the obstruction. These pathophysiologic responses to obstruction explain the possible complications of untreated SBO, namely severe dehydration, electrolyte disturbances, strangulation obstruction, sepsis, and death.

Today, initial treatment in SBO is usually nonoperative. The cornerstones of management are nasogastric decompression, i.v. fluid resuscitation, serial abdominal examinations and serial abdominal x-rays. This nonoperative approach is appropriate in most patients, once signs of strangulation and incarcerated hernias have been ruled out. This approach is ideal in the patient who has had previous abdominal surgery. Sixty-five percent to eighty percent of adhesive obstructions resolve with nonoperative management. Long intestinal tubes are now seldom used but can be helpful in recurrent cases.

Complete obstruction (signified by absence of flatus or bowel movements) and obstruction in the absence of previous surgery are much less likely to resolve with nonoperative management, and early operation is indicated (24 to 48 hours). For any patients not undergoing immediate operation, serial abdominal examinations at least every 12 hours are required. Focal tenderness, peritoneal signs, fever, leukocytosis, and hemodynamic instability indicate bowel ischemia and failure of nonoperative management.

Broad-spectrum antibiotics are indicated, as soon as the decision to operate has been established. The use of early routine antibiotics in patients who are managed nonoperatively is controversial. Some feel antibiotics may delay appropriate operative intervention by masking progression to strangulation obstruction while others argue for benefits of decreased rates of bacterial translocation, wound infection, and intraabdominal sepsis in those patients who do progress.

The abdomen may be opened via a transverse or midline incision. There may be an advantage to avoiding a previous incision site due to adhesions to the anterior abdominal wall. Slow sharp dissection is used to lyse adhesions. The point of obstruction is identified by working from distal decompressed bowel toward proximal dilated bowel. Once the obstruction is relieved by resection or lysis of adhesions at the obstructing point, further dissection is avoided, unless exploration is for recurrent SBO. Nonviable bowel must be resected, and questionable areas can be inspected with mesenteric Doppler imaging or i.v. fluorescein dye and a Wood lamp. In volvulus or other closed loop obstruction, some researchers recommend isolating the rotated segment with proximal and distal clamps before manipulating it.

Special cases of bowel obstruction include early *postoperative SBO*. SBO within 4 weeks of surgery is a special case occurring following fewer than 1% of operations. It is also due to adhesions in 90% of cases and usually will resolve with nonoperative management (75%). Small bowel contrast studies can be helpful in this situation, because 2 to 3 weeks after laparotomy is the period of densest and most vascular adhesions. Avoiding a second exploration at this time is desirable unless signs of strangulation appear.

SBO in the setting of intraabdominal *malignancy* is often due to adhesions rather than cancer recurrence. Therefore, despite the wisdom of avoiding invasive procedures in the terminally ill, one must remember that successful palliation is possible with surgical intervention in selected patients.

Gallstone ileus is a rare condition characterized by a fistulous tract between the gallbladder fundus and the duodenum. A large gallstone may then enter the intestine directly and obstruct it. Air in the biliary tree or an ectopic calcification on x-ray suggests the diagnosis. Cholecystectomy is usually not performed at the time of initial operation, in which the stone is simply removed through an enterotomy.

Functional or *neurogenic obstruction* occurs due to a lack of coordinated peristalsis, without mechanical occlusion. This may result in paralytic ileus of the small intestine or pseudoobstruction of the large intestine (Ogilvie syndrome). Paralytic ileus may be due to surgery, sepsis, electrolyte abnormalities, drugs (psychotropic, autonomic, cardiac, narcotics), ureteral and biliary colic, retroperitoneal hematoma, spinal cord injury, or myocardial infarction. Patients who present with acute or chronic ileus in the absence of surgical manipulation should be questioned about neurological and endocrine diseases, medications, and signs of infection or occult malignancy.

Postoperative ileus is the most common form of ileus and may result from unbalanced autonomic stimulation to the gut after surgery. Because GI tract secretions do not slow postoperatively, nasogastric decompression is necessary until motility returns to normal. This is signified by decreasing nasogastric tube output and flatus or bowel movements. Generally, small bowel function returns first, then stomach, then colon. Therefore, bowel sounds originating in the intestine may be present before a patient is ready for nasogastric tube removal or feeding. Ileus or delay in gastric emptying may sometimes be ameliorated with the prokinetic agents metoclopramide, cisapride, or erythromycin (a motilin agonist).

Radiation Enteritis

Radiation therapy is increasingly employed in the modern multimodal approach to malignancy. Nearly all patients who receive radiation to the abdomen will have early symptoms of radiation injury to the bowel, and 5% to 20% will develop long-term problems related to radiation enteritis. Patients receiving over 50 Gy of radiation are most likely to develop problems of radiation enteritis. Diabetes mellitus and hypertension are felt to predispose patients to radiation enteritis. Previous abdominal surgery is also a risk factor, due to adhesions that immobilize loops of bowel within the radiation field.

Ionizing radiation injures gut tissues through various mechanisms. DNA, RNA, membranes, and intracellular fibers are all injured. DNA damage appears to result in the majority of cell death. DNA damage can also result in mutations that increase the malignant potential and decrease the mitotic ability of the damaged cell. Due to this mechanism, cells that divide frequently are particularly affected by radiation damage, such as stem cells in the intestinal crypts and intestinal lymphatic cells. In addition, radiation treatment damages blood vessels, further contributing to bowel injury. Subendothelial proliferation and medial thickening of intestinal blood vessels have been found. Excessive scar tissue further blocks blood flow and limits repair mechanisms.

Pelvic malignancies, particularly gynecologic and urologic cancers, are the most common causes for abdominal radiation therapy. Therefore, the rectum and ileum are commonly injured segments of bowel. Because lymphatic tissue is particularly susceptible to radiation damage, the ileum is disproportionately affected due to the high concentration of lymphatic tissue in Peyer patches. If laparotomy is performed for primary therapy of the malignancy, exclusion of the bowel from the pelvis with mesh or other suspension material can be performed at the time of surgery to prevent radiation enteritis.

Patients may develop nausea, vomiting, diarrhea, and cramping pain during radiation therapy. These symptoms are very common, occurring in as many as 75% of patients. Long-term effects (the syndrome of radiation enteritis) can result in small bowel obstruction, malabsorption, and fistulas. Any bowel surgery in a patient with previous radiation exposure may be complicated by perforation, anastomotic dehiscence, fistula, or other complications related to the fragility of the exposed bowel.

Grossly, irradiated bowel may exhibit loss of normal vascular patterns, telangiectasias, edema, contact bleeding, ulcerations, or granularity. Chronic changes include thickening and foreshortening of the bowel, and fistula or stricture formation. Early on, endoscopy is the best study to make the diagnosis, revealing the changes noted above. In the chronic phase of radiation enteritis, oral contrast studies of the bowel, and angiography can reveal scarring, mucosal abnormalities, vascular irregularity, crowding, beading, or focal obstruction.

Therapy for radiation enteritis depends on the site of damage causing symptoms. Proctitis may be treated with supportive measures to reduce diarrhea, steroid enemas, or argon laser treatments. Rectal resection for proctitis leads to frequent and serious complications, and diverting colostomy is generally preferred if symptoms are unbearable. If the disease involves the small intestine, partial recurring SBO may occur, but an operation should be avoided whenever possible. If an operation must be performed, it is recommended that lysis of adhesions and bowel manipulation be kept to a minimum, unless an attempt to definitively resect the abnormal bowel is undertaken. Such resection may be warranted for severely symptomatic disease. When bowel resection is undertaken for radiation enteritis, all involved bowel should be resected, with the anastomosis constructed in grossly normal bowel. High rates of anastomotic leak have been reported.

Any patient undergoing elective laparotomy for radiation enteritis should have a preoperative evaluation of the entire bowel to define the extent of disease, as well as studies done to rule out recurrence of the primary malignancy. This usually includes endoscopy, small bowel contrast study, and barium enema. In some cases, preoperative evaluation of the urinary tract or placement of ureteral stents is indicated.

The following are important guidelines in the management of radiation enteritis. First, avoid surgery if possible. Preoperatively and postoperatively, nutrition should be optimized, with TPN if needed. A good mechanical and antibiotic bowel preparation should be performed before elective surgery. In the operating room, adhesiolysis and bowel trauma should be minimized. Abnormal or obstructed bowel should be resected, rather than bypassed, and fistulas should be resected, rather than simply closed. Meticulous operative technique should be used for anastomoses, using nonirradiated bowel for at least one end. Also, any anastomosis should be labeled with a radiopaque marker. One should avoid using irradiated bowel for stomas. With regard to postoperative management, long tubes for intestinal decompression, delayed feeding, and antibiotic use have all been suggested but remain controversial.

Diverticular Disease of the Small Bowel

Except for Meckel diverticula, most small bowel diverticula are acquired pulsion pseudodiverticula associated with increasing age. Like sigmoid colon diverticula, most are located on the mesenteric aspect of the bowel, at locations where blood vessels perforate the muscularis propria. They may be complicated by infection, obstruction, perforation, and bacterial overgrowth.

Acquired small bowel diverticula are most common in the duodenum. Duodenal diverticula may be extraluminal or intraluminal (windsock), and 75% of extraluminal diverticula are juxtaampullary. Perhaps due to bacterial overgrowth, they are associated with higher rates of cholelithiasis and choledocholithiasis. In contrast, jejunoileal diverticula are rare. They may be multiple and are usually asymptomatic. Associated bacterial overgrowth occasionally leads to malabsorption. Enteroclysis (small bowel enema) is the study of choice for making the diagnosis. Complications of diverticulitis, obstruction, or perforation are treated similarly to those associated with colonic diverticular disease.

Enterocutaneous Fistula

A *fistula* is an abnormal communication between two organs, usually resulting from focal injury or inflammation. Enterocutaneous fistula is one of the most lethal nonmalignant diseases in general surgery, with a mortality rate of 10% to 15%. Etiologies include postoperative (80% to 85%) due to anastomotic dehiscence or leak or due to a partial or full-thickness bowel injury; Crohn's disease (5% to 8%); cancer (3% to 5%); infection (3% to 5%); iatrogenic (2%); and radiation (1% to 2%). Enterocutaneous fistulae usually occur following abdominal surgery and present through the surgical wound. Malnutrition, metabolic abnormalities, infection, distal obstruction, and prior radiation exposure predispose to fistula formation. Measures to avoid enterocutaneous fistula formation in those at high risk are preferable and include preoperative nutritional support and a thorough bowel preparation before elective surgery.

The morbidity and mortality associated with fistulae are related to electrolyte abnormalities, malnutrition, and sepsis. A *high-output fistula* is defined as one that drains greater than 500 mL of enteric contents per day. High-output fistulae are more likely to result in complications while low-output fistulae (less than 200 mL per day) have little potential to cause electrolyte and volume problems. All fistulae may be associated with severe nutritional deficiencies, because of the accompanying inflammatory or infectious process, which increases metabolic demands.

The diagnosis of an enterocutaneous fistula is usually apparent when enteric contents are found at the site of a skin defect or a surgical wound. CT scan may help to define the etiology and anatomy of the problem and to rule out an associated abscess. Optimal management of the fistula often requires a formal GI contrast study. A UGIS with small bowel follow-through will sometimes define the exit site of a fistula and can identify leak of contrast into an associated abscess cavity. Some fistulae may be missed by an upper GI study, and a fistulogram (contrast injection through the fistula skin site) may be needed. One must wait about 7 to 10 days after formation of the fistula before performing a fistulogram, as the study can exacerbate an intraperitoneal leak if performed before the tract is well epithelialized. A fistulogram may identify the bowel exit site of the fistula or the presence of anastomotic dehiscence or distal obstruction. This study can be invaluable in planning and performing an elective fistula closure operation.

Initial treatment of an enterocutaneous fistula includes broad-spectrum antibiotics, bowel rest, skin care, and optimization of nutrition. With this conservative management, many enterocutaneous fistulae will close spontaneously. If sepsis is present and no drainable collection can be identified and promptly treated, a laparotomy is indicated, often with diverting proximal ostomy. Mortality is higher in those patients who require emergent surgery for uncontrolled sepsis.

Thirty percent to fifty percent of fistulae close with nonoperative therapy. Those less likely to close are associated with complete anastomotic disruption, distal obstruction, or an adjacent abscess cavity. Other situations in which conservative therapy frequently fails include underlying Crohn's disease or radiation enteritis, a short epithelialized tract (less than 2 cm), foreign bodies, or a bowel opening greater than 1 cm in diameter. Nutritional status, as reflected by serum transferrin level, has been found to predict which fistulae are more likely to heal: Levels of 200 mg/dL are associated with closure, and levels of 150 mg/dL fail to heal. Most patients are initially treated with 5 to 6 weeks of bowel rest, TPN, and control of sepsis.

Standard enteral feeding increases the output from enterocutaneous fistulae and helps to keep them open. Bowel rest is therefore the mainstay of nonoperative therapy. TPN has significantly improved outcomes in these patients. TPN has been proven to increase the spontaneous closure rate of enterocutaneous fistulae, but not to decrease mortality. In addition, TPN improves the nutritional status of patients who eventually require surgical fistula closure and probably improves outcome in that group as well. Some fistulae have been known to close with elemental enteral nutrition, but currently TPN is more commonly used.

Patients with fistulae have very high protein and calorie requirements. Proximal fistulae may also lead to losses of large quantities of fluid, sodium, potassium, and acetate. Antacids and somatostatin are frequently used to decrease the volume of enteral secretions. Somatostatin has not been proven to increase the percentage of fistulae that will close, but it may decrease the healing time in those that do. If a fistula fails to resolve with conservative therapy, an elective operation is performed. Often these are long and complex operations requiring "plastic surgical" abdominal wall closure. Prolonged ileus and malabsorption due to atrophic gastrointestinal mucosa may be present postoperatively, making decompressive gastrostomy tube and feeding jejunostomy tube placement helpful.

Crohn's Disease

IBD refers to a spectrum of chronic inflammatory diseases of the GI tract. Traditionally, IBD has been subdivided into Crohn's disease and ulcerative colitis (UC). More recently, the histological and clinical distinctions between these two entities have begun to blur, and individual patients may display characteristics of both diseases. Although this chapter will focus on Crohn's disease and Chapter 15 will focus on UC, they are best thought of as a continuous spectrum of chronic IBD with overlapping features.

Crohn's disease, or *regional enteritis,* is a transmural inflammatory disease that can affect any portion of the gut, from mouth to anus. The terminal ileum is most commonly affected (70%), with or without colonic involvement. The epidemiology of Crohn's disease includes a prevalence of 10 to 70 people per 100,000 population. It occurs more commonly in industrialized nations and among people of Jewish heritage. Although Mendelian inheritance patterns are absent, close relatives of patients are at an increased risk. The disease has a bimodal age distribution, with common ages at diagnosis of 15 to 30 years or 55 to 60 years. Men and women are equally affected.

The etiology of the disease is unknown, although an autoimmune or infectious etiology is most likely. Patients have been found to have multiple alterations of the immune system; however, no primary abnormality is consistently present. Lymphocyte-mediated cytotoxicity against colonic epithelial cells and antibodies against colonic cells have been discovered in patients with Crohn's disease, but not against small bowel enterocytes. One theory proposes the intestinal immune system may have disturbed immunoregulation, with insufficient suppressor T-cell function or overaggressive helper T cells. Unregulated immune responses to routine GI antigens could cause bystander injury to the gut. It is clear that the lamina propria of the gut with active Crohn's disease has a two- to threefold increase in lymphocytes, particularly IgG-producing B cells, as well as an increased number of mast cells and neutrophils.

The most common site of active disease is the *terminal ileum.* Grossly, it is characterized by grayish serosa with red, conspicuous vessels, thick-walled rubbery texture, and mesenteric fat reaching over the antimesenteric bowel wall (fat creeping). Cobble-stoning and aphthoid ulcerations of the mucosa are present. Involvement may be discontinuous (skip lesions). The mesentery is thickened, with prominent lymph nodes. Histologically, *transmural inflammation* of the bowel, with ulcerations, and lymphoid aggregates are found. Sixty percent of patients have submucosal noncaseating granulomas with occasional giant cells. Extraintestinal involvement includes joint (polyarthritis, ankylosing spondylitis), skin (erythema nodosum, pyoderma gangrenosum), and eye disease (iritis, uveitis), as well as sclerosing cholangitis. An increased incidence of gallstones

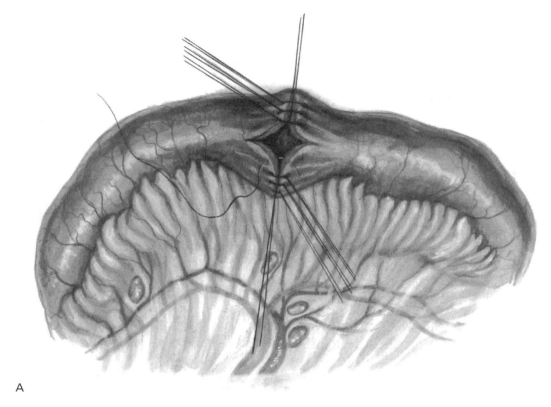

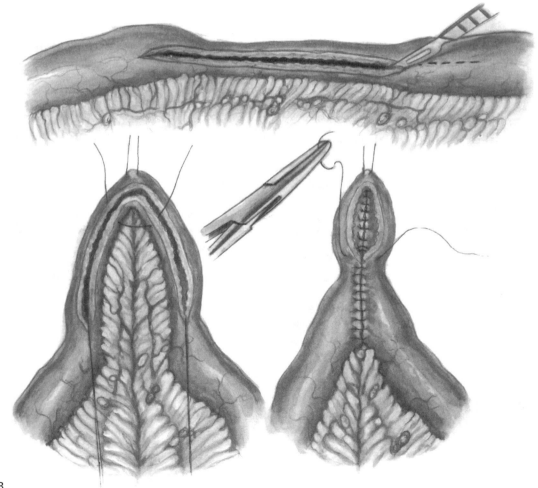

results from the failure to reabsorb bile salts with terminal ileal disease. Differentiating Crohn's colitis from ulcerative colitis may pose a difficult pathologic diagnosis.

Clinical features of Crohn's disease include abdominal pain, diarrhea, anemia, malabsorption, protein-calorie malnutrition, gallstones, vitamin B_{12} and folate deficiencies, renal oxalate stones, and short-gut syndrome in extreme cases. Complications leading to surgery include obstruction, perforation with abscess formation, fistula formation, perirectal abscess, fistula or ulceration, cancer (less common than in ulcerative colitis), and toxic megacolon. Diagnosis and workup require evaluation of the entire bowel using colonoscopy, upper endoscopy if indicated, barium enema, and UGIS with small bowel follow-through. Diagnosis is confirmed by pathologic evaluation of biopsy specimens. CT scanning is useful if fistula or abscess is suspected.

Crohn's disease is a chronic and incurable medical disease. It is characterized by remissions and flares of symptomatology; asymptomatic disease requires no treatment. Pain medication, antispasmotics, antidiarrheals, antibiotics, and antiinflammatory or immunosuppressive drugs are mainstays of therapy for active disease. The most common agents used to suppress disease flares are prednisone, topical steroids, sulfasalazine, azathioprine, 6-MP, methotrexate, and cyclosporine. Enteral or parenteral nutrition support is also crucial during flares. Modern therapy for Crohn's disease is primarily medical; surgery is reserved for serious complications only. The primary indications for operation in small bowel Crohn's disease are obstruction, fistula, perforation with abscess formation, and malignancy. The goal of surgery is to minimize the length of bowel resected.

Obstruction is the most common indication for operation, occurring in 30% to 50% of patients. It usually involves the small bowel. Acute obstruction may be due to inflammation during a disease flare and may resolve with aggressive medical treatment. Chronic obstruction may be due to a fibrous stricture at the site of previous inflammation. CT scan is nearly always indicated and is helpful in distinguishing cases that may be managed nonoperatively from those requiring urgent operation. Strictures causing partial obstruction may be multiple, and surgical therapy includes examination of the entire small bowel. This may require extensive lysis of adhesions. Because some strictures may not be apparent from the serosal bowel surface, some surgeons recommend evaluating the entire small bowel using an intraluminal balloon catheter filled with 8 mL of water to detect all strictured areas.

An obstruction may require bowel resection and reanastomosis or may be managed with stricturoplasty. Resection of the grossly diseased bowel is still considered the gold standard of treatment. Stricturoplasty is probably not a good idea in situations where an abscess or fistula is present, as well as in severe malnutrition with a serum albumin level of less than 3.0 g/dL. Nonetheless, stricturoplasty allows for conservation of bowel length and is particularly useful when multiple strictures are present. In general, if the stricture is 12 cm or longer, primary resection and reanastomosis is recommended. If less than 12 cm, stricturoplasty is performed.

The extent of resection should encompass only gross disease; the microscopic appearance of the bowel at the margins of resection is irrelevant to outcome. Also, resection of the adjacent mesentery is not required. Microscopic recurrence of disease at the ileocolic anastomosis is as high as 79% within the first year, regardless of the configuration of the anastomosis.

In general, *stricturoplasty* is used for short fibrous strictures, anastomotic strictures, duodenal strictures, and in patients with short-gut syndrome. The technique of stricturoplasty involves a longitudinal incision along the antimesenteric border of the bowel wall. Short strictures are then closed transversely using the Mikulicz pyloroplasty technique. If the incision is too long to close by this method, the Finney pyloroplasty technique is used (Fig. 14-10). There is no role for balloon dilation of strictures in Crohn's disease, and bypass of diseased segments is usually avoided because of long-term risks of cancer and bacterial overgrowth in bypassed segments.

After obstruction, fistula is the most common indication for operative intervention in Crohn's disease. However, fistulas do not always require an operation. Ileocecal fistulae are common and may be quite benign; surgery is not required unless accompanied by another operative indication. Surgery is indicated if a long segment of bowel is bypassed, giving rise to absorptive deficiency, if recurrent or ongoing abscess formation accompanies the fistula, or if peritonitis is present. Enterocutaneous fistulae usually occur through a scar, and the management of these is somewhat controversial. Some authors recommend early operation while others feel that most will resolve with conservative management. Enterovaginal and enterourinary fistulae also occur and generally require an operative repair.

Other indications for surgery in Crohn's disease include perforation, cancer, severe duodenal disease, and appendicitis. Perforation with abscess formation requires prompt drainage with resection of the perforated loop. Cancer is most common in chronic strictures of the ileum and requires routine surgical management for intestinal malignancy. Severe duodenal disease is usually treated with gastrojejunostomy, which is an exception to the general rule to resect rather than bypass diseased bowel.

FIGURE 14-10. Techniques for stricturoplasty in Crohn's disease. **A:** Mikulicz stricturoplasty. **B:** Finney stricturoplasty. (From Etala E. *Atlas of gastrointestinal surgery.* Philadelphia: Williams & Wilkins, 1997.)

Crohn's disease is sometimes discovered during exploration for presumed appendicitis. If terminal ileitis is discovered in this situation, appendectomy alone should be performed, even if preoperative suspicion of Crohn's disease was entertained. In many of these patients, the ileitis resolves spontaneously or is due to another diagnosis, such as *Yersinia* infection. If the cecum is involved, however, consideration should be given to resection of the grossly diseased bowel, to prevent postoperative fistula formation from the appendiceal stump.

Overall, patients with Crohn's disease have a 40% to 50% clinical recurrence rate within 5 years of surgery and a 75% incidence of disease recurrence at 15 years. Most recurrences occur at the neoterminal ileum. A repeated operation is required in about 30% of patients.

Short-Bowel Syndrome

Short-bowel syndrome (SBS), or *short-gut syndrome,* is defined as the condition that exists when an individual's intestinal surface is insufficient to absorb enough fluid, electrolytes, or micronutrients or macronutrients for survival without parenteral supplementation. This condition results from massive bowel resection. Fortunately, the adaptive ability of the gut is great, and patients will compensate for a loss of bowel length. With intestinal adaptation and hypertrophy, an adult can survive without TPN if a minimum of 18 inches of small bowel and an ileocecal valve are present; without the ileocecal valve, the patient usually requires somewhat more length. Overall, the prognosis for SBS is good, with up to 82% survival and up to 63% adaptation to full enteral nutrition.

The two major etiologies of SBS are *ischemic bowel* and *Crohn's disease.* Today, the most common cause of massive bowel death is a mesenteric vascular accident. The etiologies of mesenteric ischemia include arterial occlusion associated with atherosclerotic vascular disease or thromboembolic disease; abdominal trauma; or mesenteric venous thrombosis. Bowel ischemia may also result from volvulus, internal or external hernias, or SBO. Occasionally, malignancy can require massive resection and result in SBS. In children, the most common etiologies of SBS are necrotizing enterocolitis, followed by midgut volvulus and multiple intestinal atresias.

Resection of a portion of the GI tract results in loss of the specialized secretory, absorptive, immune, and hormonal functions of that segment. For example, the specialized absorptive functions of the terminal ileum in the uptake of vitamin B_{12}, fat-soluble vitamins, and bile salts are well known. The patient must have supplemental vitamin B_{12} and may need medication or specialized nutrient mixtures to treat diarrhea and malabsorption. Alternatively, decreased CCK and secretin production is due to jejunal resection. These patients must cope with altered pancreatic and biliary secretion, resulting in impaired fat and protein absorption.

As our understanding of the gut hormones improves, we may be able to significantly improve the GI function of patients with SBS by supplementing GI hormones.

SBS is associated with various severe and sometimes unique nutritional problems. Normally, protein is absorbed in the first 120 cm of the jejunum. Digestion of proteins may be severely impaired in SBS, but oligopeptides and dipeptides are more efficiently absorbed. Carbohydrates are enzymatically digested in the proximal small intestine, but patients with SBS have a shortage of disaccharidases, particularly lactase and sucrase. This will often improve with time; however, severe diarrhea and flatulence will result if excessive undigested carbohydrates reach the colon. Diarrhea in SBS results from a combination of factors, including loss of absorptive surface and decreased transit time; bile-salt malabsorption, which causes the colon to secrete more and absorb less fluid; and fat malabsorption due to bile-salt deficiency. The loss of the ileocecal valve worsens this problem, by decreasing transit time and allowing colonic flora to colonize the small bowel.

Steatorrhea in SBS results from malabsorption and eventual deficiency of bile salts. Excess intraluminal fat can bind calcium resulting in a lower concentration of free intraluminal calcium. The increased rate of nephrolithiasis in SBS is due to oxalate, a by-product of the metabolism of glycine. Oxalate is normally bound by calcium in the small intestine to form an insoluble compound that is excreted. In SBS, calcium deficiency results in excessive quantities of *unbound* oxalate reaching the colon, where it is absorbed, resulting in calcium oxalate nephrolithiasis.

Fluid and electrolyte management constitutes a major problem of SBS, separate from the nutrient problem. In normal digestion, the hyperosmolar gastric contents are diluted down to an isosmolar chyme by gastric and salivary secretion prior to entry into the small bowel. This fluid load plus pancreatic and biliary secretions may amount to 10 L per day. Normally, the small bowel and right colon reabsorb the fluid, but in patients with SBS, it may be lost, along with electrolytes. Therefore, slowing intestinal transit time is essential to treatment of SBS. Agents used are opiates, Lomotil, and Immodium.

Another problem in SBS is colonization of the small bowel with colonic bacteria, due to resection of the ileocecal valve. This may exacerbate malabsorption and lead to bacterial translocation with repeated bouts of sepsis. An increased frequency of central venous catheter infection in patients on TPN is probably due to frequent bacteriemia secondary to bacterial translocation. Some advocate monitoring the stool for overgrowth of potentially pathogenic bacteria and using selective decontamination with antibiotics.

Patients who would have previously died from SBS are now able to live with a combination of enteral and parenteral nutrition. TPN is always required early after massive bowel resection and should be accompanied by isosmolar enteral feeds as soon as possible. Enteral feeds are usually started in very low volumes and increased gradually. The goal of therapy is to encourage *intestinal adaptation* so the patient can eventually minimize parenteral nutrition. Adaptation occurs in stages. The first and most significant change is hypertrophy of intestinal villi due to an increase in enterocyte number and length. This increases the surface area for absorption. The small intestine also lengthens and dilates over time.

Intraluminal nutrients are essential for adaptation to occur. Agents thought to help in stimulation of the bowel include the fatty acid butyrate (from soluble pectin and other sources), which is the preferred colonocyte fuel, and the amino acid glutamine, which is the major metabolic fuel for enterocytes. In general, complex proteins, long-chain triglycerides, and short-chain fatty acids are felt to stimulate adaptation better than predigested component nutrients, but glutamine and butyrate are exceptions. Pancreaticobiliary secretions also promote intestinal adaptation, and several hormones also contribute to intestinal adaptation, including enteroglucagon, glucocorticoids, polamines, prostaglandin E_2, and epidermal growth factor. A 1995 study showed that a high-carbohydrate, low-fat diet supplemented with enteral glutamine and growth hormone resulted in a decrease in or complete elimination of the TPN requirement for patients with SBS. Generally 1 to 2 years or longer are needed for full intestinal adaptation.

Multiple surgical procedures have been attempted in the treatment of SBS. Procedures that have attempted to increase transit time or increase surface area include reversed intestinal segment, recirculating loop procedure, artificial ileocecal valve, and colonic interposition into the small bowel. These have been of minimal success in humans. A tapering procedure of dilated small bowel holds some promise in the prevention of stasis, bacterial overgrowth, and bouts of bacterial translocation. A split-bowel procedure in which a dilated bowel is longitudinally split into two parallel segments has also been attempted with some success.

Small bowel transplantation represents the theoretical definitive therapy for SBS; however, the current poor success rate of gut transplantation makes it a procedure of last resort. The indications for small bowel transplantation include patients whose GI tract fails to adapt despite 2 years of optimal treatment, patients developing liver disease as a result of TPN, and patients who have no remaining sites for central venous access for TPN.

SMALL BOWEL TUMORS

There are only about 3,000 cases per year of small bowel malignancies in the United States, compared to 150,000 cases of colorectal cancer. Only 2% of GI tract malignancies arise from the small bowel. There are several possible explanations for the relatively low incidence of small bowel cancer. Possible factors include the relatively rapid transit of potential carcinogens through the small bowel, the alkaline pH level and a low bacterial count, the liquid nature of the contents minimizing mechanical irritation, the detoxifying action of the enzyme benzpyrene hydroxylase, and the extensive immune system of the small intestine. The risk of developing small bowel cancer is greater with the following conditions: celiac sprue, immune deficiency such as posttransplant and human immunodeficiency virus (specifically Kaposi sarcoma and lymphoma), familial adenomatous polyposis (FAP), Crohn's disease, and in long-standing ileostomies.

The most common benign tumor of the small bowel is leiomyoma, and the most common malignant tumor is adenocarcinoma, with carcinoid the second most common. The types of malignancies that develop reflect the cell types that occur in the small intestine: adenoma and adenocarcinoma from glandular mucosa, leiomyoma and leiomyosarcoma from smooth muscle, lymphoma from enteric lymphoid tissue, carcinoid from enterochromaffin cells, lipoma and liposarcoma from fatty tissue, fibroma and fibrosarcoma from connective tissue, and neurofibroma and neurofibrosarcoma from GI neural tissue.

The clinical presentation of small bowel tumors is characteristically delayed, accounting for the high mortality rate when these are malignant. The late presentation of small intestinal tumors is due to the liquid nature of the chyme in the small bowel and the low likelihood of obstruction until the tumor is extremely large. Symptoms of benign tumors include vague pain, bleeding, or intermittent obstruction due to intussusception. Most benign tumors, however, are asymptomatic. Malignant tumors may present with abdominal pain, weight loss, or anemia. Duodenal tumors present with gastric outlet obstruction or jaundice. Occasionally, a malignant tumor will perforate the small intestine, leading to peritonitis as the initial presentation. Carcinoid syndrome is a rare presentation for this type of tumor (10%) but is characterized by flushing and diarrhea.

Diagnostic testing for small bowel tumors includes CT scanning with oral contrast, as well as enteroclysis. This provides considerably greater mucosal detail than a standard UGIS with small bowel follow-through. Enteroscopy is able to examine increasingly distal portions of the small bowel and carries the advantage of biopsy capability. Magnetic resonance imaging (MRI) is particularly good at identifying metastatic disease and involvement of adjacent organs. Multiple neuroendocrine tumors may be found within the small bowel, although only carcinoid tumors will be discussed in detail here. Endoscopy, MRI, and specialized radionuclide scans are the localizing modalities of choice.

Benign Small Bowel Tumors

The most common benign tumors are adenomas, leiomyomas, lipomas, and hamartomas. *Leiomyoma* is the most common type of small bowel tumor. If the lesion is symptomatic, a local small bowel resection may be performed. If the lesion is greater than 2 cm, a 5-cm margin should be used.

Adenomas are associated with the familial polyposis syndromes such as Gardner syndrome and FAP but may be sporadic. The duodenum is the most common site, particularly in the periampullary region. Like adenomas in the colon, adenomas in the small bowel progress into adenocarcinomas along an apparent sequence of transforming mutations. Villous adenomas will progress to cancer up to 50% of the time while tubular adenomas have a much lower malignant potential. Unlike those in the colon, the size of the lesion doesn't correlate well with the chance of malignancy. *Brunner gland adenomas* also rarely occur. Tubular adenomas and Brunner gland adenomas may be excised endoscopically, but only small villous adenomas less than 2 cm should be removed endoscopically. Larger villous lesions may be resected *trans*duodenally if the patient is not a candidate for pancreatoduodenectomy, but definitive therapy requires pancreatoduodenectomy. Management of these lesions is complicated because a frozen section diagnosis can be inaccurate for detecting foci of malignancy in the locally resected adenoma.

Lipomas are most common in the ileum but occur in all three portions of the small bowel. A lipoma may be diagnosed on CT scan as a fat-density lesion associated with the bowel. They are more common in men and in the ileum and the duodenum. Small bowel lipomas are excised only if symptomatic.

Hemangiomas are vascular neoplasms that may involve the entire GI tract and present with occult or recurrent acute bleeding. They are often multiple as in Rendu-Osler-Weber syndrome. Laser or electrocautery ablation or segmental resection may be performed.

The *Peutz-Jeghers syndrome* is characterized by *hamartomas* of the small bowel and mucocutaneous melanin spots. This is an autosomal dominant genetic disease. Despite the benign nature of the hamartomas, these patients are at increased risk of malignant tumors, including bowel adenocarcinomas, breast cancer, and genital cancers. Patients should be placed on an aggressive surveillance protocol for these cancers. The hamartomas may be complicated by intussusception or bleeding, however, extensive bowel resection for the hamartoma is not indicated.

Other benign conditions that may mimic small bowel tumors include pancreatic rests, splenosis, and endometriosis.

Malignant Small Bowel Tumors

Malignant tumors of the small bowel include adenocarcinomas, carcinoid tumors, lymphomas, leiomyosarcomas, and metastatic tumors. *Adenocarcinomas* are the most common small bowel malignancy, making up 30% to 50% of malignant small bowel tumors. Adenocarcinomas are most common in the duodenum, particularly in the periampullary region, with decreasing incidence along the

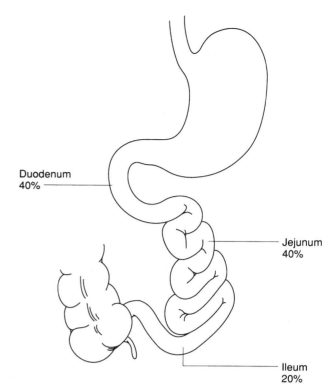

FIGURE 14-11. Distribution of small bowel adenocarcinomas. (From Greenfield LJ, Mulholland MW, Oldham KT, et al., eds. *Surgery: scientific principles and practice,* 2nd ed. Philadelphia: Lippincott-Raven Publishers, 1997, with permission.)

length of the small bowel (Fig.14-11). Pancreatic or biliary secretions may play a role in carcinogenesis. Like those in the colon, adenomas in the small bowel progress into adenocarcinomas along an apparent sequence of transforming mutations. Villous adenomas will progress to cancer up to 50% of the time, while tubular adenomas have a much lower malignant potential. Unlike those in the colon, the size of the lesion doesn't correlate well with the chance of malignancy.

Malignant duodenal tumors can not be segmentally resected. Like pancreatic and bile duct cancers, duodenal cancers require pancreatoduodenectomy, due to the shared blood supply of these structures. Periampullary adenocarcinomas may arise from the ampulla, the pancreatic or bile ducts, or the duodenum. These tumors can be differentiated by examination of the type of mucin produced. This is important due to the poorer prognosis with tumors of pancreatic origin and the better prognosis with those of duodenal origin.

Adenocarcinoma of the jejunum or ileum is resected with a 5- to 10-cm margin and a low resection of the mesentery. For terminal ileum cancer, a right hemicolectomy is often performed, due to the shared mesenteric blood supply and lymphatic drainage. Response to chemotherapy with 5-fluorouracil (5-FU) and radiation therapy is poor. The overall survival rate is 15% due to the typically late stage at presentation. This figure increases to 50% to 70% if the tumor is localized (node-negative) at presentation.

Carcinoid tumors are the second most common small bowel cancer, making up about 20% of small bowel malignancies. The small bowel is the second most common site for carcinoid tumors (13%), after the vermiform appendix (85%). Most (89%) small bowel carcinoid tumors occur in the ileum, and most (90%) are metastatic at the time of surgery. A careful search for second tumors should be undertaken during surgery, as 30% of patients have multiple primaries. Extraintestinal malignancies are also present in increased frequency in patients diagnosed with carcinoid tumor (15% to 30%, particularly colon, stomach, lung, and breast). One unique feature of carcinoid tumors is an intense local desmoplastic reaction around the site of the tumor, sometimes resulting in bowel obstruction or ischemia.

Carcinoid tumors arise from *enterochromaffin* cells, neuroendocrine cells within the crypts of Lieberkühn. These cells may produce and secrete multiple vasoactive substances and regulatory peptides, including serotonin, bradykinin, histamine, and substance P. The carcinoid syndrome, characterized by intermittent flushing and diarrhea, is presumed to result from release of these hormones by metastatic tumors, although a definite correlation of serum hormone levels with symptoms has not been proven. Serotonin and other carcinoid products are metabolized and detoxified by the liver and the lung. Therefore, the syndrome only manifests in patients with liver metastases, where products do not enter the portal circulation directly. Only 10% of carcinoid tumors present with the syndrome, despite the fact that many are metastatic to liver at the time of diagnosis. Fifty percent of patients with carcinoid tumors have elevation in serum serotonin and urine 5-HIAA (5-hydroxyindoleacetic acid). A 24-hour urine test for 5-HIAA is measured when the diagnosis is suspected. A carcinoid crisis may occur in association with general anesthesia. I.V. octreotide (somatostatin analog) may be used to treat the carcinoid crisis, and the symptoms of the syndrome are managed with octreotide or somatostatin.

Carcinoid tumors are always treated by resection, because they often have a very indolent course even when metastatic. Local complications such as obstruction can also be prevented by resection. The malignant potential of a carcinoid tumor is directly related to its size and its location. Small bowel carcinoids tumors have a worse prognosis than rectal or appendiceal carcinoid tumors. Small bowel lesions of less than 1 cm rarely metastasize while 1- to 2-cm tumors have a 50% chance of metastasis and 2-cm tumors have an 80% chance of metastasis. In contrast appendiceal and rectal carcinoid tumors less than 2 cm rarely metastasize. Treatment consists of a local excision if the lesion is smaller than 1 cm (including endoscopic resection) and a standard cancer operation for larger lesions. Prognosis is excellent if there is no distant metastatic disease, with a 90% 5-year survival rate if disease is limited to mesentery and bowel. If liver metastases are present, the 5-year survival rate ranges from 20% to 50%. Palliative resection or hepatic artery embolization is warranted in highly symptomatic patients with hepatic metastases due to improved survival and quality of life. Liver transplant has been performed with good results in the occasional patient. Chemotherapy using doxorubicin, 5-FU, and streptozocin also may provide some benefit.

Fifteen percent to twenty percent of small bowel malignancies are *leiomyosarcomas,* likely arising from the smooth muscle layers of the bowel (Fig. 14-12). These tumors tend to be large and vascular, and may present with bleeding. Because the bulk of the tumor is extraluminal, they are less likely to obstruct, contributing to their late presentation. Metastases are primarily found in the liver and lung. CT scan is useful for identifying these tumors, but CT-guided biopsy is not useful, because it may not differentiate benign from malignant disease. It may be very difficult to differentiate benign from malignant tumors on histologic section, and the number of mitoses, cellularity, nuclear atypia, tumor size, and necrosis are all features that must be examined.

Resection of the involved bowel with its adjacent mesentery is the treatment of choice, but extended lymphadenectomy is unnecessary because the spread is generally hematogenous. A small duodenal lesion with possible benign pathology may be locally excised, but a completion pancreatoduodenectomy may be required if the final pathology reveals malignancy. Again, frozen section histology may be inaccurate for definitive diagnosis. For unresectable tumors, a palliative bypass procedure or palliative primary tumor resection is indicated because survival and quality of life may be improved. Isolated liver or lung metastases are sometimes resected in an attempt at a cure. Chemotherapy and radiation therapy are generally not beneficial for this type of tumor. Overall 5-year survival is about 40% to 50%, and the grade of the tumor is the most

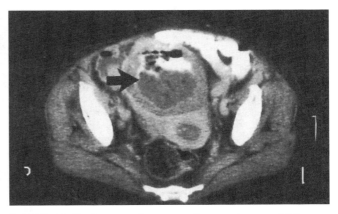

FIGURE 14-12. Computed tomography scan image of leiomyosarcoma, showing large size and central necrosis. (From Greenfield LJ, Mullholland MW, Oldham KT, et al., eds. *Surgery: scientific principles and practice,* 2nd ed. Philadelphia: Lippincott-Raven Publishers, 1997, with permission.)

important predictor. In addition to leiomyosarcomas, less common gut sarcomas may arise from any mesodermal component of the intestine, such as fat, and connective, neural, or vascular tissue.

Primary small bowel *lymphomas* comprise 10% to 15% of malignant small bowel tumors. Unlike other types of lymphoma, small bowel lymphoma is a surgical disease. Most are B-cell in origin, except lymphomas arising in the setting of celiac sprue. Special types of primary gut lymphomas include posttransplant lymphoproliferative disease, immunoproliferative small intestinal disease (heavy-chain or alpha-chain disease), found in the Mediterranean basin, and disseminated Burkitt lymphoma, found in young children. Immunosuppressed patients are at particular risk of primary bowel lymphoma. Clinical presentation is nonspecific and not characterized by fevers, night sweats, or pruritus, as in systemic lymphomas. Some may present with malabsorption secondary to diffuse intestinal involvement or with peritonitis (25%), due to perforation, obstruction, intussusception, or bleeding.

Due to the high concentration of lymphatic tissue in the ileal Peyer patches, the ileum is the most common location for small bowel lymphoma. For localized disease, the involved bowel with its mesentery should be resected and a liver biopsy and sampling of the mesenteric and paraaortic lymph nodes should be performed. If any residual disease is present, chemotherapy and radiation therapy are employed. Pancreatoduodenectomy (Whipple procedure) should be considered for duodenal lymphomas due to the high risk of perforation or significant bleeding (20%) when chemotherapy and radiation therapy are used as the primary therapy. Debulking unresectable disease is considered worthwhile. Adjuvant chemotherapy and radiation therapy are usually employed, even for low-stage disease. If the disease is fully resected, 5-year survival rate is approximately 60%, but metastatic disease carries a very poor prognosis.

Small bowel tumors rarely may be metastatic from melanoma, pancreatic cancer, colon cancer, gastric cancer, lung cancer, and others.

SUGGESTED READING

Ashcraft KW, Holder TN. *Pediatric surgery*, 2nd ed. Philadelphia: WB Saunders, 1984.

Geoghegan J, Pappas TN. Clinical uses of gut peptides. *Ann Surg* 1997;225:145–154.

Nance ML. Motility of the gastrointestinal tract. In: Savage EB, Fishman SJ, Miller LA, eds. *Essentials of basic science in surgery*. Philadelphia: JB Lippincott Co, 1993.

Reilly KJ. Endocrine function of the gastrointestinal tract. In: Savage EB, Fishman SJ, Miller LA, eds. *Essentials of basic science in surgery*. Philadelphia: JB Lippincott Co, 1993.

15

THE COLON, RECTUM, AND ANUS

EDWARD Y. WOO AND JOHN L. ROMBEAU

ANATOMY

The *large intestine* (Fig. 15-1) includes the appendix, ascending colon, transverse colon, descending colon, and sigmoid colon, and it measures approximately 1.5 m in length. The rectum and anus can be considered separately. The appendix, which arises from the base of the cecum, is approximately 8 cm long and has its own mesentery, the mesoappendix. It has a variable relation to the cecum and can be directed downward, curve behind in a retrocecal manner, or take almost any other position. The appendix has a complete longitudinal outer muscle layer formed by the converged taeniae. The arterial supply to the appendix comes from the appendicular artery, arising off the ileocolic artery. Venous drainage parallels arterial vessels and lymphatics drain to the ileocolic lymph nodes along the ileocolic artery. The celiac and superior mesenteric ganglion are the source of innervation to the appendix.

The *cecum,* the base of the ascending colon, is approximately 5 cm long and has the largest diameter of the colon. It is usually fixed to the lateral abdominal wall and is the largest part of the colon with an average diameter of approximately 7 cm. This is the most common site of perforation when the colon becomes overly distended. The ileocecal valve forms the junction of the terminal ileum and colon and functions as a one-way valve. The arterial supply to the cecum arises from the ileocolic artery and the venous and lymphatic drainage are similar to that of the appendix. The cecum also derives its innervation from the celiac and superior mesenteric ganglion.

The ascending, or right, colon, in continuation with the cecum, measures 10 to 20 cm in length. At the liver, the colon turns medially forming the hepatic flexure. The right colon is retroperitoneal lying along the posterior abdominal wall with peritoneum on its anterior border. It is important to recognize that the ureter and duodenum lie posterior and can easily be injured during mobilization of the right colon. The groove lateral to the colon is called the right paracolic gutter. The ileocolic artery and right colic artery supply blood to the right colon, and the venous drainage parallels this. Lymphatics drain first into the paracolic and epicolic nodes, then into the superior mesenteric lymph nodes. Innervation is the same as in the appendix and the cecum.

After the right colon bends at the liver, it becomes the transverse colon, which is about 45 cm long, and traverses one side of the abdomen to the other. This part of the colon is intraperitoneal and freely mobile. The transverse colon is also attached to the stomach via the gastrocolic ligament. Because of its location, it can often be involved in contiguous tumor spread from the stomach or pancreas. Its blood supply is mainly from the middle colic artery traveling in the transverse mesocolon, although blood flow also arises from the right and left colic arteries. The transverse mesocolon is a dual layer of mesentery connecting to the base of the pancreas. The superior mesenteric vein drains the transverse colon, and the lymph nodes along the middle colic artery provide lymphatic drainage. Innervation arises from both the superior and inferior mesenteric plexus.

Upon reaching the left side of the abdomen, the colon bends downward, forming the splenic flexure. Here, the colon is attached to the diaphragm via the phrenocolic ligament. This flexure is more posterior and superior than its counterpart and is often difficult to mobilize. The descending colon, 20 to 30 cm long, travels down from the splenic flexure. Like the ascending colon, it, too, is a retroperitoneal structure, with the left paracolic gutter just lateral to it. The left colic and sigmoid arteries supply blood flow, and the inferior mesenteric vein drains it. The left colic and sigmoid arteries arise from the inferior mesenteric artery, unlike the ileocolic, right colic and middle colic, which come off the superior mesenteric artery. Due to this vascular distribution, the splenic flexure is a watershed area between two sources of blood supply and is often the first area of the colon compromised by marginal blood flow. The intermediate colic lymph nodes along the left colic artery drain into the inferior mesenteric lymph nodes. Sympathetic innervation arises from the superior hypogastric plexus, and parasympathetic supply is from the pelvic splanchnic nerves.

The sigmoid colon connects the remainder of the colon to the rectum. It is approximately 40 cm in length,

---

Hospital of the University of Pennsylvania, Philadelphia, Pennsylvania

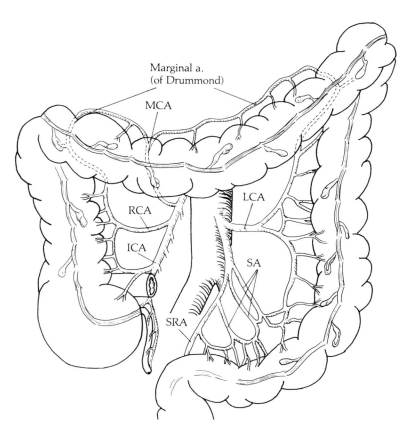

FIGURE 15-1. Arterial supply to the colon. ICA, ileocolic artery; LCA, left colic artery; RCA, right colic artery; SA, sigmoid arteries; SRA, superior rectal artery. (From Monsen H. Anatomy of the colon. In: Nyhus LM, Baker RJ, eds. *Mastery of surgery*. Boston: Little, Brown and Company, 1992:1186, with permission.)

intraperitoneal, and freely mobile. As the taeniae end, the rectum begins. This junction is approximately 15 cm from the anus. Normally, several sigmoid arteries off the inferior mesenteric artery supply blood to this portion of the colon, and the inferior mesenteric vein returns the blood. Lymphatic drainage and neural innervation are similar to those of the descending colon.

The rectum begins at the end of the sigmoid colon, approximately at the level of the third sacral vertebra (Fig. 15-2). At the anorectal junction, the puborectalis muscle forms a sling, creating a 90-degree angle, which helps preserve continence. The anterior and lateral walls have peritoneum along the superior third of the rectum, whereas only the anterior rectum is covered in the middle third and no peritoneum is on the lower third of the rectum. As the peritoneum reflects off the anterior wall, it joins the bladder in men and the vagina in women, forming the rectovesical pouch or rectouterine pouch, respectively. Posteriorly, the rectum is attached to the anterior surface of the sacrum via a fascial sheath. The inferior aspect of the rectum, the rectal ampulla, has the greatest diameter and is also easily distensible for fecal storage. The arterial supply to the rectum is very profuse. The superior rectal artery, the terminal branch of the inferior mesenteric artery, forms an anastomosis with the middle and inferior rectal arteries, which arise off the internal iliac arteries and internal pudendal arteries, respectively. This creates an abundant vascular supply to the rectum. The venous drainage parallels the arterial tree, which creates a dual drainage system. The superior rectal vein drains into the portal system, whereas the middle and inferior rectal veins drain into the systemic system. This configuration is important because very low tumors can potentially metastasize systemically without first passing through the liver and this portal/systemic venous junction forms an important area of collateral blood flow during portal hypertension. Lymphatic drainage is via the inferior mesenteric and internal iliac lymph nodes. Both the sympathetic system, off the inferior hypogastric plexus, and the parasympathetic system, off S1-4, supply innervation to the rectum.

The anal canal is approximately 4 cm long, starting at the anorectal junction and ending at the anal verge (Fig. 15-2). Within the anus are the anal columns, which consist of longitudinal folds containing the terminal branches of the superior rectal artery. The superior border of these columns is named the *anorectal line* where the rectum becomes the anus. The inferior border is the pectinate line consisting of valves, which are folds of epithelium. Above these valves are a series of sinuses that secrete mucus during defecation. The pectinate line divides the columnar epithelium above from the squamous epithelium below. The superior rectal artery supplies the anus above the pectinate line and the inferior

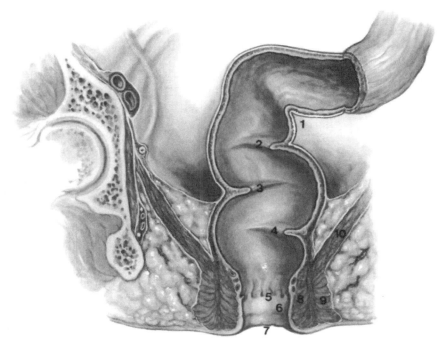

FIGURE 15-2. Coronal section of the rectum, anus, and perineum. 1, rectosigmoid junction; 2, superior valve of Houston; 3, middle valve of Houston; 4, inferior valve of Houston; 5, pectinate of dentate line; 6, pecten; 7, anal margin; 8, internal anal sphincter; 9, external anal sphincter; 10, levator ani muscle and puborectalis. (From Etala E, ed. *Atlas of gastrointestinal surgery.* Philadelphia: Williams & Wilkins, 1997: 1737, with permission.)

rectal artery supplies the anus below the pectinate line. Venous drainage parallels this. Lymphatics above the line drain into the internal iliac nodes, whereas below the line they drain into the superficial inguinal nodes. Innervation above the pectinate line is the same as that in the rectum and is only sensitive to stretch. Below the pectinate line, the inferior rectal nerves of the pudendal supply the anus and allow pain, touch, and temperature. Surrounding the anus are the internal and external anal sphincters. The internal sphincter is involuntary and is formed by the circular muscle layer. The external sphincter is voluntary and joins the puborectalis muscle. Both are necessary for continence.

The colon, rectum, and anus are not sterile organs. A dense bacterial flora exists within them, with a predominance of anaerobes such as *Bacteroides*. Thus, it is important that these organs be prepared before surgery. Nichols, in 1973, demonstrated the benefit of nonabsorbable orally administered antibiotics in addition to mechanical cleansing. This bowel preparation is widely used today.

PHYSIOLOGY

The colon is very important in fluid absorption. Approximately 1 L of water reaches the colon every 24 hours. Of this, approximately 900 mL is reabsorbed, mostly in the proximal colon. Furthermore, of the 200 mEq/L of sodium that arrives at the colon 175 mEq/L is absorbed. This occurs mostly through active transport. The colon also plays a role in the enterohepatic circulation, thus being responsible for reabsorption of bile acids along with the terminal ileum. This becomes particularly important when the terminal ileum is resected.

The primary source of energy for the colon is *n*-butyrate, a short-chain fatty acid, which is produced by fermentation of certain dietary fibers and undigested starch by intraluminal bacteria. Without this source of energy, there is decreased sodium and water absorption leading to diarrhea. Other short-chain fatty acids produced in the colon include acetate and propionate. These all participate in mucosal regeneration, acid-base status, and regulation of blood flow. Not all dietary fibers are fermented, however. For example, lignin is not fermented at all and cellulose is only partially fermented. These fibers provide bulk in the stool.

The colon also plays a role in mineral secretion. Potassium is actively secreted in part due to mineralocorticoid stimulus. This is important in conditions such as a large villous adenoma, which can lead to a high rate of potassium secretion and systemic hypokalemia. Bicarbonate is also secreted along electrochemical gradients.

In addition to absorption and secretion, the colon is important for transit. As a food bolus enters and distends the ileum, the ileocecal valve opens. Once the bolus enters the colon, the colon distends and the valve closes. Within the ascending colon are segmental propulsive and retropulsive contractions that last 12 to 60 seconds and serve to mix intraluminal contents. The left colon, in contrast, has mostly propulsive contractions, propelling the stool caudally. One to three times daily, a large peristaltic contraction moves the contents distally, up to one third the length of the colon. This is referred to a "mass movement." During this time, the bowel segments contract and the haustra disappear. The rectum for the most part stays empty because it has more segmental contractions than the sigmoid, thus propelling contents retrograde. When fecal material is forced into the rectum, the internal anal sphincter relaxes, known as the "rectosphincteral reflex." When the rectum is filled to 25% capacity, there is an urge to defecate. Defecation is prevented by contraction of the external anal sphincter via reflex neural activity from the sacral roots. As time continues and defecation does not occur, the internal sphincter begins to regain tone and the urge to defecate subsides. In the act of defecation, the external sphincter is voluntarily relaxed. Furthermore, the rectum and distal colon contract and the pelvic floor relaxes, both of which help straighten the rectosigmoid angle. Increases in intraabdominal pressure also aid in defecation.

PATHOLOGY OF THE COLON

Motility

Colonic motility is vital for removal of fecal material. Constipation refers to having fewer than three bowel movements per week, whereas obstipation refers to having no bowel movements at all. The reasons for constipation are many. Most common in the surgical population is a colonic ileus secondary to anesthetic effect and bowel manipulation. In general, the colon is the last of the gastrointestinal (GI) organs to regain its motility (the small bowel is first and the stomach second). Many other causes of constipation, however, do exist. Hirschsprung disease is a congenital neuronal deficit resulting in the absence of distal GI ganglion cells. These patients tend to present with constipation at birth or early in life. Endocrine abnormalities such as hypothyroidism or hyperparathyroidism affect motility and some systemic diseases, such as scleroderma or amyloidosis, alter normal colonic tissue. Medications, particularly narcotics and iron, can often cause poor colonic transit. Most importantly, though, an obstruction (tumor, diverticulitis, volvulus) can cause constipation and require urgent or emergent intervention.

Ogilvie syndrome deserves special mention. This syndrome was first described in 1945. It consists of a dilated colon that appears obstructed but has no underlying mechanical obstruction. The etiology of this pseudoobstruction is broad, including medication, neurological or muscular disorders, electrolyte abnormalities, hypothyroidism, and many more. Patients usually present with abdominal distension and no pain. The colon can perforate if it becomes excessively dilated. The law of Laplace correlates wall tension to intraluminal pressure and radius (tension = pressure × radius). According to this principle, the cecum is at greatest risk of perforation due to its large diameter and must be followed closely. Initial management includes nasogastric tube decompression, intravenous (i.v.) fluid hydration, and serial abdominal examination and x-ray evaluation. The presumed underlying cause should be treated. Rectal tubes are often placed with some success, although care must be taken not to injure the rectal wall. If the above measures are unsuccessful, colonoscopic decompression can be attempted. This has an 80% to 90% success rate. Ultimately, surgery may be needed, and in the absence of cecal ischemia or necrosis, a cecostomy should be adequate for decompression. However, if there is suspicion of perforation or necrotic bowel, a formal segmental resection may need to be performed.

Ulcerative Colitis

Ulcerative colitis is a form of inflammatory bowel disease of unknown etiology. It is primarily limited to the colon and rectum, although in certain circumstances it can involve the terminal ileum, known as "backwash ileitis." The disease classically has a biphasic distribution, with most patients presenting between 15 and 40 years of age and a small minority presenting after 60 years of age. There is an increased racial preponderance among whites and increased ethnic preponderance among Jewish people. Women and men are affected almost equally.

There is no known cause of ulcerative colitis and its etiology is presumed to be multifactorial. Many possibilities exist, such as genetic, infectious, dietary, vascular, or allergic factors. There is evidence that at least part of the disease is due to immunologic phenomena because the disease responds to immunosuppressive treatment. Studies of those with ulcerative colitis show elevated levels of IL-1 as well as alterations in IL-2, IL-6, IL-8, and IFN-γ, supporting its inflammatory etiology. Genetic factors also play a role because of the increased preponderance among family members. There is a greater association among monozygotic twins as opposed to nontwin siblings. Current evidence supports that ulcerative colitis is probably caused by a combination of genetic and environmental processes.

By definition, the disease is limited to the mucosa and submucosa. Grossly, the mucosa becomes hyperemic and edematous with ulcerations. Swollen tags of mucosa protrude upward forming pseudopolyps. Microscopically, there is predominance of inflammatory cells with formation of crypt abscesses. The inflammatory cells consist of neutrophils, lymphocytes, plasma cells, and mast cells. Granulation tissue forms within the ulcers, which bleed. As the epithelium becomes atrophic, sodium and water absorption decreases leading to diarrhea. Unlike Crohn's disease, there are no skip lesions, as the disease progresses proximally from the rectum in a continuous fashion.

The presentation of ulcerative colitis can range from mild to severe colonic inflammation. In about 15% of patients, the disease will initially present in an acute fulminating manner with bloody diarrhea, abdominal pain, and fever. The rest will present with milder, more chronic symptoms such as weight loss and abdominal tenderness. Most patients have disease limited to the distal colon, although as many as 20% can have pancolitis.

Systemic manifestations also occur. Some patients develop mucocutaneous lesions such as aphthous ulcers, gingivitis, and erythema nodosum. Ophthalmologic problems such as uveitis and iritis, as well joint disease, such as sacroiliitis, parallel the disease process in the colon; i.e., they worsen with more severe colonic disease. *Hepatobiliary* disease, however, is independent of colonic inflammation and ranges from mild fatty infiltration of the liver to severe sclerosing cholangitis. Unlike that of other systemic manifestations, the course of sclerosing cholangitis is not necessarily reversed after colectomy and palliative treatment of this process includes biliary stents and antibiotics while the definitive treatment is a liver transplant. Cholangiocarcinoma has also been known to develop.

Ulcerative colitis must be suspected in anyone presenting with the above symptoms. However, other diseases must also be considered, such as Crohn's disease, infectious diarrhea, ischemic bowel, and radiation-induced injury. Physical examination often reveals a tender abdomen and systemic manifestations of the disease. Proctosigmoidoscopy is often adequate to obtain tissue for diagnosis, but a full colonoscopy is needed to determine the extent of the disease. Radiographic studies can be indicative or diagnostic, such as the classic "stovepipe" appearance of the denuded colonic mucosa in advanced disease on a barium enema. However, sigmoidoscopy and colonoscopy allow for tissue sampling and definitive diagnosis.

Unlike Crohn's disease, ulcerative colitis can be cured surgically, but medical management is most often the first line of treatment. Sulfasalazine and its derivatives are the primary medication used. They exert their antiinflammatory effect by inhibiting mucosal prostaglandin synthesis. Side effects include reversible hypospermia and infertility in men, as well as headaches, nausea, anorexia, and dyspepsia. Steroids are also commonly used in both systemic and topical forms. When patients have disease limited to the rectum, steroid enemas are quite useful, avoiding systemic side effects. Studies have also shown the possible benefit of using adrenocorticotropic hormone in place of steroids. When these modalities are ineffective, other stronger immunosuppressive agents can be employed. Azathioprine and 6-mercaptopurine are purine analogs that inhibit DNA synthesis. Because they do not take immediate effect, they are not used to treat acute flares. Cyclosporin A is also used as an immunosuppressive agent with some success. However, it is usually reserved for the treatment of severe refractory disease, as it is associated with nephrotoxic and infectious complications. Finally, antibiotics, such as metronidazole, are often employed, albeit, with questionable benefit.

The definitive treatment of ulcerative colitis is surgical resection. The disease is cured upon removal of the entire colon and rectum. This procedure, however, involves a significant degree of morbidity. Indications for surgery include unrelenting hemorrhage, toxic megacolon, obstruction, suspicion/risk of cancer or dysplasia, systemic complication, and failure of medical management. In cases of surgical emergency, patients should undergo a more conservative Hartmann operation followed by a more definitive operation in the future. In an elective setting, it is important to determine whether the procedure is indeed indicated. The two situations would include intractability and cancer prevention. Failure of medical management is difficult to define. It usually entails chronic debilitation with severe disease greatly affecting the patient's quality of life. In regard to cancer prevention, the first 10 years of disease demonstrate a very low risk of cancer, approximately 2% to 3%. However, after 10 years, the risk of cancer increases 1% to 2% per year, such that after 20 years of disease, there is a 10% to 20% risk of colorectal cancer. Adenocarcinoma is most common and is multicentric in 15% of patients. Furthermore, it occurs equally throughout the colon. As a result, some surgeons believe that after 10 years of active disease, patients should have a total proctocolectomy regardless of the disease's course. Seldom, however, is this the only indication for operation this far into the disease process.

Acute toxic megacolon occurs in approximately 10% of patients with ulcerative colitis. Patients have severe abdominal pain, diarrhea, and distension. Often, however, patients on high doses of steroids will not manifest these symptoms and signs. The transverse colon becomes acutely dilated, averaging 9 cm in diameter. Treatment consists of hydration, antibiotics, and possible stress dose steroids. If the situation does not improve in 24 to 48 hours, surgery is indicated. Because morbidity and mortality in this acute setting are already high, conservative resection is often favored with a definitive resection, i.e., total proctocolectomy, at a later date.

Total proctocolectomy is a curative procedure and should be performed whenever possible. Historically, a permanent ileostomy was performed. This has complications including skin excoriation, leakage, stomal hernias, not to mention psychological ramifications. Alternatives, such as a subtotal colectomy with ileorectal anastomosis, were attempted. The mucosa of the residual rectum continues to be affected by disease and retains the risk for carcinoma. Continent ostomies were created, such as the Kock ileostomy, where a pouch of terminal ileum was brought to the skin, and a nipple valve was created by intussuscepting a piece of ileum and using it as an outflow tract. Complications included displacement of the valve leading to incontinence, bowel obstruction, and inflammation of the pouch.

In the past 15 years, the ileoanal anastomosis has been developed and improved upon. It still allows a total proctocolectomy but does not require the creation of a permanent ileostomy. The operation includes the removal of the entire colon, followed by a rectal mucosectomy or low rectal resection. Rectal mucosectomy removes all disease-bearing tissue, but some believe that the preservation of the mucosa of the anal transitional zone allows for superior fecal control. In contrast, low rectal resection leaves this transitional zone, but this tissue still bears disease and is at risk for development of carcinoma. In either case, an ileal pouch is formed as a J, S, or W pouch, and anastomosed to the anus (Fig. 15-3). Advancements in technology, such as stapling devices, have significantly improved the results of this operation. Most surgeons also create a diverting loop ileostomy, but this can be omitted in select patients. The ileostomy may help prevent leakage and anastomotic breakdown, but it necessitates a second operation for ileostomy closure. After this operation, patients generally have six to ten bowel movements a day, with some nocturnal seepage. Complications of the procedure include pouchitis, which occurs in nearly 50% of patients. Although this syndrome is not completely understood, it probably involves bacterial overgrowth with subsequent inflammation. Symptoms include abdominal pain, incontinence, fever, and malaise. Pouchitis usually responds to a single course of metronidazole, but in more chronic cases, repeated courses of antibiotics are needed. In the most severe cases, removal of the pouch may be necessary. Other complications of total proctocolectomy and ileoanal pouch anastomosis include obstruction, sexual dysfunction, and renal stones. In summary, ileoanal anastomosis provides a significantly improved alternative to permanent ileostomy. This is acknowledged by an extremely high level of patient satisfaction.

Colorectal Crohn's Disease

Crohn's disease differs from ulcerative colitis in many aspects. It, too, is an inflammatory bowel disease without known etiology. Crohn's disease, however, can affect any area of the GI tract from the mouth to the anus in a noncontinuous manner. Pathologically, the lesions are transmural and contain noncaseating granulomas. In 55% of patients, the small and large bowel are involved, and in 15% of patients, only the large intestine is involved. Abdominal pain is the most common symptom. Diarrhea is common, although it is usually not bloody. Diagnosis is made definitively by tissue biopsy, although characteristic radiographic findings can be highly suggestive. Medical therapy is similar to that used for ulcerative colitis. Surgical therapy, however, is reserved only for complications and can not be curative due to the panenteric nature of the disease. Approximately 70% of patients will ultimately need an operation, most commonly to treat an obstruction, perforation, or fistula. Segmental resection of a diseased colon can be performed in patients without proctitis or severe anorectal disease. Total proctocolectomy with ileoanal anastomosis is not indicated, as it is not curative in this disease. However, total proctocolectomy with permanent ileostomy is indicated in patients with combined refractory colonic and anorectal disease.

COLONIC POLYPS

A polyp is an abundant growth of tissue projecting from the normal surface. Polyps are caused by abnormal growths of mucosa. They can be pedunculated and have a long stalk or be sessile and flat. The important differential factor, however, is the neoplastic or nonneoplastic nature of the polyp.

There are several types of nonneoplastic polyps. *Hyperplastic polyps,* the most common type of nonneoplastic polyp, represent expanded epithelium with distended goblet cells but no cellular atypia and normal crypt architecture. Their formation may result from failure to shed proliferating cells. Although they carry no malignant potential, they can not be distinguished from neoplastic polyps grossly and should be removed for histologic examination. *Inflammatory polyps* also have no malignant potential. They arise in patients with inflammatory bowel disease or other inflammatory states due to regenerating epithelium. *Juvenile polyps* occur most often in children less than 10 years of age. They are hamartomas and most often present in the distal colon. They also have no malignant potential but can bleed and should be removed for analysis and relief of symptoms.

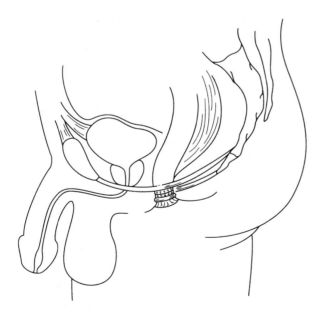

FIGURE 15-3. End-to-end ileoanal anastomosis after colectomy, mucosal proctectomy, and endorectal ileoanal pull-through. (From Becker JM. Ulcerative colitis. In: Greenfield LJ, Mulholland MW, Oldham KT, et al., eds. *Surgery: scientific principles and practice*, 2nd ed. Philadelphia: Lippincott-Raven Publishers, 1997: 1102, with permission.)

The evolution of colorectal cancer from neoplastic polyps occurs through a series of molecular changes. Alterations in protooncogenes or genes involved in repair of DNA, as well as loss of tumor suppressor genes, play a part in the sequence of steps leading to carcinoma. Mutation of the k-*ras* gene on chromosome 12p is found in approximately 65% of sporadic colorectal cancers, and it is believed to be involved in the early dysplastic changes of an adenoma. Deletions of the familial APC gene on chromosome 5q, which acts as a tumor suppressor gene, can be found in more than 60% of sporadic adenomas. Likewise, deletions in chromosome 18q, the deleted in colorectal cancer gene, as well as in the p53 gene on 17p are also found in cases of carcinoma, both of which are tumor suppressor genes. In general, there seems to be a stepwise progression that leads from normal mucosa to adenoma to carcinoma along with each mutation (Fig. 15-4).

Adenomas, themselves, can be further characterized. Tubular adenomas make up 60% to 80% of preneoplastic polyps and contain a network of adenomatous glands, whereas villous adenomas have glands extending straight down to the base. Mixed tubulovillous adenomas also exist. The extent of malignant potential is directly related to the degree of villous architecture. Dysplasia within the polyp can be defined as mild, moderate, or severe. Cases of severe dysplasia with an intact basement membrane are defined as *carcinoma in situ*. Not all polyps result in cancer, but size and histology do correlate with cancerous potential and large villous polyps present the greatest risk. In general, polyps are asymptomatic but can cause bleeding, and if very large, they can result in electrolyte disturbances such as hypokalemia.

Patients with polyps should have a full colonoscopy to rule out synchronous lesions. Endoscopic polypectomy is the preferred treatment for pedunculated lesions. The criteria for curative polypectomy of a neoplastic polyp require free margins of at least 2 mm, no evidence of vascular invasion, and a well-differentiated polyp. In the case of a sessile villous adenoma that can not be completely removed, surgical resection is indicated. It has been demonstrated that removal of adenomatous polyps decreases the rate of subsequent colon cancer and further supports the hypothesis of adenoma progression to cancer. Follow-up consists of repeated colonoscopy 3 to 6 months after a neoplastic polyp is removed to rule out recurrence. A negative follow-up result ensures a 5-year disease-free interval due to the gradual progression of dysplasia.

In some cases, polyps arise as part of a syndrome; the most common is familial adenomatous polyposis. Polyps develop at an early age and continue to form, so the colon can be covered by thousands of polyps. The entire GI tract can also be involved with polyps. Colorectal cancer develops at a mean age of 35, and screening includes sigmoidoscopy starting as early as 10 years of age, as well as DNA testing. Gardner syndrome is a variation of familial adenomatous polyposis and includes systemic manifestations such as osteomas, lipomas, and sarcomas. Turcot syndrome is a variation that includes brain tumors. All these classifications are of historic interest only because these diseases represent variable manifestations of a mutation in the same gene.

Familial adenomatous polyposis occurs as a result of a deletion on the APC gene located on chromosome 5q. Patients with known family history are typically screened by

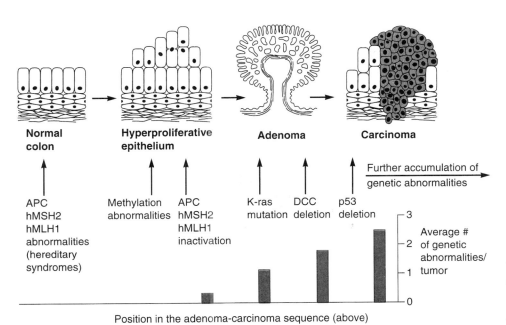

FIGURE 15-4. Molecular genetic events during the adenoma-to-carcinoma sequence. (From Bresalier RS, Toribara NW. In: Eastwood GL, ed. *Premalignant conditions of the gastrointestinal tract.* New York: Elsevier Science, 1991, with permission.)

sigmoidoscopy. A few years may elapse before polyps progress to cancer and surgery may be postponed until the patient fully matures. Total proctocolectomy is the procedure of choice, as any residual rectal mucosa is at risk for subsequent malignancy. Recently, total abdominal colectomy with rectal mucosectomy and ileoanal pouch has been used with success. Medical management may be possible, as reports have demonstrated regression of polyps on sulindac. The polyps, however, recur upon discontinuation of the drug. As a result, this is not a cure but an adjunct in patients with remaining rectal mucosa.

Hereditary nonpolyposis colorectal cancer, otherwise known as "Lynch syndrome," is a hereditary form of colorectal cancer that arises from adenomas but does not involve polyposis. This autosomal dominant disease presents early in life, between 20 to 40 years of age. It involves a mutation on chromosome 2. Genetic testing exists and involves testing of hMSH2, hMSH1, hPMS1, and hPMH2 genes in leukocytes. Other cancers associated with this syndrome include endometrial, ovarian, stomach, and urinary tract tumors. Peutz-Jeghers syndrome consists of hamartomatous polyps associated with cutaneous pigmented lesions. Intestinal obstruction is the main complication of this disease. The polyps present a very low risk for malignancy and surgical resection is not indicated. Cowden disease involves hamartomatous polyps with facial epithelial lesions. These patients also have an increased risk for breast cancer. The Cronkhite-Canada syndrome, a noninherited disorder, consists of polyps, diarrhea, alopecia, and hyperpigmentation. The polyps consist of hamartomatous lesions.

COLORECTAL CANCER

Colorectal cancer is the third most common malignancy in the world, and it is the second leading cause of cancer death. Ninety percent to ninety-five percent of cases are adenocarcinoma, and the remaining consist of squamous cell, lymphomas, sarcomas, and carcinoids. It presents equally in men and women. Other than genetic factors discussed earlier, diet plays a role in predisposition to cancer. A high-fat, low-fiber diet leads to a higher risk for colorectal cancer and other risk factors for this disease include adenomatous polyps, inflammatory bowel disease, radiation, familial polyposis syndrome, and previous ureterocolostomy. Because colorectal cancer is so prevalent in our society, screening plays a very important role in early diagnosis. In high-risk patients, such as first-degree relatives of patients with known hereditary colon cancer syndromes, colonoscopy should be performed by the age of 20 and regularly thereafter. Otherwise, the National Cancer Institute and the American Cancer Society recommend fecal occult blood testing annually and flexible sigmoidoscopy every 3 to 5 years after the age of 50.

Disease stage is a very important prognostic factor. The most common classification system is the Dukes classification with the modified Astler-Coller system. Stage A indicates involvement of the mucosa only. Stage B_1 indicates invasion but not penetration of the muscularis propria, whereas stage B_2 disease penetrates the muscularis layer. Stage C_1 and C_2 are the same as B_1 and B_2, respectively, except with lymph node involvement. Stage D represents distant metastases (Table 15-1). Survival correlates with the stage, and stages A through D have 90%, 75%, 45%, and 10% survival rates, respectively. Colon cancer typically spreads by direct invasion, lymphatic, and hematogenous routes.

Surgical resection remains the mainstay for the treatment of colorectal cancer even in metastatic disease to the liver. Preoperative studies such as liver function tests, abdominal computed tomography (CT) scan, and endoscopic ultrasound can be used to stage disease, and obtaining a carcinoembryonic antigen (CEA) level before resection offers a sensitive method to detect postoperative recurrence. Surgical resection should include the tumor with at least a 3-cm margin of normal bowel, the vascular supply to that segment, and all the respective lymphatic drainage (Fig. 15-5). Right colectomy is adequate for cecal and ascending colonic lesions. Hepatic flexure lesions require an extended right hemicolectomy, resecting the entire transverse colon along with the ascending colon. Transverse colon lesions are treated by resection of the transverse colon, and splenic flexure lesions require removal of mid transverse colon to mid descending colon. Tumors of the descending colon are removed by left hemicolectomy. Sigmoid and rectosigmoid lesions are treated by segmental resection. When the tumor involves the middle third of the rectum, 5 to 10 cm from the anal verge, a low anterior resection can be performed and a pri-

TABLE 15-1. STAGING OF COLON CANCER

Stage	TNM classification	Description
A	T1, N0, M0	Invasion into submucosa, no nodes
B1	T2, N0, M0	Invasion into muscularis propria, no nodes
B2	T3, N0, M0	Invasion through muscularis propia but not through serosa, no nodes
B3	T4, N0, M0	Invasion through the serosa, no nodes
C1	T2, N1–2, M0	Invasion into muscularis propria, positive nodes
C2	T3, N1–2, M0	Invasion through muscularis propria but not through serosa, positive nodes
C3	T4, N1–2, M0	Invasion through the serosa, positive nodes
D	Tx, Nx, M1	Distant metastases

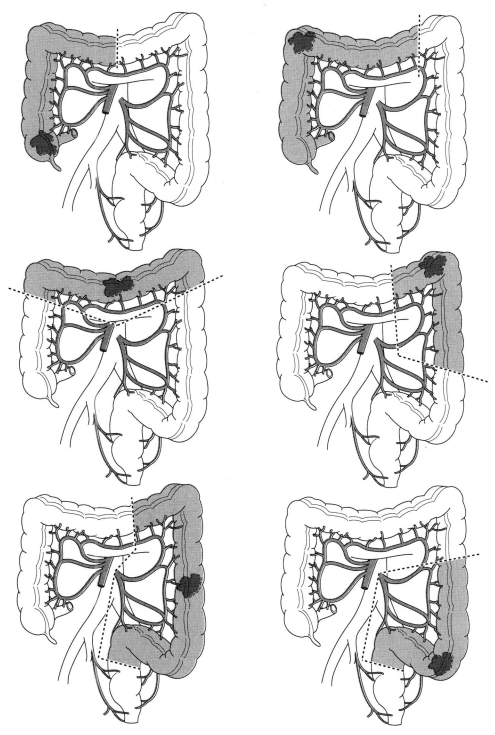

FIGURE 15-5. Segmental colonic resection including the vascular supply and lymphatics for various locations of colorectal cancer. (From Change AE. Colorectal cancer. In: Greenfield LJ, Mulholland MW, Oldham KT, et al., eds. *Surgery: scientific principles and practice*, 2nd ed. Philadelphia: Lippincott-Raven Publishers, 1997:1139, with permission.)

mary anastomosis can still be done. Tumors lower than this, however, require an abdominoperineal resection with a permanent ileostomy.

Adjuvant therapy involves radiation therapy and chemotherapy. Radiation is used mostly in rectal cancer and has been shown to decrease local recurrence. Adjuvant radiation can be delivered preoperatively, postoperatively, or as a combination of both. No clear superiority of one method over another has been documented. It is used in patients with stage II or greater disease with significant success. Chemotherapeutic agents include 5-fluorouracil (5-FU), levamisole, semustine, and vincristine. Different combinations have led to different results. The National Surgical Adjuvant Breast and Bowel Project demonstrated a significant improved survival rate with 5-FU, semustine, and vincristine versus no treatment. Furthermore, a later study showed that 5-FU and leucovorin increased survival compared to 5-FU, semustine, and vincristine. In general, the use of chemotherapy is advocated in stage III colon cancer and stage II and III rectal cancer.

Half the cancers that recur do so within 18 months of surgery and 90% of recurrences happen within 3 years. CEA level is a good marker for early recurrence. If the tumor produced CEA and levels were high prior to but normalized after resection, elevation can signify recurrence of disease. Local recurrence is common and occurs in about 20% of patients. The local lesion is the only site of disease in about one third of patients who recur and this population can be cured by reresection. Unfortunately, most cases of recurrence present as disseminated disease.

The most common location for metastatic disease is the liver. Patients who have no extrahepatic lesions, fewer than four intrahepatic lesions, and can tolerate a liver resection are candidates for removal of metastatic deposits. Because wedge resection is often adequate, anatomic resection is not indicated unless it is needed to obtain free margins. If the metastatic tumor deposits can be resected with at least 1-cm negative margins, 5-year survival rate is approximately 25% and can be as high as 45% with a detailed preoperative and intraoperative examination for other disease. Patients who are not candidates for a curative resection can benefit from chemotherapy by hepatic arterial infusion. The rationale for this treatment is based on the fact that unlike hepatocytes, metastatic liver tumors derive most of their blood supply from the hepatic artery, rather than the portal vein. Treatment with floxuridine, which has a 95% first-pass extraction from the liver, allows for high tumor exposure and low systemic exposure to the chemotherapeutic agent. In isolated metastases to the lung, pulmonary resection can be performed with as high as a 20% 5-year survival. For systemic, widely metastatic disease, resection of the metastatic foci is not indicated and 5-FU in combination with leucovorin is the treatment of choice.

A minority of tumors occurring in the colon are not adenocarcinoma. Carcinoid tumors arise from primitive ectodermal stem cells in the gut. The appendix is the most common site for carcinoid tumors and the size of the lesion determines treatment. For tumors less than 2 cm, local resection can be curative. However, carcinoid tumors larger than 2 cm have a 90% metastatic risk and require a more extensive resection such as a right hemicolectomy. Lymphoma represents less than 0.5% of colorectal cancer cases. Because it is often part of a widespread disseminated disease, primary therapy consists of chemotherapy and radiation therapy, rather than surgery. If the workup reveals a focal site of disease in the colon, surgical resection may be considered. Even rarer are sarcomas, occurring as 0.1% of colorectal malignancies. Surgical resection is the treatment of choice for localized disease.

DIVERTICULAR DISEASE

Diverticula are outpouchings of the bowel varying in size from millimeters to centimeters. True diverticula involve all layers of the bowel, whereas false diverticula (pseudodiverticuli), which are far more common, only involve mucosa and submucosa. The point of herniation usually occurs near the mesenteric vessels entering the muscularis layer (Fig. 15-6). In most patients, diverticula are located in the sigmoid colon. Many causes of diverticula have been proposed including lack of dietary fiber and motility dysfunction. There is certainly an increased prevalence among people with low-fiber diets. In general, 35% to 50% of people have diverticula with an increasing preponderance with age. There is no difference in incidence rates between men and women, and most cases of diverticulosis are asymptomatic.

It is important to understand the difference between diverticulosis and diverticulitis. *Diverticulosis* simply means outpouching of the bowel wall, whereas *diverticulitis* refers to inflammation of the diverticulum. Inflammation may result from microperforations in the bowel wall or fecal obstruction leading to pressure necrosis and inflammation. It occurs in about 20% of patients with diverticulosis and most often presents in the sigmoid colon. Diverticulitis can present with fevers or abdominal pain. Bleeding from inflamed diverticula is less likely. The microperforation is often localized and walled off but can lead to free intraperitoneal perforation. Most often, patients present with left lower quadrant pain, fever, and an elevated white blood cell count. The differential diagnosis for this disease is broad and includes inflammatory bowel disease, perforated colon cancer, ischemic colitis, as well as other colonic pathology. CT scanning can be very useful for making the diagnosis of both colonic inflammation as well as abscess and perforation. Colonoscopy is also helpful but should be avoided during active inflam-

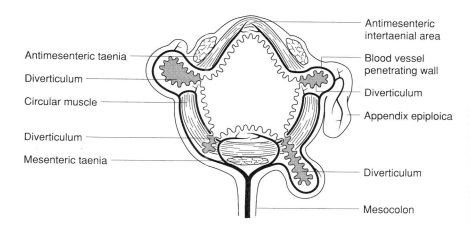

FIGURE 15-6. Colonic diverticula (pseudodiverticula or false diverticula) occur in the weak points in the colonic wall where mesenteric blood vessels penetrate the circular muscle layer. (From Telford GL, Otterson MF. Diverticular disease. In: Greenfield LJ, Mulholland MW, Oldham KT, et al., eds. *Surgery: scientific principles and practice*, 2nd ed. Philadelphia: Lippincott-Raven Publishers, 1997:1152, with permission.)

mation, as it can precipitate perforation. Patients with mild disease can be treated on an outpatient basis with oral antibiotics and a liquid diet. Those with more debilitating disease require hospitalization with bowel rest, i.v. fluids with possible parenteral nutrition, i.v. antibiotics, and pain medication. Most patients respond to this regimen. If they do not, a complication of diverticulitis must be suspected.

In general, *surgical indications* include repeat episodes, inability to rule out cancer, right-sided disease, a young patient, and complications. The complications include abscess, obstruction, fistula, and free perforation. Twenty percent of patients develop complications with their first bout of diverticulitis. In contrast, 60% have complications after their second bout. In the case of a localized abscess, CT-guided percutaneous drainage has become the treatment of choice. This allows drainage of the collection and time for the inflammation to subside, allowing for a technically easier operation. Multiple approaches to surgical resection can be performed. In the one-stage approach, the segment of diseased bowel is removed and a primary anastomosis is performed. If this can not be done, as in cases of generalized peritonitis or severely inflamed bowel, a two-stage approach can be performed. This entails resecting diseased bowel and creating a Hartmann pouch with an endcolostomy or a proximal diversion by a loop colostomy. As the patient improves, a second operation can be performed in approximately 6 weeks to take down the colostomy and perform the colonic anastomosis (Fig. 15-7). The three-stage approach is rarely used and is more of historical interest. Here, during the first operation, a drain is placed near the diseased bowel to remove the collection. At the same time, a diverting ostomy is formed. During the second stage, the diseased bowel is resected and a primary anastomosis is performed. Finally, in a third operation, the ostomy is reversed.

Obstruction is a significant complication of diverticulitis. The cause is usually a stricture that forms from inflammation and subsequent fibrosis. It is important to differentiate this from cancer, and thus, colonoscopy with biopsy should be performed. If the situation is more urgent and the patient is in need of an operation, the degree of obstruction is important. In a partial obstruction, the bowel can be prepared and a single-stage operation can be carried out. In a complete obstruction, because a bowel preparation is contraindicated, a Hartmann procedure needs to be performed.

Fistulae also occur as a complication of diverticulitis. The most common site for fistula formation is between the colon and the bladder. These patients present with urinary tract symptoms including dysuria, fecaluria, and pneumaturia. Fistulae can occur in other organs as well and can sometimes communicate with the vagina and skin. Diagnosis of the fistula can be aided by CT scan, barium enema, cystoscopy, vaginoscopy, or other tests specific for the type of fistula. Treatment usually consists of resection of the diseased bowel and closure of the fistulous opening of the connected organ. The colon can either be reanastomosed or left as an ostomy and a Hartmann pouch depending on the circumstances. A flap of omentum should be interposed between the colon and bladder or vagina.

Diverticulitis is not limited to the descending and sigmoid colon. Some 5% to 10% of diverticula are located in the cecum and ascending colon. Most right-sided diverticula are acquired pseudodiverticula, as are those on the left side, but congenital diverticula involving all layers of the bowel wall are more common in the cecum and ascending colon than in the remainder of the colon. Right-sided diverticulitis usually presents in a younger age group, around 30 to 40 years of age, and is often confused with appendicitis, as many of the symptoms are similar: fever, nausea, and right-sided abdominal pain. A CT scan can significantly improve the rate of correct diagnoses and operative strategy is the same as with left-sided diverticulitis.

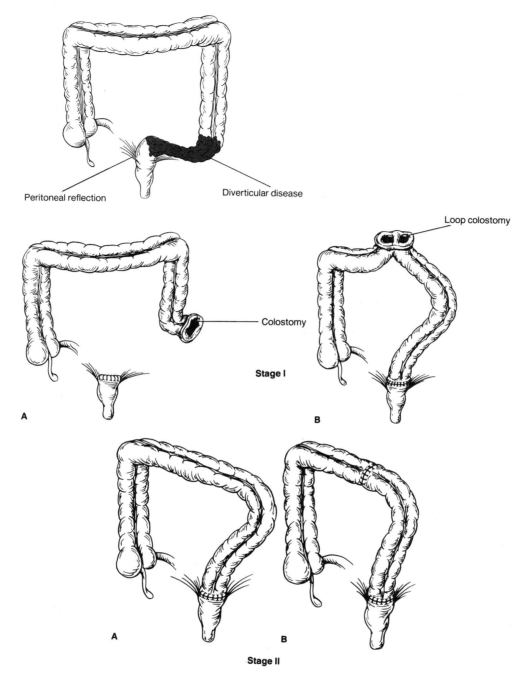

FIGURE 15-7. The two-stage operation for complicated colon diverticulitis. Stage I involves resection of the affected colon and either **(A)** a descending colostomy and rectal pouch (Hartmann operation) or **(B)** a proximal loop colostomy and colorectal anastomosis. Stage II involves **(A)** restoration of colon continuity and **(B)** takedown of the loop colostomy if necessary. (From Knol JA. Colonic diverticular disease. In: Bell RH, Rikkers LF, Mulholland MW, eds. *Digestive tract surgery: text and atlas*. Philadelphia: Lippincott-Raven Publishers, 1996:1376, with permission.)

LOWER GI BLEEDING

GI bleeding presents in many ways. A patient can have hematemesis, bright red blood per rectum, or melena. The bleeding can occur anywhere along the GI tract, but only 1% of bleeding arises from the small intestine. It is important to characterize the bleeding source. *Upper GI bleeds* are defined as those proximal to the ligament of Treitz, whereas, lower GI bleeds are distal to the ligament. Differentiation between the two depends on history, physical examination, and diagnostic studies. Causes for upper GI bleeding include peptic ulcer disease, gastritis, varices, as well as other sources. For the purpose of this chapter, only colorectal sources of bleeding will be discussed. Colorectal bleeding manifests itself as hematochezia or bright-red blood per rectum. Rarely does it present as melena, although slow transit in the colon can lead to this presentation. Patients who have acute GI bleeding must be treated quickly. Large-bore i.v. lines should be started and i.v. fluids infused. Serial hemoglobin levels should be followed while platelets and coagulation studies are obtained. If bleeding is brisk, the patient should be followed in an intensive care setting. A nasogastric tube is inserted initially to rule out an upper GI source. If bile is obtained and after saline lavage no blood is visible in the aspirate, the bleeding is unlikely to be due to an upper GI source. Esophagoduodenoscopy, however, is the only way to definitively rule out bleeding proximal to the ligament of Treitz.

If the bleeding is indeed from the lower GI tract, the first step involves ruling out anorectal bleeding. A careful rectal examination is performed to look for anorectal lesions, specifically, internal hemorrhoids. An anoscope is very helpful to visualize these lesions. The rate of bleeding will determine the next diagnostic procedure. In patients who are bleeding slowly or who have stopped bleeding, colonoscopy is helpful. It can not only diagnose the source of bleeding but can also be therapeutic by allowing electrocauterization of bleeding vessels. Patients should be prepared with cathartics if possible. In the presence of active bleeding, however, it can often be difficult to inspect the colon endoscopically. In such a case, a radionuclide scan with either technetium-labeled red blood cells or technetium-labeled sulfur colloid can help localize the bleeding site. This test can be performed in patients bleeding at a rate as slow as 0.1 mL per minute. Radionuclide scans, however, can only demonstrate the region of bleeding and offer no therapeutic potential. Furthermore, positive studies can be misleading. For example, a high transverse colon that is bleeding could be confused with an upper GI bleed, and blood from a right-sided source may pool in the left side. Angiography, on the other hand, is very selective and can pinpoint the bleeding vessel by the extravasation of blood and contrast into the colon. It can combine diagnosis with treatment by allowing embolization of bleeding vessels with thrombotic agents or injection with vasopressin. The superior mesenteric artery, inferior mesenteric artery, and their branches can be catheterized. Bleeding must also be brisk, on the order of 0.5 mL per minute, in order to be visualized. Complications of these procedures include bowel ischemia, myocardial ischemia, as well as complications related to the catheterization.

The main causes of massive colonic bleeding are diverticulosis (approximately 50%) and arteriovenous malformations (approximately 30%). Miscellaneous conditions such as cancer, ischemic colitis, and inflammatory bowel disease make up the remaining etiologies. Diverticula, as discussed previously, usually occur at the site where blood vessels penetrate the muscularis. It is at this site that the vessels can be damaged and bleed. Fifteen percent of patients with diverticula will experience at least one lower GI bleeding episode. Eighty percent of patients spontaneously stop bleeding, and less than 25% of these patients will rebleed. The rate of recurrent bleeding, however, doubles after a second episode. In 70% to 90% of cases, it is a right-sided diverticula that bleeds, most likely because the thinner less muscular colonic wall can not tamponade the bleeding. It is important to note that a diverticulum does not need to be inflamed in order to bleed and diverticulitis rarely bleeds.

Bleeding from arteriovenous malformations (AVMs) is also usually right-sided, as most AVMs occur in the right colon. The AVM consists of malformed vessels with thin friable walls. As with diverticula, most AVMs will stop bleeding spontaneously. They are readily identified by colonoscopy or angiogram. Although less common, other sources of massive colonic bleeding do occur, such as inflammatory bowel disease, irradiated bowel, colon cancer, and infectious colitis. Colon cancer is the leading cause of low-grade GI bleeding but rarely presents as a massive bleed.

The treatment for all bleeding patients is immediate resuscitation and definitive diagnosis. With invasive studies, such as colonoscopy and angiography, bleeding lesions can usually be stopped. If patients continue to bleed and nonoperative methods are unsuccessful, surgical intervention is warranted. Patients with persistent bleeding requiring greater than a 6-U blood transfusion within 24 hours will most likely need an operation. Diagnostic studies to localize the lesions are extremely important. Even a tagged red blood cell scan will at least identify the segment of bowel that needs to be removed. In the absence of localizing studies, a subtotal colectomy will need to be performed. Almost all likely sources of lower GI bleeding can be removed by this operation but a mortality of 30% to 50% can be anticipated in this situation. It is of utmost importance to rule out anorectal lesions as the source of bleeding to prevent the unnecessary removal of a patient's entire colon.

COLONIC VOLVULUS

Volvulus is a torsion of the bowel that may or may not involve the mesentery and vascular stalk. The sigmoid colon is the most common site of volvulus followed by the right colon and transverse colon. Etiology of volvulus depends upon location. Cecal volvulus is usually caused by a congenital lack of fixation to the abdominal wall. In debilitated patients and those on chronic laxatives who develop redundant colon, it is the sigmoid that usually twists and rotates upon itself.

Sigmoid volvulus usually presents in the 60- to 70-year-old age group (Fig. 15-8). The colon develops a clockwise rotation, resulting in a closed loop obstruction. This can progress to vascular compromise and ischemia. Nevertheless, only 10% of patients will present with perforation or infarction and most develop symptoms of distal colonic obstruction. Diagnostic studies include plain films (bent inner tube), barium enema (bird's beak), and colonoscopy or sigmoidoscopy. In patients who do not have symptoms of systemic illness, sigmoidoscopy or colonoscopy is used as the initial treatment to reduce the volvulus and decompress the colon. A rectal tube is inserted and left in place. There is an 80% success rate with this procedure for immediate decompression and relief of symptoms. Because endoscopic therapy does not treat the underlying redundant colon and only relieves the obstruction, a high recurrence rate of 50% to 90% can be expected. Therefore, in patients who can tolerate an operation, definitive treatment by resection of redundant sigmoid should be performed. The advantage of preoperative endoscopic detorsion is that a bowel preparation can be performed, allowing for a safer primary anastomosis. In any patient with suspicion of complications such as infarction or perforation, immediate laparotomy should be undertaken without attempts at endoscopic therapy.

The cause of cecal volvulus, as mentioned earlier, is the congenital lack of fixation to the abdominal wall. Symptoms usually occur in those 50 to 60 years of age. Volvulus can involve a clockwise rotation along the longitudinal axis (85% of cases) of the cecum or a transverse folding upon itself with the appendix pointing cephalad, otherwise known as a *cecal bascule*. Symptoms, again, are related to degree of obstruction, and diagnostic studies are the same as with a sigmoid volvulus. Treatment, however, consists of immediate operation because there has been very little success with endoscopic detorsion. Mortality is significantly higher in those with infarcted bowel and operative management consists of detorsion alone, detorsion and cecopexy, or right hemicolectomy. Detorsion alone has a recurrence rate of 13%, and it is unclear if cecopexy significantly improves this number. As a result, in any patient who can tolerate the operation, a right hemicolectomy is most appropriate.

Volvulus of the transverse colon is rare. Endoscopic detorsion is usually unsuccessful and operative intervention is indicated. As with a cecal volvulus, operative detorsion alone is associated with a high rate of recurrence, so resection or pexy should be performed.

PSEUDOMEMBRANOUS COLITIS

Pseudomembranous colitis is named after the pathologic appearance of the colonic mucosa. It is an antibiotic-associated colitis that leads to formation of exudative, pseudomembranous material on the mucosa. This exudative substance is formed of leukocytes, epithelial cells, mucus, and fibrin. The inflammatory process is usually contained within the lamina propria but can extend deeper. The lesions most commonly occur in the rectosigmoid region but can be found elsewhere.

In most instances, the pathogenic organism is *Clostridium difficile*. This in an anaerobic, spore-forming, Gram-positive rod that exists in the colon of approximately 5% of the normal population. When patients are taking antibiotics that neutralize the normal flora, *C. difficile* can cause a superinfection and resultant colitis. Patients can be on any type of antibiotic, via any route, for any length of time. Furthermore, the colitis may not develop until weeks after the antibiotic is stopped. The antibiotic most often associated with pseudomembranous colitis is clindamycin. *C. difficile*, itself, does not cause the colitis, rather a toxin that the bacteria releases is the culprit. There are two toxins, toxin A and toxin B. These toxins attack the mucosa, causing inflammation. In general, patients present with watery, green diarrhea that is associated with crampy abdominal

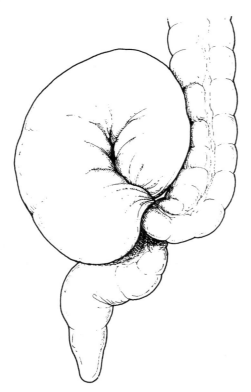

FIGURE 15-8. Sigmoid volvulus. (From Evans JT, Dayton MT. Colon, rectum, and anus. In: Lawrence PF, ed. *Essentials of general surgery*, 3rd ed. Philadelphia: Lippincott Williams & Wilkins, 2000:286, with permission.)

pain. Stools can contain blood but are rarely grossly bloody. Complications include shock from sepsis or hypovolemia, colonic dilation, or perforation.

Diagnosis depends on clinical suspicion with supporting studies. Stool can be sent for a fecal leukocyte test, but this is neither sensitive nor specific. The test most often used is an enzyme-linked immunosorbent assay, testing for the presence of toxin A or B. Multiple stool samples should be sent on different days to increase the sensitivity. Endoscopic examination can also be performed. Upon sigmoidoscopy or colonoscopy, pseudomembranes can be seen, which are diagnostic of the disease. Endoscopy, however, is expensive and can be very uncomfortable for the patient with an inflamed colon.

Treatment consists of antibiotics directed at *C. difficile*. Oral metronidazole is used initially at a regimen of 250 mg four times a day. It is the least expensive drug and most isolates of *C. difficile* are sensitive to this antibiotic. Vancomycin is used as a secondary agent because it is more expensive but rarely are any *C. difficile* isolates resistant to vancomycin. If oral intake is impossible, i.v. metronidazole can be used because it is secreted by the hepatobiliary tree into the duodenum. Many believe, however, that most of this drug is absorbed by the small intestine and never reaches the colon in therapeutic amounts. The i.v. form of vancomycin definitely does not reach the colonic mucosa in therapeutic concentration, although it is sometimes used in combination with i.v. metronidazole. In either case, the oral form should be used whenever possible. Even after successful treatment, patients may still have stool cultures positive for *C. difficile,* as they remain asymptomatic carriers.

Cholestyramine, an anion exchange resin, has also been used as a treatment for this disease. It binds toxin B and possibly toxin A. It does not affect the bacterial isolate itself and theoretically works by binding the noxious toxin while allowing the normal flora to repopulate the colon. This form of therapy is used only in the mild form of illness.

Antimotility agents should be avoided, as they may cause serious side effects, such as toxic dilation of the colon. Stool-hardening agents, such as Kaopectate, can be used because they do not alter colonic motility. Recurrence or persistence is also treated by metronidazole or vancomycin, but colonic repopulation by normal flora is the most important aspect of disease management.

APPENDIX

The appendix is believed to be a vestigial organ with no particular function in man. Appendicitis occurs due to luminal obstruction. The cause of obstruction is usually due to lymphoid hyperplasia or a fecalith and less likely due to tumors or parasites. As the appendix continues to produce mucus, it becomes distended and bacterial overgrowth occurs. As distension continues, venous and eventually arterial flow is occluded, leading to wall ischemia, necrosis, and perforation.

Diagnosis of appendicitis can follow a classic presentation. The patient complains of periumbilical pain that eventually localizes to the right lower quadrant. This represents the change from visceral peritoneal irritation to parietal peritoneal irritation. Nausea and vomiting follow the onset of pain. Anorexia is almost always present with appendicitis. On examination, the patient can have a low-grade fever and varying degrees of abdominal pain. Before perforation, the patient classically has pain at a McBurney point (two thirds the distance from the umbilicus to the anterior superior iliac spine). Other signs include a Rovsing sign (right lower quadrant pain upon palpation of the left lower quadrant), the psoas sign (pain upon extension of the right leg), and the obturator sign (pain upon internal rotation of the right leg at the hip). A rectal examination can sometimes elicit tenderness with a low-lying appendix. Confirmatory studies include laboratory evaluation, which may reveal a slightly elevated white blood cell count, as well as radiologic studies. Plain films are diagnostic if a fecalith is present, otherwise, ultrasound and CT scan are the studies of choice. Both modalities have sensitivities above 90%, but ultrasound is less expensive, uses no ionizing radiation, and is portable. It is, however, operator dependent, less useful in obese patients, and only visualizes one area. A CT scan can visualize a normal appendix and the entire abdomen. A focused appendiceal CT using rectal contrast only can be performed in less than 15 minutes with over a 98% sensitivity and specificity for appendicitis. Nevertheless, if a patient has a significant presentation for appendicitis, it is warranted to take the patient to the operating room without a radiologic examination with an acceptable 15% negative laparotomy rate.

The treatment for appendicitis is surgical removal of the inflamed appendix. An incision is made at the McBurney point and carried down to the peritoneum. The cecum is delivered into the wound and the appendix is removed, tying off the appendicular arteries. The appendiceal stump is cauterized and sometimes buried in the cecum with a pursestring or Z stitch. If upon exploration, the appendix is normal, it should still be removed to prevent future diagnostic confusion, but a search for other pathology must be undertaken. It is important to rule out a Meckel diverticulum.

In the case of a ruptured appendix, immediate or interval appendectomy can be performed. Immediate appendectomy entails the same operation, but a drain is left in place and the patient is continued on i.v. antibiotics. The skin of the wound is also left open to heal by secondary intention. If the patient has a ruptured appendix, is stable, and has a periappendiceal abscess, an interval appendectomy can be performed. The patient is maintained without oral intake and started on broad-spectrum antibiotics. If the abscess is well-contained, immediate percutaneous drainage can be carried out under ultrasound or CT guidance, and an interval appendectomy performed after 6 weeks. If at any time before appendectomy, the patient shows signs of toxicity—fever, tachycardia, hypotension—immediate operative removal is indicated. In cases in which the diagnosis is not clear, laparoscopy can be performed. This can be diagnostic for appendicitis as well as other pathologic processes. Appendectomy can subsequently be performed laparoscopically.

Occasionally, neoplasms can occur in the appendix, the most common of which is carcinoid. These tumors are often incidental findings, and their treatment and prognosis depends on the size. In carcinoid neoplasms of less than 1.5 cm, appendectomy is sufficient and rarely do these small tumors metastasize. Tumors of greater than 1.5 to 2.0 cm have increased rates of spread and a right hemicolectomy should be performed. The overall 5-year survival rate is 99% with this treatment. Other neoplasms of the appendix include cystadenoma, cystadenocarcinoma, and adenocarcinoma. The treatment of these depends on the stage of the tumor and can vary from appendectomy to right hemicolectomy.

ANORECTAL PATHOLOGY

Hemorrhoids

The anal canal consists of cushions of subcutaneous tissue containing veins and smooth muscle most commonly located in the left lateral, right anterior, and right posterior positions. These cushions support the anal canal lining during the process of defecation. When these cushions become dilated, they form internal hemorrhoids (Fig. 15-9). It is important to distinguish between internal and external hemorrhoids. External hemorrhoids are simply dilated venules below the dentate line. They can become thrombosed and cause quite a significant amount of pain. Internal hemorrhoids, however, are located above the dentate line and are painless. They are classified into four degrees. First-degree hemorrhoids simply bleed but do not protrude through the anal canal. Second-degree hemorrhoids herniate downward but spontaneously reduce. Third-degree hemorrhoids require manual reduction, and fourth-degree hemorrhoids are incarcerated and irreducible.

Depending on the type of hemorrhoid, patients will present with different symptoms. External hemorrhoids can cause pain, burning, and itching, whereas internal hemorrhoids usually present with bleeding or prolapse. With chronic hemorrhoids, mucosal prolapse can occur, causing pain and irritation. This type of prolapse needs to be differentiated from rectal prolapse, which involves all rectal layers. The diagnosis of hemorrhoids is made by physical examination and proctoscopy. External hemorrhoids can often be seen without instrumentation. Internal hemorrhoids are visualized by anoscopy or proctoscopy. Patients can be asked to strain to visualize the degree of prolapse. If the patient has too much pain to perform an adequate examination, an examination under anesthesia can be performed.

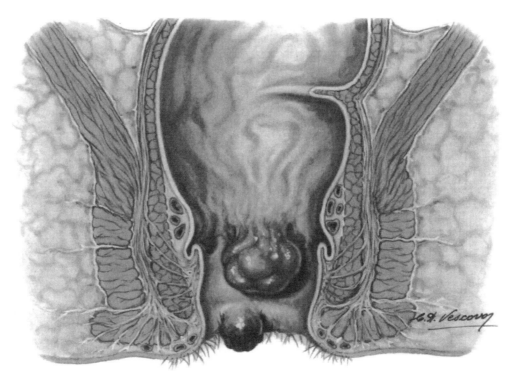

FIGURE 15-9. Internal hemorrhoids are located above the pectinate line while external hemorrhoids are located below. (From Etala E, ed. *Atlas of gastrointestinal surgery.* Philadelphia: Williams & Wilkins, 1997:2309, with permission.)

Treatment of hemorrhoids is initially medical. For both external and internal hemorrhoids, sitz baths and stool softeners can be helpful. Furthermore, dietary management can increase stool bulk and decrease straining. Thrombosed external hemorrhoids causing severe pain can be treated operatively with evacuation of clot and excision of the hemorrhoid. Second-degree internal hemorrhoids that do not respond to medical management can be treated in the office with rubber band ligation. An anoscope is inserted, the hemorrhoid is grasped, and a rubber band is then placed over the base of the hemorrhoid, causing necrosis and eventual sloughing. This should be a painless procedure, as internal hemorrhoids are located above the dentate line and have no somatic innervation. If the rubber band is misfired below the dentate line, however, the patient will have a significant amount of pain. Even with proper band placement, the patient may also have some discomfort from anal sphincter spasm. This problem can be prevented by treating only one hemorrhoidal bundle at a time. Complications of this procedure are uncommon but do include infection, necrosis, and perforation. It should be avoided in patients who are immunosuppressed due to the potential perianal sepsis.

Operative management of internal hemorrhoids is reserved for third- and fourth-degree hemorrhoids. The procedure can be performed with local anesthesia only and entails excision of the hemorrhoid from its superior margin to the perianal skin. The mucosa and submucosa are dissected off the internal sphincter with care not to disrupt this muscle. The wound may either be closed primarily or left open. Recent trials have shown that metronidazole significantly decreases postoperative pain. This is presumed to be due to a reduction of infected microthrombi.

Rectal Prolapse

As already stated, rectal prolapse, or procidentia, must be differentiated from mucosal prolapse. True rectal prolapse involves all layers of the rectum and not just the mucosa (Fig. 15-10). It is essentially a downward intussusception of the rectum and occurs mostly in patients with increased straining during defecation. Childbearing may be a predisposing factor as well, due to the weakness of the pelvic floor. Prolapse occurs more commonly in women than in men with a 5 to 6:1 ratio. Anatomic defects include deep rectovaginal or rectovesical pouch, weak pelvic floor, abnormal rectal fixation, and a redundant rectosigmoid.

Symptoms of rectal prolapse include anorectal discomfort, tenesmus, constipation, and gross prolapse. Incontinence, both fecal and urinary, can be associated with prolapse. Rectal prolapse is readily diagnosed on physical examination, particularly when it is beyond the anal verge. Endoscopy can be performed to rule out an associated lesion, such as a tumor. Other findings upon endoscopy include redness of the rectal mucosa or an anterior solitary rectal ulcer.

There are several approaches to repair. The Ripstein operation, used most commonly, incorporates a mesh sling that tacks the rectum to the presacral fascia. In another procedure, the redundant rectosigmoid is resected and reanastomosed primarily. Sometimes the remaining rectum is then fixed to the presacral fascia. Rectosigmoid resection can also be approached via a *trans*perineal method. This is preferred in patients who can not tolerate a *trans*abdominal procedure. Complications of these procedures include bleeding, particularly from the presacral venous plexus, as well as sepsis.

Fecal incontinence is not an uncommon complication of prolonged prolapse. It occurs from chronic stretching of the anal sphincters as well as the pudendal nerve. Approximately half of these patients will regain continence from repair of the prolapse, although it may take up to 1 year.

Fissure

Fissures are linear tears in the anal mucosa. The most common location for a fissure is in the posterior midline and the

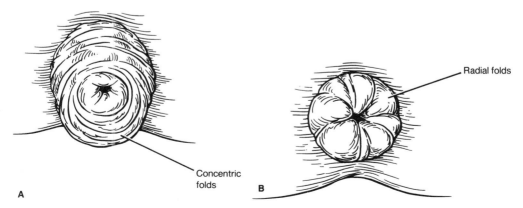

FIGURE 15-10. A: Full-thickness rectal prolapse involves more than just mucosa and is characterized by concentric mucosal folds. **B:** Rectal mucosal prolapse, however, is characterized by radial folds. (From Vernava AM III, Madoff RD. Anorectal disease. In: Bell RH, Rikkers LF, Mulholland MW, eds. *Digestive tract surgery: a text and atlas.* Philadelphia: Lippincott-Raven Publishers, 1996:1446, with permission.)

underlying cause is probably localized mucosal ischemia. Other etiologies include mucosal damage after passage of a hard stool or some underlying process, such as Crohn's disease or cancer. If this is not the case, suspicion should arise as to an underlying cause and further workup should be pursued. Pain is the most common presentation. Fissures are diagnosed by physical examination. They can be palpated on rectal examination and visualized by anoscopy. Often patients have too much pain for an office-based physical examination and must undergo an examination under anesthesia.

Anal fissures are usually managed nonoperatively. Good pain control is needed. Warm sitz baths, dietary bulking agents, and topical steroids are used. Newer medical treatments include nitric oxide ointment and injection of botulinum toxin into the internal anal sphincter. Both treatments are hypothesized to relieve internal sphincter spasm and decrease ischemia. Most fissures will heal in about 6 weeks.

Operative management is warranted for chronic fissures. Lateral internal sphincterotomy is the procedure of choice, relieves the chronic sphincter spasm, and can be done under local anesthesia. In the closed version of the procedure (Fig. 15-11), a speculum is inserted into the anus and the internal sphincter is palpated as a taut structure. On either the right or left side, a scalpel is vertically inserted along the lateral edge of the sphincter through the perianal skin to the level of the dentate line. The scalpel is then rotated 90 degrees so that the blade lies upon the sphincter, and the scalpel is withdrawn while incising the muscle. One can feel the relaxation of the sphincter. In the open method, the subcutaneous tissue is incised and the internal sphincter visualized. It is subsequently incised and the wound is closed primarily. The depth of incision of the internal sphincter should not exceed the depth of the fissure. Either procedure works well and has excellent results.

Fissures secondary to other disease processes are rarely treated operatively. The main therapy is to uncover the underlying process and treat it. The fissure is managed with local hygiene, pain control, and stool softeners and will usually heal when the underlying disease is under control.

FISTULA IN ANO AND PERIANAL ABSCESS

Abscesses often form from infection of the anal glands that line the anal canal. Localized infection can spread to the intersphincteric space as well as the perianal, ischioanal, and supralevator spaces. Patients most often complain of pain from the abscess. They can have fevers and a palpable mass as well. Upon examination, the abscess will be quite tender, possibly fluctuant, and may have an overlying cellulitis. The definitive treatment is drainage. Depending on the location, size, and condition of the patient, these abscesses can be drained at the bedside under local anesthesia or in the operating room under a more controlled environment. Certainly patients with underlying diseases, such as immunodeficiencies or diabetes, the more sterile environment of the operating room is preferred. Furthermore, antibiotics are favored in these patients, as well as those with an associated cellulitis. In contrast, in uncomplicated cases, patients do not have to be admitted and can be discharged after incision and drainage with close follow-up. At times, if local incision and drainage

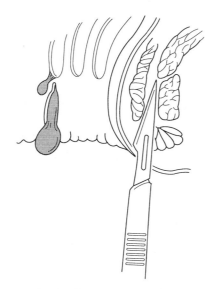

FIGURE 15-11. The closed technique of internal sphincterotomy involves selectively cutting the internal anal sphincter while the anal canal is stretched open. (From Nivatvongs S. Anorectal disorders. In: Greenfield LJ, Mulholland MW, Oldham KT, et al., eds. *Surgery: scientific principles and practice,* 2nd ed. Philadelphia: Lippincott-Raven Publishers, 1997:1196, with permission.)

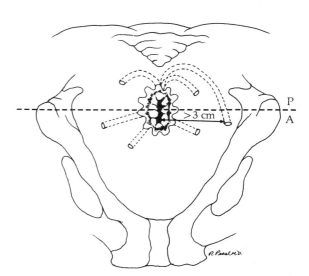

FIGURE 15-12. Goodsall's rule describes the relationship between the internal and external openings of fistula in ano. (From Abcarian H. Surgical treatment of anal disorders. In: Nyhus LM, Baker RJ, eds. *Mastery of surgery.* Boston: Little, Brown and Company, 1992:1358, with permission.)

is unsuccessful, other underlying conditions must be pursued. CT scan or MRI can be very helpful in these situations.

Fistula in ano is a version of the anorectal abscess that has formed a communication between the anal crypts and the perianal skin. That fistula occurs in close to half of the patients with perianal abscess. Goodsall's rule describes the relationship between the internal and external opening of the fistulous tract. If the external opening of the fistula is located posterior to the midline or 3 cm away from the anus, the fistula originated in a posterior anal crypt. Anterior fistulae, on the other hand, follow a direct line between the skin and the mucosa (Fig. 15-12). Fistulae are classified as intersphincteric (70%), *trans*sphincteric, suprasphincteric, and extrasphincteric (Fig. 15-13). On examination, the external opening will usually consist of raised granulation tissue along the rectal wall, and the tract can often be palpated. Anoscopy will help locate the internal opening. It is not uncommon for patients to have recurrent abscesses.

Management of fistulae consists of fistulotomy, or unroofing of the tract and drainage of any concurrent abscesses. Fistulectomy offers no advantage. Fistulotomy allows the tract to drain and the wound to heal upward, closing the tract. If the fistula traverses both sphincters, a seton must be used and a fistulotomy should not be performed because of the risk of injury to the sphincters. The seton, consisting of a vessel loop or suture, is threaded through the tract and tied down. The patient is closely followed and the seton is slowly, over weeks, tied down more and more. This transects the sphincters and unroofs the fistula while allowing the sphincter muscles to heal by fibrosis, thus preventing incontinence.

ANAL CANCER

The anal canal is lined by squamous epithelium below the dentate line and columnar epithelium above the dentate line. Adenocarcinoma may arise from the anus or extend down from the rectum. Patients present with bleeding, pain, and a mass. Local resection can be performed with lesions of less than 3 cm that are well-differentiated, have no vascular invasion, and if free margins can be obtained. Otherwise, an abdominoperineal resection is indicated.

In the case of squamous cell carcinoma, the presentation is similar, but the treatment differs. Carcinoma *in situ*, known as *Bowen disease*, can be treated with wide local excision. Invasive lesions require more extensive therapy. Chemotherapy with radiation is started first. If there is no residual disease, no further treatment is necessary. However, if cancer is present, abdominoperineal resection should be

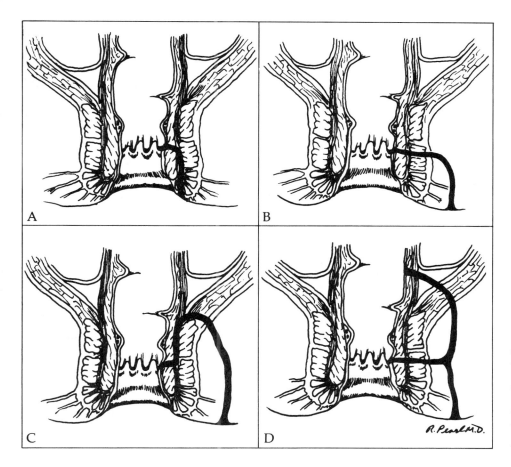

FIGURE 15-13. Classification of anal fistulae include **(A)** intersphincteric fistula, **(B)** *trans*sphincteric fistula, **(C)** suprasphincteric fistula, and **(D)** extrasphincteric fistula. (From Abcarian H. Surgical treatment of anal disorders. In: Nyhus LM, Baker RJ, eds. *Mastery of surgery.* Boston: Little, Brown and Company, 1992:1359, with permission.)

performed. Success rates as high as 90% have been reported with chemotherapy with radiation.

Malignant melanoma represents 1% of all anal cancer. The disease has usually progressed by the time of presentation. The tumors are resistant to chemotherapy and radiation. The survival rates of wide local excision and abdominoperineal resection are similar, both less than 20%.

PEDIATRICS

Imperforate Anus

Imperforate anus results from failure of the rectum to reach its full descent. The incidence of this disease is approximately 1 in 5,000 births. When the rectal descent is arrested above the pubococcygeal line, the anomaly is termed a *high imperforate anus*. This variation is twice as common in men as in women. A *low imperforate anus* nearly reaches the perineum. Associated anomalies are common and occur in as many as 70% of patients. The VATER complex consists of *vertebral* defects, *anal* atresia, *tracheoesophageal* fistula with *esophageal* atresia, and *radial* and *renal* anomalies. The VACTERL syndrome includes the above, as well as *cardiovascular* tree and *limb* buds abnormalities. Imperforate anus is usually identified at birth by examination, although a large fistula can sometimes be mistaken for the anus. In most low lesions, a perineal fistula is present. Contrast studies via the GI and genitourinary tract can be very useful in defining the anatomy.

In the case of low lesions, surgical repair is indicated early. If only a membrane is covering the anus, it can simply be excised. Posterior wall division to the external sphincter is performed for a simple fistula. With more complicated fistulae, the fistula is mobilized to the site of the external sphincter.

High imperforate lesions are also treated operatively, but a colostomy is initially performed to divert feces from the fistula. When the infant reaches 10 to 20 kg, an endorectal pull-through procedure can be done. The most common approach is the posterior sagittal anorectoplasty or Pena procedure. Division of the external sphincter and levators is done down to the rectal pouch. The pouch is then mobilized and brought to the perineum. In the process, any fistula is taken down and closed. The levators and external sphincter are then reapproximated around the neoanus, and the colostomy is left intact for diversion until the anastomosis heals.

Hirschsprung Disease

The etiology of Hirschsprung disease is unknown. It results from the failure in development of intestinal ganglion cells in the myenteric and submucosal nerve plexus. Due to the migration of ganglion cells during development, the distal colon and rectum are always affected but proximal extension of the aganglionic segment can involve a larger portion of the colon and even the small bowel. A transition zone of bowel with decreased numbers of ganglion cells is preceded by normal bowel with normal amounts of ganglion cells. The classic theory involves defective migration of neuroblasts to the intestine, but newer studies have also demonstrated a lack of nitric oxide synthase, which may be necessary for smooth muscle relaxation. In virtually all cases, Hirschsprung disease travels proximally with no skip lesions. There seems to be a dysfunction of both propulsion and relaxation, thus leading to abnormal or absent peristalsis.

The incidence is 1 in 5,000 births with a male to female ratio of 4:1. There is some familial relations, and studies suggest involvement of chromosomes 13q22, 21q22, and 10q. Trisomy 21 is associated with 5% to 15% of cases. Presentation includes abnormal to absent passage of meconium, abdominal distension, and bilious vomiting. Most cases are discovered by 2 years of age; however, milder forms are sometimes not diagnosed until after years of complaints of chronic constipation. Up to 30% of patients can develop colitis due to stasis and bacterial overgrowth. Diagnosis of Hirschsprung disease is aided by a contrast enema, which demonstrates a transition zone between dilated and nondilated bowel. Definitive diagnosis, however, is made by rectal biopsy. Suction biopsies are taken 2 to 3 cm proximal to the pectinate line and are diagnostic when the absence of ganglion cells is documented. Multiple samples must be taken to ensure the diagnosis.

A diverting colostomy is classically the first step in treatment. This allows for fecal diversion and decompression of the dilated bowel. An endorectal pull-through procedure can then be performed, although it is possible to perform both procedures at the same time. Occasionally, the pull-through can be performed as a one-step procedure without fecal diversion. The original procedure was pioneered by Swenson, where the diseased bowel was resected and proximal nondiseased bowel anastomosed to the low rectum. In the case of Hirschsprung disease involving the entire colon, an ileoanal anastomosis can be performed. In all cases, it is important to demonstrate existence of ganglion cells in the bowel proximal to the resected segment.

TRAUMA

Most cases of colorectal trauma are due to penetrating, rather than blunt, injury. The position of the colon and rectum make them less susceptible to forces of blunt trauma. When these organs are injured, the presentation can range from asymptomatic to obvious peritonitis. Penetrating injuries necessitate abdominal exploration. Blunt injuries, however, can be worked up with studies such as diagnostic peritoneal lavage and CT scan. Diagnostic peritoneal lavage is not useful for retroperitoneal areas of the colon and rectum because the perforation may not extend into the abdominal cavity. Any pelvic trauma should raise the suspicion for rectal injury as well. Morbidity and mortality are significantly decreased with early diagnosis.

Previous recommendations regarding operative treatment of colonic trauma included resecting the injured segment and creating a proximal ostomy. However, resection with primary anastomosis is now performed in select patients, particularly those with injuries of the right colon due to the decreased bacterial concentration in the proximal colon. In general cases of minor injury without gross fecal contamination, hemorrhage or hypotension are successfully treated by primary repair. Otherwise, it is safer to take a more conservative approach and resect the damaged area while creating a proximal endostomy. Subsequent reanastomosis can be performed at a later date after infectious complications resolve and other traumatic injuries are treated.

Rectal trauma is associated with significant morbidity if untreated. Any suspicion of rectal injury should be thoroughly investigated. Sigmoidoscopy is very useful in this situation. Patients should have a colostomy with debridement of necrotic tissue. Rectal wall closure should be performed if possible and copious irrigation of the pelvis performed. Finally, retrorectal drains need to be placed and the patient started on broad-spectrum antibiotics. Further debridement may be necessary.

SUGGESTED READING

Johnson LR, ed. *Essential medical physiology.* Philadelphia: Lippincott-Raven Publishers, 1998.

Zinner MJ, ed. *Maingot's abdominal operations.* Stamford: Appleton & Lange, 1997.

16

HEPATOBILIARY SYSTEM

ALLAN S. STEWART AND JAMES F. MARKMAN

ANATOMY OF THE LIVER

The liver resides in the right upper quadrant of the abdomen, immediately inferior to the diaphragm. It is invested in a peritoneal reflection (the Glisson capsule), which is continuous posteriorly with the right and left triangular ligaments and anteriorly with the falciform ligament. In the *American classification*, the liver is composed of two lobes divided by the interlobar fissure (the Cantlie line), an imaginary line between the gallbladder fossa anteriorly and the inferior vena cava (IVC) posteriorly (Fig. 16-1A). Each lobe is composed of two segments. The falciform ligament marks the left segmental fissure between the median and lateral segments of the left lobe. The right lobe is made up of anterior and posterior segments, which do not have an anatomic boundary. In the *French classification* of Couinaud, the liver is divided into eight segments, which correspond to blood supply, as well as venous and biliary drainage. Segment I is the caudate lobe, II through IV comprise the left lobe while V through VIII form the right lobe (Fig. 16-1B).

The liver receives a dual *blood supply*. Seventy-five percent of blood flow arises from the portal vein, which is formed by the confluence of the splenic vein, as well as the coronary and superior mesenteric veins. The portal vein then drains cephalad posterior to the first portion of the duodenum and becomes the most posterior structure in the porta hepatis. It branches into right and left veins, which progress into the parenchyma, where after extensive branching, a venule reaches the hepatic sinusoid. The remaining 25% of blood flow originates from the hepatic artery. The hepatic artery is a branch of the celiac axis, where it begins as the common hepatic artery. It gives off the gastroduodenal artery before progressing cephalad in the porta hepatis as the proper hepatic artery. In most people, the hepatic artery may be found anterior to the portal vein and medial to the common bile duct (Fig. 16-2). It divides into right and left branches before entering the parenchyma. In approximately 20% of patients, a replaced right hepatic artery is observed. This artery is a branch of the superior mesenteric artery and is located lateral to the common bile duct. Care must be taken during cholecystectomy to avoid ligation. In approximately 25% of patients, a replaced left hepatic artery will be observed. This artery arises from the left gastric artery and reaches the liver in the gastrohepatic ligament. It is important that liver tumors derive their nutrient blood flow from the hepatic arterial circulation. This is the rationale behind treating hepatic tumors with local administration of chemotherapy via intraarterially placed pumps or hepatic artery ligation and embolization. Blood drains from the liver to the IVC via three major vessels: the right, middle, and left hepatic veins. They course between segments and are located entirely within the hepatic parenchyma in most patients. The caudate lobe drains directly into the IVC through short posterior vessels.

STUDIES OF THE LIVER

Several *liver function tests* are available to test the synthetic, clearance, and excretory functions of the liver. Steady state function is most commonly evaluated by measuring serum protein levels such as serum albumin. A more sensitive indicator of change in function is the assessment of clotting factors, particularly the prothrombin time. The majority of clotting cascade enzymes are synthesized in the liver. Of particular importance is factor VII, which has a half-life of about 7 hours. Serum ammonia and indirect bilirubin measure excretory function. Hepatocyte injury is assessed by measurement of aspartate transaminase (also known as *serum glutamic-oxaloacetic transaminase*), alanine transaminase (also known as *serum glutamic-pyruvic transaminase*), γ-glutamyltransferase, and alkaline phosphatase.

Various *imaging modalities* can be used to evaluate patients with suspected hepatobiliary pathology. Ultrasonography is particularly useful in the diagnosis of cholelithiasis and assessment of the biliary system. It is also able to identify lesions in the liver. In addition, it is

Hospital of the University of Pennsylvania, Philadelphia, Pennsylvania

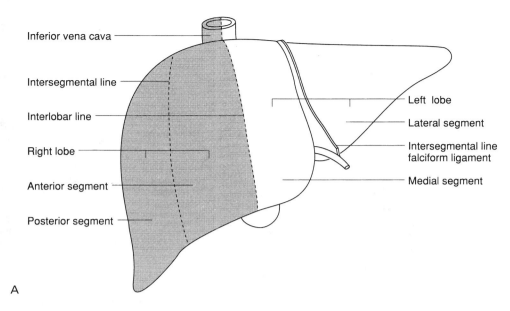

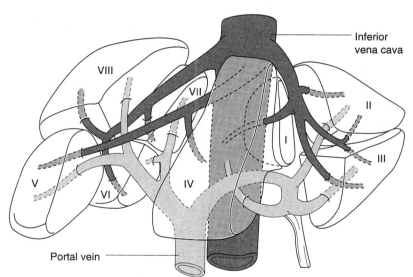

FIGURE 16-1. A: Lobar anatomy of the liver. **B:** Segmental anatomy of the liver. (From Greenfield LJ, Mulholland MW, Oldham KT, et al., eds. *Surgery: scientific principles and practice,* 2nd ed. Philadelphia: Lippincott-Raven Publishers, 1997:933, with permission.)

frequently used intraoperatively to evaluate further anatomic relations of intrahepatic lesions and in particular, the involvement of vascular structures. Computed tomography (CT) is a sensitive tool to detect primary or metastatic tumors involving the hepatic parenchyma. In many settings, magnetic resonance imaging (MRI) is also useful in diagnosing hepatic lesions, as it allows evaluation of the hepatic vasculature and biliary tree. However, MRI is not as widely available as CT and may be more expensive. One of its main applications in the evaluation of patients with hepatobiliary pathology is the differentiation of hemangiomas from other liver lesions.

BENIGN TUMORS OF THE LIVER

Hemangiomas are the most common benign tumors of the liver, second only to metastases in liver lesions overall. They occur more frequently in women than men, are usually asymptomatic, and are found on imaging studies for unrelated complaints. In a minority of cases, the mass may cause symptoms by compression of liver parenchyma (such as obstructive jaundice) or adjacent structures (such as gastric outlet obstruction). *Kasabach-Merritt syndrome* is defined as consumptive coagulopathy due to thrombosis within a large hemangioma lesion. Conservative management of asymp-

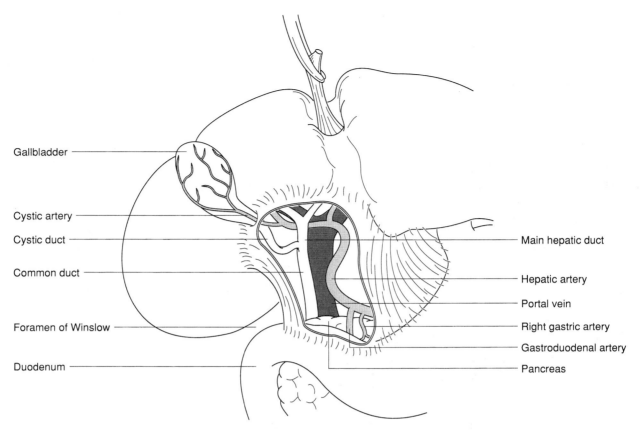

FIGURE 16-2. Anatomic relations of hepatic artery, portal vein, and common bile duct. (From Greenfield LJ, Mulholland MW, Oldham KT, et al., eds. *Surgery: scientific principles and practice*, 2nd ed. Philadelphia: Lippincott-Raven Publishers, 1997:1025, with permission.)

tomatic lesions is the rule with formal resection indicated only in symptomatic cases. On gross inspection of the resected lesion, single or multiple masses may be found. Microscopic evaluation reveals vascular lacunae lined with normal endothelial cells.

Hepatocellular adenoma is predominantly found in women and is strongly associated with oral contraceptive use. Symptoms are found in a minority of patients and include pain from stretching of the liver capsule, compression of adjacent structures, or spontaneous rupture. Spontaneous rupture presents as right upper quadrant pain and patients may demonstrate symptoms of hypovolemic shock. It carries a mortality rate of approximately 10%. Diagnosis is usually incidental, occurring when imaging for unrelated complaints. In patients who present with pain, ultrasound or CT may demonstrate a homogeneous mass, prompting biopsy to exclude malignancy. Transaminase levels are usually normal. Treatment is conservative; however, oral contraceptives should be discontinued, with anticipation of tumor regression. In patients with large tumors or in women who are fertile, resection should be considered, as pregnancy greatly increases the risk of rupture. In patients who present in extremis, treatment is directed at control of hemorrhage by hepatic artery ligation, either surgically or via embolization.

Focal nodular hyperplasia (FNH) is more frequently found in women, and there is no clear association with oral contraceptive use. Again, this mass is usually discovered incidentally. Biopsy is indicated to exclude malignancy. Microscopic examination reveals hyperplastic hepatocytes with inflammatory cells. The presence of bile-duct epithelium differentiates the mass from adenoma. A positive nuclear medicine scan is a useful diagnostic modality in distinguishing FNH from adenoma. Central stellate scars are occasionally seen in larger lesions. Unlike adenomas, these lesions are generally not associated with bleeding and their treatment is conservative.

PRIMARY MALIGNANT TUMORS OF THE LIVER

The incidence of primary *hepatocellular carcinoma* (HCC) varies geographically, with the highest number of cases seen in Africa and Asia and the lowest incidence seen in the Western world. Interestingly, the incidence of hepatocellular carcinoma corresponds directly to hepatitis B virus (HBV) and hepatitis C virus (HCV). The risk of chronic HBV infection increases the risk of hepatoma 200-fold. The increasing incidence of HCV during the last few decades has contributed to an increasing incidence of HCC in the United States and the Mediterranean countries of Europe. The main route of transmission of HCV is parenteral, through unscreened blood or by intravenous (i.v.) drug use. In the United States, the relative risk of HCC is 7 to 11.4 for HBV-positive patients and 10.5 to 23.2 for HCV-positive patients. There is evidence that coinfection of HCV and HBV, or either infection with associated heavy alcohol consumption, may have a synergistic effect. Other conditions associated with hepatoma are cirrhosis, hemochromatosis, schistosomiasis, and environmental exposures. Examples of exogenous carcinogens include aflatoxin (produced by *Aspergillus flavus* and found on foods such as peanuts), Thorotrast radiologic dye, carbon tetrachloride, vinyl chloride, and nitrosamines.

HCC often presents with dull pain in the right upper quadrant. It is accompanied by nonspecific, constitutional symptoms such as fever, malaise, and jaundice. Physical examination reveals hepatomegaly, a tender abdominal mass, and findings associated with cirrhosis such as caput medusae, varices, or ascites. Liver function test results are usually nonspecifically abnormal; however, the tumor marker α-fetoprotein (AFP) level is elevated in approximately 80% of cases. Diagnostic studies include right upper quadrant ultrasound, CT scan, and MRI to determine resectability.

Hepatoma occurs as a solitary mass or as multiple masses. Local invasion, most commonly into the diaphragm, is common, as is distant metastasis, most commonly to the lung. The *fibrolamellar variant* of HCC, which is characterized histologically by fibrous ingrowth, affects primarily younger patients and carries a more favorable prognosis.

Surgical treatment includes biopsy for tissue diagnosis and laparotomy to assess resectability. Intraoperative ultrasound is useful to assess intraparenchymal vascular invasion. With resection, the 5-year survival rate is approximately 20%. In lesions found to be unresectable, the average survival time is approximately 4 months. Patients with child's class B or C liver failure are usually not candidates for resection, unless the mass is small and peripheral. Resection in these patients includes total hepatectomy and transplantation. Results for this modality are currently inconclusive. Attempts to induce tumor necrosis by hepatic artery ligation have been disappointing; however, there are preliminary data supporting hepatic artery infusion of chemotherapeutic agents. Five-year survival rate after hepatic resection for the fibrolamellar variant is much higher, at approximately 50%.

Hepatoblastoma is the most common malignant liver tumor in children. It presents with abdominal distension, failure to thrive, and constitutional symptoms of liver failure. Histologically, this tumor is composed of immature hepatocytes. AFP level is elevated in most patients. Treatment is surgical, with inoperable tumors treated with radiation and chemotherapy. Results are uniformly poor.

Cholangiocarcinoma is a tumor arising from bile-duct epithelium and represents between 5% to 30% of all liver tumors. Patients present with right upper quadrant pain, jaundice, and occasionally a palpable right upper quadrant mass. At operation, the tumor is a hard, gray mass that on microscopic examination is adenocarcinoma of the biliary epithelium. Metastases are common and are found within the regional nodes and liver parenchyma. The etiology is attributed to exposure to Thorotrast radiologic dye, exposure to the parasite *Clonorchis sinensis,* or a history of primary sclerosing cholangitis. Treatment is resection when possible, but the overall results are poor.

Angiosarcoma is a highly malignant tumor composed of spindle cells lining the lumen of vascular spaces. It is aggressive in course and rapidly fatal. The most common etiology is exposure to vinyl chloride, Thorotrast, arsenic, organochloride pesticides, or androgens.

METASTATIC TUMORS OF THE LIVER

Metastatic tumors of the liver are far more common than the primary liver tumors (ratio 20:1). The liver is the most common solid organ site for metastatic involvement from primary gastrointestinal malignancies. Over 66% of colon tumors ultimately involve the liver, and over 50% of tumors with primaries outside the abdomen metastasize to the liver. Synchronous colorectal metastases are reported in 15% to 25% of patients while metachronous metastases are found in up to 40% of patients with colorectal cancer. The liver is the most common organ of hematogenous spread.

No single laboratory test can effectively diagnose a liver metastasis. Liver function test results are often elevated, but in no characteristic manner. Carcinoembryonic antigen level is elevated in patients with colorectal malignancies; however, the test lacks specificity. The best method of diagnosis is by imaging studies such as CT scan, MRI, and hepatic ultrasound. Resection is the mainstay of treatment for colorectal metastasis. Left untreated, colorectal metastasis survival rates have been reported at 31% at 1 year, 8% at 2 years, and 2.5% at 3 years. Resection increases the reported 1-year survival rate to more than 90% in patients with solitary metastasis and to more than 50% in patients with multiple lesions confined to one lobe. This treatment is limited to patients who have unilobar disease and enough viable liver to survive resection. Surgical resection of hepatic metastases should aim to obtain adequate margins of at least 1 cm and to preserve as much liver parenchyma as possible. Peripherally located metastatic lesions can be excised by nonanatomic wedge resection with a margin of at least 1 cm. Anatomic resections can be employed for centrally located lesions that involve vascular structures. For patients who are unresectable, alternatives include radiation, chemotherapy, and hepatic artery embolization. Radiation and systemic chemotherapy have been disappointing; however, early results with hepatic artery infusion therapy are encouraging. Hepatic artery ligation and embolization have demonstrated only transient benefits to tumor shrinkage.

HEPATIC ABSCESSES AND CYSTS

Bacterial abscesses are the most common hepatic abscesses in the Western world. Bacteria may reach the liver parenchyma by systemic spread, ascending biliary infection, or via portal venous drainage. They usually arise from intraabdominal infections such as cholangitis, diverticulitis, or appendicitis. Abscesses may also arise from hematogenous seeding such as from endocarditis. The most common organisms isolated are Gram-negative rods, predominantly *Escherichia coli* and *Bacteroides fragilis*; however, with endocarditis, Gram-positive rods predominate.

Patients present with fever, chills, leukocytosis, and less commonly right upper quadrant pain, septicemia, and hemobilia. Liver function test results will be abnormal, with a pronounced elevation of alkaline phosphatase. Hepatic ultrasound and CT scan are diagnostic. The standard treatment is surgical drainage and culture directed antibiotic therapy. Alternatively, good results have been reported with CT-guided aspiration and closed drainage. Patients are followed with periodic sinography to assess resolution of the abscess. Multiple abscesses are treated initially with antibiotics, before invasive therapy. The mortality rate for hepatic abscess is as high as 40%, most commonly because of a delay in diagnosis. Additional factors contributing to the high mortality rate are patients with multiple abscesses, as well as confounding factors such as malnutrition and septicemia.

Amebic abscesses are the second most common cause of hepatic abscesses in the United States and are the most common cause in the Third World. In the United States, amebic abscesses are more common in homosexual men with acquired immunodeficiency syndrome. The organism *Entamoeba histolytica* is a protozoan that infects the colon and reaches the liver through the portal vein. The abscess is usually solitary and is predominantly found in the right lobe.

Patients present with nonspecific symptoms consistent with hepatic abscess. Liver function test results, again, are nonspecific. However, indirect hemagglutination titer levels are elevated in more than 98% of patients with active hepatic infection. Treatment is conservative, with metronidazole. Cysts are aspirated if they are large, are adjacent to vital structures, or are not responsive to antibiotics.

The *hydatid cyst* of the liver results from infection with the parasite *Echinococcus granulosum,* a parasite found in dogs. Dogs shed parasites in stool, which can secondarily infect intermediate hosts, particularly people, sheep, and cattle. The parasite is endemic in areas where sheep are raised, predominantly Southern Europe, South America, and the Middle East.

The cysts can develop anywhere in the body but have a predilection for the liver. The cyst and its lining contain live parasites, which can propagate the infection. The outer layer, ectocyst, is composed of compressed liver parenchyma and an inflammatory peel. This layer is not infective and should not be removed during cystectomy. The natural history of disease is expansion of the cyst with rupture. A ruptured cyst may cause extensive spread of infection, and urticaria, eosinophilia, or frank anaphylaxis and death. Patients who have been infected will present with right upper quadrant pain, fever, chills, and a history of travel or close contact with a traveler to the endemic areas. Differential blood count may reveal eosinophilia. Ultrasound and CT scan are the most frequently used diagnostic imaging modalities. The treatment is surgical with controlled rupture of the cyst, followed by removal. The operative field is isolated with towels soaked in 3% NaCl, followed by aspiration of the cyst. The cyst is then peeled off the ectocyst lining and removed. The residual cavity is sterilized with silver-nitrate solution. No drains are placed.

Viral Hepatitis

Viral hepatitis can cause acute or chronic inflammation of the liver. Hepatitis A virus is an RNA virus that is transmitted through the fecal-oral route. It often remains asymptomatic and is generally not associated with chronic disease. In rare instances, however, patients can deteriorate into fulminant liver failure, which frequently reverses spontaneously. HBV is a DNA virus, which is transmitted through blood or sexual contact. It can lead to chronic infections and is associated with the development of cirrhosis and HCC. Acute infection can be diagnosed by the presence of HBV surface antigen or the IgM isotype of the HBV core antibody. The presence of hepatitis E antigen indicates active infection. Hepatitis surface antibody indicates immunity or prior immunization. Patients who have been exposed to HBV should receive the HBV vaccine and HBV immunoglobulin. HCV is an RNA virus that is most frequently transmitted parenterally. It can lead to chronic infection and is associated with the development of cirrhosis and HCC. In the United States, the increased incidence of HCV is thought to be contributing to an increased incidence of HCC. The calculated population-attributed risk for HCV developing HCC is 9% to 36%. Hepatitis D virus (HDV) is composed of RNA and is only seen in association with HBV. Simultaneous infection with HBV and HDV can lead to fulminant courses of disease.

Hepatic Trauma

Opening the abdomen in a patient with severe liver trauma requires a coordinated approach between the surgeon and the anesthesiologist. Temporary control may be achieved with manual compression with lap pads in the right upper quadrant. This will allow the resuscitative effort to correct hypovolemia and acidosis before proceeding to definitive therapy. In the event that the bleeding can not be controlled with compression, the hepatoduodenal ligament may be compressed (Pringle maneuver) (Fig. 16-3). The Pringle maneuver effectively eliminates inflow into the liver and may be employed for up to 1 hour without untoward effects. In addition to minimizing hemorrhage, this maneuver may be diagnostic. Further bleeding implies "back bleeding" from the vena cava. Ninety percent of penetrating injuries and 60% of blunt injuries may be managed conservatively by packing, clotting factor resuscitation, topical hemostatic agents, and suture ligation of bleeding vessels. Liver injuries are graded according to severity. Grade I and II injuries are simple injuries that are not bleeding at the time of exploration or that require only simple suture ligature to control hemorrhage. A grade III injury involves severe hemorrhage and requires the Pringle maneuver for control. Grade IV injuries involve major lobar destruction while grade V involves the IVC. Complete avulsion of the liver from its blood supply is considered a grade VI injury and is incompatible with life in the absence of emergent transplantation.

Management of grades III through V involves portal compression and hepatotomy via the finger-fracture technique to identify the bleeding vessel(s) (Fig. 16-4). Placement of omental packing is appropriate in penetrating and burst injuries after definitive ligation of bleeding vessels. In patients with severe coagulopathy and hypotension, "damage control" of the abdomen with placement of perihepatic packing can be effective. All major hepatic injuries should be drained with closed suction drains. In the event of caval involvement, efforts should be made to control the hemorrhage by extensive mobilization of the liver and the institution of atriocaval bypass or venovenous bypass, if necessary.

Hemobilia is defined as bleeding into the biliary tract. It is due to a connection between a vascular structure and the biliary system. Arteries are more commonly responsible for hemobilia than veins. The most frequent etiology for hemobilia is iatrogenic, after biopsy or percutaneous transhepatic cholangiography. Other causes include trauma, infection, malignancy, aneurysms, gallstones, and extrahepatic diseases, including pancreatitis and peptic ulcer disease. Hemobilia is associated with a classic triad of gastrointestinal bleeding, jaundice, and right upper quadrant pain. The most useful diagnostic modality is arteriography. Because blood loss can be substantial, patients should be resuscitated aggressively. Definitive management is based on the severity of bleeding and the general condition of the patient. Nonoperative approaches include observation or selective

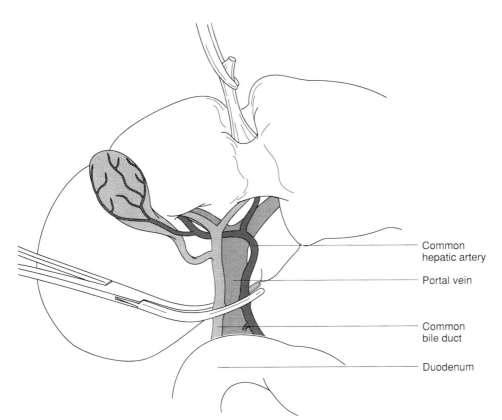

FIGURE 16-3. Pringle maneuver. (From Greenfield LJ. *Surgery: scientific principles and practice*, 1st ed. Philadelphia: Lippincott-Raven Publishers, 1997:299, with permission.)

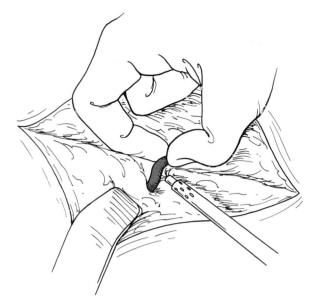

FIGURE 16-4. Identification of vessels via the finger-fracture technique. (From Bell RH, Rikkers LF, Mulholland MW. *Digestive tract surgery: a text and atlas.* Philadelphia: Lippincott-Raven Publishers, 1996:726, with permission.)

embolization of the bleeding vessel. Operative interventions include vascular ligation and hepatic resection.

PORTAL HYPERTENSION

Portal hypertension is an abnormal elevation of portal venous pressure (normal 5 to 6 mm Hg). It has traditionally been defined as an elevation of portal venous pressure of more than 5 mm Hg compared to the pressure in the IVC. This increased portal pressure, which generally exceeds 20 mm Hg, opens venous collaterals and permits blood to bypass the portal system. Sites of collateralization are in areas where the portal and systemic venous circulations are in close proximity (Fig. 16-5). The most clinically significant collateral network is through the coronary and short gastric veins to the azygous system because it results in the formation of esophagogastric varices. Other sites include a recanalized umbilical vein from the left portal vein to the epigastric venous system, retroperitoneal collateral vessels, and the hemorrhoidal venous plexus. The veins of Sappey are diaphragmatic veins that drain portal blood to the umbilicus when the portal circulation is congested. Additionally, a fair amount of portal venous flow passes through both anatomic and physiological shunts. As a rule, as hepatic portal perfusion decreases, the flow through the hepatic artery increases.

Portal hypertension results most commonly from an increased *resistance to flow*. Classifications of this disorder are therefore generally based on the site of elevated resistance. In addition to increased portal resistance, an increased portal inflow secondary to a hyperdynamic systemic circulation or splanchnic hyperemia can lead to portal hypertension. However, portal hypertension secondary to increased portal vein flow is relatively rare. Etiologies include intrahepatic or extrahepatic arteriovenous fistulae, which can be congenital such as in patients with Rendu-Osler-Weber syndrome or more commonly acquired secondary to trauma or ruptured hepatic artery aneurysms. Massive splenomegaly can lead to increased flow in the splenic vein, which can cause elevation of pressures in the portal vein. Glucagon and a decreased sensitivity to catecholamines are thought to play a role in splanchnic hyperemia.

The most important cause of *prehepatic portal hypertension* is portal vein thrombosis. This accounts for approximately 50% of cases of portal hypertension in the pediatric age group. In the absence of liver disease, collaterals develop to restore portal perfusion (hepatopetal circulation). This phenomenon is known as *cavernous transformation* of the portal vein. Portions of the portal confluence may become thrombosed secondary to inflammation or tumor. The most common example is splenic vein thrombosis secondary to pancreatitis. The result is gastrosplenic, or sinistral, hypertension with prominent esophageal varices, secondary to high flow through the left gastroepiploic vein. Although intrahepatic causes of portal hypertension are divided into presinusoidal, sinusoidal, and postsinusoidal causes, most disease processes involve more than one level. The most common cause of presinusoidal portal hypertension, worldwide, is obstruction by schistosomiasis. Portal hypertension develops when parasitic ova in small portal venules cause obstruction. In the Western world, most of the nonalcoholic etiologies of cirrhosis begin as presinusoidal portal hypertension. Alcoholic cirrhosis, however, begins as sinusoidal obstruction, secondary to collagen deposition in the space of Disse. As the process evolves, postsinusoidal obstruction ensues secondary to regenerating nodules compressing small hepatic veins. Postsinusoidal causes are rare and include the Budd-Chiari syndrome (hepatic vein thrombosis), right heart failure, and constrictive pericarditis.

A consequence of shunting blood around the liver is a reduction in "detoxification" of portal blood. *Encephalopathy* may develop in patients with cirrhosis or presinusoidal obstruction. Initially, ammonia was implicated in the pathophysiology of hepatic encephalitis; however, current data do not implicate a direct correlation between levels and severity of presentation. Patients may present with *malnutrition*, particularly in the case of alcoholic cirrhotic patients. Helpful indices include albumin, prealbumin, transferrin, and hematocrit. *Ascites* is a common symptom of portal hypertension and is secondary to hepatic sinusoidal hypertension, hypoalbuminemia, and hyperaldosteronism. *Splenomegaly* is a common sign in patients with portal system congestion and is a sign of the hypersplenism syndrome, which is associated

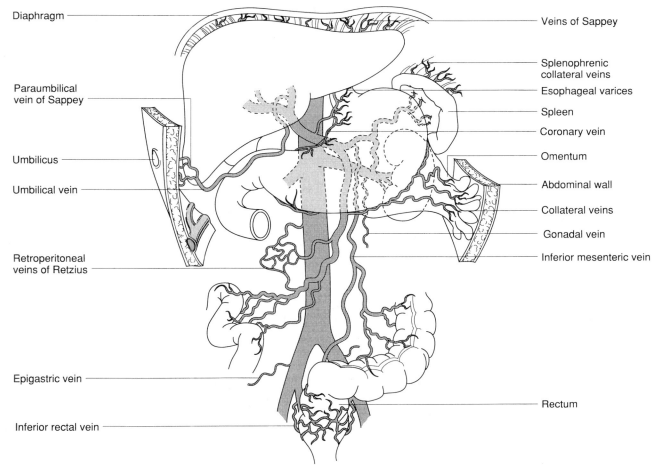

FIGURE 16-5. Sites of collateralization in portal hypertension. (From Greenfield LJ. *Surgery: scientific principles and practive,* 1st ed. Philadelphia: Lippincott-Raven Publishers, 1997:888, with permission.)

with pancytopenia or thrombocytopenia. Superficial signs of portal hypertension and/or cirrhosis include hemorrhoids, caput medusae, and gynecomastia. Perhaps the most concerning manifestation of portal hypertension is the onset of acute variceal hemorrhage. Between 30% and 50% of patients die from their first variceal hemorrhage without definitive treatment.

Patients who present with acute variceal hemorrhage should initially be resuscitated with the placement of two large-bore catheters in the antecubital fossae. Six units of packed red blood cells should be typed and cross-matched for expectant transfusion. Platelets should be transfused when their level is lower than 50,000 per mm^3. Prolonged prothrombin times should be treated with fresh frozen plasma. Central monitoring with a Swan-Ganz catheter and a Foley catheter to assess urinary output should be considered. *Gastroesophagoscopy* should be performed urgently, in concert with resuscitative efforts, to identify the source of bleeding and determine the presence of varices. The etiology of upper gastroesophageal hemorrhage in cirrhotic patients in decreasing order of frequency is as follows: gastritis in 20% to 60%, varices in 20% to 50%, peptic ulcer disease in 5% to 20%, and Mallory-Weiss tears in 5% to 10%.

Initial management includes octreotide, balloon tamponade, and sclerotherapy. *Octreotide* is a potent vasoconstrictor that lowers portal pressure by mesenteric arterial vasoconstriction with resultant diminished mesenteric blood flow. It is administered in patients with known varices as a bolus dose of 20 U over 20 minutes, followed by an infusion over 0.4 U per minute. Patients should be monitored for adverse effects including hypertension, bradycardia, coronary ischemia, and ischemic bowel. In an effort to prevent these side effects, many centers place the patient on both vasopressin and a low-dose nitroglycerin infusion. Vasopressin is effective in controlling up to 50% of variceal hemorrhages; however, it is not a definitive therapy and is indicated only in short-term control of bleeding. *Balloon tamponade* is accomplished with a Sengstaken-Blakemore tube. It has an effectiveness of 85% and is immediately available for insertion in most institutions. The main disadvantage is that it does not provide definitive therapy. There is a high rate of bleeding upon deflation, a higher rate of esophageal perforation than with esophagoscopy, and an added complication of esophageal necrosis with balloon overinflation. Balloon tamponade, therefore, is a useful temporizing therapy but should be used with caution and with the recognition that a definitive treatment such as *trans*jugular intrahepatic portosystemic shunt (TIPS), sclerotherapy, or surgery will be required. *Injection sclerotherapy* is the most commonly used therapy for both emergent management and prevention of recurrent hemorrhage. Endoscopists employ a flexible endoscope and inject sodium morrhuate or sodium tetradecyl, both into and around the bleeding varix. Alternatively, the varix may be controlled by placement of a rubber band. Complications of emergent sclerotherapy include esophageal perforation, exacerbation of bleeding, and aspiration. Bleeding is controlled in approximately 85% of patients at first presentation. A patient is said to have *failed sclerotherapy* when two sessions fail to control the bleeding.

Patients who continue to bleed despite the maneuvers discussed above may require therapy with interventional radiology or surgery. TIPS involves placement of a stent between a hepatic vein and portal vein, via a parenchymal tract. TIPS is associated with a high in-hospital mortality and with failure rates in both the acute (incomplete control of bleeding) and long-term (50% stent occlusion at 1 year). TIPS has not been demonstrated to reduce the incidence of encephalopathy in comparison to surgical shunting. TIPS, however, is indicated as a less invasive palliative treatment in patients who are not transplant candidates (survival is unlikely to outlast the TIPS), and as a means of reducing portal pressure in patients who are awaiting a transplant. Emergent surgery is indicated in patients who fail acute endoscopic therapy or hemorrhage from varices inaccessible by endoscopy (gastric varices). Operative intervention is indicated when transfusion exceeds 6 U of packed red blood cells within 24 hours. Surgery is contraindicated in patients with severe coagulopathy, encephalopathy, and end-stage liver disease.

Emergent surgery is focused on control of the bleeding source or decompression of the portal system. Interruption of varices is accomplished by direct suture ligature or esophageal transection and reanastomosis. Ligation is associated with an operative mortality rate exceeding 30% and a rebleeding rate of greater than 80% at 6 months in survivors. Esophageal transection and reanastomosis can be accomplished with an end-to-end anastomosis (EEA) stapler through a gastrotomy or alternatively through a Sugiura operation. The Sugiura operation may be performed in one or two stages (Fig. 16-6). In the first stage, a transthoracic devascularization is performed. Four to six weeks later, a laparotomy is performed and the proximal gastric fundus is devascularized, followed by selective vagotomy, pyloroplasty, and splenectomy. The Japanese quote mortality and rebleeding rates of less than 5%; however, these data have

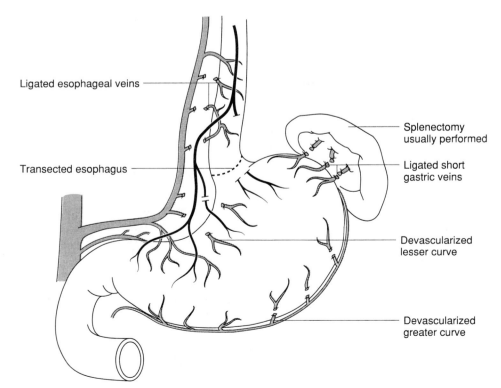

FIGURE 16-6. Sugiura procedure. (From Greenfield LJ, Mulholland MW, Oldham KT, et al., eds. *Surgery: scientific principles and practice*, 2nd ed. Philadelphia: Lippincott-Raven Publishers, 1997:1005, with permission.)

not been duplicated in disease-matched patients in the United States. This procedure is used rarely and only in select cases in the United States.

The most commonly performed emergency shunting procedure is a portacaval shunt because it effectively and rapidly decompresses the portal system. However, operative mortality rates exceed 25% and there is a high incidence of postoperative hepatic failure related to the acute reduction of portal blood flow.

ELECTIVE MANAGEMENT OF ESOPHAGEAL VARICES

Preoperatively, the patient should undergo esophagoscopy to prove that the source of bleeding was esophageal varices. In addition, the patient should be evaluated for acute alcoholic hepatitis, because operative mortality rates exceed 50% in this group of patients. Operation should be delayed in these patients until liver enzymes and liver function return to baseline. Additionally, each patient should be assigned a Child's classification to assess operative risk (Table 16-1). The Child's classification categorizes liver failure patients based on serum bilirubin level, serum albumin level, nutritional status, ascites, and mental status. The Child's classification is widely used to assess hepatic reserve in liver-failure patients and was developed as a prognostic indicator of postoperative outcome of liver-failure patients who undergo placement of portosystemic shunts. Finally, the patient should undergo radiographic assessment of portal venous anatomy. The most helpful study is a splenic and superior mesenteric arteriography followed by delayed phase imaging of the venous anatomy.

There are various shunting procedures employed by consideration of surgeon preference and patient pathophysiology (Fig. 16-7). They are designated as selective or nonselective depending on the amount of portal blood diverted. Nonselective shunts include the portacaval and mesocaval shunts. In an end-to-side *portacaval shunt,* the hepatic end of the portal vein is ligated and the proximal portion is anastomosed in an end-to-side fashion into the infrahepatic IVC (Fig. 16-7C). The result is a dramatic decrease in portal pressure and a rebleeding rate of less than 5%. However, portal blood flow into the liver is eliminated, which leads to a high rate of acute hepatic failure and a reduction in blood detoxification by the liver, with a resultant increase in encephalopathy. In circumstances where the liver must be decompressed, as in Budd-Chiari syndrome, the portacaval shunt may be performed as a side-to-side shunt (Fig. 16-7D). The effect is to reverse portal flow into an outflow vessel, replacing the thrombosed hepatic veins. Due to the high incidence of hepatic failure by eliminating portal blood flow, eliminating portal blood flow reserves this procedure for refractory ascites and variceal hemorrhage. The *mesocaval shunt* involves a functional side-to-side H-graft anastomosis connecting the superior mesenteric vein to the IVC (Fig. 16-7E). The shunt function is therefore unpredictable. In the most ideal case, the portal system will be decompressed enough to allow a reduction in rebleeding, without an adverse effect on liver function and portal blood detoxification. However, a most adverse outcome is the total reversal of portal blood flow direction, resulting in a hepatic steal phenomenon. In this circumstance, the risk of hepatic failure may be higher than in the portacaval shunt. An additional disadvantage is that the institution of Gortex material into the peritoneum increases the risk of graft infection.

Selective portosystemic shunts decrease the pressure in the gastroesophageal bed only and reduce the risk of variceal bleed by shunting gastroesophageal venous drainage into the systemic circulation. The advantage is a reduction of variceal bleeding without the risk of encephalopathy or hepatic steal. The most common selective shunt performed is the distal splenorenal (Warren) shunt (Fig. 16-7B). The procedure involves ligation and division of the splenic vein at its junction with the superior mesenteric vein. The proximal end (closest to the hilum) is anastomosed to the left renal vein. All portosystemic connections to the esophagus and proximal stomach are ligated: coronary vein, right gas-

TABLE 16-1. CHILD'S CLASSIFICATION OF LIVER FAILURE (ONE MODIFICATION)[a]

Criterion	Class A (good risk)	Class B (modest risk)	Class C (poor risk)
Serum bilirubin (mg/100 mL)	<2.0	2.0–3.0	>3.0
Serum albumin (g/100 mL)	>3.5	3.0–3.5	<3.0
Ascites	None	Easily controlled	Not easily controlled
Encephalopathy	None	Minimal	Advanced
Nutrition	Excellent	Good	Poor

[a]From Meyers WC, Jones RS. Textbook of liver and biliary surgery. Philadelphia: JB Lippincott, 1990;213, with permission.

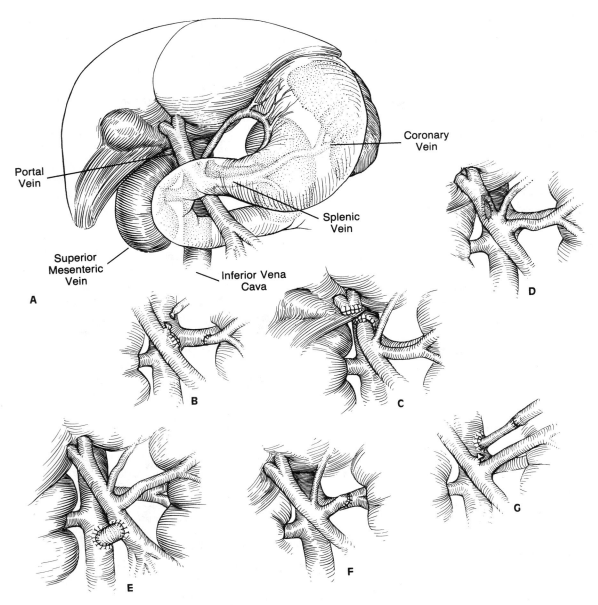

FIGURE 16-7. Portosystemic shunts. **A:** Intact portal venous anatomy. **B:** Distal splenorenal (Warren) shunt. **C:** End-to-side portacaval shunt. **D:** Side-to-side portacaval shunt. **E:** Mesocaval (H) shunt. **F:** Proximal splenorenal shunt. **G:** Coronary caval shunt. (From Meyers WC, Jones RS. *Textbook of liver and biliary surgery.* Philadelphia: JB Lippincott Co, 184, with permission.)

troepiploic, and any visible venous branches. This procedure does not reduce global portal flow, so the incidence of ascites is unchanged. The second most common selective shunt is the left gastric vena caval shunt (Fig. 16-7G). The distal end of the coronary vein is anastomosed to the IVC directly or connected through an interposition graft. This shunt selectively decompresses esophagogastric varices. However, the small size of the coronary vein translates into a higher degree of technical difficulty. The proximal splenorenal shunt involves a splenectomy and an anastomosis of proximal splenic vein to the left renal vein (Fig. 16-7F). However, unlike the distal splenorenal shunt, this shunt is not selective and is associated with complications comparable to those of portacaval shunts.

ANATOMY OF THE BILIARY STSTEM

Bile is secreted by the hepatocytes into the bile canaliculi, which are formed by a groove of the lateral plasma membrane between two hepatocytes, the diameter of which is approximately 1 μm (Fig. 16-8). The hepatocyte plasma membrane is oriented in three domains: the sinusoidal (facing the blood sinusoids), the canalicular, and the intracellular. These

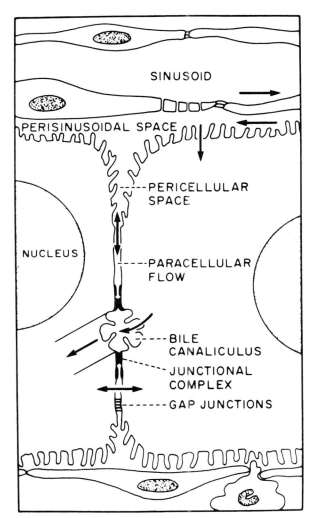

FIGURE 16-8. Microscopic architecture of hepatocytes. (From Arias IM, Popper H, Jakoby WB, et al. *The liver: biology and pathobiology.* Philadelphia: Raven Press, 1988:5, with permission.)

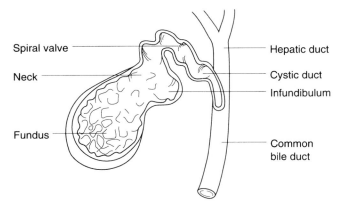

FIGURE 16-9. Gallbladder and cystic duct. (From Greenfield LJ, Mulholland MW, Oldham KT, et al., eds. *Surgery: scientific principles and practice,* 2nd ed. Philadelphia: Lippincott-Raven Publishers, 1997:1026, with permission.)

domains have functional significance in the composition of bile. A plasma substrate may enter *canalicular bile* in one of two ways: the transcellular pathway or the paracellular pathway. In the transcellular pathway, the substrate enters the hepatocyte through the sinusoidal membrane, crosses the hepatocyte, and enters the canaliculus through the canalicular membrane. A substrate may also enter via the paracellular pathway, where it crosses intercellular tight junctions. Bile formation is generally divided into two fractions. Bile-acid–dependent flow describes the correlation between bile-acid output and bile flow, while bile-acid–independent flow refers to bile flow in the absence of bile-acid output. Gastrointestinal hormones such as glucagon are thought to regulate bile-acid–independent flow.

Canalicular bile is transferred through the intrahepatic ductules, which ultimately form the right and left hepatic ducts. The confluence of the right and left bile duct forms the common bile duct (3 to 5 cm in length). The common bile duct gives off the cystic duct, which allows for storage of bile in the gallbladder. Distal to the cystic duct is the common bile duct (10 cm in length, 5 to 10 mm in diameter). The common bile duct is lateral to the common hepatic artery and anterior to the portal vein. The flow of bile progresses caudally in this lateral position of the porta hepatis, flows behind the head of the pancreas, until it enters the duodenum through the ampulla of Vater. The sphincter of Oddi surrounds the common bile duct as it traverses the ampulla and controls the secretion of bile.

The hepatic arteries supply the hilar ducts within the liver. The blood supply to the supraduodenal common bile duct is via the three o'clock and nine o'clock arteries, named for their orientation on the bile duct as a clock's face. The gallbladder is located on the inferior aspect of the liver and resides in the fossae, which marks the division of the liver into right and left lobes (Fig. 16-1). The gallbladder proper is divided into a fundus, body, infundibulum, and neck (Fig. 16-9). The neck is the portion that connects the gallbladder with the cystic duct. The blood supply is via the cystic artery, which is a branch of the right hepatic artery. The artery is usually located inferior to the cystic duct. There is no named venous branch draining the gallbladder. Cystic veins drain both directly into the portal system and into the gallbladder fossae. Lymphatic drainage is both into the gallbladder fossae and into the hilar nodes.

Bile Acids and Canalicular Bile Flow

Bile is the exocrine secretion of the liver. It is composed of water and inorganic electrolytes, bile acids (principally bilirubin), cholesterol, phospholipids (principally lecithin), and small amounts of protein. The human liver secretes about 600 to 1,000 mL of bile each day. The secretion of bile serves two functions: excretion of certain organic solutes such as bilirubin and cholesterol and facilitation of absorption of lipids and fat-soluble vitamins. Bile-acid molecules are amphipathic, containing both hydrophobic and hydrophilic ends. In combination with phospholipids, bile acids form *micellar solutions* with their hydrophilic ends oriented outward and the hydrophobic ends pointing inward. This is important for the transport of cholesterol, which is dissolved in the hydrophobic center of these mixed micelles (Fig. 16-10).

Bile acids are characterized as primary or secondary. *Primary bile acids* are steroid molecules synthesized in the liver from cholesterol. In humans, there are two primary bile acids: cholic acid and chenodeoxycholic acid. *Secondary bile acids* are formed in the intestine by bacterial dehydroxylation of the primary bile acids. Dehydroxylation of cholic acid generates deoxycholic acid and lithocholic acid is formed from chenodeoxycholic acid.

Primary bile acids are synthesized and undergo conjugation with the amino acids taurine and glycine in the liver, secreted into the biliary system, concentrated and stored in the gallbladder, and then delivered to the duodenum after gallbladder contraction. Bile acids are predominantly absorbed in the terminal ileum. Conjugated bile acids are predominantly ionized while in the intestinal lumen and are, therefore, relatively lipid insoluble. They are resistant to passive reabsorption and are absorbed predominantly by

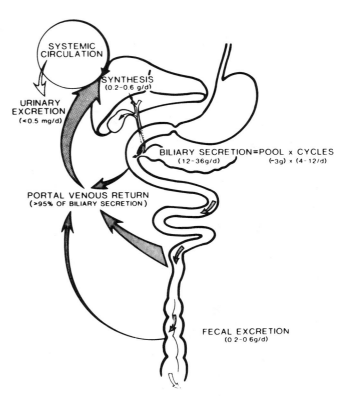

FIGURE 16-11. Enterohepatic circulation. (From Arias IM, Popper H, Jakoby WB, et al. *The liver: biology and pathobiology.* Philadelphia: Raven Press, 1988:576, with permission.)

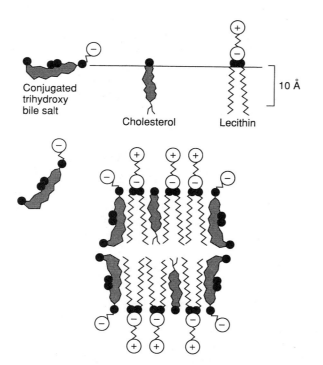

FIGURE 16-10. Mixed micelle. (From Greenfield LJ, Mulholland MW, Oldham KT, et al., eds. *Surgery: scientific principles and practice,* 2nd ed. Philadelphia: Lippincott-Raven Publishers, 1997:1036, with permission.)

active transport. Bacterial deconjugation occurs in the distal small bowel and large intestine. Deconjugation facilitates passive absorption by nonionic diffusion.

After reabsorption, both primary and secondary bile acids are transported via the portal circulation to the liver. The unconjugated bile acids are then reconjugated and resecreted. Hepatic bile, then, contains a mixture of primary and secondary bile acids. Primary bile acids, however, comprise 60% to 90% of the bile-acid pool.

The liver has an extraction efficiency for bile acids of approximately 90% to 95% (Fig. 16-11). The symport mechanism for bile-acid uptake is the electrochemical sodium gradient between sinusoidal blood and the cytoplasm of the hepatocyte. The bile-acid pool (2 to 4 g) circulates approximately 4 to 12 times per day. Approximately 0.3 to 0.6 g of bile salts are lost in stool per day. The bile-acid pool remains constant, however, because the liver synthesizes 0.2 to 0.6 g of bile salts per day. The synthesis of bile salts is the major mechanism of cholesterol degradation. This is how cholesterol-lowering drugs such as cholestyramine function. The drug binds bile salts, preventing their reabsorption. The result is a loss in the bile-salt pool that stimulates the liver to increase the rate of synthesis, thereby increasing the degradation of cholesterol.

Cholelithiasis

Risk factors for the development of gallstones include female gender, childbearing age and/or estrogen therapy, and obesity. Most gallstones are composed predominantly of cholesterol, with lesser quantities of calcium and bilirubin. The solubility of cholesterol in bile depends on its relative concentration, in terms of bile salts and lecithin. Lecithin and cholesterol are insoluble in aqueous solutions but dissolve in bile-salt–lecithin micelles (Fig. 16-10). Cholesterol will precipitate out of solution when the concentrations of bile salts or lecithin are decreased (Fig. 16-12). Exploiting this relationship, medical management is aimed at increasing the concentrations of lecithin and bile salts to improve the solubility of cholesterol (chenodeoxycholic acid therapy). Unlike cholesterol stones, pigment stones have generally low concentrations of cholesterol. They are classified as either black or brown. Heme, which is derived from the breakdown of senescent red blood cells, is converted to biliverdin through the enzyme heme oxygenase. Biliverdin reductase then converts biliverdin into bilirubin. This relatively insoluble unconjugated bilirubin is conjugated to glucuronic acid by glucuronosyltransferase in the liver. Patients with hemolytic diseases such as spherocytosis and sickle cell anemia have increased concentrations of unconjugated bilirubin in their gallbladder bile and are predisposed to the development of *black pigment stones*. *Brown pigment stones* are generally associated with states of infection when the concentrations of biliary calcium as well as β-d-glucuronidase are increased. Calcium binds to the unconjugated bilirubin and precipitates out of solution. Although black stones are typically located in the gallbladder, brown stones are frequently encountered in the common bile duct.

There are a variety of presentations of cholelithiasis, ranging from asymptomatic cholelithiasis to chronic cholecystitis. Nondiabetic patients with asymptomatic cholelithiasis may be managed with dietary restriction alone. Approximately 50% of these patients will develop symptoms related to gallstones. Diabetic patients, however, require cholecystectomy because of higher morbidity and mortality rates associated with stones (15% mortality from acute cholecystitis).

Acute cholecystitis originates from an impacted stone in the cystic duct or gallbladder neck. Gallbladder contraction against this obstruction leads to increased pressure within the gallbladder wall. The result is increased wall tension, tissue ischemia, and venous congestion. The patient presents with right upper quadrant and epigastric pain, nausea, and vomiting. The pain may radiate to the back or right shoulder. The gallbladder may be palpable, but pressure will elicit a Murphy sign (tenderness over the region of the gallbladder upon deep inspiration). Liver enzymes are not diagnostic and plain abdominal radiographs will not visualize 85% of stones. Right upper quadrant ultrasound will reveal stones and an edematous gallbladder wall, with perhaps some surrounding fluid. Approximately 75% of patients will have bacteria present in the bile; the most common organisms are the enteric bacteria *E. coli, Klebsiella, Enterobacter,* and *Enterococcus*. Oral cholecystography (OCG) and hepatobiliary iminodiacetic acid (HIDA) scans will fail to visualize the gallbladder. Treatment is cholecystectomy during the hospital admission of presentation. Some surgeons have advocated a 6-week "cooling off" period before operation. However, with the improvement in laparoscopic technique and the understanding that many patients will require readmission with recurrent symptoms, the standard of care is to operate within 72 hours of the onset of symptoms.

Chronic cholecystitis presents with a history of right upper quadrant pain exacerbated by consumption of fatty foods. HIDA scan and OCG may reveal a filling defect and ultrasound will reveal stones. The treatment is elective cholecystectomy. Approximately 75% of patients will be relieved of symptoms while 25% will present with further complaints. This postcholecystectomy syndrome is often due to nonbiliary causes such as hiatal hernia, pancreatitis, food intolerance (particularly lactose), or peptic ulcer disease. Biliary causes, however, include biliary stricture, sphincter of Oddi stenosis, common bile-duct stone, or a stone in the ligated cystic duct.

Several complications can arise from cholecystitis. *Emphysematous cholecystitis* arises from the presence of gas-

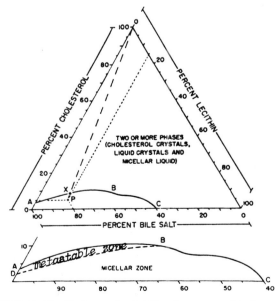

FIGURE 16-12. Cholesterol solubility decreases with decreasing bile-salt or lecithin concentration. (From Schoenfield LJ, Marks JW. Formation and treatment of gallstones. In: Schiff L, Schiff ER, eds. *Diseases of the liver*, 6th ed. Philadelphia: JB Lippincott Co, 1987:1268, with permission.)

forming organisms in the gallbladder wall such as *Clostridium perfringens*. It is more prevalent in diabetic patients, more common in men, and associated with a higher mortality rate than that of acute cholecystitis. Treatment is emergent cholecystectomy. This process must be differentiated from enterobiliary fistula by radiographic study. An abdominal film will reveal gas bubbles within the gallbladder wall in the absence of any connection to the bowel.

Enterobiliary fistula is the result of a stone eroding through the gallbladder wall and into the bowel. It may be complicated by gallstone ileus. Gallstone ileus occurs when a stone passes through the fistula and obstructs the distal ileum. The patient presents with symptoms of bowel obstruction, which can be associated with a history of previous right upper quadrant pain. Radiographs will reveal small bowel obstruction with air in the biliary tree. HIDA scans may visualize the fistula. Treatment is directed at the bowel obstruction with elective fistula repair to occur concomitantly if the patient is not particularly ill or at a later time.

Choledocholithiasis, or common bile-duct stone, is found in up to 20% of patients undergoing cholecystectomy. Patients present with jaundice, acholic stool, right upper quadrant pain, and bilirubinuria. Liver enzyme tests will reveal an elevation of total and direct bilirubin and alkaline phosphatase. Radiographic studies include right upper quadrant ultrasound, which will reveal an enlarged common bile duct, *trans*hepatic cholangiography, or HIDA scan. Cholangiography is indicated during laparoscopic cholecystectomy when there is an increase in the size of the common bile duct, a history of cholangitis or pancreatitis, a history of jaundice, or a large cystic duct. The treatment is cholecystectomy, common duct exploration (either laparoscopically or via open choledochotomy depending on the surgeon's ability), stone removal, T-tube placement, and T-tube cholangiogram.

Recurrent stones after common duct exploration may be treated by chemical dissolution through the T tube, extraction via interventional radiology, endoscopic sphincteroplasty, or choledochoduodenostomy.

Cholangitis is an infection within the bile ducts. It is most commonly due to ascending infection with *E. coli*. The patient may present with a Charcot triad: right upper quadrant pain, fever, and jaundice. More severe cases can present with a Reynold's pentad, which is defined as right upper quadrant pain, jaundice, fever, hypotension, and mental status changes. The treatment is i.v. antibiotics, fluid resuscitation, and surgical decompression. The prognosis is related to the cause of obstruction and time from presentation to treatment. Survival is the rule when obstruction is due to stones and benign stricture. However, rate of mortality increases when the obstruction is due to neoplasm.

Primary sclerosing cholangitis is a disease of unknown origin that affects the biliary tree. It begins as progressive stricturing and fibrosis of both the extrahepatic and intrahepatic biliary system. The natural history of this disease involves biliary cirrhosis and liver failure. Patients with inflammatory disorders, particularly ulcerative colitis, are predisposed to primary biliary cholangitis. They may present with right upper quadrant pain or painless jaundice. The diagnosis is made with endoscopic retrograde cholangiopancreatography (ERCP) or *trans*hepatic cholangiography. Treatment is surgical and involves biliary drainage. Depending on the level of disease, patients may undergo a choledochoenteric anastomosis or a hepaticojejunostomy, if necessary. Patients with intrahepatic progression of disease will ultimately require liver transplant for survival. Attempts to establish external drainage through a T tube are successful in the short-term but ultimately lead to cholangitis.

Benign bile-duct strictures are usually the consequence of iatrogenic injury to the bile ducts. The incidence of bile-duct injuries has increased with the widespread application of laparoscopic cholecystectomies. The risk of bile-duct injuries is increased in cases of severe inflammation, aberrant anatomy, and inexperience of the surgeon. Several inflammatory conditions such as chronic pancreatitis, cholangitis, and duodenal penetrating ulcers can also predispose to the development of bile-duct strictures. Most iatrogenic bile-duct injuries are recognized in the early postoperative period. The classic injury during laparoscopic cholecystectomies is complete transection and segmental resection of the common bile duct or the common hepatic duct. Primary reanastomosis is usually associated with tension at the anastomosis and a high degree of stricturing due to ischemic changes and is therefore not the surgical treatment of choice. The most commonly performed surgical procedure for bile-duct injuries that are recognized in the postoperative period is restoration of enterobiliary continuity with a Roux-en-Y hepaticojejunostomy.

Choledochal Cysts

There are five types of choledochal cysts (Fig. 16-13). Type I, a fusiform dilation of the common bile duct, accounts for approximately 80% to 90% of all choledochal cysts. Type II is a diverticulum of the common bile duct and type III is a choledochocele involving the intraduodenal portion of the common bile duct. These types are relatively rare. Type IV is defined as a combination of multiple cysts usually involving both intrahepatic and extrahepatic ducts. It has an incidence of approximately 10%. Type V cysts, known as Caroli disease, are uncommon. This type is characterized by intrahepatic cystic dilation and can be associated with hepatic fibrosis. Most choledochal cysts are diagnosed before 20 years of age. The most common presentation is with intermittent jaundice secondary to a partial obstruction of the distal common bile duct. Right upper quadrant ultrasound is diagnostic. HIDA scan may be used to better

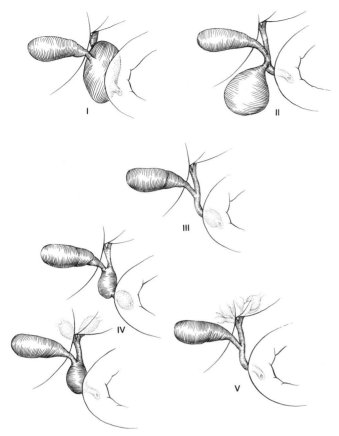

FIGURE 16-13. Choledochal cysts. (From Meyers WC, Jones RS. *Textbook of liver and biliary surgery*. Philadelphia: JB Lippincott Co, 1990;313, with permission.)

define the anatomy. Treatment is with cyst excision to prevent the increased incidence of malignancy. Type I cysts are treated with cholecystectomy, cyst excision, and Roux-en-Y choledochojejunostomy. Type II cysts are managed with diverticulectomy. Type III patients are treated with *transduodenal sphincteroplasty* or *choledochoduodenostomy*. Intrahepatic cystic dilation in types IV and V is usually not amenable to surgical resection and may require treatment with liver transplantation.

Biliary Cancers

Carcinoma of the gallbladder is the most common cancer of the biliary tract but accounts for less than 5% of all carcinomas. Predisposing factors include age and female gender. Although the vast majority of patients with gallbladder cancer have gallstones, only 2% of patients who have gallstones develop cancer of the gallbladder. Some studies suggest that large gallstones may be associated with an increased risk of developing gallbladder cancer. This may be related to mechanical irritation of the gallbladder mucosa. Metastases occur early and involve direct extension into the liver and via the lymph drainage of the portal triad. The 5-year survival rate is less than 5%. Only those cancers found incidentally, at the time of cholecystectomy, are compatible with a high chance of survival. Recommended surgical treatment for resectable tumors is a radical cholecystectomy, which involves a wide hepatic wedge resection and regional lymphadenectomy.

Carcinoma of the bile duct is associated with exposure to Thorotrast, schistosomiasis, sclerosing cholangitis, choledochal cysts, and the presence of gallstones. Diagnosis is with tissue biopsy obtained with ERCP. Known as *cholangiocarcinoma*, these tumors are adenocarcinomas. Metastatic spread of these tumors is slow and not responsible for patient demise. Patients usually succumb to progressive biliary cirrhosis, sepsis, cachexia, and persistent intrahepatic abscess formation. When the tumor involves the confluence of the right and left bile ducts, it is known as a Klatskin tumor. Less than 10% of cholangiocarcinomas are resectable at the time of laparotomy. Patients who are unresectable should be treated with a palliative biliary stent. Distal common bile-duct tumors are treated with pancreatoduodenectomy, whereas more proximal lesions are treated with resection and enterobiliary anastomosis.

SUGGESTED READING

Meyers WC, Jones RS. *Textbook of liver and biliary tract surgery*. Philadelphia: JB Lippincott Co, 1990.
University of Texas, Southwestern Medical Center at Dallas Texas. *Selected Readings in General Surgery. Portal Hypertension*. Vol 24. No 6 and 7, 1997.

17

NUTRITION, DIGESTION, AND ABSORPTION

WILSON Y. SZETO AND GORDON P. BUZBY

Digestion and nutrient metabolism are processes essential to survival. The gastrointestinal (GI) tract is the major organ system involved with these processes. The primary component of the GI tract is an epithelialized canal with an enormous surface area, across which the body interfaces with its external environment. Through the processes of digestion and absorption, the GI tract must efficiently provide for the assimilation of carbohydrates, lipids, proteins, vitamins, and trace minerals.

Over the past decades, we have achieved a better understanding of the basic physiology of the GI tract and its role in clinical nutrition. This chapter will review the overall function of the GI tract and the basic physiology of digestion, absorption, and metabolism. In addition, we will review the metabolic processes involved with altered states such as starvation, trauma, and sepsis. Finally, we will review the methods of nutritional support and their complications.

DIGESTION AND ABSORPTION

Mouth and Pharynx

The *mouth* and the *pharynx* contain salivary glands that produce approximately 1,000 to 1,500 mL of saliva daily. The functions of saliva are to lubricate the oral cavity and to moisten food material for the ease of swallowing. Limited digestion occurs in the oral cavity. Saliva contains amylase, which begins the digestion of starch. Other enzymes found in saliva include RNase, DNAse, lysozyme, peroxidase, and lingual lipase. Lastly, saliva has a protective function as a germicide.

The major glands in the mouth responsible for the secretion of saliva are the parotid, submaxillary, and sublingual glands. The parotid glands are the largest, and they are located at the temporomandibular angle. Their secretions are serous and lack mucins. The submaxillary and sublingual glands are mixed glands, and they secrete a viscous saliva containing mucins. Structurally, these salivary glands resemble the exocrine glands of the pancreas. This structural architecture permits these glands to secrete the enormous volume of saliva that occurs daily.

In humans, saliva is almost always hypotonic relative to plasma. Compared to those in plasma, Na^+ and Cl^- concentrations in saliva are lower, and K^+ and HCO_3^- concentrations are higher. The secretion of saliva is commonly described as a two-stage model (Fig. 17-1). The end pieces of each gland produce an amylase-containing secretion that is isotonic to plasma. The amylase is secreted via the process of exocytosis as zymogen granules. Modification of the ionic content with reabsorption of Na^+ and Cl^- and secretion of K^+ and HCO_3^- during passage through the excretory ducts leads to hypotonicity of the saliva. Consequently, the saliva becomes less hypotonic with increases in flow rate.

The salivary secretion is controlled through the autonomic nervous system. Unlike most other parts of the GI tract, the autonomic nervous system has no hormonal component. Although both the parasympathetic and the sympathetic system have roles in the stimulation of the salivary glands, the parasympathetic component appears to be more significant. The effects of the parasympathetic system appear to be longer lasting and more vigorous. Parasympathetic stimulation increases blood flow to the salivary glands and augments glandular metabolism and growth, which leads to secretion of saliva that is rich in amylase and mucins. Parasympathetic stimulation also increases the rate of HCO_3^- secretion but inhibits the reabsorption of Na^+ and K^+. Atrophy of the salivary glands can result from a lack of parasympathetic innervation.

On the other hand, while the sympathetic system also stimulates salivary secretion, its interruption causes no significant dysfunction of the salivary glands. Sympathetic stimulation results in secretion of saliva rich in amylase, K^+, and HCO_3^-. It stimulates contraction of the myoepithelial cells around the acini and constriction of blood vessels. In contrast to the parasympathetic arm, sympathetic stimulation results in decreased blood flow and metabolism of the salivary glands.

Hospital of the University of Pennsylvania, Philadelphia, Pennsylvania

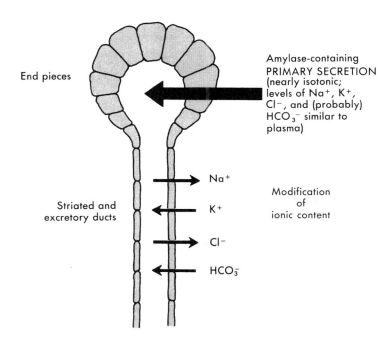

FIGURE 17-1. Salivary secretion. (From Berne RM, Levy MN, eds. *Physiology*, 2nd ed. St. Louis: Mosby, 1988, with permission.)

Esophagus

The *esophagus* serves as a conduit for food from the oropharynx to the stomach. It begins at the upper esophageal sphincter, where it is formed by striated muscles of the cricopharyngeus and inferior pharyngeal constrictor. It ends at the lower esophageal sphincter, a physiologic barrier at the most distal 1 to 2 cm of the esophagus.

Swallowing begins with a voluntary initiation, followed almost entirely by reflex control. The swallowing reflex is a sequence of events that propels food from the oropharynx to the stomach while inhibiting respiration. There are three phases of swallowing: the oral or voluntary phase, the pharyngeal phase, and the esophageal phase (Fig. 17-2).

The oral or voluntary phase is initiated by voluntary contraction of the musculature of the floor of the mouth and tongue, which results in propulsion of the food bolus to the hypopharynx. Upon entering the hypopharynx, the bolus stimulates tactile receptors that initiate the next phase, the pharyngeal phase.

The pharyngeal phase is a complex sequence of events that ensure the proper passage of the bolus into the esophagus proper in less than 1 second with reflex inhibition of respiration. The soft palate contracts upward to prevent reflux of food into the nasopharynx, and the epiglottis covers the opening of the larynx to prevent aspiration of food into the trachea. Contraction of the superior pharyngeal muscles propels the food bolus through the coordinated relaxation of the upper esophageal sphincter. The upper esophageal sphincter, 2.5 to 4 cm in length, is closed at rest with a mean pressure between 20 and 60 mm

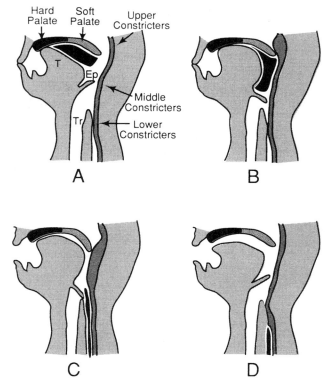

FIGURE 17-2. The oral and pharyngeal phases of swallowing involve the **(A)** separation of the bolus of food between the tongue, the soft and hard palate and **(B)** advancement of the bolus into the oropharynx. As respiration is inhibited, the bolus of food is propelled through the **(C)** pharynx by the sequential peristalsis of the superior, middle, and inferior constrictor muscles and advanced into the **(D)** upper esophagus, initiating the esophageal phase of swallowing. (From Johnson LR. Motility. In: Johnson LR, ed. *Essential medical physiology.* Philadelphia: Lippincott-Raven Publishers, 1999:432, with permission.)

Hg. The upper esophageal sphincter is predominantly innervated by the vagus nerve, with minor contributions from the glossopharyngeal and accessory nerves. The relaxation of the upper esophageal sphincter is coordinated via the dorsal vagal nuclei and nucleus ambiguus in the medulla and lower pons. Disruption of this coordinated relaxation with the contraction of the pharyngeal muscles may cause elevation of the intrapharyngeal pressure, which may have a role in the pathogenesis of pharyngoesophageal (Zenker) diverticulum.

The esophageal phase begins with the propulsion of food beyond the relaxed upper esophageal sphincter. The upper esophageal sphincter constricts, and a peristaltic wave initiates just below the upper esophageal sphincter and transverses the esophagus in 10 seconds. This initial wave, or primary peristalsis, serves to propel food into the stomach. If food remains in the esophagus, a secondary peristalsis will initiate at the site of distention. These peristaltic waves relax the lower esophageal sphincter, allowing entrance of food particles into the stomach.

The lower esophageal sphincter is a physiologic barrier between the esophagus with its negative intrathoracic pressure and the stomach with its positive intraabdominal pressure. The sphincter is constricted at rest with a resting pressure of approximately 30 mm Hg, and it serves to prevent reflux of gastric contents into the esophagus. The tonic contraction is mainly regulated by neural mechanisms mediated through vagal cholinergic innervation. Hormonal regulation via a complex endocrine control has also been suggested. Agents that have been shown to decrease lower esophageal sphincter pressure include atropine, isoproterenol, prostaglandins E_1 and E_2, secretin, calcium channel blockers, tobacco, ethanol, and caffeine. A decrease in the tone of the lower esophageal sphincter may be manifest as gastroesophageal reflux disease. At the other end of the spectrum, an increase in the tone of the sphincter, or failure of relaxation, plays a major role in the pathogenesis of achalasia and esophageal spasm syndrome. Lower esophageal sphincter pressure can increase due to cholinergic or α-adrenergic stimulation.

Stomach

The *stomach* is a temporary reservoir for food. The storage capacity may exceed 1,000 mL. It mixes the food with its acid secretions into a semifluid mixture, or chyme, and regulates the discharge of this chyme into the duodenum. The stomach also plays important roles in the initial steps of proteolysis, absorption of simple molecules, and the metabolism of vitamin B_{12} via the secretion of intrinsic factor.

The stomach is anatomically divided into the cardia, fundus, body, and antrum (Fig. 17-3). From a physiologic standpoint, only two major zones exist: the body and the antrum. The gastric mucosa of the body, which includes the cardia and the fundus, is covered by columnar epithelial cells and gastric pits, into which gastric glands empty. Within these gastric glands are mucous neck cells, parietal or oxyntic cells, and chief or peptic cells. Mucous neck cells are located at the neck of the gland and secrete mucus that serves to protect the gastric epithelium from the acidic environment. The parietal cells, located deeper in the gland, secrete HCl and intrinsic factor. The chief cells secrete pepsinogen, which when activated by HCl, serves to initiate the digestion of protein. The antrum, or pyloric region, contains few parietal and chief cells. It is dominated by mucus-producing cells, as well as G cells, which secrete gastrin.

The stomach has a minimal role in digestion and absorption. Initiation of proteolysis is achieved by pepsin, which is activated from pepsinogen by HCl. Pepsin has its highest activity at a pH level of 3 or lower, and it can digest as much as 20% of the protein in a meal. However, pepsin is not essential in normal digestion, and protein digestion can be completed by pancreatic proteases. In the alkaline environment of the duodenum, pepsin is inactivated. Minimal absorption occurs in the stomach. This includes the absorption of water and certain simple molecules such as alcohol

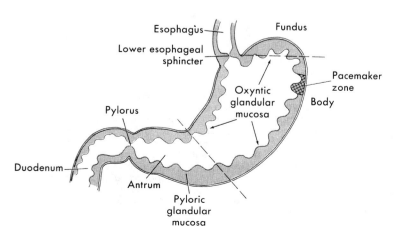

FIGURE 17-3. The stomach. (From Berne RM, Levy MN, eds. *Physiology,* 2nd ed. St. Louis: Mosby, 1988:633, with permission.)

and poisons (cyanide or arsenic). Intrinsic factor is secreted by parietal cells and is essential in the absorption of vitamin B_{12}. Intrinsic factor binds vitamin B_{12}, and this complex is absorbed in the terminal ileum. The intrinsic factor–B_{12} complex is highly resistant to digestion within the GI tract.

Acid secretion is one of the major functions of the stomach. Its acid secretion dissolves soluble foods, brings the chyme osmolality close to plasma, and acts as a bactericide. The ionic composition of the gastric secretion varies with the rate of secretion and among individuals. At low rates of secretion, the fluid is low in H^+ and high in Na^+. As the rate increases, the concentrations of H^+ and Cl^- also increase (Fig. 17-4). Basal gastric acid secretion is normally in the range of 1 to 5 mEq per hour and can rise to as high as 6 to 40 mEq per hour. When compared to normal individuals, patients with gastric ulcers secrete less HCl and patients with duodenal ulcers secrete more HCl, although substantial overlap exists.

Parietal cells are responsible for secretion of gastric acid and are tightly regulated through a combination of neural and humoral mechanisms. The neural mechanism is effected through the vagus nerves while the humoral mechanism is effected through the antral hormone gastrin. This regulation of acid secretion can be divided into three phases: (i) cephalic, (ii) gastric, and (iii) intestinal.

The *cephalic phase* begins with the sight, smell, thought, or taste of food. This results in the stimulation of the vagus nerves. The vagus nerves, through an acetylcholine-mediated process, directly stimulate the parietal cells, causing a rise in gastric secretion. Acetylcholine also indirectly increases acid secretion by releasing the hormone gastrin from the G cells in the antrum. Because the cephalic phase is entirely vagal-mediated, bilateral truncal vagotomy abolishes this phase.

The entry of food into the stomach initiates the *gastric phase*. The major stimulus to acid secretion during this phase is gastric distention. When the stomach is distended, mechanoreceptors are stimulated. This results in local and vagovagal reflexes, which stimulate the parietal cells and the antral G cells. The majority of acid secretion in response to a meal is during this phase.

The *intestinal phase* begins with the entry of gastric chyme into the duodenum, which initially stimulates and later inhibits gastric acid secretion. In the early intestinal phase, gastric chyme has a pH level of more than 3 and stimulation of acid secretion dominates. Distention of the duodenum causes the release of gastrin from duodenal G cells, thus further stimulating acid secretion. A second hormone, enterooxyntin, is also released from the duodenum and acts to stimulate the parietal cells to secrete HCl.

In the late intestinal phase, the pH level of gastric chyme falls to less than 3 and inhibition of acidic secretion dominates. Inhibition of acid secretion is triggered by intragastric acid and the presence of acid or fat in the duodenum. Low gastric pH level decreases the release of gastrin. Acid and fat in the duodenum result in the release of the hormone secretin into the bloodstream. Secretin inhibits the release of gastrin, as well as the effect of gastrin on the parietal cells. Fat in the duodenum results in the release of gastric inhibitory peptide (GIP). GIP suppresses acid secretion by inhibiting gastrin release and HCl production by the parietal cells.

Another important physiologic aspect of the stomach is its *motor function*. Not only must the stomach distend to accommodate the volume of food that has been ingested, but at the same time, it also must be able to mix the ingested food and empty it into the duodenum at a controlled rate. With each swallow and the subsequent distention during filling of the stomach, proximal gastric relaxation occurs. This receptive relaxation allows the stomach to increase in volume with only a minimal increase in intragastric pressure. This process appears to be mediated through the vagus, as vagotomy decreases the distensibility of the proximal stomach. The midportion, or body, of the stomach is more motile and is responsible for mixing of the chyme. The pacemaker of the stomach is probably located in this region. The wave of peristalsis progresses, forcing the chyme vigorously toward the antrum. A vigorous backward motion of the chyme, or retropulsion, occurs, resulting in effective mixing of the chyme and acid.

Gastric emptying is a complex process, regulated by both neural and hormonal processes (Fig. 17-5). The mechanism of this interplay is not well understood. However, the physical and chemical characteristics of the ingested food appear to play a dominant role. Osmolarity appears to be a factor affecting gastric emptying, for osmoreceptors exist in the duodenum and the jejunum. Hyperosmolar solutions appear to decrease gastric emptying by releasing an uniden-

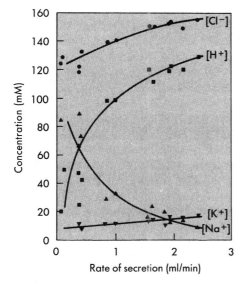

FIGURE 17-4. Ionic composition of gastric secretion. (From Berne RM, Levy MN, eds. *Physiology*, 2nd ed. St. Louis: Mosby, 1988:660, with permission.)

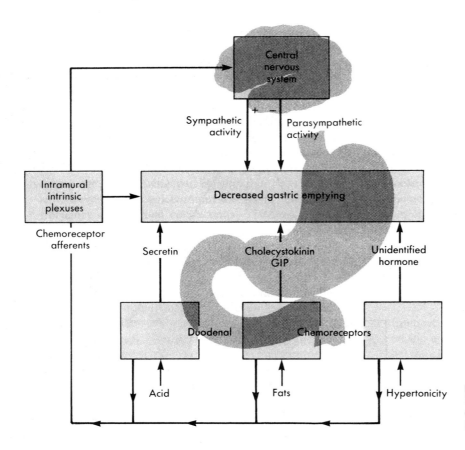

FIGURE 17-5. Regulation of gastric emptying. (From Berne RM, Levy MN, eds. *Physiology*, 2nd ed. St. Louis: Mosby, 1988:639, with permission.)

tified hormone. In addition, there may also be a neural component. Acidity of the solution also appears to be a factor affecting gastric emptying. Acid in the duodenum results in the slowing of gastric emptying. Studies in dogs have shown that this response may be vagal-mediated, as vagotomy abolishes this response. Intraduodenal acidity also results in the release of secretin, which has been shown to decrease gastric emptying. Other factors including fat and amino acids appear to have a role in the regulation of gastric emptying. Fatty acids in the duodenum cause the release of cholecystokinin (CCK) and GIP while amino acids cause the release of gastrin. All three hormones (CCK, GIP, and gastrin) appear to suppress the rate of gastric emptying. The processes discussed above ensure that the chyme is emptied into the duodenum at a rate that the chyme can be efficiently processed.

Pancreas

The *pancreas* is a small organ, weighing approximately 100 g in the adult. However, its secretion can be up to 2 L per day. The pancreas has endocrine and exocrine secretory functions. It is the enormous secretory capability of the pancreas that is essential to the process of digestion.

Pancreatic juice has two components important to the process of digestion. The aqueous component, rich in bicarbonate, helps to neutralize gastric chyme as it enters the duodenum. The enzymatic component contains enzymes for the digestion of carbohydrates, lipids, and amino acids. Both hormonal components and local factors play a major role in the regulation of pancreatic secretion. Acidic chyme in the duodenum is the primary stimulus for the secretory function of the pancreas. Secretin stimulates the secretion of the aqueous component, and CCK stimulates the secretion of the enzymatic component.

The acinus is the secretory unit of the exocrine pancreas. The acinus is made up of columnar cells, called "acinar cells," draining into collecting systems of tubules, called the "intercalated ducts." These intercalated ducts empty the secretory contents into larger ducts that eventually drain into the main pancreatic duct and enter the duodenum via the biliary tract (Fig. 17-6). Acinar cells are highly polarized and have a distinct apical membrane oriented toward the ductal lumen. The orientation of the intracellular organelles reiterates the cellular polarity and reflects the secretory properties of these cells.

The two components of the pancreatic secretion are produced in different regions of the acinus. The columnar ductal cells appear to be responsible for the secretion of the aqueous component. This component contains bicarbonate and serves to neutralize the acid chyme that enters the duodenum. The fluid is clear and colorless, and remains iso-

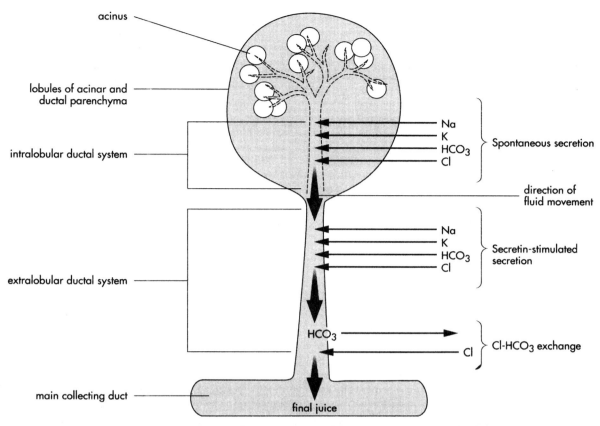

FIGURE 17-6. Pancreatic secretion. (From Savage E, Fishman S, Miller L. *Essentials of basic science in surgery.* Philadelphia: JB Lippincott Co, 1993:189, with permission.)

tonic to plasma. The major cations are Na^+ and K^+, and their concentrations remain similar to that of plasma irrespective of the rate of flow. The major anions are bicarbonate and chloride and their concentrations are reciprocal with respect to the rate of flow. When secreted by the ductal cells, the aqueous solution has a high bicarbonate concentration. As the solution flows distally, the bicarbonate is exchanged for chloride anions. As a consequence, the concentration of the bicarbonate anion correlates with the flow rate (Fig. 17-7).

The enzymatic component appears to be the product of the terminal acinar cells. This component contains numerous enzymes important for the digestion of carbohydrates, lipids, and proteins. Secreted in inactive forms called

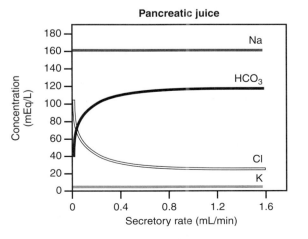
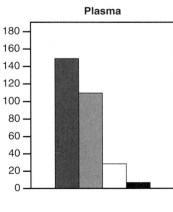

FIGURE 17-7. Ionic composition of pancreatic secretion. (From Greenfield L, ed. *Surgery: scientific principles and practice*, 1st ed. JB Lippincott Co, 1993:784, with permission.)

"zymogens," the major pancreatic proteases are trypsin, chymotrypsin, and carboxypeptidase. The inactive form of trypsin is trypsinogen, and it is activated to trypsin by enterokinase, which is secreted in the duodenum. Trypsin then activates its own precursor trypsinogen, as well as chymotrypsinogen and procarboxypeptidase, the precursors of chymotrypsin and carboxypeptidase, respectively. This process causes a cascade of events resulting in the activation of multiple pancreatic enzymes. A trypsin inhibitor in the pancreatic juices prevents premature activation within the pancreatic ducts.

Other pancreatic enzymes include amylase, lipases, and nuclease. Amylase is secreted in its active form, and it cleaves polysaccharides at a specific site to initiate digestion of carbohydrates. Numerous lipases are found in pancreatic juice, and they cleave at specific ester bonds to initiate the digestion of fat, resulting in free fatty acids and monoglyceride. Ribonuclease and deoxyribonuclease reduce RNA and DNA, respectively. The nucleotides produced are further reduced to nucleosides by brush-border enzymes in the intestine.

The regulation of pancreatic exocrine secretion is achieved through hormonal and neural mechanisms. Secretin and CCK stimulate the secretion of the aqueous and enzymatic components of the pancreatic secretion, respectively. Parasympathetic stimulation via vagal branches increases the rate of pancreatic secretion while the sympathetic counterpart has the opposite effect. The regulation of the exocrine function of the pancreas, similar to that of the stomach, can be categorized into three phases: (i) cephalic, (ii) gastric, and (iii) intestinal.

The cephalic phase results from the sight, smell, or taste of food. Low volume of pancreatic juice with high enzymatic content is secreted, likely the result of gastrin release in response to a vagal-mediated event. Although gastrin is in the same family of peptides as CCK, it is much less potent as a pancreatic stimulant. Conditions that decrease gastrin secretion, such as acidity in the duodenum, also suppress the cephalic phase of pancreatic secretion.

The gastric phase begins with the entry of food into the stomach, resulting in gastric distention. This continues to stimulate the release of gastrin, thus producing low volumes of pancreatic juice with high enzymatic content. Gastrin has an indirect role in the stimulation of pancreatic secretion. Gastrin-induced gastric acid secretion stimulates the release of secretin and CCK, resulting in the secretion of pancreatic juices.

The intestinal phase begins when food enters into the duodenum. Acidity stimulates the release of pancreatic juice high in bicarbonate and low in enzymes. This response is mediated through the hormone secretin, released by the mucosa of the duodenum when the pH level is lower than 4.5. Secretin directly stimulates the ductal cells to secrete pancreatic juices high in bicarbonate. The presence of peptides and fatty acids in the duodenum elicits the release of pancreatic secretion high in enzymatic component. CCK is the primary mediator of this response, resulting in the direct stimulation of the acinar cells to secrete their enzymatic products. Secretin and CCK potentiate each other's effect on the ductal and acinar cells, respectively. Neural factors also appear to have a role in the regulation of pancreatic secretion. Vagotomy suppresses the magnitude of the response, as well as the rapidity of the pancreatic response to acidic chyme in the duodenum. These responses are probably augmented by enteropancreatic vagovagal reflexes.

Inhibition of pancreatic secretion is less well understood. Feedback inhibition appears to play a role in bicarbonate secretion. Products from the endocrine pancreas, such as somatostatin, glucagon, and pancreatic polypeptide, appear to inhibit the exocrine function of the pancreas. However, the exact mechanism is not well understood.

Gallbladder and Liver

The *liver* has a major role in the digestion and metabolism of nutrients. Its role in metabolism will be discussed in a later section. Bile secretion, the principal digestive function of the liver, will be discussed in this section. The gallbladder, a reservoir for the liver's bile secretion, and its role in bile secretion and fat digestion will also be discussed.

Bile contains bile acids, cholesterol, lecithin, and bile pigments, and it is produced by the liver's hepatocytes at a rate of 500 to 1,500 mL per day. Bile serves to emulsify lipids, allowing the lipolytic enzymes of the pancreas to function. The exocrine function of the liver is similar in some respects to that of the pancreas. They both secrete a solution isotonic to plasma and subsequently modify it. Collected into ducts called "bile canaliculi," the bile is eventually secreted into the common bile duct and to the duodenum. The hormonal mechanisms regulating bile secretion are similar to those regulating pancreatic secretions. Although CCK stimulates the release of bile, secretin stimulates the secretion of the bicarbonate component of the bile.

Between meals, bile is diverted to the gallbladder as a consequence of the tonic contraction of the sphincter of Oddi. Bile is concentrated by the gallbladder by the removal of water and salts. With meals, the gallbladder is stimulated to contract by the release of CCK. At the same time, CCK also causes relaxation of the sphincter of Oddi. Approximately 250 to 1,500 mL of bile enters the duodenum daily.

Bile acids or bile salts are the major component of bile, constituting about 65%. Formed from cholesterol by hepatocytes, these primary bile acids include cholic acid and chenodeoxycholic acid. They are secreted after conjugation with glycine or taurine, these conjugated bile acids are more water soluble than their unconjugated counterparts. Bacterial dehydroxylation in the GI tract converts these primary bile acids into the secondary bile acids deoxycholic acid and lithocholic acid.

The major digestive functions of the bile salts are to emulsify lipids and to transport lipids via the formation of micelles. By emulsification, bile acids increase the surface area of the lipids available to the lipases, then micelles are formed from bile acids and the products of lipid digestion. These micelles are highly polarized, with the hydrophobic poles oriented toward the center, allowing hydrophobic elements such as cholesterol and lipids to aggregate. This permits lipids to be transported in an aqueous environment and to be absorbed eventually across the mucosa of the GI tract.

As stated above, the primary stimulus for the secretion of bile and the contraction of the gallbladder is CCK. In addition, the rate of bile secretion and synthesis is also influenced by the intestinal absorption of bile acids and the enterohepatic circulation (Fig. 17-8). As chyme travels distally into the distal ileum, fat absorption is almost complete. Here, the epithelial cells take up bile acids avidly and return the bile acids to the liver via the portal system. Typically, only about 0.5 g of bile acids, or 15% to 35% of the total pool, is lost via feces. This loss is replaced by hepatic synthesis of bile acids. The rate of return of bile acids to the liver, or the enterohepatic circulation, regulates bile acid secretion and synthesis (Fig. 17-9). Bile acids returning to the liver during digestion are a potent stimulus, resulting in further secretion of bile acids. During a meal, the entire pool may circulate twice through the enterohepatic circulation. Bile acids returning to the liver inhibit the neosynthesis of bile acids. Hence, during a meal when the bile return

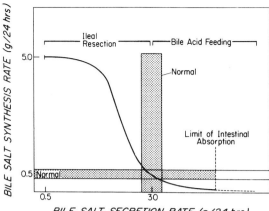

FIGURE 17-9. Regulation of bile acid secretion and synthesis. (From Carey MC, Cahalane MJ. In: Arias IM, et al. *The liver: biology and pathobiology*, 2nd ed. New York: Raven Press, 1988, with permission.)

is high, recirculation is stimulated and synthesis is inhibited. After a meal, when the portal return of bile acids is low, secretion is not stimulated, allowing slow filling of the gallbladder. Low return of bile acids such as after ileal resection results in an increase in hepatic synthesis of bile acids.

Small Intestine

The *small intestine* in an adult ranges from 700 to 800 cm in length with a surface area of approximately 7,600 cm^2. This large surface area is further amplified by two anatomical features: the presence of circular concentric folds, or plicae circulares, and the fingerlike epithelial projections, or villi. The major role of the small intestine is the absorption of nutrients, including simple molecules such as water, electrolytes, carbohydrates, lipids, proteins, minerals, and vitamins.

The small intestine is a semipermeable membrane with an enormous capacity for secretion and absorption. Approximately 9 L of fluid reach the small intestine daily. Of the 9 L, approximately 7 L are of endogenous origin (i.e., salivary, gastric, hepatic, and pancreatic secretion) and 2 L from ingestion. Of the 9 L that reach the small intestine per day, the cecum receives only 500 mL to 1,000 mL of fluid. Water absorption across the intestinal mucosa is very effective, and it is usually coupled to the absorption of other solutes (i.e., Na$^+$, Cl$^-$) and nutrients (sugars, amino acid). The jejunum is the most active site of water absorption (Fig. 17-10).

The *absorption of electrolytes* across the mucosa occurs through three mechanisms: (i) passive diffusion, (ii) solvent drag, and (iii) active transport. Passive diffusion is the simple diffusion of electrolytes down an electrochemical gradient across the mucosal barrier via a protein channel or between the cells. This process is energy independent and is most pronounced in the jejunum. Solvent drag is the coupling of the absorption of electrolytes to that of water. This

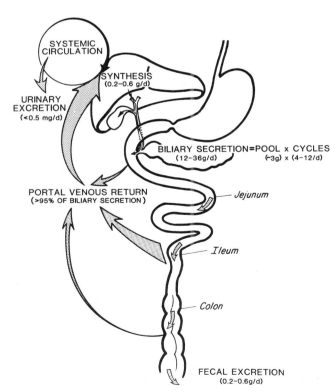

FIGURE 17-8. Enterohepatic circulation of bile acids. (From Carey MC, Cahalane MJ. In: Arias IM, et al. *The liver: biology and pathobiology*, 2nd ed. New York: Raven Press, 1988, with permission.)

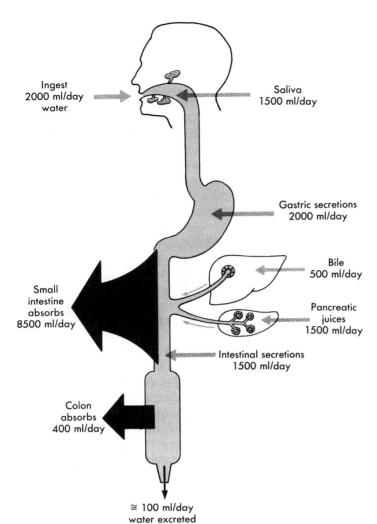

FIGURE 17-10. Fluid balance in the gastrointestinal tract. (From Berne RM, Levy MN, eds. *Physiology,* 2nd ed. St. Louis: Mosby, 1988:697, with permission.)

process is similar to that seen with water and electrolyte absorption in the proximal tubules of the kidney. Active transport involves energy-dependent mechanisms that allow movement of ions against electrochemical gradients. The sodium-potassium adenosine triphosphatase (ATPase) pump, located at the basolateral membrane of the mucosal cells, is an important active-transport mechanism for the absorption of water and electrolytes (i.e., Na^+). Na^+ transported into the intercalated space by the ATPase pump causes hyperosmolarity in that region, resulting in the absorption of water from the lumen into the intercalated space. The decreased intracellular concentration of Na^+ causes influx, or absorption, of Na^+ from the lumen into the cells. A carrier mediating the cotransport of sugar or amino acid with Na^+ ensures near-total absorption of Na^+, and hence water.

Constituting approximately 30% to 40% of a western diet, carbohydrates provide a major portion of our energy source. There are two major forms of carbohydrates, poly-saccharides and disaccharides. Polysaccharides, or starch, consist of amylose and amylopectin. Disaccharides, or simple sugars, include sucrose, maltose, and lactose. Digestion of carbohydrates begins with salivary amylase in the oral cavity. Salivary amylase, similar to pancreatic amylase, cleaves starch at the $\alpha_1,4$ glucose-glucose links. Once in the small intestine, carbohydrates are exposed to pancreatic amylase, and the result is a mixture of oligosaccharides. Digestion of the carbohydrates is completed by the surface oligosaccharidases located on the brush border of the intestinal mucosa. These are highly efficient enzymes, and most carbohydrates are hydrolyzed to glucose.

The monosaccharides produced during digestion are too large to be absorbed by simple diffusion, and their absorption requires specific transport mechanisms. Glucose and galactose absorption are coupled to an active-transport mechanism, as described earlier. An Na^+-K^+ ATPase pump actively displaces Na^+ into the intercalated space, creating an electrochemical gradient. Luminal Na^+ diffuses into the cell through a carrier coupled to glucose and galactose transport. In contrast, fructose is absorbed via a passive mechanism involving a carrier-mediated facilitated diffusion (Fig. 17-11).

Deficiencies of carbohydrate digestion are uncommon in surgical patients. Carbohydrate intolerance usually results from a deficiency of brush-border enzymes. Lactose intolerance is an example of this deficiency, and it appears to be genetically determined. Most adults of Asian descent as well as African Americans are lactose intolerant, exhibiting symptoms of distention, bloating, and diarrhea upon ingestion of lactose-containing food products. In contrast, most adults of Northern European descent tolerate lactose-containing food.

Lipids in our diet are primarily long-chain triglycerides. The process of digestion and absorption of long-chain lipids is complex, as it requires the coordination of hepatobiliary secretion and the absorptive properties of the intestinal mucosa. Also, lipids are water insoluble and pose a special problem to the GI tract.

Bile, in particular bile salts, plays a vital role in the digestion and absorption of lipids. Bile salts emulsify fats, increasing their surface to the action of the pancreatic lipases. The majority of fat digestion occurs in the proximal small intestine. Long-chain triglyceride is hydrolyzed into monoglyceride and two fatty acids. These products aggregate with bile salts to form micelles. The formation of micelles is essential to the absorption of fat. As stated in a previous section, micelles are highly polarized entities with hydrophobic elements in the center. The water-insoluble products of the lipolytic enzymes are enveloped within the micelles while the exterior hydrophilic component of the micelles allow their solubility in the aqueous environment of the GI tract. These micelles are essential to the transport of lipid digestive products to the absorptive surfaces of the mucosa. Once in contact with the mucosal brush border, lipid products are absorbed across the mucosa in a passive manner, leaving the remaining micelle (Fig. 17-12).

Once absorbed into the intestinal mucosal cell, the lipid products are resynthesized into triglycerides and processed into chylomicrons. The formation of chylomicrons is important in the transport of long-chain lipids to the body for utilization. Chylomicrons are absorbed into the lymphatic system via intestinal lacteals. There, they will eventually return to the central circulation via the thoracic duct for peripheral utilization. In contrast, short-chain and medium-chain triglycerides are small enough to be absorbed directly into the capillary system. These triglycerides are more easily

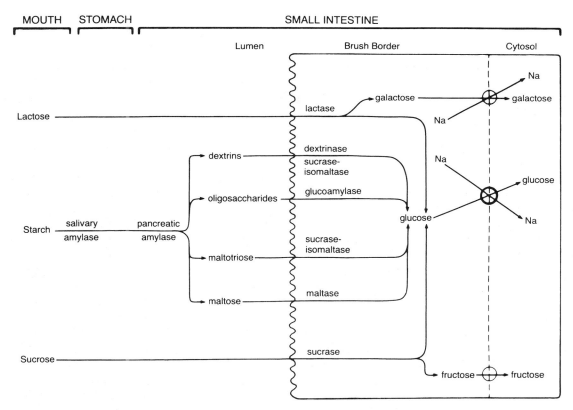

FIGURE 17-11. Carbohydrate digestion in the gastrointestinal tract. (From Rombeau JL, Caldwell MD, eds. *Clinical nutrition: enteral and tube feeding,* 2nd ed. Philadelphia: WB Saunders, 1990:25, with permission.)

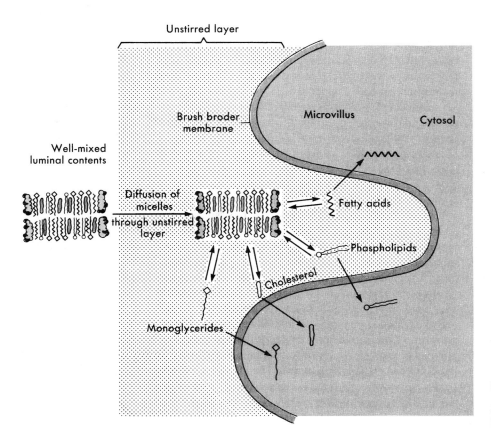

FIGURE 17-12. Lipid absorption. (From Berne RM, Levy MN, eds. *Physiology*, 2nd ed. St. Louis: Mosby, 1988:712, with permission.)

digested and can aid in the management of patients with lipid malabsorption.

Digestion and absorption of protein is also very efficient in the human. The amount of protein ingested can vary greatly among individuals with different dietary habits. Nevertheless, almost all ingested protein is digested and absorbed. The small amount of protein lost in feces is primarily from colonic bacteria or desquamated cells.

Digestion of protein begins in the stomach. As described earlier, pepsin is secreted by the chief cells in its inactive form, pepsinogen. The activity of pepsin is variable, and it is responsible for only a minority of protein digestion. Pancreatic proteases are very efficient, and they play a critical role in the digestion of protein. These proteases, secreted in an inactive form, are activated in a cascade of events described in a previous section. Enterokinase, found in the duodenal mucosa, activates trypsinogen into trypsin, which in turn activates trypsinogen, chymotrypsinogen, and procarboxypeptidase. All these enzymes are highly efficient, and 50% of the protein ingested is digested and absorbed in the duodenum. The remaining oligopeptides produced by the pancreatic proteases are hydrolyzed by a number of peptidases found in the brush border of the small intestine. These peptidases further reduce the oligopeptides to smaller peptides and amino acids in preparation for absorption.

The absorption of peptides is an active process requiring energy. Using a carrier-mediated mechanism similar to that of glucose absorption, the absorption of peptide and amino acids is very efficient. Interestingly, this process prefers dipeptides to amino acids, which are absorbed variably depending on the amino acid. Once absorbed into the cytosol of the mucosal cell, the peptides are transported across the basolateral membrane via other transport systems. Protein absorption can be accomplished in most segments of the small intestine. Hence, protein malabsorption is rare even with extensive resection.

Minerals and *vitamins* are essential components of our diet. Even though the volume of minerals and vitamins ingested is small when compared to that of macronutrients, their deficiencies have major clinical sequelae. This section will briefly discuss the mechanisms for digestion and absorption of minerals and vitamins.

Calcium absorption is most active in the duodenum and the jejunum, and vitamin D is essential to this process. Calcium is absorbed across the brush border of the mucosa and binds to a specific cytosolic transport protein, or calcium-binding protein (CaBP). The calcium is transported to the basolateral membrane of the mucosal cell. where two proteins (Ca^{++}ATPase and Na^+/Ca^{++} exchanger) can actively transport calcium across the basal membrane. Vitamin D stimulates all aspects of calcium absorption. It enhances the absorption at the brush border, and acting as a hormone, it stimulates the production of proteins involved in the transport of calcium. Even though calcium is mostly absorbed in the upper small intestine, extensive resection will result in only temporary malabsorption. Over time, the ileum can adapt to provide near-complete calcium absorption.

Iron stores in people are fairly constant. Although an average daily diet provides an adult with approximately 20 mg of iron, only 1 to 1.5 mg are absorbed. The mechanism of iron absorption is not completely understood, and it appears that the majority of iron absorption occurs in the duodenum. In food, iron exists in the form of ferric iron (Fe^{3+}), which is insoluble in solution with a pH level of more than 3. Gastric HCl reduces Fe^{3+} to ferrous iron (Fe^{2+}), making it soluble and therefore more easily absorbable. In the lumen, a protein called transferrin binds iron. Through the process of endocytosis, the transferrin-iron-receptor complex is engulfed into the cytosol of the mucosal cell. In a poorly understood manner, the iron is released from this complex, and it is transported across the basolateral membrane, where it again binds to the plasma form of transferrin. In times of iron excess, iron is bound to ferritin within the intestinal epithelial cell. Once bound, iron is not available for absorption and is lost when the cell is desquamated.

Magnesium, zinc, copper, and selenium are other minerals that are important in our diet. Their specific mechanisms of absorption are not well understood. Magnesium absorption appears to occur along the entire length of the small intestine. The site of zinc absorption has not been clearly defined, but its absorption appears to be an active process. Copper appears to be absorbed most actively in the upper small intestine. Its mechanism of absorption may be nonspecific and other ions such as zinc may be competitive.

Vitamins are essential in human metabolism because they serve as important cofactors in chemical processes. This brief discussion of vitamin absorption will be divided into fat-soluble versus water-soluble vitamins. Fat-soluble vitamins (A, D, E, and K), like lipids, are nonpolar and require the formation of bile acid micelles for their absorption. Once absorbed across the brush border, like lipids, fat-soluble vitamins are incorporated into chylomicrons for transport to the lymphatic system via the lacteals. Like lipids, fat-soluble vitamins depend on bile acids for their absorption. In general, water-soluble vitamins (B complex, C, D, niacin, folate, biotin, and pantothenic acid) are absorbed across the brush border either by simple diffusion or via carrier-mediated processes. For vitamin B_{12}, absorption occurs mainly in the terminal ileum. As discussed earlier, intrinsic factor released by the chief cells in the stomach is essential to the absorption of vitamin B_{12}. In the stomach, vitamin B_{12} is released with the digestion of proteins by pepsin. Once free, vitamin B_{12} binds to gastric intrinsic factor, making it resistant to digestion and absorp-

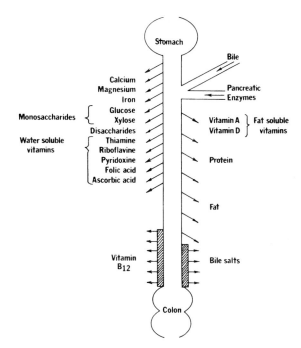

FIGURE 17-13. Absorptive sites. (From Rombeau JL, Caldwell MD, eds. *Clinical nutrition: enteral and tube feeding,* 2nd ed. Philadelphia: WB Saunders, 1990:19, with permission.)

tion. In the terminal ileum, receptors for this specific B_{12}-IF complex facilitate absorption.

As described, the small intestine is a highly specialized organ for the absorption of essential nutrients, vitamins, and minerals. The sites of absorption for each specific component of our diet are summarized in Fig. 17-13.

Colon

The *colon* is approximately 1.5 m long, and it is the last organ in the aerodigestive tract. The colon's major functions in the digestive process are the absorption of water and electrolytes and the storage of nonabsorbable fecal matter for eventual disposal. As stated earlier, approximately 1 L of chyme reaches the cecum on a daily basis. However, only about 100 to 200 mL of water is lost from the feces daily.

The mechanism of water and electrolyte absorption in the colon is similar to that in the small intestine. This process is dependent on the basolateral membrane Na^+/K^+ ATPase. The electrochemical gradient created enables Na^+ and Cl^- to be actively absorbed in exchange for K^+ and HCO_3^-, respectively. As in the small intestine, water absorption is coupled to the absorption of electrolytes.

As described, the GI system is highly efficient and organized for the roles of digestion and absorption. In the next section, we will discuss how the body utilizes these vital nutrients through its efficient metabolic pathways and adaptations.

NUTRITION AND METABOLISM

Assessment

Malnutrition is a major and common problem seen in the surgical population. Because malnutrition has been shown to predispose patients to postoperative complications, identification of this group of patients can be helpful. Studies have suggested that adequate nutritional support may reduce this risk.

The first step of assessment is a thorough history and physical examination. This method of assessment has been proven to be of significant value. A thorough history should include dietary habits and recent weight changes. Recent history of surgery or trauma and chronic medical issues may provide insight regarding treatment. Other issues (such as tobacco use and drug and alcohol abuse) that may have significant nutritional impact should be elicited. The physical examination should be meticulous because signs of malnutrition can be subtle. The height and weight of the patients should be assessed, and the patient's weight relative to normal (for age, height, and sex) standards should be determined. Also, the overall appearance should be appreciated. Decreases in subcutaneous fat in the extremities and the buttocks could be a sign of decreased caloric intake. Severe caloric deficiency, or *marasmus,* produces a cachectic appearance with signs of protein wasting. Protein wasting can be manifested by temporal wasting and decrease in extremity bulk and strength. Patients with *kwashiorkor,* or isolated protein malnutrition, often are obese, and they can be difficult to identify. Peripheral edema and changes in skin turgor should be sought. Abdominal examination for evidence of ascites and liver enlargement should be performed. Changes in skin and nail texture can be informative. Vitamin and trace-mineral deficiency can be manifested by neurological changes.

Estimation of protein and fat reserves in the body can be enhanced by laboratory and special anthropometric measurements (midarm muscle circumference and triceps skin fold). Serum albumin level provides the best simple estimate of visceral protein reserve. Because of the long half-life of albumin (18 days), other proteins with shorter half-lives, such as transferrin (8.5 days), prealbumin (1.3 days), and retinol-binding protein (0.4 days) may provide a better estimate in periods of acute changes. Total lymphocyte count and antigen skin testing are other estimates of visceral protein reserve. Measures of midarm circumference and triceps skin fold, when compared with normal values for the patient's age and sex, can be used to estimate skeletal protein reserve and total body fat reserve, respectively.

By measuring nitrogen balance, nitrogen synthesis and breakdown can be evaluated. Nitrogen intake is simply the amount of nitrogen delivered to the body, either through the enteral or parenteral route. Nitrogen output is the sum of all excretions and secretions that may contain nitrogen, such as urine, feces, or fistula drainage. Commonly, the output is estimated by measuring the total nitrogen output in urine in a 24-hour period. One gram of nitrogen composes 6.25 g of protein. In addition, a correction factor (4 g per 24 hours) is used to estimate nonurinary nitrogen losses such as diarrhea or bleeding, which are usually minimal.

$$\text{nitrogen balance} = \text{protein intake}/6.25 - (\text{urinary urea nitrogen} + 4)$$

Though not very precise, the nitrogen balance estimation may be essential to patients receiving nutritional support. Over an extended period, this estimate may reveal clinical trends to which management can be adjusted. In general, a positive nitrogen balance signifies adequate protein intake while a negative balance represents protein wasting, or loss.

Metabolism in the Basal State

Caloric Requirements

The body requires caloric intake to provide an energy source to perform work and to fuel its vital metabolic pathways. Energy is derived primarily from carbohydrate and fat. There are three ways to estimate an individual's total energy requirement, also known as the "resting energy expenditure" (REE). The simplest way is to estimate REE based on the weight of the patient. For maintenance of weight in simple unstressed starvation, the REE is approximately 30 Kcal/kg per day. This estimate should be adjusted in cases of severe stress (such as trauma, burn), where the REE can be as high as 40 to 50 Kcal/kg per day.

The second method estimates basal energy expenditure (BEE), utilizing the Harris-Benedict equation. BEE is about 10% less than REE and reflects energy expenditure

TABLE 17-1. CORRECTION FACTOR APPLIED TO BASAL METABOLIC RATE FOR VARIOUS CONDITIONS

Condition	Stress factor
Mild starvation	0.85–1.00
Postoperative recovery (no complications)	1.00–1.05
Cancer[a]	1.10–1.45
Peritonitis[a]	1.05–1.25
Severe infection or multiple trauma[a]	1.30–1.55

[a]Proportional to the extent of the disease

upon first awakening, fasting, and at rest. By multiplying the BEE by a factor, the energy expenditure estimate can be adjusted to the different clinical scenarios (Table 17-1).

$$BEE \text{ (women)} = 655 + (9.6W) + 1.8(H) - (4.7A)$$
$$BEE \text{ (men)} = 66 + (13.7W) + (5H) - (6.8A),$$

where W is weight in kilograms, H is height in centimeters, and A is age in years.

The third technique, indirect calorimetry, calculates energy expenditure by measuring oxygen consumption and carbon dioxide production. By having the patient breathe into a spirometer for gas analysis (metabolic cart), this technique is the most accurate in measuring caloric requirement. The process of collecting gas for analysis can be difficult. However, if gas is correctly collected and calculated, this process can provide an accurate estimate of energy expenditure.

$$\text{metabolic rate (Kcal/m}^2\text{/h)} = [3.9 \times VO_2(L/min)] \\ + 1.1 \times VCO_2 \text{ (L/min)} \\ \times 60 \text{ (min/h)/body surface area (M}^2)$$

In addition, this technique can provide information on substrate utilization through the respiratory quotient (RQ). The RQ is the ratio of carbon dioxide production to oxygen consumption. For glucose oxidation, the RQ is 1.0. For protein and fat, they are 0.8 and 0.7, respectively. The RQ can provide information on the type of substrates that are being used at a point in time.

Carbohydrate

Glucose is a major energy source for metabolic processes and to fuel muscular work. Approximately 30% to 40% of the caloric content of the typical western diet is made up of carbohydrates. Once absorbed into the cell, glucose is converted to glucose 6-phosphate (G6P). G6P is polymerized to glycogen (glycogenesis) or catabolized via glycolysis yielding energy in the form of adenosine 5'-triphosphate (ATP). During conditions of excess, glycogen synthetase converts G6P to *glycogen* for storage. Once glycogen stores are repleted, glucose is converted to lipids. During conditions of need, glycolysis converts G6P to pyruvic acid. Pyruvic acid is converted to acetyl-CoA, where it passes to the *tricarboxylic acid* (TCA) cycle to yield hydrogen, electrons, CO_2, and water. These products are then used to provide the substrate for the electron transport chain in the mitochondria, yielding energy in the form of ATP. The oxidation of glucose yields approximately 4 Kcal/g. This second phase of aerobic reaction is the common pathway for the oxidation of amino acids, fatty acids, and glucose (Fig. 17-14).

Certain tissues, such as the brain and red blood cells, prefer glucose for energy and require a minimal amount of glucose even in times of stress. The minimum requirement

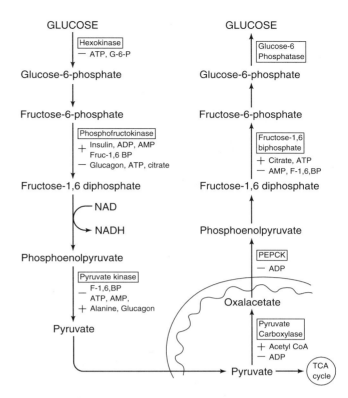

FIGURE 17-14. Glycolysis, gluconeogenesis.

for the brain and red blood cells is 100 to 150 g per day. Our body reserve of carbohydrate, in the form of glycogen, is approximately 300 to 400 g. Approximately 100 g is stored in the liver, and 200 to 250 g in skeletal muscles. Only the liver store is available for systemic use. The skeletal glycogen, however, can be used by the skeletal muscle for its own energy use. This form of body energy reserve is relatively small and is depleted after only 24 hours of starvation. The body must then rely on lipolysis and proteolysis for energy production.

During the time of glycogen depletion and the absence of carbohydrate intake, gluconeogenesis occurs to provide glucose for these tissues. Gluconeogenesis occurs mostly in the liver, but to some extent in the kidneys. Gluconeogenesis is more than a simple reversal of glycolysis because of three irreversible reactions. It requires the conversion of pyruvate to oxaloacetate, which occurs in the mitochondria. Oxaloacetate is converted to malate for its transport into the cytosol. Once transferred to the cytosol, malate is converted back to oxaloacetate for its conversion to phospho-*enol*pyruvate (Fig. 17-14).

It is important to note that the major substrates for gluconeogenesis are gluconeogenic amino acids from proteolysis. The glycerol backbone generated from lipolysis provides a small fraction of the substrate for this process because acetyl-CoA from fatty acids can not be converted back to pyruvate. In essence, the body can convert glucose to fat in time of excess, but it is unable to convert fat to glucose during the time of glucose depletion. Proteolysis, therefore, provides most of the substrates for gluconeogenesis.

Lipids

Fat provides 30% to 40% of the daily caloric intake in the western diet. Fat is the most efficient form of energy storage in the body, and the oxidation of fat generates 9 Kcal/g. Fat reserve is in the form of triacylglycerol in the adipose tissues. Triglycerides are made up of a glycerol backbone with three fatty acids covalently bound. Fatty acids are a major fuel for the heart, liver, and skeletal muscle. During a time of starvation, ketone bodies are derived from fatty acids for utilization by the heart, skeletal muscle, and the brain.

In the well-fed state, triglyceride is formed for the storage of energy. Unlike lipid breakdown, the synthesis of fatty acids occurs in the cytosol. The rate-limiting step is the conversion of acetyl-CoA to malonyl-CoA. By elongating malonyl-CoA with two carbon units derived by acetyl-CoA sequentially, fatty acids are formed.

During times of dietary deficiency, triglycerides are mobilized from the adipose tissue for lipolysis. Released from triglyceride, fatty acids are absorbed by cells for energy utilization. Once absorbed, a reaction with coenzyme A and ATP activates fatty acids to fatty acyl-CoA for oxidation. Because oxidation occurs in the mitochondria of cells, fatty acyl-CoA must be transported into the mitochondria through a reaction with carnitine. Once inside the mitochondria, the carnitine is released, and the fatty acyl-CoA is ready for oxidation. Beta-oxidation of fatty acyl-CoA is a series of reactions that results in the generation of acetyl-CoA and an acyl-CoA that is two carbon atoms shorter with each pass (Fig. 17-15). The acetyl-CoA generated can enter the TCA cycle for complete oxidation. As stated earlier, the acetyl-CoA generated can not be converted to pyruvate for gluconeogenesis. This is because the conversion of pyruvate (from the glycolysis pathway) to acetyl-CoA is irreversible. However, the glycerol generated from triglycerides can be converted to pyruvate for gluconeogenesis.

Ketone bodies are synthesized in the liver when glucose availability is low and are transported to other tissues for energy. Ketone bodies are particularly important during times of starvation for tissues, such as the brain, that have obligate glucose needs. During starvation when the oxaloacetate level is low, acetyl-CoA is shunted away from the TCA toward the formation of ketones (i.e., acetoacetate and β-hydroxybutyrate). The remaining available oxaloacetate is shunted toward the gluconeogenesis pathway.

Protein

Protein comprises about 15% of our total ideal body weight. None of this exists as a storage form, as all proteins in humans have biological function. Adults require approximately 0.8 to 1 g of exogenous protein per kilogram daily. Nonessential amino acids can be synthesized from nitrogenous precursors while essential amino acids must be ingested in the diet. The major role of amino acids is to serve as substrates to be incorporated into proteins, but some amino acids can also serve nonprotein functions. For example, the carbon skeleton of some amino acids (such as alanine, glutamate, the gluconeogenic amino acids) is important in gluconeogenesis and the TCA cycle, and glutamine plays a major role in the transport of nitrogen between organs.

Gluconeogenesis from amino acids occurs during starvation after glycogen stores are depleted. Rates of gluconeogenesis are increased during stress due to increased caloric requirements and impaired utilization of ketones. The amino group must be removed from amino acids prior to gluconeogenesis. This involves four steps: (i) transamination, (ii) deamination, (iii) ammonia transport, and (iv) the urea cycle. Through the process of transamination, a pair of amino acids and a pair of α-keto analogs are interconverted. Usually, α-ketoglutarate or pyruvate is the amino group receptor, and glutamate and alanine are produced. Alanine is transported to the liver, where it is deaminated to form pyruvate, which can be used for gluconeogenesis. The amino group generated from the deamination must be eliminated, and this is achieved through the urea cycle. α-ketoglutamate or pyruvate is regenerated from

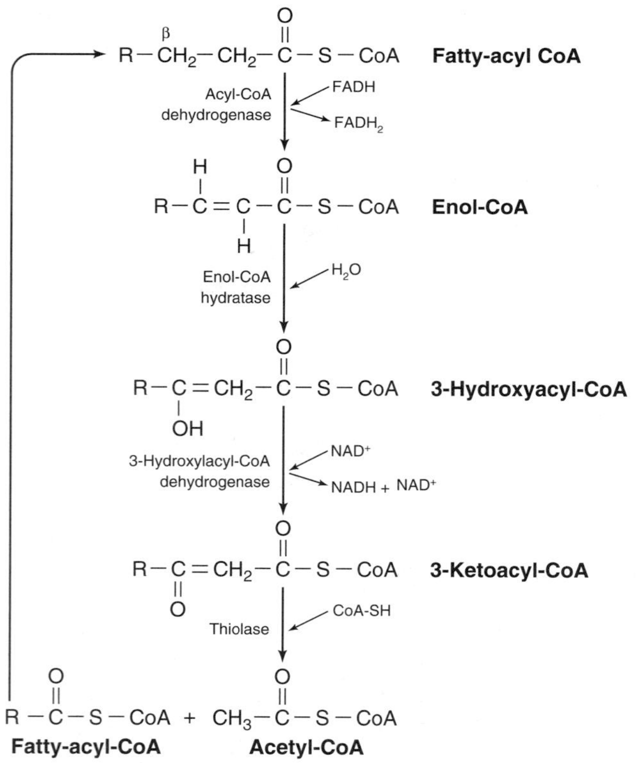

FIGURE 17-15. Fatty acid beta-oxidation.

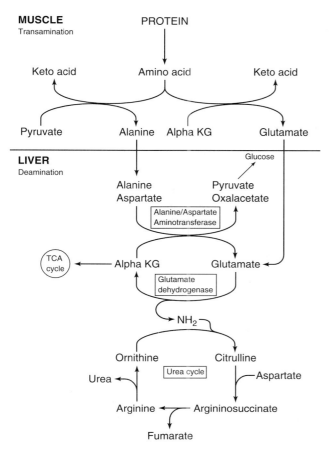

FIGURE 17-16. Protein metabolism.

glutamate or alanine, respectively, producing ammonia via another deamination reaction. The ammonia molecule generated enters the urea cycle and is excreted into the urine (Fig. 17-16).

Vitamins, Minerals, Trace-element Requirements

Vitamins are an essential component of our diet. They cannot be synthesized by the body, and vitamins serve as important cofactors in many biochemical pathways. The function, deficiency state, and toxicity of important vitamins are listed in Table 17-2.

As described in an earlier section, vitamins are categorized as fat soluble or water soluble. Fat-soluble vitamins are stored in body fat. Measuring a low serum level is diagnostic of vitamin deficiency and should be treated. Vitamin D, which is important in the control of calcium and phosphate metabolism, is formed from a derivative of cholesterol by the action of ultraviolet light. Conversion of vitamin D_3 (cholecalciferol) into the active form calcitriol ($1\alpha,25$-Dihydroxycholecalciferol) requires hydroxylation steps that take place in the liver (25) and kidneys (1). Water-soluble stores are limited, except for vitamin B_{12}, so that during states of deficiency, water-soluble vitamins are more likely to be depleted.

Minerals play major roles in numerous metabolic processes. Calcium, the most abundant cation, plays a major role in skeletal muscle and cardiac muscle contraction, neuronal excitability, coagulation, and other processes. Bone is the largest store of calcium, and calcium homeostasis is pre-

TABLE 17-2. VITAMINS

Vitamin	Function	Deficiency state
Fat soluble		
A (retinol)	Rhodopsin synthesis	Xerophthalmia, keratomalacia
D (cholecalciferol)	Intestinal calcium absorption, Bone remodeling	Rickets (children), osteomalacia (adults)
E (α-tocopherol)	Antioxidant	Hemolytic anemia, neurologic damage
K (naphthoquinone)	τ-Carboxylation of glutamate in clotting factors	Coagulopathy (deficiency in factors II, VII, IX, X)
Water soluble		
B_1 (thiamide)	Decarboxylation and aldehyde transfer reactions	Beriberi, neuropathy, fatigue, heart failure
B_2 (riboflavin)	Oxidation-reduction reactions	Dermatitis, glossitis
B_5 (niacin)	Oxidation-reduction reactions	Pellagra (dermatitis, diarrhea, dementia, death)
B_6 (pyridoxal phosphate)	Transamination and decarboxylation reactions	Neuropathy, glossitis, anemia
B_7 (biotin)	Carboxylation reactions	Dermatitis, alopecia
B_9 (folate)	DNA synthesis	Megaloblastic anemia, glossitis
B_{12} (cyanocobalamin)	DNA synthesis, myelination	Megaloblastic anemia, neuropathy
C (ascorbic acid)	Hydroxylation of hormones, hydroxylation of proline in collagen synthesis, antioxidant	Scurvy

TABLE 17-3. TRACE ELEMENTS

Trace element	Function	Deficiency
Chromium	Promotes normal glucose utilization in combination with insulin	Glucose intolerance, peripheral neuropathy
Copper	Component of enzymes	Hypochromic microcytic anemia, neutropenia, bone demineralization, diarrhea
Fluorine	Essential for normal structure of bones and teeth	Caries
Iodine	Thyroid hormone production	Endemic goiter, hypothyroidism, myxedema, cretinism
Iron	Hemoglobin synthesis	Hypochromic microcytic anemia, glossitis, stomatitis
Manganese	Component of enzymes, essential for normal bone structure	Dermatitis, weight loss, nausea, vomiting, coagulopathy
Molybdenum	Component of enzymes	Neurologic abnormalities, night blindness
Selenium	Component of enzymes, antioxidant	Cardiomyopathy
Zinc	Component of enzymes involved in metabolism of lipids, proteins, carbohydrates, nucleic acids	Alopecia, hypogonadism, olfactory and gustatory dysfunction, impaired wound healing, acrodermatitis enteropathica, growth arrest

dominantly under the control of the parathyroid hormone. The recommended daily allowances (RDA) for calcium is 800 mg, but certain populations such as postmenopausal women may need as much as 1.2 to 1.5 g per day.

Magnesium serves as a cofactor for numerous enzymes and as a regulator of neuromuscular excitability. The RDA for magnesium is 350 mg per day, and magnesium can be detected by a low serum level. Magnesium deficiency can be seen in patients with rapid intestinal transit, fat malabsorption, pancreatitis, and nephritis, as well as with diuretic use. Low serum levels respond adequately to parenteral doses of magnesium.

Phosphorous plays crucial roles as metabolic intermediates (ATP, cyclic AMP, nucleic acids) and in skeletal structure. The RDA for phosphorus is 800 mg per day. Deficiency in phosphorous can have deleterious effects on glycolysis, gluconeogenesis, oxygen transport, and cardiac and muscular contractility. Parenteral therapy with close monitoring should be instituted for deficiency.

Trace elements, although generally less than 0.1% of the diet, play important roles in metabolism, immunology, and wound healing. Their deficiencies can have major clinical sequelae and should be treated immediately. Some of the trace minerals, their functions, and signs of deficiency are listed in Table 17-3. Trace elements should be an integral part of nutrition support and a significant factor in the choice of enteral as well as parenteral formulas.

Metabolism in Starvation

Simple *starvation* is one of the most common situations surgical patients must face. Many patients are exposed to starvation either waiting for an operation or a diagnostic study or due to inadequate oral intake secondary to their illness or therapy. An understanding of the metabolic processes in starvation is vital to providing adequate nutritional support.

During the first 24 hours of starvation, glycogen stores are rapidly depleted. Because tissues such as the brain and red blood cells have obligate glucose needs, a second glucose source must be available. As insulin levels fall in response to the fall in serum glucose, stimulation for protein and lipid synthesis is diminished. The combination of a rise in glucagon secretion and the fall in insulin release results in triglyceride breakdown. The glycerol released from triglyceride breakdown and the amino acids available from decreased protein synthesis and increased proteolysis provide the substrates for hepatic gluconeogenesis. The process of gluconeogenesis is energy dependent, with energy provided by the fatty acids released from the breakdown of triglycerides.

During early starvation, urinary nitrogen loss can be 8 to 12 g per day, or approximately 340 g per day of tissue. At this rate, protein stores would be depleted rapidly and the patient would not survive beyond a month. Yet, unstressed patients with chronic starvation can survive up to 2 to 3 months and more. Survival is achieved by decreasing overall energy expenditure and specifically the utilization of glucose by tissues normally dependent on glucose, particularly the brain. After several days, the brain changes its preference for glucose as its major energy source to ketone bodies. With this adaptation, protein breakdown for gluconeogenesis is reduced. Free fatty acids generated by increased lipid breakdown continue to serve as an energy source for peripheral tissues. Adaptation to chronic starvation enables the body to conserve body protein and to enhance the utilization of triglyceride stores for energy.

Metabolism in Stress/Injury/Sepsis

Injury to the body activates neural as well as endocrine stress responses that alter the adaptation of metabolism seen in simple starvation. Energy expenditure increases dramatically, and the protein sparing seen in late starvation is abolished. Carbohydrate metabolism is affected producing glucose intolerance, and lipolysis is continued at an accelerated rate. Simply put, the body's response to injury is a neuroendocrine event.

Cuthbertson described the altered metabolism following injury as two phases: (i) the ebb phase and (ii) the flow phase (Fig. 17-17). The *ebb phase* involves the initial hours following injury, where normal to reduced energy expenditure, hyperglycemia, and restoration of tissue perfusion are seen. The *flow phase*, usually lasting from days to weeks, follows the ebb phase, and it is characterized by hypermetabolism, negative nitrogen balance, glucose intolerance, and lipolysis. Later modified by Moore, the flow phase was further divided into two phases, the catabolic and the anabolic phase. The *catabolic phase* can continue despite correction of the underlying injury. The *anabolic phase* that follows results in protein synthesis and restoration of fat stores.

Resting energy expenditure can increase dramatically after injury, in contrast to the chronic adaptation (decrease in resting energy expenditure) seen in simple starvation. The extent of increase in metabolism depends on the type of injury, with routine postoperative REE approximately 10% above resting state. The most severe changes occur with extensive thermal burn, where it can be as high as 100% above resting state. This hypermetabolic state appears to be due to increased sympathetic nervous system discharge and the release of catecholamines.

The *neuroendocrine response* seen after injury creates increases in the levels of adrenocorticotropic hormone, cortisol, catecholamines, glucagon, and growth hormone. As a result, a state of hyperglycemia is commonly seen in patients with injury or sepsis. The insulin level during the initial ebb phase is low, but it rises as the body approaches the flow phase. Despite high levels of insulin, the body continues to be in a state of hyperglycemia. This is a result of increased glucose production and inhibition of its use peripherally. High levels of glucagon are believed to drive the high production of glucose by the liver. Elevated levels of cortisol and catecholamines favor gluconeogenesis and inhibit peripheral glucose use. As a result, profound insulin resistance and glucose intolerance occurs.

Protein metabolism is severely altered in states of injury or sepsis. Unlike simple starvation, extensive nitrogen loss continues because protein catabolism is often accelerated with no adaptation to ketone utilization (known as a "failure to ketoadapt"). Glucose administration fails to suppress the protein catabolism, as seen in simple starvation (known as the "protein-sparing effect of glucose"). Amino acids from muscle proteolysis are a major source of substrate for oxidative fuels, gluconeogenesis, and new protein synthesis.

During times of stress, energy production is increasingly protein dependent. Only the glycerol backbone generated from lipolysis can be used for gluconeogenesis. This leaves proteins as the major source of carbon skeletons for gluconeogenesis. Glutamine and alanine appear to have a pivotal role in protein metabolism involving gluconeogenesis in the liver during times of stress. Glutamine and alanine are criti-

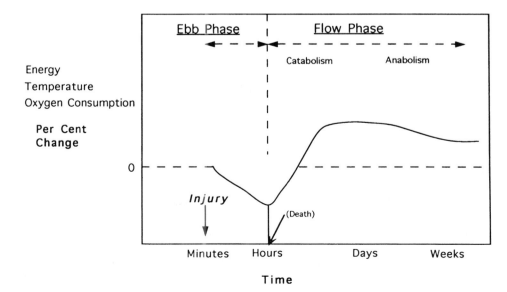

FIGURE 17-17. Metabolism following injury. (From Schwartz SI, Shires GT, Spencer FC, eds. *Principles of surgery*, 7th ed. New York: McGraw Hill, 1994: 27, with permission.)

cal substrates in the transfer of nitrogen from skeletal muscles to visceral organs. The transfer of these amino acids ensures a reliable hepatic source of glucose that is essential for the hematopoietic cells involved in wound healing and infection.

The need for protein synthesis by the liver, the bone marrow, and the wound further drives the obligate protein loss seen in injury or sepsis. The synthesis of acute phase proteins involved with the complement cascade, coagulation, and opsonization is accelerated in injury or sepsis and further contributes to protein losses elsewhere. In addition, protein synthesis is also required for wound healing and for eventual return of function. This combination of increased utilization of structural and visceral proteins as energy substrates and increased synthesis of proteins necessary for survival can increase exogenous protein requirements up to threefold during periods of stress.

Fat remains a major source of energy during times of injury or sepsis. The accelerated lipolysis seen in injury states is most likely due to increased sympathetic discharge. However, lipid metabolism in injury or sepsis is different from that of starvation. Fatty acid levels may stay close to normal despite the increased turnover rate. The plasma-free fatty acid level is a reflection of the balance between production and clearance. In a hypermetabolic state such as sepsis, the fatty acid level may stay normal, demonstrating the high metabolic rate. In contrast to simple starvation, ketone production is decreased after major injury or sepsis. This is most likely the result of increased insulin level, glucagon, glucose, alanine, and lactate. These molecules all appear to inhibit metabolic pathways of ketogenesis.

Burns

Thermal injury has a substantial effect on metabolism because of the extensive injury and the prolonged state of neuroendocrine stimulation. Burns can raise the REE as much as 100% to 200% above baseline with urinary nitrogen losses exceeding 30 to 40 g per day. The major drive behind this hypermetabolic state is the sympathetic discharge and catecholamine release. Inflammatory mediators such as tumor necrosis factor and IL-1 appear to have major roles as well.

The hypermetabolic state in burn patients appears to return to baseline only when skin coverage is complete. Therefore, it is essential to immediately address the tremendous increase in caloric requirement found in burn patients. In addition to maintenance needs, 40 Kcal per percentage of total body surface area burned is required. During the initial phase of burn injury, fat metabolism is compromised and the majority of caloric requirement should be in the form of carbohydrates. Following the initial phase, fat metabolism should return to baseline. The obligate protein catabolism seen in burns is similar to that seen in sepsis. Similarly, caloric infusion in the form of carbohydrates does not suppress protein catabolism.

Cancer

Malnutrition is a major component of the disease process found in cancer patients. Reports of REE in cancer patients have been conflicting. Although most cachectic patients demonstrate low REE as expected during hypocaloric feeding, some malignancies are associated with increases in REE of 20% to 30%. This increase in REE can even be found in some cancer patients with severe cachexia, which would usually produce a significant decrease in REE during simple starvation.

A variety of mechanisms have been proposed to explain this hypermetabolism seen in some cancer patients. In some patients, tumor tissue continues to achieve a state of hypermetabolism at the expense of the host despite the host's starvation. In others, metabolic derangements involving lipids, carbohydrates, and protein are seen, similar to that found in injury or septic states. Glucose intolerance, increase in gluconeogenesis, and increase in lipolysis may be present. Negative nitrogen balance may occur as the tumor tissue acts as a nitrogen trap, continuing to synthesize proteins while the host organism is catabolizing protein. Nutritional support of cancer patients may or may not correct these specific metabolic derangements seen in this minority of cancer patients. However, the wasting and weight loss associated with cancer (so-called "cancer cachexia") in most patients is not due to metabolic derangements but to decreased nutrient intake. Appropriate nutrient intake will prevent or correct cancer cachexia in these patients.

NUTRITION SUPPORT

Routes of Administration

Once the decision to provide nutritional support has been made, the route of administration must be determined. Enteral and parenteral routes of administration are both viable means, each with its own advantages and complications.

Enteral nutrition

Enteral nutritional support provides more physiologic utilization of nutrients and helps to maintain the gut-barrier function. Compared to parenteral nutrition, enteral nutrition may be less expensive, easier to administer, and may have fewer complications. Whenever possible, enteral nutrition should be the first line of therapy. However, GI function may be impaired in surgical patients. The presence of ileus, obstruction, hemorrhage, and other processes that prohibit the function of the GI tract can be a contraindication to enteral nutritional support.

For patients who require temporary nutritional support, a *nasoenteric tube* placed distal to the pylorus can serve as a route of administration for 4 to 6 weeks. It is generally placed under fluoroscopic guidance to confirm position. A position distal to the pylorus decreases the risk of aspiration pneumonia and its devastating effect on critically ill patients.

In patients with low aspiration risk, a *gastrotomy tube* can be a viable option for long-term enteral access. The gastrotomy tube can be placed either percutaneously under endoscopic guidance or open during an abdominal operation. The percutaneous endoscopic gastrostomy tube has become a popular method with minimal morbidity and mortality.

In patients who are neurologically compromised or at high risk for aspiration, enteral access distal to the ligament of Treitz is preferred. At the time of laparotomy, a *jejunostomy tube* can be placed using the Witzel technique. A segment of jejunum 20 to 30 cm distal to the ligament of Treitz is selected for placement. This can provide a long-term method of therapy with minimal risk of aspiration pneumonia.

Aspiration pneumonitis is a devastating complication of enteral therapy. Placement of access distal to the ligament of Treitz is one of the best methods to prevent this complication. Other serious complications involve the technical aspects of the placement of the tube, such as bowel obstruction, volvulus, perforation, and ischemia.

Parenteral Nutrition

When enteral support is contraindicated, parenteral therapy should be used to provide optimal nutritional support. Parenteral therapy is less physiologic, more expensive, and less effective in maintaining gut integrity. Relative to enteral feeding, it may be more difficult to manage, and the complication rates may be higher. Parenteral therapy can be used to supplement enteral therapy when only a suboptimal level of enteral support is tolerated.

The preferred site of access for parenteral support is usually the subclavian vein. Care of the catheter in this region is easier (as compared to the internal jugular vein or femoral vein), resulting in lower infection rates and improved patient comfort. Numerous types of catheters have been devised, and some can provide safe access for months to years when tunneled underneath the skin.

The safety of parenteral therapy is mainly dependent on the control of catheter-related infection and sepsis. Studies have shown that factors increasing access to the catheters (such as phlebotomy, piggyback infusion, and multiple lumina) increase the rate of infection. Pneumothorax associated with catheter placement can be life threatening, and all catheters should be placed under the guidance of an experienced operator. All line placements should be followed immediately by a chest radiograph to confirm placement and rule out pneumothorax.

Nutrition and metabolism are important aspects in the management of all surgical patients. Significant improvements and better understanding of nutrition support have been achieved since its beginning. Enteral and parenteral nutritional support have allowed the clinician to provide optimal nutritional support in the debilitated patient.

SUGGESTED READING

Berne RM, Levy MN, eds. *Physiology,* 2nd ed. St. Louis: Mosby, 1988.

Rombeau JL, Caldwell MD, eds. *Enteral nutrition,* 2nd ed. Philadelphia: WB Saunders, 1990.

Rombeau JL, Caldwell MD, eds. *Parenteral nutrition,* 2nd ed. Philadelphia: WB Saunders, 1993.

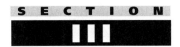

CARDIOVASCULAR AND RESPIRATORY SYSTEMS

18

HEMOSTASIS AND THROMBOSIS

T. SLOANE GUY AND L. HENRY EDMUNDS

Humans maintain the fluidity of blood and integrity of the vascular system by continuously balancing procoagulants and anticoagulants in a biochemical tug-of-war that defines an equilibrium between fluid and gel. Normally, small adjustments between procoagulants and anticoagulants maintain a balance, but in response to disease, trauma, or surgery, procoagulants and/or anticoagulants increase or decrease and shift the "flag" toward thrombosis or bleeding. As long as the flag remains near the equilibrium point, intravascular blood flows and extravascular blood clots. When it does not, complications develop.

Four separate plasma protein systems and three blood cells are primarily involved in maintaining the fluidity of blood and the integrity of the vascular system. The protein systems are the *contact proteins, intrinsic* and *extrinsic coagulation pathways,* and the *fibrinolytic system.* The major cells involved in coagulation are the *endothelial cell, platelets, monocytes,* and to a minor extent *neutrophils.* The coagulation proteins are designed to amplify and accelerate the production of thrombin and fibrin with each enzymatic step in the cascade. The cells contribute procoagulants and anticoagulants and provide phospholipid surfaces and specific membrane receptors to hasten the process. By analogy, blood coagulation is like a city fire: It starts with a match but ends with a conflagration. The system is complex but can be understood in general terms by focusing on the major reactions.

Understanding the fundamental structure of the hemostatic mechanism is relevant to surgical practice in that both minor and major alterations in hemostasis by acquired and congenital diseases are seen every day in the operating room and wards. Successful surgery and optimal management of severe trauma require a working knowledge of the coagulation system, screening tests for preoperative patients, and replacement products.

PARTICIPANTS IN CLOT GENERATION AND LYSIS

The majority of plasma coagulation proteins are glycoproteins. The liver produces all factors except VIII and von Willebrand factor (vWF), which are produced by endothelial cells. Factors II, VII, IX, and X are produced in the liver through a vitamin K–dependent reaction. Carboxylation of precursors form γ-carboxylated glutamic acid residues that bind to phospholipid membranes via a calcium cofactor. These residues are negatively charged and are linked to the negatively charged membrane by positively charged calcium ions. This γ-carboxylation is blocked by warfarin.

Plasma proteins circulate as inactive zymogens; active forms are either serine proteases or cofactors. By convention, the active protein is designated by a lowercase "a" after the Roman numeral. Zymogens are activated by cleavage of peptide bonds. Cofactors of the coagulation cascade include calcium, high molecular weight kininogen (HMWK), prekallikrein, tissue factor (TF), and factors V and VIII. Chelators of calcium such as EDTA and citrate inhibit clotting by binding calcium; calcium is an important cofactor for both the intrinsic and extrinsic coagulation pathways. Factor VIII and vWF combine to form a large protein, factor VIII/vWF; vWF is a carrier protein for factor VIII. The factor VIII/vWF complex primarily exists within the endothelium, where it helps to maintain the integrity of the vascular system.

The coagulation cascade is divided into the *contact* and *intrinsic coagulation systems* and the *extrinsic coagulation pathway.* Both systems produce activated factor Xa, which is the gateway enzyme of the common coagulation pathway that produces thrombin and fibrin (Fig. 18-1). When blood initially contacts a nonendothelial cell surface, plasma proteins are adsorbed onto that surface. If the surface is a wound, most of the cells in the wound express tissue factor (TF), which initiates the extrinsic coagulation cascade. If heparinized or nonanticoagulated blood touches a biomate-

---

Hospital of the University of Pennsylvania, Philadelphia, Pennsylvania

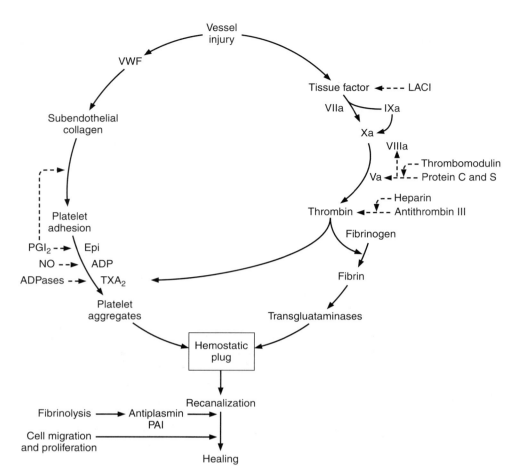

FIGURE 18-1. Overview of hemostasis. (From Coleman RW, Hirsh J, Marder VJ, et al. *Hemostasis and thrombosis: basic principles and clinical practice.* Philadelphia: JB Lippincott Co, 1994, with permission.)

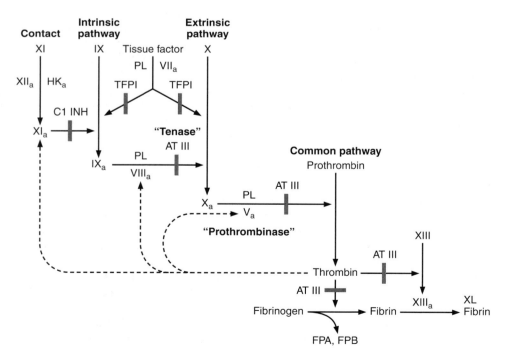

FIGURE 18-2. The clotting cascade (see text for details). (From Coleman RW, Hirsh J, Marder VJ, et al. *Hemostasis and thrombosis: basic principles and clinical practice.* Philadelphia: JB Lippincott Co, 1994, with permission.)

rial or nontissue surface (as in the heart-lung machine or cell-saver), plasma proteins are instantaneously adsorbed onto the surface as a monolayer that is densely packed and immobile. Concentrations of surface-adsorbed proteins differ from those found in bulk plasma and are influenced by the physical and chemical attributes of the surface. However, it is not possible to predict or control the protein topography of the surface; so called "thromboresistant" biomaterials are discovered empirically. Fibrinogen is selectively adsorbed when heparinized blood touches a biomaterial. Once on the surface, adsorbed proteins may undergo conformational changes to expose reactive sites. Adsorbed factor XII is activated in this way, as is complement protein C3.

Contact Activation System

Four zymogens constitute the contact proteins: factor XII (Hageman factor), prekallikrein, high molecular weight kininogen (HMWK) and factor XI (Fletcher factor). Upon contact with an activating surface, factor XII is converted into XIIa and XIIf in the presence of cofactors HMWK and prekallikrein (Fig. 18-2). Factor XIIa then cleaves prekallikrein to kallikrein, an important agonist for activating neutrophils. Factor XIIa also cleaves HMWK to produce bradykinin, a vasodilator and inflammatory mediator. Importantly, factor XIIa catalyzes cleavage of factor XI to XIa to initiate the intrinsic coagulation pathway. Congenital absence of factor XII, prekallikrein or HMWK does not produce symptoms. Absence of factor XI causes a mild bleeding disorder.

Intrinsic Coagulation Pathway

Factor XIa activates factor IX to factor IXa. Factor IX in combination with factor VIIIa, Ca^{2+} and a phospholipid surface forms the tenase complex, which cleaves factor X to factor Xa. Factor VIII is activated by thrombin, as are factors V and VII. Phospholipid surfaces greatly accelerate reactions between coagulation proteins and are primarily provided by platelets, monocytes, and endothelial cells. Activated factor X in the presence of cofactors Va and Ca^{2+} on a phospholipid surface (the prothrombinase complex) cleaves prothrombin to thrombin (factor II). In the process, a useful marker, prothrombin fragment F1.2, is formed. Thrombin then cleaves fibrinopeptides A and B from fibrinogen to form polymerized fibrin. Thrombin also activates factor XIII, which cross-links fibrin molecules. Thrombin is a powerful procoagulant and directly activates platelets and factors V, VII, and VIII. Thrombin also induces TF expression in both monocytes and endothelial cells. Thrombin is regulated by antithrombin.

Extrinsic Coagulation Pathway

TF, which is membrane-bound protein that is constitutively expressed in an active form on cells of most tissues (muscle, fat, adventitia, epicardium, etc), initiates the extrinsic coagulation pathway. TF in the presence of factor VIIa, Ca^{2+}, and a phospholipid surface directly cleaves factor X to factor Xa. The combination of TF, factor VIIa, Ca^{2+}, and a phospholipid surface also activates factor IX and leads to the formation of the tenase complex, which cleaves factor X to factor Xa. Thus, factor Xa is produced by both the intrinsic and extrinsic coagulation pathways, but the extrinsic pathway is by far the most important in most surgical procedures and trauma victims. Interleukin-1 (IL-1) and tumor necrosis factor (TNF) increase TF synthesis in many cells.

Fibrinolysis

Plasmin is produced from plasminogen by cleavage of a specific disulfide bond and is the active enzyme that hydrolyzes fibrin, fibrinogen, and factors V and VIII. Initially, both plasminogen and tissue plasminogen activator (TPA) assemble on the surface of fibrin; plasminogen is first cleaved to produce plasmin, then fibrin is hydrolyzed into fibrin-degradation products. TPA is the primary signal for fibrinolysis and is produced by endothelial cells in the presence of thrombin. It is regulated by plasmin activator inhibitor-1 (PAI-1). *Urokinase* is produced by fibroblasts, epithelial cells, and monocyte/macrophages, but the source of circulating urokinase is unknown. Unlike TPA, which binds avidly to fibrin, urokinase binds poorly and therefore plays a much smaller role in fibrinolysis. Fibrin cross-linking inhibits but does not prevent degradation of the polymer. Fibrin-degradation products are produced from the breakdown of fibrin and include D dimer, a useful indicator of fibrinolysis.

Therapeutic fibrinolysis is induced by recombinant TPA, urokinase, or recombinant streptokinase. Streptokinase activates plasminogen by forming equimolar complexes with the protein. Acylated plasminogen streptokinase activator complex represents an altered form of streptokinase that has a longer half-life and can be given by bolus injection. Epsilon amino caproic acid inhibits fibrinolysis by competitively blocking the critical binding site of plasminogen.

Plasmin does not normally circulate. α_2-antiplasmin is the primary regulator of fibrinolysis but is not effective when plasmin is bound to fibrin. α_2-macroglobulin also inhibits plasmin, but this reaction is much slower than that with α_2-antiplasmin.

CELLS

The *endothelial cell* is the only known nonthrombogenic surface and helps to maintain the fluidity of blood and the integrity of the vascular system by producing at least nine procoagulants and nine anticoagulants (Table 18-1). Endothelial cells and vascular smooth muscle cells also regulate vascular tone and capillary permeability and separate

TABLE 18-1. PROCOAGULANTS AND ANTICOAGULANTS PRODUCED BY ENDOTHELIAL CELLS

Procoagulant	Anticoagulant
Produces types IV, V, and VIII collagen	Produces PGI2, nitric oxide
Produces laminin, thrombospondin, fibronectin	Produces heparan sulfate, dermatin sulfate
Produces von Willebrand factor, factor V	Produces protein S
Produces plasminogen activator inhibitor-1	Inactivates platelet-secreted adenosine diphosphate, adenosine triphosphate
Produces platelet-activating factor	Produces thrombomodulin
Produces endothelin-1, renin, and angiotensin-converting enzyme	Produces tissue factor pathway inhibitor
Activates platelets	Produces tissue plasminogen activator
Expresses tissue factor	Produces protease nexin-1
Binds von Willebrand factor, factor IXa, factor Xa, high molecular weight kininogen vibronectin	
Inactivates bradykinin	

blood cells and proteins from basement membrane and the interstitial space. Whereas both endothelial cells and platelets are negatively charged and therefore resist adhesion, subendothelium contains adhesive proteins that make up basement membrane and the extracellular matrix. These include collagen and TF, fibronectin and vWF, which couples with platelet GPIb and GPIIb/IIIa receptors. Thus, the subendothelium plays a large role in developing the "platelet plug" when the endothelial cell barrier is breached.

Procoagulant activity by endothelial cells is stimulated by thrombin, cytokines (IL-TNF and γ-INF), and endotoxin and other mediators resulting from surgery, trauma, or infection. These agonists induce expression of TF and production and release of PAIs, which regulate TPA. They also stimulate expression of various integrin-adhesive receptors for fibronectin, collagen, laminin, and vitronectin. Endothelial cells express P and E selectin, which bind leukocytes. The powerful vasoconstrictor, endothelin 1, is produced by endothelial cells.

Anticoagulant activities of endothelial cells include production of heparitin sulfate and dermatan sulfate, proteins C and S, thrombomodulin, TF protein inhibitor, TPA, and protease nexin 1. Endothelial cells inactivate platelet-secreted adenosine 5'-triphosphate (ATP) and adenosine 5'-diphosphate (ADP) and produce adenosine.

Prostacyclin (PGI$_2$) is a product of cyclooxygenase and arachidonic metabolism and is primarily produced by endothelium. Prostacyclin causes vasodilation and inhibits platelet activation and adhesion. PGI$_2$ is synthesized and secreted at the borders of hemostatic plugs, preventing intravascular platelet aggregation. Thrombin, epinephrine, and trauma increase PGI$_2$ synthesis.

Nitric oxide (NO) is produced by endothelial cells and is a product of l-arginine metabolism. NO functions as a potent local vasodilator and platelet inhibitor. The chemical inhibits platelet function by raising cyclic guanosine 3',5'-monophosphate (cGMP). NO has a very short half-life (less than 1 second).

The *platelet* is a complex structure that has a central role in hemostasis. Platelets are produced in the bone marrow by megakaryocytes. An individual megakaryocyte produces over 1,000 platelets by fragmentation. Blood normally contains approximately 150,000 to 400,000 platelets per microliter, but approximately one third are sequestered within the spleen. Platelets have life spans from 9 to 12 days and an average of 35,000 platelets per microliter turnover each day. Platelet functions include adhesion to sites of injury, adhesion to exposed subendothelial surfaces, secretion of important procoagulatory and wound-healing molecules, formation of platelet aggregates, expression of receptors for procoagulatory proteins, inducing clot retraction, and secretion of mitogenic factors to facilitate wound healing (Fig. 18-3).

Platelets circulate as biconvex disks measuring 3 to 4 μ in diameter. Without a nucleus, platelets can not synthesize certain important enzymes such as cyclooxygenase and instead carry chemicals and proteins within granules. The disk shape of the platelet is maintained by an intracellular matrix composed of microtubules, microfilaments, and intermediate filaments. A system of canaliculi, which functions much like the sarcoplasmic reticulum in muscle cells, regulates rapid influx of calcium into the cytoplasm and provides for rapid secretory product egress. Contractile proteins including actin and myosin mediate shape change and cause centralization of granules when platelets are activated.

The major agonists for activation of platelets are ADP, thromboxane A$_2$, collagen, thrombin, epinephrine, and platelet-activating factor. ADP may be released from damaged red cells and/or endothelial cells or activated platelets. Platelet membranes have specific receptors for these physiologic agonists, which control platelet function by raising or lowering adenosine 3',5'-cyclic monophosphate (cAMP) or cGMP. Cyclic AMP and cGMP concentrations are regulated within platelets by three classes of phosphodiesterases that either inhibit or stimulate metabolism of the cyclic nucleotides. When activated, platelets express pseudopods (shape change) and membrane receptors and release granule contents in accordance with the strength of the stimulus.

Various glycoprotein receptors on the membrane surface are expressed with activation and interact with other platelets and subendothelial structures to produce aggregation and adhesion. These receptors include GPIb, GPIIb, GPIIIa, GPIV, and GPV, which interact with vWF, fibrino-

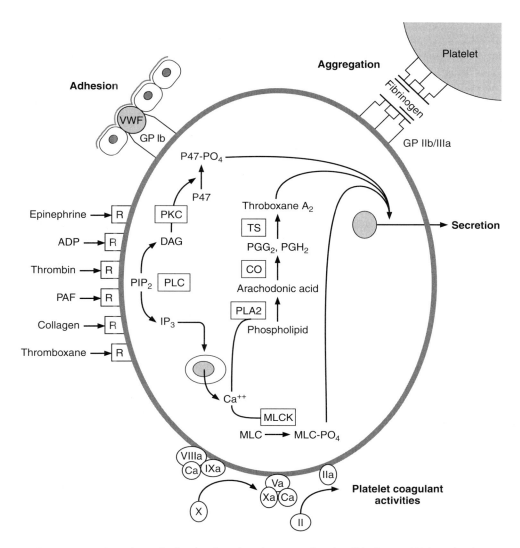

FIGURE 18-3. Overview of platelet function (see text for details). Factor VII has the lowest plasma concentration, thus explaining why warfarin affects the extrinsic pathway initially, demonstrated by an increase in prothrombin time. (From Coleman RW, Hirsh J, Marder VJ, et al. *Hemostasis and thrombosis: basic principles and clinical practice.* Philadelphia: JB Lippincott Co, 1994, with permission.)

gen, fibronectin, vibronectin, and collagen. Platelets also express receptors for procoagulant proteins including thrombin and facilitate formation of both the tenase and prothrombinase complexes in producing thrombin.

Each platelet contains several types of granules; granules contain various chemicals and proteins that participate in coagulation and wound healing. Dense bodies contain serotonin, calcium, ATP, ADP, and pyrophosphate. α granules contain fibrinogen, vWF, factor V, HMWK, fibronectin, α_1-antitrypsin, β-thromboglobulin, platelet factor 4, platelet-derived growth factor, thrombospondin, fibrinogen, and P selectin. Platelets also contain lysosomes, which store and release various acid hydrolases. Elevated cytoplasmic calcium level causes granules to fuse with intracellular canaliculi to release granular contents into the surrounding environment.

Platelets produce thromboxane A_2 (TXA$_2$), which is a short-acting, powerful vasoconstrictor and platelet agonist. TXA$_2$ is a product of arachidonic acid metabolism and the cyclooxygenase pathway. This pathway also produces PGD$_2$, a modulator of platelet activities. Platelets do not contain prostacyclin synthetase and therefore do not produce PGI$_2$. PGD$_2$ and PGI$_2$, produced by endothelial cells, stimulate adenylate cyclase to increase intracellular cAMP. Cyclic AMP removes calcium from the cytosol via phosphorylation of an ATP-dependent calcium pumping system and thus inhibits platelets.

The formation of a hemostatic plug begins with platelet activation by ADP, epinephrine, thrombin, subendothelial collagen, and perhaps other agonists. Activation expresses membrane adhesive receptors, particularly GPIb, and

GPIIb/IIIa. GPIb with vWF binds to subendothelial structures. Platelet GPIIb/IIIa binds to fibrinogen, fibronectin, vWF, and vibronectin. GPIIb/IIIa receptors also bind platelets together into aggregates using fibrinogen bridges. The GPIV receptor with thrombospondin stabilizes platelet aggregates. ADP and TXA_2 both induce platelet adhesion and cross-linking. Secreted platelet granules provide local epinephrine, serotonin, and calcium. Platelets also provide phospholipid surfaces for assembly of the tenase (VIII, IXa, Ca^{2+}) and prothrombinase (Va, Xa, Ca^{2+}) complexes. All of these reactions focus production of fibrin and aggregation and adhesion of platelets at the site of vascular injury to quickly stem the entrance of blood into the extravascular space.

Monocytes are activated by relatively high concentrations of thrombin as may occur in a wound, complement protein C5a, immune complexes, endotoxin, and IL-1β. Monocyte chemotactic protein 1 is a powerful monocyte agonist that is produced by monocytes and several other cells. The procoagulant activity of monocytes is primarily in expression of TF. Monocytes also express Mac-1 and L selectin and form aggregates with platelets.

Neutrophils do not have an important role in blood coagulation, but have weak procoagulant activity that involves expression of membrane Mac-1 and fibrinogen receptors.

NATURAL INHIBITORS OF THE COAGULATION CASCADE

Thrombomodulin is a potent inhibitor of thrombin. It binds to thrombin and inhibits its ability to cleave fibrinogen or activate factors V and VIII. It also enhances thrombin's ability to activate protein C, which degrades factors V and VIII. Protein S is a cofactor for protein C and acts by stabilizing protein C on a phospholipid membrane. Antithrombin III is a large protease inhibitor that primarily inhibits thrombin and to a lesser extent factors IXa, Xa, XIa, and XIIa but does not inhibit thrombin within clots. Heparin accelerates the reaction time of antithrombin III 1,000-fold. Heparin cofactor II inactivates thrombin in the presence of heparin. C1 inhibitor modulates the contact system by neutralizing factors XIIa and kallikrein. α_2-antiplasmin inactivates unbound plasmin and unbound activated coagulation factors. α_1-antitrypsin inactivates factor IXa. α_2-macroglobulin inactivates many coagulation factors and fibrinolytic enzymes, including kallikrein, thrombin, and plasmin, and acts as a secondary inhibitor for most of these reactions. TF pathway inhibitor inhibits factor VIIa/TF.

CLINICAL TESTING AND PREOPERATIVE SCREENING
Functional Tests of Coagulation

Whole blood coagulation is performed by collecting venous blood and agitating it at 37°C until a clot forms. Normally a clot forms within 4 to 8 minutes. A 50% reduction in clot volume at 1 hour is normally observed. Prolonged clot formation or poor contraction of clot volume are gross indicators of problems with platelet number (thrombocytopenia), function (thrombasthenia), or coagulation cascade. Ragged clots or clot breakdown suggest fibrinolysis.

Bleeding time is obtained by making a standard skin incision on the volar forearm with a lance and template. Blood is then blotted with filter paper every 30 seconds until all bleeding ceases, at which time the bleeding time is recorded. With the Ivy method, a 40 mm Hg tourniquet is applied proximal to the incision. Normal bleeding time ranges from 3 to 9 minutes. Standard deviations within individuals are small, but standard deviations between individuals are relatively large. Therefore, serial measurements are more meaningful than screening studies. Elevation of the bleeding time suggests platelet dysfunction or thrombocytopenia.

Prothrombin time (PT) is a measure of extrinsic and common coagulation pathway function. Citrated plasma is added to thromboplastin (animal TF) and calcium to activate factor VII. If the patient's blood contains fibrinogen, prothrombin, and factors V, VII, and X, factor Xa is formed with eventual production of thrombin and clot. PTs normally range from 11 to 14 seconds but differ from lab to lab because of different batches and sources of thromboplastin. The international normalized ratio (INR) is used to adjust for different PTs performed at different times or in different laboratories. INR values permit comparisons of PT values.

The PT is affected by low concentrations of fibrinogen, prothrombin, and factors V, VII, X, and II but is most sensitive to changes in factor VII because of normally low plasma concentrations. PT is used to monitor anticoagulation with warfarin because the drug inhibits γ-carboxylation of vitamin K–dependent coagulation factors in the liver. This inhibition is particularly effective for factor VII because of its short half-life in plasma.

Activated partial thromboplastin time (aPTT) measures intrinsic and common coagulation pathway function. This test is performed by adding plasma, calcium, and phospholipid to tubes containing celite or kaolin. These compounds provide a nonendothelial cell surface that activates contact and intrinsic coagulation pathways. Deficiencies in all clotting factors except factors VII and XIII may prolong the aPTT. The aPTT is used to monitor heparin dosing because of that drug's inhibitory effect on thrombin, factor IX, and factor XI. The presence of lupus anticoagulant protein, misnamed because it is a procoagulant, interferes with the aPTT. A simple method of determining whether a prolonged aPTT is due to a factor deficiency or a circulating anticoagulant is to mix the sample with normal plasma. In the case of a factor deficiency, the aPTT proportionally improves while the presence of an anticoagulant continues to prolong the aPTT time.

Thrombin time (TT) is obtained by adding thrombin to plasma and measuring the time to clot formation. The test primarily measures the quantity and function of fibrinogen and is prolonged in the presence of fibrin inhibitors such as heparin or fibrin-degradation products. With the advent of direct fibrinogen and fibrin-split product testing, the TT is rarely used.

The *activated clotting time* (ACT) represents the whole blood clotting time with the addition of celite, a clay surface that reduces the standard deviation of the test. A normal ACT is less than 110 seconds. Clinically, the ACT is used to monitor the degree of heparin effect during and after cardiopulmonary bypass or vascular procedures.

Fibrin-degradation products are measured as fibrin-split products or the marker of fibrinolysis, D-dimer. More sophisticated tests of various coagulation protein concentrations and activities and antibodies and substances that affect coagulation are usually available in well-staffed and well-equipped clinical hematology laboratories.

Preoperative Screening

Preoperative evaluation of surgical patients for bleeding disorders begins with a thorough history. A history of bleeding during dental procedures, previous surgery or trauma, and any history of excessive bruising should arouse suspicion. A review of the patient's medications may reveal important anticoagulants. A history of recent aspirin use is the most common cause of coagulation impairment. The presence of purpura, petechia, hepatomegaly, splenomegaly, joint deformities, or occult gastrointestinal tract bleeding also raise the possibility of a deficiency in clot formation. Any history of problems (venous or arterial thrombosis, pulmonary embolism, etc) with prior heparin exposure should prompt investigation for heparin-induced antiplatelet antibodies.

If minor surgery is proposed and the history and physical examination results are unrevealing, no further evaluation is needed. If major surgery is proposed and the history and physical examination results are normal, a platelet count and aPTT are obtained. An unexpected low platelet count, particularly in cardiac patients who have received heparin, raises the possibility of heparin-induced thrombocytopenia and the possibility of devastating heparin-induced thrombocytopenia and thrombosis if more heparin is given. A prolonged aPTT raises the possibility of a circulating anticoagulant or a defect in the intrinsic coagulation system such as factor XI deficiency that may not be uncovered by a bleeding history.

A *one-stage prothrombin time* (PT) and a test of clot solubility to screen for factor XIII deficiency is added to the platelet count and aPTT in patients with a history or physical examination results suggestive of bleeding tendencies or in patients undergoing surgery that is frequently associated with coagulation problems (cardiopulmonary bypass, prostatectomy, expected large blood loss, etc). A prolonged aPTT or PT requires workup for a coagulation deficiency; consultation with a hematologist may be helpful.

Drugs Affecting Platelet Function

Aspirin inhibits platelet function for the life of the platelet by inhibiting cyclooxygenase and thromboxane A_2 production. The inhibition is irreversible but does not inhibit activation of platelet membrane receptors and the thrombin receptor. Aspirin prolongs template bleeding times. Aspirin also inhibits cyclooxygenase in endothelial cells and formation of prostacyclin. However, endothelial cells can produce new cyclooxygenase and more prostacyclin. Low-dose aspirin (80 mg per day) is effective in permanently blocking platelet arachidonic metabolism and is usually used for long-term platelet inhibition to reduce side effects. Nonsteroidal antiinflammatory medications reversibly inhibit cyclooxygenase; thus, platelets recover full function in 2 to 3 days after the last dose.

Dipyridamole is a weak nonspecific phosphodiesterase inhibitor that partially inhibits platelets and has a half-life in plasma of 100 minutes. High doses (400 mgm per day), which cause unwelcome side effects, are needed to fully inhibit platelets. Phosphodiesterases metabolize cAMP; therefore, inhibition of the enzyme increases cAMP concentration and inhibits platelets. Iloprost increases platelet cAMP concentration by stimulating adenyl cyclase. Iloprost and other prostanoids, including prostacyclin, are also potent vasodilators. This property has limited their clinical use. NO and nitroprusside increase platelet cGMP concentration, which in low concentrations increases cAMP. NO has a very short half-life in plasma (less than 1 second), is given by inhalation, and is primarily used to reduce pulmonary vascular resistance.

Abciximab (Repro) is a chimeric monoclonal antibody against the platelet GPIIb/IIIa (fibrinogen) receptor. Onset of inhibition is rapid, but blockade of platelet function is long lasting (more than 12 hours). Tirofiban (Aggrastat) is a nonpeptide RGD mimetic that reversibly inhibits the platelet GPIIb/IIIa complex and has a half-life in plasma of approximately 1.6 hours. Eptifibatide (Integrilin), a synthetic cyclic heptapeptide, also reversibly inhibits the platelet GPIIb/IIIa receptor complex and has a half-life of 60 to 90 minutes.

Ticlopidine and *clopidogrel* inhibit platelet aggregation induced by ADP by inhibiting the platelet ADP receptor. Both drugs prolong bleeding times, inhibit platelet aggregation, and delay clot retraction.

Drugs Affecting the Coagulation Cascade

Coumadin (warfarin) blocks vitamin K–dependent carboxylation of amino-terminal glutamate residues on precursors of factors II, VII, IX, and X, as well as proteins C and S. These proteins require the presence of vitamin K during synthesis within the liver. Rarely, initiation of Coumadin without prior heparin anticoagulation may cause skin necrosis secondary to small vessel thrombosis. This may be due to the high sensitivity of proteins C and S to Coumadin inhibition and loss of anticoagulant activity. Vitamin K is a fat-soluble vitamin that antagonizes the effect of Coumadin. Fresh frozen plasma is a safer and faster means to reverse the effect of Coumadin anticoagulation.

Heparin is a catalyst that accelerates the covalent binding of antithrombin III to thrombin and to activated coagulation factors of the intrinsic coagulation pathway: factors IXa, Xa, XIa, and XIIa. The primary substrate is circulating thrombin; the drug does not inhibit thrombin bound to fibrin and is a relatively weak inhibitor of the intrinsic coagulation pathway proteins. The drug is given intravenously or subcutaneously, and its effect is monitored by aPTT. Protamine binds to heparin and reverses its anticoagulant activity. Low molecular weight heparin avidly inhibits both thrombin and factor Xa and has a long half-life in plasma. Protamine does not effectively inhibit low molecular weight heparin.

D-deoxy desmopressin arginine vasopressin (desmopressin acetate, DDAVP) is a polypeptide with chemical structure homology to vasopressin (antidiuretic hormone [ADH]). DDAVP promotes vWF release from endothelium. It is used to treat hemophilia A, von Willebrand disease and uremic coagulopathy.

SELECTED DISEASE STATES

Disseminated intravascular coagulation (DIC) results from widespread activation of coagulation, which produces intravascular generation of thrombin and fibrin. The consumptive coagulopathy can deplete platelets and soluble coagulation proteins to cause severe bleeding. The syndrome is most commonly associated with sepsis, massive trauma with major wounds and/or head injury, certain uncontrolled cancers, severe immunologic disorders, and reactions to snake venom and other toxins. These stimuli cause a massive increase in the generation of thrombin and simultaneous suppression of natural anticoagulants including antithrombin III. Fibrinolysis is impaired. The clinical diagnosis is made by the presence of an initiating condition, platelet count below 100,000/μL, prolonged prothrombin and activated thromboplastin times, and the presence of fibrin-degradation products (such as fibrinopeptide A) in plasma. A low concentration of antithrombin III strengthens the diagnosis. Successful management requires control of the underlying cause. For example, DIC can not be controlled if an abscess remains undrained. Heparin is sometimes used to inhibit thrombin activity but under some conditions (e.g., large fresh wounds) is prohibited. Bleeding caused by platelet and/or coagulation factor deficiencies is treated with replacement therapy.

Cardiopulmonary bypass (CPB) requires the use of heparin. Despite high doses of heparin, thrombin is continuously formed both in the wound and perfusion circuit. Fibrinolysis also occurs; thus, CPB produces a consumptive coagulopathy despite doses of heparin that raise activated clotting times to 400 to 500 seconds. CPB activates platelets and causes platelet loss and dysfunction that prolongs template bleeding times after heparin is reversed by protamine. Although soluble coagulation factors are diluted during CPB and open heart surgery, concentrations are sufficient to maintain clot formation with only rare exception. In patients with congenital coagulation deficiencies, concentrations of coagulation proteins 5% to 30% above normal levels are adequate to prevent symptoms.

Hemophilia A is an X-linked recessive bleeding disorder consisting of decreased factor VIII levels. It accounts for 80% of hemophilia cases. Hemophilia B is also X-linked recessive and is caused by reduction in factor IX levels. The clinical manifestations of hemophilia A and B include joint and muscle hemorrhage, easy bruising, lack of excessive bleeding from minor cuts (normal platelet function), and severe postoperative hemorrhage. Laboratory abnormalities include elevated aPTT and reduced factor VIII or IX levels. Other basic coagulation studies are usually normal. Transfusions to 80% to 100% of normal concentrations of these factors should be obtained for surgery or life-threatening hemorrhage. Hemophilia A treatment may also include vitamin K.

The vWF participates in platelet adhesion to collagen and is a carrier protein for factor VIII. *Von Willebrand disease* may be transmitted as autosomal dominant (heterozygous) or autosomal recessive (homozygous). There are many variations. Clinical manifestations include epistaxis, menorrhagia, and subcutaneous bleeding. Bleeding into joints or muscle is more rare than with hemophilia A or B. Laboratory abnormalities include prolonged aPTT, prolonged bleeding time, decreased factor VIII activity, decreased vWF level, and abnormal platelet aggregation as measured by ristocetin. Treatment involves delivery of cryoprecipitate, DDAVP, or factor VIII concentrates, which contain vWF.

BLOOD PRODUCT AND TRANSFUSION THERAPY

Most stored blood is anticoagulated with CPD (citrate-phosphate-dextrose) along with adenine and dihydroxyacetone. The pH level of stored blood is initially around 7.2 but falls to approximately 6.5 after 1 month. This is partially due to the citrate. ATP, important in maintaining red cell membrane integrity, is gradually reduced with time. 2,3-diphosphoglyceric acid (2,3-DPG), which shifts the oxygen-hemoglobin disassociation curve to the right (favoring oxygen delivery), is reduced. After 1 month, 1% of erythrocytes lyse, potassium increases to around 8 mEq/dL, and ammonia accumulates. Free hemoglobin and other microparticles increase over time.

Whole fresh blood is unique in that is retains the labile factors V and VIII if used within hours. It also has a higher level of 2,3-DPG, less potassium, and is less acidic. Washed packed red blood cells have a hematocrit of around 70%. They contain few of the harmful metabolic products contained in stored whole blood but lack coagulation factors or platelets. Platelet concentrates have half-lives of around 4 days. Fresh frozen plasma provides soluble coagulation factors. Cryoprecipitate is the best source of factor VIII and fibrinogen. Many factor concentrates are also available for use.

Complications of transfusion include nonfatal hemolytic reactions (1 in 6,000), fatal hemolytic reactions (1 in 600,000), viral hepatitis (1 in 50,000), human immunodeficiency virus (1 in 420,000), and bacterial infections. Significant febrile reactions occur in approximately 1 in 100. Platelets, which are normally stored at room temperature, are culture positive for bacteria in 1 in 500 U. Massive transfusion is associated with dilutional coagulopathy. It also causes hypothermic coagulopathy.

SUGGESTED READING

Coleman RW, Hirsh J, Marder VJ, et al. *Hemostasis and thrombosis: basic principles and clinical practice*. Philadelphia: JB Lippincott Co, 1994.

Edmunds, L.H. Hemostatic problems in surgical patients. In: Colman RW, Clowes AW, Hirsh J, et al., eds. *Hemostasis and thrombosis: basic principles and clinical practice*. Philadelphia: JP Lippincott Co, in press.

Greenfield LJ. *Surgery: scientific principles and practice,* 2nd ed. Philadelphia: JB Lippincott Co, 1997.

Hillman RS, Ault K. *Hematology in clinical practice: a guide to diagnosis and management,* 2nd ed. New York: McGraw Hill, 1998.

Hoffman R, Blanz EJ, Jr., Shattil SJ, eds. *Hematology: basic principles and practice,* 3rd ed. New York: Churchill Livingstone, 2000.

Levi M, ten Cate H. Disseminated intravascular coagulation. *N Engl J Med* 1999;341:586–592.

Smythe WR, Fishman SJ. Hemostasis and thrombosis. In: Savage EB, Fishman SJ, Miller LD. *Essentials of basic science in surgery.* Philadelphia: JB Lippincott Co, 1993.

19

CARDIOVASCULAR PHYSIOLOGY

FRANK W. BOWEN AND ROBERT C. GORMAN

The function of the heart is to provide adequate cardiovascular support to the body. This includes the supply of oxygen and nutrients, as well as the removal of waste products and carbon dioxide. The complex structure and function of the heart is tightly regulated by both intrinsic mechanisms and the autonomic nervous system. Understanding these regulatory mechanisms is paramount to managing cardiovascular disease.

EMBRYOLOGY

The cardiovascular system is the first system to function in the embryo as blood begins to circulate by the end of the third week of gestation. This early development is necessary because the rapidly growing embryo outgrows its ability to obtain nutrients through diffusion; thus, the embryo needs an efficient method of acquiring nutrients and disposing waste products. The cardiovascular system is derived from angioblastic tissue, which arises from the mesenchyme, an aggregation of mesenchymal cells. Primitive blood vessels can not be distinguished from arteries or veins but are named according to their future fates and relationship to the heart.

The cardiovascular system begins to develop during the third week, and the first heart beats occur at 21 to 22 days. Isolated cell clusters, derived from mesoderm, develop into endothelial tubes that join to form the primitive vascular system. Paired endocardial heart tubes develop in the cardiogenic area and fuse to form the primitive heart. This primordium consists of four chambers (sinus venosus, atrium, ventricle, and bulbus cordis). The truncus arteriosus is continuous caudally with the bulbus cordis and enlarges cranially to form the aortic sac. As the heart tube grows, it enlarges and bends to the right. By the fourth to seventh week, the heart becomes partitioned into four chambers (Fig. 19-1).

Three paired systems of veins drain into the primitive heart. These include (i) the vitelline system, which becomes the portal system, (ii) the cardinal veins, which form the caval system, and (iii) the umbilical system, which involutes after birth. The aortic arches develop during the fourth to fifth week from the aortic sac and penetrate the branchial arches. By the sixth to eighth week, this primitive aortic arch pattern is transformed into the mature carotid, subclavian, and pulmonary arteries.

Formation of the ventricles begins during the fourth week when swellings called "endocardial cushions" form on the ventral and dorsal walls of the atrioventricular canal. During the fifth week, mesenchymal cells invade these cushions and they approach each other and fuse. This divides the atrioventricular canal into right and left atrioventricular canals.

Until the end of the seventh week, there is usually a crescentic interventricular foramen between the free edge of the interventricular septum and the fused endocardial cushions. The interventricular foramen usually closes by the end of the seventh week as the bulbar ridges fuse. Closure of the interventricular foramen results from the fusion of tissue from (i) the right bulbar edge, (ii) the left bulbar edge, and (iii) the endocardial cushions.

The primitive atrium is divided into right and left atria by the formation and subsequent modification and fusion of two septa, the septum primum and the septum secundum. The septum primum is a thin, crescent-shaped membrane that grows from the dorsocranial wall (roof) of the atrium (Fig. 19-1). As this septum grows, a large opening, the foramen primum, forms between its crescentic free edge and the endocardial cushions. The foramen primum becomes smaller and disappears when the septum primum fuses with the endocardial cushions (atrioventricular septum).

Toward the end of the fifth week, another crescentic membrane, the septum secundum, grows from the ventrocranial wall of the atrium immediately to the right of the septum primum. As this septum grows, it gradually overlaps the septum primum. The septum secundum forms an incomplete partition, forming an oval opening called the "foramen ovale."

Formation of the pulmonary artery and aorta involves active proliferation of mesenchymal cells in the bulbus

Hospital of the University of Pennsylvania, Philadelphia, Pennsylvania

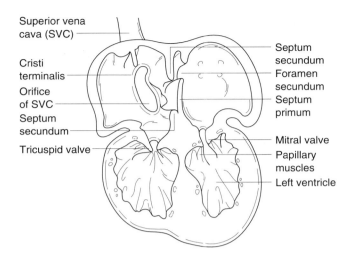

FIGURE 19-1. After about 8 weeks, the heart is partitioned into four chambers. Well-oxygenated blood bypasses the pulmonary circulation through the foramen secundum. (From The cardiovascular system. In: Moore KL, Persuad TVN. *The developing human,* 6th ed. Philadelphia: WB Saunders, 1998:362, with permission.)

cordis during the fifth week. Fusion of truncal ridges (from the truncus arteriosus) with the bulbar ridges gives rise to the spiral aortopulmonary septum. This septum separates two channels, the aorta and the pulmonary trunk (Fig. 19-2).

The fetal circulation system is designed to serve prenatal needs and to permit modifications at birth to establish good postnatal oxygenation and circulation. Well-oxygenated blood returns from the placenta in the umbilical vein. About half of the blood from the placenta passes through the hepatic sinusoids, whereas the remainder bypasses the liver through the ductus venosus into the inferior vena cava. Blood then enters the right atrium. Most blood from the inferior vena cava is diverted by the inferior border of the septum secundum, through the foramen ovale into the left atrium. Here, it mixes with the small amount of deoxygenated blood returning from the lungs via the pulmonary veins. From the left atrium, the blood passes into the left ventricle and leaves via the ascending aorta.

A small amount of oxygenated blood from the inferior vena cava remains in the right atrium. This blood mixes with deoxygenated blood from the superior vena cava and coronary sinus and passes into the right ventricle. This "medium saturation" blood is ejected through the pulmonary trunk. Because of the high pulmonary vascular resistance, most blood bypasses the pulmonary circulation and enters the aorta through the patent ductus arteriosus. Forty percent to fifty percent of blood from the descending aorta passes into the umbilical arteries and is returned to the placenta for reoxygenation.

At birth, important circulatory changes occur as the placental circulation ceases and the infant's lungs begin to function. Aeration of the lungs is associated with a dramatic fall in pulmonary vascular resistance and an increase in pulmonary blood flow. Because of the increased pulmonary blood flow, left atrial pressure is increased and the foramen ovale closes as the valve of the foramen ovale presses against the septum secundum.

The ductus arteriosus usually constricts at birth and becomes functionally closed 10 to 15 hours after birth. However, in premature infants and in those with persistent hypoxia, it may remain open much longer. The patency of the ductus before birth is controlled by locally produced prostaglandins. Cyclooxygenase inhibitors that reduce the production of prostaglandin, such as indomethacin, can cause constriction of a patent ductus arteriosus in the premature infant.

ANATOMY

The normal anatomy of the adult human heart is complex. The *atrioventricular valves* include the mitral and tricuspid

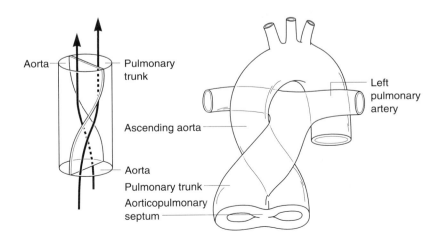

FIGURE 19-2. Partitioning of the truncus arteriosus by the aortopulmonary septum separates the aorta from the pulmonary trunk. (From The cardiovascular system. In: Moore KL, Persuad TVN. *The developing human,* 6th ed. Philadelphia: WB Saunders, 1998:373, with permission.)

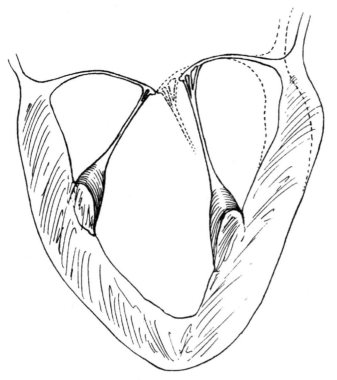

FIGURE 19-3. Chordae tendineae tether the leaflets of the mitral and tricuspid valves, allowing precise coaptation during systole. (From Chitwood WR Jr. Mitral valve repair: ischemic. In: Kaiser LR, Kron IL, Spray TL, eds. *Mastery of cardiothoracic surgery.* Philadelphia: Lippincott-Raven Publishers, 1998:312, with permission.)

valves. They provide for a systolic pressure gradient between the atria and ventricles. The *semilunar aortic* and *pulmonary valves* affect the diastolic gradient between the ventricles and systemic circulation.

The tricuspid and mitral valves are fibrous structures lined by endocardia. The tricuspid valve consists of a large anterior leaflet attached to the anterior wall of the heart, a posterior leaflet at the right margin, and a septal leaflet attached to the septum. The mitral valve, at the orifice of the left ventricle, consists of a large anterior leaflet in continuity with the posterior wall of the aorta and a smaller posterior leaflet. Chordae tendineae tether the leaflets to the anterior and posterior papillary muscles and allow for precise coaptation during systolic contraction (Fig. 19-3).

The aortic and pulmonary valves are positioned at the orifices of the two ventricles. The aortic valve consists of three leaflets. The leaflets are named according to the origin of the coronary arteries in the sinus of Valsalva and include the right coronary, left coronary, and noncoronary leaflet (Fig. 19-4). The pulmonary valve also consists of three leaflets, including the right, left, and noncoronary.

The left main coronary artery originates from the left sinus of Valsalva and passes posteriorly between the pulmonary artery and the left atrial appendage, where it divides into the left anterior descending artery and the circumflex coronary artery. The left anterior descending artery continues down the anterior wall along the interventricular septum to the apex of the left ventricle. It has two branching systems: (i) septal branches that supply the anterior two thirds of the interventricular septum and (ii) diagonals that

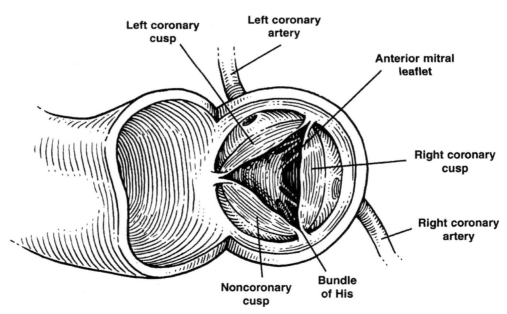

FIGURE 19-4. Normal aortic valve from a surgeon's point of view. (From Damiano RJ. Aortic valve replacement: prosthesis. In: Kaiser LR, Kron IL, Spray TL, eds. *Mastery of cardiothoracic surgery.* Philadelphia: Lippincott-Raven Publishers, 1998:362, with permission.)

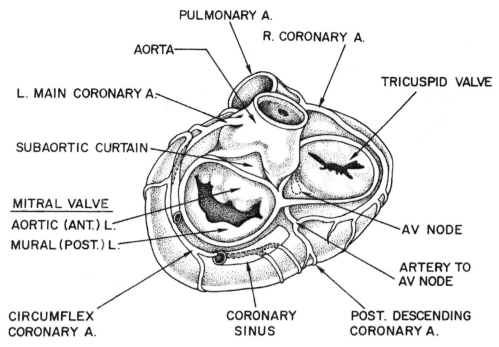

FIGURE 19-5. Normal cardiac and coronary artery anatomy, as seen from the base of the heart. (From Buchanan SA, Tribble RW, Tribble CG. Reoperative mitral replacement. In: Kaiser LR, Kron IL, Spray TL, eds. *Mastery of cardiothoracic surgery*. Philadelphia: Lippincott-Raven Publishers, 1998:351, with permission.)

supply the anterior-lateral wall of the left ventricle. The circumflex coronary artery runs posteriorly in the atrioventricular groove and provides marginal branches that supply the posterior left ventricle. In approximately 10% of patients, the circumflex coronary artery ends in a posterior descending artery, which supplies the posterior one third of the interventricular septum and the atrioventricular node. If the posterior descending artery arises from this position, it defines a left-side-dominant circulation (Fig. 19-5).

The *right coronary artery* arises from the anterior right sinus of Valsalva and passes along the atrioventricular groove between the right atrium and the right ventricle. It provides blood supply to the right ventricle. In approximately 85% of patients, the posterior descending artery arises from the right coronary artery and defines a right-side-dominant circulation. In approximately 5% of patients, a balanced pattern exists in which the circumflex coronary artery and the right coronary artery supply the posterior descending branches to the septum and atrioventricular node. (Fig. 19-5).

CARDIAC PHYSIOLOGY

The cardiovascular system consists of two subsystems, each with a pump and a circuit. The pulmonary circulation serves one organ, the lung. The systemic circulation supplies all other organs (and a small component to pulmonary parenchyma) in series. The pulmonary circulation contains a blood volume of about 0.5 L. It operates at low pressure with low resistance to blood flow. Control mechanisms for blood flow including PO_2 and CO_2 regulate the vascular resistance. The systemic circulation has a blood volume of approximately 5.5 L. It operates at a high pressure with a high resistance to blood flow. Regulation within organs of the systemic circulation involves a combination of local, neural, and circulating hormonal factors.

The operation of the ventricle is cyclic. The ventricle fills with blood during diastole and pumps blood into the arteries during systole. Therefore, pressure fluctuations are seen in the arterial circulation throughout the cycle. The distribution system for blood flow consists of branching arterial structures. The aorta, large arteries, and small arteries offer little resistance to the flow of blood. The high pressure and pulsatile nature of the blood flow provided by ventricular ejection is maintained throughout the systemic circulation due to aortic and arterial elasticity. Small arteries give rise to arterioles, which are small thick-walled structures with a large amount of vascular smooth muscle. The *arterioles offer the principal resistance* within the systemic circuit; therefore, the largest pressure drop within the circuit occurs at the level of the arterioles (Fig. 19-6). As we move out through the circuit from the aorta to large artery and then to capillaries and vena cava, pressure is dissipated, overcoming the resistance to blood flow through the vasculature. Therefore, blood flow occurs down a pressure gradient from high to low.

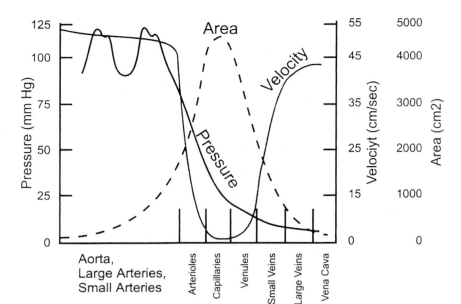

FIGURE 19-6. Pressure, area, and velocity relationship across the systemic circulation.

As the arterial structures branch out from the aorta, the cross-sectional area of the vascular bed continues to increase until it reaches the capillary bed. From the capillary bed, the venous structures begin to coalesce into larger structures, and the total cross-sectional area of the vascular bed declines. Velocity of blood flow is inversely related to the cross-sectional area: velocity (cm per second) equals flow (cm^3 per second) divided by area (cm^2). As the cross-sectional area increases from aorta to capillary bed, the velocity of blood flow decreases (Fig. 19-6). The increased surface area of the capillary bed and the decreased velocity of blood flow provides conditions suitable for the exchange of oxygen between the tissues and capillary blood.

CARDIAC ELECTROPHYSIOLOGY

The electrocardiogram gives an overall interpretation of the electrical activity of the heart. The electrical activity of atrial and ventricular depolarization is represented by the respective P and QRS complexes. Ventricular repolarization is represented by the T wave.

Individual cells within the heart demonstrate two types of action potentials: fast and slow. *Fast cardiac action potentials* occur in normal myocardial fibers of atria, ventricle, Purkinje fibers, and His bundle. These action potentials have five different phases, 0 to 4. The shape of the fast action potential of a Purkinje fiber and the temporal changes in membrane ion conductance due to concentration gradient changes are summarized in Fig. 19-7.

After a cardiac myocyte has been stimulated, it becomes partially or completely refractory to a second stimulation until it has recovered from the first stimulation. There are several *refractory periods,* depending on the stimulus needed to elicit the second stimulation (Fig. 19-7). The *effective refractory period* (ERP) is the period in the cardiac cycle during which no stimulus, regardless of strength, can produce a propagated response. This period occurs during phase 1, phase 2, and the early part of phase 3 when the inactivation gates are still closed. The *relative refractory period* (RRP) occurs during the later part of the phase 3, during which a propagated response can be elicited but the stimulus required is greater than that normally needed. The *supranormal period* (SNP) is the period during which the threshold for stimulation is slightly lower than normal. The *period of normal excitability* extends from the end of the supranormal period to the beginning of the next action potential.

In addition to fast cardiac action potentials, slow cardiac action potentials occur in the sinuatrial and atrioventricular node. The slow cardiac action potential consists of three phases as demonstrated in Fig. 19-8.

The rate of firing of the pacemaker is dependent on the magnitude that occurs during phase 3 to 4 of the slow action potential. The greater the hyperpolarization, the longer it will take for the pacemaker to reach threshold and the slower the heart rate. In addition, the rate of firing is dependent on the rate (slope) of depolarization. The faster the rate of depolarization, the sooner threshold voltage will be reached and the faster the heart rate. Increases in the rate of depolarization can be induced by hypokalemia, β-adrenergic stimulation, fiber stretch, and acidosis. The threshold voltage also influences the rate of pacemaker firing. The more negative the threshold voltage, the sooner the pacemaker will reach threshold and initiate depolarization.

The pacemaker is influenced by both the sympathetic and the parasympathetic nervous system. The parasympathetic nervous system lowers heart rate by increasing potassium conductance, thereby increasing the magnitude of hyperpo-

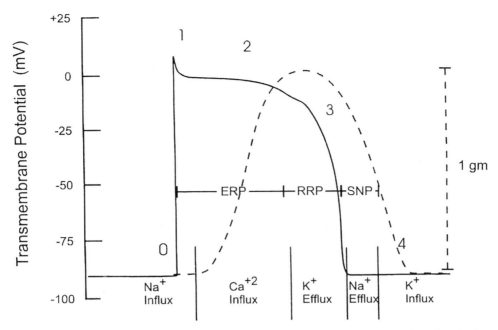

FIGURE 19-7. Schematic fast action potential of human ventricular myocardium (*solid*) with electrolyte movements, refractory periods (see text) and force generated (*dashed line*). The five phases of fast cardiac action potential are indicated as numbers. *Phase 4:* the resting membrane potential. Potassium conductance is high and sodium conductance is low. *Phase 0:* Upstroke of the action potential due to membrane depolarization. An increase in sodium conductance due to the opening of voltage dependent fast sodium channels causes depolarization. There is a simultaneous decrease in potassium conductance. *Phase 1:* Period of partial repolarization due to a dramatic decrease in sodium conductance and a brief increase in chloride conductance. *Phase 2:* Plateau phase during which changes in potassium efflux (conductance decreases and then plateaus) is matched by calcium influx (conductance increases and then plateaus). *Phase 3:* Membrane repolarization phase due to an increase in potassium efflux (increased potassium conductance) and a decrease in calcium influx (decreased calcium conductance).

larization, and by decreasing the rate of closure of potassium channels, which reduces the rate of depolarization during phase 4. The sympathetic nervous system increases heart rate by increasing the rate of depolarization during phase 4.

The *sinuatrial node* is the normal pacemaker of the heart. This structure lies within the wall of the right atrium in the sulcus terminalis, at the junction of the superior vena cava and the right atrium. The action potential is transmitted from the sinuatrial node to the atrioventricular node via internodal pathways. Additionally, there are interatrial pathways that conduct the action potential from the right to left atrium. Finally, there are conductions between one atrial myocyte and another via gap junctions and nexus.

The *atrioventricular node* is a specialized area of tissue located in the lower border of the interatrial septum near the coronary sinus and above the tricuspid valve. The atrioventricular node functions to protect the ventricles from excessive atrial rates. The atrioventricular node also allows adequate time for the ventricles to relax and fill prior to ventricular systole. The bundle of His is a specialized pathway that conducts the action potential from the atria to ventricles. It divides into left and right branches and then divides into Purkinje fibers which pass over the subendocardial surfaces of the heart. The pattern allows the depolarization of the subendocardial surfaces prior to the epicardial surface. In addition to Purkinje fibers, the cardiac action potential is transmitted from one ventricular myocyte to another via gap junctions.

The properties of cardiac muscle cell membranes are basically similar to those in other excitable cells. However, specific differences in ionic channels give rise to action potentials of different time courses in various regions of the heart.

In cardiac muscle, the sarcoplasmic reticulum is less extensive than in skeletal muscle, with smaller cisternae at the cell surface adjacent to T tubules. The cardiac myocyte has a diameter of 20 μm compared to 100 μm in skeletal muscle fibers. Therefore, the diffusion of substances from the extracellular space to the myocyte interior occurs more readily. In cardiac muscle, some calcium for contraction is derived from the sarcoplasmic reticulum and the extracellular fluid including the T-tubule lumen, whereas in skeletal muscle, contraction depends critically on calcium released from the sarcoplasmic reticulum.

In a cardiac ventricular fiber, Ca^{2+} enters the fiber during the plateau phase of the action potential. The cardiac action potential has a long duration of about 250 milliseconds, and there is considerable overlap of the action potential, ele-

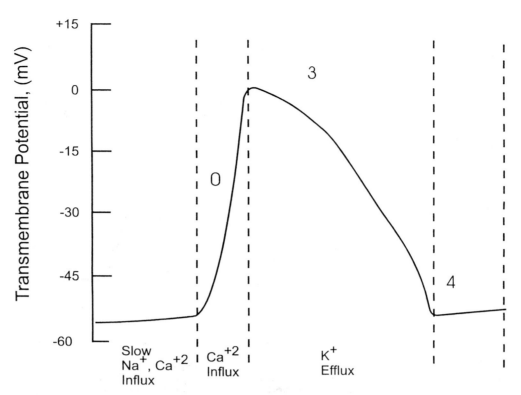

FIGURE 19-8. Phases of slow cardiac action potentials that occur in the sinuatrial and atrioventricular nodes. *Phase 0:* Period of depolarization. Depolarization during phase 0 is due to an influx of calcium through slow channels and the closure of potassium channels. Cells that have slow cardiac action potentials have resting membrane potentials that are less negative (i.e., –60 mV) than cells that have fast action potentials (–90 mV). In addition, the upstroke of the action potential (dV/dT) due to membrane depolarization occurs more slowly. Finally, the overshoot of the action potential is less in these cells. *Phase 3:* Period of repolarization due to an efflux of potassium as conductance increases. *Phase 4:* The resting membrane potential is not as negative and not as stable as for cells that have the fast action potential. There is a slow depolarization of the membrane during phase 4 due to several factors including a time-dependent decrease in potassium efflux due to a decrease in potassium conductance. A slow influx of sodium and a slow influx of calcium. When membrane potential depolarizes to threshold voltage, the action potential (phase 0) begins. This slow depolarization during phase 4 is referred to as a "pacemaker potential" and explains why the heart beat potential reaches threshold in the sinuatrial node first.

vation in myoplasmic calcium, and the contractile event. Calcium enters the cardiac muscle fiber through Ca^{2+} channels in the sarcolemma (cell membrane) and T tubules. The binding of this Ca^{2+} to the sarcoplasmic reticulum Ca^{2+} release channel is required to induce opening of the sarcoplasmic reticulum Ca^{2+} release channels and further increase the intracellular calcium concentration. This process is called "calcium-induced calcium release."

Most of the Ca^{2+} that enters during excitation is taken up by the sarcoplasmic reticulum and then causes the release of a large quantity of Ca^{2+} from the sarcoplasmic reticulum. Thus, changes in the duration of the action potential do not affect the strength of the accompanying beat but affect the subsequent beat. Calcium influx during excitation serves to load the sarcoplasmic reticulum so that the calcium is available for later release. Once calcium is released from the sarcoplasmic reticulum, it serves to facilitate cycling of actin-myosin crossbridging through binding of troponin C. The adenosine 5'-triphosphate–dependent (ATP) cycling of actin-myosin cross bridges serves to generate the force of contraction (Fig. 19-9).

For cardiac muscle to relax between beats, the intracellular free calcium concentration must be rapidly reduced. This is accomplished by a Ca-ATPase located in the longitudinal tubules of the sarcoplasmic reticulum and in the sarcolemma, as well as by the sodium/calcium exchange mechanism in the sarcolemma that extrudes Ca^{2+} using energy derived from the Na^+ gradient. In the steady state, the amount of Ca^{2+} pumped back into the sarcoplasmic reticulum must equal the amount that entered through the cell membrane.

The *parasympathetic system* is important in the control of pacemaker cells of the sinuatrial node. Release of acetylcholine by nerve endings of the parasympathetic system

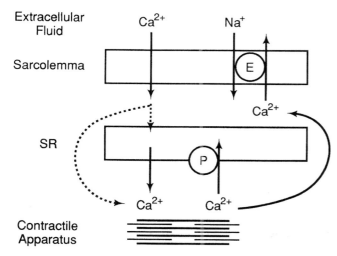

FIGURE 19-9. Excitation contraction coupling in a cardiac myocyte. (From Johnson LR. *Essential medical physiology.* New York: Raven Press, 1992:170, with permission.)

simulates muscarinic receptors, which produce an intracellular stimulatory G protein that opens acetylcholine-gated potassium channels. This leads to hyperpolarization of the sinuatrial nodal cells. In addition, parasympathetic stimulation also inhibits the formation of cyclic AMP (adenosine 5'-monophosphate), which inhibits the opening of calcium channels. These two effects lead to a slowing of the sinuatrial pacemaker potential. Decreased conduction through the atrioventricular node is also caused by these changes.

There are two types of β-*adrenergic receptors*. $β_1$-receptors predominate in the heart and $β_2$-receptors are present in the liver and lungs. The β-adrenergic receptor couples with adenocyclase. When the receptor is occupied by a catecholamine, a stimulatory G protein is formed that combines with guanosine 5'-triphosphate (GTP). This activated G protein–GTP complex then increases the activity of adenocyclase, leading to the production of cyclic AMP. This increase in cyclic AMP promotes calcium channel opening in the sarcoplasmic reticulum, leading to increased uptake of calcium.

The increased activity of calcium channels has several effects on cardiac function. First, there is an increased discharge rate of the sinuatrial node and accelerated conduction through the atrioventricular node. Second, the increased cytosolic concentration of calcium leads to a positive ionotropic effect. Finally, the increased activity of the sarcoplasmic reticulum calcium pump results in a more rapid removal of the calcium from the cell after systole, leading to rapid relaxation (lusitropic effect).

CARDIAC MECHANICS

The function of the heart is to convert chemical energy into mechanical energy. This provides blood flow for the rapid distribution of oxygen and nutrients to the body while removing waste products such as carbon dioxide. Within normal physiologic parameters, the heart functions as a sump pump. The Frank-Starling relationship describes the interplay between diastolic volume and contractility. As ventricular filling is increased, the strength of ventricular contraction increases as sarcomere are stretched to their optimal length. In addition, stretching of the right atrium leads to an increase in heart rate, which contributes to the hearts ability to pump blood. With sympathetic stimulation, the heart contracts more forcefully with every beat (ionotropic). Importantly, it also exhibits chronotropic, dromotropic, and lusitropic effects to this stimulation.

The *preload* of the left ventricle is the intracavitary volume or pressure immediately prior to contraction. The compliance (distensibility) of the ventricle is defined as the change in volume divided by the change in pressure. The stiffness is the reciprocal of compliance. Fibrosis and hypertrophy both increase stiffness. Fibrosis causes a change in the collagen network. Hypertrophy causes an increase in the stiffness of noncontractile components. Relaxation is an active process that is increased by catecholamine stimulation but impaired by ischemia, hypothyroidism, and chronic congestive heart failure.

The *afterload* of the ventricle is the pressure against which it must eject during systole. This is determined by the aortic pressure gradient. The greater the afterload, the more mechanical energy the heart must generate to achieve adequate ejection into the pulmonary artery or aorta.

Pressure-volume loops are a graphical depiction of function over the entire cardiac cycle (Fig. 19-10). The diastolic component of the pressure-volume loop is determined by the diastolic (preload) relationship. The shape of the loop during systole is determined by the contractility of the ventricle and the afterload against which it has to eject. As systole begins, pressure builds during isovolumic contraction until the pressure in the ventricle exceeds the pressure in the aorta. Once aortic pressure is overcome by the ventricle, the aortic valve opens and the ventricle ejects. As the pressure falls during ejection, the aortic valve closes when aortic pressure exceeds ventricular pressure at the end of systole. During the period of isovolumic relaxation, the volume in the ventricle stays the same as the ventricle relaxes. Once the ventricular pressure is less than the right atrium pressure, the mitral valve opens and blood fills the left ventricle from the atrium.

Many factors affect the pressure-volume relationship of the heart. Increasing afterload moves the pressure-volume loop slightly up and to the right. Adrenergic stimulation combines a positive ionotropic and lusitropic effect to lead to a decrease in end-diastolic pressure, a shift of the pressure-volume loop to the left, and an increase in ejection fraction.

The circumferential stress or *tension in the wall of the ventricle* is determined by the pressure within the chamber and the geometry of the ventricle. If the ventricle is approx-

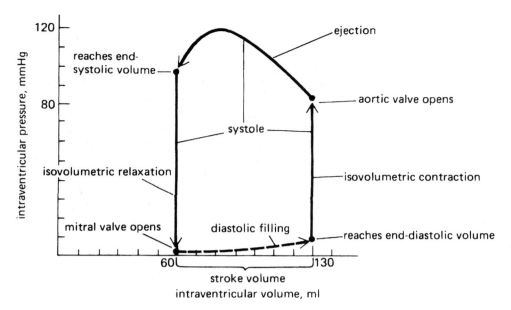

FIGURE 19-10. Pressure-volume loop of one cardiac cycle. (From Mohrman DE, Heller LJ. *Cardiovascular physiology*, 3rd ed. New York: McGraw Hill, 1991:54, with permission.)

imated as a sphere, the wall tension is proportional to the pressure times the radius. This relationship is known as the law of Laplace. Increasing the wall thickness decreases the tension because a greater number of muscle fibers reduces the tension on each fiber. Therefore, tension is proportional to pressure times radius divided by wall thickness.

The major chemical fuels of the heart are carbohydrates including glucose and lactate, and nonesterfied free fatty acids. In the fasting state, lipids may account for as much as 70% of fuel utilized by the heart. During the well-fed states when glucose and insulin levels are high, carbohydrates will account for close to 100% of cardiac fuel.

Sixty percent to seventy percent of the ATP synthesized in the heart is used to fuel systolic contraction. An additional 10% to 15% is used to maintain the concentration gradients across the cell membranes (Na-K ATPase). The remaining ATP is used to maintain glycogen stores and the synthesis of triglycerides.

Changes in the rate of oxygen consumption of the heart are directly related to the changes in the contraction cycle. Energy utilization and oxygen consumption are proportional to the workload of the heart. Factors that effect the workload of the heart include heart rate, increasing stroke volume, and a rise in afterload (aortic pressure). With increasing workload, myocardial oxygen consumption will increase. If myocardial supply is inadequate to meet demand such as in coronary atherosclerosis, ischemia will result in the affected myocardial distribution.

Resting *coronary blood flow* is approximately 1 mL/g of heart muscle per minute. During exercise, myocardial blood flow can increase three to four times the normal rate. This increase is accomplished by vasodilation of the penetrating arteries and recruitment of additional capillaries. Maximal coronary blood flow occurs primarily during diastole when the heart is relaxed and the myocardial wall tension is at its lowest. Local control of coronary blood flow is regulated by several factors. *Adenosine* in the primary mediator of the metabolic vasodilator system. It is produced by cardiac myocytes whenever local nutrient flow is insufficient to meet metabolic demands. It functions to act directly on the smooth muscle cells in the arterioles to cause relaxation. The *sympathetic nervous system* acts through α-receptors (vasoconstriction) and β-receptors (vasodilation). There is a direct inervation of large conductance vessels and smaller resistance vessels. α-receptors predominate over β-receptors, and the release of norepinephrine from nerve endings facilitates vasoconstriction.

The last factor that regulates coronary blood flow is the *vascular endothelium*. This regulation is a balance between two factors produced by the endothelium: endothelium-derived relaxing factor (nitric oxide) and endothelial-derived constricting factor (endothelin). Nitric oxide generation is stimulated by adenosine, acetylcholine, and sheer stress from increased intraluminal blood flow. Nitric oxide leads to significant vasodilation of the resistance vessels and increased coronary blood flow.

MECHANICAL CARDIAC ASSISTANCE

Dr. John Gibbon performed the first successful open heart operation with cardiopulmonary bypass in 1953 at Jefferson Medical Collage in Philadelphia, when he repaired an atrial septal defect in a young woman. Since that time, *cardiopulmonary bypass* is now used in more than one million cases per year. The basic components of the bypass machine include a venous reservoir that provides storage of blood from the right atrium. Oxygenation and elimination of carbon dioxide from the blood is provided by either a bubble or membrane oxygenator. A heat exchanger is used to cool the blood for myocardial protection and for rewarming. In addition, either a roller or centrifugal pump returns blood to the body via the ascending aorta or femoral artery.

Myocardial protection is provided during cardiopulmonary bypass by perfusing the coronary arteries with either cold hyperkalemic solution consisting of blood or crystalloid. Blood cardioplegia provides increased myocardial protection for up to 3 hours of aortic cross clamp. The cardioplegia solution may be delivered into the aortic root, into the coronary ostia, or into the coronary sinus via a retrograde technique.

The *intraaortic balloon pump* has been labeled as the ultimate ionotrope. It is positioned just below the left subclavian artery in the descending aorta. It inflates during diastole to improve coronary blood flow and deflates during systole to decrease afterload. This reduces myocardial workload and myocardial oxygen consumption. The current indications and contraindications for its use are summarized in Table 19-1.

In 1963, Dr Michael DeBakey, at Baylor College of Medicine, implanted the first ventricular assist device. Since that time, research funded by the National Heart, Lung, and Blood Institute has lead to the development of several devices for long-term circulatory support. Currently, the Thoratec ventricular assist system, the Novacor left ventricular assist device, and the Heartmate left ventricular assist device are available on an acute and chronic basis. The ventricular assist device may be univentricular or biventricular. These circuits incorporate centrifugal or impeller pumps and do not contain an oxygenator. Access usually requires cannulation of the heart or great vessels. These devices function to bypass the failing ventricle and provide "assistance" to augment systolic flow. The major advantage is that they volume unload the ventricle and function to reduce both end-systolic and end-diastolic volume. The major indications for use of a ventricular assist system include postcardiotomy shock and the need for a bridge to cardiac transplantation. Relative inclusion criteria are summarized in Table 19-2. Complications from use of the devices include perioperative bleeding, infection, and stroke. In addition, the blood surface activation and sheer stress may lead to thromboembolism and hemolysis. Because of this, chronic anticoagulation and serial transfusion may be necessary.

TABLE 19-1. INDICATIONS AND CONTRAINDICATIONS FOR PLACEMENT OF AN INTRAAORTIC BALLOON PUMP

Indications	Contraindications
Refractory unstable angina	Aortic insufficiency
Complications of myocardial infarction	Acute aortic dissection
Mitral regurgitation	Cardiomyopathy
Ventricular septal defect	Peripheral vascular disease (relative)
Refractory arrhythmias	Abdominal aortic or thoracic aneurysm (relative)
Ventricular aneurysm	
Cardiogenic shock	
Severe left main coronary disease prior to revascularization	
Pump failure after cardiac surgery	
Septic shock (rare cases)	

TABLE 19-2. RELATIVE INDICATION FOR PLACEMENT OF A VENTRICULAR ASSIST DEVICE

Left ventricular failure	Right ventricular failure
Cardiac index <1.8 L/min/m^2	Cardiac index <1.8 L/min/m^2
Left atrial pressure >20 mm Hg	Right atrial pressure >20 mm Hg
Peak systolic aortic pressure <90 mm Hg	Left atrial pressure <15 mm Hg
Poor tissue perfusion	

20

CARDIOVASCULAR PATHOPHYSIOLOGY AND TREATMENT

HOWARD K. SONG AND TIMOTHY J. GARDNER

Cardiovascular diseases are the predominant cause of disability and death in industrialized nations. In the United States, cardiovascular diseases account for approximately 40% of all deaths, almost twice the number of deaths caused by all forms of cancer combined. Diseases of the cardiovascular system encompass a diverse array of pathologic processes, including congenital malformations, acquired lesions of the coronary circulation and aorta, valvular diseases, and inflammatory and autoimmune processes. Because of the importance of the cardiovascular system for perfusion of all tissues of the body, clinical presentation of many of these disorders can be precipitous and severe. Cardiovascular surgery has evolved to achieve prompt correction or replacement of anatomic lesions represented by these disorders. This chapter reviews the major cardiovascular disorders and their surgical management.

CONGENITAL HEART DISEASE

Congenital heart defects occur in 4 to 9 per 1,000 livebirths. A useful classification system organizes the congenital heart defects into three general physiologic disturbances: left-to-right shunt, right-to-left shunt, and ventricular outflow obstruction. In addition, there are several complex congenital defects that can be classified as bidirectional shunts.

Left-to-right Shunts

This condition is characterized by the absence of cyanosis and increased pulmonary blood flow. Communication between pulmonary and systemic circulations may occur at the level of the atria, ventricles, or great vessels. Lesions leading to this condition are common and represent 40% of anomalies diagnosed in the first year of life.

Hospital of the University of Pennsylvania, Philadelphia, Pennsylvania

Atrial Septal Defect

Atrial septal defect (ASD) is one of the most common congenital heart anomalies. It accounts for 10% to 15% of patients with congenital heart disease and is the most common congenital heart lesion in adults. ASDs are commonly observed with other heart anomalies, including ventricular septal defects, pulmonary stenosis, patent ductus arteriosus, coarctation of the aorta, and mitral stenosis, and are associated with genetically determined syndromes such as Down, Turner, Marfan, and Ehlers-Danlos. Maternal rubella exposure or ingestion of thalidomide is also associated with development of ASDs. The male to female ratio is approximately 1:2.

Approximately 20% of healthy individuals have a patent foramen ovale. This usually is of no consequence because the flap mechanism formed by the septum primum prevents interatrial shunting unless there are high right atrial pressures. Defects or deficiencies in the septum primum lead to ostium secundum–type ASDs (Fig. 20-1). Sinus venosus or superior vena cava–type ASDs occur at the junction of the superior vena cava and the right atrium and low or inferior vena cava ASDs are located between the orifice of the inferior vena cava and the inferior limbic septum. Rare types of ASDs include unroofed coronary sinus and common or single atrium, which results from failure of development of the entire atrial septum.

Blood flow across an ASD depends on the size of the defect and the compliance of the left and right ventricles during diastole. Small ASDs result in limited left-to-right shunting. With defects larger than 1 to 2 cm^2, atrial pressures equalize, the high compliance of the right ventricle leads to significant left-to-right shunting, and pulmonary blood flow may be increased two to four times systemic flow. Volume overload is generally well tolerated by the pulmonary vasculature for long periods, but after the third or fourth decade, medial hypertrophy and intimal proliferation lead to pulmonary hypertension and right heart failure in as many as half of all patients.

Secundum ASDs typically present in asymptomatic children who have a cardiac murmur on routine physical exami-

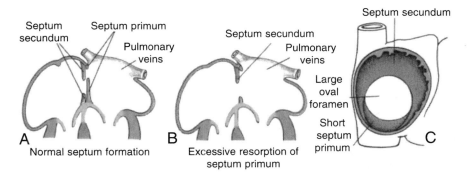

FIGURE 20-1. Normal atrial septum formation **(A)** and ostium secundum type atrial septal defect caused by excessive resorption of the septum primum **(B, C)**. (From Sadler TW. *Langman's medical embryology,* 5th ed. Baltimore: Williams & Wilkins, 1985, with permission.)

nation. Rarely, large ASDs may present in infants with severe heart failure, mandating early surgical repair. Otherwise, diagnosis may be delayed until adulthood when patients present with dyspnea and decreased exercise tolerance. Physical examination findings include a prominent right ventricular impulse and a systolic murmur along the left sternal border. The electrocardiogram shows evidence of right ventricular hypertrophy and right atrial enlargement. The diagnosis may generally be confirmed by echocardiography with cardiac catheterization reserved for complex cases or to determine the extent of pulmonary vascular disease.

Spontaneous closure of ASDs is rare after 2 years of age. Operative closure of ASDs by primary repair or with a pericardial or prosthetic patch is indicated in patients with $Q_p:Q_s$ ratio of greater than 1.5. Closure should be performed at 2 to 4 years of age. Occasionally, infants with congestive heart failure refractory to medical management will require earlier repair.

Cor Triatriatum

Cor triatriatum is an uncommon congenital anomaly in which the pulmonary veins drain into an accessory atrial chamber. Classically, the accessory chamber receives all return from the pulmonary vasculature, and blood must then pass through a fibromuscular membrane into the left atrium. Cor triatriatum is thought to result from failure of incorporation of the embryonic common pulmonary vein into the left atrium and is therefore felt to be related to anomalies of pulmonary venous return. Cor triatriatum is commonly associated with an ASD, which may lead to a large left-to-right shunt. More rarely, it is associated with complex congenital lesions such as transposition of the great vessels or tetralogy of Fallot.

Cor triatriatum may cause obstruction of pulmonary venous return, which leads to pulmonary congestion, pulmonary hypertension, and right heart failure. Presentation varies with the degree of obstruction of pulmonary venous return, with most patients having symptoms such as dyspnea and frequent respiratory infections within the first few years of life. Physical examination may reveal a loud pulmonary component to the second heart sound, a right ventricular heave, and signs of right-sided heart failure such as liver congestion, ascites, and peripheral edema. Cardiac catheterization is useful for demonstration of the accessory atrial chamber. Surgical repair consisting of excision of the anomalous membrane and repair of any associated ASD or anomalous pulmonary venous return is indicated for all symptomatic patients.

Ventricular Septal Defect

Ventricular septal defect (VSD) is the most common congenital heart lesion and accounts for approximately one fourth of all congenital heart defects. It is present as an isolated anomaly approximately once in every 1,000 livebirths. In addition, approximately half of patients with a VSD have associated anomalies such as patent ductus arteriosus, coarctation of the aorta, aortic stenosis, pulmonary stenosis, and other complex lesions.

VSDs are categorized by their anatomic location in the ventricular septum (Fig. 20-2). Conoventricular or perimembranous VSDs occur in the membranous septum immediately below the aortic valve ring and represent 70% to 80% of all VSDs. Conal septal or outlet defect VSDs represent 5% to 10% of all VSDs and are located immediately below the pulmonary valve. Inlet VSDs are also called atrioventricular (A-V) canal–type defects and result from incomplete fusion between the endocardial cushions and the muscular ventricular septum. Muscular or trabecular VSDs are defined by their muscular margins and may occur in the inlet septum where they are usually single or in the trabecular septum where they may be multiple.

A VSD is considered large when its diameter is equal to or greater than the diameter of the aortic valve ring. In the setting of low pulmonary vascular resistance after the first few months of life, a large defect may lead to high pulmonary blood flow ($Q_p:Q_s$ ratio of greater than 2), left ventricular diastolic overload, and congestive heart failure. Ultimately, high pulmonary blood flow results in medial thickening of the pulmonary vasculature, pulmonary hypertension, and right heart failure.

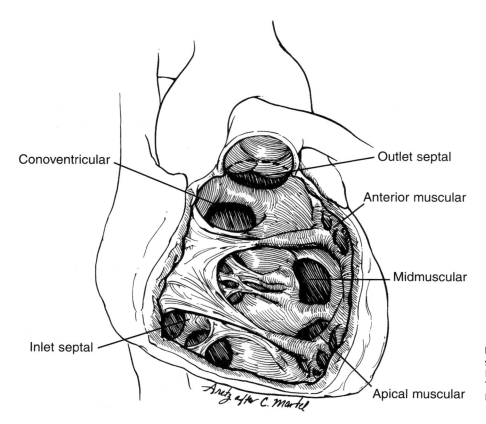

FIGURE 20-2. Major types of ventricular septal defects categorized by anatomic location. (From Kaiser LR, Kron IL, Spray TL, eds. *Mastery of cardiothoracic surgery*. Philadelphia: Lippincott-Raven Publishers, 1998, with permission.)

The clinical presentation of a VSD is highly dependent on its size. Patients with small defects are asymptomatic. Infants with large defects may present with tachypnea, failure to thrive, and congestive heart failure. Physical examination reveals a harsh pansystolic murmur and thrill over the fourth left intercostal space. Chest roentgenograms show left atrial enlargement and left ventricular hypertrophy in addition to prominent central and peripheral pulmonary arteries secondary to increased pulmonary blood flow. Echocardiography is useful for determining the site of the defect and the magnitude of the associated shunt. Cardiac catheterization is essential to confirm the diagnosis of VSD and determine the size of the defect, its location, the shunt volume, the pulmonary vascular resistance, and to inspect for associated anomalies.

Early surgical repair is indicated for infants with large defects ($Q_p:Q_s$ ratio of greater than 2) who have severe symptoms. Otherwise, repair of large defects is usually deferred until between 1 and 2 years of age. Repair of moderate-size defects ($Q_p:Q_s$ ratio of 1.5 to 2) is generally done in childhood because of the likelihood of spontaneous size reduction or closure. Surgery is contraindicated in patients with severely increased pulmonary vascular resistance (greater than 10 U/m^2) and resulting small left-to-right shunt. Pulmonary banding as a palliative procedure to reduce pulmonary blood flow is currently reserved for symptomatic infants with multiple muscular defects for whom risk of early primary repair is significant. Otherwise, primary repair of VSDs by patch closure is routinely carried out.

Patent Ductus Arteriosus

Patent ductus arteriosus (PDA) is a common congenital heart lesion, particularly in premature infants where the incidence may exceed 15%. For this reason, PDA is not considered to be abnormal until after 3 months of age. Maternal exposure to rubella, high-altitude living, polygenic inheritance, prematurity, neonatal hypoxia, and respiratory distress of the newborn have all been found to be associated with this lesion. The male to female ratio is approximately 1:2.

The function of the ductus arteriosus in fetal life is to divert blood away from the nonventilating lungs to the descending aorta. Shortly after birth, the ductus arteriosus normally constricts as soon as the P_{O_2} exceeds 20 mm Hg. Functional closure usually occurs within the first day of life while anatomic closure may take 1 to 12 weeks. Failure of this closure is thought to be due to immaturity of the thick medial layer of smooth muscle of the ductus arteriosus and biochemical unresponsiveness to stimuli. The decrease in pulmonary vascular resistance combined with the increase in systemic vascular resistance that occurs shortly after birth leads to reversal of blood flow through a PDA and left-to-right shunting.

The symptoms and signs related to a PDA vary with its size. Small PDAs are asymptomatic. Moderate-size or large PDAs may lead to physical underdevelopment, susceptibility to respiratory infections, and exercise limitation. Congestive heart failure is rare. Physical examination findings include a continuous systolic-diastolic machinery murmur at the left sternal border, a systolic thrill in the second left intercostal space, a hyperdynamic cardiac impulse, and bounding femoral pulses. Chest roentgenography may show increased vascular markings and mild cardiomegaly in infants with large PDAs. Echocardiography is useful to confirm the diagnosis, with cardiac catheterization generally reserved for patients with suspected pulmonary hypertension and pulmonary vascular disease.

Newborn infants with cyanotic heart disease associated with decreased pulmonary blood flow, such as pulmonary atresia, pulmonary stenosis, and hypoplastic right ventricle with intact septum may require patency of the ductus for survival. In addition, in infants with aortic arch anomalies, the PDA may function to provide blood flow to the lower half of the body. In these groups of patients, patency of the ductus arteriosus may be maintained by prostaglandin E_1 infusion. Otherwise, closure of a PDA in newborns can be attempted medically with prostaglandin synthase inhibition using acetylsalicylic acid or indomethacin. If this fails, operative division via a posterolateral thoracotomy is indicated in all patients whether they are symptomatic or not because of the long-term risk for development of medial hypertrophy of the pulmonary vasculature and subsequent pulmonary hypertension. Older age is not a contraindication to operative repair as long as pulmonary hypertension is not present.

Aorticopulmonary Septal Defects

Aorticopulmonary septal defect (or aorticopulmonary window) is a rare congenital anomaly involving communication between the great vessels. Type I defects are located between the posterior ascending aorta and the lateral main pulmonary artery and result from incomplete fusion of the aortopulmonary septum. Type II defects are more cephalad and arise between the posterior ascending aorta and origin of the right pulmonary artery. Type III defects result from anomalous origin of the right pulmonary artery from the posterolateral ascending aorta. Associated anomalies include inclusion of the coronary artery in the origin of a type I defect, PDA, VSD, and ASD.

Aorticopulmonary septal defect leads to a left-to-right shunt and has a clinical presentation often indistinguishable from that of a large PDA. A machinery murmur is present on physical examination and the chest roentgenogram often shows a large cardiac shadow and increased pulmonary vascular markings. Cardiac catheterization is required for definitive diagnosis of this anomaly. Findings include a large pulmonary artery step-up in oxygen saturation, high right-sided chamber pressures, and demonstration of the anatomy and type of defect by retrograde aortography.

Surgical correction of aorticopulmonary septal defects is indicated at the time of diagnosis regardless of patient age because of the risk of medial hypertrophy of the pulmonary vessels and pulmonary hypertension, as in patients with a large PDA. Repair of type I and II defects is commonly performed through a *trans*aortic approach while for type III defects, excision of the anomalous right pulmonary artery from the lateral aorta and connection to the main pulmonary artery is the procedure of choice.

A-V Septal Defects

A-V septal defects (endocardial cushion defects or atrial ventricular canal defects) comprise a spectrum of congenital anomalies that result from deficiencies of the A-V septal structures immediately above and below the A-V valves (tricuspid and mitral). These defects share a common embryologic origin, namely, failure of the major endocardial cushions to fuse and contribute to development of the lower portion of the atrial septum, the posterosuperior portion of the ventricular septum, and the septal leaflets of the tricuspid and mitral valves. A-V septal defects can be classified as partial, complete, and complete with absent interatrial communication. "Partial A-V septal defect" refers to an ostium primum–type ASD, which is commonly associated with a cleft anterior mitral leaflet with or without mitral regurgitation. A complete A-V septal defect has defects of the atrial septum above and ventricular septum below a common A-V valve. The rare complete A-V septal defect with absent interatrial communication has all the features of complete A-V septal defect including a common valve orifice but has an intact primum septum.

Presentation of A-V septal defects depends on the degree of left-to-right shunting and the degree of A-V valvular incompetence. Generally, there is a large left-to-right shunt present with increased pulmonary blood flow. Left A-V valve regurgitation is also frequently present. Symptoms include dyspnea, failure to thrive, and repeated respiratory infections. Patients with isolated ostium primum defects may be asymptomatic for many years. Physical examination reveals a prominent pulmonic flow murmur and wide fixed splitting of the second heart sound. The electrocardiogram may be highly suggestive of this disorder, with left axis deviation, large P waves, and a prolonged PR interval. Echocardiography may be diagnostic when atrial and ventricular septa and valvular abnormalities are clearly delineated. Cardiac catheterization is reserved for patients with equivocal findings on noninvasive tests or when pulmonary vascular resistance must be evaluated.

Surgical repair of A-V septal defects is indicated to eliminate left-to-right shunting of blood flow and subsequent risk for development of medial hypertrophy of the pulmonary vasculature and pulmonary hypertension. Treatment for a partial A-V septal defect entails closure of the ostium primum ASD, with additional repair of an associated cleft anterior mitral leaflet in patients with mitral regurgitation. For a complete A-V septal defect, atrial and ventricular septa can be repaired using either a single or two-part patch technique and the common A-V valve is reconstructed to form separate left and right A-V valves.

Right-to-left Shunts

This condition results from obstruction of pulmonary blood flow in combination with an intracardiac defect that leads to right-to-left shunting and systemic hypoxia.

Tetralogy of Fallot

Tetralogy of Fallot is the most common of the cyanotic congenital heart lesions, accounting for up to 50% of such lesions. In most cases, the cause of the condition is not known. However, the condition has been associated with maternal exposure to rubella and thalidomide and diabetic embryopathy. Tetralogy also occurs in association with Down, XXX, Turner, Klippel-Feil, and Noonan syndromes. There is a slight preponderance of men affected by this lesion.

Tetralogy of Fallot consists of VSD, right ventricular outflow tract obstruction, an overriding aorta, and right ventricular hypertrophy (Fig. 20-3). Tetralogy may be associated with a number of other congenital malformations. The additional presence of an ASD is referred to as "pentalogy" of Fallot. Right-sided aortic arch is present in 25% of patients and abnormalities of the coronary circulation, such as origin of the left anterior descending coronary artery from the right coronary artery, are present in 5%.

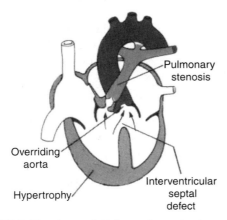

FIGURE 20-3. Tetralogy of Fallot: schematic drawing. (From Sadler TW. *Langman's medical embryology,* 5th ed. Baltimore: Williams & Wilkins, 1985, with permission.)

The hemodynamic effects of tetralogy depend on the degree of right ventricular outflow obstruction. With severe obstruction, there is significant early right-to-left shunting with greatly reduced pulmonary blood flow that is dependent on a patent ductus arteriosus. With mild obstruction, there may be mixed intracardiac shunting initially with left-to-right predominance, resulting in increased pulmonary blood flow and only mild oxygen desaturation. This has been referred to as the "pink" tetralogy. In severe cases, most patients present with cyanosis within the first 6 months. Older children with tetralogy may squat for relief of symptoms or develop "blue spells," which are thought to result from spasm of the right ventricular outflow tract. Physical examination reveals a systolic murmur over the left sternal border and an accentuated aortic second heart sound. A common finding on electrocardiogram is right axis deviation and right ventricular hypertrophy. Chest roentgenograms usually show reduced pulmonary vascular markings and a "boot-shaped" heart due to right ventricular hypertrophy. Findings on echocardiography include infundibular stenosis, pulmonary artery hypoplasia, VSD, and right ventricular hypertrophy. Cardiac catheterization is still considered necessary for preoperative evaluation. Findings include high right-sided pressures, left ventricular and aortic desaturation, and important anatomic information including the nature of the right ventricular outflow obstruction, the size of the pulmonary artery, the size and location of the VSD, the degree of aortic overriding, and associated cardiac anomalies.

Surgical treatment of tetralogy of Fallot is indicated because of the long-term risk for congestive heart failure, cerebrovascular accidents secondary to polycythemia, and bacterial endocarditis. Early definitive correction is increasingly being carried out in young patients without the intervening step of a palliative systemic-to-pulmonary shunt (e.g., the Blalock-Taussig shunt). Several groups now reserve palliation for young infants who present with severe cyanosis and extensive obstruction of the right ventricular outflow tract. Systemic-to-pulmonary shunts have been demonstrated to improve pulmonary artery hypoplasia and decrease pulmonary vascular resistance in this group of patients, making complete repair of tetralogy at a later date more feasible.

Tricuspid Atresia

Tricuspid atresia is characterized by lack of communication between the right atrium and ventricle. Associated anomalies include interatrial communication, enlargement of the mitral valve and left ventricle, and right ventricular hypoplasia. Tricuspid atresia is the third most common cyanotic heart lesion, following tetralogy of Fallot and transposition of the great arteries. It is classified into three types, depending on the relationship of the great arteries with the ventricles. In type I, there is concordance between the great arteries and ventricles, whereas in type II and type III, d-transposition and l-transposition are found, respectively.

Because there is complete mixing of systemic venous return and pulmonary venous return, the degree of systemic arterial desaturation depends upon the volume of pulmonary blood flow, which varies with patient anatomy. Most patients (71%) present with reduced pulmonary blood flow and cyanosis, whereas a smaller proportion have unobstructed pulmonary blood flow and no cyanosis but present with congestive heart failure and subsequent pulmonary vascular disease. Chest roentgenogram findings are variable. Classically, there is a flattened right heart border, a tall blunt left heart border, a high apex, and a concave arc at the aorta–lower segment junction. Echocardiography confirms absence of the tricuspid valve, the size and type of interatrial communication, enlargement and hypertrophy of the left ventricle, and hypoplasia of the right ventricle. Cardiac catheterization is useful for confirmation of the diagnosis and identification of the source of pulmonary blood flow. Systemic-to-pulmonary artery collateral vessels identified at the time of catheterization are occluded with coils and other interventional devices in preparation for definitive surgical repair.

Surgical therapy is indicated because of the poor prognosis, even for patients with near-normal pulmonary blood flow. Palliative procedures are often performed to allow growth and development of the patient before definitive repair. These include balloon or blade septostomy for restrictive interatrial communication, systemic-to-pulmonary shunting to increase pulmonary blood flow, and pulmonary artery banding for patients with excessive pulmonary blood flow. All palliative procedures are planned with the goal of preparing the patient for definitive repair by the Fontan procedure. The Fontan procedure is typically performed electively in asymptomatic patients between the ages of 5 and 10 years. Relative exclusion criteria include increased pulmonary vascular resistance and poor left ventricular performance. The Fontan procedure achieves separation of the pulmonary and systemic circulations by diverting systemic venous return directly to the lungs, relying on the right atrium to provide pulmonary perfusion pressure. This results in increased systemic arterial saturation and decreased left ventricular work.

Ebstein Anomaly

Ebstein anomaly is a rare malformation of the tricuspid valve, accounting for less than 1% of all congenital heart lesions, and is characterized by downward displacement of the septal and posterior leaflets, which are thickened, shortened, and adherent to the wall of the right ventricle. This downward displacement leads to reduced right ventricular contractility and leaves a portion of the right ventricle above the tricuspid valve to form part of the right atrium (atrialized ventricle). The anterior leaflet is typically large and billowy and may be fused to the septal and posterior leaflets. A dilated right ventricle and ASD are commonly found in association with Ebstein anomaly.

Hemodynamic alterations resulting from Ebstein anomaly vary greatly with anatomic lesions; however, there is almost always right-to-left shunting through the ASD that is exacerbated by severe tricuspid incompetence. Infants typically present with marked cyanosis and congestive heart failure while patients beyond infancy experience fatigue, dyspnea, and cyanosis. On physical examination, heart sounds are soft and a systolic tricuspid regurgitation murmur may be heard along the left sternal border. The electrocardiogram may show right bundle branch block, right axis deviation, and large P waves. The classic chest roentgenogram finding is a globular-shaped heart. The diagnosis of Ebstein anomaly can be made definitively by echocardiography, which gives detailed information on the anatomy and function of the tricuspid valve, right atrium, and right ventricle. Surgical repair or replacement of the tricuspid valve is indicated because all patients develop progressive congestive heart failure and cyanosis by young adulthood if treated medically.

Pulmonary Stenosis

Pulmonary valve stenosis (PVS) with intact ventricular septum is the most common cause of right ventricular outflow tract obstruction and makes up 8% to 10% of all congenital heart defects. PVS can be inherited in an X-linked dominant fashion and also has been associated with hemophilia. Anatomically, PVS is characterized by three well-formed leaflets that are fused into a domelike shape with a fixed central opening. A patent foramen ovale (PFO) is almost always present.

The hemodynamic effects of this lesion depend on the severity of the stenosis and vary from "trivial" to "critical." Patients with critical PVS present in infancy with severe cyanosis due to right-to-left shunting through the PFO and congestive heart failure. Physical exam usually reveals a systolic pulmonary outflow murmur, best heard in the second left intercostal space. A chest roentgenogram can be normal or show cardiomegaly or decreased pulmonary vascular markings. Echocardiography can be used to definitively diagnose PVS, although cardiac catheterization may be necessary in cases of critical PVS to distinguish it from pulmonary atresia. Simple PVS can be treated effectively by percutaneous balloon dilatation, which has been shown to have long-term durability matching that of surgical valvotomy. Surgery is reserved for infants presenting with "critical" PVS who require emergency valvotomy and patients with associated congenital heart lesions that require repair.

Pulmonary Atresia

Pulmonary atresia with intact ventricular septum is a rare cause of right ventricular outflow tract obstruction and makes up only 1% to 3% of all congenital heart defects. The lesion typically is characterized by three thickened leaflets with fused commissures. The pulmonary artery is usually confluent with normal diameter, although in rare cases, there is complete absence of the main pulmonary artery. Pulmonary atresia leads to right-to-left shunting via a patent foramen ovale and pulmonary blood flow is dependent on a patent ductus arteriosus. Most patients present within the first few days of life with cyanosis and congestive heart failure. Prostaglandin E_1 infusion is used initially to maintain ductal patency and allows for preoperative stabilization and diagnostic procedures. Early surgical intervention is necessary for survival in almost all patients with pulmonary atresia with intact ventricular septum. Surgical treatment varies with individual patient anatomy and may consist of a right ventricular outflow patch alone, a systemic-to-pulmonary shunt alone, or a systemic-to-pulmonary shunt with pulmonary valvotomy.

Eisenmenger Syndrome

Longstanding left-to-right shunting of blood flow, as occurs with VSD, can lead to medial hypertrophy of the pulmonary vasculature and a progressive increase in pulmonary vascular resistance. Subsequent reversal of blood flow through the shunt causes cyanosis and decreased pulmonary blood flow. Repair of the underlying defect at this stage is usually contraindicated because of the likelihood of right heart failure.

Ventricular Outflow Obstruction

This group consists of congenital heart anomalies that cause obstruction to right and/or left ventricular outflow.

Aortic Stenosis

Congenital aortic stenosis collectively describes all lesions that cause left ventricular outflow obstruction and includes supravalvar stenosis, valvar stenosis, subaortic stenosis, and left ventricular outflow obstruction. All of these forms of aortic stenosis occur predominantly in men, with a ratio of approximately 4:1. Idiopathic hypertrophic subaortic stenosis and to a lesser extent supravalvar aortic stenosis have been recognized to occur in families and are, in some cases, thought to have a genetic component. Most cases of valvar aortic stenosis present as an isolated lesion; however, these lesions may also be associated with coarctation of the aorta, mitral valve anomalies, and left ventricular hypoplasia.

Supravalvar stenosis accounts for 11% to 21% of cases of aortic stenosis. Three anatomic types have been described: a localized, diagphramlike obstruction, a localized hourglass narrowing, and a diffuse narrowing of the ascending aorta. Valvar stenosis accounts for 45% to 59% of cases of aortic stenosis and typically results from a bicuspid or unicuspid valve with thickened leaflet(s). Subvalvar stenosis accounts for 7% to 30% of cases of aortic stenosis and typically results from a discrete ring of fibrous tissue just below the aortic valve annulus. Evidence suggests that such subvalvar rings may in some cases develop after birth.

Severe left ventricular outflow obstruction caused by aortic stenosis leads to pulmonary congestion, pulmonary venous hypertension, systemic hypoperfusion, and metabolic acidosis. Patients presenting in childhood may have infective endocarditis, left ventricular failure, and sudden death. On physical examination, aortic stenosis is characterized by a systolic murmur over the aortic area. Chest roentgenogram findings include left ventricular and aortic enlargement and pulmonary venous congestion. Echocardiography is useful for confirmation of the diagnosis and noninvasive follow-up examinations. Cardiac catheterization provides pressure gradient measurements, allows calculation of valve areas, and reliably distinguishes between the different anatomic types of aortic stenosis.

Aortic valvotomy is indicated for young children with severe aortic stenosis (gradient greater than 75 mm Hg) whether or not they are symptomatic. It may also be indicated for older children with moderate aortic stenosis (gradient between 50 and 75 mm Hg) who have angina, syncope, exercise intolerance, or evidence of left ventricular hypertrophy with strain on electrocardiogram. Follow-up with serial echocardiography is generally recommended for patients with mild to moderate aortic stenosis who are asymptomatic because of the frequent need to perform valve replacement in patients who have undergone valvotomy early in life.

Mitral Stenosis

Congenital mitral stenosis occurring as an isolated lesion is rare, accounting for only 0.6% of congenital heart lesions. Mitral valve malformations are more commonly found in association with other lesions and in these instances may contribute to complex anomalies such as hypoplastic left heart syndrome, complete A-V canal, and double inlet ventricle. Although congenital mitral stenosis may result from abnormalities of the leaflets, papillary muscle abnormalities are a more common cause of mitral valve obstruction. The parachute deformity of the mitral valve results from insertion of the chordae into a single papillary muscle. The thickened and shortened chordae associated with this lesion lead to impaired mobility of the valve leaflets, which leads to obstruction of flow. Rarely, mitral valve atresia can occur, but it is usually seen in association with hypoplastic left heart syndrome.

Patients with congenital mitral stenosis present with fatigue, recurrent pulmonary infections, growth retardation, tachypnea, and central cyanosis. Physical examination usually reveals a diastolic murmur. Chest roentgenograms show left atrial enlargement and increased pulmonary vessel markings. Echocardiography is useful for identifying leaflet and papillary muscle abnormalities and supravalvar fibrous rings. Cardiac catheterization is necessary to thoroughly investigate for associated lesions such as intracardiac shunts.

Surgical intervention is limited by the lack of satisfactory procedures for many of the anatomic lesions causing mitral stenosis. Open commissurotomy of fused leaflets can be performed but frequently does not relieve obstruction at the level of the chordae that may accompany valvar lesions. Splitting of chordae and the papillary muscle to relieve this obstruction and to correct parachute deformity is only partially effective and mitral insufficiency is often produced, necessitating subsequent mitral valve replacement. Mitral valve replacement is associated with increased morbidity and mortality in children, and to avoid this and the long-term risks of anticoagulation, repair is usually attempted and valve replacement is generally reserved for patients with intractable congestive heart failure.

Coarctation of the Aorta

Coarctation of the aorta is characterized by a discrete narrowing or hypoplasia of the proximal descending thoracic aorta at the site of entrance of the ductus arteriosus. It is a relatively common lesion and accounts for 5% to 8% of all congenital heart anomalies. It may be associated with VSD, congenital aortic stenosis, hypoplastic left ventricle, and congenital mitral valve stenosis. In addition, bicuspid aortic valve is reported to be present in about one third of patients with coarctation.

Coarctation has historically been categorized into two groups: infantile and adult. In infantile coarctation, the aortic obstruction is most often preductal and leads to separation of left ventricular flow, which is directed to the head and arms, from pulmonary artery flow, which is directed to the lower body. This type of coarctation results in early left ventricular failure and death if not surgically corrected. The more common adult type of coarctation is postductal and leads to proximal hypertension and eventual congestive heart failure over time, although patients may remain asymptomatic and appear healthy into adulthood.

Approximately 15% of patients with coarctation present with severe congestive heart failure requiring early surgical intervention within the first few months of life. In the remainder, coarctation is most frequently detected during workup for a heart murmur or for hypertension noted during routine physical examinations. Patients who are symptomatic at the time of presentation may complain of dyspnea, headache, and nosebleeds. Physical examination findings include upper extremity systolic hypertension, absent or decreased lower extremity pulses, prominent pulsations at the sternal notch, and a systolic heart murmur over the left sternal border that may be transmitted to the back. Chest roentgenograms may reveal rib notching by the age of 10 years secondary to enlarged intercostal artery collaterals. Other x-ray findings include an indentation over the left border of the heart at the site of coarctation, which gives the "3" sign.

Patients presenting early with severe congestive heart failure are treated with prostaglandin E_1 to maintain ductal patency, which improves blood flow to the descending aorta until surgical repair can be attempted. Subclavian flap repair is preferred in neonates and infants to avoid late restenosis, which may complicate end-to-end anastomosis. In older children, end-to-end anastomosis is appropriate. Repair in adults may be hazardous because of the presence of large, friable intercostal artery collaterals. Bypass using a prosthetic tube graft may be performed in this setting and also in the case of recurrent coarctation.

Anomalous Origin of the Left Coronary Artery from the Pulmonary Artery

This lesion is the most common congenital abnormality of the coronary vessels. Despite this, it remains a rare condition, accounting for only 0.25% of congenital heart lesions. In this condition, the left coronary artery arises from the main pulmonary artery while the right coronary artery arises normally from the aorta. After the neonatal period, when the pulmonary artery pressure decreases, forward flow in the left coronary artery decreases, creating a strong stimulus for development of collaterals from the right coronary circulation. Reversal of flow through the left coronary artery through these collaterals leads to a coronary arteriovenous fistula and myocardial ischemia. Approximately 65% of patients die within the first year of life due to heart failure related to anterolateral myocardial infarction, left ventricular fibrosis, and mitral insufficiency secondary to papillary muscle dysfunction.

Clinical features include dyspnea, pallor, fatigue, and a semblance of pain. Signs of heart failure are apparent on physical examination and chest roentgenogram. A systolic mitral insufficiency murmur is frequently present. Although echocardiography has been successfully used to demonstrate the anomalous coronary artery, a definitive diagnosis is usually made by cardiac catheterization and coronary angiography. Early surgical repair is indicated because of the high mortality associated with this condition. Simple ligation of the anomalous left coronary artery eliminates A-V shunting and improves myocardial perfusion; however, this procedure alone is of little value for patients with poorly developed collaterals and no retrograde flow. In most cases, establishment of a two coronary artery circulation is optimal. This has been accomplished by aortic reimplantation of the anomalous coronary artery, creation of a tunnel using a portion of the anterior pulmonary artery to establish aortocoronary continuity, or coronary artery bypass grafting using saphenous vein grafts, internal mammary artery grafts, and subclavian artery grafts. Mitral valve replacement or repair may be necessary for treatment of mitral insufficiency.

Bidirectional Shunts

These complex congenital defects have also been termed *admixing lesions* because they result in both left-to-right and right-to-left shunts. Patients with these lesions commonly present with congestive heart failure because of increased pulmonary blood flow and volume overload.

Transposition of the Great Arteries

Transposition of the great arteries is the most frequent congenital heart lesion causing cyanosis in the newborn period and accounts for 8% to 10% of all congenital heart defects. There is a distinct male preponderance in patients presenting with this condition. In complete transposition, the aorta arises anteriorly from the right ventricle and the pulmonary artery arises posteriorly from the left ventricle (Fig. 20-4). The venous-atrial and A-V connections are normal. Patent ductus arteriosus, VSD, and patent foramen ovale are usually associated with transposition.

The physiologic effect of complete transposition is separation of the pulmonary and systemic circulations so that they exist in parallel rather than in series. Absence of intracirculatory shunts that allow admixture of oxygenated pulmonary circulation blood with deoxygenated systemic circulation blood is incompatible with life. The most common clinical features of complete transposition are cyanosis, which is usually present at birth, and congestive heart failure, which develops in the neonatal period as the pulmonary vascular resistance decreases. Physical examination reveals a systolic murmur and loud single second heart sound. Classic chest roentgenogram findings are an oval or egg-shaped heart, a narrow superior mediastinum, and increased pulmonary vascular markings. Definitive diagnosis of complete transposition can be made by echocardiography, with cardiac catheterization reserved for patients with inadequate intracirculatory shunting or complex associated anomalies.

Balloon atrial septostomy (Rashkind procedure) has been used successfully to achieve palliation in small infants

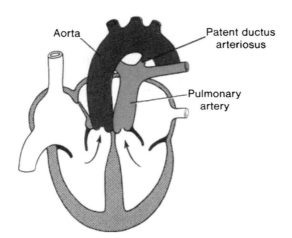

FIGURE 20-4. Transposition of the great vessels: schematic drawing. (From Sadler TW. *Langman's medical embryology*, 5th ed. Baltimore: Williams & Wilkins, 1985, with permission.)

by increasing pulmonary and systemic venous blood admixture at the atrial level. Successful physiologic correction of complete transposition by use of an intraatrial baffle was first reported in 1964 by Mustard. This procedure uses the right ventricle as the source of systemic flow but at late follow-up has been associated with progressive right ventricular failure. This finding has led to the increasing use of the arterial switch procedure, which involves switching the great vessels to their appropriate ventricles and reimplanting the coronary arteries into the neoaorta.

Truncus Arteriosus

Truncus arteriosus describes a condition in which a solitary arterial trunk exits the heart through a semilunar valve and supplies the systemic, pulmonary, and coronary arterial systems. The single vessel overlies a large VSD and receives the entire outflow from both ventricles. Truncus arteriosus results from failure of septation of the embryonic truncus arteriosus and conal septum, which normally separates the trunk into aortic and pulmonary components. It is an uncommon congenital lesion, accounting for 0.4% to 2.8% of all cases.

The hemodynamic effects of truncus arteriosus are determined by the amount of pulmonary blood flow and the competence of the truncal valve. As the pulmonary vascular resistance falls in the neonatal period, pulmonary flow increases and patients present after the first week of life with congestive heart failure. Patients with severe truncal valve insufficiency may present with severe heart failure. Symptoms at presentation include dyspnea, poor feeding, pallor, and failure to thrive. Cyanosis is an uncommon finding. On physical examination, there is evidence of congestive heart failure, a single second heart sound, and systolic and early diastolic heart murmurs. The diagnosis can be made definitively by echocardiogram; however, cardiac catheterization and angiography are still necessary to delineate pulmonary artery anatomy and to measure hemodynamic parameters.

Early surgical intervention is indicated because of the high (75% to 85%) 1-year mortality rate associated with this lesion. Pulmonary artery banding has been largely abandoned as a palliative procedure because of inconsistent results and the increasing success of complete intracardiac repair in infants. This consists of detachment of the pulmonary arteries from the truncus, closure of the VSD, and connection of the right ventricle to the pulmonary arteries using a valve homograft.

Double Inlet Ventricle

Double inlet ventricle or single ventricle describe a diverse group of anomalies in which both atrial chambers empty into the same ventricle. In this condition, the atria can be connected with a left, right, or solitary and indeterminate ventricle. Double inlet ventricle has a range of clinical presentations, depending on the amount of pulmonary blood flow. Most commonly, patients present with cyanosis and severe congestive heart failure within the first months of life. Definitive diagnosis is made by echocardiography. Cardiac catheterization and angiography remain useful for delineation of the systemic and pulmonary arterial pathways. Surgical correction of double inlet ventricle can proceed via two pathways. Septation of the ventricle to form two chambers, one supplying the pulmonary circulation and one supplying the systemic circulation, may be difficult and is usually reserved for patients with elevated pulmonary vascular resistance. A Fontan-type procedure is more commonly used to separate the pulmonary and systemic circulations by directing systemic venous return away from the ventricle and directly to the pulmonary artery.

Total Anomalous Pulmonary Venous Connection

Total anomalous pulmonary venous connection (TAPVC) describes a condition in which the pulmonary veins do not communicate with the left atrium but rather with the right atrium, coronary sinus, or a major systemic vein. The left atrium receives blood via a patent foramen ovale or ASD in those patients who survive beyond birth. A patent ductus arteriosus is also present in 25% to 50% of cases. The male to female ratio among patients with this lesion is nearly 2:1. TAPVC and other severe congenital heart defects may be associated with the asplenia syndrome. In approximately 50% of cases of TAPVC, the site of pulmonary venous connection is supracardiac, most commonly a left anomalous vertical vein draining to the innominate vein. In approximately 25% of cases, the connection is intracardiac, with the coronary sinus being the most common site of connection in this group.

The anomalous connection leads to obligatory mixing of systemic and pulmonary venous blood. If there is a large ASD and the anomalous connection is not obstructed, there may be adequate flow to the left atrium, high pulmonary blood flow, and only mild systemic cyanosis. On the other hand, patients with obstructed TAPVC present within the first few weeks of life with tachypnea, cyanosis, and low cardiac output. On physical examination, the right ventricle is prominent, the second heart sound is split and fixed, and a parasternal systolic heart murmur is present. Electrocardiogram reveals right ventricular hypertrophy and right axis deviation. In patients with obstructed TAPVC, chest roentgenograms show pulmonary venous congestion. Cardiac catheterization can be helpful in delineating the site of pulmonary venous return and hemodynamic measurements. Over 80% of infants born with TAPVC die before the age of 1 year. Early surgical intervention is therefore indicated, even in those patients with unobstructed connections and only mild cyanosis. Surgical repair involves redirecting flow from the pulmonary venous chamber to the left atrium and, if successful, is associated with only rare long-term complications.

Hypoplastic Left Heart Syndrome

Hypoplastic left heart syndrome is a complex anomaly characterized by marked hypoplasia or atresia of the left ventricle, hypoplasia of the ascending aorta, intact ventricular septum, and mitral valve atresia or hypoplasia. The cause of hypoplastic left heart syndrome in most cases is felt to be severe underdevelopment of left ventricular outflow secondary to isolated aortic valve atresia or double outlet right ventricle with aortic valve atresia. Hypoplastic left heart syndrome is relatively common, making up 7% of congenital heart malformations presenting in the first year of life.

In this condition, the left ventricle is nonfunctional and the systemic circulation is dependent on a patent ductus arteriosus. Newborns typically present within the first 24 to 48 hours of life with cyanosis and tachypnea. As the ductus closes, systemic perfusion decreases and metabolic acidosis develops. Physical examination reveals a dominant right ventricular impulse, a single loud second heart sound, and a soft systolic murmur over the left sternal border. Definitive diagnosis of this lesion is made by echocardiography. Cardiac catheterization is generally not indicated for diagnostic or therapeutic purposes.

Initial management consists of prostaglandin E_1 infusion to maintain patency of the ductus arteriosus and allow systemic perfusion through this structure. Early surgical intervention is required because this lesion is uniformly fatal without reconstructive surgery or heart transplantation. The Norwood procedure involves application of a Fontan-like reconstruction to this malformation in two stages. Two stages are required because the pulmonary vascular resistance of the newborn is prohibitively high for an immediate Fontan procedure. In the first stage, the main pulmonary artery is divided and the proximal stump anastomosed to an augmented proximal aorta and aortic arch. The distal pulmonary artery stump is oversewn and an aortic-pulmonary artery shunt is formed to provide pulmonary blood flow. The second stage (modified Fontan procedure) is performed at 12 to 18 months of age after evaluation of pulmonary vascular resistance. Systemic venous return is diverted from the right ventricle to the pulmonary circulation via a right atrial–distal pulmonary artery anastoamosis. Because of the high mortality associated with this procedure, particularly the first stage, cardiac transplantation has been advanced as a potential alternative for the management of this syndrome. This strategy is limited by the inadequate supply of donor hearts, the need for chronic immunosuppression, and unknown long-term outlook.

TABLE 20-1. NEW YORK HEART ASSOCIATION FUNCTIONAL CLASSIFICATION[a]

Class I: Patients with cardiac disease but without resulting limitation of physical activity.
Class II: Patients with cardiac disease resulting in slight limitation of physical activity. Ordinary physical activity causes fatigue, palpitations, dyspnea, or angina. No symptoms at rest.
Class III: Patients with cardiac disease resulting in marked limitation of physical activity. Less than ordinary physical activity results in fatigue, palpitations, dyspnea, or angina. No symptoms at rest.
Class IV: Patients with cardiac disease who are unable to carry on any physical activity without discomfort. Symptoms of cardiac insufficiency or angina may be present even at rest. Any physical activity increases discomfort.

[a]From Braunwald E. The history. In: Braunwald E, ed. *Heart Disease: a textbook of cardiovascular medicine*, 5th ed. Philadelphia: WB Saunders, 1997:1–14, with permission.

ACQUIRED HEART DISEASE

Functional classification has been useful in stratifying patients with acquired heart disease for prognostic and therapeutic purposes. The two most commonly used classification systems are the New York Heart Association (NYHA) functional classification, which is a general subjective classification of symptoms (Table 20-1), and the Canadian Cardiovascular Society functional classification, which classifies angina symptoms related to coronary artery disease (Table 20-2).

Coronary Artery Disease

Coronary artery disease is the leading cause of death in the United States. It is caused by atherosclerotic narrowing of the arteries. Risk factors include inappropriate diet, hypertension, diabetes, smoking, sedentary lifestyle, and family history. Men are at higher risk for developing premature coronary artery disease than women, for whom the risk after menopause increases to that of men. Anatomically, the most severe atherosclerotic changes occur in the proximal third of the coronary arteries, making therapeutic bypass of such lesions feasible. Diffuse atherosclerotic disease of the coronary arteries does occasionally occur, however, and may be associated with diabetes mellitus and hyperlipidemia disorders.

Patients with coronary artery disease may present with angina pectoris, myocardial infarction, or sudden death secondary to ventricular arrhythmias. Severe manifestations of this disease are not necessarily preceded by angina. Indeed, half of all fatal heart attacks occur in previously asymptomatic individuals. Individuals at risk for cardiac events can be identified by use of stress electrocardiogram and thallium tests, stress echocardiography, or intravenous (i.v.) dipyridamole thallium-201 scintigraphy (DTS). The ability to identify patients at high risk for cardiac events is of particular interest to surgeons, as the leading cause of death after major surgery is cardiac. It has been estimated that more than 10% of patients undergoing surgical procedures in this country are at risk for coronary disease, and up to 15% of these patients suffer significant cardiac morbidity. The group at highest risk for cardiac morbidity are patients undergoing surgery for peripheral vascular disease. This group has been found to have associated severe coronary artery disease in up to one third of patients.

I.V. DTS is now thought to be the best preoperative noninvasive screening test for patients at risk for cardiac events. It is particularly useful for patients who are unable to undergo exercise stress testing due to peripheral vascular, orthopedic, neurological, or other debilitating conditions. The finding of positive DTS results (an initial myocardial perfusion defect followed by delayed reperfusion of this region) is associated with increased risk for cardiac events and should be followed by coronary angiography and appropriate therapy. Conversely, negative DTS results are associated with a low incidence of perioperative cardiac events.

Clinical risk factors associated with increased risk for significant coronary artery disease include history of angina, Q waves on electrocardiogram, age greater than 70 years, ventricular ectopy requiring medical therapy, diabetes mellitus, and clinical evidence of left ventricular failure. Patients with none of these risk factors have been found to have a 3% incidence of perioperative cardiac events versus a 50% incidence for patients with three or more clinical risk factors. DTS has been found to be most useful as a screening tool for patients with one or two clinical risk factors who are at intermediate risk. In this group, patients with negative DTS results had a 3% incidence of cardiac events versus 30% for patients with positive DTS results.

TABLE 20-2. CANADIAN CARDIOVASCULAR SOCIETY FUNCTIONAL CLASSIFICATION[a]

Class I: Ordinary physical activity does not cause angina. Angina may occur with strenuous or prolonged exertion.
Class II: Slight limitation of ordinary activity. Angina may occur with walking or climbing stairs rapidly, walking uphill, walking or stair climbing after meals or in the cold, in the wind, or under emotional stress, or walking more than two blocks on the level or climbing more than one flight of stairs under normal conditions at a normal pace.
Class III: Marked limitation of ordinary physical activity. Angina may occur after walking one or two blocks on level ground or climbing one flight of stairs under normal conditions at a normal place.
Class IV: Inability to carry out any physical activity without anginal discomfort; angina may be present at rest.

[a]From Braunwald E. The history. In: Braunwald E, ed. *Heart disease: a textbook of cardiovascular medicine*, 5th ed. Philadelphia: WB Saunders, 1997:1–14, with permission.

Indications for Revascularization

General indications for revascularization of the coronary circulation include increasing symptoms, to prevent myocardial damage in high-risk patients, and to prolong life. Because the long-term benefits of coronary artery bypass grafting (CABG) decrease with time, surgery is usually not recommended for patients presenting with mild to moderate symptoms who do not have evidence of life-threatening coronary artery disease and do not have left ventricular dysfunction. These patients can be treated medically until symptoms become unmanageable.

Patients with progressive or unstable angina despite maximal medical therapy frequently have significant amounts of myocardium at risk and are candidates for urgent revascularization. For one- or two-vessel disease, percutaneous transluminal coronary angioplasty (PTCA) is frequently attempted, with surgery reserved for patients with early failure. In most centers where angioplasty is a common procedure, the incidence of patients requiring emergency surgery after early PTCA failure is less than 3%. In addition to early failure, an additional 20% to 30% of patients with initially successful angioplasties develop restenosis within 6 to 12 months, requiring further intervention.

Indications for elective CABG have been developed on the basis of results of large randomized trials of CABG versus medical therapy (Table 20-3). Improved survival with surgery has led to the following clear indications for CABG: NYHA class III or greater angina unresponsive to medical therapy, unstable angina, left main coronary artery disease, symptomatic patient with three-vessel disease or two-vessel disease where the LAD has a severe obstruction proximal to the first septal perforator, and failed PTCA. Possible indications for CABG are postmyocardial infarction patients with positive stress test results at low workload and patients in cardiogenic shock.

The decrease in long-term benefits of CABG over time is primarily related to development of vein graft disease. After 10 years, only 50% to 60% of saphenous vein grafts remain patent. In contrast, the internal mammary artery appears to be relatively resistant to late atherosclerosis and graft disease, leading to a greater than 95% patency rate even after 20 years. Significant improvement in survival and freedom from cardiac events has been demonstrated in patients receiving internal mammary artery bypass grafts to the LAD. Long-term benefits of CABG are also limited by progression of atherosclerotic changes in the native vessels. Postoperative care therefore includes patient education, diet control, cessation of smoking, control of hypertension, and use of cholesterol-lowering agents if indicated.

Myocardial Infarction

Current management of acute myocardial infarction includes early reperfusion within the first 3 to 6 hours after onset. Thrombolytic therapy with recombinant tissue–type plasminogen activator has yielded reperfusion rates as high as 66%. In patients for whom such therapy is contraindicated because of risk of bleeding, angioplasty of the infarcted vessel may be successful in approximately 95% of cases.

Although CABG has not been shown to prolong survival for patients who are asymptomatic after recovery from myocardial infarction, studies have identified subgroups of patients who are at high risk for death in the postinfarction period and who may benefit from bypass surgery. For postinfarction patients who have positive stress test results at a low workload or patients with cardiogenic shock, CABG may prolong survival and in some instances be lifesaving. An important factor in the immediate and long-term prognosis of such patients for whom surgery is considered is the amount of residual functioning myocardium that remains after the patient has sustained an infarction. Early results in patients with left ventricular ejection fractions of less than 25% have been discouraging.

Surgical Complications of Myocardial Infarction

Myocardial infarction may lead to a number of sequelae that require surgical intervention in the early or late postinfarction period. Papillary muscle infarction may lead to dysfunction or rupture and acute mitral regurgitation, necessitating mitral valve replacement. Infarction of the ventricular septum may cause a VSD and left-to-right shunt, which usually leads to rapid deterioration without surgical intervention. Left ventricular aneurysms are a late complication of myocardial infarction. Indications for resection include congestive heart failure, embolism, or recurrent ventricular tachyarrhythmia.

Acquired Valve Disease

Aortic Stenosis

Obstruction of the left ventricular outflow tract may occur at the subvalvular, valvular, and supravalvular levels. In the

TABLE 20-3. INDICATIONS FOR CORONARY ARTERY BYPASS GRAFTING[a]

New York Heart Association class III angina unresponsive to medical therapy
Unstable angina
Left main coronary artery disease
Symptomatic patient with three-vessel coronary artery disease
Failed percutaneous transluminal coronary angioplasty
Postmyocardial infarction patient with positive stress test results at low workload
Acute myocardial infarction with cardiogenic shock

[a]From Franco KL, Hammond GL. Surgical indications for coronary revascularization. In: Baue AE, Geha AS, Hammond GL, et al., eds. *Glenn's thoracic and cardiovascular surgery,* 6th ed. Stamford: Appleton & Lange, 1996:2073–2079, with permission.

adult population, most patients present with obstruction at the valvular level, which results from congenital or degenerative abnormalities of the aortic valve. A bicuspid configuration is generally responsible for the congenital type and has an incidence of 0.9% to 2.0% in the general population and about 50% in patients with aortic stenosis. Both congenital and degenerative aortic stenosis are associated with progressive calcification and loss of cusp mobility.

The common hemodynamic effect of these lesions is decreased valvular area, which necessitates a large *trans*valvular gradient to maintain left ventricular outflow. Most patients become symptomatic at valve areas of less than 1.0 cm^2, and areas of less than 0.7 cm^2 represent critical stenosis (normal aortic valve area equals 2.5 to 3.5 cm^2). The adaptive response of the left ventricle to outflow obstruction is progressive hypertrophy, which is accompanied by decreased diastolic compliance. Because of the capacity of the left ventricle to adapt to the outflow obstruction, gradients as high as 90 to 120 mm Hg may be present in severe aortic stenosis. Eventually, the ventricle is unable to compensate and dilates, which results in decreased cardiac output, increased pulmonary artery pressures, and congestive heart failure. Left ventricular changes associated with aortic stenosis also may lead to myocardial ischemia, even in the presence of normal coronary arteries. Myocardial oxygen demand is increased with increased ventricular mass and high systolic pressure while oxygen delivery is decreased by high end-diastolic pressures. This mismatch in myocardial oxygen supply and demand may lead to effort-related angina or an anginal equivalent, such as dyspnea.

Because of the capacity of the left ventricle to adapt for long periods to the demands of outflow obstruction, patients may remain asymptomatic for many years. As the valve area progressively decreases, however, they typically experience congestive heart failure, angina, or syncope. After the appearance of symptoms, the clinical course of aortic stenosis may become progressively severe. Aortic stenosis is the most frequently fatal valvular lesion and sudden death may occur in up to 20% of patients. Physical examination reveals a loud, harsh systolic aortic murmur, which may be transmitted to the neck. The second heart sound is usually split. An S_4 is commonly heard with decreased left ventricular compliance and adaptive left atrial hypertrophy. The electrocardiogram demonstrates left ventricular hypertrophy and left atrial enlargement. Chest roentgenogram results may be normal or reveal left ventricular prominence; however, end-stage patients have gross cardiomegaly and evidence of congestive heart failure. The aortic root may show calcification and poststenotic dilation. Echocardiography is useful in demonstrating the configuration of the aortic valve and motion of the leaflets; however, cardiac catheterization is necessary to directly measure pressure and flow across the valve. The valve area can be calculated by the Gorlin formula. Coronary arteriography is also recommended even in patients without ischemic symptoms to assess the need for combined valve replacement and coronary bypass. Indications for aortic valve replacement are patients with aortic stenosis who have symptoms of angina, congestive heart failure, or syncope, and asymptomatic patients with severe aortic stenosis demonstrated by an aortic valve area of less than 0.7 cm^2.

Aortic Regurgitation

Aortic regurgitation (AR) most commonly results from rheumatic fever, which accounts for up to half of patients requiring aortic valve replacements. Progressive fibrosis and thickening lead to retraction and abnormal coaptation of the cusps. In addition, there are numerous nonrheumatic causes of AR including infective endocarditis, cuspal avulsion or laceration following blunt chest trauma, myxomatous degeneration, rheumatoid arthritis, and systemic lupus erythematosus. AR can result from dilation of the aortic root in the presence of a histologically normal aortic valve, as occurs with tertiary syphilis and Marfan syndrome, which is an autosomal dominant (rarely autosomal recessive) disorder characterized by a basic defect in the formation of elastic fibers. Acute aortic dissection may cause detachment of the valve cusps, leading to AR.

The size of regurgitant orifices leading to significant AR range from 0.5 to 1.0 cm^2. Up to 60% to 70% of stroke volume in such cases may regurgitate into the left ventricle during diastole. To maintain normal forward flow, the left ventricle increases stroke volume and work. Chronic changes include hypertrophy, which is followed by the gradual onset of ventricular dilation. Patients with moderate or severe AR may remain asymptomatic for many years because of left ventricular adaptation. Eventually, however, ejection fraction and cardiac output decrease and patients experience symptoms of congestive heart failure. In contrast to that of aortic stenosis, the course of AR after the onset of symptoms is prolonged, and 50% of patients may survive 10 years. Physical examination reveals a widened pulse pressure and a blowing diastolic murmur along the left sternal border. An S_3 may be present in patients with deteriorating ventricular function. Electrocardiograms and chest roentgenograms demonstrate left ventricular hypertrophy and left atrial enlargement in some cases. Echocardiography is useful in documenting the degree of dilation and hypertrophy of the left ventricle but does not accurately quantitate the degree of regurgitation. The best method for demonstrating the dynamics and severity of AR is by aortography, which should be performed with cardiac catheterization and coronary angiography when aortic valve replacement is considered.

Aortic valve replacement is indicated for symptomatic patients with AR. Asymptomatic patients should be treated medically until they experience symptoms or noninvasive studies demonstrate significant left ventricular dilation or deteriorating function. Patients with severe acute AR and congestive heart failure should be operated on as soon as possible.

Idiopathic Hypertrophic Subaortic Stenosis

Idiopathic hypertrophic subaortic stenosis (IHSS) is an asymmetrical obstructive hypertrophic cardiomyopathy in which anatomic and physiologic obstruction of the left ventricular outflow tract results in presentation similar to that of aortic stenosis. The male to female ratio is approximately 2:1. In some cases, IHSS has been demonstrated to be inherited in an autosomal dominant pattern. Anatomically, IHSS results in marked thickening of the middle and upper ventricular septa. Histologic examination reveals a bizarre, whorled configuration of myocytes and connective tissue elements described as myocardial disarray.

Left ventricular outflow obstruction is dynamic, increasing with factors that decrease ventricular volume, such as inotropes, or that decrease afterload, or decrease venous return. In patients who are symptomatic, dyspnea and angina are common. IHSS may also present as sudden death, which accounts for over 50% of deaths in patients with this condition. On physical examination, a systolic murmur usually is heard over the left sternal border. Electrocardiograms and chest roentgenograms show left ventricular hypertrophy. Echocardiograms display various patterns of hypertrophy and mitral valve function. Cardiac catheterizations provide pullback gradient measurements across the outflow tract as well as coronary arteriograms.

Symptomatic patients usually can be treated medically with β blockers and calcium channel blockers. Surgery is reserved for patients with severe symptoms and resting or provocative gradients despite maximal medical therapy and patients who have survived sudden death episodes and have significant resting or provocative gradients. Surgical treatment of IHSS may involve left ventricular myotomy and myomectomy by Morrow technique or in certain cases elimination of systolic anterior motion of the mitral valve by mitral valve replacement.

Mitral Stenosis

Despite its dramatic decrease in incidence in most western countries, chronic rheumatic disease remains the most common cause of mitral stenosis. Approximately 55% of patients have a documented history of group A streptococcal pharyngitis. Although the pathogenesis of rheumatic heart disease remains unclear, patients typically have high antistreptolysin O (ASO) titers, and valvular lesions are felt to result from autoimmune damage. Rare causes of mitral stenosis include degenerative calcification in the elderly, myxoma, malignant carcinoid, systemic lupus erythematosus, and rheumatoid arthritis.

Anatomically, rheumatic mitral valve stenosis is due to fibrous fusion of the valve commissures. In advanced cases, fibrosis progresses to involve the leaflets and chordae, giving the valve a funnellike appearance. The hemodynamic effect of mitral stenosis is chronic pulmonary venous obstruction. Left atrial pressures are elevated, and in severe cases, reactive pulmonary hypertension, right ventricular enlargement, and congestive heart failure may develop. If there is a documented history of acute rheumatic fever, symptoms typically develop after a long asymptomatic latent period. The most common presenting symptom is dyspnea, which initially occurs with exertion but then progresses to occur at rest. Classic physical examination findings are an opening snap, a loud first heart sound, and a diastolic rumble. Signs of right heart failure may be present. Electrocardiograms frequently show atrial fibrillation and chest roentgenograms show left atrial enlargement. Echocardiography is useful in delineating anatomy and flow dynamics across the mitral valve. Cardiac catheterization is reserved for patients for whom noninvasive studies are inadequate or coronary angiography is indicated.

The normal mitral valve area is 4 to 6 cm^2. Patients typically develop symptoms secondary to mitral stenosis when valve areas reach 1.5 to 2 cm^2. Valve areas of less than 1.0 cm^2 are usually associated with severe symptoms. Surgery is indicated for patients with hemodynamically significant valve obstruction and NYHA class III to IV symptoms, onset of atrial fibrillation regardless of symptoms, increasing pulmonary hypertension, episodes of systemic embolization, or infective endocarditis. Choice of procedure is highly dependent on individual valvular anatomy and includes open commissurotomy, more complex valve repair techniques, and mitral valve replacement.

Mitral Regurgitation

Mitral valve competence depends on the coordinated function of the annulus, leaflets, chordae tendineae, papillary muscles, and ventricular wall. Disease processes affecting any of these elements may lead to valvular incompetence. Rheumatic heart disease is still the most common cause of mitral regurgitation. Progressive fibrosis and retraction of leaflets and fusion and shortening of the chordae lead to mitral regurgitation, which is commonly associated with mitral stenosis. Other etiologies include myxomatous degeneration, ischemia, infective endocarditis, and cardiomyopathies. Blunt chest trauma may also led to chordal rupture and mitral regurgitation.

As in mitral stenosis, left atrial pressures are elevated and lead to chronic pulmonary venous obstruction. Reactive pulmonary hypertension may ensue, and in severe cases, there may be right heart failure and functional tricuspid incompetence. In contrast to mitral stenosis, the left ventricle is subject to chronic volume overload, which may cause left ventricle dilation, diminished ejection fraction, and left heart failure. Symptoms, which typically include dyspnea, occur when the regurgitant volume approaches 50% of stroke volume. Physical examination reveals an apical pansystolic murmur, which is accompanied in severe cases by an S_3 gallop. Chest roentgenograms show enlargement of cardiac chambers, and electrocardiograms frequently indicate atrial fibrillation. As in mitral stenosis, echocardiography provides useful information on valvular anatomy, flow dynamics across the mitral valve, and ventricular function.

Surgical intervention is indicated for patients with hemodynamically significant lesions who have symptoms that compromise their lifestyle (usually NYHA class III or IV). For asymptomatic patients, surgery is recommended for progression of pulmonary hypertension, onset of atrial fibrillation, or left ventricular dilation. Acute mitral regurgitation resulting from infective endocarditis or myocardial ischemia leads to rapid clinical deterioration and urgent operation is indicated. Prosthetic ring annuloplasty, complex mitral valve repair, or mitral valve replacement may be performed depending on the patient's valve anatomy and clinical setting.

Tricuspid and Pulmonary Valves

Acquired tricuspid valve disease most commonly occurs in the setting of annular dilation leading to tricuspid incompetence. More rarely, rheumatic involvement leads to tricuspid stenosis, which may be associated with regurgitation as in rheumatic disease of the mitral valve. Acquired pulmonary valve disease is rare, although rheumatic involvement can occur. Valve fibrosis secondary to carcinoid syndrome most commonly affects right-sided valves.

Infective Endocarditis

Invasion of the endocardium of the heart by microorganisms most commonly occurs on the valves. The infectious agent can be bacterial, fungal, or viral. Predisposing factors for development of infective endocarditis include previous congenital or acquired heart lesions, immunocompromised status, i.v. catheters, and i.v. drug abuse. The male to female ratio is 2:1. Gram-positive organisms remain the most common cause of bacterial endocarditis, specifically *Streptococcus viridans, Staphylococcus aureus,* and *Staphylococcus epidermis*. With the increasing use of broad-spectrum antibiotics in the treatment of critically ill patients, Gram-negative bacterial endocarditis has increased in frequency in recent years. Broad-spectrum antibiotics, prosthetic valve endocarditis, nosocomial infection, and i.v. hyperalimentation are all factors in the increasing frequency of fungal endocarditis as well.

Fever, weakness, night sweats, and anorexia are common presenting complaints. Physical examination commonly reveals a cardiac murmur; splinter hemorrhages, Osler nodes, Janeway lesions, and Roth spots are classic findings. Blood cultures are positive in 85% to 95% of patients due to persistent bacteremia from seeding of the bloodstream from vegetations, which can be visualized by echocardiography in many cases. Cardiac catheterization is useful for demonstration of hemodynamic and anatomic abnormalities caused by infective endocarditis; however, catheterization is generally not necessary for patients with acute hemodynamic instability and may cause embolization in patients with aortic valve endocarditis. Medical management with appropriate i.v. antibiotics is the treatment of choice for most patients with infective endocarditis. Valve replacement is reserved for prosthetic valve endocarditis, failure of medical management, life-threatening emboli, severe valvular insufficiency or obstruction, and congestive heart failure.

Valve Prostheses

The three general types of prosthetic valves used for valve replacement are (i) mechanical valves, which include caged ball, tilting disk, and bileaflet designs, (ii) tissue heterograft valves, which include glutaraldehyde-preserved native porcine valves and fabricated bovine pericardial prostheses, and (iii) aortic valve homografts, which are cryopreserved after being harvested from human cadaveric hearts. In general, the advantages of mechanical valves reside in their durability, and in the case of tilting disk and bileaflet designs, the advantages lie in the low profile of the prosthesis. Disadvantages of mechanical valves include a higher incidence of thromboembolic events, anticoaguation-related complications, hemolysis, and perivalvular leaks. In contrast, tissue valves may not require permanent anticoagulation and have fewer thromboembolic and perivalvular leak complications but degenerate over time and have a tendency to calcify. Many tissue heterograft valves will require replacement after 10 to 14 years. Calcific degeneration is accelerated in younger patients and use of valves is generally contraindicated in pediatric and adolescent patients for this reason.

Current recommendations are that tissue valves be reserved for patients with a limited life expectancy (those older than 70 years) or for those who have contraindications for permanent anticoagulation. The St. Jude mechanical valve (bileaflet design) is recommended for pediatric and young adult patients because of durability and superior hemodynamics. Homograft valves are commonly used for the repair of complex congenital malformations or in patients with native or prosthetic valve endocarditis. Long-term follow-up of patients with cryopreserved homograft valves is limited; however, durability of these grafts up to 15 years has been reported.

Valve Repair

The significant consequences of valve replacement with prostheses including thromboembolism, valve dysfunction, infection, anticoagulation, bleeding, and hemolysis have led to efforts to develop techniques for valve repair. Currently, tricuspid and mitral valvuloplasty are considered preferable to valve replacement when technically feasible because of lower morbidity and mortality. Operative repair and bal-

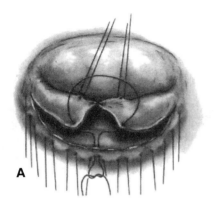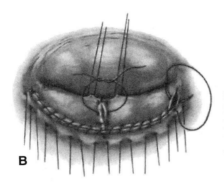

FIGURE 20-5. Quadrangular resection of the posterior mitral valve leaflet and mitral valve annuloplasty for mitral valve prolapse. The free edges of the resected margin are reapproximated in the midline and the posterior valve is sutured to the annulus. (From Kaiser LR, Kron IL, Spray TL, eds. *Mastery of cardiothoracic surgery.* Philadelphia: Lippincott-Raven Publishers, 1998, with permission.)

loon valvuloplasty of the aortic valve, on the other hand, have had disappointing results.

Prosthetic ring annuloplasty is a central technique for valve repair and is required in most cases of mitral insufficiency. The basic principle is to reduce the size and restore the shape of the dilated annulus. More complex repairs involving chordal transposition, cuneiform resection of elongated papillary muscles, and resection of secondary or marginal chordae are tailored to the individual lesion. Figure 20-5 illustrates a quadrangular resection of the posterior leaflet of the mitral valve and annuloplasty to correct mitral valve prolapse. Competency of repaired valves is tested by saline injection and intraoperative transesophageal echocardiography, allowing immediate evaluation and revision of repairs at the same operation.

A number of factors are thought to contribute to the lower morbidity and mortality associated with valve repair. The ability to perform valve repair, as opposed to valve replacement, has prompted earlier referrals, which allows better long-term results. Left ventricle function is improved with valve repair possibly because continuity between the mitral valve and the ventricular wall is maintained via the chordae and papillary muscles, which is thought to play an important role during isometric contraction and results in increased stroke volume. Endocarditis and thromboembolism are rare following valve repair and anticoagulation is not required. Long-term follow-up has demonstrated that mitral valve repair is durable, particularly for patients with myxomatous or degenerative disease, as compared to patients with rheumatic valve disease who tend to have more subvalvular scarring and patients with ischemic mitral regurgitation in whom papillary muscle or regional ventricular wall dysfunction may be seen.

Arrhythmia Surgery and Pacemakers

Endocardial catheter and surgical procedures have been developed for the treatment of medically refractory supraventricular and ventricular tachyarrhythmia. Although diagnosis of these arrhythmias can frequently be made by routine electrocardiogram, further electrophysiologic evaluation is generally necessary before intervention. Supraventricular tachycardia involving an accessory A-V connection (Wolff-Parkinson-White Syndrome), A-V nodal reentry, enhanced A-V nodal conduction, ectopic automatic atrial tachycardia, Mahaim fibers, or concealed accessory connections that conduct retrograde may require ablation of aberrant connections using endocardial catheter or open surgical techniques.

Ventricular arrhythmias potentially amenable to direct surgical treatment include monomorphic ventricular tachycardia and ventricular fibrillation evolving from monomorphic ventricular tachycardia. Surgical treatment may involve excision or ablation of tissue responsible for initiating the arrhythmia, implantation of an automatic implantable cardioverter defibrillator that terminates the arrhythmia, revascularization of ischemic myocardium that is demonstrated to initiate or sustain the arrhythmia, or a combination of the above. Thorough preoperative evaluation is therefore critical to establish the indication for surgery and to guide the choice of the most appropriate procedure.

Insertion of a permanent pacemaker is frequently necessary for the treatment of patients with bradyarrhythmia. Generally accepted indications for permanent pacing are

TABLE 20-4. INDICATIONS FOR PERMANENT PACEMAKER INSERTION[a]

Sick sinus syndrome
Symptomatic type II arteriovenous block
Complete arteriovenous block
Bilateral bundle branch block following acute myocardial infarction
Bifascicular or trifascicular block with symptomatic bradycardia or with intermittent type II arteriovenous block
Carotid sinus syncope
Intractable low cardiac output syndrome benefited by temporary pacing

[a]From Lowe JE, Wharton JM. Cardiac pacemakers and implantable cardioverter-defibrillators. In: Sabiston DC Jr, Spencer FC, eds. *Surgery of the chest,* 6th ed. Philadelphia: WB Saunders, 1995:1763–1813, with permission.

given in Table 20-4. The most commonly used pacing systems are VVI and DDD systems. VVI (ventricular-demand) systems sense and pace only the ventricle and therefore lack A-V synchrony, which may not be important in patients with slow atrial fibrillation and who are not able to respond to increased physiologic stress by increasing heart rate. DDD systems sense and pace both chambers and therefore maintain A-V synchrony, which has been associated with a 20% to 25% increase in cardiac output, and which can increase heart rate with increasing physiologic demand.

Cardiac Neoplasms

Primary cardiac neoplasms are rare, with an incidence of less than 0.25% in autopsy series. Nevertheless, because they represent one of the potentially curable forms of cardiac disease, their early diagnosis and management has assumed increasing emphasis.

Approximately 70% to 80% of primary cardiac neoplasms are benign, with myxoma being by far the most common lesion in this group except in children. Myxomas account for approximately 75% of benign cardiac neoplasms and 50% of all primary cardiac tumors. They are derived from multipotential mesenchymal cells and grossly present as polypoid masses projecting into the cardiac chamber from the endocardium. Approximately 75% of myxomas occur in the left atrium, typically arising from the limbus of the fossa ovalis. Twenty percent of myxomas occur in the right atrium, and 5% in more than one chamber. Myxomas arising from the ventricles are extremely rare. These tumors have been reported in all age groups; however, they are most frequently seen in women in the fourth, fifth, and sixth decades. Rarely, familial forms may be inherited in an autosomal dominant fashion. The most frequent presentation is with mitral valve obstruction and embolism. Surgical resection is indicated after diagnosis is confirmed, usually by echocardiography. Preoperative coronary angiography should be considered in patients older than 40 years if the clinical setting allows. Rhabdomyomas account for approximately 20% of benign cardiac neoplasms and are the most common tumor in pediatric populations. These lesions are typically of ventricular origin, poorly encapsulated, multicentric, and may not be resectable.

Almost all malignant primary cardiac neoplasms are sarcomas. The most common types are angiosarcoma, rhabdomyosarcoma, and fibrosarcoma. These tumors tend to grow rapidly with invasion and displacement of cardiac and mediastinal structures leading to progressive congestive heart failure. Metastases are present at the time of diagnosis in up to 80% of cases. The prognosis for this disease is poor, with the median survival in surgically treated patients being less than 1 year. Metastatic tumors to the heart are the most common cardiac neoplasms. The major types secondarily invading the heart are bronchogenic carcinoma, melanoma, leukemia, lymphoma, and carcinoma of the breast.

Cardiovascular Trauma

Penetrating Cardiac Injury

Penetrating cardiac injury is a highly morbid event, with 50% to 80% of patients dying before presentation to an emergency room. Mortality is higher for gunshot injuries than stab wounds. The most commonly injured structure is the right ventricle, followed by the left ventricle, right atrium, and left atrium. The intrapericardiac superior vena cava, inferior vena cava, or great vessels are involved in approximately 5% of cases. Intrapericardiac injury to any of these structures may cause cardiac tamponade, which presents with systemic hypotension, distended neck veins, and narrowed pulse pressure. Pericardiocentesis and removal of as little as 20 mL of blood from the pericardium may allow stabilization before definitive repair is attempted. For patients arriving at the emergency room in extremis, emergent left anterolateral thoracotomy may be performed as a resuscitative and therapeutic measure. For patients presenting with associated intraabdominal injury, cardiac repair precedes laparotomy. Injuries to major coronary arteries can be bypassed but will require standard cardiopulmonary bypass in most cases. Injuries to the distal third of the LAD can be ligated. Valve injuries and VSDs may present later, depending on the hemodynamic significance of the lesions.

Blunt Cardiovascular Trauma

Automobile accidents are the most common cause of blunt trauma leading to cardiovascular injury. Blunt chest trauma can cause cardiac contusion, which may resolve or lead to myocardial infarction. Electrocardiogram findings in cardiac contusion include ventricular arrhythmias, supraventricular tachyarrhythmia, bundle branch block, Q waves, ST segment elevation, heart block, or cardiac standstill. Valve injuries more commonly follow blunt trauma than penetrating injuries. Echocardiography is useful to evaluate valve function and ventricular contractility. Patients diagnosed with cardiac contusion should be monitored for 24 to 48 hours with serial cardiac enzyme measurements and electrocardiograms.

Blunt trauma to the chest can cause injury to the thoracic aorta as well. The most commonly affected regions are the areas of the ligamentum arteriosum and the pericardial reflection over the ascending aorta. Patients with free aortic rupture die at the scene of the accident. Approximately 15% to 20% of patients with aortic injuries may survive to be evaluated at the hospital. Chest roentgenograms show widening of the mediastinum in most cases and should be followed by aortogram, chest computed tomography (CT), or transesophageal echocardiogram.

Surgical repair of contained aortic rupture generally requires replacement of the involved segment with a prosthetic graft. Circulatory management during aortic repair may involve the clamp-and-sew technique, heparin-bonded shunt, or partial cardiopulmonary bypass, depending on the clinical circumstances. Paraplegia resulting from spinal cord ischemia remains an important complication of thoracic aortic surgery and has a higher incidence in the setting of traumatic rupture because of the absence of collateral circulation.

Aortic Dissection

Aortic dissection refers to development of a hematoma within the middle to outer third of the media of the aorta. In approximately 95% of cases, this hematoma originates from a tear in the aortic intima and media and can extend around the circumference of the aorta as well as proximally and distally from the site of the tear. Aortic dissection commonly is associated with cystic medial necrosis, which is a tissue factor defect associated with Marfan syndrome that may also occur sporadically. Dissection of the aorta also is associated with aortic stenosis, particularly the bicuspid type, and a history of hypertension. The most common symptom of dissection is severe back pain. Occlusion of arteries by extension of the hematoma can lead to loss of pulses, stroke, and limb or end-organ ischemia.

Aortic dissections are classified by duration and anatomy. Acute dissections are defined as being less than 2 weeks old, whereas chronic dissections have occurred 2 weeks or more earlier. The most useful anatomic classification system is the Stanford system, because initial surgical versus medical management generally follows this system. In the Stanford classification, type A dissections involve the ascending aorta and type B dissections do not (Fig. 20-6). Emergent surgical repair of acute type A dissections is indicated because of the high mortality associated with this

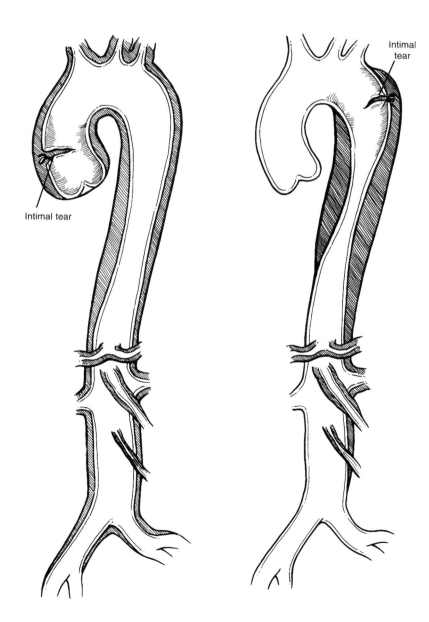

FIGURE 20-6. The Stanford classification of aortic dissections. (From Kaiser LR, Kron IL, Spray TL, eds. *Mastery of cardiothoracic surgery*. Philadelphia: Lippincott-Raven Publishers, 1998, with permission.)

lesion. Approximately 80% of these patients die within the first week because of free rupture, pericardial tamponade, myocardial infarction secondary to extension to the coronary ostia, or massive aortic insufficiency and congestive heart failure. Acute type B dissections are initially treated medically with control of hypertension unless there is evidence of aortic rupture into the left chest or severe major organ or limb ischemia from aortic branch obstruction.

The indications for surgical repair of chronic dissections differ. Type A dissections, which are not diagnosed acutely, are repaired for late development of aortic insufficiency and congestive heart failure or aneurysmal dilation of the ascending aorta exceeding 5 cm. Chronic type B dissections are repaired for aneurysmal dilation of the descending aorta greater than 6 cm.

A goal of surgical repair is to replace the segment of aorta containing the intimal tear with a prosthetic graft whenever possible. For acute type A dissections, aortic replacement is limited to the ascending aorta and proximal aortic arch, even when the dissection extends distally. This procedure effectively eliminates the causes of death related to type A dissection without exposing the patient to the hazards of replacement of the entire aorta. Lifetime follow-up with serial magnetic resonance imaging (MRI) or CT scans is necessary to identify the 5% to 10% of patients who develop aneurysmal dilation of the aorta at other points of reentry distal to the original intimal tear.

Aneurysms of the Thoracic Aorta

Ascending and Arch Aneurysms

Ascending and arch aneurysms of the aorta result from atherosclerosis, chronic dissection, and cystic medial necrosis. Ascending aortic aneurysms are repaired on cardiopulmonary bypass and may require a valved conduit with reimplantation of the coronary ostia into the graft when there is associated annuloaortic ectasia. Repair of arch aneurysms typically necessitates a period of total circulatory arrest under profound hypothermia (14° to 15°C core temperature). Retrograde cerebral perfusion via the superior vena cava during this period may decrease the incidence of central nervous system ischemic complications.

Descending Thoracic and Thoracoabdominal Aneurysms

Descending thoracic and thoracoabdominal aneurysms result from atherosclerosis or degenerative disease in most cases. Other etiologies include chronic dissections, contained traumatic transections, cystic medial necrosis, and aortitis. Commonly, descending thoracic aneurysms originate at the left subclavian artery and terminate above the diaphragm. Patients may be asymptomatic or present with upper back pain or hoarseness when the aneurysm compresses the recurrent laryngeal nerve. Aortogram, CT, MRI, and transesophageal echocardiography are used to delineate the anatomic extent of the lesion.

The size indications for surgical repair are controversial; however, repair is usually recommended for asymptomatic patients with aneurysms greater than 6 to 8 cm in diameter. This is because of the poor prognosis of patients after diagnosis of descending thoracic aneurysm. Up to 60% to 70% of patients with aneurysms larger than 6 cm die within 2 years of diagnosis and at least half of these deaths result from rupture. Symptomatic aneurysms should be repaired irrespective of size.

Circulatory management during repair typically involves some method of distal perfusion. This may be accomplished with the use of left atrial to femoral artery bypass or a heparin-bonded shunt to the distal aorta or femoral artery. A major source of morbidity is spinal cord ischemia leading to paraplegia. The arteria magna provides most of the blood supply to the region of the spinal cord at risk and arises variably between the T-8 and L-4 vertebral bodies. Because of this, every attempt is made to preserve all large intercostals not involved in the aneurysm. Use of the clamp-and-sew technique has been associated with a higher incidence of spinal cord ischemia, particularly when clamp times exceed 30 minutes. Intraoperative spinal cord monitoring by measurement of somatosensory or motor evoked potentials has been used in an attempt to limit this complication. Thoracoabdominal aortic aneurysms are repaired using a branch inclusion technique with direct anastomosis of branch vessels to the graft.

SUGGESTED READING

Alexander RW, Schlant RC, Fuster V, eds. *Hurst's the heart, arteries and veins,* 9th ed. New York: McGraw Hill, 1998.

Baue AE, Geha AS, Hammond GL, et al., eds. *Glenn's thoracic and cardiovascular surgery,* 6th ed. Stamford: Appleton & Lange, 1996.

Braunwald E, ed. *Heart disease: a textbook of cardiovascular medicine,* 5th ed. Philadelphia: WB Saunders, 1997.

Kaiser LR, Kron IL, Spray TL, eds. *Mastery of cardiothoracic surgery.* Philadelphia: Lippincott-Raven Publishers, 1998.

Sabiston DC Jr, Spencer FC, eds. *Surgery of the chest,* 6th ed. Philadelphia: WB Saunders, 1995.

21

VASCULAR DISEASE AND VASCULAR SURGERY

DAVID G. NESCHIS AND MICHAEL A. GOLDEN

BASIC VASCULAR ANATOMY AND PHYSIOLOGY

Atherosclerosis remains the most significant cause of death and serious morbidity in the Western world. Fifty percent of all deaths in the United States are attributed to atherosclerosis. This disease can affect any artery; however, prime targets include the aorta, the lower extremities, and the coronary and cerebral systems. Atherosclerosis is slowly progressive, with plaques developing insidiously until end-organ damage manifests itself often in the form of ischemic symptoms or actual infarction involving the heart, brain, extremities, or internal organs.

Atherosclerosis is the most common form of arteriosclerosis, or "hardening of the arteries." *Arteriosclerosis* refers to a group of disorders that are distinguished by thickening and loss of elasticity of the arterial wall.

Atherosclerosis is characterized by the formation of atheromas, fibrofatty plaques consisting of a raised focal plaque within the intima, having a core of lipid separated from the lumen by a covering fibrous cap.

Mönckeberg medial calcific sclerosis is characterized by calcification of the media of muscular arteries.

Arteriolosclerosis is distinguished by proliferative or hyaline thickening of the walls of small arteries and arterioles.

Normal Structure of the Vessel Wall

The structure of the vascular wall is organized into several layers (Fig. 21-1).

The *tunica intima* is composed of a lining of endothelial cells with underlying subendothelial connective tissue consisting of collagen, proteoglycans, elastin, and numerous other matrix glycoproteins. The boundaries of the intima are the vessel lumen and the internal elastic lamina, a longitudinally oriented layer of elastic fibers. This layer is not continuous but is interrupted by fenestrae, through which smooth muscle cells may migrate into the intima.

Hospital of the University of Pennsylvania, Philadelphia, Pennsylvania

The *tunica media* is made up of concentric layers of smooth muscle cells alternating with layers of fine elastic fibers. These elastic fibers condense as a poorly defined external elastic membrane, forming the outer boundary of the tunica media. The medial smooth muscle cells are dispersed in a matrix made of elastin, collagen, and proteoglycan. The media is, in general, poorly vascularized, with the inner layers relying mostly on diffusion of nutrients from the lumen. In arteries with greater than 28 elastic layers, a microvasculature known as the "vasa vasorum" penetrates the media from the adventitial side. The vasa vasorum provide nutrient blood flow to the inner media.

The *tunica adventitia* lies outside the external elastic lamina and consists of a poorly defined layer of connective tissue in which elastic and nerve fibers are dispersed.

Arteries can be divided into three categories. Large or elastic arteries include the aorta, brachiocephalic, subclavian, and the beginnings of the common carotid and pulmonary arteries. The larger vessels are rich in elastin, providing these vessels with resilience that aids in the forward propulsion of blood in diastole. This elasticity is progressively lost during the aging process, predisposing these vessels to stretching and elongation, leading to tortuosity in older age groups. Histologically, the internal elastic lamina is not as distinct as in the medium-size arteries. The medium-size, or muscular, arteries have well-defined elastic laminae separating the three layers. The adventitia of these vessels is particularly rich in nerve fibers, likely related to the role they play in the autonomic regulation of blood flow. In the small arteries, there is a progressive loss of both the internal elastic membrane and the external elastic membrane, so by the prearteriolar level, the distinction between layers is lost. The arterioles are richly supplied by nervous tissue, being the major site of autonomic control of vascular flow. The anatomical and histological distinction between these types of arteries is important in that the pattern of pathology in each class of vessel is distinct. For instance, atherosclerosis is generally a disease of the large and muscular arteries while hypertension is often associated with changes in the smaller arteries and arterioles.

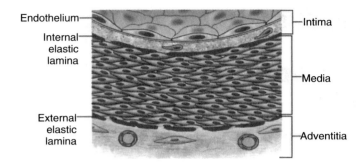

FIGURE 21-1. Structure of the vascular wall. (From *Robbins, Pathologic basis of disease*, 6th ed. Philadelphia: WB Saunders, 1999:494, with permission.

In general, the *veins* are thin-walled vessels with indistinct layers and relatively large lumina. The thin walls predispose these vessels to dilation, compression, and tumor invasion. Many veins, particularly those of the extremities, possess valves that help maintain the unidirectional flow of blood back to the heart.

Lymphatics are very thin walled structures lined by endothelium. These channels are involved in the return of extracellular fluid to the circulation. The largest lymphatic channels possess a thin muscular wall as well as valves.

It is clear that the *vascular endothelium* is not simply a passive nonsticky surface; rather, it is a dynamic, multifunctional cell layer. Endothelial cells produce various substances that affect smooth muscle including the vasodilators prostaglandin I_2 and E_2, adenosine, and endothelium-derived relaxing factor (EDRF) and the potent vasoconstrictor endothelin. The predominant EDRF is nitric oxide, which is derived from the breakdown of arginine. Factors that stimulate endothelial cells to secrete EDRF include thrombin, acetylcholine, bradykinin, serotonin, and products of platelet release. These same, often thrombogenic, substances, which cause vasodilation in the presence of endothelium, cause vasoconstriction when the endothelium is either absent or dysfunctional. It appears that endothelial cells can sense changes in blood velocity and shear and respond in order to maintain a consistent flow. A common pattern is the ability of diseased arteries to dilate in response to luminal narrowing by either stenosis or an atherosclerotic plaque. This vasodilation is felt to be mediated by the above mentioned substances such that luminal diameter is maintained. Once the plaque occupies over 40% of the luminal cross-sectional area, the ability to vasodilate is overcome and pathological luminal narrowing occurs.

The bulk of the vessel wall consists of *smooth muscle cells* and the surrounding *extracellular matrix*. The vascular smooth muscle cells are regulated by a multitude of substances. Platelet-derived growth factor (PDGF) is produced mainly by platelets, but other cells including endothelial and smooth muscle cells as well as leukocytes can express the PDGF gene. PDGF is felt to be an important chemoattractant, particularly stimulating the migration of medial smooth muscle cells to the tunica intima in response to vascular injury. A powerful mitogen for smooth muscle cells is fibroblast growth factor (FGF), particularly basic FGF (bFGF), which is felt to be released by injured smooth muscle cells, thereby stimulating smooth muscle cell proliferation in response to vascular injury. Other growth factors, such as transforming growth factor β, may be important in regulating the production of extracellular matrix surrounding the smooth muscle cells. Additionally, there is neuroendocrine control of smooth muscle growth. For example, serotonin, neurokinin A, substance K, and substance P all can affect smooth muscle cell hypertrophy and proliferation.

Risk Factors for Arterial Occlusive Disease

Age

The earliest lesions are seen even in childhood. Death rates from ischemic heart disease rise with each decade, even up to 75 to 85 years. Interestingly, death rates from myocardial infarction seem to decline after age 75.

Sex

Death rates from ischemic heart disease for men outweigh those for women between 75 and 85 years, at which time both genders appear to be affected equally. Myocardial infarction in a premenopausal woman is quite rare.

Family Predisposition

This appears to be a risk factor independent of families merely sharing similar diet and health habits.

Hyperlipidemia

There is a large body of evidence to suggest that hypercholesterolemia is a major risk factor for atherosclerosis. It is evident that atheromatous plaques are rich in cholesterol, and that such plaques can be produced routinely in various experimental animals, including primates, by feeding them a high-cholesterol diet. Children with genetic hyperlipidemia develop severe atheromatous plaques early in life without possessing other risk factors. Population studies have shown that groups with higher levels of blood cholesterol have higher rates of ischemic heart disease.

Hypertension

It is clear that elevated blood pressure is associated with accelerated growth of atherosclerotic plaques and subsequent end-organ damage such as ischemic heart or cerebrovascular disease. It would also appear that the higher the blood pressure, the greater the risk. This risk correlates best with diastolic pressure and after age 45, appears to be a greater risk factor than hypercholesterolemia.

Cigarette Smoking

The death rate in male smokers (one or more packs per day) can be as high as 200% that of nonsmokers. The recent increase in the death rate from ischemic heart disease in women correlates with increased cigarette smoking as well. It has been demonstrated that men at high risk can reduce their risk of dying of ischemic heart disease by smoking cessation.

Diabetes

Diabetes is associated with a twofold increase in the incidence of myocardial infarction and an 8-fold to 15-fold increased frequency of gangrene of the lower extremities.

Other Risk Factors

Other risk factors include sedentary lifestyle, type A personality, stress, obesity, use of oral contraceptives, hyperuricemia, and high carbohydrate intake. Clearly a combination of risk factors significantly increases the risk, with patients having three or more major risk factors having a seven times greater risk of developing myocardial infarction.

Lipid Metabolism

All lipids circulate in combination with protein. "Apoprotein" is the term used for the protein moiety of a conjugated protein or protein complex. The major plasma lipoproteins can be divided by their varying densities.

Chylomicrons have the lowest density of the lipoproteins, are composed of 80% to 95% dietary triglycerides, are found in the plasma only after a meal, and are associated with apolipoproteins C, A-I, A-II, and B-48. Chylomicrons are involved in the exogenous pathway of cholesterol transport (Fig. 21-2). In this pathway, dietary triglycerides and cholesterol are incorporated with the above mentioned apolipoproteins into chylomicrons within the intestinal epithelial cells. These chylomicrons, via intestinal lymphatics, reach peripheral capillaries, where endothelial lipoprotein lipase, activated by apolipoprotein C-II, hydrolyzes the chylomicron to liberate fatty acids for adipose and muscle tissue. The remaining chylomicron remnant is now rich in cholesterol. Chylomicron remnant receptors in the liver recognize the B-48 apoprotein and take up the remnant by pinocytosis. The result is that chylomicrons, via the exogenous pathway, transport dietary cholesterol to the liver and triglycerides to the adipose and muscle tissue.

The main function of *very low density lipoproteins* (VLDLs) is to transport triglycerides that have been synthesized in the liver. They are made up of 45% to 65% endogenous triglyceride and 25% endogenous cholesterol and are associated with apolipoproteins C, E, and B-48.

Intermediate density lipoproteins (IDLs) are composed of 45% cholesterol and are associated with apolipoproteins B-100 and E. They are remnants following the hydrolysis of VLDL by endothelial lipoprotein lipase (activated by apolipoprotein C-II on VLDLs).

Low density lipoproteins (LDLs) are made up of 70% cholesterol and are the primary transporters of endogenous cholesterol. They are associated with apoprotein B-100.

High density lipoproteins (HDLs) are composed of less than 25% cholesterol and are also a major transporter of endogenous cholesterol. HDLs are associated with apolipoproteins A-I and A-II.

The endogenous pathway of cholesterol transport refers to the cholesterol that is produced in the liver. In this pathway, VLDL, containing triglycerides and apolipoproteins E, C, and B-100, is secreted by the liver. Hydrolysis by lipoprotein lipase yields triglycerides for muscle and adipose tissue, and via the formation of IDL, forms LDL. LDL is associated with a single apolipoprotein, B-100, which is recognized by the LDL receptors on hepatic and extrahepatic cells. Two thirds of the LDL is taken up and metabolized by various cells while the remaining third is degraded by non-LDL-receptor–dependent mechanisms. HDL transports unesterified cholesterol derived for cell membrane turnover to the plasma, after which time the action of lecithin-cholesterol acyltransferase (LCAT) delivers cholesterol from HDL to LDL. Apolipoprotein A-I appears to be the activator of LCAT. It is felt that the inverse relationship between high levels of HDL and the development of atheromatous plaques is due to the ability of HDL to clear cholesterol from the plaque and deliver it to the liver, where is may be excreted rather than utilized.

Pathogenesis of Atherosclerosis

The principal lesion of atherosclerosis is the *atheromatous plaque.* The plaque is made up of a superficial fibrous cap and a deeper necrotic core. The fibrous plaque consists of smooth muscle cells, leukocytes, and dense connective tissue with an underlying more cellular layer containing a mixture of macrophages, smooth muscle cells, and T lymphocytes. Deep to this is a necrotic core containing necrotic debris, extracellular lipid, primarily cholesterol and cholesterol ester, lipid laden foam cells, fibrin, and various plasma proteins. The lipid-laden foam cells are mostly smooth muscle cells and macrophages (Fig. 21-3).

Atheromatous plaques become most significant clinically when they develop into complicated plaques. They may become calcified, rendering the affected vessel brittle and noncompliant. The plaque may become ulcerated and rup-

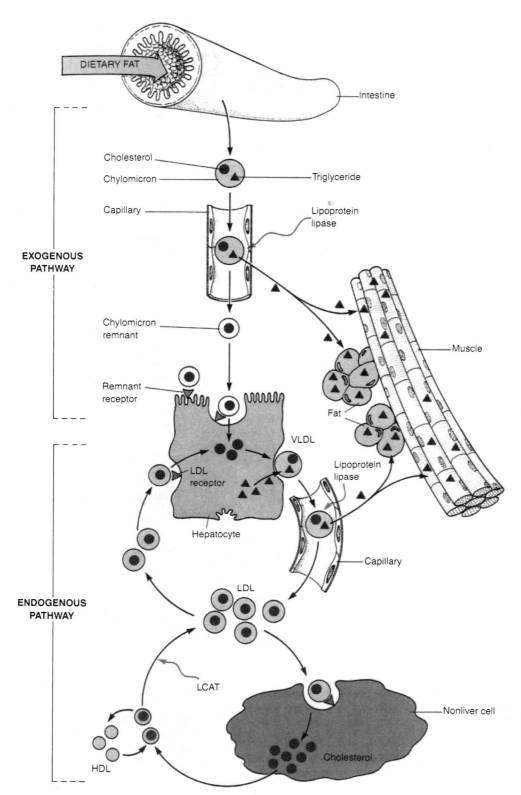

FIGURE 21-2. Cholesterol transport pathways. (From Benditt EP, Schwartz SM. Blood vessels. In: Rubin E, Farber JL, eds. *Pathology*, 2nd ed. Philadelphia: JB Lippincott Co, 1994:477, with permission.)

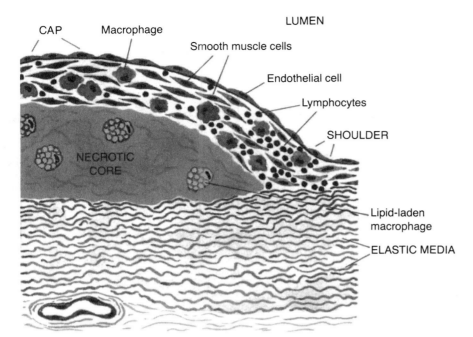

FIGURE 21-3. Plaque in atherosclerosis. (From Benditt EP, Schwartz SM. Blood vessels. In: Rubin E, Farber JL, eds. *Pathology,* 2nd ed. Philadelphia: JB Lippincott Co, 1994:472, with permission.)

ture, leading to the discharge of emboli into the circulation. Atherosclerotic lesions are prone to superimposed thrombosis, often leading to the most devastating complications in affected end organs. Hemorrhage into the plaque can also occur with subsequent luminal occlusion.

Atheromatous plaques are generally found in consistent locations. Common sites of plaque formation include the coronary arteries, the femoral arteries, the popliteal arteries, the descending thoracic aorta, the abdominal aorta, the internal carotid arteries, and major intracranial vessels. The abdominal aorta is more frequently affected than the thoracic aorta, and aortic lesions are generally found at the ostia of major branches.

Current Theories of Atherosclerosis

Reaction to Injury Hypothesis

This theory assumes that the initial event in the formation of an atherosclerotic lesion is injury to the endothelium or endothelial dysfunction resulting in increased permeability. Such injury can be due to deposition of immune complexes, irradiation, or chemical causes. Frank denudation of the endothelium is not necessary. Risk factors such as hypertension and smoking may also cause endothelial injury or increased permeability. Hemodynamic forces such as turbulence and sheer stress may also have a role and might help explain the propensity for lesions to develop at sites of arterial bifurcation. Endothelial injury and increased permeability allow adherence of platelets and monocytes to the vessel wall. Adherent platelets become activated and express growth factors such as PDGF that stimulate medial smooth muscle cells to migrate to the intima, where they may proliferate and deposit extracellular matrix. These processes are mediated by other growth factors such as bFGF and transforming growth factors. Additionally, monocytes that have invaded the vessel wall transform into macrophages, which take up cholesterol, which undergoes

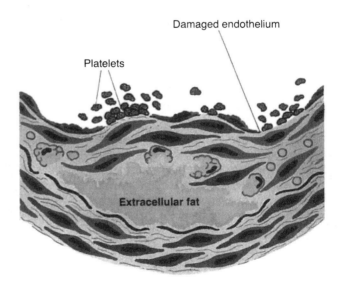

FIGURE 21-4. Reaction to injury. (From Benditt EP, Schwartz SM. Blood vessels. In: Rubin E, Farber JL, eds. *Pathology,* 2nd ed. Philadelphia: JB Lippincott Co, 1994:469, with permission.)

hydrolysis and reesterification followed by storage in lipid-laden droplets, thus forming the foam cells characteristic of the atherosclerotic lesion (Fig. 21-4).

Other Theories of Atherosclerosis

Other theories of atherosclerosis are generally based on the hypothesis that smooth muscle proliferation in the absence of endothelial injury may be the initiating event, with endothelial injury being a secondary phenomenon. Inflammation has also been thought to cause the arterial changes observed in atherosclerosis. Some theories suggest that elevated levels of lipids or oxidized lipids may reach the smooth muscle cells, resulting in smooth muscle cell injury or another trigger of proliferation. The monoclonal hypothesis of atherogenesis has been spurred by the observation that some human plaques seem to be composed of the progeny of a single cell. These observations suggest that smooth muscle cell growth may be similar to other forms of neoplastic proliferation, potentially initiated by genetic mutation. Exogenous chemicals or viruses may cause such mutations. It is likely that most clinically significant lesions are the result of multiple origins.

Arterial Hemodynamics

The major components of the arterial wall include collagen, elastin, and smooth muscle cells. Collagen is mainly responsible for the wall strength of the vessel and increases in content with increasing vessel diameter. Elastin is highly deformable and is responsible for vascular compliance. The larger central arteries are rich in elastin, allowing expansion in systole and recoil during diastole, thereby buffering changes in systemic pressure during the cardiac cycle. In more distal medium to large vessels, the muscular content relative to elastin increases, leading to decreased compliance. Although the resting tone in these vessels does not contribute greatly to peripheral resistance, it does augment systolic pressure and pulse-wave propagation. In the smaller arteries and arterioles, the high muscular content creates a high wall-thickness to lumen ratio, which makes these vessels the prime determinants of peripheral resistance.

Fluid Pressure

The pressure of a fluid system is defined as force per unit area (given in dynes per square centimeter). Intravascular arterial pressure (P) is the additive sum of three components including the dynamic pressure produced by the contracting heart, the hydrostatic pressure, and the static filling pressure. The hydrostatic contribution results from the weight of a column of blood between the heart and the position of pressure measurement—i.e., the hydrostatic component is additive in areas below the heart in the erect individual and negative in sites above the heart.

Hydrostatic pressure is defined as $P(\text{hydrostatic}) = -\rho g h$, where ρ is the specific gravity of blood (approximately 1.056 g/cm^3), g is the acceleration of gravity (980 cm/s^2), and h is the height in centimeters of the site of measurement above the point of reference (heart).

The static filling pressure represents the residual pressure existing in the absence of arterial flow. The volume of blood and elastic properties of the vessel wall determine this pressure (usually 5 to 10 mm Hg).

Fluid Energy

Total fluid energy (E) is the sum of the potential energy (E_p) and the kinetic energy (E_k). The components of potential energy are intravascular pressure (P) and gravitational potential energy. The components of intravascular pressure are described above. Gravitational potential energy is generated from the same factors as the hydrostatic pressure but with an opposite sign, i.e., $+\rho g h$. The result is that the hydrostatic pressure and the gravitational potential energy usually cancel each other out, and the main component of potential energy is produced by cardiac contraction. Potential energy can be expressed as

$$E_p = P + (\rho g h)$$

Kinetic energy represents the ability of the blood to do work on the basis of its motion. This is proportional to the specific gravity of blood and the square of its velocity, in centimeters per second.

$$E_k = \tfrac{1}{2} \rho v^2$$

Therefore, the total fluid energy per unit volume of blood (in ergs per cubic centimeter) is as follows:

$$E = P + (\rho g h) + \tfrac{1}{2} \rho v^2$$

In an idealized system, these formulas can be combined into the *Bernoulli principle* of the conservation of energy between two separate points along a single tube, this being

$$P + (\rho g h)_1 + \tfrac{1}{2} \rho v_1^2 = P + (\rho g h)_2 + \tfrac{1}{2} \rho v_2^2$$

This relationship explains the consistent flow of a fluid in a tube in which there is a change in the diameter of the tube. The increase in potential energy attributed to an increase in pressure is matched by a similar decrease in kinetic energy due to decreased velocity. Therefore, the total energy in the system remains the same. This relationship can be simplified such that flow (Q), which must remain constant, is the product of the fluid velocity (v) and cross-sectional area (A) such that

$$Q = v \times A = v \times \pi r^2,$$

where r is the tube radius.

Principles of Blood Flow

An ideal fluid is one in which there is no internal friction between layers of the fluid—i.e., no viscosity (discussed below), no friction with the conduit, and all fluid particles flowing at the same velocity. This would result in a flat

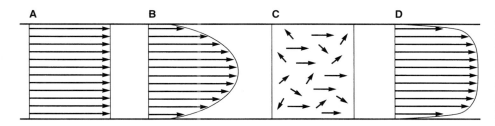

FIGURE 21-5. A: Flat profile. **B:** Parabolic profile. **C:** Chaotic profile. **D:** Blunted profile. (From Cronenwett JL. Arterial hemodynamics. In: Greenfield LJ, Mulholland MW, Oldham KT, et al., eds. *Surgery: scientific principles and practice*, 1st ed. Philadelphia: JB Lippincott Co, 1993:1515, with permission.)

velocity profile (Fig. 21-5A). In a real system, there are invariably cohesive forces with the conduit wall, with layers of fluid in contact with the conduit approaching zero velocity and a gradient of increasing velocity with increasing distance from the conduit wall. This results in a parabolic profile for laminar flow (Fig. 21-5B). Because arteries are not straight smooth tubes but have multiple branches and lesions, laminar flow is disrupted, resulting in *turbulence*. At any point, the velocity of the fluid particles would appear chaotic (Fig. 21-5C). However, when averaged over time, the mean velocity profile is similar to true laminar flow, only with a blunted appearance (Fig. 21-5D).

Turbulence can be expressed as a dimensionless quantity called the "Reynolds number" (Re), which is the ratio of inertial forces to viscous forces acting on the fluid.

$Re = dV\rho/\eta$,

where d is the tube diameter in centimeters, V the mean velocity, ρ the specific gravity of the fluid, and η the fluid viscosity.

In flowing blood, it is at Reynolds numbers greater than 2,000 when inertial forces may disrupt laminar flow and produce turbulence. In most normal arteries, Reynolds numbers are less than 2,000.

Shear stress (τ) is the stress, or force (F), per unit area (A) required to overcome the friction between adjacent fluid layers, where

$\tau(dyn/cm^2) = F/A$

Shear rate (D) is defined as the velocity gradient (dv) that develops between fluid layers divided by the distance (radius or dr) between adjacent layers.

$D(s^{-1}) = dv/dr$

Viscosity (η) describes the resistance to blood flow that arises because of the intermolecular attractions between fluid layers. Viscosity is measured in pois or $dyn/s^{-1}/cm^2$. Viscosity is defined as the ratio of sheer stress to shear rate.

$\eta = \tau/D = (F \times dr)/(A \times dv)$

Fluids with strong intermolecular attractions offer a high resistance to flow and have high coefficients of viscosity. Elevations in the hematocrit, plasma-protein concentrations and a decrease in shear rate (or velocity) increase the viscosity of blood. The hematocrit is the most important determinant of blood viscosity. At low sheer rates, blood viscosity increases very rapidly. On the other hand, at high sheer rates, blood viscosity approaches a constant value, so that in most vessels with diameters greater than 1 mm, blood viscosity is essentially constant.

Fluid Energy Losses

Energy losses in a fluid such as flowing blood are due to friction secondary to viscosity or can be attributed to changes in velocity or direction of flow. The former is termed *viscous energy loss* and the latter *inertial energy loss*. As heat is generated by the friction between layers of a fluid, energy lost is in proportion to the fluid's viscosity. This relationship can be described as

$\Delta P = Q \times 8L\eta/\pi r^4$,

where ΔP equals the pressure gradient between two points, Q equals the flow, L equals the tube length between the points, η equals the coefficient of viscosity, and r equals the tube radius. Because the term $8L\eta/\pi r^4$ represents the resistance to flow in this system, the equation can be simplified to $P = QR$, or pressure equals flow times resistance.

This equation is analogous to Ohm's law of electrical circuits, where electromotive force (volts) equals current times resistance.

Although these formulas would predict pressure gradients in a newtonian fluid flowing in a rigid cylindrical tube, they can only estimate the minimum pressure gradient or viscous energy losses that may be expected in arterial flow. In the living artery, additional energy losses related to inertia (ΔE) are proportional to a constant (K), the specific gravity of blood (ρ), and the square of the blood velocity.

$\Delta E = K \frac{1}{2}\rho v^2$

Because velocity has components of both speed and direction, these inertial energy losses are most significant in small-caliber vessels and at sites of tortuosity and branching (Fig. 21-6).

Boundary Layer Separation

In fluid flowing in a tube, the portion of the fluid adjacent to the conduit wall is referred to as the "boundary layer." During normal flow, the velocity of the fluid–vessel interface is essentially zero. At a bifurcation, the laminar velocity profile changes, being skewed with higher velocities toward

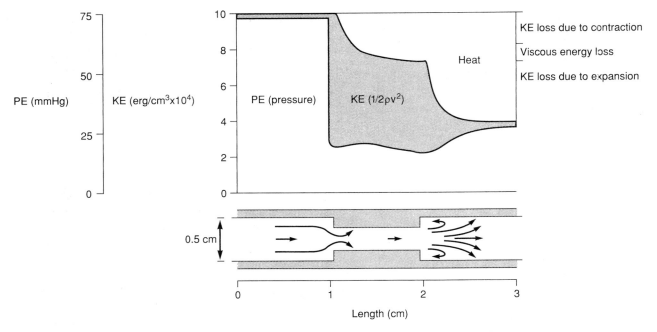

FIGURE 21-6. Kinetic and potential energy losses during passage of blood through a 1-cm stenosis. (From Rutherford RB. *Vascular surgery,* 4th ed. Philadelphia: WB Saunders, 1995:24, with permission.)

the central flow divider. The pressure gradients thus created cause the boundary layer to stop or reverse direction. This complex localized, low-flow pattern is known as an "area of flow separation" or a " separation zone." Clinically, these areas of low flow, and therefore low sheer stress, have been found to correlate with the development of atherosclerotic lesions. A dramatic example of this is at the carotid bifurcation, where the lesion develops at the site of stagnant flow along the outer wall of the internal carotid artery sparing the actual flow divider, which is a site of high sheer stress (Fig. 21-7).

Arterial Stenoses

Energy losses across a stenosis are due to both viscous and inertial energy losses. As described above, the viscous energy losses are proportional to the stenotic length and inversely proportional to the fourth power of the radius. Therefore, the radius of a stenotic segment will have a much greater effect on viscous energy losses than its length. Inertial energy losses occur at the entrance (contraction effect) and exit (expansion effect). These energy losses are proportional to the square of the blood velocity. The most significant energy losses are due to sudden expansion and dissipation of energy as heat at the exit of a stenosis. Energy lost at an arterial stenosis is proportional to the fourth power of the change in radius and second power of the velocity within the normal artery. Therefore, energy lost at any stenosis increases exponentially with increasing blood flow or velocity. The viscous losses are small and occur only within the length of the stenosis.

A *critical stenosis* is defined by the degree of narrowing that is required to produce a significant reduction in blood pressure or flow. This degree of narrowing is usually reached at a 75% to 90% reduction of the luminal cross-sectional area. This is equivalent to a 50% to 70% reduction in diameter. As described above, the energy loss (pressure drop) across a stenosis varies with the flow rate. Hence, a stenosis that might not be critical at a lower flow rate might become critical at a high flow rate. This is the basis for the term "subcritical stenosis." This is apparent clinically when a patient may be asymptomatic at rest and shows no pressure changes across a subcritical stenosis but may become symptomatic and demonstrate a significant pressure drop across a stenosis during exercise.

Because atherosclerosis is a diffuse process, it is rare to have a single isolated stenosis. The circulation of the patient with atherosclerotic disease consists of multiple parallel channels (collaterals) consisting of vessels with frequently multiple stenotic areas (Fig. 21-8).

The total resistance (R_T) in a single vessel with multiple stenoses in series can be described as

$R_T = R_1 + R_2 + R_3$

As already discussed, the inertial losses are independent of stenosis length and are particularly prominent at the exit of a stenosis. Therefore, energy losses across multiple stenotic areas are far more significant than those across a

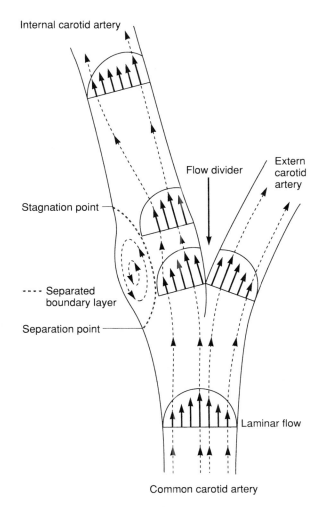

FIGURE 21-7. Flow separation in carotid arterial bifurcation. (From Rutherford RB. *Vascular surgery*, 4th ed. Philadelphia: WB Saunders, 1995:34, with permission.)

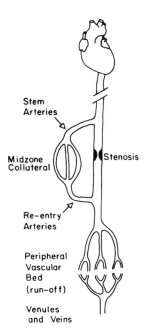

FIGURE 21-8. Arterial circuit with stenotic main artery and collateral channels. (From Rutherford RB. *Vascular surgery*, 4th ed. Philadelphia: WB Saunders, 1995:26, with permission.)

single stenosis of the same total length. Additionally, it is therefore possible that multiple subcritical stenoses can have the same effect as a single critical stenosis. The formula for resistances in parallel is

$1/R_T = 1/R_1 + 1/R_2 + 1/R_3$

Initially collateral arteries may dilate in response to a stenosis in a major artery. Over time, this leads to dilation and possibly proliferation of collateral vessels. Although collateral vessels can for a time compensate for a significant stenosis, a large number of vessels are required to compensate for a stenosis in a major artery. For example, as resistance is an inverse function of the radius to the fourth power, a 50% stenosis in a 0.5-cm artery would require 625 collateral arteries of 1-mm diameter to compensate completely. It is this inability to develop such numerous collateral vessels that results in the requirement for direct intervention.

Aneurysm Physiology

The hemodynamic contribution to aneurysm expansion and rupture is well defined. Tangential stress (τ) causes expansion, and when this stress exceeds wall tensile strength, rupture occurs. In a cylinder, circumferential wall tensile stress (τ_c) is defined as

$\tau_c = P \times r/\delta$,

where P equals pressure, r equals internal radius, and δ equals wall thickness.

As in the law of Laplace for cylinders, with negligible thickness, wall tension is proportional to the radius of the lumen ($T = P \times r$). Therefore, increased arterial blood pressure and aneurysm size are proportional to wall tensile stress and subsequently to the risk of rupture.

PRINCIPLES OF PERIPHERAL VASCULAR DISEASE

Chronic Lower Extremity Ischemia

The overwhelming majority of conditions treated by the vascular surgeon are related to lesions of atherosclerosis. In the lower extremity, most lesions remain asymptomatic until blood flow is reduced such that the metabolic demands of tissue are not met. The more common symptoms that result from chronic ischemia to the lower extremities include intermittent claudication, rest pain, and ischemic ulcers. In general, claudication alone, as will be discussed below, is rarely limb threatening. In contrast, rest pain and tissue loss will likely progress to limb loss if untreated.

Claudication, derived from the Latin word *claudico* meaning "to limp," can be defined as extremity pain, discomfort, or weakness consistently produced by the same amount of walking or equivalent muscular activity in a given patient and is promptly relieved by cessation of that activity. For the purposes of reporting, claudication can be divided into mild, moderate, or severe, depending on performance on exercise testing and ankle pressures. For the purpose of clinical management, it is more helpful to separate those patients whose claudication is "incapacitating" from the others. Incapacitating claudication is of such severity that the patient either can not work or is prevented from performing other functions they consider vital to their lifestyle.

The natural history of claudication makes the distinction of incapacitating symptoms very important. It is accepted that if untreated, only approximately 5% of patients with claudication will go on to amputation. Those that are more likely to develop limb-threatening complications are in the incapacitating category. The safety of treating most patients with claudication nonoperatively with programs of exercise, risk management, including smoking cessation and control of lipid, glucose, and blood pressure levels, medication with antiplatelet and rheologic agents, and meticulous care of the lower extremity is also well accepted. Claudication may be considered a relative indication for revascularization, warranting careful selection of low-risk patients with disabling symptoms for such procedures.

Claudication as a Result of Aortoiliac Occlusive Disease

Atherosclerotic lesions in the aortoiliac location generally begin at the bifurcation of the aorta or the common iliac arteries and can progress in either direction (Fig. 21-9). In general, patients complaining of claudication due to isolated aortoiliac disease tend to be younger than those whose claudication is due to disease of the femoropopliteal system. Additionally, the fact that lesions of the aortoiliac system are less likely to cause symptoms is a tribute to the excellent collateral system in this area. However, due to the larger number of muscle groups directly perfused by these vessels, claudication as a result of aortoiliac disease may result in greater disability. In addition, lesions of the aortoiliac system, regardless of lumen diameter, are at risk for distal embolization. This complication has been described as the "blue toe syndrome." It is for these reasons, as well as the excellent long-term results obtained with this patient population (primary unassisted patency approaching 95% at four years), that a more aggressive approach to claudication due to aortoiliac disease is taken.

It must be stressed, however, that to continue to achieve excellent functional and survival results, we must be careful

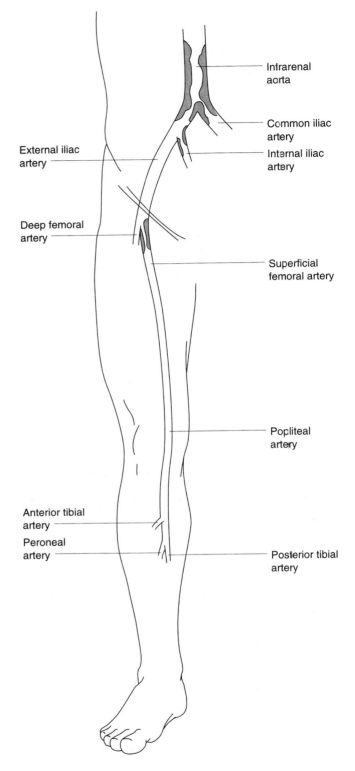

FIGURE 21-9. Atherosclerotic sites in aortoiliac region. (From Brewster DC. Aortoiliac disease. In: Greenfield LJ, Mulholland MW, Oldham KT, et al., eds. *Surgery: scientific principles and practice*, 1st ed. Philadelphia: JB Lippincott Co, 1993:1645, with permission.)

in selecting good risk patients with disabling symptoms for revascularization if the only indication is claudication.

Claudication as a Result of Infrainguinal Occlusive Disease

Intermittent calf claudication is usually due to a lesion in the superficial femoral artery. For the most part, multiple lesions at various levels are required to progress to limb-threatening ischemia. As discussed earlier, most patients complaining of intermittent calf claudication can be safely observed until symptoms of critical ischemia provide an absolute indication for revascularization. However, it is quite reasonable to consider a good risk patient with incapacitating claudication for revascularization as well.

Cumulative femoropopliteal graft patency rate for disabling claudication can be more than 90% at 2 years and more than 85% at 5 years, with minimal operative mortality. These patency rates are clearly superior to collective results of femoropopliteal graft patency performed for limb salvage. Femorotibial bypass for claudication is only rarely performed, but similar patency rates can be expected.

Although these reports demonstrate that revascularization for claudication at any level can lead to excellent durable results with a high degree of patient satisfaction, the importance of careful patient selection can not be overemphasized.

Approach to the Patient with Intermittent Claudication

As with any medical problem, evaluation begins with a careful history and physical examination. Patients with aortoiliac occlusive disease will generally complain of symptoms of the thigh, hip, buttock, or even the calf. Men may complain of difficulty achieving or maintaining an erection or both as a result of decreased perfusion through the internal pudendal arteries, which originate from the internal iliac arteries. On physical examination, these patients may have evidence of leg muscle atrophy and diminished or absent femoral pulses. This syndrome described by *Leriche* now bears his name. Patients with infrainguinal disease generally complain of symptoms in the calf or on occasion the foot. It is imperative to distinguish foot claudication, which begins after a specific degree of muscular activity, from pain that occurs at rest, is worsened by the recumbent position with associated elevation of the foot, and is improved with foot dependency.

Diminished peripheral pulses will make the diagnosis of vascular disease more likely; however, *nonvascular causes of claudication* need to be considered. The most common conflicting diagnosis is that of neurogenic leg pain. Because spinal stenosis and nerve compression can occur concomitantly with vascular occlusion, the absence of distal pulses does not rule out a spinal problem. Symptoms that begin with a change in position and are relieved only by assuming the recumbent position must be suspected to be of neurogenic origin. Additionally, a normal systolic pressure response to exercise, despite the occurrence of symptoms with exercise, effectively excludes claudication on a vascular basis. Further studies to evaluate patients with atypical symptoms thought likely neurogenic in origin include lumbosacral spine films, electromyography, lumbosacral spinal magnetic resonance imaging (MRI) or computed tomography (CT), and myelography. In addition, patients in whom symptoms do not resolve following revascularization should be evaluated for a neurogenic process.

Objective Measurement of Arterial Insufficiency

Patients with signs and symptoms suggestive of vascular disease should first undergo noninvasive testing of the arterial system. Two simple tests include the measurement of segmental systolic pressures and the ankle-brachial index (ABI). Normally, Doppler segmental pressures increase 20 mm Hg from the brachial artery to the proximal femoral artery. Any change less than a 20-mm Hg increase indicates significant aortoiliac disease. A pressure drop of more than 30 mm Hg between any two successive cuffs normally placed at the arm, proximal thigh, distal thigh, proximal calf, and distal calf signifies a significant arterial obstruction. The ABI is also a helpful test that can be performed at the bedside. The ABI is the ratio of the ankle blood pressure to the brachial blood pressure. An ABI of greater than 0.85 is considered normal. An ABI of 0.5 to 0.84 suggests that the degree of arterial obstruction is associated with claudication, and an ABI of less than 0.50 suggests severe arterial obstruction often associated with critical ischemia. A more rigid objective determination of claudication severity uses exercise testing. The standard exercise test is a treadmill test for 5 minutes at 2 mph hour on a 12% incline. Severe claudication can be defined as an inability to complete the treadmill exercise due to leg symptoms and ankle pressures of less than 50 mm Hg following exercise. Exercise testing is often required for patients with a convincing history but with normal examination results and resting ankle pressures. In these patients, segmental Doppler pressures and ABIs performed both before and after exercise may unmask the severity and location of the obstruction. Although angiography remains the gold standard for evaluation of vascular lesions, its use should be limited to only those patients who are to undergo intervention.

Limb-threatening ischemia occurs when the arterial blood supply is insufficient to meet the metabolic demands of resting muscle or tissue and is the most common indication for lower extremity arterial reconstruction. Chronic ischemia is manifested as imminent or actual tissue loss in the form of rest pain, ischemic ulcers, or gangrene. In contradistinction to the often benign natural history of mild and moderate claudication, the natural history of limb-threatening ischemia is progression to amputation unless intervention occurs with improvement of arterial perfusion.

Ischemic *rest pain* or diffuse pedal ischemia can be described as severe pain not readily controlled by analgesics, which is usually localized in the forefoot and toes of the chronically ischemic extremity. If the pain is also felt more proximally, it usually does not spare the distal sites. This pain is brought on or made worse by elevation of the extremity and is relieved or improved by dependency. Therefore, it is often experienced only at night or while reclining. Diffuse pedal ischemia is commonly associated with ankle pressures below 40 mm Hg and toe pressures below 30 mm Hg.

Ischemic ulcers are often the result of minor traumatic wounds failing to heal due to reduced blood supply insufficient to meet the increased demands of healing tissue. They are often painful and associated with other manifestations of chronic ischemia including rest pain, pallor, hair loss, skin atrophy, and nail hypertrophy. These ulcers often form at sites of increased focal pressure such as the lateral malleolus, tips of toes, metatarsal heads, and bunion area. Ischemic ulcers are usually dry and punctate and need to be distinguished from ulceration as a result of venous insufficiency. Venous ulcers are more commonly located above the medial ankle and are often moist, superficial, and diffuse. They are often associated with hemosiderin pigmentation and other evidence of venous insufficiency such as varicosities and worsening symptoms with dependency. Patients may have combined arterial and venous disease and manifest signs of both arterial and venous insufficiency.

Gangrene is characterized by cyanotic anesthetic tissue associated with necrosis due to reduction of arterial blood supply below the level necessary to meet minimal metabolic requirements. Gangrene can be described as either dry or wet. Dry gangrene is more common in patients with atherosclerotic disease that frequently results from embolization to the toe or forefoot. Wet gangrene is a true emergency, often occurring in diabetic patients who sustain an unrecognized trauma to the toe or foot. If sufficient viable tissue is present to maintain a functional foot, emergent debridement of all affected tissue usually results in a healed foot. If the wet gangrene involves an extensive portion of the foot, emergent guillotine amputation may be warranted, with revision to below-the-knee or above-the-knee amputation 72 hours later.

Acute ischemia can be manifest in the form of distal embolization of proximal atheromatous material to the toes, resulting in the blue toe syndrome, or be caused by a large embolus or sudden occlusion of a previously stenotic area, causing diffuse acute ischemia.

Blue toe syndrome consists of the sudden appearance of a cool painful cyanotic toe or forefoot in the often perplexing presence of strong pedal pulses and a warm foot. This clinical situation results most often from embolic occlusion of digital arteries with atherothrombotic material from proximal arterial sources. These episodes portend both similar and more severe episodes in the future. Therefore, location and eradication of the embolic source is usually indicated.

Diffuse acute ischemia is characterized by the sudden onset of pain progressing to numbness and finally paralysis of the extremity accompanied by pallor, coolness, and absence of palpable pulses. Acute ischemia is usually caused by embolic or thrombotic occlusions of native arteries sometimes in conjunction with previous vascular occlusions. Factors that predict a favorable prognosis include a preexisting history of claudication or other factors suggesting the formation of collaterals before the acute event, audible arterial flow at the time of presentation, and the absence of neurological changes at the time of presentation. Absence of the above factors suggests a poorer prognosis. It is important that limb-revascularization procedures in the form of thrombolysis, embolectomy, or bypass be performed early and expeditiously in the face of deteriorating clinical findings and is withheld in the face of irreversible ischemic changes with extensive gangrene.

Patient evaluation begins with a detailed history and careful physical examination. Rare is the patient complaining of limb-threatening ischemia that does not have some evidence of underlying medical disease including heart disease, diabetes, kidney disease, hypertension, chronic pulmonary disease, or extracranial cerebral vascular disease. Maximal therapy of these conditions must be provided preoperatively, intraoperatively, and postoperatively to ensure the best possible outcome. The physical examination must be complete, including a careful search for bruits, aneurysms, and malignancies. Additional time must be dedicated to the examination of the extremities for a careful evaluation of pulses, tissue changes, and evidence of prior vascular intervention.

Noninvasive Testing

Because physical examination findings are neither specific nor sensitive enough to design operative therapy, patients with evidence of peripheral ischemia should undergo objective testing. Segmental pressures and ABI are discussed above.

Pulse volume recordings (PVRs) involve placement of cuffs at the levels of the proximal and distal thigh, calf, and ankle, to help localize the site of obstructive lesions (Fig. 21-10). The PVR is a calibrated air plethysmographic waveform recording system that can also be performed at the metatarsal and toe levels, which is particularly helpful in diabetic patients with relatively incompressible proximal vessels.

Duplex imaging is a useful tool that in experienced hands can provide accurate localization and quantification of lesions, as well as help differentiate stenoses from occlusions, which is an advantage over segmental Doppler pres-

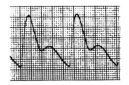 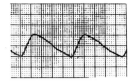

FIGURE 21-10. Normal and abnormal pulse volume recordings at ankle level. (From Rutherford RB. *Vascular surgery*, 4th ed. Philadelphia: WB Saunders, 1995:86, with permission.)

sures or PVRs. However, the time, equipment, and expertise required to perform a complete screening examination of the lower extremity vessels with duplex imaging makes it an impractical replacement for segmental pressures and PVRs. Its ability to answer precise questions about specific arterial segments and measure flow velocities in bypass grafts makes Duplex imaging a useful tool in following known lesions for evidence of progression.

Magnetic resonance angiography (MRA) is becoming increasingly popular in the evaluation of lower extremity ischemia, particularly for patients who have a contraindication to standard angiography. Its use as a replacement for angiography requires careful evaluation and significant experience with MRA.

Currently, contrast angiography remains the gold standard in the evaluation of lower extremity ischemia. A complete study of the aorta, iliac, femoral, popliteal, and runoff vessels is usually performed on both the affected and contralateral sides, as atherosclerotic disease is most commonly bilateral and occurs at multiple levels. However, angiography should be reserved for patients who are expected to undergo revascularization and do not have contraindications for this imaging modality, such as renal failure.

Therapeutic Interventions

Aortoiliac Occlusive Disease

In recent years, for patients requiring open surgery, the aortofemoral bypass graft has become the preferred method of treatment of symptomatic aortoiliac occlusive disease in good risk patients, having achieved perioperative mortality rates well under 5%. In general, approximately one fourth to one third of aortofemoral bypass grafts are performed for limb salvage with the remainder performed for severe claudication. Overall 5-year cumulative patency rates approach 88% with 10-year rates approaching 75%. When further categorized by the severity of disease, cumulative patency rates of aortofemoral bypass grafts in patients with rest pain or gangrenous tissue loss are 60% to 70% at 5 years and 50% to 60% at 10 years.

In high-risk patients, the axillobifemoral bypass graft offers a reasonable alternative. Because neither the thoracic nor the abdominal cavity is violated in performing an axillofemoral graft, the procedure usually does not interfere with the patients' ability to breathe, cough, or take oral feedings. In addition, it is possible to perform the procedure under local anesthesia in particularly poor risk patients. Cumulative graft patency of 70% at 5 years can be obtained with this procedure. These results are inferior to results for aortofemoral bypass, and therefore, axillofemoral bypass grafting is usually reserved for high-risk patients with limb-threatening ischemia and not performed for claudication alone. For patients with unilateral iliac occlusive disease, and whose aorta and contralateral iliac artery are free of disease, unilateral iliofemoral or femorofemoral bypass grafts are useful options. Femorofemoral bypass is particularly useful in high-risk patients, because it can be performed under regional anesthesia. Cumulative 5-year patency rates of over 80% can be achieved.

Femoropopliteal Tibial Occlusive Disease

Femoropopliteal bypass grafts are indicated when the superficial femoral artery or proximal popliteal artery is occluded and the patent popliteal artery has luminal continuity on arteriogram with any of its three terminal branches. In the case of a popliteal occlusion, bypass to an isolated segment of popliteal artery is effective if the segment is greater than 7 cm long. If the isolated popliteal segment is less than 7 cm, or if there is severe gangrene of the foot, a sequential bypass to the popliteal and then to a more distal vessel should be considered. Femoropopliteal bypass grafts are categorized as either above the knee or below the knee. A review of recent literature reveals primary above-the-knee femoropopliteal graft patency rates at 84% and 69% at 1 and 4 years, respectively, with reversed saphenous vein as the conduit, and 79% and 60% at 1 and 4 years, respectively, using polytetrafluoroethylene (PTFE). In the below-the-knee position, performed specifically for limb salvage, cumulative patency rates with reversed saphenous vein is 90% and 75% at 1 and 4 years, respectively, with similar results for *in situ* bypass. Secondary patency rates for PTFE grafts in the below-the-knee position for all indications is 68% and 40% at 1 and 4 years, respectively. Therefore, prosthetic material should be avoided whenever possible for infrageniculate bypass. The use of PTFE in the above-the-knee position is a far more viable alternative. Proponents of its use as the material of choice in the above-the-knee position cite similar early patency rates to autologous vein and the frequent need of saphenous vein for future coronary bypass or more distal peripheral revision. However, the argument for future vein requirements does not appear to be justified in many cases. A policy of the preferential use of autologous vein graft in any position is followed by most vascular surgeons.

Infrapopliteal bypass grafts should be performed only in situations of lower extremity ischemia, in which femoropopliteal bypass grafting is not feasible. Accepted primary patency rates for all indications with reversed saphenous vein graft are 77% and 62% at 1 and 4 years, respectively, and secondary patency rates with PTFE as the conduit of 68% and 48% at 1 and 4 years, respectively. When performed for limb salvage, cumulative patency rates for reversed saphenous vein grafts are 85% and 82% at 1 and 4 years, respectively, and for PTFE 68% and 48% at 1 and 4 years, respectively. The use of prosthetic material to bypass to infrapopliteal arteries should be avoided if at all possible.

The generally accepted order of preference for the infrapopliteal anastomosis is the posterior tibial artery, the anterior tibial artery, and lastly the peroneal artery based on the fact that the peroneal artery is not directly continuous with the pedal arteries and therefore may produce an inferior result. However, more importantly, the choice of outflow vessel should be based on the overall quality of the vessel and its runoff. If two vessels of excellent quality are available, the preference probably should go to the vessel with the greatest degree of direct continuity with the foot.

Profundaplasty is a procedure consisting of endarterectomy of the origin and proximal portion of the deep femoral artery. It is most useful when combined with an inflow procedure such as an aortobifemoral bypass or axillofemoral bypass. On occasion, it is performed as an isolated procedure, usually following graft failure, in an attempt to achieve limb salvage by less than maximal improvement in limb perfusion.

Axillopopliteal bypass is generally used as a final effort to prevent amputation. It is usually performed in a situation in which the usual options are not available whether it be due to groin infection with or without graft infection, extensive operative scarring, or extensive involvement of the iliac and femoral systems.

Fortunately, most patients presenting with even critical ischemia can be offered a reasonable attempt at limb salvage. However, there are situations in which the best option remains primary amputation. In cases in which gangrene extends into the deeper tissues of the tarsal region of the foot, primary amputation at the below-the-knee level is indicated. If the patient was previously reasonably healthy, a well-fitting prosthesis will provide excellent functionality. The functional outcome following below-the-knee amputation is far better than that following amputation at the ankle despite the higher level. In cases in which the patient has severe depression of mental status such that he or she is unable to ambulate, stand and pivot, communicate, or provide selfcare, an above-the-knee primary amputation should be considered. Severe, long-standing contractures can occur with below-the-knee amputations in this patient group, and often the below-the-knee amputation wound may break down due to contact with the mattress.

Postoperative Graft Surveillance

There are three major causes of graft failure. Failure in the immediate postoperative period (less than 30 days) is most often due to technical or judgmental errors. Other causes include inadequate outflow, infection, or an unrecognized hypercoagulable state. Failure between 30 days and 2 years is most often due to myointimal hyperplasia within the vein graft or at anastomotic sites. Late graft failure is usually due to the natural progression of atherosclerotic disease. It is estimated that strictures develop in 20% to 30% of infrainguinal vein bypasses during the first year. Careful surveillance is justified because intervention based on a duplex ultrasound surveillance protocol can result in 5-year assisted patency rates of 82% to 93% for all infrainguinal grafts studied, significantly higher than the 30% to 50% secondary patency rates of thrombosed vein grafts. A typical surveillance protocol would include duplex ultrasonography to measure flow velocity and the velocity ratio across a stenosis. Further workup would be indicated in vein grafts with less 45 cm per second flow velocity and a velocity ratio of more than 3.5 across a stenosis. In addition, ABIs can be easily measured, with a decrease of more than 0.15 between examinations considered significant. Examinations should be performed perioperatively, at 6 weeks, then at 3-month intervals for 2 years, and every 6 months thereafter.

Considerable progress has been made over the past 10 years in the treatment of limb-threatening ischemia particularly, with the success of distal bypass grafts. Patients with limb-threatening ischemia are most likely to do well if they receive an aggressive approach with revascularization if indicated.

Acute Lower Extremity Ischemia

The treatment of acute ischemia remains a challenge to the vascular surgeon. Often the etiology and precise location of an obstructing lesion is unclear. Additionally, acute ischemia occurs in patients with multiple medical comorbidities. Optimal outcome clearly depends on expedient diagnosis and management, as extremity function can be lost in a matter of hours.

The classic signs of acute ischemia are referred to as the "six *P*s," which include pain, paresthesias, pulselessness, pallor, poikilothermy, and paralysis. As ischemia continues, paresthesia progresses to anesthesia, pallor to cyanosis and mottling, and paralysis becomes more complete. Systemic effects of tissue necrosis include acidosis, hyperkalemia, and myoglobinuria.

The most common etiologies of acute lower extremity ischemia include embolism and thrombosis of an already diseased artery. Although initial treatment strategies may often be similar, it is important to make the distinction between embolus and thrombosis. Certain characteristics help sort out this diagnostic dilemma. Often patients with an embolus can pinpoint the exact time at which severe ischemic symptoms presented. Additionally, these patients may have a history of heart arrhythmias, suggesting a potential source or a history of previous emboli. Further, if the contralateral limb is without evidence of chronic vascular disease, it is more likely that the acute event is from a remote source. Conversely, patients with thrombosis of a diseased vessel will often give a history of prior chronic-type symptoms in the involved extremity, may not have an obvious source for an embolus, and will most often have some evidence of chronic vascular disease in the contralateral extremity.

The next important distinction to make concerns location. The examination should include palpation of all peripheral pulses. The most common location for a lower extremity embolus is at the femoral bifurcation. This is evidenced by the presence of a pulse in the external iliac artery when a femoral pulse is not palpable. The next most common site is at the popliteal trifurcation. The location of an embolus is important because more distal emboli are less amenable to surgical intervention and may need thrombolytic therapy. It is also important to determine the degree of ischemia, because advanced ischemia may require more immediate intervention without preoperative angiography.

The source of an embolus can be divided into cardiac and noncardiac sources. Cardiac causes include atrial fibrillation, mural thrombi following myocardial infarction, cardiomyopathy, or ventricular aneurysm, diseased or prosthetic heart valves, and atrial myxomas. Noncardiac sources include aortic and peripheral aneurysms, atherosclerotic ulcers and plaques, iatrogenic sources such as angioplasty, foreign bodies, and paradoxical sources such as venous emboli traversing a patent foramen ovale.

As mentioned above, the treatment of acute embolus and thrombosis is initially similar. As a rule of thumb, the maximum time before irreversible extremity ischemic injury occurs is about 6 hours. Clearly this varies with the degree of ischemia. Additionally, patients with chronic ischemia will often have developed significant collaterals, allowing them to tolerate an acute event for a longer period. All patients with an acutely ischemic extremity should be started on intravenous (i.v.) therapeutic doses of heparin unless there is a major contraindication. Systemic heparinization helps prevent propagation of clot adjacent to the acute lesion, helps prevent clot formation in the arterial tree distal to the obstruction, and helps prevent further embolic events. Additional maneuvers include keeping the extremity level or slightly lower than the level of the heart (reverse Trendelenburg position), avoiding the application of heat or cold, and using a regimen of skin protection including placement of the extremity on an egg crate–style pad and possible use of lamb's wool between the toes.

The next management decision to make is whether to obtain angiography with possible thrombolytic therapy or to proceed directly to the operating room. These decisions are strongly influenced by the etiology and location of the obstruction, as well as the degree of ischemia and overall operative risk to the patient. *Thrombolytic therapy* with urokinase would likely be a good choice for primary therapy of an arterial embolus in a very distal location that is surgically inaccessible. Additionally, thrombolytic therapy would be useful in a patient with mild or moderate ischemia at high risk for surgery. In the case of thrombosis, lytic therapy may help unmask the chronically diseased segment that may then be amenable to angioplasty or semielective bypass. This is particularly true in patients whose chronic changes allow additional time. Thrombolytic therapy is not indicated in the treatment of a severely ischemic extremity that requires expedient revascularization to maintain viability. Other contraindications to lytic therapy include active bleeding, recent stroke or craniotomy, pregnancy or recent delivery, uncontrolled hypertension, and recent gastrointestinal (GI) tract bleed or surgery.

The mainstay of treatment for an arterial embolus following initial heparinization is *balloon embolectomy* (Fig. 21-11). This is usually performed through a cutdown in the groin over the common femoral artery. The entire abdomen and extremity should be prepared in case a bypass or fasciotomy is required. A transverse arteriotomy allows for closure without vessel narrowing and can be used if the diagnosis of an embolus is clear. Otherwise, a longitudinal arteriotomy should be used because it can be used for a bypass if that becomes necessary. Balloon catheters are run proximally and distally until two passes are clear of clot. In cases of emboli in the infrageniculate location, embolectomy through the groin may be difficult and a below-the-knee popliteal cutdown to expose the trifurcation may be required. Fluoroscopically guided embolectomy may help avoid the need for popliteal exploration. If efforts at embolectomy fail, intraoperative lytic therapy is indicated. This is performed by infusing a dilute mixture of a thrombolytic agent directly into the involved artery and allowing it to dwell for approximately 10 to 15 minutes. This is followed by flushing the vessels with heparinized saline and reevaluation with intraoperative angiography. If flow remains inadequate, bypass, local endarterectomy, patch angioplasty, or extraanatomical femorofemoral bypass may be required.

Following revascularization, patients who have had prolonged periods of ischemia or who have signs of impending compartment syndrome should undergo fasciotomy. If fasciotomy is not performed at the initial operation, the patient needs to be followed very closely for signs of *compartment syndrome*. As most physical signs are unreliable, regular measurements of compartment pressures may need to be performed, with prompt fasciotomy if pressures exceed 30 mm Hg or signs of neurological compromise occur. Postoperatively, the patient is at risk for other complications of reperfusion including hyperkalemia, acidosis, myoglobinuria, and renal failure.

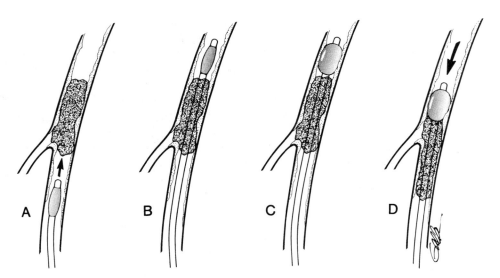

FIGURE 21-11. Balloon embolectomy. (From Rutherford RB. *Vascular surgery*, 4th ed. Philadelphia: WB Saunders, 1995:656, with permission.)

Embolectomy should not be performed if there is evidence of irreversible tissue damage with myonecrosis unless it is felt necessary to allow a subsequent amputation site to heal. Reperfusion of a necrotic extremity carries a high mortality rate with no hope of restoration of function. In this situation, the patient should be optimized for surgery and primary amputation should be performed.

After the acute ischemic event is addressed, a search for the source is indicated. In the case of an embolus, this should include an echocardiogram to help identify a cardiac source. *Trans*thoracic echocardiography can miss 30% to 50% of thrombi in the left atrium and up to 85% in the atrial appendage. Therefore, transesophageal echocardiography may be necessary to detect the offending thrombus. If an aortic plaque is believed to be the source of atheroemboli, aortography may be indicated.

ANEURYSMAL DISEASE

Abdominal Aortic Aneurysms

Abdominal aortic aneurysms (AAAs) remain a major health problem. They are the 13th leading cause of death, causing approximately 15,000 deaths per year in the United States. It is estimated that 2% to 6.5% of individuals over the age of 60 have an AAA. An *aneurysm* is defined as a focal dilation of a vessel by greater than 50% of its usual diameter. Therefore, in the case of the infrarenal aorta, this corresponds to a diameter of 3.0 to 3.5 cm.

AAAs are four to six times more common in men than in women. Ninety-five percent are infrarenal with only 5% involving the suprarenal aorta. Aneurysms in which there is no normal segment of infrarenal aorta are termed "juxtarenal." Those that involve the renal artery origins but not the superior mesenteric artery are termed "pararenal." Fifty percent of AAAs extend to involve the iliac arteries. Isolated aneurysms of the iliac arteries are uncommon and isolated aneurysms of the suprarenal abdominal aorta are extremely rare. Concomitant thoracic aortic aneurysms occur in 12% of patients with an AAA.

Risk factors for AAAs include coronary artery disease, hypertension, peripheral artery occlusive disease, smoking, and chronic obstructive pulmonary disease. Approximately 15% to 20% of first-degree relatives of patients with an AAA will be similarly affected. Inheritable connective tissue disorders also can contribute to the formation of aneurysmal dilation, e.g., Marfan syndrome and Ehlers-Danlos syndrome.

The pathophysiology of AAAs involves a degenerative process that appears to be related to aging, the exact mechanism of which remains elusive. There seems to be an association with atherosclerotic disease, but this would not explain why some aortas develop occlusive disease as opposed to becoming aneurysmal. Other causes of aneurysms include cystic medial necrosis, dissection, and syphilis. Experimental evidence would suggest abnormalities in the content and distribution of elastin and collagen layers. Hemodynamic, immune, and inflammatory mechanisms have all been implicated.

The majority (approximately 75%) of AAAs remain asymptomatic unless they rupture. Most are identified on routine physical examination, incidentally during ultrasonographic or radiographic imaging of the abdomen for an unrelated problem, during surgical exploration, or by the patients. On occasion, AAAs can cause symptoms including those of duodenal compression, hydronephrosis, venous thrombosis from iliocaval compression, or vague abdominal and back pain. The sudden onset of severe abdominal, flank, or back pain is characteristic of aneurysmal rupture or acute expansion. Other clinical findings associated with aneurysm rupture include shock and a pulsatile abdominal mass. Often the pain may radiate to the groin or thigh. On very rare occasions, the aneurysm may rupture into the vena cava, causing a major arteriovenous fistula, or into the GI tract, causing an aortoenteric fistula. However, the pain is usually nonspecific and the history is poor. Difficult diagnostic dilemmas occur when it is unclear whether the patients' pain and hypotension are due to a ruptured AAA or an ongoing myocardial infarction. In this situation, if there is any evidence of a ruptured AAA, particularly a known history of aneurysm, the patient should be taken immediately to the operating room, where transesophageal echocardiography can be used to evaluate the heart. Additionally, the presence of collapsed external jugular veins would also suggest hypotension from intraabdominal blood loss in this setting as opposed to cardiogenic shock, which is often manifested by distended external jugular veins and other signs of congestive heart failure. A stable patient with a known history of AAA presenting with new acute symptoms of impending rupture should be taken immediately to the operating room. An undue delay in treatment to obtain imaging studies often leads to aneurysm rupture and increased mortality.

A discussion of imaging studies is usually geared toward the assessment of stable asymptomatic aneurysms. The advantages of real-time B-mode ultrasound are that it is available in most hospitals, is relatively inexpensive, can be portable, and requires no ionizing radiation. It can assess the presence of an aneurysm with close to 100% sensitivity and is fairly accurate in measuring the size of an aneurysm. Disadvantages include the inability to assess the suprarenal aorta and to define the relation of the AAA and the renal arteries, and obesity, intestinal gas, or barium in the bowel impairs images. The above qualities make ultrasound useful in the acute setting to establish the presence of an AAA and for routine follow-up to determine increases in size.

CT images are useful because they provide reliable information about the entire aorta including accurate size, location, and extent (Fig. 21-12). Often, relations to major branches, venous structures, and other intraabdominal abnormalities can be assessed. Additionally, CT scans can reliably detect small leaks and contained ruptures. Disadvantages include a time requirement, although this is getting shorter with modern equipment, and additional expense when compared to ultrasound.

MRI can produce highly accurate images in longitudinal, transverse, and coronal planes without the use of ionizing radiation. However, the technology is expensive and not widely available. Additionally, the presence of intracorporeal metal cardiac pacers or monitoring equipment makes scanning impossible.

Aortography is expensive and invasive. It is well known that due to the mural thrombus present in almost all AAAs, the size of the aneurysm can not be accurately assessed by angiography. Many surgeons advocate aortography preoperatively in all patients due to the accurate information provided regarding the extent of aneurysm formation, including renal and iliac artery involvement, and information regarding associated lesions of renal and visceral vessels. Surgeons who are more selective generally recommend angiography for the following indications: suspicion of visceral ischemia, occlusive ileofemoral vascular lesions, severe hypertension suggesting potential renal artery stenosis, suspicion or history of horseshoe kidney, suspicion or history of suprarenal or thoracoabdominal aneurysm, or the presence of femoral or popliteal aneurysms.

Clearly, the primary indication for aneurysm repair is to prevent rupture. The risk of aneurysm rupture correlates well with aneurysm size. The yearly risk of rupture for aneurysms less than 5 cm is about 4.1%; for aneurysms between 5 and 7 cm, 6.6%; and for aneurysms exceeding 7 cm, 19%. Five-year rupture rates for the same categories are 20.5%, 33%, and 95%, respectively. Autopsy studies have shown that 10% of aneurysms less than 4 cm rupture. Therefore, if aneurysm repair can be performed with a minimum of morbidity and mortality, even small aneurysms may be considered for repair in good risk patients.

The major cause of perioperative mortality is related to coronary artery disease (CAD). CAD has been angiographically documented in 50% of patients with AAAs in whom CAD was suspected clinically and in 20% of patients without clinical suggestion of CAD. Therefore, prudent evaluation of the coronary arteries before elective AAA repair is critical.

The specifics of operative repair of AAAs are beyond the scope of this text; however, it should be noted that the recent advent of endovascular prosthetic exclusion of aortic aneurysms has the potential to expand therapy to patients

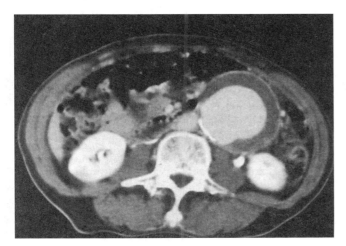

FIGURE 21-12. Abdominal computed tomographic scan demonstrating abdominal aortic aneurysm with mural thrombus. (From Goldstone J. Abdominal aortic aneurysms. In: Greenfield LJ, Mulholland MW, Oldham KT, et al., eds. *Surgery: scientific principles and practice*, 1st ed. Philadelphia: JB Lippincott Co, 1993:1715, with permission.)

who were previously considered too high a risk for conventional repair.

As with all major abdominal surgery, cardiac, pulmonary, and renal complications are not uncommon. The following section will address complications more specific to aortic surgery.

Sigmoid colon ischemia is rare but can carry a 90% mortality rate if detected late. Usually, mesenteric collateral flow is sufficient, or the IMA is reimplanted to the new graft. Sigmoid ischemia can also be addressed early by careful evaluation of the left colon before abdominal closure. Colon ischemia should be suspected postoperatively in the presence of crampy abdominal pain or early diarrhea, usually containing blood. This situation calls for prompt evaluation with flexible sigmoidoscopy to evaluate the colonic wall for evidence of mucosal necrosis. If there is evidence of transmural involvement, emergent return to the operating room for resection and colostomy is indicated. If there has been gross spillage of stool, resection of the graft with extraanatomical bypass may be required.

Lower extremity ischemia may occur following aneurysm surgery usually as a result of debris embolizing distally. Small distal emboli may cause small areas of necrosis distally that are not amenable to surgical treatment. Rarely, larger emboli may require surgical intervention.

Impotence or retrograde ejaculation may result due to injury of autonomic nerves during distal aortic dissection.

Paraplegia, due to spinal cord ischemia, occurs rarely following repair of infrarenal AAAs (less than 0.2%) but likely results when important collateral flow to the spine originates from the internal iliac arteries or when the origin of the major spinal artery is abnormally low.

Pseudoaneurysm is due to anastomotic disruption usually as a result of graft infection or arterial degeneration. The incidence of anastomotic pseudoaneurysm at 3 years is 0.2% at the aortic anastomosis, 1.2% at the iliac anastomosis, and 3% for the femoral anastomosis. The incidence of aortic pseudoaneurysm can be as high as 20% at 15 years, warranting postoperative follow-up with CT scanning long term. Once a pseudoaneurysm is identified, repair is indicated.

Graft infection is significantly less common when dissection and grafting in the groin is avoided. Aortoiliac graft infection incidence is about 0.5%, usually manifested at 3 to 4 years following implantation. The most common pathogens are *Salmonella sp.* and *Staphylococcus aureus.* Aortoenteric fistula formation is also uncommon, with an incidence of approximately 0.9%. Both complications carry a mortality risk of approximately 50%, and both require complete graft resection and extraanatomical bypass.

Inflammatory AAA is a distinct entity with an unclear etiology. The aneurysm is characterized by a markedly thickened wall containing an intense fibrotic inflammatory response. Most patients with inflammatory AAAs complain of pain, and this frequently leads to emergent exploration for presumed rupture. If detected electively, inflammatory aneurysms have characteristic features on CT scanning, which is helpful for preoperative planning. As the inflammatory process often involves adjacent structures including the ureters and duodenum, preoperative ureteral stenting is recommended. Additionally, proximal control should be obtained often at the supraceliac position, and minimal dissection of the aorta with endoaneurysmal repair should be the principles of management. Attempted dissection and mobilization of the duodenum off the aorta can lead to duodenal perforation.

Mycotic aneurysm does not refer to a fungal etiology, but rather to a mushroom-shaped false aneurysm of the arterial wall of an infectious etiology. These aneurysms usually occur as a result of bacterial or septic emboli or local extension of an infectious process. The aorta is the second most common site next to the femoral artery. These aneurysms can present with abdominal pain, fever, and a pulsatile abdominal mass. The aneurysm is usually saccular in shape and may be lobulated. If intraoperative Gram-stain results are negative and there is no evidence of purulence or bacteremia, *in situ* prosthetic repair may be considered. Otherwise, complete excision with extraanatomical bypass is indicated.

Aneurysms of Peripheral Arteries

Femoral artery aneurysms are rare but are important because of their propensity to thrombose or rupture. In addition, they are also a marker for aneurysms located elsewhere in the body. The presence of a femoral artery aneurysm is associated with a 70% chance of having a contralateral femoral artery aneurysm, an 85% chance of having an AAA, and a 40% chance of having a popliteal artery aneurysm. On the other hand, a patient with an abdominal AAA has only a 3% chance of a concomitant femoral artery aneurysm. Femoral artery aneurysms can be asymptomatic, present with acute or chronic thrombosis or with rupture.

It is generally recommended that asymptomatic femoral artery aneurysms greater than two times the diameter of the external iliac artery be repaired in good risk patients. All symptomatic femoral artery aneurysms should be considered for repair as well.

The popliteal artery is the most common site for peripheral aneurysmal disease. A patient with a *popliteal artery aneurysm* has a 50% chance of having a contralateral lesion and a 30% chance of having an AAA. Peripheral aneurysms are more common in men. Aneurysms of the popliteal artery should be repaired if their diameter exceeds 2 cm or is 1.5 times the diameter of the proximal nonaneurysmal segment. If these aneurisms are not repaired, complications such as thrombosis, distal embolization, or rupture can occur in 50% to 70% of cases, which may necessitate amputation. Thus, elective repair is warranted whenever possible.

Splanchnic Artery Aneurysms

Aneurysms of the splanchnic arteries are uncommon but are important, as a large proportion present with rupture and are associated with a high mortality rate. Splenic artery aneurysms are the most common, accounting for 60% of splanchnic artery aneurysms. They occur four times as frequently in women as in men. These lesions often can be diagnosed by calcifications in the left upper quadrant on plain x-rays. Indications for surgery include all aneurysms greater than 2 cm in diameter in acceptable risk patients, and any lesion in women of childbearing age. The reason for this is that over 90% of splenic artery aneurysms recognized during pregnancy have ruptured. In this situation, the maternal mortality rate can be 75% and the fetal mortality rate 95%. Treatment depends on aneurysm location. Lesions in the splenic hilum warrant splenectomy, whereas those located in the middle of the splenic artery may be treated by ligation and endoaneurysmorrhaphy of feeding vessels.

Hepatic artery aneurysms account for 20% of splanchnic artery aneurysms. Unlike splenic artery aneurysms, these lesions are twice as common in men. Hepatic artery aneurysms are extrahepatic in about 80% of cases and intrahepatic in 20%. Common hepatic artery aneurysms can usually be treated by aneurysmectomy or exclusion without reconstruction, as collateral circulation and portal flow provide sufficient flow to the liver. In cases of intrahepatic lesions, hepatic resection may be necessary.

Aneurysms of almost all named splanchnic vessels have been reported, including the superior mesenteric artery, celiac, gastric, and pancreaticoduodenal arteries. Details regarding these rare lesions are beyond the scope of this review.

MESENTERIC ISCHEMIA

Mesenteric ischemia usually occurs in elderly individuals. The consequences of an episode of mesenteric ischemia can be devastating and a high index of suspicion and timely intervention often offer the only hope for a successful outcome. Mesenteric ischemic syndromes can be subdivided into acute and chronic. The acute syndromes include embolus, thrombosis, nonocclusive ischemia, and venous thrombosis.

An *acute embolic occlusion* of the mesenteric vessels usually involves the superior mesenteric artery and the embolus usually originates from the heart. Risk factors for formation of thrombi in the heart include mainly atrial fibrillation and myocardial infarctions with development of ventricular aneurysms. In addition, valvular vegetations and paradoxical emboli from the venous system crossing a patent foramen ovale can be etiologic factors for acute embolic occlusion of the mesenteric vessels (Fig. 21-13). The most common site for an embolus to lodge is at the origin of the middle colic in the superior mesenteric artery, distal to the first jejunal branches (Fig. 21-14). Hence, the proximal small bowel is often spared with acute embolic mesenteric ischemia. However, smaller emboli may lodge more distally, causing more focused areas of ischemia.

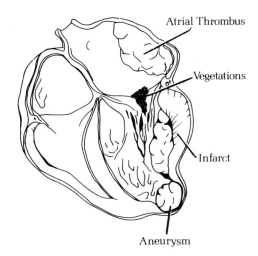

Figure 21-13. Cardiac sources of arterial emboli. (From Rutherford RB. *Vascular surgery*, 4th ed. Philadelphia: WB Saunders, 1995:648, with permission.)

The importance of a high degree of suspicion can not be overemphasized. Patients with an acute mesenteric embolus often have an underlying history of heart disease. They present with sudden periumbilical pain with associated rapid GI tract emptying in the form of diarrhea, vomiting, or both. In addition, these patients often have evidence of GI tract bleeding. Early in the disease course, patients' physical examination may be unremarkable and radiological studies and laboratory values may be nonspecific. Once the ischemia has progressed to the point of peritoneal signs, radiological changes and leukocytosis, the damage is usually irreversible and the mortality rate high.

If a high index of suspicion allows for intervention before frank peritoneal signs and the need for emergent celiotomy, mesenteric arteriography remains the diagnostic test of choice. The classic signs on an arteriogram of acute embolus include an occlusion with a meniscus several centimeters from the ostium, with nonopacification of the distal branches, and usually sparing of the first few jejunal branches (Fig. 21-14).

Following diagnosis, intervention must be immediate. The patient should be treated with aggressive fluid resuscitation, electrolyte correction, heparinization, and antibiotic coverage. The patient should then be taken to the operating room for exploration, embolectomy of the superior mesenteric artery, and resection of nonviable bowel.

Acute thrombotic occlusion occurs in about one fourth of patients with acute mesenteric ischemia. The pathophysiology in this situation is usually a sudden vascular occlusion at the site of an atherosclerotic plaque. Although the presenting symptoms are similar to those of acute embolus, these patients often have a history of chronic ischemia due to stenosis, as will be discussed later. The diagnostic study

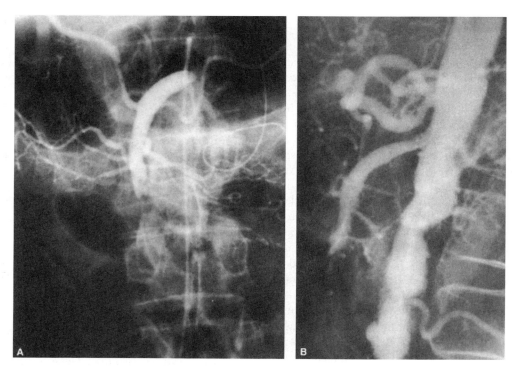

FIGURE 21-14. Angiogram demonstrating embolus in superior mesenteric artery with sparing of first few jejunal brances. (From Zelenock GB. Visceral occlusive disease. In: Greenfield LJ, Mulholland MW, Oldham KT, et al., eds. *Surgery: scientific principles and practice*, 1st ed. Philadelphia: JB Lippincott Co, 1993:1623, with permission.)

of choice is mesenteric angiography, which demonstrates occlusion of the superior mesenteric artery near or at the ostium, with evidence of atherosclerotic disease in the other visceral vessels. In the case of thrombosis, proximal jejunal branches are usually not visualized. As in the case of acute embolus, once the diagnosis is made, treatment must be immediate, which includes revascularization and resection of nonviable bowel.

Nonocclusive mesenteric ischemia is responsible for about 20% of cases of acute mesenteric ischemia. This situation is most often encountered in intensive care units in patients with severely reduced cardiac output due to heart disease and corresponding splanchnic vasospasm. The main symptom is abdominal pain. In noncommunicative patients, clues may include tube-feeding intolerance, abdominal distension, leukocytosis, metabolic acidosis, or GI tract bleeding. Angiographic findings include a patent arterial trunk that may appear to be in spasm and nonvisualization of the mesenteric arcades, also known as "pruning." Treatment includes direct injection of vasodilators such as papaverine into the mesenteric vessels, as well as aggressive treatment of the underlying disorder.

Mesenteric venous thrombosis is relatively uncommon. This disorder usually develops in younger patients without underlying atherosclerotic disease. Most patients will be found to have an underlying hypercoagulability disorder. Often, the patient may have a history of deep venous thrombosis (DVT) or pulmonary embolus. Unlike its arterial counterpart, mesenteric venous thrombosis develops initially in the distal vessels and propagates proximally with development of symptoms insidiously over days to weeks. Most frequently, patients complain of diffuse abdominal pain; however, vomiting, diarrhea, and fever may be present as well. The abdominal examination is usually not suggestive of peritonitis. The study of choice in this situation is the CT scan, which often will reveal bowel wall edema, mesenteric streaking, ascites, and an enlarged superior mesenteric vein with a dark central lucency suggestive of thrombus. Management includes fluid resuscitation, bowel rest, nasogastric decompression, and i.v. antibiotics. The patient should be heparinized and followed for development of peritonitis, which should be addressed by exploration. Usually, symptomatic relief is rapid and the patient should then be started on oral anticoagulants after several days of heparinization.

Chronic mesenteric ischemia is usually due to atherosclerotic plaques that develop at the ostia of the visceral vessels. The classic teaching is that two or more vessels need to have a significant degree of stenosis for a patient to become symptomatic. This is largely due to the ability of the mesenteric circulation to develop collaterals including the gastroduodenal and pancreaticoduodenal arcades, the marginal artery of Drummond and the meandering mesenteric artery. However, when multiple stenoses become severe enough to overwhelm the collateral reserves, ischemic symptoms ensue. The characteristic symptom is postprandial pain, often in a patient with evidence of atherosclerotic disease elsewhere. This pain creates a hesitancy to eat, resulting in weight loss. Patients are often thoroughly worked up for other conditions causing chronic abdominal pain before the diagnosis of mesenteric ischemia is entertained.

The gold standard of diagnosis remains angiography. If significant stenoses are detected in a symptomatic patient, revascularization should be prompt, as the risk of occlusion and acute infarction in this population is high.

RENAL ARTERY STENOSIS

The major indications for reconstruction of the renal arteries are renovascular hypertension, ischemic nephropathy, and as an adjunct to aortic reconstruction.

Renovascular hypertension probably accounts for 5% to 10% of all cases of hypertension. The percentage of patients with mild hypertension due to renal artery stenosis is probably negligible. Conversely, up to 40% of patients with severe diastolic hypertension (more than 118 mm Hg) may have renovascular hypertension.

The occlusive lesions of the renal artery include atherosclerotic lesions, which account for 70% of patients with renovascular hypertension and fibromuscular dysplasia. *Atherosclerotic lesions* usually occur in older patients with evidence of systemic atherosclerotic disease, are located at or near the ostium, and are more commonly encountered on the left side.

Fibromuscular dysplasia is an inclusive term involving hyperplastic and fibrosing lesions of any of the three layers of the arterial wall. The most frequent variety involving the renal arteries is medial fibrodysplasia with mural aneurysms. These lesions occur most often in women, and while most are bilateral, right-sided lesions are more common than left-sided ones.

There are two types of hypertension related to the kidneys, *renin-dependent hypertension* and *volume-dependent hypertension*. In the case of a unilateral lesion, decreased flow, as detected by the juxtaglomerular apparatus, results in increased renin production, which in turn results in the production of angiotensin I by conversion of angiotensinogen in the liver. Angiotensin I is converted to angiotensin II by angiotensin-converting enzyme, mostly found in the lungs. Angiotensin II is a powerful vasoconstrictor and stimulates the production of aldosterone by the adrenal glands. If the contralateral kidney functions normally, however, it compensates for the increased fluid by inducing natriuresis and thereby reducing plasma volume. In this setting, a renin-dependent angiotensin-II vasoconstrictive source of hypertension is created. If the contralateral kidney or artery is diseased, however, there is loss of the compensatory diuresis and an angiotensin-aldosteron–mediated volume-dependent hypertension is created. Renovascular revascularization should be effective in either of these situations.

Screening tests include captopril renal scanning, renal duplex sonography, MRI, and arteriography. The most commonly performed functional test is the renal vein renin assay. Lateralizing renal venous renin ratios of 1.4:1 or greater or a renal systemic renin index (RSRI) of greater than 0.48 is suggestive of renal hypertension. The RSRI is calculated by subtracting the systemic renin activity (renin level in inferior vena cava) from the individual kidney renin activity and dividing this difference by the systemic venous renin activity. An RSRI exceeding 0.48 from an individual kidney reflects renin production that exceeds hepatic clearance and suggests hyperreninemia. Renal vein renin studies are not indicated in patients with bilateral renal artery stenosis, because of failure to lateralize.

If *renal artery reconstruction* is performed in the presence of a positive functional study, an improvement in blood pressure should be expected in over 90% of cases. The ideal patient is generally younger than 55 years and has had hypertension of relatively short duration (less than 5 years).

Patients over the age of 50 who suffer from hypertension and have experienced the recent onset of renal failure or accelerated renal dysfunction with creatinine levels of 2 mg/dL or greater should undergo evaluation for ischemic nephropathy. The best candidates for renal revascularization are patients with severe (80% or greater) bilateral lesions and with critically stenotic lesions involving solitary kidneys.

Sixty percent of patients with severe bilateral lesions respond favorably to renal revascularization with improvement in renal function, although this procedure benefits 33% of patients who have only a significant unilateral lesion. Nevertheless, this should not exclude a good risk patient with unilateral disease from renal artery reconstruction.

Concomitant aortic reconstruction is probably now the most common indication for renal artery reconstruction. Aortorenal bypass as an adjunctive procedure may be required in 24% to 35% of patients undergoing aortic surgery. It is recommended to revascularize all symptomatic renal artery stenoses, and asymptomatic stenoses, that exceed 80%.

A situation may be encountered when aortic clamping is undesirable because of a diffusely diseased aorta or a frail patient. In a high-risk patient with bilateral renal vascular disease, unilateral revascularization may often be sufficient. If the indication for surgery is hypertension, the more ischemic kidney is revascularized. However, if surgery is indicated to preserve renal function, the larger kidney is revascularized. Alternative revascularization techniques to aortorenal bypasses include the splenorenal bypass for left-sided lesions and hepatorenal bypass for right-sided lesions.

Percutaneous transluminal angioplasty (PTA) has been found to yield results similar to those of open surgery in cases of short stenotic lesions that are located in the midartery. Currently, most nonostial lesions are treated by

PTA because it is less invasive than open surgery and recurrences are amenable to reangioplasty. The treatment of ostial lesions by angioplasty has been less promising to date. However, with the advent of stenting, more lesions may be amenable to percutaneous techniques. As of now, data regarding long-term outcome with renal artery stenting are not yet available.

VENOUS DISORDERS

Deep venous thrombosis (*DVT*) is not uncommon and can have serious short-term and long-term sequelae. Risk factors include age of more than 40 years, obesity, malignancy, previous episodes of DVT, prolonged bed rest, surgery, trauma, pregnancy, and hypercoagulable states. The most common presentation is unilateral swelling of the lower extremity, but a diagnosis on clinical findings alone is only accurate 50% of the time. Some important terms include *phlegmasia cerulea dolens* (swollen, blue, painful), which is due to iliofemoral venous thrombosis resulting in massive leg swelling and cyanosis. This could progress to *phlegmasia alba dolens* (swollen, white, painful), in which the leg becomes white due to compromised arterial flow.

Treatment of DVT should be prompt because material could dislodge, resulting in *pulmonary embolism*. Long-term sequelae include the postphlebitic syndrome in which venous valve destruction results in chronic reflux and venous insufficiency. Currently, duplex sonography is considered to be the study of choice for evaluation of a DVT. Once DVT is diagnosed, traditional treatment includes bed rest with leg elevation, systemic heparinization, and conversion to oral anticoagulants for 3 to 6 months. In the setting of phlegmasia cerulea dolens with impending gangrene, venous thrombectomy may be required. Alternatives to traditional treatment include treatment with thrombolytic therapy, in particular to reduce the extent of valvular damage, and more recently outpatient treatment involving the use of subcutaneous low molecular weight heparin followed by oral anticoagulants.

Patients at risk should receive DVT prophylaxis, which involves the perioperative use of subcutaneous heparin and pneumatic stockings, as well as a program of early ambulation.

In certain cases mechanical prophylaxis of pulmonary embolism in the form of *vena caval filters* is warranted. These filters are usually placed percutaneously into the infrarenal inferior vena cava and are designed to catch thromboembolic material that could otherwise enter the pulmonary vasculature. Indications for placement of a vena caval filter include, but are not limited to, DVT or pulmonary embolism in situations when systemic heparinization is contraindicated, recurrent pulmonary embolism despite therapeutic anticoagulation, bleeding problem while on heparin, propagation of thrombus while on heparin, and a free-floating iliofemoral thrombus.

Some basic concepts are important to understand and treat venous disorders. The *anatomy of the venous system* of the lower extremity includes a superficial system based on the greater and lesser saphenous veins, a deep system, and veins that perforate the fascia at right angles to the deep and superficial systems to connect them. A system of valves is arranged to keep flow in the proximal direction from ankle to thigh and from superficial to deep. Almost all venous problems of the lower extremity are due to obstruction, or reflux due to valvular insufficiency.

Varicose veins are dilations usually of superficial veins. They generally occur as a result of valve failure. The only durable treatment for severe varicosities, in which the involved vessels are tributaries of the greater saphenous vein, is stripping of the greater saphenous veins with ligation of the branch vessels at the saphenofemoral junction. However, this procedure should be reserved only for the most symptomatic patients, as the saphenous vein remains the most useful conduit for peripheral or coronary bypass surgery. Unfortunately, lesser procedures such as excision of only the involved vein segment are likely to result in recurrence. Varices that are not in communication with the greater saphenous vein may be amenable to local excision or sclerotherapy. It is imperative to rule out deep venous thrombosis in the treatment of varicose veins, as stripping of the greater saphenous vein in this setting may be eliminating the only significant route of egress of venous blood from the lower extremity.

A state of *chronic venous insufficiency* exists when elevated venous pressures persist due to either obstruction of the deep venous system or reflux of the deep venous system and perforators. Chronic venous hypertension results in transudation of fluid into the interstitial space, resulting in edema. Additionally, persistent hypertension results in deposition of hemosiderin, which leads to induration and pigmentation changes. Chronically elevated pressures and edema lead to eventual ulceration and propensity for cellulitis. Most of these patients can be treated conservatively with an aggressive program of leg elevation, compression, and wound care.

A select group of patients who are refractory to a conservative regimen and have evidence of local incompetence of the perforating veins may be candidates for perforator vein ligation. If the underlying problem is one of reflux in the major veins or obstruction and the condition is severe and refractory to conservative therapy, venous reconstructive procedures such as valve repair, valve transposition, or venous bypass might be considered. However, these procedures are currently performed at specialty centers and have not yet achieved widespread use.

SUGGESTED READING

Ernst CB, Stanley JC. *Current therapy in vascular surgery*, 4th ed. St. Louis: Mosby, 1999.
Rutherford RB. *Vascular surgery*, 5th ed. Philadelphia: WB Saunders, 1995.

22

PULMONARY PHYSIOLOGY

ERIC S. LAMBRIGHT AND JOSEPH B. SHRAGER

In the simplest of terms, the functions of the respiratory system are to extract oxygen from the atmosphere and transport it to the blood such that it may be supplied to cells, as well as to remove carbon dioxide, the by-product of aerobic metabolism, from the blood. These functions are accomplished by a combination of ventilation, perfusion, and gas exchange. *Ventilation* is the process by which air reaches the alveoli; *perfusion,* the process by which blood reaches the alveoli; and *gas exchange,* the process that occurs at the blood–gas interface within the alveoli. All components of the respiratory system—the central nervous system (CNS) regulators of respiration, the muscles of the respiratory pump, the conducting airways, the pulmonary vasculature, and alveoli—act in concert to achieve these functions. This chapter will discuss the physiology of air movement, pulmonary blood flow, and the gas–blood interface, as well as describe derangements in respiratory physiology that result in hypoxemia and/or hypoventilation. Additionally, the treatment of respiratory failure with mechanical support will be reviewed.

AIR MOVEMENT

Atmospheric oxygen can enter the bloodstream only if it is delivered to the alveoli, the basic functional unit of the lung. There, it comes into contact with the mixed venous blood in the pulmonary capillaries. Air enters through the oropharynx or nasopharynx and then travels past the larynx, into the trachea, through the conducting airways of the tracheobronchial tree, and then into the alveoli. The pressure gradient required for air movement is generated by the primary and in some circumstances, the accessory respiratory muscles. These are regulated by components of the CNS. Thus, movement of air requires several components: an intact CNS, a patent airway and conducting system, adequate respiratory musculature, and functional alveoli at the gas–blood interface.

Airways

The upper airway is composed of the mouth, pharynx, and larynx. The so-called "conducting zone" of the lung is composed of the trachea and the first 16 branchings or generations of airways. The intrathoracic trachea measures approximately 7.5 cm and extends inferiorly to the carina where it bifurcates into the left and right main bronchi. The right main bronchus gives rise to the upper lobar bronchus and the bronchus intermedius, which subsequently splits into the middle and lower lobar bronchi. On the left, the main bronchus bifurcates directly to give rise to the upper and lower bronchi. Segmental bronchi continue to divide until they reach the most distal conducting airways, which are called the "terminal bronchioles." These airways, including the oropharynx, larynx, trachea, and its branches to the terminal bronchioles, constitute the *anatomical dead space* because there is an absence of alveoli, and thus gas exchange is not possible while air dwells within them. The 17th to 19th generations consist of the respiratory bronchioles, from which the first alveoli emerge. This region is termed the "transitional zone" of the lung. Subsequent generations are lined with alveolar ducts and sacs and are known collectively as the "respiratory zone" whose primary function is the exchange of gases (Fig. 22-1). This zone will be discussed further in a later section of this chapter.

The conducting airways distal to the pharynx to the level of terminal bronchioles are lined with ciliated epithelium interspersed with mucus-secreting goblet cells (Fig. 22-2). The cilia and mucus are involved in the clearance of inhaled or aspirated particles. The mucociliary escalator carries particles in the tracheobronchial tree to the pharynx, where they are either swallowed or expectorated. Smokers demonstrate abnormalities in both mucous production and ciliary motility that contribute to their difficulties with secretion clearance. Additionally, some smokers will develop frank metaplasia in the tracheobronchial epithelium to nonciliated squamous epithelium, further compromising secretion clearance mechanisms. Cystic fibrosis is a disease in which there is markedly abnormal mucous production. Patients are unable to clear these abnormal secretions, which will

Hospital of the University of Pennsylvania, Philadelphia, Pennsylvania

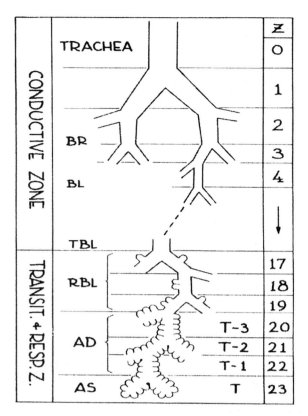

FIGURE 22-1. Lung zones. Bronchi, bronchioles, terminal bronchioles, respiratory bronchioles, alveolar ducts, and alveolar sacs. (From Weibel ER. *Morphometry of the human lung.* Berlin: Springer-Verlag, 1963:111, with permission.)

subsequently manifest in several pathological changes seen within the lungs including pneumonitis, bronchiolitis obliterans, and bronchiectasis. These pathological changes predispose patients to life-threatening bacterial pneumonia.

The structure of the airways varies markedly between levels. The trachea is supported by C-shaped cartilaginous rings anterolaterally, and its posterior wall is composed of smooth muscle oriented longitudinally. Cartilaginous plates also support the bronchi while bronchioles and alveoli lack cartilage. This lack of support renders the smaller distal airways more susceptible to collapse. This occurs in emphysema, and increased extraluminal pressure must be generated during exhalation.

Systemic disorders of cartilage, such as relapsing polychondritis, may cause collapse of the large airways. These are collectively referred to as "malacia." These disorders result in an obstruction to the movement of air that can be defined by the flow-volume loop that is seen in Fig. 22-3. Tracheomalacia most commonly results from local factors such as previous tracheostomy or prolonged intubation. To avoid this complication of tracheomalacia and tracheal stenosis, most authors recommend tracheostomy before 2 weeks of mechanical ventilation using as small a cannula as possible and careful avoidance of torque on the tracheostomy tube. The use of tracheostomy tubes with high-volume–low-pressure cuffs is now standard practice.

The histologic morphology of the respiratory zone differs markedly from the conducting and transitional zones and will be discussed further in the section on gas exchange to follow. The only component of the alveoli that is critical to air movement is the elastin that is embedded within the basal laminae in the alveolar septal interstitium. Elastin has the capability of stretching to 130% of its length while retaining its elastic recoil properties. This helps determine many of the mechanical properties of the lung. Loss of elastin is thought to be one of the primary pathogenic mechanisms leading to loss of elastic recoil and hyperexpansion of lung tissue seen in emphysema patients.

Chest Wall

The muscles of respiration and the chest wall must be intact to create the negative intrathoracic pressure that is required to establish a pressure gradient that results in the movement of air. The mechanics of ventilation are an interaction between the lungs, the chest wall, and the muscles of respiration. The anatomical components that make up the respiratory pump include: the diaphragm and accessory respiratory muscles, as well as the rib cage.

Mechanics of Ventilation

Ventilation can be achieved only if there is air movement to and from the alveoli. In clinical practice, it is assessed by the measurement of the partial pressure of arterial carbon dioxide (PCO_2). Alveolar ventilation is dependent on the depth of inspiration (tidal volume, V_T), the volume of the conducting airways (dead space, DS), and the rate of respiration (R) and is equal to $(V_T - V_{DS}) \times R$ measured as liters per minute.

Air will move down the tracheobronchial tree when a force is generated that is sufficient to overcome the combined pressures of the elastic recoil of the lung, the frictional resistance to airflow, and the inertia of the gas. At the end of a quiet exhalation, the alveolar and atmospheric pressures are equal; thus, there is no gradient for air movement. This point on the flow-volume loop is defined as the "functional residual capacity" (FRC). The outward recoil force of the chest wall is equal to the inward recoil force of the lung at FRC, resulting in a negative intrapleural pressure of 5-cm H_2O. All movement of air results from deflections from FRC resulting from active or passive properties of the respiratory muscles and chest wall.

With inspiration, the increased negative pressure generated by the respiratory muscles (chiefly the diaphragm) ini-

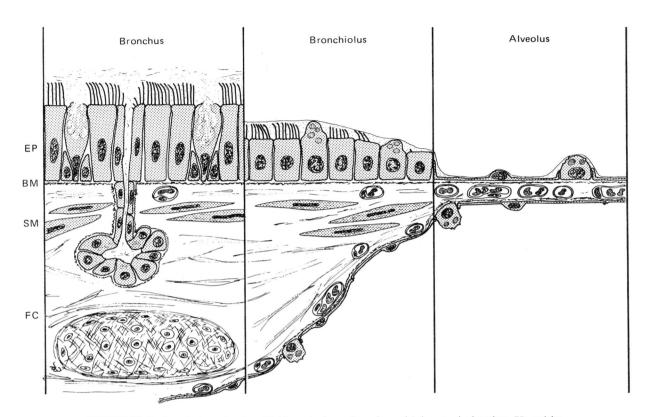

FIGURE 22-2. Respiratory tract epithelium in bronchus, bronchiolus, and alveolus. EP, epithelium; BM, basement membrane; SM, smooth muscle; FC, fibrocartilage. (From Weibel ER, Taylor CR. Design and structure of the human lung. In: Fishman AP, ed. *Pulmonary diseases and disorders,* Vol 1. 2nd ed. New York: McGraw-Hill, 1988:14, with permission.)

tially overcomes the elastic recoil of the lung. Once overcome, the alveoli will enlarge. The end of inspiration is achieved when the summed forces of the elastic recoil of the lung and chest wall equal the force generated by inspiratory muscle contraction. During normal exhalation, the muscles of inspiration relax and the elastic recoil of the lungs results in a passive decrease in alveolar volume, which produces a positive alveolar pressure. Thus, there is a pressure gradient for air to move out of the lungs until FRC is reached. Air can be forcefully exhaled until the fixed outward recoil of the chest is equal to the force exerted by the expiratory muscles (chiefly the intercostal and abdominal muscles). Exhalation will also be partially active during exercise, when there is a premium on maximizing ventilation, and in certain disease states. In emphysema, e.g., the resistance to expiratory airflow often results in the activation of expiratory muscles.

It is critical to note that at any point in the respiratory cycle, there exists a balance between forces that will collapse the lungs and pressures that maintain inflation. This balance is dependent on surfactant and the elastic nature of the lung, as well as the mechanics of the thoracic cavity. *Surfactant,* a dipalmitoyl phosphatidylcholine, reduces alveolar surface tension, a force that tends to decrease alveolar size and result in alveolar collapse. This decrease in surface tension also helps equalize pressures within alveoli of differing sizes that would have otherwise resulted in the emptying of smaller alveoli into larger ones and subsequent collapse of smaller alveoli. In normal individuals, surfactant has the beneficial effect of reducing the elastic recoil of the lung, increasing lung compliance, and thus decreasing the work of breathing. An example of a pathologic state in which surfactant is reduced is adult respiratory distress syndrome (ARDS). The loss of surfactant contributes to the decreased lung compliance characteristic of this syndrome.

The *compliance* of the lungs (defined as the change in volume divided by the change in pressure) is a measurement of the resistance of the lungs to expansion. It is very relevant in the clinical setting because the lung with decreased compliance requires the development of a larger pressure gradient to establish the same inflation. Thus, patients with decreased lung compliance have an increased work of breathing. Classically, pulmonary fibrosis results in "stiffer" lungs with decreased compliance. Additionally, pulmonary edema and atelectasis result in decreased lung compliance. In contrast, in emphysema, there is a destruction of the alveolar tissue that

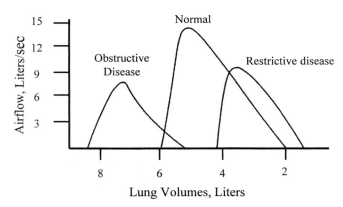

FIGURE 22-3. Maximal expiratory flow-volume curves representative of obstructive and restrictive diseases. (From Levitzky MG. *Pulmonary physiology,* 3rd ed. New York: McGraw-Hill, 1991:47, with permission.)

contains the elastin that would otherwise oppose lung expansion. This results in lungs that have increased compliance (Fig. 22-4). These patients have increased work of breathing for different reasons: alterations in lung volumes resulting in respiratory muscles that are forced to operate at a disadvantage and increased expiratory resistance.

Lung Volumes and Pulmonary Function Tests

The amount of air in the lungs is determined by the interaction of the muscles of inspiration and the mechanics of the lung and chest wall. There are four lung volumes that can be measured directly by spirometry; however, others require more complicated measuring devices such as helium dilution or body plethysmography. These measurements can each be compared to predicted values based on patient body size and age. This can give useful information regarding potential pathologic alterations.

As previously described, the FRC is the amount of air in the lungs at the end of quiet exhalation; i.e., the point at which the passive outward recoil of the chest and the inward recoil of the lungs resulting from elastin are equal. V_T is the volume of air entering the lungs in a quiet breath. Residual volume (RV) is the amount of air left in the lungs following maximal expiration. Expiratory reserve volume (ERV) is the volume of air that is expelled from the lung during maximal expiration that starts at the end of normal tidal expiration. In contrast, the inspiratory reserve volume (IRV) is the volume of gas that is inhaled during a maximal forced inspiration starting at the end of a normal tidal respiration. Routine spirometry can be used to define these lung volumes (Fig. 22-5).

There are three other standard lung capacities that are clinically relevant and reflect combinations of lung volumes. Inspiratory capacity (IC) is the amount of air that can be inhaled during maximal inspiratory effort starting at FRC (i.e., VC + IRV). Total lung capacity (TLC) is the volume of air in the lungs after maximal inspiratory effort and normally is approximately 5 L. Vital capacity (VC) is the amount of air that can be expelled from the lungs during a maximal forced expiration starting after maximal forced inspiration. Lung volumes are altered in pathologic states and can be a helpful diagnostic tool. Restrictive lung diseases such as pulmonary fibrosis and sarcoidosis typically cause a decrease in all lung volumes secondary to less-compliant lungs. With the decreased tidal volumes, respiratory

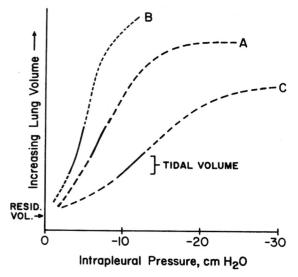

FIGURE 22-4. Compliance (change in volume divided by change in pressure) in **(A)** normal individuals, **(B)** patients with emphysema, and **(C)** patients with pulmonary fibrosis. (From Shields. *General thoracic surgery,* 3rd ed. Philadelphia: Lea & Febiger, 1989;111, with permission.)

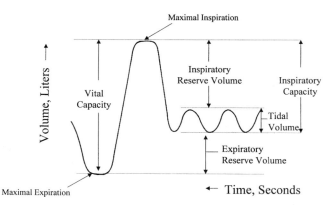

FIGURE 22-5. Determination of the tidal volume, vital capacity, inspiratory capacity, inspiratory reserve volume, and expiratory reserve volume from a spirometer. (From Levitzky MG. *Pulmonary physiology,* 3rd ed. New York: McGraw-Hill, 1991:57, with permission.)

frequency is often increased to maintain adequate alveolar minute ventilation. Chronic obstructive pulmonary diseases (COPD) cause an increased resistance to airflow. This is most pronounced on expiration that may lead to air trapping. Additionally, in emphysematous states, there is destruction of lung parenchyma at the alveolar level, leading to coalescence of alveoli into larger air spaces and decreased elastic recoil of the lung. These pathologic derangements often result in measurable increases in RV, FRC, and TLC.

In addition to the measurement of static lung volumes, dynamic characteristics of the lungs can be quantified and compared to predicted normal values as a measure of pathologic states. A common test is the forced expiratory volume (FEV), often expressed as "FEV_1," which is defined as the volume of gas exhaled in 1 second. The relationship between FEV_1 and forced vital capacity (FVC) can define normal, restrictive, or obstructive patterns. In both restrictive and obstructive lung disease, the FEV_1 and the FVC are reduced; however, in obstructive disease, the ratio is markedly reduced in contrast to restrictive disease states where the ratio may be normal or increased. $FEF_{25\%-75\%}$ (forced midexpiratory flow) is another useful measurement of the flow of air. This measurement is defined by the slope (volume vs. time) of the line between the points at 25% and 75% on the expiratory curve. To perform these flow measurements, the patient is asked to inspire maximally to TLC, and then with maximal forced expiratory effort, air is blown out of the lungs to RV. Using a spirometer, air volumes can be measured as a function of time, and FEV_1, FVC, $FEF_{25\%-75\%}$, and other volumes can be determined.

Pulmonary function tests (PFTs) are selectively used in the preoperative evaluation of the general surgical patient and routinely used in the preoperative evaluation of patients undergoing lung resection. The general surgical patient with COPD has an increased risk of postoperative pulmonary complications and must be managed aggressively. Several criteria are indicative of increased risk following lung resection: FVC less than 2 L, FEV_1/FVC less than 50%, an FVC less than 50% predicted, and a diffusing capacity less than 50% predicted. Additionally, PFTs can help define the amount of lung that may be resected with a low likelihood of postoperative respiratory insufficiency. In general, pulmonary resection can be tolerated if the postoperative FEV_1 is anticipated to be greater than 800 mL per second. Patients who have an FEV_1 measurement greater than 2 L per second can usually tolerate most pulmonary resections, including pneumonectomy. Ventilation-perfusion studies can complement the preoperative PFTs in those patients with FEV_1 measurements less than 2 L per second and can be used to predict postresection lung function. The test can determine how much of the area of planned resection contributes to overall lung function, and thus, postoperative lung function can be predicted by subtracting that quantity from initial baseline values.

Despite these guidelines, it must be noted that many of our previous concepts of adequacy of pulmonary reserve for emphysema patients undergoing pulmonary resection are currently being revised based on experience derived from lung volume reduction surgery. By this new concept, if an area of severe disease is removed from a hyperexpanded emphysematous lung, that patient's pulmonary function may actually improve. If valid, this concept renders any predictions of postoperative morbidity and mortality based on preoperative pulmonary function unreliable in this population.

PULMONARY VASCULATURE

The lung has a *dual vascular supply*: the pulmonary circulation and the bronchial circulation. The pulmonary circulation receives the entire cardiac output from the right ventricle and is composed of mixed venous blood with an approximate oxygen saturation of 68% to 76% in normal individuals. This blood consists of the systemic venous return mixed with the cardiac venous return that enters the right heart via the thebesian veins and coronary sinus. The bronchial circulation, in contradistinction, arises directly from the aorta and receives only 1% of the left ventricular cardiac output and has an oxygen saturation near 100%. The pulmonary arterial vessels are thin-walled vessels, containing much less vascular smooth muscle than the systemic vessels. This results in a vasculature that is under normal conditions, more distensible and thereby maintains relatively low pressure and low resistance within the pulmonary circulation. Normal pulmonary arterial pressures (15-30/6-12 mm Hg) are one fifth of the systemic circulation.

The main pulmonary artery quickly branches to form the right and left pulmonary arteries, which subsequently branch into the lobar, segmental, and subsegmental branches that are intimately related to the airways with one or more branches of the pulmonary artery supplying each bronchopulmonary segment. These larger elastic arteries give rise to the morphologically distinct arterioles that comprise the precapillary pulmonary vessels. The arterioles, capillaries, and venules comprise the microcirculation of the lung and establish the blood–air interface required for gas exchange. Other cellular components are important in the pulmonary microcirculation. Pericytes are found in alveolar capillaries and are thought to be phagocytic and control vascular contraction. Additionally, mast cells are found in the connective tissue of pulmonary vessels and may provide the vasoactive substances mediating pulmonary hypoxic vasoconstriction.

Blood returns from the pulmonary capillary network to the left atrium through the pulmonary veins. These veins lack valves and will drain into distinct superior and inferior pulmonary veins on either side. Some bronchial arteries will

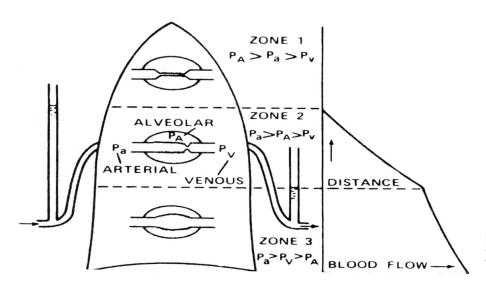

FIGURE 22-6. Lung zones. (From West JB. *Respiratory physiology: the essentials*, 4th ed. Baltimore: Williams & Wilkins, 1990, with permission.)

drain directly into the pulmonary venous system without entering the capillary network and thus contribute to physiological shunting.

It is critical to realize that the distribution of blood flow within the lung is not uniform. Gravity and alveolar pressures can influence regional lung perfusion. The relationship between perfusion (Q) and ventilation (V) is fundamental in understanding normal physiology as well as pathological states. Importantly, both V and Q increase from the top to the bottom of the lung; however, Q increases more rapidly. Classically, West described three zones of the lung based on the relationships between alveolar pressure (P_A), pulmonary arterial pressure (P_a), and pulmonary venous pressure (P_V) as affected by gravity (Fig. 22-6). Zone 1 conditions ($P_A > P_a > P_V$) are those at the apex of the lung. No blood flow can occur in this area because alveolar pressures exceed pulmonary arterial pressures. Thus, this area is alveolar dead space because it is ventilated but not perfused. Normally, zone 1 conditions do not exist. However, in situations where pulmonary arterial pressures are low (e.g., hypovolemia) or when alveolar pressures are elevated (e.g., mechanical ventilation with positive end-expiratory pressure), this physiology will be present, increasing alveolar dead space. Zone 3 conditions ($P_a > P_V > P_A$) are present at the base of the lungs. The driving pressure for flow is the difference between the pulmonary arterial and pulmonary venous pressures. Zone 2 conditions ($P_a > P_A > P_V$) prevail in the middle of the lung. The driving pressure for flow in this zone is the difference between the pulmonary arterial and alveolar pressures. These zones do not have specific anatomical boundaries but are dependent on the physiological conditions in a certain individual at a given point. Changes in cardiac output, blood volume, alveolar pressures, or body position will affect the boundaries between zones and thus the distribution of pulmonary blood flow.

The relationship between ventilation and perfusion determines alveolar and thus arterial PO_2 and PCO_2. Ideally, alveolar ventilation and perfusion should allow for complete hemoglobin saturation and removal of sufficient carbon dioxide to result in a normal pH level. This does not occur uniformly within the lung, and as described above, there are regions in which perfusion is decreased relative to ventilation (high V/Q ratios) or ventilation is decreased relative to pulmonary blood flow (low V/Q ratios) under even normal circumstances (Fig. 22-7). The extremes of these ratios are pure shunt (lung that is perfused, but not ventilated) and dead space (lung that is ventilated, but not perfused). Under relatively normal conditions, alveolar PO_2 is 100 mm Hg and a PCO_2 is 40 mm Hg. The mixed venous blood in the pulmonary arterial system has a PO_2 of about

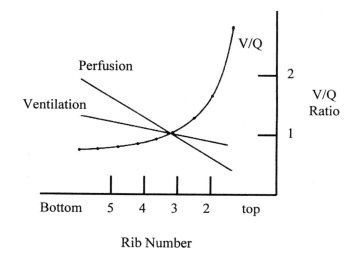

FIGURE 22-7. Distribution of ventilation and perfusion. (From West JB. *Ventilation blood flow and gas exchange*, 3rd ed. Oxford: Blackwell Science, 1977, with permission.)

40 mm Hg and a P_{CO_2} of 45 mm Hg. The resulting gradients for gas diffusion are 60 mm Hg for oxygen favoring movement toward the blood and 5 mm Hg for carbon dioxide favoring movement toward the alveoli. In the absence of alveolar ventilation, no gas exchange can occur and thus the partial pressures of oxygen and carbon dioxide in the blood will be unchanged. Similarly, any area of lung that is not perfused also can not be involved in gas exchange. Those units with low V/Q ratios will have a relatively lower P_{O_2} and higher P_{CO_2} in contrast to those areas with a high ratio, where the P_{O_2} is relatively higher and P_{CO_2} lower. The concept of V/Q mismatch will be further discussed as an etiology of hypoxia.

Pulmonary blood flow can be actively redistributed to optimize the V/Q relationship by a process called "hypoxic pulmonary vasoconstriction." Alveolar hypoxia (P_{O_2} < 70 mm Hg), hypercarbia, or collapse result in local pulmonary arteriolar vasoconstriction. The exact mechanism for this response remains unclear but may involve local release of vasoactive mediators. This vasoconstriction will divert blood from areas that will undergo little gas exchange (low V/Q) thus lowering P_{O_2} and increasing P_{CO_2} to areas that are better ventilated (relatively higher V/Q). Patients with COPD may develop pulmonary hypertension from chronic pulmonary vasoconstriction secondary to chronic alveolar hypoxia. Vasodilators, classically nitroprusside, can abolish this response. This can ultimately lead to arterial hypoxia due to the increase in the perfusion of poorly ventilated lungs, which results in a relative increase in the shunt fraction.

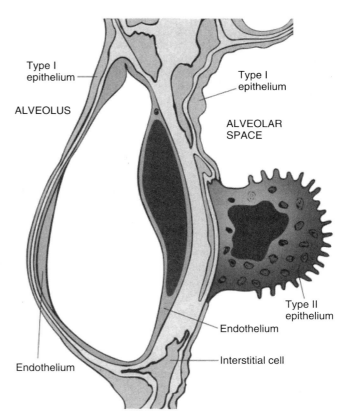

FIGURE 22-8. Alveolar septum. (Robbins RB. *Pathologic basis of disease*, 6th ed. Philadelphia: WB Saunders, 1999:698, with permission.)

GAS EXCHANGE

Gas exchange occurs at the alveolar level at the *interface of the alveolar epithelium and the capillary endothelium*. The alveoli are outpouchings of the respiratory bronchioles, alveolar ducts, and alveolar sacs. The alveolar septa are made up of a continuous flattened epithelium comprised of type I and type II alveolar epithelial cells covering a thin layer of interstitial tissue (Fig. 22-8). Type I alveolar cells cover approximately 95% of the alveolar surface and functionally are involved in resorbing pathological alveolar fluid or ingesting intraalveolar particulate material. The type II epithelial cells are the source of alveolar surfactant and are also involved in the renewal of the alveolar surface by differentiation into type I cells. A continuous basal lamina underlies both type I and type II cells and is in apposition to the underlying endothelial cell. The alveolar septal interstitium is also composed of connective tissue made of a proteoglycan matrix that is embedded with elastin and collagen. Alveolar macrophages are important in clearance of intraalveolar material, production of inflammatory mediators, and antigen presentation.

Disorders of the components of the respiratory zone occur in many different disease states, both primary pulmonary disease and pulmonary complications of systemic diseases. Alveolar epithelium is damaged by exposure to high oxygen concentrations. Type I cells are most susceptible to this oxidant injury. Sarcoidosis and idiopathic pulmonary fibrosis are classic examples of disease processes that cause alveolar lung damage due to abnormal inflammatory injury. Both diseases result in interstitial thickening secondary to inflammation and thus a decreased diffusion capacity. Chronic exposure to cigarette smoke stimulates neutrophil release of proteases. This causes significant destruction of the pulmonary interstitium, leading to emphysematous pulmonary diseases. Particulate inhalation can initiate pulmonary disease. Inhaled asbestos particles are ingested by pulmonary macrophages. The activated macrophages produce cytokines and attract neutrophils. These neutrophils induce an increased inflammatory response through the release of proteases that will result in parenchymal lung injury. These disorders will adversely affect the diffusion capacity of the lung.

After delivery of oxygen to the alveoli, it diffuses through the alveolar–capillary interface. At the blood–air interface, there are approximately 500 million alveoli with a combined surface area of 100 m², thus 120 L of air will come into contact with 25 L of blood per minute. For oxygen to be delivered to the blood, it must first dissolve into the layer of pulmonary surfactant, thus moving from the gas phase to the liquid phase. Oxygen then diffuses through the alveolar epithelium, interstitium, and capillary endothelium and into the plasma. Once in the plasma, some oxygen will remain dissolved; however, the majority of oxygen enters the erythrocyte where it becomes bound to hemoglobin. The blood carries the oxygen out of the lung and subsequently to the tissues of the body.

The rate of diffusion of a gas, governed by the Fick law of diffusion, is proportional to the area available for diffusion, the diffusion coefficient of a particular gas, and the partial pressure gradient across the barrier and is inversely proportional to the thickness of the barrier. The area available for diffusion is relatively constant; however, during exercise, additional capillaries can be recruited, thus increasing diffusion. In hypovolemia, the reverse may be true. The diffusion coefficient is proportional to the solubility of a given gas and inversely proportional to its molecular weight. When comparing oxygen and carbon dioxide, although carbon dioxide is larger than oxygen, it is about 25 times more soluble in the liquid phase and thus diffuses more rapidly through the air–blood barrier. The thickness of the alveolar–capillary barrier is about 0.2 to 0.5 μm. Pathologic states such as interstitial edema (e.g., congestive heart failure) and fibrosis (e.g., idiopathic pulmonary fibrosis) will cause thickening of the barrier and interfere with diffusion. Clinically, the *diffusing capacity* for oxygen is difficult to measure, and therefore, that of carbon monoxide is used. The diffusing capacity of carbon monoxide (DL_{CO}) can be determined by dividing the uptake of carbon monoxide by its measured arterial partial pressure. The diffusing capacity of the lung is determined from the diffusing capacity of the alveolar–capillary membrane, the reaction of carbon monoxide and hemoglobin, and pulmonary capillary blood volume.

Hypoxia

Gas exchange is best understood by looking at the factors that can cause malfunction or hypoxemia (Table 22-1). Alveolar P_{O_2} and thus arterial P_{O_2} are determined by the partial pressure of oxygen in the inspired gas as well as alveolar ventilation and O_2 consumption. Decreased alveolar ventilation results in an increased alveolar P_{CO_2} (and thus arterial P_{CO_2}) and a corresponding decrease in alveolar and arterial P_{O_2} (which defines hypoxia). This relationship is defined by the alveolar gas equation.

$P_{AO_2} = P_{IO_2} - P_{ACO_2}/0.8$,

where P_{AO_2} is the alveolar partial pressure of oxygen, P_{IO_2} is the partial pressure of oxygen in inspired air, and P_{ACO_2} is the alveolar CO_2, which approximately equals arterial CO_2. The important pulmonary physiology equations are summarized in Table 22-2.

Thus, hypoventilation is one cause of hypoxemia. Hypoventilation can be caused by CNS depressants (such as opiates, narcotics), respiratory muscle paralysis or dysfunction (e.g., neuromuscular blockade, phrenic nerve paresis), or mechanical impairments of the chest wall (such as flail chest). The equation also points out the obvious fact that hypoxia may be caused by a low concentration of oxygen in the inspired air.

Hypoxemia may also be caused by an increased diffusion gradient. Normally, the red cell has fully equilibrated with alveolar oxygen during its transit through an alveolar capillary. In some interstitial lung disease such as sarcoidosis, collagen vascular diseases, alveolar cell carcinoma, interstitial edema secondary to congestive heart failure and interstitial fibrosis, there is a failure of the red cell to equilibrate with alveolar oxygen due to an underlying diffusion impairment, and systemic hypoxemia may result. It is important to note that the equilibration of mixed venous oxygen with alveolar oxygen occurs within about 0.25 seconds, which is approximately one third of the time that blood is in a pulmonary capillary. Thus, patients who have abnormal diffusing capacity may have normal arterial oxygen at rest, but during exercise, hypoxia is present due to the relatively decreased pulmonary capillary transit time.

Shunt is another cause of hypoxemia. "Shunt," by definition, is the fraction of blood that enters the systemic arterial system without passing through a ventilated portion of

TABLE 22-1. CAUSES OF HYPOXIA

Ventilation-perfusion mismatch
Shunt
Decreased alveolar P_{O_2}
Hypoventilation
Increased diffusion gradient

TABLE 22-2. IMPORTANT PULMONARY PHYSIOLOGY EQUATIONS

Alveolar gas equation[a]	$P_{AO_2} = P_{IO_2} - P_{ACO_2}/0.8 + F$
A-a gradient (Nrl 15–20 mm Hg)[b]	$P(A-a)O_2 = P_{AO_2} - P_{aO_2}$
Shunt Equation[c]	$Q_s/Q_T = C_{cO_2} - C_{aO_2}/C_{cO_2} - C_{vO_2}$
Pulmonary vascular resistance[d]	$PVR = PA_m - LA_m/CO$
Fick's law of diffusion[e]	$V_{gas} = A \times D \times (P_1 - P_2)/T$

[a]P_{AO_2}, alveolar partial pressure of oxygen; P_{IO_2}, partial pressure of oxygen in inspired air; P_{ACO_2}, alveolar CO_2 = arterial CO_2; F, correction factor (ignored).
[b]P_{AO_2}, alveolar partial pressure of oxygen; P_{aO_2}, arterial partial pressure of oxygen.
[c]Q_s/Q_T, shunt; C_{cO_2}, content of capillary oxygen; C_{aO_2}, content of arterial oxygen; C_{vO_2}, content of venous oxygen.
[d]PA_m, mean pulmonary artery pressure; LA_m, mean left atrial pressure; CO, cardiac output.
[e]A, area available for diffusion; D, diffusion coefficient; $P_1 - P_2$, pressure gradient of the gas across the diffusion barrier; T, thickness of the barrier.

the lung, i.e., lung that is perfused, but not ventilated. Shunt can be seen in pathological states such as intracardiac right-to-left shunts or congenital heart diseases, arteriovenous malformations, and in states in which there is lung consolidation (such as pneumonia, atelectasis). Shunt is the only cause of hypoxemia that can not be corrected by the administration of oxygen.

Ventilation/perfusion (V/Q) mismatch is the most common cause of hypoxemia, as discussed above. V/Q mismatch can be considered "partial shunting." In patients with pulmonary disease, the lung will have alveoli with varying V/Q ratios (those tending toward shunt and those toward dead space). The hyperventilatory response to hypoxia, which results from chemoreceptors at the carotid bifurcation and below the aortic arch, is more effective in correcting hypercarbia than hypoxia. Thus, the net result of V/Q mismatch is hypoxemia and hyperventilation. The diagnosis of V/Q mismatch as the cause of hypoxia is often by exclusion of other etiologies.

MECHANICAL VENTILATION

The first description of positive pressure ventilation was by Vesalius in 1555. Negative pressure ventilators (iron lungs) were used extensively during the polio epidemic of the 1950s. The prototypes for today's positive pressure ventilators were first used at the Massachusetts General Hospital also in the 1950s. Positive pressure ventilators have become increasingly sophisticated with various potential modes of support.

Indications for Mechanical Ventilation

Although a number of criteria have been proposed as guides, it should be emphasized that indications for the institution of mechanical ventilatory support are subjective and require clinical judgment. Support may be indicated secondary to derangements in any component of the respiratory system: CNS, chest wall, airway, respiratory muscles, or alveoli. Patients with CNS depression secondary to narcotic overdose or closed head injury often require intubation for airway protection and respiratory support. Abnormalities of the chest wall such as a flail chest, open pneumothorax, or marked scoliosis may require mechanical support. Respiratory muscle fatigue is thought to play a role in respiratory failure requiring support in COPD. Intubation is often required in patients with facial trauma, anaphylaxis, or atelectasis from endobronchial masses or foreign bodies. Respiratory failure due to the alveolar component may be secondary to multiple causes including cardiogenic or noncardiogenic pulmonary edema and extensive pneumonia. Mechanical support may be indicated in these settings for hypercapnia ($PaCO_2$ >45 mm Hg) or life-threatening hypoxia (PaO_2 <55 mm Hg) despite maximal oxygen therapy. Others have suggested a respiratory rate greater than 35 as a criterion. However, the most common indication for intubation and mechanical ventilation is the judgment of an experienced clinician that the overall clinical condition of the patient requires it.

Modes of mechanical support

There are multiple modes of mechanical ventilatory support and no strategy is inherently better than any other. The most common modes include assist-control (AC) ventilation, intermittent mandatory ventilation (IMV), pressure support (PS), and pressure control (PC) ventilation. In AC ventilation, the ventilator will deliver a breath at a preset interval provided there is no patient-initiated breath. Any patient-triggered respiratory effort will result in the delivery of a breath at a preset tidal volume. In intermittent mandatory ventilation, the patient receives breaths at a preset tidal volume and rate. Any spontaneous respiration by the patient is not mechanically supported and additional minute ventilation is patient dependent. Synchronized intermittent mandatory ventilation (SIMV) differs from IMV only in that delivered breaths are initiated only after the patient exhales completely (Fig. 22-9). PS ventilation is a mode that is pressure cycled, unlike assist-control and intermittent mandatory ventilation, which are volume cycled. A preset positive pressure will support each patient-initiated breath. The tidal volume achieved with each inspiration is dependent on the amount of PS, the patient effort, and the compliance of the lungs. In PC ventilatory support, the inflation pressure (peak airway pressure), inspiratory time, and respiratory rate are set. The delivered tidal volume is determined by pulmonary compliance. This mode can be used in patients with ARDS in an attempt to minimize the barotrauma that may result from elevated peak airway pressures. Positive end-expiratory pressure (PEEP) can also be used in mechanical ventilatory support. PEEP can help decrease V/Q mismatch by increasing FRC, which can allow for a reduction in inspired oxygen, and PEEP is also useful in a patient with ARDS.

Positive pressure ventilation affects cardiac performance and entails a significant risk of developing complications. The increase in intrathoracic pressure from mechanical ventilation results in both compression of the superior vena cava and distention of the alveoli. The right heart thus has a decreased preload (decreased venous return) and increased afterload (increased pulmonary vascular resistance secondary to compression of alveolar vessels), resulting in decreased cardiac output. These changes in the right ventricle produce a leftward shift of the interventricular septum and affect left ventricular compliance. This altered physiology, which results in decreased cardiac performance, is most pronounced in hypovolemic patients. In addition to alterations in hemodynamic parameters, other complications of mechanical ventilation include oxygen toxicity with pro-

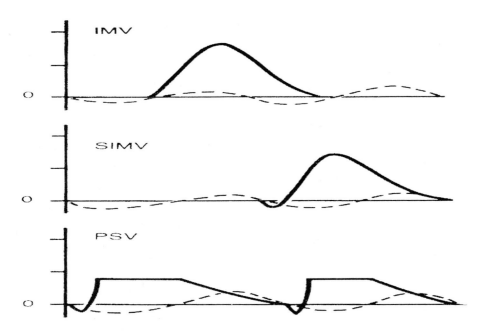

FIGURE 22-9. Ventilation modes. IMV, intermittent mandatory ventilation; SIMV, synchronized intermittent mandatory ventilation; PSV, pressure support ventilation. Dashed lines indicate spontaneous breaths, and solid lines indicate augmented breaths. (From Marino PL. *The ICU book*, 1st ed. Philadelphia: Lea & Ferbiger, 1991:373, with permission.)

longed use of 70% or greater FIO_2, endotracheal tube complications —tracheal stenosis, laryngeal injury, tracheomalacia, and tracheoinnominate fistulae—barotrauma including tension pneumothorax, and infection including sinusitis and pneumonia. These potential complications suggest that mechanical support should be discontinued as promptly as possible.

The weaning of mechanical ventilation is as much trial and error as science. Discontinuation of mechanical support is not considered in those patients who have an inadequate neurological or airway status or hemodynamic instability. Weaning from assist control is often achieved by increasing periods without support, until the patient can support adequate ventilation. IMV weaning is achieved by decreasing the number of breaths per minute, requiring the patient to maintain adequate minute ventilation with progressively more unsupported breaths. In PS weaning, the amount of positive PS is decreased until the patient is maintaining adequate ventilation in the absence of support. Many criteria have been used to predict successful extubation. Both lung mechanics and the ability to maintain oxygenation must be assessed. Mechanically, a minute ventilation less than 10 L per minute, a VT greater than 5 mL/kg, a vital capacity > 10 mL/kg, and a negative inspiratory force greater that 20 cm H_2O are useful data to support extubation. A PaO_2 > 60 mm Hg on a FIO_2 < 40% and an A–a gradient ($\frac{PaO_2}{FIO_2}$) better than 300 mm Hg suggest adequate gas exchange to support extubation.

SUMMARY

We have reviewed respiratory physiology in the context of its three major components: ventilation, perfusion, and gas exchange. The anatomical and physiological determinants of these three key functions have been detailed. Air movement has been seen to depend on the conducting airways and the dynamic properties of the respiratory muscles, lung, and chest wall. We have described lung volumes and pulmonary function testing as they relate to these properties of pulmonary mechanics. Pulmonary blood flow has been described in normal and pathophysiologic states, and its complex relationship to ventilation and the concept of V/Q mismatch has been presented. Gas exchange at the alveolar–arterial interface has also been touched upon. We have attempted throughout to provide common clinical scenarios that highlight the value of these basic concepts in daily practice.

23

THORACIC PATHOPHYSIOLOGY AND MALIGNANCIES

SETH D. FORCE AND LARRY R. KAISER

Although normal thoracic physiology contributes toward healthy daily respiratory function, alterations in this physiology can lead to dramatic consequences. Clinical knowledge of the proper management of thoracic pathophysiology and diseases is a must for all physicians.

BENIGN LUNG DISEASE

Bronchiectasis is the abnormal dilation of the bronchi usually found beyond the subsegmental bronchi. This process can result from congenital disorders such as primary ciliary dysmotility (Kartagener syndrome), α_1-antitrypsin deficiency, and cystic fibrosis, but most cases are due to lung infections, which cause impaired clearance of airway secretions and lead to bronchial injury.

Most patients present in childhood with a persistent productive cough, fetor oris, hemoptysis, and recurrent pulmonary infections. Physical examination may reveal rales over the involved areas, osteoarthropathy, and clubbing. Although chest radiographs usually show nonspecific findings of increased lung markings, atelectasis, or cystic areas, computed tomography (CT) scans demonstrate more specific findings of bronchial dilation within the lung parenchyma. Bronchoscopy should be included in the diagnostic regimen to rule out obstructing lesions, and pulmonary function tests should be performed in surgical candidates to assess the adequacy of pulmonary reserve.

The majority of patients with bronchiectasis can be treated successfully with antibiotics, cessation of cigarette smoking, and pulmonary toilet during periodic exacerbations. Pulmonary resection of the involved lung parenchyma is reserved for patients who do not respond to conservative management. Patients who have bilateral lung involvement benefit most if the side with the more severe disease is operated on first. This, in turn, may lead to improvement in the contralateral lung disease.

Pulmonary tuberculosis is the number one infectious disease cause of death in the world. The decline of the disease in the Western world has been halted by the emergence of human immunodeficiency virus (HIV) infection. Atypical mycobacteria disease also is on the rise secondary to HIV, the use of immunosuppressants in transplant recipients, and patients with autoimmune disease, and the use of chemotherapy in cancer patients. Among all the mycobacteria, *Mycobacterium tuberculosis* is the most commonly seen pathologic organism in the lung.

Mycobacterial infection is spread by a respiratory route via aerosolization. Patients who become infected initially (primary tuberculosis) develop a necrotizing pneumonia. The mycobacteria eventually spread to the hilar lymph nodes, where they form caseous granulomas. The disease usually is halted at this point by a vigorous cell-mediated immune response, but occasionally, the mycobacteria can enter the bloodstream, leading to disseminated or miliary tuberculosis.

Treatment of pulmonary tuberculous infections center around the use of antimycobacterial drugs and includes either 2 months of isoniazid, rifampin, and pyrazinamide followed by 4 months of isoniazid and rifampin or 9 months of isoniazid and rifampin (for individuals who can not take pyrazinamide). Ethambutol is added to each regimen until drug sensitivities can be determined. Due to the ocular toxicity of ethambutol, streptomycin is used in its place for children who are too young to be monitored effectively. Surgical resection rarely is required and is limited to the following situations: (i) positive sputum samples plus cavitary lung lesions after more than 5 months of treatment with two or more drugs, (ii) severe or recurrent hemoptysis, (iii) bronchopleural fistula not responsive to treatment with chest tube drainage, (iv) a persistently infected space (empyema), (v) a mass found in the area of the lung infected with *M. tuberculosis,* and (vi) disease caused by drug-resistant atypical mycobacteria such as *M. avium-intracellulare.*

Hospital of the University of Pennsylvania, Philadelphia, Pennsylvania

LUNG CANCER

Incidence, Epidemiology, Molecular Biology

Lung cancer is the most common cause of cancer-related deaths in both men and women and second in prevalence only to breast cancer in women and prostate cancer in men. Although men make up over 60% of all patients with lung cancer, the percentage of women being diagnosed is quickly climbing secondary to the increased incidence of smoking in women. Although smoking is a clearly defined risk factor, most people who smoke do not develop lung cancer while others who have no history of tobacco use are diagnosed with the disease. Accordingly, the mechanism behind lung cancer appears to be multifactorial. Epidemiological studies show an increase in familial cases while environmental toxins, such as asbestos, chromium, and radon gas have also been linked to the development of lung cancers.

Several genetic mutations are linked to the development of lung cancer. K-ras mutations are the most common oncogene abnormalities seen in non–small cell lung cancer (NSCLC) and are associated with a decreased survival rate. Mutations in the tumor suppressor genes, p53 and Rb, are also associated with the development of lung cancer. Other associations with lung cancer include the growth factors epidermal growth factor receptor (EGFR), vascular endothelial growth factor (VEGF), and transforming growth factor-α (TGF-α), lack of A- and H-related blood group antigens and nonexpression of the bcl-2 protein.

Seventy-five percent to eighty percent of primary lung cancers are NSCLC, with small cell lung cancer (SCLC) making up the remaining 25% to 30%. Most NSCLCs are adenocarcinomas, followed by squamous cell, and large cell carcinomas. Two thirds of patients who develop lung cancer present with disseminated disease and thus are inoperable. Of the remaining one third of patients, approximately two thirds have potentially resectable disease.

NSCLC is staged according to the TNM staging criteria, which is summarized in Table 23-1 and Fig. 23-1. Most patients present with an asymptomatic pulmonary nodule on chest radiograph. Although many benign lesions can appear on a chest radiograph, a solitary pulmonary nodule is assumed to be lung cancer until proven otherwise. The management of a patient with an asymptomatic solitary pulmonary nodule depends on many factors including age, history of cigarette use, size of the nodule, and change in size of the nodule. Young patients or patients with nodules that have been stable in size over many years do not necessarily warrant a biopsy but can be managed with serial chest radiographs. However, patients who are older, have a history of cigarette use, or have a significant increase in size of the nodule warrant a definitive tissue diagnosis. Additionally, symptomatic patients who present with chronic nonproductive cough, pneumonia, hemoptysis, or chest pain also warrant a thorough cancer workup, including biopsy of any pulmonary nodules.

All patients with pulmonary nodules and significant risk factors or pulmonary symptoms should undergo either an open biopsy or a thoracoscopic wedge biopsy followed by definitive resection if cancer is found. Transthoracic or computed tomography (CT) guided needle biopsy can also be employed in patients who can not tolerate an operation, who are suspected to have recurrent lung cancer, or who are thought to have SCLC. One drawback of needle biopsy is that it has a significant false-negative rate and thus a negative biopsy can not completely exclude the presence of carcinoma.

Bronchoscopy, along with bronchial brushing, washing, and biopsy, is another technique that can be used to obtain a tissue diagnosis from pulmonary nodules. Bronchial washings and brushings of bronchoscopically visible tumors supply a diagnosis 75% of the time, versus 50% of the time when the tumor is not visible. When tissue biopsy is added to this procedure, the diagnostic yield is increased to 94% for visible tumors and 60% for tumors that are not visible.

Magnetic resonance imaging (MRI) and positron emission tomographic (PET) scanning have also been used in the preoperative workup of a patient with a solitary pulmonary nodule. MRI is primarily used to evaluate masses and nodal spread in patients who can not tolerate intravenous contrast. PET scanning uses fluoronated glucose uptake to differentiate benign masses from malignant masses. This technique is highly sensitive, with rates ranging from 94% to 98%, but it is limited in its specificity. False-positive results occur mainly with inflammation from mycobacterial or other pulmonary infections.

Once a diagnosis of NSCLC has been made, a preoperative evaluation of the patient should be performed, including a complete history and physical examination, anterior posterior (AP) and lateral chest x-ray, complete blood count, chemistry panel, liver function tests, and CT scan of the chest and abdomen, with particular attention to the adrenal glands. Other studies that may help rule out metastatic disease include a CT scan of the brain and a bone scan.

Mediastinoscopy is another essential tool in ruling out advanced stage disease. Mediastinoscopy can be used in conjunction with CT scanning to help identify nodal disease or to rule out lymphadenopathy secondary to benign or reactive processes. Patients who have peripheral lesions and CT scans negative for mediastinal disease have only a 10% chance of having nodal disease and do not require a mediastinoscopy. However, patients with more centrally located tumors or mediastinal lymph nodes of more than 1 cm, seen on CT scan, require mediastinoscopy to rule out nodal disease. Approximately 90% of the mediastinal lymph nodes can be sampled with this technique.

Pulmonary function testing is also essential for patients undergoing resection for lung cancer. Most patients will be able to tolerate surgery as long as their postoperative forced expiratory volume (FEV$_1$) is $\geq$ 800 mL per second. Patients

TABLE 23-1. CLASSIFICATION OF LUNG CANCER

Stage	TNM classification
IA	T1 N0 M0
IB	T2 N0 M0
IIA	T1 N1 M0
IIB	T2 N1 M0, T3 N0 M0
IIIA	T1 N2 M0, T2 N2 M0, T3 N1 M0, T3 N2 M0
IIIB	Any T N3 M0, T4, Any N M0
IV	Any T Any N M1

Primary tumor

T1	• Tumor ≤3 cm
	• No bronchoscopic evidence of invasion into main bronchus
T2	• Tumor >3 cm
	• Involvement of main bronchus
	• ≥2 cm from the carina
	• Invasion of visceral pleura
	• Associated atelectasis or obstructive pneumonitis extending into the hilar region but not entire lung
T3	• Any size tumor invading chest wall (includes superior sulcus tumors), diaphragm, mediastinal pleura, parietal pericardium
	• Tumor >2 cm from the carina, without carinal involvement
	• Atelectasis or pneumonitis of the entire lung
T4	• Any size tumor invading mediastinum, heart, great vessels, trachea, esophagus, vertebral body, carina
	• Separate tumor nodules in the same lobe
	• Malignant pleural effusion

Regional lymph Nodes

N0	• No lymph node metastases
N1	• Ipsilateral peribronchial or hilar metastases
	• Ipsilateral intrapulmonary nodes involved by direct extension
N2	• Ipsilateral mediastinal and/or subcarinal lymph node metastases
N3	• Contralateral mediastinal or hilar lymph node metastases
	• Ipsilateral or contralateral scalene or supraclavicular lymph node metastases

Nodal levels

N	Level/nodes
N2	1/ highest mediastinal
	2/ upper paratracheal
	3/ pretracheal and retrotracheal
	4/ lower paratracheal, including azygous nodes
Aortic	5/ subaortic (aortopulmonary window)
	6/ paraaortic (ascending aortic or phrenic)
Inferior	7/ subcarinal
mediastinal	8/ paraesophageal (below carina)
nodes	9/ inferior pulmonary ligament
N1	10/ hilar
	11/ interlobar
	12/ segmental
	13/ subsegmental

Distant metastases

M0	No distant metastases
M1	Distant metastases, including synchronous nodules in a different lobe

with marginal lung function may require a ventilation-perfusion scan to determine how much of the involved lung parenchyma is adding to overall lung function. Additionally, preoperative P_{CO_2} level of more than 50 mm Hg also identifies patients at a higher risk.

Non–Small Cell Lung Cancer

A complete discussion about therapy for lung cancer, including adjuvant and neoadjuvant therapy, is complex and dependent on many factors, such as the physical condition of the patient, tumor histology, tumor size, and lymph node status. *Surgical resection* is the *mainstay* of therapy for stage I and II NSCLCs (Fig. 23-1, A–D). Most patients will undergo a lobectomy or pneumonectomy to achieve negative margins, depending on the location of their tumor. Segmentectomy and wedge resection may be appropriate for patients with marginal lung reserve who would not tolerate larger resections, but these procedures are associated with higher recurrence rates than either lobectomy or pneumonectomy.

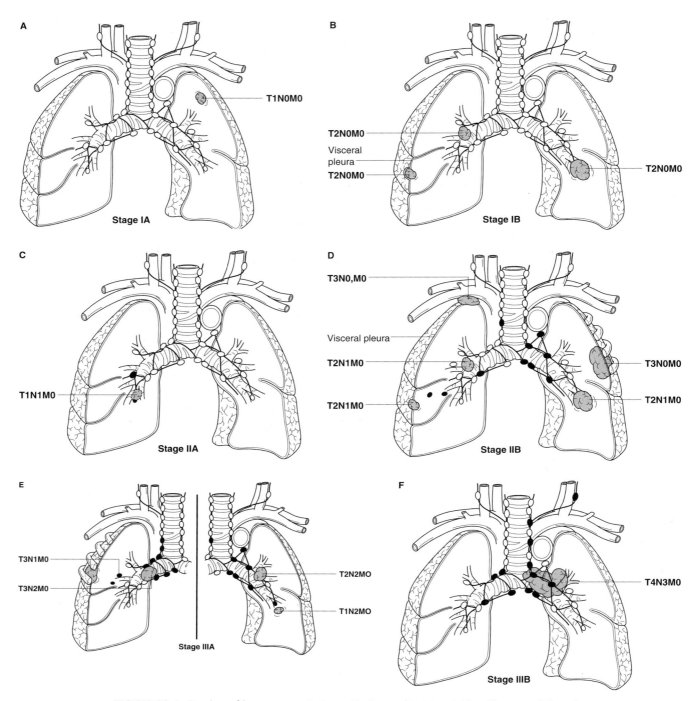

FIGURE 23-1. Staging of lung cancer. **A:** Stage IA disease (T1 N0 M0) identifies a small (less than 3-cm) tumor surrounded by lung parenchyma. **B:** Stage IB disease (T2 N0 M0) includes larger tumors that invade the visceral pleura or the main bronchi, or that have evidence of atelectasis/pneumonitis extending to the hilar regions. No metastatic disease is present with stage I tumors. **C:** Stage IIA (T1 N1 M0) identifies small tumors with TI characteristics (less than 3 cm) involving the peribronchial or hilar nodes by extension or metastasis. **D:** Stage IIB disease includes larger tumors (more than 3 cm) involving the peribronchial or hilar lymph nodes (T2 N1 M0) or tumors with limited extrapulmonary extension such as involvement of the chest wall or the pericardium (T3 N0 M0) but no evidence of metastasis. **E:** Stage IIIA describes tumors with localized extrapulmonary extension and involvement of peribronchial or hilar lymph nodes (T3 N1 M0) as well as any T1, T2, or T3 tumors with metastasis to the ipsilateral mediastinal and subcarinal lymph nodes (T1, T2, or T3 N2 M0). **F:** Stage IIIB describes either extensive extrapulmonary tumor invasion (T4 any N M0) or metastasis to the contralateral mediastinal and hilar lymph nodes as well as ipsilateral and contralateral supraclavicular/scalene lymph nodes. (From Mountain CF. The international system for staging lung cancer. *Semin Surg Oncol* 2000;18:106–115, with permission.)

Resection for stage IIIA is performed with the objective of resecting all pulmonary disease and lymph node disease (Fig. 23-1E). Survival rates of 25% to 40% can be achieved in patients with resected T3 or N1 disease. Current practice regarding N2 disease centers around operative diagnosis utilizing mediastinoscopy and bronchoscopy. Patients with documented N2 metastases are treated with neoadjuvant chemotherapy followed by surgical resection if the treatment is successful. This aggressive method of treatment has been shown to increase the median survival of patients with N2 disease.

Patients with *stage IIIB disease* are generally *not considered operative candidates* (Fig. 23-1F). This is particularly true in the case of positive contrateral lymph nodes. One study, however, by the Southwest Oncology Group, did show a benefit to surgical resection in these patients. They were able to achieve a 63% resectability rate and a 39% 2-year survival rate in patients with stage IIIB disease who received neoadjuvant chemotherapy/radiation therapy.

Adjuvant Therapy

Adjuvant chemotherapy or *radiation therapy* is generally not used for patients with stage I disease. Three prospective trials were carried out by the Lung Cancer Study Group (LCSG) to evaluate the use of adjuvant therapy for stage II and III lung cancers. The first of these studies showed an increase in disease-free and overall survival in patients treated with postoperative chemotherapy versus intrapleural BCG plus oral levamisole. The BCG group did not have a survival advantage over the surgery alone group and the increase in survival in the adjuvant chemotherapy group was limited to 7 months, the duration of the chemotherapy.

In the second study, patients with incompletely resected lesions were randomized to receive postoperative chemotherapy either alone or in combination with radiation. The group that received both modalities had a significant increase in disease-free survival and an increase in overall survival that was not statistically significant. In the third LCSG trial, patients with stage III disease who received postoperative chemotherapy did not show any increase in overall survival. In summary, adjuvant chemotherapy for stage II and III lung cancer has not been shown to increase overall survival and therefore is not generally accepted.

Postoperative radiation therapy was also evaluated by the LCSG in the late 1970s and early 1980s. Similar to their findings concerning adjuvant chemotherapy, they found no survival advantage in stage II and III patients treated with adjuvant radiation over surgery alone. The studies did show that local recurrence was decreased, and that therefore, radiation may have some role in patients with incompletely resected cancers.

Most *lung cancer recurrences* appear as metastatic lesions rather than local disease. The majority of patients with stage II and III who develop recurrences do so within 2 years, and nearly 100% within 5 years of diagnosis. Although the brain is the most common site of recurrence for tumors of all stages, recurrences may also be found in almost any organ including the bones, adrenal glands, lung, liver, kidney, and heart.

Survival depends most on the stage of the tumor at the time of diagnosis, with lymph node status having the greatest effect on long-term survival. Five-year survival rates are 60% to 80% for stage I tumors, 40% to 50% for stage IIA tumors, 22% for stage IIIA tumors, and 5% for stage IIIB tumors and stage IV tumors. The effect of lymph node status can be seen in stage IIB tumors. Stage IIB T3 N0 tumors have a 40% 5-year survival rate. This rate falls to 15% with N1 disease.

Small Cell Lung Cancer

SCLCs are grouped as APUD (amine precursor uptake, decarboxylase) tumors because of their ability to produce and secrete neuroendocrine peptides. These aggressive tumors rarely present as resectable lesions, with fewer than 10% of all patients presenting with T1 to T2 or N0 to N1 lesions. Primary treatment involving chemotherapy can achieve response in up to 80% of patients with any stage disease. Despite the good response of SCLC to chemotherapy, the 5-year survival rate is a dismal 10%. Most patients will receive a combination of chemotherapy and radiation therapy even though the addition of radiation only seems to improve disease-free survival and not overall survival. Patients who do present with limited disease can be treated with a combination of surgical resection and adjuvant chemotherapy/radiation therapy, achieving 5-year survival rates of 30% to 50%.

Resection of Pulmonary Metastases

The lungs represent the primary, and possibly sole, location for metastases from various tumors. Pulmonary metastatectomy, initially performed in the late 1920s, has now become an excepted aid to treatment of many cancers. Most patients with pulmonary metastases present with asymptomatic lesions on follow-up chest radiographs. Further investigation of the lesions with CT scans may be necessary, but it is important to mention that CT scan results are unreliable in quantitating the number of metastases and up to 25% of pulmonary metastases may be missed by standard chest CT scanning.

Although particular contraindications to resection are under debate, several guidelines for resection include control of the primary cancer, absence of extrathoracic metastases, adequate health and pulmonary function, and lack of an efficacious systemic therapy.

The largest study of patients to undergo pulmonary metastatectomy was performed by the International Registry of Lung Metastases. It reported on over 4,000 cases of metastatic germ-cell tumors, epithelial tumors, sarcomas, and melanomas in the *Journal of Thoracic and Cardiovascular Surgery* in 1997. Five-, ten-, and fifteen-year actuarial survival rates for completely resected metastases were 36%, 26%, and 22%, respectively. This contrasted to 5- and 10-year actuarial survival rates of 13% and 7% for incompletely resected tumors. A better prognosis was seen in patients with germ-cell tumors, disease-free interval of more than 36 months, and single metastases. Among all patients with tumors, patients with resections for metastatic Wilms tumors had the best prognosis, and those with melanoma the worst.

Carcinoid Tumors: Typical and Atypical

Carcinoid tumors are neuroendocrine tumors that arise from bronchial epithelial cells. They make up only 2% of all lung carcinomas and over 80% of all pulmonary adenomas. Although usually associated with serotonin production, these tumors can produce and secrete various neuroendocrine peptides, such as bradykinin, glucagon, insulin, vasopressin, melanocyte-stimulating hormone, and calcitonin. Unlike typical carcinoids, which rarely metastasize, atypical tumors are associated with lymph node metastases in 50% of patients. Carcinoid tumors usually present with pulmonary symptoms (hemoptysis, dyspnea, obstructive pneumonia) while the true carcinoid syndrome is only seen in 2% of patients who have metastatic disease. Treatment centers around complete surgical resection of the tumor. Five-year survival is 90% for typical carcinoids and 60% for atypical carcinoids.

Bronchial Adenomas

The term "bronchial adenomas" encompasses a group of tumors that includes adenoid cystic carcinoma, mucoepidermoid carcinoma, and mucous gland adenoma (some sources will include carcinoid tumor in this group). The last of these, mucous gland adenoma, represents the only benign tumor in the group. These tumors are very slow growing, requiring years of growth to produce pulmonary symptoms.

Adenoid cystic carcinomas, also known as "cylindromas," arise from the submucosal glands in the bronchi and trachea and resemble salivary gland tumors. These tumors, although slow growing, invade the submucosal plane along the perineural lymphatics, and therefore, upon resection, they may be found to extend well past their gross margin. The mainstay of therapy for these lesions is resection of the tumor and involved trachea followed by postoperative radiation therapy. When lesions prove unresectable, palliation can be obtained with endobronchial laser therapy and radiation. The slow growth of these tumors allows for long-term survival, even in patients with unresectable tumors.

Mucoepidermoid carcinomas are rarely seen and account for less than 5% of all bronchial adenomas. These tumors can vary in degree of malignancy from low to high grades, and have features of salivary glands on histology. Treatment for these lesions involves surgical resection. High-grade lesions can be treated as bronchogenic carcinomas with regard to resection and survival.

BENIGN LUNG TUMORS

Benign lung masses may arise from epithelial, mesenchymal, or endothelial tissue. The most common of these lesions is the hamartoma. Hamartomas usually present as asymptomatic solitary pulmonary nodules that exhibit a slow rate of growth. On chest radiographs, they may be seen as discrete rounded nodules, often with "popcorn calcifications." Rarely, hamartomas cause symptoms secondary to obstruction or erosion into a bronchus. More often, however, these lesions present as diagnostic dilemmas and must be resected to rule out malignancy.

CHEST WALL TUMORS

Chest wall tumors are relatively uncommon tumors that may arise from bone, cartilage, or soft tissue. A little over half of these lesions are primary tumors, with the rest being metastatic lesions from the genitourinary tract, colon, or thyroid. Approximately 60% of chest wall tumors are malignant and are composed of, in decreasing order of frequency, chondrosarcomas, fibrosarcomas, multiple myeloma, Ewing's sarcoma, and osteosarcoma. The most common benign tumors are fibrous dysplasia of bone, chondromas, and osteochondromas.

Most patients present with an enlarging chest wall mass. Preoperative workup includes AP and lateral chest radiographs to look for rib involvement, metastases, or pleural effusion. Chest CT scans are important to evaluate the relationship of the mass to other thoracic structures and to rule out adenopathy or pulmonary metastases. Abdominal CT scans should also be obtained to rule out hepatic metastases and to search for possible primary renal or colonic tumors. A bone scan is also essential to rule out the involvement of other bony sites in the event of a metastatic lesion.

Tumors smaller than 4 cm can be excised with wide margins as definitive management. Larger lesions will require either excision biopsy or core needle biopsy before surgical resection. Contrary to prior beliefs, preoperative biopsy can provide adequate tissue for a diagnosis and does not increase the risk of local recurrence or distant spread. The biopsy incision should be performed as to allow for scar excision upon definitive resection of the mass.

Malignant Chest Wall Tumors

Bone/Cartilage

Most rib tumors are malignant, the most common of these being chondrosarcomas. Chondrosarcomas are usually seen in adult patients and present as painful slowly growing solitary masses involving the first four ribs. Chest radiographs may show a lobulated mass with poorly defined margins and the presence of bony destruction. Local excision with a 4- to 5-cm margin is the treatment for these lesions. Resection can achieve 10-year survival rates of over 90%. Negative predictors of survival include metastases, age over 50 years, and incomplete resection.

Ewing sarcomas are vascular tumors that are usually seen in male children or adolescents. The tumors commonly present as painful chest wall masses often associated with pleural effusions. Patients may also experience fever, leukocytosis, and an elevated erythrocyte sedimentation rate. Radiographically, these lesions take on an "onion skin" appearance due to periosteal elevation and new bone formation. There may also be areas of bone destruction on the x-rays. The radiographic findings in conjunction with a fever can be mistaken for osteomyelitis, requiring a biopsy for definitive diagnosis. Treatment with radiation, surgical resection, and chemotherapy yields 10-year survival rates of 40% to 50%. Approximately half of the patients with Ewing sarcoma present with metastases to the lungs or brain.

Osteogenic sarcoma, like Ewing sarcoma, usually affects male children or adolescents. Typically, these lesions present as painful rapidly growing chest wall masses. Chest radiographs may show a characteristic "sunburst" pattern along with bony destruction and soft tissue involvement. Patients commonly present with pulmonary metastases secondary to vascular invasion. Treatment consists of excision with wide margins and chemotherapy. Even with this combined approach, the 5-year survival rate is a disappointing 15% to 20%.

Plasmacytomas are most commonly seen in men in their 40s to 60s who have been diagnosed with multiple myeloma. These tumors usually present with pain, and an associated mass may or may not be present. Patients will also commonly have fever, malaise, anemia, elevated erythrocyte sedimentation rates, an abnormal serum protein electrophoreses, hypercalcemia, and Bence Jones proteinuria. Chest radiographs show lytic "punched out" rib lesions and soft tissue involvement. These tumors can be diagnosed by identifying plasma cells in a biopsy specimen. Because these tumors usually occur with multiple myeloma, treatment centers around chemotherapy, prednisone, and radiation therapy. Surgical resection is reserved for the rare isolated chest plasmacytoma. The 5-year survival rate in these patients has been reported at 20% to 40%.

Soft Tissue

Soft tissue sarcomas comprise 20% of chest wall tumors and include fibrosarcomas, leiomyosarcomas, liposarcomas, synovial sarcomas, neurofibrosarcomas, and malignant fibrous histiocytomas. Ten percent of these tumors will recur locally after excision, and early metastases, usually to the lungs, is the rule.

Benign Chest Wall Tumors

Osteochondromas are the most common benign bony chest wall tumors. These tumors are most commonly seen in men during childhood and tend to grow slowly. Due to their slow growth, osteochondromas may be treated with observation during childhood. Painful tumors in children may signify malignant degeneration and should be resected. Osteochondromas arising in adults should also be resected to rule out malignancy.

Chondromas are slow-growing tumors that usually arise from the costochondral junction. These tumors may be difficult to differentiate from chondrosarcomas and therefore require excision for definitive diagnosis.

Fibrous dysplasia is a cystic disease of the rib caused by replacement of the rib marrow with fibrous tissue. These tumors occur with equal prevalence in men and women but may also present as part of Albright syndrome along with other bone cysts, dark pigmentation, and precocious puberty in girls. These tumors occur most commonly on the posterolateral aspect of the ribs. Resection is reserved for symptomatic tumors or tumors found in adults. Asymptomatic tumors in children can be observed and usually stop growing by puberty.

Histiocytosis X is one of several reticuloendothelial disorders that include eosinophilic granuloma, Letterer-Siwe disease, and Hand-Schueller-Christian disease. All of these diseases may present with rib tumors. The most common bone tumors in histiocytosis X occur in the skull, but rib tumors can also be seen. Histology of these tumors shows eosinophilic and histiocytic infiltration into the bone marrow. Solitary lesions can be treated with excision while radiation therapy is reserved for multiple lesions.

Chest Wall Resection/Reconstruction

The principles guiding chest wall resection follow those of general oncology: resection of all tumor and adequate margins (Fig. 23-2). All biopsy scars should be resected along with 4-cm margins and one normal rib above and below the tumor. Reconstruction may involve the use of Marlex, Gortex, or Marlex methyl methacrylate patches. Muscle flaps can also be used to provide coverage of the chest wall defect. Posterior defects that underlie the scapula may not require any coverage. Overall, reconstruction should provide protection of the intrathoracic organs, good cosmetic results, and prevention of paradoxical chest movements.

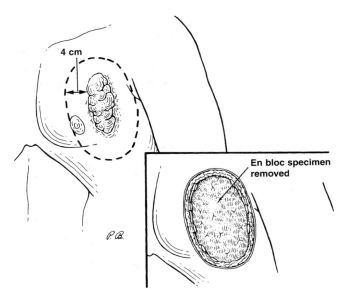

FIGURE 23-2. Planned en block resection of a chest wall tumor should include a 4-cm margin of tissue and one normal rib above and below the tumor. (From Miller JI. Surgical resection of the chest wall including sternum. In: Kaiser LK, Kron IL, Spray TL, eds. *Mastery of cardiothoracic surgery*, Philadelphia: Lippincott-Raven Publishers, 1998:190, with permission.)

DISEASE OF THE PLEURA AND PLEURAL SPACE

The pleural surface is a mesothelial layer that is composed of the parietal pleura, which covers the chest wall, diaphragm, and mediastinum, as well as the visceral pleura, which covers the lungs. The arterial and venous blood supply of the parietal pleura is derived from the intercostal, internal mammary, superior phrenic, and anterior mediastinal arteries. The visceral pleural receives its blood from the bronchial and pulmonary arteries while its venous flow is via the pulmonary veins alone. There is also an extensive lymphatic network within the pleura. The pleura and its components are subject to the same benign and malignant processes that affect epithelial tissues throughout the body.

Benign Pleural Disease

A *pleural effusion* can be a sign of a localized or systemic process stemming from a wide variety of etiologies. Classically, effusions are divided into transudates and exudates. A transudate is caused by either increased production or decreased absorption of pleural fluid and is not necessarily indicative of a primary pulmonary process. Exudates, on the other hand, are indicative of pleural disease or pleural lymphatic disease. The need to differentiate an exudative effusion from a transuded one is crucial because almost half of exudates are due to malignant processes while most transudates are secondary to congestive heart failure.

Generally, a transudate will have a specific gravity less than 1.016 and a protein content of less than 3 g/dL. This may not be true for long-standing transudates. Most transudates are either clear or straw colored and odorless. A bloody effusion, when trauma and pulmonary embolus have been ruled out, is secondary to malignancy in approximately 90% of cases. Findings that may also be seen include elevated amylase level in pancreatitis, malignancy or esophageal rupture, and a glucose level of more than 60 mg/dL in tuberculosis, malignancy, rheumatoid disease, and parapneumonic effusions. Additional tests that should be sent include culture, cell count, lactate dehydrogenase (LDH), cytology and fat content in the case of a milky white effusion.

Effusions can usually be diagnosed by chest x-ray, but occasionally, ultrasound or CT scan may be necessary to differentiate them from masses and to further characterize them. Treatment focuses on diagnostic thoracentesis followed by reversing the underlying process. In the case of malignant pleural effusions in which the primary cancer is not amenable to chemotherapy or radiation therapy, the only possibly therapy may be chemical pleurodesis with talc or bleomycin.

Spontaneous pneumothorax has an incidence of approximately 10 cases per 100,000 people with a 3:1 male to female ratio. Classically patients have a tall, thin body habitus and are often in their early 20s or 30s. The source of the pneumothorax is usually rupture of a bleb located in the apex of the upper lobe or the superior segment of the lower lobe and occurs more commonly in the right lung. Although the exact cause of spontaneous pneumothoraxes is unknown, cigarette smoking has been linked to an increased incidence. Occasionally, pneumothoraxes are diagnosed in relation to women's menstrual cycles. These catamenial pneumothoraxes are thought to be caused by endometrial implants on the lung.

Patients who have experienced a spontaneous pneumothorax complain of a sudden onset of chest pain and shortness of breath. These patients may subsequently develop subcutaneous emphysema, pneumomediastinum, a continuous air leak, hemopneumothorax, and rarely tension pneumothorax. Approximately 30% of these patients will have a recurrence after their initial presentation and over 60% of those who experience a second pneumothorax will experience a subsequent one.

Spontaneous pneumothoraxes are successfully treated in most patients with chest tube placement, and most air leaks will stop by 24 hours. Surgical intervention is mandated by a persistent air leak (3 to 5 days), a massive air leak for 24 hours, failure of the lung to reexpand, history of previous pneumothorax, bilateral pneumothoraxes, patients with occupations that could lead to life-threatening pneumothoraxes (pilot, diver), location far from any medical facility, and large pulmonary bullae. In these situations, treatment involves either open or thoracoscopic mechanical pleurodesis alone or in combination with blebectomy. Occasionally, young patients who have experienced a spontaneous pneumothorax and are asymptomatic can be watched and followed with serial chest x-rays until the lung is completely reexpanded.

Hemothorax refers to a collection of blood in the pleural space. This is usually secondary to a traumatic injury to the chest, but it may also occur with pulmonary emboli/infarction, tumors, heparinization, and after thoracic surgery. Diagnosis can usually be made with an upright chest x-ray along with the patient's history, physical examination, and vital signs. Small hemothoraxes, which may not even be diagnosed, often resolve without intervention. Larger collections can be successfully treated with tube thoracostomy in up to 85% of patients. Surgical intervention is required for hemothoraxes that drain over 1,500 mL upon tube thoracostomy placement or for ongoing chest tube output greater than 250 mL per hour for 3 or more hours.

Two problems that can arise from undrained or incompletely drained hemothorax are empyema and fibrothorax with entrapped lung. Empyema requires urgent surgical management, which is discussed latter in this chapter. Fibrothorax and entrapped lung result when undrained blood in the chest fibroses, leading to a functional reduction in the volume of the hemithorax. Therapy involves removing the fibrous peel on the chest wall and lung to allow full lung expansion. Although this procedure used to be performed through a thoracotomy, video-assisted thoracoscopy is gaining wide popularity as the method of choice.

Chylothorax is due to the leakage of chyle from an injured thoracic duct. The thoracic duct originates in the abdomen as the cisterna chyli, just to the right of the aorta. From here, the duct passes through the diaphragmatic hiatus, into the chest, finally crossing over to the left of the aorta, at the level of T4-5, where it ultimately empties into the confluence of the left subclavian vein and internal jugular vein. Although often depicted as a single conduit, in actuality, the thoracic duct has a variable course that involves many branches and connections with the azygous vein.

Chyle is a milky white, alkaline, odorless liquid with a specific gravity of 1.012 to 1.025 and a lymphocyte count of 400 to 6,800 cells per µL. Approximately half of adult chylothoraxes are due to tumors, of which lymphoma is most commonly seen. Other etiologies may include trauma, violent coughing, iatrogenic injury (thoracic surgery, central line placement), and infection. Once the thoracic duct is injured, chyle continues to fill the mediastinum until it ruptures into one or both of the pleural spaces. Chylothoraxes can be distinguished by a cholesterol/triglyceride ratio of less than 1 and a triglyceride level of more than 110 mL/dL. In addition, fat in the chyle can be stained with Sudan red to secure the diagnosis. In postoperative patients who have persistent high-volume serous chest tube output, chyle leaks can be diagnosed by feeding the patients a high-fat substance and observing if the color of the chest tube output changes to a milky white.

Treatment of chylothoraxes can involve either conservative or invasive management. Conservative therapy uses chest tube drainage along with a low-fat hyperalimentation regimen. This is more often successful for isolated thoracic duct injuries than for leaks secondary to tumor infiltration where congestion and multiple leakage sites are seen. Conservative therapy can be attempted initially, but prolonged treatment in the absence of decreasing chyle output can lead to severe nutritional depletion and lymphopenia. For adults with chyle leaks greater than 1 L per day for 1 week or for leaks that last longer than 2 weeks, conservative management should not be continued. The goal of surgical therapy is closure of thoracic leak or ligation of the duct at the level of the diaphragm. Due to the difficulty of identifying the thoracic duct, this latter technique may require ligation of all of the tissue between the azygous vein and the aorta.

An *empyema* is defined as the accumulation of pus in the pleural space. These collections have a pH level of less than 7.0, glucose less than 40 mg/dL, LDH more than 1,000 IU/L, and a positive Gram stain. Additional findings include a white blood cell (WBC) count of more than 15,000 cells per µL, protein more than 3 g/dL and a specific gravity more than 1.016. Most empyemas are secondary to pneumonia while others are attributed to surgical procedures involving the chest or mediastinum and thoracic extension of subphrenic abscesses. The most common organism cultured from an empyema is *Staphylococcus aureus,* but *Streptococcus,* Gram-negative and anaerobic organisms are also found in these infections.

Empyema can present in any of three phases, as defined by the American Thoracic Society: acute/exudative, transitional/fibrinopurulent, and chronic/organizing. The fluid of the acute/exudative phase is thin and has a low WBC count, low LDH level, and low glucose level with a normal pH level. The next phase is the transitional/fibrinopurulent phase, which is hallmarked by a turbid fluid with a chemistry profile that resembles classic empyema fluid. During this phase, a fibrinous layer forms on the parietal and visceral pleural that can begin to limit lung expansion. The third and final phase, the chronic/organizing phase, is seen after 4 to 6 weeks. The fibrinous layer eventually becomes infiltrated with new blood vessels and the fluid contains a large amount of sediment.

Patients with empyema may present with any array of symptoms including overt sepsis and pleuritic chest pain accompanied by cough, fever, pneumonia, or lung abscess. In the later stages, patients can develop empyema necessitans where the empyema erodes through the chest wall and presents as a soft tissue abscess, draining sinus, or disseminated infection. Diagnosis is made with an AP and lateral chest x-ray and thoracentesis. Chest CT scans may be helpful in defining the size of the empyema and ruling out invasion of the chest wall, mediastinum, and other adjacent structures.

Treatment of empyema involves eradicating the primary infection, evacuating the infected fluid, and reexpanding the lung. When the pleural fluid has a pH level of more than 7.20, glucose more than 40 mg/dL, and an LDH of less than 1,000 IU/L, thoracentesis alone may prove therapeutic and chest tube placement is not required. Purulent collections, reaccumulation of the aspirated fluid, or systemic toxicity, on the other hand, will require the placement of a large chest tube for ideal drainage. Some patients are not able to be adequately drained by tube thoracostomy alone and require more extensive procedures such as video-assisted thoracoscopic drainage and decortication or rib resection along with vigorous irrigation and chest tube placement for drainage of the abscess. In this latter procedure, the chest tube is then gradually removed over a period of 3 to 4 weeks to allow the cavity to close around the tube. If the lung fails to expand once the chest tube has been removed, decortication or marsupialization (Eloesser flap) of the cavity may be required.

Lytic agents, first introduced in the 1950s, have regained some popularity due to a rising emphasis on less-invasive approaches toward empyema. Streptokinase, the most widely used agent can be mixed with saline with a concentration of 250,000 U/100 mL of normal saline and inserted into the thoracic cavity via a chest tube. The chest tube is then clamped for several hours and the procedure is performed daily for 2 weeks. Success rates of up to 90% have been reported with minimal systemic absorption and toxicity.

Malignant Pleural Disease

Pleural malignancies most commonly present as metastases from lung, breast, gastric, and pancreatic cancers. Primary malignant tumors of the pleura also occur but are far less common than metastatic disease. The most common primary pleural tumor, *malignant mesothelioma,* is found in the chest in over 80% of the cases, although it may also occur in the pericardium, peritoneum, testes, and ovaries. There are approximately 3,000 cases of malignant pleural mesothelioma per year in the United States, and most of these are linked to asbestos exposure. Approximately 20% of patients with malignant mesothelioma are either unaware of or deny exposure to asbestos.

Malignant mesothelioma can be separated into three subtypes based on histology: epithelial, sarcomatous, and a mixed/biphasic tumor that is a combination of the other two subtypes. The epithelial variant is most commonly seen followed by the mixed and then the sarcomatous subtype. The disease usually affects older men, as the latency period from time of asbestos exposure to onset of the disease is about 30 to 40 years. Patients typically present with nonpleuritic chest pain, dyspnea, cough, fever, and weight loss. Chest radiograph may show classic pleural plaques or pleural thickening, and most patients will develop a pleural effusion at some time during the course of their disease.

Mesothelioma may be difficult to distinguish from adenocarcinoma metastatic to the pleural cavity. Definitive diagnosis is achieved only by biopsy of the tumor. Certain characteristics that distinguish malignant mesotheliomas from other tumors include large length to diameter ratio of microvilli on electron microscopy, negative test results for carcinoembryonic antigen (CEA), positive staining results for keratin, negative staining results for LEU M1 antigen, and the presence of hyaluronic acid in the absence of any other acid mucins.

Patients diagnosed with malignant mesothelioma have a dismal prognosis with a median survival of 8 to 14 months. Positive prognostic indicators include early stage disease, epithelial subtype, age of less than 55 years, female sex, and the absence of malignant cells in the pleural fluid. Surgical treatment options include biopsy with pleurodesis, pleurectomy/decortication, and extrapleural pneumonectomy. The lack of response to single modality therapy has created interest in multimodal therapy. Trimodal therapy combining extrapleural pneumonectomy and postoperative chemotherapy and radiation therapy has been used with some success in selected patients. A 5-year survival rate of 45% has been achieved in patients with the epithelial subtype and no nodal disease. However, the perioperative morbidity and mortality from this approach are 30% and 4.6%, respectively. The poor response to treatment in malignant mesothelioma has led to research efforts evaluating adenoviral-based suicide gene therapy, photodynamic therapy, and immunotherapy. None of these approaches have yet proven efficacious.

THORACIC OUTLET SYNDROME

Thoracic outlet syndrome (TOS) refers to a constellation of symptoms caused by compression of the subclavian artery or vein, axillary artery or vein, or the brachial plexus (Fig. 23-3). Symptoms secondary to neural compression are found in most (more than 90%) cases. Compression may occur at many points, including between the anterior and middle scalene muscles, between the anterior scalene muscle and the clavicle, at the level of the first rib, or between the first rib and clavicle, at the pectoralis minor fascia, at congenital cervical ribs, at a long transverse process of C-7, or secondary to clavicular deformities caused by old fractures.

Most patients present with symptoms of pain and paresthesias in the neck, upper arm, or hand, but unless a cervical rib is present, there is no discrete anatomical abnormality that can be identified. The symptomatic area is specific to the portion of the brachial plexus that is being compressed. Arterial compression can present as ischemia, arm fatigue or weakness, and cold intolerance. Thrombosis and embolization can also be seen with arterial compression. Venous compression can present as arm pain or edema and

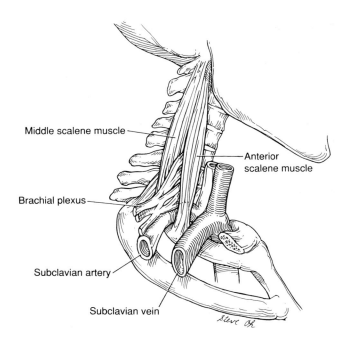

FIGURE 23-3. Structures passing through the thoracic outlet include the subclavian artery, vein, and brachial plexus. Symptoms secondary to neural compression of brachial plexus structures are most common. (From Gerken MV. First rib resection for thoracic outlet syndrome. In: Scott-Conner C, Dawson DL, eds. *Operative anatomy.* Philadelphia: JB Lippincott Co, 1993:207, with permission.)

may be associated with a feeling of heaviness in the affected extremity.

The diagnosis must be made carefully, as many pathologic processes, including arthritis, cervical disk disease, peripheral nerve entrapment, malignancy, arteriosclerosis, and thrombophlebitis, may mimic TOS. A detailed history and physical examination that includes a good neurovascular examination is essential. Certain diagnostic maneuvers that may be helpful, but not definitive, in diagnosing vascular compression include: (i) the Adson maneuver, diminished radial pulse with a deep breath, neck extension, and head rotation toward the examined side; (ii) the costoclavicular compression maneuver, diminished radial pulse with shoulders thrust backward (military posture); and (iii) the hyperabduction maneuver, diminished radial pulse with passive hyperabduction of the arm.

Diagnostic studies may include arteriography or venography to identify areas of obstruction and rule out aneurysmal disease. Duplex ultrasound has also been found to be useful in evaluating the blood vessels in the thoracic outlet while MRI is useful in evaluating neural structures. Nerve conduction studies tend to be variable and are more useful in ruling out peripheral nerve compression. Another neurodiagnostic test, somatosensory evoked potentials, can be useful in identifying patients that will benefit from surgery and in following postoperative nerve dysfunction. There is no definitive diagnostic study that secures the diagnosis of TOS, which remains a clinical impression.

The initial treatment for TOS involves nonoperative management including weight loss, exercise, and targeted physical therapy. This regimen will lead to improvement in symptoms in over half of patients with TOS. Patients who show no improvement after 4 months of conservative management or those who present with signs and symptoms of vascular compression are candidates for surgical management. Surgery involves resection of a cervical rib, if present, and most commonly complete resection of the first rib. Patients who have postcompression arterial dilation can be treated with resection of the compressing structures, but if dilation has progressed to a frank aneurysm or if there is evidence of emboli, arterial resection and reconstruction is required. Venous thrombosis is usually treated with lytic therapy followed by resection of the compressive structures. Occasionally, axillary-jugular venous bypass may be required.

MEDIASTINAL DISEASE

The mediastinum can be conceptualized into three anatomical divisions, anterior/superior, middle, and posterior, based on their relation to the pericardium (Table 23-2). Some have further divided the anterior mediastinum into a separate superior portion. The anterior mediastinum includes all structures anterior to the pericardium and the great vessels. The middle mediastinum is bounded by the anterior and posterior pericardial reflections while the posterior mediastinum includes everything posterior to the posterior pericardial reflections

One process that can affect any area of the mediastinum is *mediastinitis*. Bacterial contamination of the mediastinum can lead to a rapidly progressive infection that is associated with a high morbidity and mortality rate if it is not recognized and treated immediately. Mediastinitis may be secondary to esophageal perforation or contamination after a surgical procedure, or it may descend from an infectious process in the posterior pharynx. Patients often present with fever, tachycardia, chest pain, or overt sepsis. Subcutaneous emphysema may also be present if the source is a perforation in the esophagus, trachea, or main bronchi. Pharyngeal abscesses can also spread to the mediastinum and present in patients as erythema and pain over the anterior neck and chest (Ludwig angina).

Standard AP and lateral chest radiographs often show air or air–fluid levels in the mediastinum or chest. Chest CT scan is helpful in identifying fluid and gas in the mediastinum and in localizing infectious sources in the neck or chest. Bronchoscopy, esophageal endoscopy, and water-soluble contrast studies are other important tests in identifying tracheal and esophageal perforations. Treatment of mediastinitis involves rapid identification followed by reversal of

TABLE 23-2. MEDIASTINAL STRUCTURES

Anterior	Middle	Posterior
Thymus	Heart	Esophagus
Aorta/great vessels	Pericardium	Vagus nerves
Lymphatics	Phrenic nerves	Sympathetic nerve plexus
Fatty areolar tissue	Carina	Thoracic duct
Upper trachea	Main bronchi	Descending aorta
Upper esophagus	Pulmonary hila lymph nodes	Azygous vein
		Hemiazygous vein
		Paravertebral lymphatics
		Fatty areolar tissue

TABLE 23-3. MEDIASTINAL MASSES

Anterior mediastinal masses	Middle mediastinal masses	Posterior mediastinal masses
Thymoma (31%)	Cysts (61%)	Neurogenic (52%)
	Lymphomas (20%)	Cysts (32%)
Lymphoma (23%)	Mesenchymal (8%)	Mesenchymal (10%)
	Carcinoma (6%)	Endocrine (2%)
Germ cell tumors (17%)	Other (5%)	Other (4%)
Carcinoma (13%)		
Cysts (6%)		
Other (10%)[a]		

[a]Includes teratoma, lipoma, lymphangioma, hemangioma, parathyroid adenoma/carcinoma, thyroid adenoma/carcinoma/goiter.

the inciting cause usually with drainage in conjunction with broad-spectrum antibiotic therapy. Gross contamination due to an esophageal perforation requires wide debridement and drainage followed by definitive repair. Postoperative sternal infection with mediastinitis usually requires sternal debridement along with flap closure (usually with the pectoralis major muscle).

A rare cause of mediastinitis results from granulomatous disease in the mediastinal lymph nodes. Histoplasmosis, the most common pathogen identified in this disease, is treated with antimycobacterial drugs and occasionally surgical debridement of the involved lymph nodes. Some surgeons have recommended the routine resection of all acutely inflamed lymph nodes to avoid granulomatous mediastinitis, but this is controversial.

Mediastinal Masses

The most common mediastinal masses include neurogenic tumors, thymomas, primary cysts, lymphomas, and germ-cell tumors. The most common site for these masses is the anterior mediastinum (54%), followed by the posterior mediastinum and then the middle mediastinum. Between 25% and 40% of mediastinal masses are malignant and these most commonly are found in the anterior mediastinum (Table 23-3).

Patients may present with symptoms due to localized compression or with syndromes associated with specific tumors. Diagnosis of a mediastinal mass can often be made with an AP and lateral chest radiograph. Chest CT or MRI is useful in further delineating the origin of the mass and in identifying whether it is cystic or solid in nature. Other tests that may also be useful include arteriography, endoscopy, radioisotope scanning, and needle biopsy.

Thymomas are the most common tumors found in the anterior mediastinum and rank only behind neurogenic tumors, found in the posterior mediastinum, as the second most common of all mediastinal tumors. These tumors, which are more common in adults and rarely seen in children, usually present with local symptoms such as dyspnea, cough, hemoptysis, or chest pain. Patients may also present with one of many paraneoplastic syndromes including myasthenia gravis, Cushing syndrome, lupus, rheumatoid arthritis, and hypercoagulopathy. These tumors may appear as irregular central masses on chest radiograph, but either CT scan or MRI better delineate the tumors.

Thymomas are classified histologically as either epithelial or lymphocytic, but it is the presence of either gross or microscopic invasion of either the capsule or adjacent structures that defines a thymoma as "malignant" (Table 23-4). Although 65% of thymomas are benign, it may be possible to overlook occult malignancy in an otherwise benign-appearing thymoma. During resection of any thymoma, care must be taken not to violate the capsule thereby preventing the spread of any cancer cells. The treatment for thymoma is total thymectomy usually via a median sternotomy or a thoracotomy. Adjuvant radiation therapy is recommended for stage II and III tumors while chemotherapy is reserved for patients with stage IV disease or those with recurrent disease.

Myasthenia gravis occurs in approximately 35% of patients who have thymomas, but only 10% to 20% of patients with myasthemia gravis will have a thymoma.

TABLE 23-4. STAGING AND 5-YEAR SURVIVAL RATES FOR MALIGNANT THYMOMAS

Stage	5-year survival
I (encapsulated, no evidence of gross or microscopic capsular invasion)	85%–100%
II (pericapsular invasion into mediastinal fat, pleura, or pericardium)	60%–80%
III (invasion into adjacent organs or intrathoracic metastases)	40%–70%
IV (extrathoracic metastases)	50%

The disease is thought to result from the stimulation of thymic lymphocytes resulting in the production of anti-acetylcholine antibodies to acetylcholine receptor–like antigens in the thymus. Clinically, patients present with progressive skeletal muscle weakness that tends to involve the ocular muscles first but may progress to involve the respiratory muscles, leading to respiratory failure. Diagnosis is suggested by clinical muscle weakness and usually confirmed with a Tensilon test in which transient muscle strength is regained after the administration of a short-acting acetylcholinesterase inhibitor. Single fiber electromyography may be required in some cases to confirm the diagnosis.

The mainstay of treatment for myasthenia gravis are acetylcholinesterase inhibitors and immunosuppressants. Thymectomy is also beneficial in many patients with myasthenia gravis, with more than 80% of patients having some clinical improvement in their disease after resection and over 40% of patients requiring no further therapy. Positive predictors of a good response to thymectomy include short duration of disease before thymectomy, female sex, milder forms of myasthenia, and absence of a thymoma.

The *mediastinum* is *frequently* the *site of diffuse lymphoma*, however, in 5% to 10% of patients, it is the only site of disease. Patients with Hodgkin and non-Hodgkin lymphomas can present with dyspnea, hoarseness, chest pain, and superior vena cava (SVC) obstruction, as well as fever, chills, and weight loss. Chest x-ray often identifies an anterior or anterosuperior mass in the patient, but MRI and CT scan are necessary to further delineate the lesion. Definitive diagnosis must be made with tissue obtained usually from an open biopsy because fine needle aspirates do not supply sufficient material.

Hodgkin lymphoma is separated by histology into nodular sclerosing, lymphocytic predominant, lymphocyte depleted, and mixed celluarity. Stages I and IIA are treated with radiation therapy with a 10-year survival rate of 90%. Stages IIB, III, and IV are treated primarily with chemotherapy (Chapter 5). Treatment for non-Hodgkin lymphoma is systemic chemotherapy. Surgery occasionally is of value for a subset of patients with primary mediastinal lymphoma of the B-cell type that presents solely with mediastinal disease, but this is distinctly unusual. Surgical resection is used in combination with chemotherapy for these patients.

Primary *mediastinal germ-cell tumors* usually are found in the anterior mediastinum but occasionally can arise in the posterior mediastinum. These tumors are histologically identical to tumors that arise in the gonads and are separated into teratomas/teratocarcinomas, seminomas, embryonal cell carcinomas, choriocarcinomas, and endodermal cell tumors. Teratomas are tumors made up of cells derived from multiple embryonic germ-cell layers. Over 80% of teratomas are benign, the most common being the dermoid cyst, and those that are not benign are often associated with elevated CEA and α-fetoprotein (AFP) levels.

Teratomas felt to be benign require resection to rule out malignancy and to prevent local compressive symptoms. Malignant teratomas can be diagnosed with needle biopsies and then treated with a combination of neoadjuvant chemotherapy and surgery. Preoperative CEA and AFP levels should be obtained on all patients with malignant teratomas.

Malignant germ-cell tumors can be classified as seminomatous and nonseminomatous. These tumors usually arise in men in their 20s and 30s, and on presentation, these individuals may complain of chest pain, cough, dyspnea, or hemoptysis. Lesions visualized on chest x-ray are further characterized on MRI and CT scan. A male patient diagnosed with a mediastinal germ-cell tumor should have a thorough examination of the testes as well as a testicular ultrasound, and any mass identified should be sampled to rule out a primary gonadal cancer. Patients suspected of having a germ-cell tumor should also have β-HCG (human chorionic gonadotropin) and AFP levels drawn because elevation of one or both of these markers makes the diagnosis and allows the oncologist to follow the response of the tumor to treatment.

Seminomas comprise about one half of all malignant germ-cell tumors. These tumors rarely secrete β-HCG or AFP and thereby can be distinguished from nonseminomatous lesions. Seminomas usually spread within the mediastinum although late metastases may occur via the lymphatic and blood vessels. The most common sites of metastases are the lung and bone followed by the brain, spleen, tonsils, and subcutaneous tissue. Surgical resection alone is the treatment for these tumors when possible. When tumors are unresectable, radiation is used for tumors confined to the mediastinum while chemotherapy is reserved for patients with distant metastases, large intrathoracic tumors unlikely to respond to radiation therapy alone, and recurrences.

Malignant nonseminomatous tumors, including choriocarcinoma, embryonal cell carcinoma, malignant teratoma, and endodermal sinus tumors (yolk sac), tend to be more aggressive than seminomas, produce β-HCG or AFP, and are less radiosensitive. Patients usually present with cough, dyspnea, chest pain, fevers/chills, and occasionally SVC syndrome with a large mediastinal mass. Similar to patients with seminomas, most patients with nonseminomatous tumors are men, although slightly older, in their 30s and 40s. These tumors occasionally are found in association with chromosomal abnormalities (Klinefelter and trisomy syndromes) as well as rare hematological malignancies.

Nonseminomatous tumors often involve the chest wall and tend to metastasize early to the brain, lung, liver, and bone. Surgical resection rarely is possible and the surgeon usually is involved in making a tissue diagnosis and resection of residual disease in patients who have responded to chemotherapy and have negative tumor markers. Chemotherapy followed by surgical resection has yielded a

36% long-term survival rate in some studies, but patients with recurrent disease have a mean survival time of less than 6 months regardless of therapy. Some nonseminomatous tumors may also contain an adenocarcinoma or sarcomatous component that is not responsive to chemotherapy and thus is associated with a worse prognosis.

Primary mediastinal carcinoma makes up approximately 5% of all mediastinal masses. Although the origin of the tumors is unknown, most of these masses are composed of undifferentiated large cells. The most important aspect in diagnosing these tumors is to differentiate them from other mediastinal tumors such as lymphomas and metastatic cancers. Most patients have symptoms secondary to local mass effect, and when found, these tumors tend to have thoracic spread as well as distant metastases. Most lesions are not resectable and even with chemotherapy and radiation therapy, patients' survival time is less than 1 year.

The most common *mediastinal cysts* include bronchogenic cysts and esophageal duplication cysts, which are part of the spectrum of bronchopulmonary foregut abnormalities that present as pulmonary sequestrations. These cysts contain cartilage and mucous glands and are lined with epithelium, the exact type being responsible for the cyst classification. They usually do not communicate directly with the bronchus or esophagus. Most patients are asymptomatic, but when symptoms do occur, they are usually secondary to local compression or infection. Surgical resection is required to rule out malignancy and to prevent complications later in life. Malignant degeneration is often mentioned but probably occurs rarely if ever in these cysts.

Pericardial cysts are the next most frequently found lesions in the middle mediastinum. They usually occur at the pericardiophrenic angles with a predilection for the right side. Some patients have been managed with simple needle aspiration, but surgical resection is generally recommended to rule out malignancy. Usually, this may be accomplished with a video-assisted thoracoscopic procedure. Care must be taken to avoid injury to the phrenic nerve during resection.

Neurogenic tumors are the most common mediastinal tumor and usually are located in the posterior mediastinum. The cells that make up these tumors are derived from neural crest cells and have the ability to secrete various hormones but rarely do. The tumors can form in any of the mediastinal neural tissue including sympathetic ganglia, paraganglia cells, and intercostal nerves. Most neurogenic tumors that occur in adults are benign, unlike those that are found in children, and are more likely to be malignant. Neurogenic tumors that can arise in the posterior mediastinum include neuroblastomas, ganglioneuroblastomas, ganglioneuromas, neurilemomas (schwannomas), neurofibromas, neurosarcomas, and paragangliomas, with neurilemomas being the most common.

Patients usually present asymptomatically with a mass having been noted on a chest radiograph obtained for some other reason. Respiratory and neurological symptoms may arise from local compression of the tumors and invasion of the spinal canal by way of the neural foramen. These latter tumors are called "dumbbell tumors" because of the characteristic appearance of their intraspinal and extraspinal portions (Fig. 23-4). Any patient with a posterior mediastinal mass and either radicular pain or symptoms of vertebral destruction should be worked up for a dumbbell tumor with a myelogram or MRI . Failure to recognize a tumor

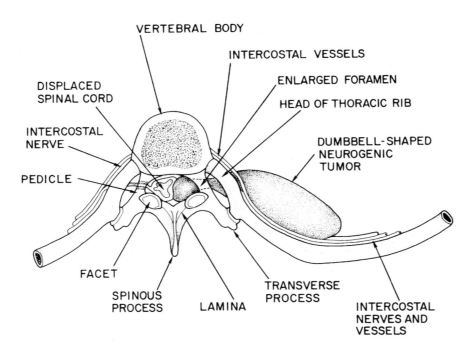

FIGURE 23-4. A neurogenic dumbbell tumor resulting in spinal cord compression, enlargement of the neural foramen, and a large posterior mediastinal mass. (From Kern JA, Daniel TM. Resection of posterior mediastinal tumors. In: Kaiser LK, Kron IL, Spray TL, eds. *Mastery of cardiothoracic surgery*, Philadelphia: Lippincott-Raven Publishers, 1998:114, with permission.)

within the spinal canal can result in disastrous complications at the time of resection if the tumor is cut and bleeding occurs in the intraspinal portion; spinal cord compression and paraplegia may result.

Neurilemomas are tumors that arise from Schwann cells and represent the most common neurogenic tumors. These tumors are most commonly seen in adults and along with neurofibromas can occur as part of neurofibromatosis. The treatment for both of these tumors is surgical resection. Neurosarcomas can arise in children with neurofibromatosis as well as in adults with no other associated illnesses. These tumors tend to be very aggressive, and if not completely resected, they carry a very poor prognosis.

Neuroblastomas are most commonly seen in children less than 4 years of age. Although most of these tumors arise in the retroperitoneum, 10% to 20% are found in the posterior mediastinum. Neuroblastomas are aggressive tumors that tend to metastasize early. Many patients present with neurological symptoms due to spinal cord compression and occasionally one of the several paraneoplastic syndromes that are associated with these tumors. Surgical resection is the definitive therapy for noninvasive stage I disease. Invasive tumors (stage II) require resection plus radiation therapy while tumors with spread to the opposite hemithorax or distant metastases (stages III and IV) are treated with a combination of surgical debulking, radiation therapy, and chemotherapy. Positive prognostic indicators include age less than 1 year and lack of the N-*myc* amplification.

Ganglioneuroblastomas can be broken down into two types based on their cellular composition. *Composite ganglioneuroblastomas* are made up mostly of well-differentiated neuroblasts while *diffuse ganglioneuroblastomas* contain a mixture of well-differentiated and poorly differentiated neuroblasts. Patients with the composite type of tumor have a much worse prognosis, with over 60% developing metastatic disease. Surgical resection is reserved for patients with stage I or II diffuse type disease. Patients who are older than 3 years, who have stage III/IV disease, or who have composite type tumors are treated with chemotherapy. Ganglioneuromas are benign tumors that arise from the sympathetic chain. These tumors are less common than neurilemomas and are treated with complete surgical resection.

Pheochromocytomas are tumors derived from chromaffin cells that actively secrete catecholamines. Ninety percent of these tumors are found in the adrenal medulla while only 2% are found in the chest. Extraadrenal pheochromocytomas, also called "paragangliomas," most commonly are found in the organ of Zuckerkandl. Mediastinal paragangliomas usually develop in the paravertebral area in the posterior mediastinum, but they may also be found in the pericardium in the middle mediastinum.

Unlike adrenal pheochromocytomas, which usually produce epinephrine and norepinephrine, tumors found in extraadrenal locations usually do not produce epinephrine and often do not produce any hormones. Patients who do present with symptoms typically have uncontrollable hypertension along with palpitations and weight loss. Urinary catecholamines, metanephrines, and vanillylmandelic acid levels usually are elevated and clinch the diagnosis. Tumor localization can be accomplished with chest CT, and if hormonally active, iodine-131 MIBG scan. The treatment for these tumors is surgical resection. In the 3% of patients who present with metastatic disease, α-methyltyrosine can be used to prevent catecholamine synthesis and reduce some of the symptoms.

THORACIC TRAUMA

Thoracic injuries account for approximately 25% of all trauma-related deaths. These injuries can be due to either penetrating trauma or blunt trauma. Penetrating injuries to the chest usually will lead to a hemothorax or a pneumothorax, and injury to all of the intrathoracic and mediastinal structures must be ruled out. Injuries that involve the heart or great vessels may present initially as life-threatening hemorrhage while injuries involving the trachea, bronchi, esophagus, or minor blood vessels (intercostal, internal mammary) may not be as obvious. Blunt injury to intrathoracic structures results either from a direct blow or from a rapid deceleration.

Initial treatment of any patient with thoracic trauma involves examining the patient's airway, breathing, and circulation. Patients who appear anxious or combative may require supplemental oxygenation or endotracheal intubation. Careful auscultation of the chest should be performed, looking for any change in breath sounds. Additionally, the chest should be palpated for soft tissue or bony crepitus, signaling a possible airway injury or fracture, respectively. Any decreased breath sound over the hemithorax of an unstable patient should alert the physician to the possibility of a tension pneumothorax, and immediate tube thoracostomy should be performed. Tension physiology with rapid hemodynamic compromise and an inability to ventilate the patient should always be considered. However, because all pneumothoraxes or hemothoraxes do not necessarily present with early clinical signs and symptoms, all patients with thoracic trauma should have an early chest x-ray (upright if possible). Throughout the examination and resuscitation, airway stability and oxygenation should be continuously checked and rechecked.

An emergency thoracotomy has been shown to be beneficial in patients who suffer penetrating thoracic trauma and present to the emergency room with sign of life. For patients who present after suffering blunt thoracic trauma, the need for emergency thoracotomy is associated with almost a 100% mortality. Patients who do undergo the procedure should receive a left thoracotomy with four main goals in mind: (i) evacuation of any pericardial fluid that could be causing acute tamponade, (ii) control of any exsanguinating thoracic hemorrhage, (iii) cross-clamping of the descending aorta to increase coronary and cerebral perfusion, and (iv) open cardiac massage. If a patient does respond to any of these maneuvers, he or she should immediately be transported to the operating room for definitive surgical repair of their injuries and closure of the chest.

Chest Wall Injuries

Rib fractures are the most common chest wall injury incurred following blunt chest trauma and their significance is often overlooked. The diagnosis is made with a combination of physical examination, looking for decreased breath sounds, tenderness, and bony crepitus, and chest x-ray. Rib fractures not only represent significant bony injuries but also may imply injury to underlying or nearby structures, particularly the lungs. Twenty percent of patients with fractures of ribs 9 to 11 on the left will have a splenic injury while fractures of the first rib imply an injury of such significance that it is often associated with aortic and subclavian artery injuries.

By far, the major morbidity associated with rib fractures is the development of atelectasis and pneumonia caused by the pain associated with these injuries that produces splinting. Significant pain leads to a decreased inspiratory effort and cough, resulting in atelectasis, retained secretions, and ultimately pneumonia. This is particularly true for elderly patients and patients with underlying respiratory disease. The treatment for rib fractures is pain control, pulmonary toilet, and prompt recognition of any infectious pulmonary process. Epidural analgesia as well as patient-controlled analgesia have been shown to greatly decrease morbidity due to rib fractures in patients with significant pain. The practice of "taping" the fractured ribs is of historical interest only and can actually harm the patient by further limiting respiratory excursion. Patients who otherwise are healthy and who have good pain control on oral analgesics and who have an isolated injury usually do not require hospital admission.

Sternal fractures occur when a significant force is placed on the anterior chest. These injuries are only seen in 5% of trauma patients with chest wall injuries. The major morbidity and mortality from these injuries is secondary to associated cardiac, aortic, and tracheobronchial injuries. These fractures can be diagnosed with palpation and a lateral chest x-ray or sternal films. As with rib fractures, the primary treatment for these fractures is pain control and pulmonary toilet. Occasionally, sternal fractures with severe posterior displacement are repaired with open reduction and fixation.

Flail chest is defined as an unstable portion of the thoracic cavity created by unilateral anterior and posterior fractures of four or more ribs or bilateral anterior or costochondral fractures of four or more ribs. These fractures result in paradoxical movement of the flail segment during inspiration. In the past, these injuries were treated with stabilization of the rib fractures. However, we now know that the major cause of respiratory failure in these patients is due to the underlying pulmonary contusion, not the rib fractures.

Pulmonary contusions are seen in most patients with severe chest trauma and are particularly associated with flail chest. The pathophysiology involves the rupture of capillaries and subsequent hemorrhage into the pulmonary parenchyma and alveoli. Although most of these injuries appear on chest x-ray within the first hour after injury as a haziness over the involved lung, some injuries may not be visible for 4 to 5 hours. Treatment for flail chest follows the guideline of all chest fractures: pain control and pulmonary toilet. Epidural analgesia may be useful for pain control. If the injury prevents adequate oxygenation and ventilation, then the patient should be mechanically ventilated. The use of positive end-expiratory pressure to increase lung volumes and the judicious use of intravenous fluids are both helpful in supporting the patient. With early diagnosis and aggressive pulmonary support, the mortality rate due to flail chest has been reduced to 5% and even this mortality is due to associated injuries.

An *open pneumothorax,* also known as a "sucking chest wound," occurs when an injury creates a large defect in the chest wall with the loss of the physiologic negative intrathoracic pressure. When the cross-sectional area of the wound is greater than the cross-sectional area of the larynx air will begin to preferentially enter the chest wound. Open pnuemothoraxes are immediate life-threatening injuries because they quickly lead to hypoventilation. Once these injuries are diagnosed, the initial treatment is coverage of the wound with an impermeable dressing followed by the placement of a chest tube. Definitive treatment can take place when the patient is stable and involves operative repair of the chest wall defect.

Lung Injuries

Pulmonary parenchymal injuries can appear as lacerations, hematomas, and pneumatoceles. Lacerations usually are caused by penetrating trauma although occasionally result from the sharp edge of a fractured rib. Most lacerations can be treated with chest tube placement and observation. The bleeding from a pulmonary laceration usually will stop on its own as the pulmonary circulation is a low-pressure circulation. Persistent or massive hemorrhage signals a more severe injury and operative exploration is required. In addition, patients with hemoptysis or large air leaks require bronchoscopy to rule out a ruptured bronchus. Surgical repair of a parenchymal injury, if required, can usually be performed as a simple stapling procedure or resection of the injured area. A formal lobectomy is required in less than 1% of all penetrating lung injuries. Bleeding from a bullet hole in the lung parenchyma may be managed by creating a tractotomy with a mechanical stapler. This opens the tract and allows for direct ligation or cauterization of bleeding vessels.

Pulmonary hematomas usually occur from mechanisms similar to those involved with pulmonary contusion. Most of these injuries can be managed conservatively with pain control and pulmonary toilet. When patients with pulmonary hematomas develop fever, infected clot or abscess needs to be ruled out. CT scan of the chest is performed to look for any pulmonary collections. Antibiotic therapy combined with drainage by way of the bronchus, often facilitated by bronchoscopy, usually results in resolution. Occasionally, percutaneous catheter drainage or resection is required.

A pneumatocele forms when significant trauma causes the rupture of a small airway, forming an air-filled cavity. The diagnosis can be made with a chest x-ray showing a round air-filled lesion and CT scan is helpful in further defining the cavity. Once other disease processes such as tuberculosis, abscess, and cancer have been ruled out, management can proceed with pulmonary toilet and observation. Most pneumatoceles will resolve spontaneously within 4 months.

Tracheobronchial injuries occur in less than 1% of patients with blunt trauma and are more commonly seen with penetrating injuries to the neck and chest. Deceleration injuries can cause disruption of one or both main bronchi or carinal injury while compression of the thorax against a closed glottis can lead to a "blow out" type injury. Patients with tracheobronchial injuries may present with hemoptysis, dyspnea, stridor, and crepitus over the neck and chest. Chest x-ray often reveals subcutaneous emphysema sometimes associated with a pneumothorax.

Treatment depends on the severity of the injury and the condition of the patient. Patients with a pneumothorax should undergo immediate chest tube placement. All patients suspected of having a tracheobronchial injury should undergo urgent bronchoscopy. Injuries that involve less than one third of the tracheal circumference, in an otherwise stable patient, can be managed conservatively, but operative repair may be necessary. Larger injuries, such as massive continuous air leaks or large pneumothoraxes unresponsive to chest tube drainage, usually require surgical repair. Occasionally the larynx or trachea may be too distorted from the injury to be able to place an endotracheal tube. In these situations, either intubation over a bronchoscope or emergent cricothyroidotomy may be necessary. Cricothyroidotomy is the emergency procedure of choice to establish an airway in the patient with significant head or neck trauma.

A *tension pneumothorax* can occur anytime air is allowed to enter the thoracic cavity without being allowed to exit. This is usually due to a lung injury with an ongoing air leak where air escapes from the lung into the chest, but it may also occur with chest wall injuries that act as one-way valves, allowing air to enter the chest without leaving. As more air begins to enter the thoracic cavity, the affected lung and the mediastinum begin to shift to the opposite side, leading to a decrease in lung ventilation and a decrease in venous return to the heart, effectively decreasing cardiac output and leading to shock.

Patients with tension pneumothoraxes present in extremis, with hypotension, cyanosis, tracheal deviation away from the affected side, and absent breath sounds over the affected hemithorax. The initial treatment involves converting the tension pneumothorax to an open pneumothorax by placing a large bore catheter into the affected chest, usually at the midclavicular line of the second or third intercostal space. Once the hemithorax has been decompressed and the patient is stable, a chest tube can be placed and the catheter removed.

Diaphragmatic Injuries

Traumatic diaphragmatic injuries present as lacerations much more commonly than ruptures. Herniation of abdominal organs into the chest can occur either at the time of injury or months to years later. When herniation occurs at the time of injury, the diagnosis can be made with a chest x-ray that shows opacification over the involved hemithorax along with intestinal gas pattern and often a nasogastric tube if the stomach has herniated. However, when the herniation is delayed, these injuries tend to be overlooked unless they are found inadvertently during abdominal exploration or on a chest radiograph.

Before the use of CT scanning, most of these injuries were thought to occur on the left side, but several studies using abdominal and chest CT scans have shown than diaphragmatic injuries may be more evenly distributed between the right and the left side than previously thought. Injuries on the right side, however, tend to lead to herniation less often because the liver is present, preventing herniation of other abdominal viscera. Treatment involves reduction of the hernia and closure of the diaphragmatic defect. This can be best accomplished via an abdominal approach that allows other intraabdominal injuries to be ruled out in the acute situation. Even in a chronic diaphragmatic hernia, the abdominal approach is preferable.

SUGGESTED READING

Kaiser LK, Kron IL, Spray TL, eds. *Mastery of cardiothoracic surgery.* Philadelphia: Lippincott-Raven Publishers, 1998.

SECTION IV

GENITOURINARY SYSTEM, HEAD AND NECK, AND MUSCULOSKELETAL SYSTEM

24

GENITOURINARY SYSTEM

JONATHAN MASOUDI AND KEITH N. VAN ARSDALEN

The urinary tract is fully contained within the retroperitoneal space and pelvis and interfaces with the gonads and external genitalia. Knowledge of the anatomy of the urinary tract and its relations to other structures is essential for the surgeon during intraabdominal exploration.

ANATOMY

The *kidneys* are derived embryologically from the metanephric blastema. They are bean-shaped organs positioned in the high retroperitoneum and are protected from trauma by the lower rib cage and overlying musculature. The hilum of the kidney is located medially and is the entry/exit point for the renal pelvis, artery, and vein. The right kidney is closely related to the liver, right adrenal gland, psoas muscle, duodenum, and the ascending colon. The left kidney is closely related to the spleen, left adrenal gland, the tail of the pancreas, and the descending colon (Fig. 24-1). The right kidney is usually more caudal than the left because of the large size of the liver. The kidneys and the perirenal fat are contained within the Gerota fascia, a layer that also invests the adrenal gland superiorly and the ureter and gonadal vessels inferiorly. This fascia serves as a possible barrier to the spread of infection and malignancy from the kidney to other retroperitoneal structures. It may also act to tamponade potentially life-threatening hemorrhage originating from the kidney or the adrenal gland.

The arterial supply to the kidneys is derived directly from the aorta, inferior to the superior mesenteric artery. The right renal artery takes off from the aorta superior to the left renal artery and travels caudally and posterior to the vena cava to reach the hilum. The left artery is shorter than the right because of the kidney's proximity to the aorta. The renal artery usually is single but may be paired, leading to considerations during cadaveric or living renal donation. The renal artery branches into the segmental, lobar, arcuate, and interlobular arteries. The interlobular arteries in turn supply blood to the glomeruli via the afferent arterioles (Fig. 24-2).

Glomerular blood drains from the efferent arterioles into interlobular, arcuate, interlobar, and segmental veins, which join to form the main renal vein. The renal vein is located anterior to the artery and is shorter on the right side because of the kidney's proximity to the vena cava. The left renal vein typically drains the left adrenal vein, the left gonadal vein, and lumbar branches. Failure to ligate these branches can lead to significant intraoperative hemorrhage during nephrectomy. Lymphatic drainage of the kidneys follows the venous drainage.

The *adrenal* gland usually is located within the Gerota fascia supermedially to the kidney. However, it is derived independently from neuroendocrine origins, and in cases of renal ectopia, the adrenal gland will preserve its absolute location rather than its relation to the kidney. Similarly, absence of the kidney is not associated with absence of the ipsilateral adrenal gland. The adrenal gland is composed of a cortex and medulla. The cortex is divided into three zones: the zona glomerulosa, the zona fasciculata, and the zona reticularis. These zones produce mineralocorticoids, glucocorticoids, and sex steroids, respectively. The adrenal medulla produces epinephrine under the control of the sympathetic nervous system. The blood supply to the adrenal gland is via three locations: the aorta, the renal artery, and the phrenic artery. The adrenal vein on the left drains into the renal vein, and on the right, it drains directly into the vena cava. The branch on the right may be difficult to control and can be a source of significant intraoperative bleeding. Lymphatic drainage follows the venous channels.

Urine drains from the collecting ducts to the pyramids, which drain into minor calyces. These are joined to form the major calyces, which drain via infundibula to form the renal pelvis. The renal pelvis is located posterior to the renal vein and artery, and it drains into the ureter at the ureteropelvic junction. The ureter is a tubular structure whose function is the low-pressure transfer of urine in an antegrade fashion to the bladder. The collecting system and ureter are lined with a transitional cell epithelium. Surrounding this layer is a muscular layer and an adventitial layer. The ureter courses along the posterior psoas muscle and enters the bony pelvis at the level of the bifurcation of the iliac vessels. It passes posterior to the cecum and ascend-

---

Hospital of the University of Pennsylvania, Philadelphia, Pennsylvania

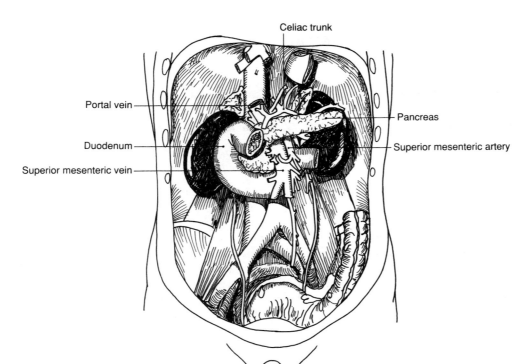

FIGURE 24-1. Relations of the kidney to adjacent organs. (From Scott-Connor C, Dawson DL, eds. *Operative anatomy.* Philadelphia: Lippincott Williams & Wilkins, 1993;511, with permission.)

ing colon on the right and to the sigmoid and descending colon on the left, then it enters the bladder posterolaterally. There are three relative narrowings of the ureteral lumen: at the ureteropelvic junction, at the level of the iliac vessels, and at the ureterovesical junction. It is at these three sites that ureteral calculi will most commonly lodge.

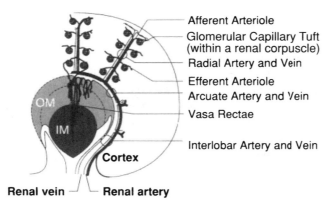

FIGURE 24-2. Schematic diagram of the major blood vessels supplying the kidney. All the glomeruli are located in the cortex and are supplied by the afferent arteriole arising as a branch of the renal artery. The peritubular capillary network arising from the glomeruli in the outer regions of the cortex remains confined to the cortex while the capillary network of the glomeruli located next to the corticomedullary junction penetrates deep into the medulla (OM, outer medula; IM, inner medula) in a series of hairpin loops known as "vasa recta." (From Johnson LR. *Essential medical physiology.* Philadelphia: Lippincott Williams & Wilkins, 1998:309, with permission.)

The blood supply to the ureter is derived from many arteries, most commonly the renal artery, the gonadal artery, the aorta, the hypogastric artery, and the vesical arteries. The blood supply approaches the ureter from the medial side proximally and from the lateral side distally. When the ureter is mobilized, care must be taken not to disrupt the adventitia, where distal branches of the arterial supply of the ureter anastomose.

The *urinary bladder* is a pelvic muscular organ whose function is twofold: (i) low-pressure filling and storage of urine and (ii) low-pressure expulsion of urine at a socially opportune time. The bladder is derived from the urogenital sinus, and during development, it is connected to the umbilicus by the urachus, which obliterates to form the median umbilical ligament during normal development. The umbilical arteries likewise obliterate to form the lateral umbilical ligaments. The bladder is lined with a transitional epithelium and has a thick muscular layer made up of inner and outer longitudinal and middle circular layers. The serosa of the bladder is surrounded by the perivesical fascia, which is proximate to the peritoneum cephalad, the space of Retzius anteroinferiorly, and the rectum posteriorly in men. In women, the vagina is posterior, with the uterus lying posterior and superior. The bladder has a rich blood supply derived mainly from the superior and inferior vesical arteries, both branches of the internal iliac (hypogastric) artery. Obturator, gluteal, uterine, or vaginal branches may also supply the bladder. Venous drainage is via the vesical plexus into the internal iliac (hypogastric) vein. Lymphatic drainage is primarily to the external iliac chain but may also include obturator and internal iliac chains. The innervation of the smooth muscle of the bladder is autonomic, with sacral parasympathetic innervation initiating the contraction of the bladder. Extensive perivesical dissection during pelvic surgery (e.g., abdominoperineal resection) can lead to bladder atony and resultant urinary retention.

The *prostate* is a small organ located deep in the male pelvis. It abuts the bladder at its outlet and surrounds the prostatic urethra. Its anatomical relations are the bony pelvis anteriorly (puboprostatic ligaments), the rectum and seminal vesicles posteriorly, and the bladder cephalad. The verumontanum is the exit point of the ejaculatory duct, which empties sperm and seminal fluid from the vas deferens and the seminal vesicles, respectively.

The prostate can be divided into several zones. The most common sites of pathology are the transition zone (most frequent site of benign prostatic hyperplasia [BPH]) and the peripheral zone (most frequent site of adenocarcinoma of the prostate).

The blood supply of the prostate is mainly from the inferior vesical artery, and the venous drainage is via the pelvic plexus of Santorini. The venous drainage of the penis, the deep dorsal venous complex, travels anterior to the prostate, and its careful ligation is necessary during radical retropubic prostatectomy. The lymphatic drainage of the prostate is to the obturator and external iliac lymph nodes. This explains the common practice of pelvic lymph node dissection prior to radical prostatectomy.

The *penis* is composed of the two erectile bodies: the *corpora cavernosa* (homologues of the labia minora), which fuse at the base of the penis and join the *corpus spongiosum,* which contains the urethra and is contiguous with the glans penis (homologue of the clitoris). The corpora derive their blood supply from the internal pudendal artery.

The *male urethra* can be divided into two portions: posterior (prostatic and membranous) and anterior (bulbar, penile, and glanular). The prostatic urethra includes the portion from the bladder neck to the verumontanum. The membranous urethra continues to just past the external urinary sphincter and is the most common site of urethral disruption in pelvic trauma. These portions are derived from mesodermal origin and are lined with transitional cell epithelium. The bulbous urethra is the most common site of post–gonococcal urethral stricture. It is somewhat dilated and continues until the corpus spongiosum becomes adherent to the underside of the fused corpora cavernosa. The penile urethra continues along the length of the penile shaft, where the glanular urethra dilates at the fossa navicularis. The bulbar and penile urethra are derived from endodermal origins and are lined with stratified columnar epithelium, and the fossa is derived from ectodermal origins and is lined with squamous cell epithelium. The blood supply to the posterior urethra is from the inferior vesical artery, and the anterior urethra from the bulbar branch of the internal pudendal artery. Lymphatic drainage of the posterior urethra is to obturator and iliac nodes, and the anterior urethra to superficial and deep inguinal nodes.

The *scrotum* (male equivalent of labia majora) is a pouchlike structure inferior to the penis that serves to maintain the homeostasis of the testes, which are contained in the two separate compartments of the scrotum. The muscular dartos layer of the scrotum is continuous with the Colles fascia in the perineum and with the Scarpa fascia in the abdominal wall. Fournier gangrene may track via these fascial planes but virtually never affects the testes. Blood supply to the scrotum is via the external pudendal artery. The scrotum is innervated by the ilioinguinal and genitofemoral nerves. Inadvertent injury of the genitofemoral nerve during inguinal hernia repair presents as numbness of the lateral scrotum and medial thigh.

The *testes* are paired egg-shaped organs normally located in the scrotum, whose function is the production of sperm for transport through the epididymis and vas deferens into the urethra during ejaculation. The tubules of the testis are surrounded by a dense layer of tissue called the "tunica albuginea." The blood vessels and nerves supplying the testis travel in the spermatic cord. The testis is supplied by the gonadal artery, deferential artery, and cremasteric artery.

The parenchyma of the testis consists of Leydig cells, Sertoli cells, and seminiferous tubules. Leydig cells are responsible for the production of testosterone under the influence of gonadotropins. The Sertoli cells function as support cells in spermatogenesis. The seminiferous tubules serve as the location of spermatogenesis and connect to the rete testis, which connects to the epididymis. Sperm travel through the epididymis into the vas deferens, where they travel for weeks until they are expelled into the posterior urethra during emission.

RENAL PHYSIOLOGY

The kidney is an organ with myriad functions. Its main purpose is homeostatic, and the kidney is integral in the regulation of intravascular volume, salt and water balance, and control of blood pressure. It acts to rid the body of acids and other by-products of normal metabolism, and it degrades exogenous substances, including many pharmacologic agents. It serves as an endocrine organ, secreting several hormones, including erythropoietin and renin.

The most obvious function of the kidney is urine production. The kidneys filter about 1,440 L of blood per day to create a glomerular filtrate of about 170 L per day. This filtrate is acted upon by passive and active forces along the length of the nephron to create 1 to 2 L of urine per day.

Renal blood flow (RBF) travels through the renal artery into the interlobar, arcuate, interlobular, and afferent arterioles before entering the glomerulus, where the plasma is filtered. The filtration fraction, or renal plasma flow (RPF) divided by glomerular filtration rate (GFR) is dependent on the oncotic and hydrostatic forces acting in the glomerulus (g) and the Bowman space (bs), which determine the pressure for ultrafiltration (P_{uf}). Increased hydrostatic forces (P) within the glomerulus increase P_{uf}, and increased P within the Bowman space decreases P_{uf}. Because the glomerular basement membrane is impermeable to most proteins, oncotic forces also play a role in filtration, and increased oncotic pressure (π) within the glomerulus decreases P_{uf} while increased π within the Bowman space increases P_{uf}. In general, $P_{uf} = [(P_g - P_{bs}) - (\pi_g - \pi_{bs})]$. Because the act of filtration changes the P and π along the glomerulus, the fraction of the plasma filtered per unit length decreases.

The GFR is the volume of plasma that is filtered into the Bowman space per unit time. Given a substance that is freely filtered at the glomerulus and neither secreted nor absorbed, the GFR is equal to the clearance of that solute, defined as the volume of plasma that is cleared of that substance per unit time, or $GFR = U_{cr}V/P_{cr}$. Creatinine is a plasma solute that is for practical purposes neither secreted nor absorbed, and thus creatinine clearance is an excellent proxy for GFR. Knowing the patient's age, weight (in kilograms), and plasma creatinine concentration, one can estimate creatinine clearance with a simple formula: $GFR = [(140 - \text{age}) \times (\text{body weight})]/(72 \times P_{cr})$.

The glomerular filtrate flows through the various segments of the nephron, where all but a fraction of 1% of the filtrate is reabsorbed. In the proximal convoluted tubule (PCT), almost three fourths of the glomerular filtrate is reabsorbed by passive diffusion. In the loop of Henle, energy is consumed to reabsorb salt in greater proportion than water in order to make a relatively dilute urine and to create the medullary gradient necessary for countercurrent exchange and urine concentration. In the distal convoluted tubule (DCT), the fine-tuning of salt and water reabsorption occurs, and the final urine may be as dilute as one third or as concentrated as fourfold the osmolality of plasma.

Several hormones and neural stimuli act on the nephron to regulate electrolytes and blood pressure. The *renin/angiotensin/aldosterone* series of hormones is interdependent and sensitive to volume status. Renin is produced in the juxtaglomerular apparatus in response to stimuli caused by decreased intravascular volume, namely decreased hydrostatic pressure in the afferent arteriole, decreased salt delivery to the macula densa of the distal tubule, and increased sympathetic tone. Renin cleaves angiotensinogen to form angiotensin I. This peptide is metabolized to form angiotensin II in the lung. Angiotensin II is a peripheral vasoconstrictor and a constrictor of the efferent arteriole. This effect leads to decreased delivery of sodium to the collecting duct. Angiotensin II also acts on the zona glomerulosa of the adrenal gland to stimulate secretion of aldosterone, a potent mineralocorticoid that increases sodium reabsorption and potassium secretion in the collecting duct. Increased plasma potassium level is also a stimulus for aldosterone secretion.

Increased *sympathetic tone* causes afferent arteriolar vasoconstriction, leading to decreased RBF and GFR. Furthermore, increased sympathetic tone promotes renin secretion and proximal tubular reabsorption of sodium. These changes cause decreased delivery of salt and water to the distal nephron.

Atrial natriuretic factor (ANF) is a polypeptide secreted by the atrium in response to stretch, increased sodium concentration, and other stimuli related to hypervolemia. It causes a salt and water diuresis as well as a significant peripheral vasodilation, and it inhibits antidiuretic hormone (ADH) action.

ADH is released by the posterior pituitary gland (neurohypophysis), mainly in response to osmotic stimuli on the hypothalamus, although some regulation by volume stimuli has also been recognized. ADH makes the collecting duct permeable to water, which is reabsorbed into the medulla because of the high concentration of medullary solutes. Without the medullary concentration gradient, ADH cannot function and the concentrating ability of the kidney is hampered. The syndrome of inappropriate ADH secretion causes an inappropriately concentrated urine in the face of plasma hyposmolality. Diabetes insipidus, or a lack of ADH action, leads to polyuria from a defect in renal concentration ability.

Homeostasis

The aforementioned agents act in concert with several other factors to regulate the electrolyte homeostasis. The balance of *sodium* is regulated by factors affected primarily by intravascular volume. An increase in intravascular volume triggers baroreceptors and receptors in the juxtaglomerular apparatus, leading to the following changes, which increase the excretion of sodium:

1. Increased RBF, RPF, and glomerular hydrostatic pressure, all of which lead to increased GFR.
2. Decreased renin and aldosterone levels, which cause decreased reabsorption of sodium in the PCT and collecting duct, respectively.
3. Increased ANF level, which leads to increased sodium excretion by increasing delivery of salt to the distal tubule and by inhibiting ADH action.
4. Decreased sympathetic tone, which leads to increased GFR, decreased PCT sodium reabsorption, and increased delivery of sodium to the distal nephron.

Water balance is responsible primarily for the sodium concentration and osmolality of the plasma, and it is appropriately regulated by osmoreceptors in the hypothalamus. The osmolality of the plasma is a function of the concentration of solutes that do not freely cross the cell membrane. The main determinants of the osmolality of plasma are sodium and glucose. Plasma osmolality can be estimated using the simple formula $2 \times [Na^+] + [glucose]/18 + [urea]/2.8$.

Increased osmolality triggers the osmoreceptors, leading to increased thirst for free water, as well as the release of ADH from the anterior pituitary. ADH acts to make the collecting duct permeable to water, thus allowing the urine to equilibrate with the medullary concentration gradient. This causes reabsorption of free water and concentration of the urine.

Potassium is mainly an intracellular ion. Plasma potassium concentration in the short term is mainly dependent on shifts of the extracellular store of potassium into and out of the intracellular store. Factors that cause a shift of potassium into cells, thus decreasing the plasma potassium level are as follows:

1. Alkalosis, by driving protons out of the cell. This increases the positive charge gradient for potassium to move into the cell.
2. Insulin level, by increasing the active cotransport of glucose and potassium into cells.

Factors that may cause a shift of potassium out of the intracellular space, thus increasing plasma potassium, include the following:

1. Acidosis, by driving protons into the cell. This decreases the positive charge gradient for potassium to move into the cell.
2. Cell lysis, by rapidly releasing intracellular potassium. This may occur during certain pathologic states such as transfusion reaction and rhabdomyolysis.

The total body store of potassium is dependent on intake and excretion. The excretion of potassium by the kidney is almost solely dependent on two factors. They are as follows:

1. Aldosterone level. Aldosterone makes the collecting duct permeable to potassium, leading to passage of potassium from the cells of the collecting duct into the urine.
2. Urine flow rate in the collecting duct. The increased flow of urine leads to a washout of the potassium gradient in the collecting duct, causing an increase in the secretion of potassium at this site.

By-products of normal metabolism lead to a significant *acid load,* which must be excreted each day. This is accomplished by the secretion of hydrogen ions, the reabsorption of bicarbonate, and the buffering of the urine with ammonium in the distal tubule. In response to acid loads, the body maintains *acid-base homeostasis* in several ways. The pH level of the plasma is dependent on the concentration of bicarbonate and carbon dioxide. In response to an acid load, the body has a short-term and a long-term response. In the short term, the acid load is buffered by the bicarbonate buffer system. Furthermore, increased ventilation causes a decrease in plasma carbon dioxide concentration. In the long term, acid loads are neutralized by increased bicarbonate reabsorption in the kidney, a process that is dependent on a sodium-proton exchange and on carbonic anhydrase.

The kidney is responsible for significant regulation of calcium balance. It metabolizes 25-hydroxy vitamin D to its highly active form, 1,25-dihydroxy vitamin D. Furthermore, under the regulation of parathyroid hormone (PTH), it excretes most of the daily calcium load. PTH causes an increased secretion of calcium and phosphate ions by the kidney.

Erythropoietin is secreted by the kidney in response to decreased oxygen delivery to the renal cortex. This hormone acts on the bone marrow to increase the production of erythrocytes. Patients with chronic renal failure may have anemia responsive to exogenous erythropoietin because of their decreased viable renal parenchyma. Erythropoietin secretion by renal cell carcinoma may cause a paraneoplastic polycythemia.

Acute Renal Failure

Renal failure may be classified according to its various causes as prerenal, intrarenal, or postrenal. *Prerenal failure* (prerenal azotemia) is caused by a decreased blood flow to the kidneys. This may be secondary to decreased intravascular volume, decreased cardiac output, or relative vasodilation of the peripheral vasculature. Decreased renal blood flow leads to the conservation of salt via an increased sympathetic tone and increased renin/angiotensin II/aldosterone activity by decreasing the amount of glomerular filtrate but increasing the filtration fraction, and thus the reabsorption in the PCT. The increase in resorption by the PCT (which resorbs blood urea nitrogen (BUN) but not creatinine) is greater than the decrease in GFR; thus, the BUN level rises faster than the creatinine level. A BUN/creatinine ratio of greater than 20:1 is typical in prerenal azotemia.

Intrarenal failure is caused by reversible or irreversible insults to the kidneys. Hypoxia, drug toxicity, myoglobinuria, profound hypotension, and sepsis are but a few of the potential causes of this type of renal failure. Intrarenal failure may cause oliguria but rarely causes complete anuria.

Postrenal failure is caused by urinary tract obstruction. This obstruction may occur at any level of the collecting system, ureter, or bladder outlet. Causes of obstruction include stones, tumors, extrinsic compression by tumor or retroperitoneal fibrosis, and bladder outlet obstruction from prostatism, urethral stricture, or detrusor failure. Complete acute obstruction of one ureter usually leads to a temporary increase of the serum creatinine level followed by a gradual return to the baseline caused by contralateral renal compensation. True anuria in a patient with two normal kidneys suggests bladder outlet obstruction or bilateral ureteral obstruction, which is rare. In cases of suspected postrenal failure, the passage of a Foley catheter should confirm or exclude the possibility of bladder outlet obstruction.

Renal ultrasound can suggest upper tract obstruction by showing hydronephrosis and hydroureter. Obstruction can be confirmed by diuretic renogram, intravenous urogram, or by antegrade/retrograde pyelography. Prompt relief of acute obstruction usually leads to a return to normal renal function. Upper tract obstruction may be relieved percutaneously or by retrograde placement of ureteral stents. Bladder outlet obstruction may be relieved by placement of a Foley or suprapubic catheter.

Relief of bilateral upper tract obstruction may lead to a brisk postobstructive diuresis. A temporary concentrating defect in the kidney leads to derangements in serum electrolytes and volume status. Most patients who are alert and have relatively short-term obstruction may be followed as outpatients, as their thirst and hunger mechanisms will compensate for renal losses of sodium, potassium, and water. Obtunded, elderly, or demented patients, as well as those with long-term obstruction, require intravenous fluids and close monitoring of electrolytes.

Diuretics

Diuretics cause the excretion of salt and water in addition to what the kidney would excrete under normal physiologic conditions. There are several classes of diuretics. *Loop diuretics* (such as furosemide) work by inhibiting the active transport of sodium in the thick ascending limb. This deactivates the medullary concentration gradient (rendering ADH ineffective) and increases the delivery of salt to the collecting duct. The result is a salt and water diuresis. Chronic use of loop diuretics can cause hypokalemia because of the increased secretion of potassium secondary to increased urine flow in the collecting duct.

Thiazide diuretics (such as hydrochlorothiazide) act in the distal nephron. Their mechanism of action is incompletely understood. *Osmotic diuretics* (such as mannitol) are osmotically active particles that are filtered but not reabsorbed by the kidney. The osmotic pressure within the nephron causes an obligate loss of free water.

Potassium-sparing diuretics (such as spironolactone and amiloride) inhibit aldosterone action. This causes an increase in sodium excretion and a decrease in potassium excretion. Often a loop diuretic is formulated with a potassium-sparing diuretic to mitigate the potassium wasting effects of the former.

GENITOURINARY TRAUMA

Genitourinary (GU) trauma may result from blunt or penetrating trauma to the chest, abdomen, or pelvis. Over 15% of patients with blunt or penetrating abdominal trauma have injuries to the GU tract. In the management of the trauma patient, it is important to identify patients at risk for GU trauma and evaluate them appropriately with further imaging of the urinary tract. After initial evaluation and institution of resuscitation, secondary and tertiary surveys, as well as adjunct imaging, may identify patients with specific GU trauma.

Urine should be obtained and examined for microscopic or gross blood in all trauma patients who may have GU injuries. A Foley catheter should be placed unless there is suspicion of a urethral injury, as catheter placement may convert a partial urethral tear to a complete tear. Blood at the urethral meatus following trauma is a contraindication to catheter placement until the urethra is properly imaged. Radiographic imaging should be performed in all patients with gross hematuria as well as those with microscopic hematuria whose physical findings or mechanism of injury strongly suggests trauma to GU structures. All pediatric patients with hematuria should be imaged. Management is directed in the short term to the patient's resuscitation and stabilization and in the long term, to preserving renal function and maintaining or restoring the integrity of the GU tract.

Radiographic Studies

Radiographic imaging studies are commonly used in evaluating for GU trauma. *Intravenous urography* (IVU) has historically been the preferred first study in stable patients with suspected renal or ureteral trauma, although computed tomographic (CT) scanning has played a larger role in recent years because of its immediate availability in most trauma centers. It is performed by injecting a high dose (2 mg/kg) of radiopaque contrast material that is concentrated and excreted by the kidneys. A scout film and a subsequent series of images at timed intervals show the contour of the renal parenchyma and the internal architecture of the collecting system and ureters. Incomplete visualization of the renal contour, extravasation of contrast, or a persistent nephrogram raise the possibility of injury to these structures. Failure of a kidney seen on the scout film to take up contrast indicates a probable pedicle injury of the kidney. A one-shot intravenous pyelography (IVP) on the operating room table may be used in the unstable patient who is explored before imaging in order to confirm the presence of a functioning contralateral kidney if nephrectomy is considered.

CT is useful for staging renal trauma as well as for delineating other intraabdominal injuries in the trauma patient. CT should be used for patients in whom the IVP raises the suspicion for renal injury, as well as the patient with suspected multiple intraabdominal injuries. As noted above, CT is now often the first and only study used to assess renal trauma and function in patients with abdominal injuries.

Angiography may be used to identify renovascular injuries but has been largely supplanted by CT, which is usually more readily available and is less invasive.

Ultrasound is not commonly used to diagnose intraabdominal GU injuries. However, it may be useful in the evaluation of the scrotum and testes. *Cystogram* may be used to identify pelvic trauma patients with rupture of the bladder, as IVU is specific but not sensitive for bladder injury. A Foley catheter is placed and 50 mL of contrast material is instilled. Extravasation at this stage indicates a severe rupture of the bladder. If no extravasation is seen, 300 mL is instilled and predrainage/postdrainage films obtained to show extravasation in case of smaller rupture. CT cystogram may be performed following CT of the abdomen if other injuries are suspected. The Foley catheter is clamped and images of the bladder full of contrast are obtained. The catheter is then unclamped and postdrainage views are obtained. If CT cystogram is nondiagnostic, conventional cystogram should be performed.

Retrograde urethrogram may be used to identify urethral trauma in patients with physical findings or injury mechanism consistent with urethral trauma. A small Foley catheter is inflated with 3 mL of water in the fossa navicularis and 5 to 10 mL of contrast material is injected. A film during the injection will show the contour and integrity of the urethra. Contrast must be seen in the bladder to ensure full visualization of the urethra.

RENAL TRAUMA

The kidney is involved in about one of ten abdominal injuries in spite of the fact that it is well-protected anatomically. Most renal injuries occur as a result of blunt trauma. The clinician must quickly decide whether a patient needs radiographic imaging and how to treat a given renal injury once it is identified. Most blunt renal injuries can be managed conservatively.

The mechanism of injury, if available from witnesses or the patient, is important in determining the probability of significant renal injury. Rapid deceleration injury (MVA, fall from a considerable height) raises a suspicion for blunt renal trauma. History of removal or congenital absence of one kidney may alter management significantly.

The physical examination may raise suspicion for renal injury. Flank hematoma or penetrating flank trauma will alert the clinician to a high likelihood of injury of the kidney. Patients with systolic blood pressure of less than 90 mm Hg unresponsive to vigorous resuscitation should be assumed to have a renal injury unless the urine is microscopically free of red blood cells.

Any stable trauma patient with gross hematuria or microscopic hematuria, coupled with a history or physical examination consistent with renal injury, should undergo imaging. Furthermore, all patients with penetrating abdominal trauma and all pediatric patients with microscopic hematuria or suspicious physical findings should undergo imaging. If other significant intraabdominal injuries are suspected, CT with intravenous contrast may be substituted for IVP. In the case of abnormal or indeterminate findings on IVU, CT will be of use in staging renal injury.

Blunt renal trauma is staged according to a simple system outlined in Fig. 24-3. Grade I is a simple contusion; grade II is a minor laceration of the cortex without involvement of the collecting system; grade III is a major laceration without involvement of the collecting system; grade IV is a deep fracture with involvement of the collecting system; and grade V is a shattered kidney or a major pedicle injury.

Treatment of renal injuries is controversial, but the consensus is that most renal injuries can be managed conservatively. Serial CT scanning can be used to follow grade II, III, and even grade IV injuries if the extravasation is minimal and there is no other indication for exploration. The indications for operative intervention are grade V injury, devitalization of a significant portion of the renal parenchyma (20%), and expanding retroperitoneal hematoma. If a patient is to be explored for other injuries, a grade IV renal laceration with minimal extravasation should be repaired at this time. All patients with hypovolemic shock should be explored immediately for a presumed source of surgical bleeding. Most patients with penetrating abdominal trauma will require exploratory laparotomy.

After other associated injuries have been repaired and the presence of a contralateral functioning kidney has been confirmed, exploration of the retroperitoneum to identify and repair renal injuries should be performed. In the case of severe uncontrolled bleeding from the kidney, this repair should obviously take precedence. Control of the renal artery and vein should be accomplished early in case life-threatening bleeding necessitates immediate nephrectomy. After the vessels are controlled, the Gerota fascia is entered and injuries are identified. Parenchymal injuries should be debrided and the capsule reapproximated with chromic suture. Defects in the collecting system should be closed with chromic suture as well. Shattered kidney or severe pedicle injuries usually require nephrectomy. Closed suction drains are mandatory, particularly in the case of significant extravasation.

URETERAL TRAUMA

Ureteral trauma is relatively rare compared to other GU traumas. Its main causes are penetrating wounds, particularly gunshot wounds, and iatrogenic injury at the time of operative procedures. In the short term, the priority in management of ureteral injury is the drainage of the upper urinary tract. In the long term, the priority is the preservation of the renal function on the affected as well as the unaffected side with the smallest number of interventions to reestablish continuity.

All patients with penetrating trauma to the lower abdomen should be suspected of having ureteral trauma. Intravenous pyelography and CT scanning with contrast should identify more than 90% of ureteral injuries. Patients

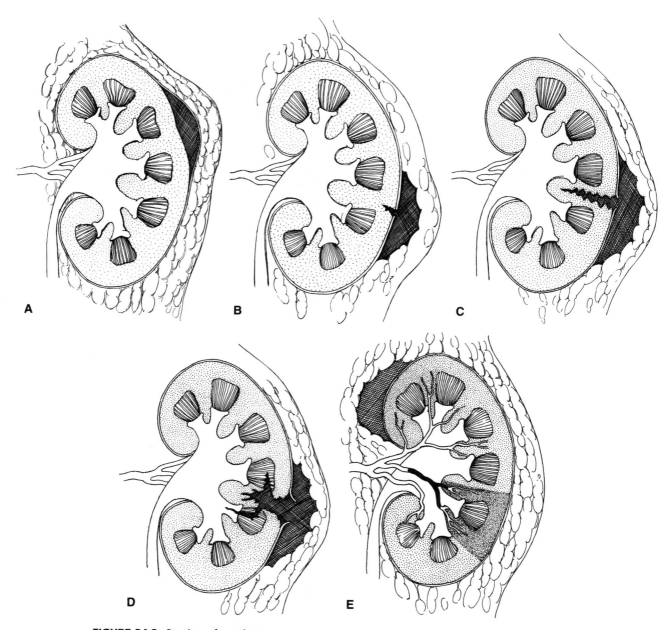

FIGURE 24-3. Staging of renal trauma. **A:** A grade I injury is defined as a contusion or a subcapsular hematoma without parenchymal laceration. **B:** A grade II injury is defined as a nonexpanding or confined perirenal hematoma or cortical laceration less than 1 cm deep without urinary extravasation. **C:** A grade III renal injury involves a parenchymal laceration extending more than 1 cm into the cortex without urinary extravasation, and **(D)** a grade IV injury is defined as a parenchymal laceration extending through the corticomedullary junction with urinary extravasation. **E:** A grade V injury involves a shattered kidney or major parenchymal injury. (From Krane RJ, Sirosky MB, Fitzpatrick JM, eds. *Clinical urology*. Philadelphia: JB Lippincott Co, 1994:400, with permission.)

who are taken to the operating room immediately without such imaging can be confirmed to have ureteral injury by direct visualization or by intravenous administration of indigo carmine. Rarely, retrograde pyelography can be used intraoperatively if these methods fail and a high level of suspicion remains. When an injury is detected early, surgical repair should be attempted. Upper and middle ureteral injuries can be managed with debridement and end-to-end anastomosis. Distal injuries should be managed with ureteral reimplantation with a psoas hitch or a Boari flap. In case of multiple injuries or loss of a large segment of ureter, ileal ureter, nephrectomy, or autotransplantation to the pelvis should be considered. Transureteroureterostomy should be rarely performed because of the risk it may place on the unaffected renal unit, particularly in patients with a history of kidney stone disease or transitional cell carcinoma of the ipsilateral unit. All ureteral repairs should be coupled with urinary diversion with a ureteral stent or a percutaneous nephrostomy tube. In patients who are too unstable at the time of exploration to undergo immediate repair, ureteral clipping and percutaneous nephrostomy may serve as a temporizing measure.

Iatrogenic injury occurs most commonly during abdominal hysterectomy or vascular procedures, but it may also occur during other operations for inflammatory bowel disease, diverticulitis, pelvic malignancy, or during ureteroscopy. Uncontrolled blood loss and inflammatory or neoplastic processes involving the ureter are obvious risk factors. Preoperative imaging and ureteral stenting can reduce risk of injury. Principles of repair are similar to those for external trauma, and as always, the condition of the patient as well as other complicating factors should be considered. For instance, for injury during a vascular procedure with fresh prosthetic material, nephrectomy should be strongly considered, particularly if the contralateral kidney has normal function. If primary reanastomosis is performed, an omental wrap will reduce the risk of a significant leak.

If a clip is placed on the ureter and immediately recognized, it may be removed and treated with only ureteral stenting. If there is any question about the severity of a crush injury to the ureter, urology consultation should be obtained. Excision of the affected segment and reanastomosis may be necessary.

BLADDER TRAUMA

Trauma to the bladder is relatively rare because of its well-protected position in the bony pelvis. The bladder is usually injured as a result of pelvic fracture, but penetrating trauma may also cause a significant number of injuries as well. Bladder injury virtually always presents with hematuria but will not usually be shown on IVU. Thus, patients with pelvic injuries raising suspicion for bladder injury should undergo three-phase cystogram or CT cystogram as described above. In cases of suspected urethral trauma, a retrograde urethrogram should be performed prior to placing the catheter into the bladder.

When a bladder injury is diagnosed, treatment depends on the severity of the injury, the location of the extravasation (intraperitoneal vs. extraperitoneal), as well as the presence of other injuries that may require exploration. Small extraperitoneal leaks may be managed with temporary catheter drainage. If a bladder injury is explored, the bladder should be opened widely in order to inspect its entire mucosal surface. All devitalized tissue should be debrided and the bladder wall should be closed in two layers with absorbable suture. A suprapubic tube ensures maximal drainage of the healing bladder, and a surgical drain should be used until the healing of the injury can be confirmed with a cystogram 1 to 2 weeks postoperatively.

URETHRAL TRAUMA

Trauma to the posterior urethra involves almost exclusively the membranous urethra and most commonly results from pelvic fracture. Trauma patients with blood at the urethral meatus or a high-riding prostate on physical examination should undergo retrograde urethrography before placement of a catheter. Although patients with a minimal amount of extravasation may benefit from temporary Foley catheter drainage of the bladder, any significant disruption should be treated with either immediate debridement and repair (if a concurrent injury is to be repaired immediately) or with suprapubic cystostomy and delayed repair. Placement of a Foley catheter through a partial disruption of the urethra may cause a complete tear and make the repair more difficult.

The injured urethra should be approached through a perineal incision. The ends of the urethra are identified and spatulated, then reanastomosed with absorbable suture. The corpus spongiosum is closed over the urethra. The long-term complications of pelvic fracture with urethral injury are stricture (more than 50%), impotence (10%), and incontinence (less than 5%).

PENILE TRAUMA

The penis may be injured during sexual intercourse (penile fracture) or from penetrating trauma (gunshot, traumatic amputation). Penile fracture should be managed immediately with degloving of the penis and closure of the rupture of the tunica albuginea of the corporal body. Urethral injury should be ruled out with retrograde urethrography unless the urine is microscopically free of blood.

Penetrating trauma should be managed similarly, with debridement of the corporal edges. Delayed urethral injury may result from the blast effect of a gunshot wound. Penile amputation may be managed with reattachment if medical attention is sought within a few hours, but neurological function is poor postoperatively.

SCROTAL TRAUMA

Avulsion of the scrotal skin should be treated immediately by closure of the remaining skin or by placement of the testes into temporary thigh pouches. Blunt scrotal trauma may be managed conservatively, but if there is significant scrotal hematoma, exploration may be warranted, as ultrasound is not sensitive for testicular rupture in this setting. Penetrating trauma to the scrotum should be explored to evaluate testicular injury. The testicular tubules should be debrided and the tunica albuginea closed primarily in both types of injuries.

EMERGENCY ROOM UROLOGY

Urologic emergencies are rare but torsion of the testis, priapism, and Fournier gangrene can often present in an acute fashion and lead to significant morbidity if not treated properly. Torsion of the testis is a surgical emergency. It typically occurs in young adolescents, but it may occur in any age group. The etiology is a congenital defect of the gubernaculum of the testis and of the insertion of the spermatic cord on the testis (the "bell clapper" deformity). The typical patient will present in the emergency room with a brief history of the sudden onset of unilateral testis pain relieved by nothing. The pain is often associated with nausea and vomiting. Physical examination is difficult because of the pain but will show a tense testis that is high riding in the scrotum, as well as a "knot" in the spermatic cord. The cremasteric reflex is invariably absent in torsion of the testis. Urinalysis is typically negative for blood or white blood cells.

The differential diagnosis of acute scrotal pain includes intermittent torsion, torsion of an appendix testis, and epididymo-orchitis. History of fevers, sexually transmitted diseases (STDs), urethral discharge, or white blood cell on urinalysis strongly suggest an infectious process but do not rule out torsion. Patients with torsion of an appendix testis will have point pain and tenderness and may have a dark spot on the testis visible through the scrotal skin (the "blue dot sign"). Radiographic imaging may be useful in cases where the diagnosis is in question. Doppler ultrasound will show a lack of blood flow to the torsioned testis. Nuclear scan will show a photopenic area in the hemiscrotum of the torsioned testis.

Although manual detorsion may be attempted in the emergency room, the definitive treatment of testicular torsion is immediate exploration. The affected side is explored first and detorsion performed. If there is question of viability of the testis, it is placed to the side in a moist sponge while the other testis is exposed. The contralateral testis is fixed to the scrotum in three spots with nonabsorbable suture because of the risk of subsequent contralateral torsion. After the contralateral orchiopexy, the torsioned testis is either removed (if nonviable) or fixed to the scrotal wall in a similar fashion.

Priapism is defined as a prolonged erection, not necessarily related to arousal, that will not detumesce in response to climax. There are two types of priapism: low flow and high flow. Low-flow priapism is an ischemic state due to venous congestion and may be idiopathic or due to sickle cell disease, malignancy, drugs, neurological disorders, or even total parental nutrition administration. The patient usually complains of a painful erection of several hours' duration. Timely detumescence is important because of a rising risk of corporal fibrosis in untreated priapism.

The immediate treatment involves aspiration of hypoxic blood from the corporal bodies and injection of an alpha agonist (often phenylephrine) to cause vasospasm of the corporal arteries. A 19-gauge butterfly needle is inserted laterally into the base of the penis and aspiration of blood from the corpora is performed until bright red blood is aspirated (collaterals between the corpora will drain both bodies). One mL of a dilute solution of phenylephrine (1 mg in 40 mL of normal saline) is injected so that about 250 µg are used. This may be repeated once or twice. Detumescence should quickly ensue. Patients with recurrent priapism can be given a standing dose of oral pseudoephedrine (Sudafed) for prophylaxis. Severe recurrent priapism can be treated with antiandrogen therapy or surgically with a shunt from the corpus cavernosum to the corpus spongiosum.

High-flow priapism is usually caused by trauma and results from rupture of a cavernous artery. Treatment involves angiography and embolization of the involved artery. Because this is a nonischemic state, aspiration will reveal bright red blood and fibrosis is usually not a complication.

Fournier gangrene is a serious infection arising in the external genitalia and/or the perineal tissues that may be fulminant and even fatal. Fournier gangrene is more commonly seen in older patients with diabetes and is usually caused by genital or perineal infection that may be precipitated by urethral stricture, trauma, perirectal abscess, surgical incision, or STDs. The patient usually presents with fever and progressive scrotal swelling. The scrotum is markedly swollen and ecchymotic, and areas of necrosis or crepitus may be present. Plain film, ultrasonography, or CT may show air in the affected areas. The offending organism is usually *Escherichia coli*.

If Fournier gangrene is allowed to progress, it tracks along the Colles fascia of the perineum and may extend to Scarpa fascia of the abdomen. Broad-spectrum antibiotics are helpful, but surgery is the definitive treatment and consists of aggressive debridement and drainage, with repeated trips to the operating room as needed for further debridement. The prognosis for these patients is poor, and as many as 20% will die.

UROLOGIC NEOPLASMS

Many benign and malignant neoplasms arise from the GU organs. Those that are encountered most frequently by the general surgeon include benign and malignant renal masses, transitional cell carcinoma, tumors of the testis, adenocarcinoma of the prostate, and BPH.

Renal masses may be found during imaging for hematuria or flank pain or more commonly as incidental findings during imaging for nonurological reasons. The incidence of renal mass increased severalfold after the advent of cross-sectional imaging. Most renal masses are cysts, which may be simple, with an imperceptible wall and without septations, or complex, a term describing cysts with wall thickening, septations, or calcifications. Increasing complexity of a cyst correlates with an increasing probability of malignancy. Simple cysts are derived from proximal tubular epithelium and are truly benign entities that need no follow-up. Moderately complex cysts may be followed with cross-sectional imaging every 3 to 6 months. Significantly complex cysts should be removed because of a high probability of renal cell carcinoma.

Although most solid renal masses are malignant, benign tumors, including *angiomyolipoma* and *oncocytoma* are seen as well. Angiomyolipoma is a hamartoma of the kidney whose hallmark is fat within the tumor. It may occur sporadically, usually in women, or as a part of the syndrome of *tuberous sclerosis,* which in its most serious form consists of mental retardation, seizure disorder, hamartomas of the brain, lung, and kidney, and adenoma sebaceum. Angiomyolipoma may be an incidental finding or may present with flank pain with or without hypotension from an acute retroperitoneal hemorrhage. CT scan will show a well-circumscribed mass with fat within (less than 0 Hounsfield units). Treatment of angiomyolipoma is based on the size of the lesion and the symptomatology. Asymptomatic lesions may be treated conservatively, but lesions that are symptomatic, particularly those over 4 cm, should be treated with angioinfarction or partial nephrectomy when possible. Furthermore, asymptomatic lesions that grow significantly during follow-up should be considered for excision.

Oncocytoma is a benign tumor that may be difficult to distinguish from renal cell carcinoma by imaging alone. It is a tumor thought to be derived from distal tubular cells and it tends to be asymptomatic and discovered incidentally. Grossly, it may be large and have a central scar that extends to the periphery in a stellate pattern. Histologically, oncocytoma is well differentiated and highly eosinophilic, with significant mitochondrial hyperplasia and rare mitoses. On cross-sectional imaging, there is no reliable way to differentiate this tumor from renal cell carcinoma, but angiography may show a typical "spoke wheel" appearance caused by the stellate scar. Although these tumors are benign, excision remains the standard of care because of the difficulty in definitive diagnosis. For small lesions or in patients with large or bilateral lesions, partial nephrectomy may be attempted while radical nephrectomy remains the standard of care for large (more than 4-cm) unilateral lesions.

Renal cell carcinoma is the most common primary renal malignancy but is relatively rare compared to other adult solid tumors. About 30,000 new cases of renal cell carcinoma are reported each year, and there are over 10,000 deaths a year from the disease. The tumors are usually sporadic but may be familial or associated with von Hippel-Lindau disease. Known risk factors for renal cell carcinoma include male sex, smoking, and acquired cystic kidney disease associated with hemodialysis in end-stage renal disease patients. Most patients are affected in the fifth through seventh decades of life, although significantly younger patients have been reported.

On a molecular level, chromosomal abnormalities in the short arm of chromosome 3 have been most consistently identified, including in several familial cases. Activation of several protooncogenes, most commonly c-*myc*, c-*erb*-b1, and *erb*-b2 have also been associated with renal cell carcinoma. Overexpression of transforming growth factors TGF-α and TGF-β and epidermal growth factor receptor have also been identified in many cases of renal cell carcinoma.

Patients with renal cell carcinoma may be asymptomatic at the time of presentation or may present with one or more of the symptoms of the "classic triad," namely flank pain, abdominal mass, and hematuria. Only 10% of patients will present with all three of these symptoms. Fever, weight loss, and hypertension may also be presenting features. Certain paraneoplastic syndromes have been associated with renal cell carcinoma. Hypercalcemia may be related to tumor production of parathyroid hormone-related peptide. Stauffer syndrome, namely hepatic dysfunction not related to metastatic disease, is a transient elevation of liver function tests that resolves following tumor excision. Reappearance of the abnormality may herald recurrence of tumor. Polycythemia may be related to inappropriate production of erythropoietin by the tumor.

Physical examination is rarely useful in the diagnosis, as most patients will have a normal physical examination until the tumor is locally advanced. Radiography is the mainstay of diagnosis. Renal ultrasound will show a solid renal mass. CT scanning should be performed before and after intravenous contrast administration. A solid mass that enhances more than 20 Hounsfield units after administration of intravenous contrast is pathognomonic for renal cell carcinoma. For patients unable to receive contrast or in those in whom CT is nondiagnostic, MRI with gadolinium may be used in a similar fashion. CT and MRI have the added advantage in detecting extension into the renal vasculature or surrounding structures as well as distant metastases to the liver or bone.

Staging of renal cell carcinoma is commonly based on the TNM staging system or the modified Robson classification and is based on local extent of the tumor as well as on spread to local lymph nodes, vascular involvement, and distant metastases (Table 24-1).

The most common sites of metastases are lung, liver, and bone. Staging workup includes CT of the abdomen to evaluate for local extent and evaluation of the abdominal organs. Any question of involvement of the renal vein or vena cava with thrombus should be imaged with MRI. Chest x-ray is used to screen for lung metastases. Bone scan is often used to evaluate for bony metastases, although its use in patients without bone pain is controversial. Chemistry panel and liver function tests are performed as well, and patients with

TABLE 24-1. THE TNM AND MODIFIED ROBSON CLASSIFICATIONS

Primary tumor (T)
- TX   primary can not be assessed
- T0   no evidence of primary tumor
- T1   tumor ≤2.5 cm, limited to the kidney
- T2   tumor >2.5 cm, limited to the kidney
- T3   tumor extends into veins, adrenal or perinephric tissue
- T3a adrenal or perinephric tissue
- T3b Renal vein(s) or vena cava
- T4   Tumor outside Gerota fascia

Lymph node status (N)
- NX   Nodes can not be assessed
- N0   No nodal metastases
- N1   Single nodal metastasis, ≤2 cm
- N2   One node ≥2.5 cm and ≤5 cm, or multiple nodes ≤5 cm
- N3   Any node ≥5 cm

Metastasis (M)
- MX   Metastases can not be assessed
- M0   No metastases
- M1   Distant metastases

Stage grouping Robson		TNM		
I	=	T1	N0	M0
II	=	T2	N0	M0
III	=	T1-2	N1	M0
		T3	N0-1	M0
IV	=	T4	N0-2	M0
		T0-4	N2-3	M0
		T0-4	N0-3	M1

abnormal renal function may benefit from split-function renal scan if partial nephrectomy is considered.

Renal cell carcinoma is truly a surgical disease. The only effective treatment is extirpation of all tumor mass. Surgery is usually reserved for those with tumor localized to the kidney. Radical nephrectomy is the most effective treatment and consists of removal of the entire kidney with the surrounding Gerota fascia and the adrenal gland. Partial nephrectomy may be considered in patients with small tumors, particularly if they are exophytic and do not invade the collecting system. Partial nephrectomy is especially attractive for patients with a solitary kidney, poor renal function, or bilateral disease. Patients with thrombus extending as far as the right atrium may be treated with radical nephrectomy and removal of the tumor thrombus. This may involve consultation with vascular or cardiothoracic surgeons and can require cardiopulmonary bypass. Select patients with a single metastasis may benefit from concomitant radical nephrectomy and excision of the metastasis.

Patients with widely metastatic disease at the time of diagnosis have a poor prognosis. There is no effective medical therapy for renal cell carcinoma although limited success (about 15% complete response) has been seen with immunotherapy using IL-2 and IFN-α with 5-fluorouracil chemotherapy.

Transitional cell carcinoma may occur anywhere in the urinary tract from the collecting system of the kidney to the proximal urethra. Transitional cell carcinoma is diagnosed in approximately 50,000 new patients a year and causes about 11,000 deaths. It is about three times more prevalent in men than in women. The disease is thought to be the result of multiple epithelial mutations caused by carcinogens in the urine. As the entire urothelium is bathed by the same urine, transitional cell carcinoma is often multifocal, an example of a "field change." Known bladder carcinogens are aniline dyes and several aromatic amines from occupational exposure, nitrosamines and aromatic amines from cigarette smoke, and phenacetin. Furthermore, cyclophosphamide chemotherapy is a risk factor for transitional cell carcinoma because of the mutagenic properties of a metabolite, acrolein. This risk can be minimized by the concomitant administration of mesna, a substance that complexes with acrolein. External beam radiation is also a risk factor for transitional cell carcinoma. Substances suspected but never proven to cause bladder cancer are caffeine, artificial sweeteners, and metabolites of tryptophan.

The progression from normal urothelium to superficial or invasive transitional cell carcinoma is complex and involves several mutations. These mutations can be classified as (i) conversion of protooncogenes to oncogenes, (ii) loss of tumor suppressor genes, and (iii) amplification of growth factor action. Implicated in transitional cell carcinoma are oncogenes p21 *ras*, c-*myc*, erb-b2, and c-*jun*. Tumor suppressor genes include the retinoblastoma gene, p15, p16, and p53. The latter has been extensively studied and has a strong association with aggressive and invasive cancers. Mutations in the receptor of the epithelial growth factor and amplification of its expression have also been correlated with more aggressive tumors.

The patient with transitional cell carcinoma usually presents with hematuria. IVU, urine culture and cytology, and cystoscopy should be performed in all patients with hematuria. The IVP evaluates the upper urinary tracts for filling defects (3% of patients with transitional cell carcinoma of the bladder will have an upper tract lesion). Positive urine culture results do not eliminate the possibility of malignancy. The sensitivity of urine cytology increases as the grade of the lesion increases. Cystoscopy will identify any lesions in the bladder or urethra.

Patients with upper tract lesions should have brush biopsy or ureteroscopic biopsy of the tumor. Patients with bladder lesions should undergo complete transurethral resection including a portion of the underlying detrusor muscle. When the diagnosis is confirmed, staging workup consists of IVU, chest x-ray, CT scan of the abdomen and pelvis, and bone scan. The commonly used staging systems for bladder cancer are outlined in Table 24-2.

Treatment of transitional cell carcinoma depends on the grade, stage, and location of the lesion, as well as the overall health of the patient. In general, superficial disease (Ta

TABLE 24-2. STAGING FOR BLADDER CANCER

Extent of involvement	Stage
Marshall modification of Jewett-Strong classification	
Mucosa	0
Lamina propria	A
Superficial muscle	B1
Deep muscle	B2
Perivesical tissue	C
Pelvic lymph nodes	D1
Distant metastases	D2
Union Internationale Contre le Cancer Classification	
Carcinoma *in situ*	Tis
Mucosa	Ta
Submucosal invasion	T1
Superficial muscle invasion	T2
Deep muscle invasion	T3a
Perivesical fat invasion	T3b
Invasion of contiguous organs	T4
Regional lymph nodes involved	N1-3
Distant metastases	M1

and T1) is treated conservatively with resection, surveillance cystoscopy, and intravesical therapy when needed. When superficial disease recurs, it usually remains noninvasive. Muscle invasive bladder cancer, on the other hand, is generally treated more aggressively with partial or radical cystectomy, or with a bladder-sparing protocol of external beam radiation and chemotherapy.

In the bladder, unifocal superficial lesions (Ta) can be treated with surveillance cystoscopy every 3 to 6 months. Intravesical chemotherapy (BCG, mitomycin, thiotepa) and surveillance cystoscopy every 3 to 6 months are used for multifocal tumors, as well as those associated with carcinoma *in situ*, a flat, dysplastic lesion that is at risk for disease progression. Higher grade superficial lesions and those with invasion of the lamina propria (T1) are treated similarly with intravesical therapy but tend to be more aggressive than Ta lesions and thus need careful follow-up. Although it is not currently the standard of care, some advocate early cystectomy for T1 lesions (particularly if recurrent or multifocal) because of the high risk of progression and death from bladder cancer.

The mainstay of truly invasive disease without distant metastases (T2+, NX, M0) is radical cystectomy with pelvic lymph node dissection and urinary diversion. Patients with solitary invasive tumors away from the trigone may be treated with partial cystectomy with a 2-cm cuff of normal bladder around the tumor. Patients who refuse cystectomy or who are poor anesthetic risks may be treated with a bladder-sparing protocol of radiation therapy and MVAC chemotherapy (mitomycin, vinblastine, adriamycin, and cisplatin). Patients with metastatic disease (M1) at the time of diagnosis have a poor prognosis and should be treated with MVAC chemotherapy.

There are several methods of urinary diversion used following radical cystectomy. These include jejunal, ileal or colon conduit, continent catheterizable pouch, and orthotopic neobladder, which is connected to the native urethra and most closely approximates the normal anatomy. Stomal stenosis, ureteral stricture, pyelonephritis, and stone formation can complicate urinary diversion. In addition, several metabolic abnormalities have been observed in patients with intestinal urinary diversion. The type and severity of the metabolic abnormality depends on the segment of intestine used and the type of diversion. Jejunal segments typically cause a hyperkalemic, hypochloremic metabolic acidosis while ileum and colon cause a hyperchloremic metabolic acidosis. Although not commonly used for primary urinary diversion, gastric segments are sometimes used for bladder augmentation and may be complicated by a hypochloremic metabolic acidosis. Continent reservoirs have an increased contact time with the urine and thus lead to more severe metabolic abnormalities. These diversions should not be used in patients with significant preoperative renal insufficiency.

Transitional cell carcinoma of the upper urinary tract is usually treated with nephroureterectomy or partial ureterectomy except in those patients with lesions in a solitary kidney, those with chronic renal insufficiency, those who are poor surgical risks, or those in whom endoscopic or percutaneous resection is feasible. Transitional cell carcinoma limited to the renal pelvis or proximal ureter is generally treated with nephroureterectomy, as there is a significant risk of downstream recurrence. Transitional cell carcinoma of the distal ureter can be managed with distal ureterectomy and ureteral reimplantation. Depending on the length of ureter excised, a psoas hitch, Boari flap, or ileal ureter may be necessary to bridge the gap from the kidney to the bladder.

Postoperative management of patients with transitional cell carcinoma includes interval IVU, chest x-ray, and urinary cytology. Positive surgical margins or lymph nodes and recurrent disease are typically treated with MVAC chemotherapy.

Other bladder neoplasms include squamous cell carcinoma, which is associated with indwelling urinary catheters and *Schistosoma haematobium* infection. Small cell carcinoma and carcinosarcoma are rare and have a poor prognosis. Rhabdomyosarcoma is typically a pediatric disease and is usually treated with radiation and chemotherapy with good results.

Testicular cancer is relatively rare, but because it affects a young patient population and because it is one of the most treatable cancers, its early diagnosis and effective treatment is of obvious social and economic benefit. The incidence of testis tumors is about 5,000 to 6,000 per year in the United States. In spite of this number, fewer than 300 patients die per year of the disease, largely due to the effectiveness of available treatment. Testis tumors most often affect young men in their 20s and 30s, although young children and older men may also be affected.

The main risk factor for testis cancer is cryptorchidism, and the risk correlates with the severity of maldescent. The risk of developing cancer in a high scrotal testis is approximately 1 of 100 while the risk in an intraabdominal testis is about 1 of 20. There is an associated but smaller risk in the contralateral testis if it is normally descended, and although the risk of malignancy is not diminished by orchiopexy, the operation is recommended in part because it aids in future self-examination for tumor.

Testis tumors are almost always (more than 95%) derived from germinal elements, and *germ-cell tumors* are classified as *pure seminoma* or as *nonseminomatous germ-cell tumors* (NSGCTs). NSGCTs are further characterized as embryonal carcinoma, yolk sac tumor, teratoma, or choriocarcinoma. NSGCT also includes mixed seminoma with nonseminomatous elements. This distinction is important in treatment, as pure seminoma tumors are highly sensitive to radiation while NSGCTs are highly sensitive to chemotherapy. A testis tumor usually presents as a hard, painless scrotal mass in a young man. Although the patient may report a sudden increase in size or a recent trauma, the mass usually will have been present for several months. The differential diagnosis of testis mass includes hydrocele, hernia, hematoma, orchitis, and spermatocele. Scrotal ultrasound should easily differentiate among these diagnoses if the history and physical examination leave any doubt. In case of testis tumor, ultrasound will show a hypoechoic, often hypervascular mass in the testis.

Patients with testis tumors should undergo inguinal orchiectomy as soon as possible. Scrotal orchiectomy is not performed because of the theoretical risk of contamination of scrotal lymphatics with tumor cells. Because testis tumors metastasize most commonly to the retroperitoneum and mediastinum via lymphatics and to the lungs hematogenously, the staging workup includes CT of the retroperitoneum and chest. Staging is based on the histology of the primary specimen and on the imaging results and is outlined in Tables 24-3 and 24-4. Tumor markers α-fetoprotein (AFP) and human chorionic gonadotropin (hCG) are useful in the determination of tumor type, tumor volume, and response to treatment. AFP (half-life about 6 days) is produced by yolk sac tumors but not by choriocarcinoma or by seminoma. Presence of AFP rules out a pure seminoma. hCG (half-life about 24 hours) is produced by choriocarcinoma and embryonal carcinoma. Although hCG is not produced by seminoma directly, it is produced by syncytiotrophoblasts within the tumor. Elevation of hCG thus can be seen in seminoma, but this elevation is rarely greater than two times the normal level.

Treatment consists of removal of the primary tumor with prophylactic sterilization of the retroperitoneum in stage 1 and early stage 2 disease. This is accomplished with radiation therapy for seminoma and with *retroperitoneal lymph node dissection* for NSGCT. Patients who are well motivated and willing to undergo surveillance may be followed for recurrence of NSGCT. However, the schedule for surveillance (chest x-ray every month, CT and tumor markers every 2 months) is so rigorous that few patients actually

TABLE 24-3. STAGING CLASSIFICATION FOR NONSEMINOMATOUS GERM CELL TUMORS[a]

Boden and Gibb, 1951	Logothetis (MD Anderson Cancer Center), 1990	Bose, et al. (Memorial Sloan-Kettering Cancer Center), 1983	Einhorn (Indiana University), 1988
A (I) confined to testis	I confined to testis	I confined to testis	I confined to testis
B (II) spread to retroperi RPLN	IIa negative clinical and positive surgical RPLN or elevated markers after archiectomy	II grossly negative, pathologically positive N_1 N_{2a} grossly positive <6 nodes, all <2 cm N_{2b} >6 nodes or any one >2 cm N_3 extranodal extension N_4 incompletely resectable	IIa negative clinical and positive surgical RPLN (<2 cm, <6 nodes) IIb RPLN mass <5 cm IIc RPLN mass >5 cm III Minimal: ↑ markers only cervical nodes unresectable RPLN <5 lung metastases, all <2 cm *Moderate:* Palpable RPLN mass 5–10 lung metastases, all <3 cm or solitary metastasis >2 cm *Advanced:* >10 cm lung metastases or multiple metastases >3 cm palpable RPLN and supradiaphragmatic disease liver, bone, or central nervous system metastasis
	IIb RPLN mass <2 cm IIc RPLN mass <5 cm IId RPLN mass <10 cm		
C (III) spread beyond RPLN	IIIa supraclavicular nodes IIIb$_1$ elevated marker after RPLN dissection IIIb$_2$ pulmonary disease (minimal or advanced) IIIb$_3$ advanced abdominal disease (mass >10 cm) IIIb$_4$ visceral disease other than lung IIIb$_5$ βhCG > 50,000 IU ± IIIb$_2$, IIIb$_4$	III spread beyond RPLN Low risk: total metastatic sites <2 minimal elevation of HCG High risk: total metastatic sites >2 elevated LDH or hCG extragonadal origin	

[a]RPLN, retroperitoneal lymph node; hCG, human chorionic gonadotropin; LDH, lactate dehydrogenase.

TABLE 24-4. STAGING CLASSIFICATION FOR SEMINOMAS

Stage I
  Confined to testicle
Stage II
  Retroperitoneal disease only
   a. Mass ≤10 cm
   b. Mass ≥10 cm
Stage III
  Supradiaphragmatic or visceral disease
   a. Supradiaphragmatic nodal disease
   b. Visceral metastases

comply. Persistently elevated markers following retroperitoneal lymph node dissection suggest distant metastases that should be treated with adjuvant chemotherapy.

In both seminoma and NSGCT, bulky retroperitoneal disease should be treated first with chemotherapy. Residual NSGCT should be treated with retroperitoneal lymph node dissection if markers normalize and with salvage chemotherapy if they do not normalize. The treatment of residual seminoma is controversial.

Retroperitoneal lymph node dissection is performed through a midline incision. Pericaval and periaortic nodes are dissected from the level of the renal vessels to the bifurcation of the iliac vessels. The main risk of the procedure is loss of emission and ejaculation from disruption of sympathetic fibers. Through the use of modified templates of dissection based on the side of the tumor and by using a nerve-sparing approach, these effects have been minimized.

Prostate cancer is the most common tumor and the second most common cause of cancer death in men. About 250,000 new cases of prostate cancer are diagnosed each year, and about 45,000 men die each year of the disease. Prostate cancer is usually diagnosed between the ages of 45 and 75; although it may occur in younger men, it certainly occurs commonly in older men who eventually die *with* prostate cancer rather than *of* prostate cancer. Major risk factors include advancing age, history of prostate cancer in a first-degree relative, and race (blacks have a 30% higher incidence than whites). Potential minor risk factors include high-fat diet and high serum testosterone level, although neither of these has been definitively proven. Certain vitamins such as vitamins A, D, and selenium have been proposed as possible preventatives.

The molecular basis of prostate cancer is complex and many putative oncogenes and tumor suppressor genes have been proposed. Among the tumor suppressor genes, the most common are genes on 8p, 16q, and the retinoblastoma gene. P53 mutations have been associated with aggressive disease. Furthermore, the *ras* oncogene and mutations in the androgen receptor have been associated with the development of prostate cancer.

Because low-stage prostate cancer is asymptomatic, screening for prostate cancer using the prostate-specific antigen (PSA) and digital rectal examination is used widely. Although there is some controversy surrounding the utility of screening for prostate cancer, in the United States, men are generally screened once yearly between the ages of 50 and 70. African Americans and those with a family history of prostate cancer generally begin screening at age 40. Patients with an abnormal serum PSA level (more than 4.0 ng/mL) or digital rectal examination (DRE) undergo transrectal ultrasound-guided biopsy of the peripheral zone of the prostate, as this is the most common site of tumor formation. Biopsies are graded using the Gleason scoring system. The tumor growth pattern is graded from 1 to 5 (least dysplastic to most dysplastic) and a score of 2 to 10 is assigned by adding the two most common patterns. A Gleason score of 7 or higher suggests a poor prognosis.

The TNM staging system of prostate cancer is shown in Table 24-5. The most common sites of metastasis of prostate cancer are bone and pelvic lymph nodes. The staging workup for prostate cancer is somewhat controversial and may involve several radiographic examinations. Radionuclide bone scan may detect bony metastases. CT of the pelvis may detect obturator or iliac lymph node metastases in the pelvis. MRI with an endorectal coil can be useful in the detection of extension of the tumor beyond the capsule of the prostate, a finding that significantly alters the treatment of choice. Elevation in the PSA level alone is useful for predicting stage, as most men with low PSA levels (less than 10) have organ-confined disease while those with significant elevations in PSA have extraprostatic disease.

The treatment of prostate cancer depends on the grade and stage of the lesion, as well as on the overall condition of the patient. The various treatments, from least to most invasive, are as follows:

1. Watchful waiting consists of following the PSA level and DRE for signs of progression with treatment only for advancing lesions. This is used predominantly in patients older than 70 with minimal disease.

2. Antiandrogen therapy consists of either injection of a luteinizing hormone-releasing hormone (LHRH) agonist (Zoladex, Lupron) or surgical castration. This therapy is usually reserved for older patients and for patients with widely metastatic disease, or for treatment failures. Side effects include impotence, decreased libido, and hot flashes.

3. Brachytherapy with radioactive seeds, which may include palladium, iodine, or iridium. This therapy is usually used in patients with low-grade organ-confined disease. Its side effects are limited to irritative urinary symptoms with limited effects on potency and continence.

4. External beam radiation. This therapy is typically used in men with a life expectancy of less than 10 years and may be used for those with T3 or T4 disease, and with N+ disease. Compared to the aforementioned therapies, it has more adverse effects, including radiation cystitis and proctitis, fistula, impotence, and incontinence.

TABLE 24-5. 1992 AMERICAN JOINT COMMITTEE ON CANCER/UNION INTERNATIONALE CENTRE TNM STAGING CLASSIFICATION[a]

Stage	Definition
Primary tumor (T)	
TX	primary tumor can not be assessed
T0	no evidence of primary tumor
T1	clinically inapparent tumor not palpable or visible by imaging
T1a	tumor incidental histologic finding in 5% or less of tissue resected
T1b	tumor incidental histologic finding in more than 5% of tissue resected
T1c	tumor identified by needle biopsy (e.g., because of elevated prostate-specific antigen)
T2	tumor confined within the prostate[b]
T2a	tumor involves half of a lobe or less
T2b	tumor involves more than half a lobe but not both lobes
T2c	tumor involves both lobes
T3	tumor extends through the prostatic capsule[c]
T3a	unilateral extracapsular extension
T3b	bilateral extracapsular extension
T3c	tumor invades the seminal vesicle(s)
T4	tumor is fixed or invades adjacent structures other than the seminal vesicles
T4a	tumor invades any of bladder neck, external sphincter, or rectum
T4b	tumor invades levator muscles and/or is fixed to the pelvic wall
Regional lymph nodes (N)	
NX	Regional lymph nodes can not be assessed
NX	no regional lymph node metastasis
N1	metastasis in a single lymph node, 2 cm or less in greatest dimension
N2	metastasis in a single lymph node, more than 2 cm but not more than 5 cm in greatest dimension; or multiple lymph node metastases, none more than 5 cm in greatest dimension
N3	metastasis in a lymph node more than 5 cm in greatest dimension
Distant metastases[d] (M)	
MX	presence of distant metastasis can not be assessed
M0	no distant metastasis
M1	distant metastasis
M1a	nonregional lymph node(s)
M1b	bone(s)
M1c	other site(s)

[a]From Beahrs OH, Henson DE, Hutter RVP, et al. *Manual for staging of cancer*, 4th ed. Philadelphia: JB Lippincott Co, 1992, with permission.
[b]Tumor found in one or both lobes by needle biopsy, but not palpable or visible by imaging, is classified as T1c.
[c]Invasion into the prostatic apex or into (but not beyond) the prostatic capsule is not classified as T3 but as T2.
[d]When more than one site of metastasis is present, the most advanced category (pM1c) is used.

5. Transperineal cryoablation of the prostate is an experimental therapy that is fraught with complications and today is rarely used.

6. Radical prostatectomy is the definitive surgical treatment in men with a life expectancy of more than 10 years and with organ-confined disease. It is statistically the most durable cure for localized disease. It may be performed via a retropubic or perineal approach. Major complications include bleeding, rectal injury, impotence, and incontinence.

There is no effective chemotherapy for prostate cancer, although strontium may be palliative for patients with bone metastases and bony pain. Follow-up for treated prostate cancer consists of serial PSA determinations and DRE with repeated radiographic imaging performed as clinically indicated. Most patients with PSA recurrences following definitive treatment can receive antiandrogen therapy. Although this therapy will reduce the serum PSA level, there is no definite evidence that it will extend life.

Benign prostatic hypertrophy (BPH) is a common condition resulting from adenomatous hyperplasia of the transition zone of the prostate. Although it is by definition a benign process, it may cause significant lower urinary tract obstruction, which if left untreated may lead to life-threatening complications such as urosepsis or renal failure. BPH affects men with an increasing frequency as they age. The prevalence in autopsy studies ranges from less than 20% in men younger than 40 to more than 90% in men older than 80. A large portion of men with BPH are asymptomatic and thus never come to the attention of a clinician.

There are several theories as to the etiology of BPH and the bladder outlet obstruction that results. Most would agree that hyperplasia is largely mediated by the action of dihydrotestosterone (DHT), and indeed inhibitors of the production of DHT have been shown to decrease and even reverse BPH. Finasteride, a 5α-reductase inhibitor, inhibits the formation of DHT from testosterone and has been shown to significantly decrease the volume of the prostate in men with BPH. Bladder outlet obstruction results from increased prostate size as well as from an increased amount and tone of smooth muscle in the prostate and bladder neck. This muscle is rich in α_1-adrenergic receptors, and α_1-adrenergic antagonists such as terazosin can cause significant improvement in lower urinary tract symptoms.

Symptoms of prostatism result from many factors, including detrusor hypertrophy, increased voiding pressures, and incomplete emptying. Lower urinary tract symptoms can be separated into obstructive symptoms (such as hesitancy, straining, decreased stream, postvoid dribbling, etc) and irritative symptoms (such as urgency, frequency, and nocturia). The American Urologic Association symptom index score total symptomatology based on the severity of several obstructive and irritative symptoms and ranges from 0 to 35 with higher scores indicating more severe symptoms. This score can be valuable in assessing the effects of treatment.

Treatments of symptomatic BPH include the following:

1. Watchful waiting for mildly symptomatic cases.
2. Medical therapy, including α_1 blockade and antitestosterone agents such as finasteride and LHRH agonists.
3. Clean intermittent catheterization for patients with elevated postvoid residuals complicated by infection or significant symptoms, who have failed or refused medical and surgical therapies. This may be the only viable option for some with detrusor failure from long-standing obstruction.
4. Transurethral resection of the prostate (TURP) is a highly effective treatment reserved for patients who have failed medical therapy or for those who present with significant complications including upper tract degeneration, gross hematuria, acute urinary retention, and bladder stone. This operation requires a 1- to 2-day hospital stay and has a significant side-effect profile including bleeding, infection, incontinence, and retrograde ejaculation. Extended TURP lasting more than 1 hour may lead to significant absorption of the glycine irrigant used during the procedure. The post-TURP syndrome that results consists of a combination of hyponatremia, fluid overload, and mental status changes. Alternative techniques to debulk the surgical outlet have been developed more recently and may be considered less invasive. These include microwave therapy, thermotherapy, laser ablation, and transurethral incision of the prostate. All must be compared to TURP, the gold standard.
5. Open prostatectomy. The indications for open prostatectomy are similar to those for TURP, but open surgery is performed in those with glands too large for TURP (usually more than 60 g). The operation is performed suprapubically by opening the bladder or retropubically by incising the capsule of the prostate. This operation causes the greatest relief in symptomatology of all treatments but also requires a 4- to 6-day hospital stay and may have significant complications, as can all major pelvic surgery.

Many patients, particularly men, will experience urinary retention following nonurologic procedures. This retention may be due to several factors, including underlying BPH, anticholinergic effects of certain medications, and bladder atony secondary to the effects of anesthesia. Furthermore, certain radical surgeries, most notably APR, may interrupt autonomic pathways mediating normal voiding function. The treatment of postoperative urinary retention consists of assisted bladder drainage (Foley catheter, or preferably clean intermittent catheterization) with or without adjuvant pharmacologic therapy until emptying function has returned. In rare instances, normal voiding will not resume, and surgical therapy or prolonged catheter drainage is required.

SUGGESTED READING

Gillenwater JY, Howards S, Grayhack JT, et al., eds. *Adult and pediatric urology,* 3rd ed. St. Louis: Mosby–Year Book, 1996.

Krane RF, Sirosky MB, Fitzpatrick JM, eds. *Clinical urology.* Philadelphia: JB Lippincott Co, 1994.

Walsh PC, Retik AB, Darracott Vaughn E Jr, et al., eds. *Campbell's urology,* 7th ed. Philadelphia: WB Saunders, 1998.

FEMALE REPRODUCTIVE SYSTEM

SALLY Y. SEGEL AND SARA J. MARDER

The specialty of obstetrics and gynecology focuses on the female reproductive system. This chapter will review the anatomy, physiology and pathology of the female genital tract. Because the female pelvis contains reproductive, gastrointestinal, and genitourinary systems, the differential diagnoses for many lower abdominal complaints include both surgical and gynecologic disease processes. As a result, the general surgeon should be familiar with the anatomy and pathophysiology of the female reproductive system.

EMBRYOLOGY

Until 8 weeks of gestation, the human embryo is ambisexual and has precursors of both male and female reproductive tracts. The female reproductive tract is derived from the müllerian duct system (paramesonephric duct) and the male reproductive tract is derived from the wolffian duct system (mesonephric duct). If the embryo possesses a Y chromosome, testicular differentiation from the indifferent gonad occurs during gestational weeks 6 through 9. The testes produce testosterone and müllerian inhibiting factor (MIF), which cause the regression of the müllerian system during the eighth week of gestation. In the absence of testicular differentiation and the production of testosterone and MIF, the müllerian duct system persists and the wolffian system regresses. By 10 weeks of gestation, the müllerian ducts fuse and form the fallopian tubes, the uterus, and the upper two thirds of the vagina (Fig. 25-1). Remnants of the wolffian system can form paratubal cysts anywhere along the length of the fallopian tubes.

There are two kinds of defects related to the embryological development of the female genital tract: defects in fusion and defects in canalization. Fusion defects are responsible for duplications in the organs such as a bicornuate uterus, and uterus didelphys. Canalization defects are responsible for vaginal septi and incomplete formation of the uterine cavity or cervical canal. These defects may cause a teenager to seek medical attention for primary amenorrhea, an abdominal mass, or cyclic abdominal pain. As a result of obstruction to menstrual flow, there is a buildup of sloughed endometrium and blood in the vagina (hematocolpos) and the uterus (hematometra). Magnetic resonance imaging of the abdomen and pelvis demonstrates an enlarged vagina and uterus filled with blood.

ANATOMY

The vulva is the hair-bearing skin and adipose tissue of the external genitalia. The vulva consists of the labia majora and the labia minora. Between the labia minora are the vestibule of the vagina, the urethra, and the clitoris. The erectile bodies and their associated muscles lie underneath the subcutaneous tissue and above the fascial layer.

The fascial layer consists of the perineal membrane. This membrane is a dense sheet of fibromuscular tissue that spans the anterior portion of the pelvic outlet. The perineal body is a condensation of connective tissue between the lower vagina and the anus. The perineal membrane connects the vagina and the perineal body. The perineal membrane supports the pelvic floor against increases in intraabdominal pressure.

The nerves, arteries, and veins supplying the external genitalia travel through the pelvis together, and these are responsible for the innervation and blood supply of the anterior and posterior triangles of the external genitalia. The pudendal nerve (S2-4) contains the sensory and motor components. The pudendal artery and vein are branches of the anterior division of the internal iliac vessels. The nerve, artery, and vein leave the pelvis through the greater sciatic foramen, wrap around the ischial spine, and the sacrospinous ligament, and then reenter the pelvis through the Alcock canal and the lesser sciatic foramen. There are

Hospital of the University of Pennsylvania, Philadelphia, Pennsylvania

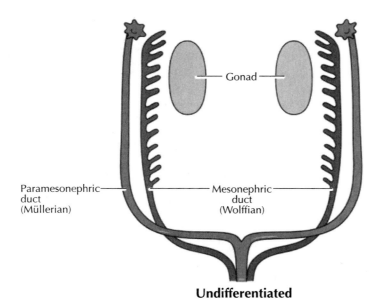
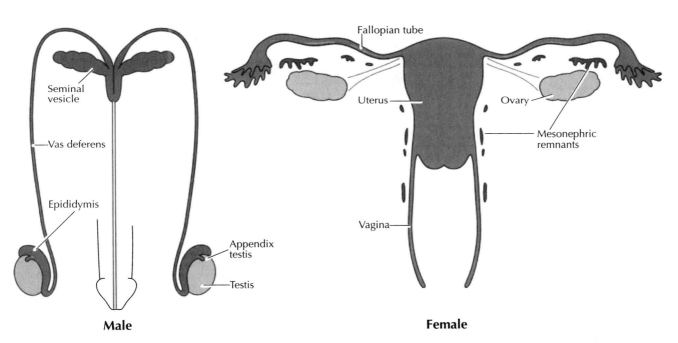

FIGURE 25-1. Develoment of the normal male and female reproductive tract. (From Speroff L, Glass RH, Kase N, eds. *Clinical gynecologic endocrinology and infertility,* 5th ed. Baltimore: Williams & Wilkins, 1994:323, with permission.)

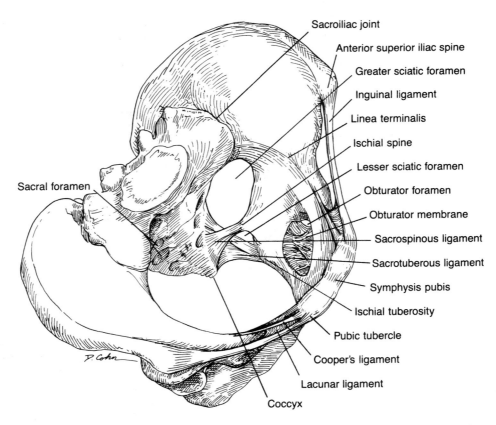

FIGURE 25-2. The female pelvis. (From Berek JS, Adashi EY, Hillard PA, eds. *Novak's gynecology,* 12th ed. Baltimore: Williams & Wilkins, 1996:72, with permission.)

three main branches of both the vessels and the nerve: clitoral, perineal, and inferior hemorrhoidal.

Lymphatic drainage of the external genitalia is through the inguinal system. Tissues external to the hymenal ring are drained by a series of lymphatics that coalesce into a few trunks lateral to the clitoris. These lymphatic channels drain into the superficial inguinal nodes. The urethral lymphatics also drain into superficial inguinal nodes. These superficial lymph nodes drain into deep inguinal lymph nodes, which are found under the fascia cribrosa in the femoral triangle.

The *pelvis* is formed by the union of the sacrum and coccyx with the ilium, the ischium, and the pubis (Fig. 25-2). The sacrospinous and sacrotuberous ligaments create the greater and lesser sciatic foramina. The main muscles of the pelvic floor are the levator ani. The levator ani muscles consist of pubococcygeal, iliococcygeal, puborectal, and coccygeal muscles and form a *U*-shaped layer. The urethra, vagina, and rectum run through the opening of the *U*. The region of the levator ani between the anus and the coccyx is the raphe anococcygea. This raphe forms a supportive shelf on which the rectum, upper vagina, and uterus rest (Fig. 25-3).

Defects in pelvic support are responsible for pelvic organ prolapse. Damage to the anterior levator ani paravaginal support can lead to a cystocele, in which the bladder prolapses into the anterior vagina. This condition usually presents as urinary incontinence. Damage in the rectovaginal septum causes the development of a rectocele, where the rectum prolapses into the vagina. This condition usually presents as difficulty in stool evacuation.

The *pelvic organs* include the vagina, uterus, fallopian tubes, and ovaries. The vagina bends at an angle of 120 degrees by traction from the levators at the junction of the lower one third and upper two thirds. The uterus is a fibromuscular organ composed of the upper muscular corpus and the lower fibrous cervix. In most women, the normal position of the uterus is anteverted over the dome of the bladder. The fallopian tubes are paired structures with four portions: interstitial, isthmic, ampullary, and fimbria. The fimbria ovarica bring the fimbria and the ovary close together at the time of ovulation.

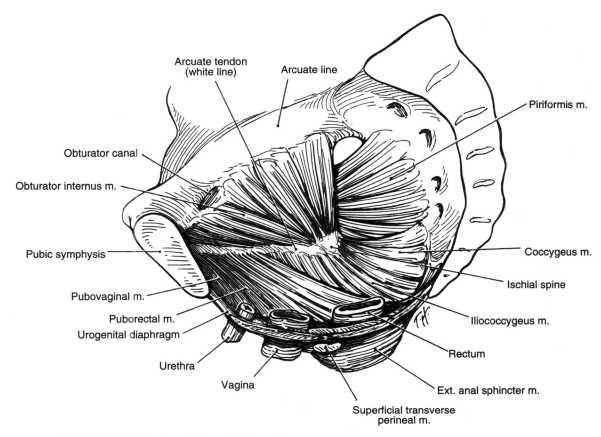

FIGURE 25-3. Muscles of the pelvic floor. (Berek JS, Adashi EY, Hillard PA, eds. *Novak's gynecology*, 12th ed. Baltimore: Williams & Wilkins, 1996:77, with permission.)

Other organs in the pelvis have important relationships to the reproductive organs. The rectum lies behind the uterus and posterior to the cul-de-sac. The bladder rests posteriorly on the lower uterine segment, cervix, and upper vagina. The ureters are intimately associated with many components of the female pelvis. The ureter passes over the bifurcation of the common iliac vessels and descends within the pelvis. Its connective tissue sheath is attached to the lateral pelvic sidewall and to the medial leaf of the broad ligament. The ureter then runs underneath the uterine artery in the cardinal ligament and lies 1 cm from the anterolateral surface of the cervix. The ureter then passes on the anterior vaginal wall and proceeds for another 1.5 cm through the bladder wall (Fig. 25-4).

The *ligaments of the internal pelvic organs* provide structural support and contain the major blood vessels of the pelvis. The broad ligament is a series of peritoneal folds continuous with the abdominal peritoneum that cover the fallopian tubes and the ovaries. The broad ligament that covers the fallopian tubes is known as the "mesosalpinx," and the broad ligament that covers the ovaries is known as the "mesovarium." The round ligament is contained within the anterior broad ligament. It is an extension of the uterine musculature and arises at the anterolateral aspect of the uterus, enters the inguinal canal at the internal inguinal ring, and exits the canal to insert into the subcutaneous tissue of the labia majora. The infundibulopelvic ligaments, also known as the "suspensory ligaments of the ovary," are derived from the broad ligament at the lateral aspect of the fallopian tube and ovary to attach these structures to the pelvic sidewall. These ligaments contain the ovarian artery and vein. The uterosacral ligaments run from the posterior cervix to the second, third, and fourth segments of the sacrum. The cervix is held posteriorly in the pelvis over the levator plate by these ligaments. Finally, the cardinal ligaments run from the lateral wall of the cervix and vagina to the pelvic sidewall and provide the primary support for the uterus in the pelvis. The uterine artery and vein are found within the cardinal ligaments.

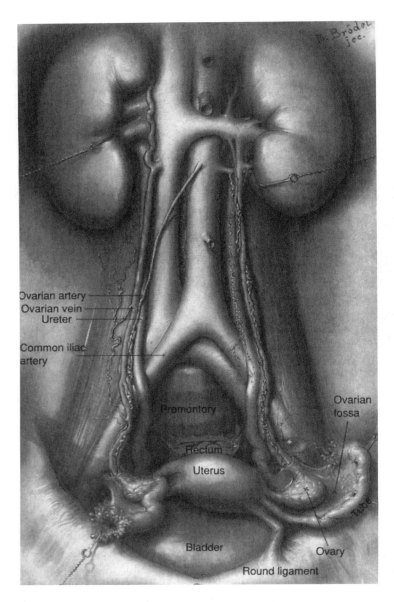

FIGURE 25-4. The relationship of the ureters to the female reproductive organs. (From Rock J, Thompson JD, eds. *TeLinde's operative gynecology,* 8th ed. Philadelphia: Lippincott-Raven Publishers, 1997:82, with permission.)

The *ovarian arteries* arise from the aorta just below the level of the renal arteries. These vessels run in the infundibulopelvic ligaments. Although the right ovarian vein follows the artery and drains into the inferior vena cava, the left ovarian vein drains into the left renal vein. The uterine arteries are branches of the anterior division of the internal iliac. These vessels course through the cardinal ligaments at the junction of the uterine corpus and cervix. These arteries flow into the marginal arteries that run lateral to the uterus and anastomose with the ovarian arteries in the mesosalpinx (Fig. 25-5).

The *primary lymphatic drainage* of the upper two thirds of the vagina and the uterus is to the obturator, internal, and external iliac lymph nodes. The lymphatic channels then proceed to the common iliac lymph nodes and the paraaortic lymph nodes. Accessory channels also include uterine drainage from the round ligaments to the superficial inguinal lymph nodes and from the posterior surface of the uterus along the uterosacral ligaments to the lateral sacral lymph nodes. The lymphatic channels of the ovaries follow the course of the ovarian vessels and drain into the paraaortic lymph nodes.

The presacral space contains the *autonomic nerves of the pelvis.* The uterus receives its innervation from the uterovaginal plexus (Frankenhäuser ganglion), which is one of three divisions from the superior hypogastric plexus. This plexus is found within the connective tissue of the cardinal ligament. The fallopian tubes and ovaries receive their innervation from the plexus of nerves that accompany the ovarian vessels. These specific nerves originate from the renal plexus.

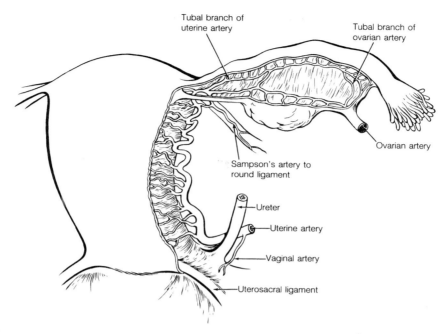

FIGURE 25-5. The vascular supply of the female pelvis. (From Rock J, Thompson JD, eds. *TeLinde's operative gynecology,* 8th ed. Philadelphia: Lippincott-Raven Publishers, 1997:73, with permission.)

ENDOCRINOLOGY OF THE HYPOTHALAMUS/PITUITARY/OVARIAN AXIS

Gonadotropin-releasing hormone (GnRH) is produced in the hypothalamus and transported to the pituitary gland. The amplitude and frequency of the pulsatile secretion of GnRH vary throughout the menstrual cycle. Follicle-stimulating hormone (FSH) and luteinizing hormone (LH) secreted from the anterior pituitary are responsible for estrogen and progesterone production from the ovary and the corpus luteum. Depending on the time of the cycle, FSH and LH may have negative and positive feedback relationships with the hypothalamus and the pituitary and therefore affect the levels of GnRH, FSH, and LH.

The *normal menstrual cycle* lasts from 21 to 35 days with 2 to 6 days of flow and an average blood loss of 20 to 60 mL. The cycle has two phases: follicular and luteal. During the follicular phase, hormonal feedback promotes the development of a single dominant follicle. This phase has an average length of 10 to 14 days. During the luteal phase, the endometrium is prepared for the possibility of pregnancy. This phase lasts 14 days and encompasses the events from ovulation to the first day of menstrual flow.

The hormonal, ovarian, and endometrial changes of the menstrual cycle are depicted in Fig. 25-6. The cycle begins with the demise of the corpus luteum and a rising FSH level. The increase in FSH recruits a cohort of ovarian follicles. These follicles secrete estrogen, which is the stimulus for endometrial proliferation. Increased estrogen levels in this phase have a negative feedback on pituitary FSH secretion and a positive feedback on pituitary LH secretion. After sufficient estrogen stimulation, there is an LH surge that causes ovulation 24 to 36 hours later. At the same time as the development of a dominant follicle, there is progressive mitotic growth of the superficial two thirds of the endometrium in response to increasing levels of estrogen. During this period, the endometrial glands become long and tortuous.

The estrogen level declines through the early luteal phase and rises again at the end of the luteal phase as a result of corpus luteum secretion. In addition to estrogen secretion, the corpus luteum also secretes significant amounts of progesterone. Both estrogen and progesterone levels remain elevated throughout the lifespan of the corpus luteum and their levels wane with its demise. This fall in gonadal steroids permits the increase in FSH level and the beginning of the next cycle.

As the corpus luteum develops, the endometrial secretory phase begins. The rise in progesterone causes the release of the glycogen vacuoles into glandular lumina. Seven days after ovulation, the spiral arteries lengthen and coil and there is an increase in stromal edema. Two days prior to menstruation, polymorphonuclear cells infiltrate the vascular system. Without implantation, there is destruction of the corpus luteum and a significant decrease in

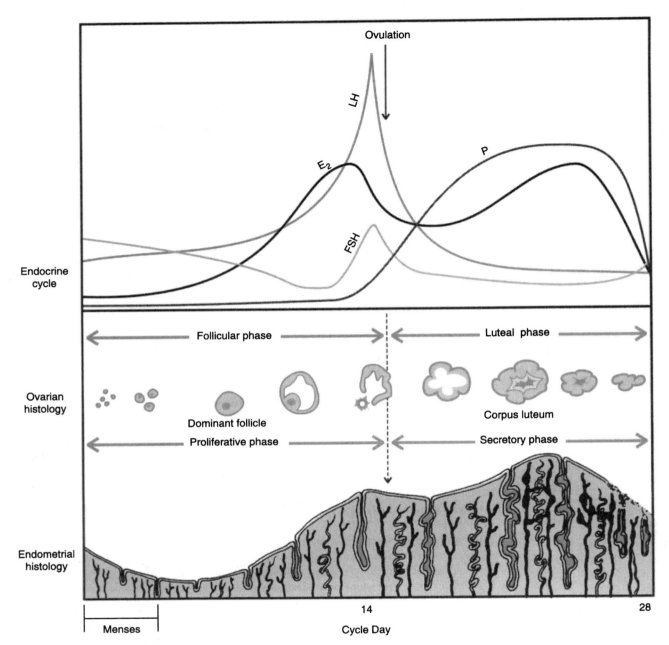

FIGURE 25-6. The menstrual cycle. (From Berek JS, Adashi EY, Hillard PA, eds. *Novak's gynecology,* 12th ed. Baltimore: Williams & Wilkins, 1996:160, with permission.)

estrogen and progesterone levels. These falling levels cause the breakdown of the superficial endometrium and the beginning of menstrual flow.

PATHOLOGY

Pelvic inflammatory disease (PID) results from the infection of the endocervix with bacteria that ascend to the endometrium and the fallopian tubes. The principal organisms are *Neisseria gonorrhea* and *Chlamydia trachomatis.* The cervicitis allows anaerobic and aerobic vaginal organisms to ascend to the upper genital tract, which causes polymicrobial infection and inflammation.

The signs and symptoms of PID are pelvic pain, purulent vaginal discharge, fever, nausea, and vomiting. Gonococcal PID has an abrupt onset of the pain, which worsens with movement. Chlamydial PID can have a more insidious course. The diagnosis of PID is usually based on the triad of abdominal tenderness with or without peritoneal signs,

TABLE 25-1. CURRENT RECOMMENDATIONS FOR TREATMENT OF PELVIC INFLAMMATORY DISEASE[a,b]

Outpatient
   A. cefoxitin 2 g i.m. plus probenecid 1 g PO *or* ceftriaxone 250 mg i.m. *and* doxycycline 100 mg PO b.i.d. for 14 days
   B. ofloxacin 400 mg PO b.i.d. for 14 days *and* clindamycin 450 mg PO q.i.d. *or* metronidazole 500 mg PO b.i.d. for 14 days

Inpatient
   A. cefoxitin 2 g i.v. q6° *or* cefotetan 2 g i.v. q12° *and* doxycycline 100 mg i.v. q12°
   B. clindamycin 900 mg i.v. q8° *and* gentamycin 2 mg/kg i.v. load then 1.5 mg/kg i.v. q8°

[a]From Berek JS, Adashi EY, Hillard PA, eds. Novak's gynecology, 12th ed. Baltimore: Williams & Wilkins, 1996, with permission.
[b]I.M., intramuscular; PO, per os; b.i.d., twice a day; q.i.d., four times a day.

cervical motion tenderness, and adnexal tenderness. Sheets of leukocytes on a wet-mount microscopic examination, fever, leukocytosis, increased erythrocyte sedimentation rate, and the presence of Gram-negative diplococci confirm the diagnosis.

Treatment of this disease requires broad-spectrum antibiotics. Both outpatient and inpatient treatment options exist (Table 25-1). Indications for inpatient therapy include nulliparity with the desire for future childbearing, pregnancy, presence of an intrauterine device, persistent nausea and vomiting precluding compliance with oral medication, or failure to respond to an outpatient regimen after 48 hours of treatment. Intravenous therapy is continued until there is complete resolution of abdominal pain and the patient has been afebrile for 48 hours.

PID may occur early in the first trimester of pregnancy. By 12 weeks of gestation, the fetal membranes have sealed over the internal cervical os, protecting the upper genital tract from infection. However, gonorrhea and chlamydia may cause cervicitis throughout pregnancy.

A *tuboovarian abscess* (TOA) is the end-stage process of acute PID. The agglutination of inflamed fallopian tubes, ovaries, and bowel with inflammatory exudates forms a palpable complex. Diagnosis requires finding a palpable mass in a woman with PID. A TOA is initially treated with a parenteral combination of ampicillin, gentamycin, and clindamycin. Seventy-five percent of patients treated with triple antibiotics will respond to therapy with resolution of fever and abdominal pain. Treatment failure requires surgical exploration for possible abscess drainage or hysterectomy and bilateral salpingo-oophorectomy.

Endometriosis is the ectopic growth of endometrial tissue outside the uterine cavity. The most prevalent site is the pelvis. Other sites include the bowel, bladder, omentum, umbilicus, and lungs. This condition is found in 7% of reproductive age women and may present as pelvic pain, infertility, dysmenorrhea, or dyspareunia. There does not appear to be a correlation between the degree of endometriosis and the severity of pelvic pain and dyspareunia. The typical lesions present as black, brown, or blue nodules surrounded by various degrees of fibrosis. Also, ovarian cysts, called "chocolate cysts," containing thick, viscous, brown fluid, may occur as a result of endometriosis.

Extrapelvic endometriosis is suspected when a palpable mass, associated with pain that occurs in a cyclic monthly pattern, is found outside the pelvis. The most common site for extrapelvic endometriosis is the intestinal tract, particularly the colon and rectum. These patients usually present with abdominal pain, back pain, abdominal distension, and cyclic rectal bleeding. Other less common sites of involvement include the ureters, bladder, umbilicus, and lungs.

Cancer antigen 125 (CA125) is a marker for the derivatives of coelomic epithelium. It is used primarily to assist in the diagnosis and to follow the treatment of ovarian cancer. However, the level of CA125 can be elevated in women with endometriosis, and the level is higher in women with moderate to severe disease.

There are two forms of treatment for endometriosis: medical and surgical. Medical treatment involves hormonal manipulation that suppresses estrogen synthesis and promotes atrophy of the endometrial implants. Drugs that have been used with variable success include continuous low-dose oral contraceptive pills, progesterone, and GnRH agonists. Surgical therapy includes both laparoscopy and laparotomy. Laparoscopy involves the ablation of the endometrial implants using bipolar coagulation, CO_2 laser, potassium-titany laser, or the argon laser. The goal is to remove all implants and adhesions in an attempt to restore the pelvis to its normal anatomy. Laparotomy is reserved for severe cases in which fertility is not a concern; a total abdominal hysterectomy and bilateral salpingo-oophorectomy with lysis of adhesions is performed.

Benign Pelvic Masses

Most adnexal tumors occur during a woman's reproductive years (19 to 40). Eighty percent to eighty-five percent of adnexal masses are benign. Masses that are unilateral, cystic, mobile, and smooth are usually benign while masses that are solid, fixed, irregular, and associated with ascites and cul-de-sac nodules may be malignant. These masses can cause abdominal distension, pain, pelvic pressure, urinary symptoms, or gastrointestinal tract symptoms. Acute abdominal pain and peritoneal signs in the presence of an adnexal mass can result from adnexal torsion, rupture of a cyst, or bleeding into a cyst.

The differential diagnosis of an adnexal mass depends on the patient's age. Until age 19, the most common benign pelvic mass is a benign cystic teratoma. The differential diagnosis of benign pelvic masses includes a Wilms tumor and neuroblastoma in young girls and imperforate hymen, agenesis of the vagina, and vaginal septum in adolescents.

Some controversy exists as to what is the most common adnexal mass in women aged 20 to 44. Most textbooks report that serous cystadenomas are found most commonly. However, benign cystic teratomas have also been reported to be the most common tumor in this age group. From age 45 to 74, the most common adnexal mass remains a serous cystadenoma. However, the incidence of malignant lesions, both primary and metastatic to the adnexa, become more frequent. In women aged 20 to 74, the differential diagnosis of adnexal masses also includes mucinous cystadenomas, adenofibromas, endometriomas, and Brenner tumors.

In addition to persistent adnexal masses, functional ovarian cysts must also be considered in the differential diagnosis in all menstruating women. Functional ovarian cysts include follicular cysts and corpora lutea. Follicular cysts are more common and usually less than 8 cm. They are often asymptomatic, found incidentally during a pelvic examination, and resolve within one or two menstrual cycles. Occasionally, they can rupture and cause acute abdominal pain and peritoneal signs. A corpus luteum is called a cyst when its size exceeds 3 cm. If a luteal cyst does not resolve in subsequent menstrual cycles, it can also rupture, causing hemoperitoneum and sometimes requiring surgical intervention. If either of these masses do not resolve spontaneously, they can be successfully treated with combination oral contraceptive pills.

Serous cystadenomas are benign multilocular cysts with papillary components. Surface epithelial cells secrete the straw-colored fluid contained within these cysts. Histologic examination demonstrates psammoma bodies, which are granular calcifications scattered throughout these masses. The calcifications sometimes allow detection of these masses on radiologic studies. Intraoperatively, a frozen section must be performed to distinguish between benign, borderline, and malignant tumors, which determines further surgical management.

Benign cystic teratomas (dermoids) result from neoplastic growth of totipotent cells, which cause a mass composed of any or all of the following: skin, bone, teeth, hair, and dermal tissue. In 10% of cases, dermoids are bilateral. Because of the high fat content within these tumors, they have a 15% incidence of torsion. Malignant transformation occurs in less than 2% of these masses. More than 75% of these transformations will occur in women older than 40. In all women for whom fertility is an important consideration, the surgical procedure of choice is an ovarian cystectomy with conservation of as much normal ovarian cortex as possible.

In addition to masses of ovarian origin, adnexal masses can also originate from tubal elements. Tuboovarian abscesses, ectopic pregnancies, and remnants of the wolffian ducts can all present as adnexal masses.

Uterine Malignancies

Endometrial carcinoma is the most common pelvic malignancy in the United States. There are 34,000 new cases and 6,000 deaths due to endometrial carcinoma annually. This malignancy is primarily a disease of postmenopausal women and becomes increasingly lethal with increasing age at presentation. In general, exposure to unopposed estrogen increases a woman's risk for endometrial carcinoma. More specifically, the most common risk factors for endometrial carcinoma include nulliparity, infertility with a history of irregular menses, menopause after age 52, obesity, prolonged estrogen exposure from polycystic ovaries or ovarian tumors, use of estrogen replacement without concurrent use of progesterone during menopause, tamoxifen use, and diabetes.

There are three oncogenes associated with endometrial carcinoma: K-ras, HER-2/neu, and p53. Mutations in codon 12 or 13 of the K-ras oncogene have been reported in 10% to 20% of endometrial adenocarcinomas. Overexpression of HER-2/neu oncogene is present in 10% to 15% of endometrial adenocarcinomas. Alterations of the p53 gene have been associated with the papillary serous cell type of endometrial carcinoma and presentation with advanced stage disease. Presence of any alterations in these oncogenes is a predictor of a poor prognosis.

The classification of endometrial carcinoma includes eight different variants: endometrioid, adenocarcinoma, mucinous carcinoma, papillary serous carcinoma, clear cell carcinoma, squamous carcinoma, undifferentiated carcinoma, and mixed type. The endometrioid variant accounts for 80% of all endometrial carcinoma, and these tumor glands resemble normal endometrial glands. Less-differentiated tumors contain more solid elements and less glandular elements.

Ninety percent of women with endometrial carcinoma present with vaginal bleeding or discharge; however, only 10% of women with these symptoms actually have endometrial carcinoma. Other diagnoses to consider in these patients include endometrial atrophy, endometrial polyps, irregular bleeding from estrogen-replacement therapy, and endometrial hyperplasia. The first diagnostic study to perform is an office endometrial biopsy, where a small piece of endometrial tissue is removed from the uterus. This biopsy has a diagnostic accuracy of 98%. A transvaginal ultrasound may be an adjunctive study. A sonographic endometrial thickness of greater than or equal to 5 mm or a polypoid endometrial mass are considered suspicious findings for endometrial carcinoma. The Papanicolaou (Pap smear) test is an unreliable outpatient test, which has a diagnostic accuracy of only 30% to 40%.

If an endometrial biopsy returns with a diagnosis of hyperplasia, the next diagnostic study is a hysteroscopic dilation and curettage to ensure the absence of carcinoma. If the endometrial biopsy results return with carcinoma, the patient begins evaluation for future surgical staging. The initial preoperative evaluation includes a chest roentgenogram and routine laboratory tests. Magnetic resonance imaging may provide preoperative information regarding

TABLE 25-2. STAGING AND GRADING OF ENDOMETRIAL CARCINOMA[a]

1988 FIGO surgical staging for endometrial carcinoma[b]
Stage	Grade	Description
Stage Ia	G123	tumor limited to endometrium
Ib	G123	invasion to less than one half of the myometrium
Ic	G123	invasion to more than one half of the myometrium
Stage IIa	G123	endocervical glandular involvement only
IIb	G123	cervical stromal invasion
Stage IIIa	G123	tumor invades serosa and/or adnexa and/or positive peritoneal cytology
IIIb	G123	vaginal metastases
IIIc	G123	metastases to pelvic and/or paraaortic lymph nodes
Stage IVa	G123	tumor invasion of bladder and/or bowel mucosa
IVb		distant metastases including intraabdominal and/or inguinal lymph nodes

1971 FIGO clinical staging for endometrial carcinoma
Stage	Description
Stage 0	carcinoma *in situ*
Stage I	the carcinoma is confined to the corpus
Stage Ia	the length of the uterine cavity is 8 cm or less
Stage Ib	the length of the uterine cavity is more than 8 cm

Stage 1 cases should be subgrouped with regard to the histologic grade of the adenocarcinoma as follows:

Grade 1	highly differentiated adenomatous carcinoma
Grade 2	moderately differentiated adenomatous carcinoma with partly solid areas
Grade 3	predominantly solid or entirely undifferentiated carcinoma
Stage II	the carcinoma has involved the corpus and the cervix but has not extended outside the uterus
Stage III	the carcinoma has extended outside the uterus but not outside the true pelvis
Stage IV	the carcinoma has extended outside the true pelvis or has obviously involved the mucosa of the bladder or rectum. A bullous edema as such does not permit a case to be allocated to stage IV
Stage IVa	spread of the growth to adjacent organs
Stage IVb	spread to distant organs

[a]From Berek JS, Adashi EY, Hilland PA, eds. *Novak's gynecology*, 12th ed. Baltimore: Williams & Wilkins, 1996:1069, with permission.
[b]FIGO, International Federation of Gynecology and Obstetrics.

the degree of myometrial invasion and may assist in the decision to proceed with lymph node sampling. In endometrial carcinoma, elevated CA125 levels may be used as a marker for extrauterine disease.

Endometrial carcinoma is surgically staged (Table 25-2). The procedure requires sampling of peritoneal fluid for cytology, excision of any extrauterine lesions, total abdominal hysterectomy, and bilateral salpingo-oophorectomy. The uterus is examined for tumor size and the extent of myometrial invasion, and a frozen section is performed to determine histologic type and grade. Clear cell carcinoma, papillary serous carcinoma, squamous carcinoma, any grade 3 lesion, myometrial invasion greater than one half of the myometrial thickness, isthmic/cervical extension, tumor size greater than 2 cm, or extrauterine disease are indications for selective pelvic and paraaortic lymph node sampling.

The primary treatment of endometrial carcinoma is surgical. Women with stage I disease and superficial invasion, or any grade 3 lesion, require postoperative radiation therapy. Almost all patients receive radiation to the upper vagina. This treatment decreases the risk of local recurrence from 15% to 1% or 2%. External beam radiation therapy is indicated for cervical involvement, pelvic lymph node metastases, or pelvic disease outside the uterus. Women with paraaortic lymph node metastases receive extended field radiation therapy to include the common iliac and paraaortic lymph nodes. Abdominal radiation therapy is reserved for women with stage III or IV disease. Chemotherapy is not indicated as a primary treatment but reserved for palliation of recurrent disease.

Disease recurrence is found in 25% of patients with endometrial carcinoma. Greater than 50% of the recurrences are discovered within the first 2 years after diagnosis. The most common sites of recurrence include local pelvic recurrence, lung, abdomen, lymph nodes, liver, brain, and bone. Patients with isolated regional recurrence are best treated with external beam radiation therapy followed by vaginal radiation brachytherapy. Progesterone therapy is currently recommended for all patients with recurrent endometrial carcinoma.

Sarcomas represent a small percentage of uterine malignancies. Women who have received pelvic irradiation are at increased risk for developing uterine sarcomas. There are three histologic variants: endometrial stromal sarcoma, leiomyosarcoma, and malignant mixed müllerian tumor. Endometrial stromal sarcoma produces an enlarged uterus with a soft yellow-gray necrotic and hemorrhagic mass. Leiomyosarcoma is differentiated from a leiomyoma by the number of mitotic figures per high-power field. Malignant mixed müllerian tumor is a mixture of carcinomatous and sarcomatous elements. Carcinomatous elements are glandular. Sarcomatous elements may resemble normal endometrial tissue (homologous) or may resemble tissue foreign to the uterus (heterologous). Uterine sarcoma is treated with total abdominal hysterectomy, bilateral salpingo-oophorectomy, and either lymph node dissection or radiation therapy. Adjuvant chemotherapy with doxorubicin or dimethyl triazenoimidazole carboxamide as the main component decreases the risk for distant metastases. Fifty percent of the recurrences are localized to the pelvis. The most common site of distant disease is the lung.

Cervical Malignancies

The squamocolumnar junction is the boundary of the columnar epithelium of the cervical canal with the squamous epithelium of the ectocervix. During the reproductive years, the columnar epithelium undergoes squamous metaplasia, and this region is known as the "transformation zone." Most neoplastic changes of the cervix occur in the transformation zone. The premalignant changes of the cervix are considered a continuum from mild to severe cytologic atypia. There are two descriptive pathologic systems used to describe these changes, the cervical intraepithelial neoplasia (CIN) system and the Bethesda system. The CIN system classifies the premalignant changes into mild (grade 1), moderate (grade 2), severe (grade 3), and carcinoma *in situ* (CIS). The Bethesda system classifies premalignant changes into low-grade squamous intraepithelial lesion (LGSIL) and high-grade squamous intraepithelial lesion (HGSIL). LGSIL includes koilocytotic change and mild dysplasia. HGSIL includes moderate and severe dysplasia and CIS.

The major risk factors for cervical neoplastic changes include early age at first sexual intercourse, multiple sex partners, early marriage, early childbearing, prostitution, sexually transmitted diseases, and immunocompromised states. In addition, human papillomavirus (HPV) plays a major role in premalignant conditions of the cervix. HPV types 16, 18, 31, 33, 35, 39, 45, 51, 52, 56, and 58 are more virulent and have been associated with cervical carcinoma.

The Pap smear is the primary screening test for cervical dysplasia. If a Pap smear demonstrates abnormal cytology, a colposcopy should be performed. The colposcope is a binocular microscope that can magnify the cervix 10 to 16 times. The cervix is cleaned with acetic acid and the colposcope is used to identify the abnormal lesions that require biopsy. If the colposcopy results are unsatisfactory, if there is a question of invasive disease, if the biopsy results return with CIN grade 2 or greater, or if there is a discrepancy between the colposcopic impression and the biopsy results, then excision therapy must be performed. The goal of excision therapy is complete eradication of all abnormal tissue with clear margins on the specimen. There are two main techniques used for excision therapy, a cold knife cone biopsy or a loop electrocautery excision procedure.

Cervical carcinoma is the third most frequently occurring gynecologic malignancy in the United States. There are 16,000 new cases and 5,000 deaths due to cervical carcinoma annually. Most women present with abnormal bleeding or brown vaginal discharge after intercourse or between menstrual cycles. The diagnosis of cervical carcinoma is made by biopsy of the tumor, and the extent of cervical involvement is determined by a cone biopsy of the cervix.

Eighty-five to ninety percent of cervical carcinomas are squamous cell carcinoma. This malignancy infiltrates locally and disease spreads from the cervix to the vagina and paracervical and parametrial tissues. Hematogenous metastases are a late complication of cervical carcinoma and most commonly involve lung, liver, and bone.

Cervical carcinoma is staged clinically (Table 25-3). The stage is primarily determined by physical examination and the status of the ureters. Initial evaluation of cervical carcinoma includes the history and physical examination, laboratory studies, an intravenous pyelogram, or computed tomography (CT), and a chest x-ray. An examination under anesthesia, cystoscopy, and sigmoidoscopy are then performed. These examinations provide information about the spread of disease to the parametrial tissues, bladder, and rectum. Once the evaluation has been completed, the patient is assigned a clinical stage and therapy is determined by this stage.

Women with stage IA_1 or IA_2 cervical carcinoma have microinvasive disease and are treated with a simple hysterectomy. Women with stage IB or IIA are treated with either radical hysterectomy and lymph node dissection or radiation therapy. If examination of the lymph nodes demonstrates metastatic disease, then postoperative external pelvic radiation is required. As a primary treatment, radiation therapy consists of both external beam radiation and brachytherapy. Women with stage IIB or greater are treated with radiation therapy as definitive treatment. Recently released results from the National Cancer Institute have demonstrated that adding cisplatin-based chemotherapy regimens to radiation therapy has decreased the death rate from cervical cancer by 30% to 50%.

One third of patients have recurrence of disease 6 months or more after primary treatment. Fifty percent of recurrences occur in the pelvis. Other common sites for recurrent disease include periaortic lymph nodes, lung, liver, or bone. Surgical failures are treated with radiation alone or chemotherapy in combination with radiation therapy. If the cervical carcinoma was treated initially with radiation therapy, surgical resection should be considered, because further radiation is usually contraindicated. Palliative chemotherapy regimens that include cisplatin and 5-fluorouracil may also be used as treatment for recurrent disease. Pelvic exenteration may be considered for patients with a central pelvic recurrence and a preoperative evaluation that fails to demonstrate disease.

Ovarian Malignancies

In the United States, ovarian carcinoma is the second most common gynecologic malignancy after endometrial carcinoma. However, ovarian carcinoma is the most frequent cause of death from any pelvic malignancy. There are 26,700 new cases and approximately 14,800 deaths caused by this disease annually. Ovarian carcinoma occurs more frequently in industrialized nations and is more common in whites than in African Americans or Asians. A mutation in the tumor suppressor gene, BRCA1, on the short arm of chromosome 17, has been associated with hereditary ovarian cancer. However, over 90% of ovarian carcinomas develop sporadically in women with a normal copy of this gene.

There are many risk factors that increase the chance of developing ovarian cancer. In general, prolongation of a woman's number of ovulatory cycles increases the risk of

TABLE 25-3. STAGING OF CARCINOMA CERVIX UTERI[a]

Preinvasive carcinoma

Stage 0	carcinoma *in situ*, intraepithelial carcinoma (cases of stage 0 should not be included in any therapeutic statistics)
Invasive carcinoma	
Stage I[b]	carcinoma strictly confined to the cervix (extension to the corpus should be disregarded)
Stage Ia	preclinical carcinomas of the cervix, i.e., those diagnosed only by microscopy
Stage Ia1	lesions with ≤3-mm invasion
Stage Ia2	lesions detected microscopically that can be measured. The upper limit of the measurement should show a depth of invasion of >3–5 mm taken from the base of the epithelium, either surface or glandular, from which it originates, and a second dimension, the horizontal spread, must not exceed 7 mm. Larger lesions should be staged as Ib
Stage Ib	lesions invasive >5 mm
Stage Ib1	lesions ≤4 cm
Stage Ib2	lesions larger than 4 cm
Stage II[c]	the carcinoma extends beyond the cervix but has not extended onto the wall the carcinoma involves the vagina, but not the lower one third
Stage IIa	no obvious parametrial involvement
Stage IIb	obvious parametrial involvement
Stage III[d]	the carcinoma has extended onto the pelvic wall. On rectal examination, there is no cancer-free space between the tumor and the pelvic wall. The tumor involves the lower one third of the vagina. All cases with hydronephrosis or nonfunctioning kidney
Stage IIIa	no extension to the pelvic wall
Stage IIIb	extension onto the pelvic wall and/or hydronephrosis or nonfunctioning kidney
Stage IV[e]	the carcinoma has extended beyond the true pelvis or has clinically involved the mucosa of the bladder or rectum. A bullous edema, as such, does not permit a case to be allotted to stage IV
Stage IVa	spread of the growth to adjacent organs
Stage IVb	spread to distant organs

[a]From Berek JS, Adashi EY, Hilland PA, eds. *Novak's gynecology*, 12th ed. Baltimore: Williams & Wilkins, 1996:1120, with permission.
[b]The diagnosis of both stage Ia1 and Ia2 should be based on microscopic examination of removed tissue, preferably a cone, which must include the entire lesion. The depth of invasion should not be more than 5 mm taken from the base of the epithelium, either surface or glandular, from which it originates. The second dimension, the horizontal spread, must not exceed 7 mm. Vascular space involvement, either venous or lymphatic, should not alter the staging but should be specifically recorded as it may affect treatment decisions in the future. Lesions of greater size should be staged as Ib. As a rule, it is impossible to estimate clinically whether a cancer of the cervix has extended to the corpus. Extension to the corpus should therefore be disregarded.
[c]A patient with a growth fixed to the pelvic wall by a short and indurated, but not nodular, parametrium should be allotted to stage IIb. At clinical examination, it is impossible to decide whether a smooth, indurated parametrium is truly cancerous or only inflammatory. Therefore, the case should be assigned to stage III only if the parametrium is nodular to the pelvic wall or the growth itself extends to the pelvic wall.
[d]The presence of hydronephrosis or nonfunctioning kidney due to stenosis of the ureter by cancer permits a case to be allotted to stage III even if, according to other findings, it should be allotted to stage I or II.
[e]The presence of the bullous edema, as such, should not permit a case to be allotted to stage IV. Ridges and furrows into the bladder wall should be interpreted as signs of submucous involvement of the bladder if they remain fixed to the growth at palpation (i.e., examination from the vagina or the rectum during cystoscopy). A cytologic finding of malignant cells in washings from the urinary bladder requires further examination and a biopsy specimen from the wall of the bladder.

developing ovarian carcinoma. For example, frequent ovulation, late menopause, nulliparity, late childbearing, and ovulation-inducing drugs increase a woman's risk of this malignancy. In contrast, breast-feeding, the use of oral contraceptive pills, tubal ligation, and hysterectomy with ovarian conservation decrease a woman's risk for this disease.

There are three major histologic types of ovarian carcinoma: epithelial, germ cell, and sex cord stromal. Epithelial tumors arise from ovarian surface epithelial cells and account for 65% of all ovarian malignancies. Germ-cell tumors originate from embryonic and extraembryonic tissues and are responsible for 20% to 25% of ovarian malignancies. They have the capacity to stimulate sex steroid hormone secretion or may themselves be hormonally inactive. Sex cord stromal tumors contain elements that recapitulate the ovary or the testes and account for 6% of ovarian malignancies. Gonadoblastomas are tumors composed of both sex cord elements and germ-cell elements. They are found in dysgenic gonads particularly when a Y chromosome is present in the patient's karyotype. Women with these genotypic abnormalities require removal of their gonads to prevent this rare tumor.

TABLE 25-4. STAGING OF PRIMARY CARCINOMA OF THE OVARY[a,b]

Stage I	growth limited to the ovaries
Stage Ia	growth limited to one ovary; no ascites containing malignant cells
	no tumor on the external surface; capsule intact
Stage Ib	growth limited to both ovaries; no ascites containing malignant cells
	no tumor on the external surfaces; capsules intact
Stage Ic[c]	tumor either stage Ia or Ib but with tumor on the surface of one or both ovaries; or with capsule ruptured; or with ascites present containing malignant cells; or with positive peritoneal washings
Stage II	growth involving one or both ovaries with pelvic extension
Stage IIa	extension and/or metastases to the uterus and/or tubes
Stage IIb	extension to other pelvic tissues
Stage IIc[c]	tumor either stage IIa or stage IIb but with tumor on the surface of one or both ovaries; or with capsule(s) ruptured; or with ascites present containing malignant cells or with positive peritoneal washings
Stage III	tumor involving one or both ovaries with peritoneal implants outside the pelvis and/or positive retroperitoneal or inguinal nodes; superficial liver metastasis equals stage III; tumor is limited to the true pelvis, but with histologically proven malignant extension to small bowel or omentum
Stage IIIa	tumor grossly limited to the true pelvis with negative nodes but with histologically confirmed microscopic seeding of abdominal peritoneal surfaces
Stage IIIb	tumor of one or both ovaries with histologically confirmed implants of abdominal peritoneal surfaces, none exceeding 2 cm in diameter; nodes negative
Stage IIIc	abdominal implants >2 cm in diameter and/or positive retroperitoneal or inguinal nodes
Stage IV	growth involving one or both ovaries with distant metastasis; if pleural effusion is present, there must be positive cytologic test results to allot a case to stage IV; parenchymal liver metastasis equals stage IV

[a]From Berek JS, Adashi EY, Hilland PA, eds. *Novak's gynecology*, 12th ed. Baltimore: Williams & Wilkins, 1996:1170, with permission.
[b]These categories are based on findings at clinical examination and/or surgical exploration. The histologic characteristics are to be considered in the staging, as are results of cytologic testing as far as effusions are concerned. It is desirable that a biopsy be performed on suspicious areas outside the pelvis.
[c]In order to evaluate the impact on prognosis of the different criteria for allotting cases to stage Ic or IIc it would be of value to know if rupture of the capsule was (i) spontaneous or (ii) caused by the surgeon and if the source of malignant cells detected was (i) peritoneal washings or (ii) ascites.

Epithelial ovarian carcinoma has five major subtypes: serous, mucinous, endometrioid, clear cell, and Brenner. Ovarian carcinoma spreads along peritoneal surfaces to both parietal and visceral surfaces of the abdomen. Because the ovaries are intrapelvic organs and ovarian tumors are usually asymptomatic, the disease has usually spread beyond the ovaries before any signs or symptoms of the malignancy are present. Patients may complain of a distended abdomen and physical examination may reveal ascites and a pelvic mass. The preoperative evaluation includes basic laboratory studies, a CA125 level, CT scan of the abdomen and pelvis, and a barium enema.

Staging of ovarian carcinoma requires a surgical procedure (Table 25-4). During this procedure, ascites or peritoneal washings are sent for cytologic examination, the undersurface of the diaphragm is sampled, all suspicious nodules are removed, and a total abdominal hysterectomy, bilateral salpingo-oophorectomy, and infracolic omentectomy are performed. If there is no gross disease outside of the pelvis, a pelvic and paraaortic lymph node dissection is completed. It is critical that staging is correctly performed at the time of the initial exploratory laparotomy to provide important prognostic information so that the appropriate postoperative treatment may be carried out.

Twenty percent of all ovarian epithelial carcinomas are borderline. These tumors consist of malignant cells that are not invasive. Women with this condition require an appropriate staging procedure. A unilateral salpingo-oophorectomy can be performed if the tumor is confined to one ovary, the contralateral ovary appears normal, and biopsy results of the omentum and peritoneal surfaces are negative. This is particularly important for young patients when preservation of fertility is desired. With resection alone, the 5-year survival rate approaches 90%. Adjuvant chemotherapy and radiation therapy are reserved for patients whose malignancy is invasive or has cytologic atypia.

The primary management for all stages of epithelial ovarian carcinoma is removal of all resectable disease and reduction of nonresectable lesions to less than 1 cm during the staging laparotomy. Patients with stage IC disease or higher or whose histology demonstrates poorly differentiated carcinoma benefit from adjuvant postoperative chemotherapy. This chemotherapeutic regimen consists of taxol and cisplatin administered every 3 weeks for six cycles. Patients are followed with serial physical examinations, CT examinations, and CA125 tests. Exponential regression of a patient's CA125 level suggests response to this regimen.

Germ-cell tumors comprise 20% to 25% of all ovarian tumors; however, only 2% to 3% are malignant. These tumors originate from the primitive germ cells and differentiate into embryonic (endoderm, mesoderm, and ectoderm) or extraembryonic (yolk sac or trophoblast) tissues. Dysgerminomas account for 45% of all malignant germ-cell tumors, and immature teratomas and endodermal sinus tumors are the next most frequently occurring malignant germ-cell tumors.

Dysgerminomas are composed of primitive germ cells infiltrated by lymphocytes. They represent approximately 1% of all ovarian malignancies. Dysgerminomas are found primarily in women less than 30 years old. In 10% of the patients, they are found on both ovaries. These tumors are very sensitive to both radiation therapy and multiagent chemotherapy with cisplatin and bleomycin plus etoposide or vinblastine. Chemotherapy generally is used as the first line of treatment.

Less than 1% of all ovarian malignancies are immature teratomas. They are composed of immature embryonic structures admixed with mature elements. Immature neuroepithelium is one of the primary immature elements found in this tumor. Metastatic disease or any tumor with grade 2 or grade 3 elements requires adjuvant chemotherapy with vincristine, actinomycin D, and cyclophosphamide.

Endodermal sinus tumors (yolk sac tumors) account for approximately 10% of malignant germ-cell tumors. This tumor resembles the extraembryonic tissue of the yolk sac and secretes α-fetoprotein (AFP), which is used as a marker to follow disease progression and response to treatment. Before the development of multiagent chemotherapy, endodermal sinus tumors were universally fatal. At present, they may be successfully treated with vincristine, actinomycin D, 5-fluorouracil, and cyclophosphamide.

Choriocarcinoma is a highly malignant rare form of germ-cell tumor. This tumor resembles the extraembryonic tissue of the cytotrophoblast and the syncytiotrophoblast. Human chorionic gonadotropin (hCG) is the tumor marker used to follow disease progression and response to treatment. In the past, choriocarcinoma was also a universally fatal disease, however, multiagent chemotherapy now provides improved response rates for this disease.

The histology of *sex cord stromal tumors* resembles the sex cord and specialized stroma of the developing gonad. In the ovary, the granulosa cells represent the sex cord tissue and the theca cells represent the specialized stroma. Granulosa theca cell tumors are a low-grade malignancy, and these tumors often secrete estrogen. This additional supply of estrogen can be responsible for a range of symptoms from precocious puberty to postmenopausal bleeding. These tumors are identified histologically by the presence of Call-Exner bodies, which are eosinophilic bodies surrounded by granulosa cells. Sertoli-Leydig tumors are also low-grade malignancies that replicate testicular elements. In 75% to 80% of patients, these tumors produce androgens. As a result, women present with amenorrhea, breast atrophy, acne, hirsutism, clitoromegaly, deepening of the voice, and male pattern baldness. Treatment for both of these tumors requires surgical excision followed by multiagent chemotherapy. The regimen for granulosa/theca cell tumors includes cisplatin and doxorubicin or actinomycin D, 5-fluorouracil, and cyclophosphamide while the regimen for Sertoli-Leydig cell tumors includes vincristine, doxorubicin, and cyclophosphamide. Once a patient has completed childbearing, the contralateral ovary should be removed.

Malignancies Metastatic to the Ovary

Most tumors metastatic to the ovary originate from malignancies of other pelvic organs such as the uterus or the fallopian tube. The most common distant sites of origin include the breasts and the gastrointestinal tract. A Krukenberg tumor is a specialized type of gastrointestinal tumor metastatic to the ovary. This tumor contains signet ring cells filled with mucin in an acellular stroma. The stomach and the large intestine are the most common sites of origin.

Vaginal Carcinoma

Vaginal carcinomas are rare and make up less than 2% of all gynecologic malignancies. Eighty percent of these carcinomas are squamous cell and the remaining are adenocarcinomas, melanomas, and sarcomas. For women with a history of cervical or vulvar carcinoma, a vaginal lesion appearing at least 5 years after the initial malignancy is considered a primary vaginal cancer and not a recurrence of their original disease. Most women present with abnormal vaginal bleeding or abnormal vaginal discharge. This malignancy spreads by direct extension to the pelvic soft tissues. Hematogenous dissemination to the lungs, liver, and bone occurs late in the disease. The diagnosis is confirmed by a directed biopsy of the vaginal lesion. The mainstay of treatment is radiation therapy to the vagina with surgical therapy, an option only for young women whose disease is limited to the upper vagina.

Vulvar Carcinoma

Squamous cell carcinoma accounts for 90% of vulvar malignancies. Five percent of vulvar malignancies are melanomas. Another 5% are adenocarcinomas, verrucous carcinomas, basal cell carcinomas, and sarcomas. Most women complain of perineal bleeding and a lesion that fails to heal. On physical examination, a polypoid mass may be found on the vulva. This tumor spreads via the lymphatic system to the superficial inguinal femoral lymph nodes to the deep pelvic, obturator, and iliac lymph nodes. The diagnosis is confirmed by a directed biopsy of the lesion. Treatment consists of a radical vulvectomy and bilateral inguinal lymph node dissection. If the superficial lymph nodes are found to contain metastatic disease, then a course of radiation therapy is given to the deep pelvic and iliac lymph nodes.

Carcinoma of the Fallopian Tube

Primary fallopian tube malignancy is the rarest gynecologic cancer and represents only 0.3% to 1.1% of all gynecologic cancers. These lesions usually are adenocarcinomas when they originate from the tube; however, 80% to 90% of fallopian tube malignancies are metastatic from other sites, which include the ovary, uterus, and gastrointestinal tract. The classic signs and symptoms in women with this malignancy include abnormal vaginal bleeding and discharge, lower abdominal pain, and an adnexal mass. The diagnosis is made during surgical exploration. The operative strategy and staging for this disease are identical to those for epithelial ovarian carcinoma. Adjuvant chemotherapy with platinum-containing regimens or radiation therapy are appropriate for advanced stage disease.

Gestational Trophoblastic Disease

Gestational trophoblastic disease (GTD) is composed of a rare spectrum of tumors that includes complete hydatidiform mole, partial hydatidiform mole, placental site trophoblastic tumor, and choriocarcinoma. In the United States, the incidence of GTD is 0.6 to 1.1 per 1,000 pregnancies. Risk factors for GTD include maternal age greater than 35, a low dietary intake of carotene, and vitamin A deficiency.

Complete hydatidiform moles contain chorionic villi with hydatidiform swelling and trophoblastic hyperplasia, and lack fetal tissue. The karyotype is 46XX; however, all of the chromosomes are of paternal origin. Partial hydatidiform moles have chorionic villi with focal hydatidiform swelling and trophoblastic hyperplasia. Identifiable fetal parts may be present with this form of GTD. Partial moles have a triploid karyotype and the extra set of chromosomes is of paternal origin.

Complete and partial molar pregnancies usually present with abnormal bleeding. Molar pregnancies may also present with excess uterine size, hyperemesis gravidarum, hyperthyroidism, and prominent theca lutein ovarian cysts. An abnormally elevated β-hCG level and a transvaginal ultrasound usually confirm the diagnosis. A complete mole has a characteristic vesicular sonographic pattern while a partial mole has cystic spaces in the placental tissue and an increase in the transverse diameter of the gestational sac. To preserve fertility, the uterus is evacuated with suction curettage. Women are followed after uterine evacuation with serial β-hCG levels. If the β-hCG level does not fall to zero or begins to increase, the patient is presumed to have persistent disease and may be at risk for distant metastases. In complete moles, local invasion occurs in 15% of the patients and metastases occur in 4% of the patients. In contrast, partial molar gestations will have a persistent nonmetastatic tumor in 4% of the patients. Single-agent chemotherapy with actinomycin D or methotrexate has achieved excellent remission rates in both nonmetastatic and low-risk GTD. Metastatic and high-risk GTD is treated with etoposide, methotrexate, actinomycin D, cyclophosphamide, and vincristine.

SURGICAL ISSUES IN PREGNANCY

In the United States, there are 16 *ectopic pregnancies* per 1,000 pregnancies annually. Ectopic pregnancy is responsible for 15% of all maternal deaths in this country, with adolescents having the highest mortality rate. After a woman has one ectopic pregnancy, there is a 50% to 80% chance of subsequent intrauterine pregnancy and a 10% to 25% risk of another ectopic pregnancy at the next conception.

The major risk factors for ectopic pregnancy are tubal damage from tubal inflammation, infection, or prior abdominal surgery. Therefore, previous PID, prior ectopic pregnancy, previous tubal surgery (tubal ligation or tubal reanastomosis), and current intrauterine device use are risk factors for ectopic pregnancy. Some chlamydial infections of the cervix are very indolent and can cause a silent ascending salpingitis without the clinical features of PID. This type of chlamydial infection leads to tubal inflammation and damage, which predisposes the patient to future tubal pregnancy.

The presentation of this disease is variable, ranging from no symptoms to hemorrhagic shock. However, common symptoms include amenorrhea, abdominal cramping, and abnormal vaginal bleeding. Serial β-hCG measurements and transvaginal ultrasound are helpful in establishing the diagnosis. In a normal intrauterine pregnancy, the β-hCG level increases by at least 66% every 48 hours. Up to 85% of patients with an ectopic pregnancy will develop a plateau in their β-hCG levels. When the β-hCG level is approximately 1,500 to 2,000 IU/mL, the earliest evidence of an intrauterine pregnancy can be visualized by a transvaginal ultrasound. If the diagnosis remains uncertain following these tests in a hemodynamically stable patient, serial β-hCG levels may be followed and ultrasound examinations repeated until the condition of pregnancy is clear. However, emergent laparotomy is indicated for evidence of hemodynamic instability. The differential diagnosis includes early normal intrauterine pregnancy, abnormal intrauterine pregnancy, and completed abortion. The natural progression for an ectopic pregnancy may lead to expulsion from the fimbriated end of the fallopian tube (tubal abortion), involution of the conceptus within the tube, or tubal rupture.

Treatment for an ectopic pregnancy can be either medical or surgical therapy. Medical management with methotrexate requires fulfillment of strict clinical criteria. Surgical intervention includes linear salpingostomy or salpingectomy via laparoscopy or laparotomy.

Appendicitis is one of the most common general surgical conditions occurring in pregnancy, with an incidence of 1 in 2,000 pregnancies. The diagnosis may be more difficult to confirm because of the physical changes and symptoms due to pregnancy. Typical symptoms of pregnancy that may confuse the diagnosis include nausea, vomiting, and abdominal discomfort of early pregnancy. In addition, upward displacement of the appendix may affect the typical clinical picture of appendicitis.

A pregnant woman with appendicitis may initially present with periumbilical pain. In the first trimester, the pain may localize to the right lower quadrant. However, after 16 weeks, the appendix is pushed upward and laterally by the expanding uterus. At 24 weeks, the appendix is found above the iliac crest, and at 32 weeks, the appendix is found at the right costal margin. One to two hours after developing pain, the patient may develop anorexia, nausea, and vomiting. Fever usually accompanies these symptoms. Tenderness of the right lateral rectus muscle is commonly found and movement of the uterus usually intensifies the pain. Positioning the patient on her left side will displace the uterus and may help differentiate pain of uterine origin from that of an appendiceal source. Elevations in white blood cell count should be interpreted with caution because of the physiologic leukocytosis of pregnancy. The differential diagnosis includes pyelonephritis, round ligament pain, placental abruption, ovarian torsion, degenerating fibroids, pancreatitis, and cholecystitis.

Treatment of this condition is appendectomy via laparotomy. If the appendix ruptures and peritonitis ensues, there is an increased risk for preterm labor or spontaneous abortion depending on the gestational age at presentation. With increased clinical suspicion, early diagnosis and surgical intervention is crucial to prevent the high perinatal mortality associated with appendicitis in pregnancy.

Cholecystitis complicates approximately 1 in 4,000 pregnancies. Risk factors for this disease include increasing age, increasing gravidity, and a history of previous attacks. Because of the high level of progesterone during pregnancy, the gallbladder's ability to contract is inhibited, and thus, new gallstones are formed during gestation, leading to this condition.

Patients present with biliary colic, nausea, and vomiting. Presence of a stone in the common bile duct may lead to persistent pain that radiates to the subscapular area. Usually a pregnant woman has right subcostal tenderness, increased temperature, and an increasing leukocytosis. An ultrasound confirms the presence of stones and evidence of gallbladder inflammation. In most cases, treatment with broad-spectrum antibiotics, nasogastric suction, intravenous hydration, and analgesics will suffice. Common bile duct obstruction or the development of pancreatitis requires a cholecystectomy or cholecystotomy.

Trauma in Pregnancy

During pregnancy, the most common types of injuries are blunt trauma secondary to automobile accidents and falls or penetrating injuries. As the uterus becomes an abdominal organ later in gestation, there is an increased likelihood of injury during trauma. The fetus is usually well protected by the amniotic fluid. The biggest risk to the pregnancy results from placental separation (placental abruption), which may result in preterm labor and delivery or an intrauterine fetal demise.

After a traumatic injury, maternal evaluation includes examination of the airway management and cardiopulmonary support. Once these organ systems have been assessed, a fetal ultrasound is performed to determine gestational age, weight, and presentation of the fetus. In addition, serial vital signs, necessary radiographic procedures, and the required blood tests are performed, including a complete blood count (CBC), type and screen, coagulation tests, and a Betke-Kleihauer test. The CBC and coagulation studies are used as indicators for disseminated intravascular coagulation, which can result from placental abruption while the Betke-Kleihauer test is an indicator for fetal/maternal hemorrhage. Once the maternal condition has been secured, the obstetric evaluation includes fetal assessment and uterine monitoring. Before fetal viability at 24 weeks of gestation, fetal heart tones are checked and continuous uterine monitoring is performed for at least 4 hours. After 24 weeks of gestation, continuous fetal heart rate monitoring and uterine contraction monitoring are employed for at least 4 hours. With continuous monitoring, determinations about the development of preterm labor and fetal well being are made. Both preterm labor and nonreassuring fetal heart rate tracing can be indicators of placental abruption. Placental abruption may present with severe abdominal pain, vaginal bleeding, regular uterine contractions, and possible nonreassuring fetal monitoring. Evidence of a significant placental abruption may indicate the need for emergent delivery.

Fetal and maternal outcome are closely linked after a traumatic injury. If there is a maternal cardiorespiratory arrest that is not corrected after 4 minutes of cardiopulmonary resuscitation, an emergent cesarean section should be considered. If an exploratory laparotomy is required and the gestational age is appropriate, a cesarean section during the operative procedure should be considered.

SUGGESTED READING

Berek JS, Adashi EY, Hillard PA, eds. *Novak's gynecology,* 12th ed. Baltimore: Williams & Wilkins, 1996.

Gabbe SG, Niebyl JR, Simpson JL, eds. *Obstetrics normal & problem pregnancies,* 3rd ed. New York: Churchill Livingstone, 1996.

Mishell DR Jr, Stenchever MA, Droegemueller W, et al., eds. *Comprehensive gynecology,* 3rd ed. St. Louis: Mosby, 1997.

Rock J, Thompson JD, eds. *TeLinde's operative gynecology,* 8th ed. Philadelphia: Lippincott-Raven Publishers, 1997.

Speroff L, Glass RH, Kase N, eds. *Clinical gynecologic endocrinology and infertility,* 5th ed. Baltimore: Williams & Wilkins, 1994.

26

OTORHINOLARYNGOLOGY

STEVEN J. WALL AND ARA A. CHALIAN

ANATOMY AND PHYSIOLOGY OF THE AUDITORY SYSTEM

The anatomy of the ear serves to transduce disturbances in atmospheric pressure into electrical impulses that are carried to the central nervous system (CNS). The human auditory system is most sensitive to impulses in the 250- to 10,000-Hz spectrum, with typical speech exhibiting frequencies in the 500- to 4,000-Hz range. Sound intensities are measured on a logarithmic scale from 0 to 120 dB. An individual with normal hearing has a threshold for perception of sounds at 0- to 20-dB intensity. Normal conversational speech is in the 20- to 50-dB range. Painful levels of noise occur in excess of 80 dB while exposure to elevated sound intensity for protracted periods may result in permanent hearing loss. The system responsible for perception of auditory stimuli consists of a *conductive portion* (external ear, external auditory canal, tympanic membrane, and ossicles) and a *sensorineural portion* (cochlea and cochlear nerve). Acoustic stimuli produce vibrations of the tympanic membrane, which are transferred via the *middle-ear bones* (malleus, incus, and stapes) to the footplate of the stapes (Fig. 26-1). Amplification of signal is accomplished due to the ratio of vibrating tympanic membrane area to stapes footplate area (17:1). The acoustic impedance matching is also enhanced by the ratio of the lengths of the long processes of the malleus and incus (1.3:1). These two factors yield an approximate 25-fold amplification of signal intensity delivered at the footplate, which rests in the oval window of the cochlea.

Conductive hearing losses occur secondary to cerumen, tympanic membrane perforation, middle-ear effusion, and ossicular discontinuity. In addition, ossicular fixation (*otosclerosis*) is a common familial disorder affecting young individuals (less than 35 years of age) and women more commonly than men (2:1 ratio). Valuable information regarding hearing loss is gained from an audiogram. For example, individuals with otosclerosis have a flat tympanogram with a characteristic notch at 2,000 Hz. In this case, management would include an attempt to divide adhesions of the middle-ear bones or to replace them with ossicular prosthetic devices. Additional information about the conductive loss can be gained by presentation of an air pressure stimulus in a sealed external auditory canal. The magnitude of reverberated impulse provides information about the integrity and mobility of the tympanic membrane. Defects in the conduction system are often amenable to improvement (e.g., cerumen disimpaction, repair of tympanic membrane perforation, and drainage of fluid).

In contrast, sensorineural hearing loss is more difficult to diagnose and correct. Exposure to loud noise at a particular frequency can be identified by a notch in the audiogram corresponding to the frequency of the insult. Evidence of an asymmetric sensorineural loss on audiogram merits workup, including radiologic studies of the temporal bone and internal auditory canal. These examinations are required to rule out the presence of a mass causing compression of the nerve, which would need to be addressed surgically (e.g., acoustic neuroma, meningioma, etc). An additional form of sensitivity testing involves delivery of stimuli to the ear while recording regional brain activity via surface electrodes (auditory brainstem response). This form of testing is valuable for auditory screening in the neonate with suspected hearing loss, in whom interactive means of testing are not possible.

In 85% of sensorineural loss patients, an etiology is not identified, although causes include iatrogenic injury due to exposure to pharmocologic agents. For example, aminoglycoside antibiotics (amikacin and neomycin) are toxic to outer hair cells at the base of the cochlea and are associated with high-frequency hearing loss (5% to 10%). Other well-described ototoxic agents include salicylates and cisplatin. The loop diuretics (ethacrynic acid, bumetanide, and furosemide) cause ototoxicity through actions on the stria vascularis of the cochlea. Interestingly, other aminoglycosides are more frequently the cause of vestibular toxicity (gentamycin, tobramycin, and streptomycin). Potential for toxicity is increased in the setting of impaired renal function or dehydration. In the at-risk patient, a premedication audiogram documenting baseline hearing is advisable.

Hospital of the University of Pennsylvania, Philadelphia, Pennsylvania

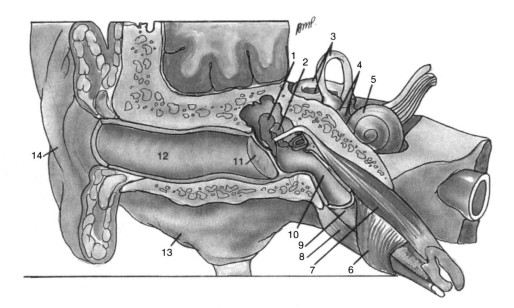

FIGURE 26-1. Structures of the ear: (1) malleus, (2) incus, (3) semicircular canals, (4) utricle and saccule, (5) cochlea, (6) dilator tubae muscle, (7) tensor tympani muscle, (8) levator veli palatini muscle, (9) cartilaginous auditory tube, (10) eustachian tube, (11) tympanic membrane, (12) external auditory canal, (13) mastoid, and (14) pinna. (From Bailey BJ, ed. *Head and neck surgery: otolaryngology.* Philadelphia: JB Lippincott Co, 1993, with permission.)

Treatable etiologies of hearing loss need to be excluded. For example, if an indolent bacterial infection is implicated (such as syphilis, Lyme disease, and tuberculosis), appropriate antibiotic therapy is initiated, which may result in partial recovery of hearing. In other cases, the patient will have a positive history of autoimmune processes (lupus, Cogan syndrome, Behçet disease), which warrants a trial of immunosuppressive medication (such as steroids and methotrexate). In many patients who experience an acute onset of sensorineural hearing loss, a history of viral prodrome can be elicited. One third of patients will achieve total recovery in a matter of weeks, one third will have partial recovery, and the remaining third will have permanent hearing deficit.

In instances of stable, idiopathic, sensorineural hearing loss (such as presbyacusis in the elderly), hearing amplification devices can be worn in one or both ears. In specialized cases (such as congenital deafness or trauma in the adult), serious sensorineural hearing loss can be improved by use of cochlear nerve implants. These devices employ a wire that is threaded into the cochlea. Specific channels activated along the length of the wire transmit electrical impulses to hair cells corresponding to the desired frequencies for amplification. Activation of selected channels can be tailored to accommodate the deficits identified in a particular individual. Success in cochlear nerve implants is influenced by the candidates. Optimal candidates are the postlingual deaf adult and the prelingual deaf child.

BALANCE AND THE VESTIBULAR SYSTEM

The perception of position, spatial orientation, acceleration, and rotation is accomplished through synthesis of sensory input from peripheral muscles and ocular cues, as well as from the vestibular structures of the inner ear. The *otolithic organs* refer to the *saccule* and *utricle,* which are filled with *endolymph* produced by the *stria vascularis.* The sensory component of each organ (*macula*) is made up of hair cells attached to a membrane composed of crystals of *calcium carbonate* (*otoconia*). Changes in gravity and linear acceleration result in displacement of the membrane, producing discharge in hair cells and a neural impulse. This information is processed with impulses generated in the *ampulla,* or in the sensory component of the *right* and *left semicircular canals.* These three structures are oriented at 90 degrees to each other in x, y, and z planes. The semicircular canals respond to angular acceleration. Movement of endolymph within a semicircular canal produces traction on a gelatinous membrane (*cupula*), resulting in discharge in vestibular hair cells. Because the right and left canals exist in a mirror orientation, changes in inertia will produce deflection of endolymph toward the ampulla on one side and away from the ampulla on the contralateral side. Proportional discharge of right and left vestibular systems allows assignment of motion direction. Asymmetric firing of right and left vestibular systems produces the subjective sensation of rotation, or vertigo. This firing pattern can be the result of viral infection (*vestibular neuritis*), vascular compromise, or displacement of otoconia in the posterior semicircular canal. The latter event results in episodic vertigo over a period of weeks elicited when the head assumes specific positions (e.g., lying down with head to the right). This syndrome is called "benign paroxysmal positional vertigo," or cupulolithiasis, which can be reversed by a series of head motions (Dix-Hallpike maneuvers) that direct the crystals back to the utricle. An additional entity associated with vertigo is Menière disease, which represents a "diagnosis of exclusion." The syndrome consists of sudden attacks of vertigo, tinnitus, aural fullness, and hearing loss lasting

30 to 120 minutes. Seventy percent of cases are unilateral while 30% develop contralateral symptoms within several years. Progressive sensorineural hearing loss occurs. Many medical and surgical treatments have been described to address the most distressing symptoms associated with intractable vertigo. These techniques have not had significantly better results than placebo treatments, with the exception of vestibular nerve division, which is reserved for debilitating vertigo.

Alternatively, a central lesion involving vestibular nuclei can result in vertiginous symptoms. Objectively, the patient presents with nystagmus (repetitive jerky movements of the eyes that have a fast and slow component). The direction of the slower component of nystagmus indicates the hypofunctioning side, although the direction of the fast component is used to describe the phenomenon, e.g., "right-beating" nystagmus. Brief episodes of nystagmus can be induced in the office by placement of warm and cold water into the external canal. This maneuver alters the flow rate of endolymph within the vestibular organs, thus producing asymmetric neural discharge. With the introduction of cold water, a nystagmus is produced in the direction of the contralateral ear, whereas the introduction of warm water produces discharge in the direction of the ipsilateral ear (cold, opposite; warm, same).

Otologic Infection

Infections of the external, middle, and inner ear are common. With respect to the external ear, the type of infection typically depends on the patient population. Otitis externa is an inflammatory condition that typically develops following water exposure (swimmer's ear). The acidic cerumen, which serves a bacteriostatic role, is removed. The patient presents with symptoms of otalgia and foul-smelling drainage (*otorrhea*). The causative organisms are usually *Pseudomonas aeruginosa* and *Staphylococcus aureus*. Management includes oral antibiotics. In addition, a cotton wick is inserted into the edematous canal impregnated with antibiotic drops for direct topical control.

Additional infections are seen in the immunocompromised population. In the poorly controlled diabetic patient, *malignant otitis externa* is a potentially life-threatening development. The pseudomonal infection spreads medially to involve the mastoid facial nerve (cranial nerve [CN] VII) and the base of the skull. Management includes diabetic control, antibiotics, and extensive debridement of necrotic tissue. *Otomycosis* refers to a fungal infection of the external auditory canal that develops in the setting of high temperature, poor hygiene, and immunosuppression. Mycelia are visible on otoscopy. Debridement is followed by topical application of antifungal agents, including 4% boric acid or nystatin powder.

Infections of the middle ear result from fluid buildup due to eustachian tube dysfunction. In the pediatric population, the eustachian tube has a horizontal orientation that becomes vertically oriented with growth. Regurgitation of food or chronic intermittent infection due to day care facility exposure increases bacterial content adjacent to the eustachian tube orifice. Retrograde bacterial growth extends to middle-ear fluid and results in infection. The causative organisms of acute otitis media include *Streptococcus pneumoniae, Haemophilus influenzae,* and *Moraxella catarrhalis.* Chronic otitis media is associated with Gram-negative organisms including *Pseudomonas aeruginosa, Proteus* spp., and *Escherichia coli.* In children with chronic middle-ear fluid or frequent episodes of otitis media, a myringotomy with tube placement should be considered. Indications include relief of frequent infections and correction of the conductive hearing loss due to middle-ear fluid. This hearing deficit between ages 2 and 4 can negatively impact speech development.

Chronic ear infections can lead to the development of a *cholesteatoma,* an epithelial cyst containing desquamated keratin. Growth leads to erosion of middle-ear bones and severe conductive hearing loss. Chronic infection also can lead to infections of the mastoid cavity (mastoiditis) and meningitis. Surgical resection of the cholesteatoma with reconstruction of middle-ear bones and tympanic membrane is required to restore functional hearing. Additional infections of the ear include viral infections harbored in CN ganglia. The most serious is caused by herpes zoster oticus, which is associated with Ramsay Hunt syndrome. Herpetic lesions are present in the external canal and in a seventh CN distribution. Facial nerve edema with associated paresis is often noted. The infections typically respond well to antiviral agents and oral steroids.

Otologic Neoplasms

Neoplastic processes affecting the inner ear are rare. Benign tumors (neuromas) arising in the internal auditory canal can compress any of four nerves that travel via this canal to the CNS: the facial nerve, the cochlear nerve division of CN VIII, or the inferior and superior vestibular nerve divisions of CN VIII. Other tumors of the cerebellopontine angle include gliomas, meningiomas, epidermoid cysts, and arachnoid cysts. Again, compression of CN VII or CN VIII divisions can produce various symptoms, necessitating diagnostic evaluation. Surgery includes extirpation of tumors with an attempt at preserving nerve function. Paragangliomas represent a tumor of chromaffin-producing cells located within the head and neck at the carotid bifurcation, jugular bulb, and middle ear. Growth of these neoplasms can result in hearing loss and cranial neuropathies. Rare malignant transformation of paragangliomas has been reported, as has catecholamine-secreting ability. Thus, resection or radiotherapy of tumors has been recommended. Preoperative assessment for hypertension and urine catecholamines is indicated.

Neoplasms of the external ear and external auditory canal are rare. The overwhelming majority are squamous cell and basal cell carcinomas developing secondary to sun exposure. Management includes wide-margin resection of involved portions of the pinna. If the canal is involved, removal of portions of the mastoid bone (mastoidectomy) and draining lymph node chains is typically required. Sacrifice of CN VII and/or CN VIII is common. Of note, tumors of the external canal can spread anteriorly via bony fissures to the parotid gland and its lymph nodes. Postoperatively, the patients require radiation therapy.

SALIVARY GLAND PHYSIOLOGY AND PATHOLOGY

There are three major paired groups of salivary glands: parotid, submandibular, and sublingual. The largest of these (20 g) is the *parotid gland* located over the masseter muscle of the cheek. The parotid gland is enclosed by deep cervical fascia and extends from its superior most point at the zygoma to an inferior point that curves around the angle of the mandible (Fig. 26-2). Saliva is directed through the Stensen duct into the oral cavity via an orifice located opposite the second upper molar. The parotid gland is divided into superficial and deep lobes by the facial nerve, which exits the stylomastoid foramen as a single trunk before dividing into five principal divisions at a point called the "per anserinus." All surgery performed on the parotid gland places the facial nerve at risk. The *temporal* and *mandibular divisions* are injured most frequently in surgery.

The *submandibular gland* (10 g) courses around the mylohyoid muscle and is enclosed by the deep cervical fascia. The mandibular division of the facial nerve lies superficial to the submandibular gland and must be identified during any procedure affecting the gland. Saliva produced in this gland is directed via the Wharton duct to an orifice on the ipsilateral side of the floor of the mouth adjacent to the frenulum (the midline attachment between the ventral tongue and the floor of the mouth). The remainder of saliva is produced by approximately 500 minor salivary glands distributed in the cheek, lips, and hard and soft palates.

Each salivary gland consists of multiple secretory units. Proximal acinar cells produce enzymatic secretions that are transported distally through the intercalated duct, striated duct, and excretory ductal components propelled by the contractions of myoepithelial cells. Each gland is also associated with lymphoid structures arranged diffusely or within nodes. The quantity of saliva produced daily is influenced by various cues but normally ranges between 500 to 1,500 mL.

Dysfunction within the salivary glands can be divided into nonneoplastic and neoplastic groups. The former includes multiple infectious processes. Acute suppurative infections cause erythema, tenderness, and swelling. Purulent discharge can frequently be expressed intraorally with gentle pressure on the gland. Bacterial organisms responsible for acute infections include *S. aureus* and *S. pneumoniae*. These disorders are more commonly observed in the debilitated, dehydrated, elderly nursing home population; however, they are also identified in younger immunocompromised patients with human immunodeficiency virus (HIV) seroreactivity. Management includes appropriate antibiotics, hydration, and sialagogues. Viral inflammation may involve the parotid gland (viral parotitis or mumps). The most frequently identified etiologic agent is the *Paramyxovirus*, although this entity has become less common with the introduction of mumps vaccinations. Additional infectious disorders include granulomatous agents and actinomycosis. Again, these disorders are more prevalent in the HIV-positive population.

Nonneoplastic salivary disease includes sialolithiasis, or ductal stones, which are commonly found in the submandibular glands (80%). Of parotid calculi, 65% are radiolucent while 65% of submandibular gland stones are radiopaque. Painful swelling is temporally associated with meals. Numerous methods exist for stone destruction and extraction (e.g., lithotripsy); however, recurrent sialolithiasis may necessitate gland removal. Autoimmune processes frequently involve the salivary glands. *Sjögren syndrome* is a disorder seen in the middle-aged and the elderly, with

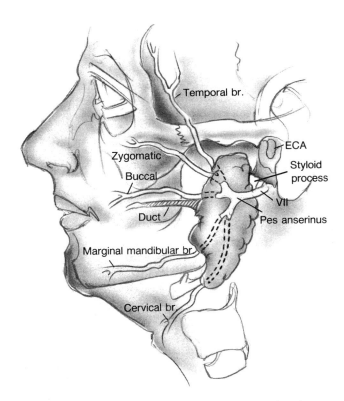

FIGURE 26-2. Anatomy of the parotid gland and facial nerve. (From Bailey BJ, ed. *Head and neck surgery:* otolaryngology. Philadelphia: JB Lippincott Co, 1993, with permission.)

women outnumbering men by a ratio of 9:1 (Fig. 26-3). Symptoms include dry mouth (xerostomia), keratoconjunctivitis sicca (dry eyes), glandular swelling and papillary atrophy of the tongue. Sjögren syndrome frequently presents as a symptom within a larger group of connective tissue disorders. Diagnosis is made on the basis of salivary gland biopsy, which demonstrates plasma cell and histiocytic infiltration with acinar atrophy. Laboratory studies include antibody screening for autoantibodies against nuclear protein antigens (SS-A and SS-B) as well as rheumatoid factor and antinuclear factor. An elevated sedimentation rate is present. Pharmacologic agents causing xerostomia must be included in the differential diagnosis (anticholinergics, diuretics, antihistamines, psychotropics, antispasmodics, and parkinsonian agents).

Neoplastic disorders include benign and malignant entities of the salivary glands and account for approximately 1 in 20 tumors arising in the head and neck. Overall, the incidence of tumors is approximately 2 per 100,000. With respect to site distribution, 65% of tumors are localized to the parotid gland and 20% to the submandibular gland. The remaining 15% originate in minor salivary glands of the hard and soft palates and the cheeks and lips. Benign entities progress slowly, are painless, and rarely cause facial nerve dysfunction. In contrast, malignant tumors are suspected in cases of rapid growth, facial nerve paresis or pain (associated with perineural invasion). Mitotic nuclei have been identified at all levels within the ductal apparatus, suggesting that neoplasms may arise from any portion of the glandular unit. Many of these cells are pluripotential in nature, and as a result, histologic classification is complicated with at least 30 described neoplasms identified in the pathology literature (Armed Forces Institute of Pathology).

With respect to benign entities, the *pleomorphic adenoma (benign mixed tumor)* is the most common salivary tumor (approximately 50%). There is a slight female preponderance in affected individuals, with peak occurrence in the fifth and sixth decades. Histologically, mucoid, osseous, chondroid, and myxoid elements can be identified. Malignant degeneration is not observed. Although these tumors can be observed, patient apprehension will frequently prompt surgical excision. Resection involves complete removal of the superficial and if indicated, deep lobes, rather than simple enucleation. Preservation of the facial nerve (CN VII) is indicated in all cases unless pathologic confirmation of malignancy is made on a permanent section. The suspicion of malignancy on frozen section does not warrant sacrifice of facial nerve. Simple extirpation of the tumor can result in unacceptably high rates of recurrence. A second group of tumors includes the *monomorphic adenomas*, which are identified in 4% of parotid masses. Histologically, they resemble pleomorphic tumors, however, only a single morphologic class is present. Subcategories include basal cell adenoma, trabecular adenoma, canalicular adenoma, and tubular adenoma, although management is not influenced by these classifications.

Warthin tumors (papillary cystadenoma lymphomatosum) represent the second most common type of the salivary neoplasms (Fig. 26-4). They represent 5% of all salivary tumors (10% of parotid tumors) with a marked male to female predilection (5:1). Again, they are most commonly identified in the fifth and sixth decades. Warthin tumors are multicentric in 12% of individuals and bilateral in 6%. Microscopically, they possess a biphasic composition with lymphoid sheets interspersed with oncocytic cells demonstrating high concentrations of mitochondria. The *oncocytoma* is the fourth most frequently identified benign salivary tumor (less than 2%) and is localized most commonly to the parotid gland. The oncocytoma exhibits a slow growth rate and multicentricity is common. A fifth entity affecting the salivary glands is the *benign lymphoepithelial lesion of Godwin*. This disorder is characterized by lymphocytic infiltration of the glands causing bilateral cystic masses that require frequent aspiration or gland excision. Association with HIV infection has been noted, and in 10% of affected individuals, this condition will progress to lymphoma.

The *malignant tumors* of the salivary gland constitute approximately 35% of all salivary masses. The likelihood of malignancy is inversely proportional to the size of the sali-

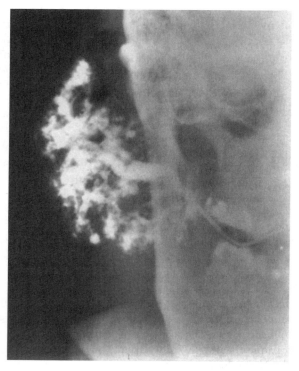

FIGURE 26-3. The end stage of Sjögren syndrome in a 36-year-old woman. The sialogram shows multiple, irregular contrast collections replacing the parotid gland. (From Bailey BJ, ed. *Head and neck surgery:* otolaryngology. Philadelphia: JB Lippincott Co, 1993, with permission.)

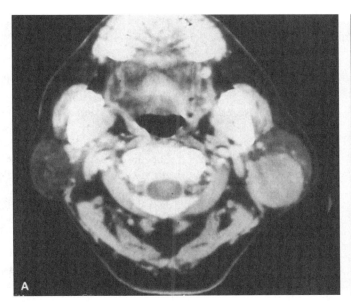 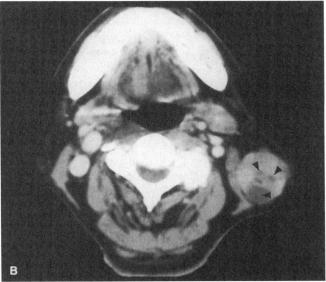

FIGURE 26-4. Computed tomography scan of a Warthin tumor. **A:** A large, well-defined mass involves the superficial lobe of the left parotid gland. The mass enhances diffusely. **B:** At the level of the parotid tail, areas of lower density (*arrowheads*) are consistent with the cystic components of the mass. (From Bailey BJ, ed. *Head and neck surgery:* otolaryngology. Philadelphia: JB Lippincott Co, 1993, with permission.)

vary gland: parotid (32%), submandibular (41%), and minor (60%). Of the minor salivary gland neoplasms, approximately 40% arise in the palate. The most common malignant tumor of the salivary gland is the *mucoepidermoid carcinoma*. These unencapsulated neoplasms arise in the third through fifth decades. Patients note a slowly enlarging painless mass with rare CN VII involvement and 35% of patients present with lymph node metastases. Of the salivary malignancies, this group is most commonly associated with prior exposure to radiation. High-grade, medium-grade, and low-grade histologic malignancies are described, with poor prognosis carried by those with progressively higher grades of differentiation.

Additional malignant tumors include *malignant mixed tumors* (6%) and *adenocarcinoma* (4%). The latter group demonstrates frequent facial nerve involvement (20%) and pain (15%). *Adenoid cystic carcinoma* accounts for 30% of minor salivary tumors and is the most common tumor of the submandibular and minor salivary glands. Classically, this tumor is associated with bone involvement and aggressive spread along nerves (perineural invasion). *Acinic cell carcinoma* arises only in the parotid gland in individuals in their fifth and sixth decades. Histologically, they are notable for the presence of amyloid. The remaining 1% of parotid malignancies fall within various cell types including squamous cell carcinoma, salivary duct carcinoma (which resemble breast cancer), and lymphomas. Metastases to the parotid gland are rare and are secondary to spread by melanoma and squamous cell carcinoma.

The diagnosis of parotid neoplasms incorporates elements of patient history (pain, paresis, and progress of growth), physical examination (tenderness, compressibility, fixation, erythema, and edema), pathology (histologic evidence from fine needle aspiration), and radiologic evaluation on computed tomography (CT) and magnetic resonance imaging (MRI) (enhancing, cystic, perineural tracking). Additional diagnostic studies of salivary function have been described (sialography and radiosialography) but are less frequently employed. Despite these factors, uncertainty with respect to malignancy may exist and most salivary tumors are ultimately excised. Superficial parotidectomy is indicated for all parotid tumors, unless deep lobe extension is noted, in which case, total parotidectomy is performed with sparing of the facial nerve. Due to the presence of pseudopod extensions from neoplasms, enucleation alone carries a higher rate of recurrence (10%). Malignant neoplasms may require excision of all or part of the mastoid bone if retrograde tracking along facial nerve branches is noted. Submandibular and minor salivary gland tumors require gland excision. Management of minor salivary gland tumors also requires wide surgical margins (more than 1 cm). Malignant masses are removed *en bloc* with nodal dissection (all or part of neck nodal levels I to VI) corresponding to the appropriate levels for preferred metastasis.

Postoperative radiation is recommended for intermediate and high-grade mucoepidermoid carcinoma, malignant mixed tumor, adenocarcinoma, adenoid cystic carcinoma, high-grade acinic cell carcinoma, squamous cell carcinomas, and malignant tumors greater than 2 cm in diameter. Protocols involving adjuvant chemotherapy are currently under investigation. Failure rates are highest for adenoid cystic and acinic cell carcinomas. Both of these entities frequently exhibit lung metastasis. The 5-year survival rate for all salivary cancers is approximately 70%, with a lower survival rate (30%) observed in instances of distal metastasis.

Complications of salivary gland surgery typically occur as sequelae of surgery on the parotid gland. Temporary facial nerve paresis is not unusual (15% to 30%) and most often involves the temporal and mandibular branches. The integrity of the nerve is assessed at the termination of the procedure with a nerve stimulator. If intact, return to normal function can be predicted with confidence. When tumor involvement requires sacrifice of CN VII (less than 5%), nerve grafting to distal branches is recommended. Grafts are obtained from the sural nerve, or alternatively, CN XII to CN VII anastomoses can be performed. Grafts are able to tolerate postoperative radiation; therefore, grafting is advised at the time of resection. Time to maximal recovery is approximately 6 to 12 months, although complete return of function is rare. The most common complication of parotid surgery is Frey syndrome or gustatory sweating (50% to 85%). Severed parasympathetic fibers synapse inappropriately with autonomic fibers directed at sweat glands of the face. When eating, facial sweating is detected. Diagnosis is made by patient history or by application of a light coat of methylene blue and starch (Minor iodine test). Treatment involves topical anticholinergic creams (scopolamine) and Teflon or fat interposition between parotid bed and skin. In recent years, botulinum toxin injection, which targets presynaptic, cholinergic terminals, has gained favor as a means for providing long-term symptomatic relief.

ORAL CAVITY AND OROPHARYNX

The oral cavity is involved in three principal functions: phonation, food ingestion, and breathing. Anatomically, it is defined as the area including the lips, lower and upper alveolar ridges, buccal mucosa, floor of the mouth, retromolar trigone, hard palate, and anterior two thirds of the tongue (defined by the circumvallate papillae). The oral cavity contains 20 deciduous teeth in the child and 32 permanent teeth in the adult. Motor functions of the oral cavity are provided by the tongue and the masticatory muscles. The muscles of mastication are innervated by CN V^3 and include the masseter, temporalis, lateral pterygoid, and medial pterygoid. The tongue receives motor innervation from the *hypoglossal nerve* (CN XII). Tactile sensory of the tongue is provided by the *lingual nerve* (CN V^3) while taste is provided by the *chorda tympani* (CN VII) (anterior two thirds) and *glossopharyngeal nerve* (CN IX) (posterior two thirds). Six ducts (Stensen, Wharton, and Rivinus ducts) open into the oral cavity from the parotid, submaxillary, and sublingual glands, respectively. Up to 1,500 mL of saliva is produced each day.

The pharynx includes three distinct regions. The *nasopharynx* extends from the base of the skull to the level of the junction of hard and soft palates. Anteriorly, it begins at the most posterior extent of the septum. Laterally, it includes the region defined by the fossa of Rosenmuller adjacent to the openings to the eustachian tubes. Proceeding inferiorly, the oropharynx begins at the undersurface of the soft palate. The lateral walls encompass the tonsils and tonsillar fossae. The base of the tongue is defined as tissue posterior to the circumvallate papillae. The *oropharynx* also includes the vallecula (the recess located between the base of the tongue and epiglottis). The final division of the pharynx is the *hypopharynx*, which extends from the level of the floor of the vallecula and pharyngoepiglottic folds to the inferior border of the cricoid cartilage. Important structures of the hypopharynx include the pharyngoesophageal junction and piriform sinuses (the funnel-shaped recessed areas located on either side of the larynx).

Multiple benign processes may produce inflammation of the oral cavity and pharynx. These include bacterial, viral, and fungal infections, autoimmune disorders, nutritional deficiencies (iron, B_{12}, riboflavin, and vitamin C), and toxin or chemical exposure. Certain entities are seen rarely in developed countries. Thus, acute necrotizing ulcerative gingivitis (Vincent angina or trench mouth associated with *Treponema vincentii* infection) is mentioned for historical purposes only. In contrast, herpetic infections are the most common of oral cavity infections. Other viral infections (rubeola) are encountered only rarely in the postimmunization era. Oral candidiasis, or thrush, is seen frequently in the HIV population and in postirradiation patients with diminished salivary production. The most concerning infections are those that can lead to airway compromise. Odontogenic infections can spread rapidly to the floor of the mouth, tongue base, and submandibular space (Ludwig angina), necessitating tracheostomy to secure the airway until resolved (Fig. 26-5). Bacterial collections adjacent to the tonsils (peritonsillar abscess) can cause compromise with submucosal extension inferiorly to the larynx. Common symptoms of peritonsillar abscess include trismus (oral cavity opening of more than 2 cm), dysphagia, dehydration, "hot potato" voice, uvular deviation to the contralateral side, presence of pus in tonsillar crypts, or bleeding from inflamed or necrotic tonsils.

Management includes broad-spectrum antibiosis against the Gram-positive, Gram-negative, and anaerobic flora of the oral cavity. Needle aspiration of the peritonsillar abscess in the emergency room frequently provides immediate diminution of discomfort. The preferred time for tonsillectomy is approximately 6 weeks postinfection. However, the "quinsy tonsillectomy" can be performed in the immunocompromised patient, those who are not responding ade-

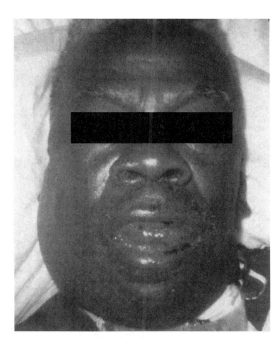

FIGURE 26-5. Ludwig angina. Note the cuff of bilateral submandibular and submental swelling enveloping the upper neck and elevation of the floor of the mouth causing protrusion of the tongue. (From Bailey BJ, ed. *Head and neck surgery: otolaryngology.* Philadelphia: JB Lippincott Co, 1993, with permission.)

quately to antibiotics, or those with airway compromise. Other noninfectious lesions that can lead to dehydration include recurrent aphthous ulcer, erythema multiforme, pemphigus vulgaris (intraepidermoid bullae), and pemphigoid (subepidermoid bullae).

Malignant Lesions of the Oral Cavity and Pharynx

Approximately 31,000 new cancers of the oral cavity and pharynx are diagnosed each year in the United States (representing 2.7% of newly diagnosed cancers in men and 1.6% in women). Overall, these tumors constitute 65% of all malignancies of the head and neck. Despite advances in radiotherapy and chemotherapy protocols, survival rates are little improved from those of the 1960s, with a 5-year survival rate of 50% documented for the oral and pharyngeal cancer patient. Factors implicated in the etiology of these carcinomas include tobacco use (cigarettes, cigars, and chewing products), excessive alcohol consumption, and human papillomavirus exposure. Exposure to ultraviolet light has been associated with carcinomas of the lower lip. In parts of the world where other oral stimulants are used (e.g., betel nut in India), significantly higher incidences of the disease are noted.

Lesions of the oral cavity present at varying levels of differentiation. Commonly identified lesions include leukoplakia, which presents as a superficial, hyperkeratotic, mucosal plaque. These white lesions demonstrate epithelial hyperplasia in approximately 80% of cases and should be biopsied to rule out carcinoma in situ or frank invasion. The overwhelmingly predominant histology identified in tumors of these areas is squamous cell carcinoma. These cancers can exhibit high, low, or moderate degrees of differentiation. Molecular biologic techniques have demonstrated a high percentage with mutations of the tumor suppressor gene p53. Clinically, the level of differentiation does not significantly influence management when compared to factors such as location of primary tumor locale and nodal status. Distal metastasis (lung, liver, and bone) is evident in advanced disease and diagnostic workup should include chest x-ray. In more advanced disease, a CT scan of the chest and abdomen, as well as a bone scan are warranted. Operative evaluation is performed in two stages. Direct laryngoscopy, bronchoscopy, and esophagoscopy are advocated because of the 5% incidence of synchronous primary lesions of the aerodigestive tract. Postoperatively, these patients carry an elevated risk of developing a second tumor (approximately 4% per year). If extensive resection is anticipated, or if radiation therapy to the head and neck region is planned, many surgeons advocate tracheostomy, insertion of gastric feeding tube, and complete teeth extraction before performing a definitive resection. These procedures are indicated due to concern over radiation-induced edema of the airway and esophagus and induction of dental caries and osteoradionecrosis of the mandible and maxilla. Moreover, reconstruction of airway/pharynx limits oral intake of nutrition or medication.

Early carcinomas of the oral cavity and pharynx (stages T1 and T2) exhibit comparable responses to either radiation or surgical modalities. However, carcinoma of the oral cavity and pharynx frequently presents as advanced disease (Table 26-1). This has been explained on the basis of the patient profile, which includes high alcohol consumption and lower socioeconomic status. Prolonged exposure of tobacco and alcohol in the gingivobuccal sulcus and the floor of the mouth regions are thought to contribute to the distribution of these cancers. Lesions are frequently painless, and abundant soft tissue of the tongue and floor of the mouth permit significant tumor growth before detection. Presenting symptoms may include altered tongue mobility, dysphagia, and dysarthria. However, more commonly, the patient will present with a mass in the neck that represents advanced nodal disease. In tumors of the hypopharynx, greater than 50% of patients will complain of ear pain.

Management of cancers of the oral cavity and pharynx are among the most challenging of surgical oncologic procedures. Resection typically includes partial or complete glossectomy and resection of involved mandibular segments. *Ipsilateral dissection* of neck lymph nodes is indicated

TABLE 26-1. CLINICAL CLASSIFICATION OF SQUAMOUS CELL CARCINOMA OF THE ORAL CAVITY[a]

Primary tumor	Regional lymph nodes	Distant metastases
T	N	M
TX carcinoma in situ	NX unassessable	MX unassessable
T1 tumor 2 cm or less in greatest dimension	N0 no nodal metastases	M0 no distant metastases
T2 tumor 2–4 cm	N1 single ipsilateral node, 3 cm or less	M1 distant metastases
T3 tumor >4 cm	N2 single ipsilateral node 3–6 cm; or multiple ipsilateral nodes, none >6 cm; or bilateral or contralateral nodes, none >6 cm	
T4 tumor invades adjacent structures (through cortical bone, deep tongue musculature, maxillary sinus, skin)	N2a single ipsilateral node 3–6 cm	
	N2b multiple ipsilateral nodes, none >6 cm	
	N2c bilateral or contralateral nodes, none >6 cm	
	N3 node >6 cm	

[a]From American Joint Committee on Cancer. Manual for staging of cancer, 4th ed. Philadelphia: JB Lippincott. 1992:29, with permission

in the absence of clinical nodal disease. Bilateral neck dissection is indicated if palpable or radiologic evidence of disease is present. Approximately one in three patients with cancer of the tongue or piriform sinus will have occult metastasis. If extension to the vallecula is noted, partial or complete laryngeal resection may also be required.

Advances have been made in reconstructive surgery, allowing creation of bulk in the oral cavity with pedicle muscle flaps and free muscle flaps to permit deglutition. In addition, mandibular reconstruction can be accomplished with titanium plates or harvested bone from the fibula and iliac crest. Nevertheless, the inability to recreate delicate motor movements performed by the tongue carry significant morbidity with respect to speech and swallowing competency.

Nasopharyngeal Carcinoma

An interesting subset of pharyngeal tumors occurs in the nasopharynx. These cancers comprise only 0.2% of newly diagnosed malignancies in the United States. However, in certain regions of China, these cancers represent 25% of all diagnosed cancers. This disparity in incidence is thought to be related to environmental exposure to specific types of Epstein-Barr virus (EBV) and to prevalence of specific human leukocyte antigen genotypes. Demographically, peak incidence occurs in the fifth decade, although 20% of patients are under the age of 30 at diagnosis. Histologically, the World Health Organization has described three classes of nasopharyngeal carcinomas. Type I (25%) is associated with keratin bridges and no association with EBV. Type II (12%) lesions are also known as "transitional cell carcinomas" and have no keratin staining. Type III (63%) tumors are notable for enlarged nuclei and clear cytoplasm. Five-year survival rates range from 10% for type I tumors to 50% for type II and type III lesions.

Tumors are located in the fossa of Rosenmuller, immediately adjacent to the eustachian tube orifice causing obstruction (Fig. 26-6). For this reason, persistent unilateral otalgia or serous otitis media in the adult represents nasopharyngeal carcinoma until proven otherwise. Delayed diagnosis can have significant negative impact with respect to prognosis. Other presenting symptoms may include nasal congestion, eye pain, hyperesthesia in the CN V^1 or V^2 distribution, epistaxis, and headache secondary to intracranial extension. Diplopia secondary to abducens (CN VI) paresis is the most commonly observed of the cranial neuropathies. Endoscopic nasopharyngoscopic examination may not detect submucosal spread, therefore, MRI examination should be ordered if uncertainty persists. The mainstay of treatment is radiotherapy, because tumor location renders these lesions unresectable. In addition, a cisplatin-based chemotherapy regimen increases disease-free survival time and overall survival. Because nasopharyngeal tumors frequently present with involvement of the level V or posterior neck nodes (60%), postirradiation dissection of neck nodes is recommended by many authors.

HEAD AND NECK NEOPLASMS

Additional cancers of the head and neck include lymphomas. Two thirds of patients with Hodgkin lymphoma have lymph node involvement throughout the cervical chain. Non-Hodgkin lymphomas typically are identified in the upper cervical nodes. Histologic classification systems for Hodgkin disease include favorable (lymphocyte predominant and nodular sclerosing), guarded (mixed cellular), and unfavorable (lymphocyte depleting). Non-Hodgkin lymphoma classifications include favorable (nodular and well-differentiated lymphocytic) and unfavor-

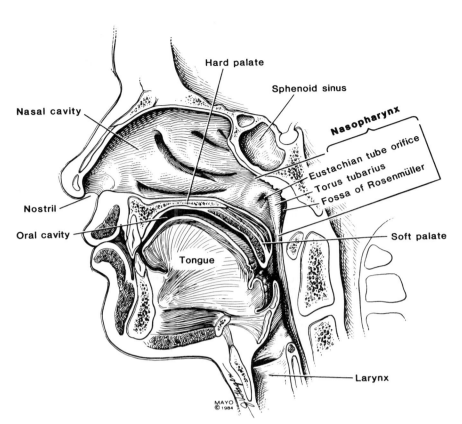

FIGURE 26-6. The nasopharynx and its anatomical relationships. (From Weiland LH, Neel HB III, Pearson GR. Nasopharyngeal carcinoma. *Curr Hematol Oncol* 1986;4:379, with permission.)

able (diffuse poorly differentiated lymphocytic, diffuse histiocytic, diffuse undifferentiated, and nodular histiocytic). Diagnosis is made on the basis of excision biopsy of the node. Specimens should also be sent for flow cytometry to identify atypical lymphocytes, which increases diagnostic accuracy.

Additional rare tumors of the head and neck include those arising from chemoreceptor tissue (carotid body tumors, glomus jugular tumors, and glomus tympanicum tumors). Less than 5% are malignant and surgical excision is recommended. Rare malignant lesions of the head and neck include angiosarcomas, which arise from vascular endothelial cells; these aggressive lesions commonly arise in the scalp and treatment requires complete excision. Hemangiopericytomas arise from Zimmermann cells around capillaries. Approximately 30% arise in the head and neck and treatment requires excision.

In the pediatric population, developmental anomalies can account for additional neck masses. *Branchial cleft cysts* (types I to IV) are typically found along the anatomical line that extends from the external auditory canal inferiorly along the anterior border of the sternocleidomastoid muscle. A patent ductal remnant frequently communicates with the aerodigestive tract, resulting in intermittent swelling associated with upper respiratory tract infections. Treatment involves excision of the cyst along with the duct. The thyroglossal duct cyst represents a midline ductal remnant, which is found along the course of descent of the thyroid gland, i.e., from the foramen cecum at the base of the tongue to the anterior neck. Again, swelling and tenderness occur with upper respiratory tract infections. Management includes extirpation of the *entire cyst* and the *midportion of the hyoid bone* (through which the embryonic thyroid gland passes). A preoperative ultrasound of the neck should be ordered to ensure that normal thyroid tissue is present. In rare instances, the lingual thyroid represents the only functioning thyroid tissue in the individual and therefore should not be resected. Lymphatic and venous malformations are frequently diagnosed in the pediatric population and are managed conservatively, provided there is no airway compromise.

LYMPHATICS OF THE HEAD AND NECK

Management of tumors involving the head and neck requires understanding of staging algorithms that incorporate size of primary tumor, nodal status, and presence of metastases. Review of surgical pathology of otolaryngeal malignancies indicates that neoplasms localized to each region of the head and neck have a predictable pattern of spread to specific lymph node chains (Fig. 26-7). This pattern is influenced by size and histologic features of the tumor. By utilizing MRI or CT scanning, it is frequently possible to identify pathologic lymph nodes that may be undetectable clinically. (Normal nodes in the neck should

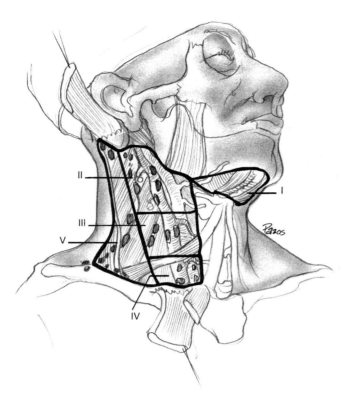

FIGURE 26-7. Lymph node regions of the neck. (From Bailey BJ, ed. *Head and neck surgery: otolaryngology.* Philadelphia: JB Lippincott Co, 1993, with permission.)

not exceed 1 cm in size with the exception of the jugulodigastric lymph node, which may be as large as 1.5 cm.) By identifying suspicious nodes, and by having a knowledge of metastatic patterns, the surgeon can plan resection of the tumor with the associated lymph nodes most likely to be involved.

The term *neck dissection* refers to procedures for surgical excision of lymph nodes from any or all of six regions defined in the neck. Multiple procedures have been described to accomplish resection. The most extreme procedure is the radical neck dissection, which requires sacrifice of lymph node chains and (i) internal jugular vein, (ii) sternocleidomastoid muscle, and (iii) accessory nerve (CN XI). Predictably, this procedure carries the highest morbidity. In recent years, efforts have been made to spare one or more of these vital structures to lessen morbidity (modified radical neck dissection). Furthermore, attention has focused on limiting nodal dissection to only those groups most likely to be involved in tumor (e.g., supraomohyoid node dissection). Six lymph node groups have been defined in the neck (Fig. 26-7). Level I nodes are located in the submental and submandibular triangles and drain the oral cavity and submandibular gland. Three nodal groups are closely associated with the internal jugular vein. The most superior group, level II, extends from skull base to carotid bifurcation at the hyoid bone. Drainage from nasopharynx, oropharynx, the parotid gland, and supraglottic structures first involves these nodes. Intermediate, or level III, nodes are located between the carotid bifurcation and the intersection of the omohyoid muscle. Level III nodes drain the oropharynx, hypopharynx, and supraglottic larynx. Level IV nodes are present inferior to the omohyoid and extend to the level of the clavicles. These nodes drain the subglottic larynx, hypopharynx, esophagus, and thyroid masses. The level V (posterior triangle) node group is located in the region located posterolateral to the sternocleidomastoid muscles. This group is a frequent site of metastasis of tumors from the nasopharynx and oropharynx. The level VI (parathyroid) nodes are located between the lateral borders of the strap muscles and drain thyroid and parathyroid malignancies.

Although authors agree that neck dissection is indicated in cases with palpable adenopathy or radiologically proven abnormal nodes, controversy exists over the management of the clinically negative or N0 neck. Ipsilateral neck dissection is advocated by authors in instances where the primary tumor is associated with a high incidence of occult nodal metastasis (e.g., tongue, floor of the mouth, and piriform sinus have approximately a 30% risk). In tumors associated with a lower risk (such as buccal mucosa with 9% incidence of occult nodes), some would recommend close observation in the postoperative period, rather than elective neck dissection.

With respect to combined therapy, radiation therapy can either precede or follow surgical resection of the primary malignancy and lymph node. Radiation therapy is directed at the site of the primary tumor and bed of involved lymph nodes. The role of chemotherapy as an adjuvant to surgery and radiation is currently under investigation. Although squamous cell carcinomas do not respond as well as certain other carcinomas, chemotherapy may enhance survival for patients with extracapsular tumor spread.

THE LARYNX

The larynx is composed of a cartilaginous tube that projects into the hypopharynx. Anatomically, the larynx is described as having three divisions: *supraglottis, glottis,* and *subglottis* (Fig. 26-8). The glottis serves as a sphincter to protect the airway from aspiration and to provide phonation. It is composed of the true vocal cords and the vocal processes of the arytenoid cartilages, consisting of the cuneiform and corniculate cartilages (Fig. 26-9). The structures are enclosed by the cricoid and thyroid cartilages, from which the intrinsic muscles of the glottis are suspended. The actions of six paired muscles serve to open and close the vocal cords, thereby permitting ventilation and cord vibration. Motor innervation to the glottis is supplied by divisions of the vagus nerve (CN X). The superior laryngeal nerve provides sensory innervation to the supraglottic area. Stimulation in

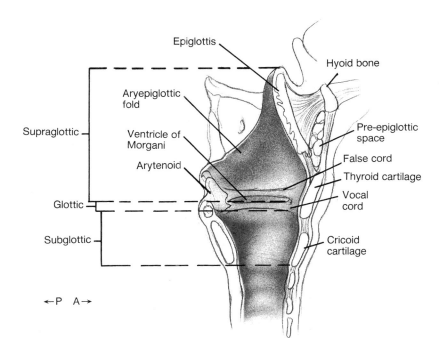

FIGURE 26-8. Midline sagittal section of the larynx, demonstrating the supraglottic and glottic regions, as well as the preepiglottic space. (From Bailey BJ, ed. *Head and neck surgery: otolaryngology.* Philadelphia: JB Lippincott Co, 1993, with permission.)

this region triggers a strong cough reflex. Inability to detect sensation in this area places an individual at great risk for aspiration. The superior laryngeal nerve also provides motor innervation to the cricothyroid muscle, which lengthens the vocal cords and deepens the voice.

The vagus nerve travels inferiorly in the carotid sheath and gives off the recurrent laryngeal nerve branches. These nerves provide innervation to the remaining intrinsic muscles of the larynx, which adduct and abduct the true vocal cords. Weakness of the vocal cords is caused by nerve compression secondary to tumors of the jugular foramen, thyroid gland, lung, or schwannomas. Strokes involving the nucleus ambiguous of the brain can also result in vocal cord weakness or paralysis. Other systemic processes can cause vocal cord weakness including polio, Guillain-Barré syndrome, or Lyme disease.

The primary events associated with management of the airway involve respiration and phonation. Patients may present with hoarseness, stridor, or dyspnea. In each case, historical information may provide clues to diagnosis. Recent thyroid surgery or lung surgery may have resulted in recurrent laryngeal nerve injury. Recent intubation is frequently associated with ulceration of the posterior glottis because of endotracheal tube positioning in the supine patient. Often this can present as delayed scarring and progressive hoarseness. In all cases, the examination of the vocal cords is necessary. Visualization is accomplished indirectly (nasopharyngolaryngoscopy, or mirror examination) and directly with laryngoscopy under general anesthesia.

With respect to sudden onset of stridor, principal causes include infectious etiologies, foreign bodies, and angioedema. Viral or bacterial infections can be managed with humidification, appropriate antibiotics, and steroids. Angioedema is an unusual entity presenting as rapid onset of swelling in all or selected parts of the oropharynx, (e.g., lips, tongue, or epiglottis). It occurs most commonly in response to food allergy or medications (particularly angiotensin-converting enzyme inhibitors). Management includes racemic epinephrine, intubation, and steroids for 24 to 48 hours to allow for edema to abate. An additional frequent cause of acute onset stridor is the foreign body. In the pediatric population, an inhaled portion of food represents the most common foreign body of the tracheo-

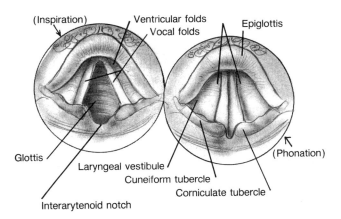

FIGURE 26-9. Endoscopic view of the larynx. (From Bailey BJ, ed. *Head and neck surgery: otolaryngology.* Philadelphia: JB Lippincott Co, 1993, with permission.)

bronchial tree. Because organic matter is often radiopaque, direct laryngoscopy and bronchoscopy is required to rule out foreign bodies as a source of wheezing or stridor. A chest x-ray is often helpful in identifying hyperinflation due to ball-valving on the affected side. In addition, operative extraction is necessary to secure a patent airway. (Similarly, the ingested foreign body, such as a coin in the pediatric population, will require esophagoscopy and visualized extraction.)

Chronic changes in voice are more commonly the result of inflammation secondary to gastroesophageal reflux disease (GERD), inflammatory neoplasms of the vocal cords, or vocal cord abuse. Reflux can be diagnosed on the basis of history and evidence of erythema and edema of the arytenoids and the posterior cricoid region (entrance to the esophagus). Vocal cord abuse is evidenced by hoarse voice and presence of vocal cord polyps or granulomas. The latter two entities can be managed with voice rest or resection. Because certain benign lesions can resemble squamous cell carcinomas on inspection (e.g., blastomycosis), a tissue biopsy is necessary to rule out malignancy. Benign neoplasms of the larynx include papillomas, chondromas, and hemangiomas. Management may include surgical or laser resection. Sarcoid is also known to affect the larynx, with epiglottic involvement being the most common. If medical management is not successful at improving the airway, partial or complete epiglottidectomy may be performed.

Additional causes of hoarseness, shortness of breath, or "breathy voice" include vocal cord paralysis due to recurrent laryngeal nerve dysfunction. Video stroboscopy permits evaluation of vocal cord motion and is diagnostic. Etiologies include central (stroke), nerve transection during surgery (e.g., thyroidectomy), compression (lung cancer or neck mass), viral (polio), degenerative (amyotrophic lateral sclerosis), autoimmune (Guillain-Barré, sarcoidosis), or trauma. In instances of permanent vocal cord paralysis, various procedures are available to medialize the affected vocal cord. This maneuver (thyroplasty) allows the functional cord to contact the mucosal surface of the contralateral cord which permits phonation and minimizes the risk of aspiration.

With respect to the pediatric population, respiratory obstruction can be the result of supraglottic or infraglottic pathology. The most common etiology of neonatal airway compromise is immature tracheal cartilage resulting in inspiratory collapse of the trachea and epiglottis. Management includes observation because children typically outgrow this difficulty. In rare instances, compromise of the trachea is due to vascular malformations (e.g., Vascular Rings) which compress the trachea. Additional offending lesions include airway cysts and hemangiomas. Management requires marsupialization of cysts. Hemangiomas typically will enlarge in the first few months of life, producing symptoms of airway compromise. Continued growth occurs for approximately 3 to 4 years before involution. The preferred treatment involves observation. In cases of severe airway compromise, tracheostomy or laser resection can be used to secure the airway. Lastly, congenital anomalies may include subglottic stenosis (70% anterior), which requires dilation, stent placement, or cartilaginous transplants to widen the stenotic region (laryngotracheoplasty).

Cancers of the Larynx

Approximately, 11,000 laryngeal cancers are diagnosed each year in the United States representing approximately 3% of all new carcinomas. Peak incidence occurs in the sixth and seventh decades with men affected more commonly than women (8:1). Principal risk factors include tobacco and alcohol products. Presenting symptoms include hoarseness, dyspnea, dysphagia, or odynophagia. A palpable neck mass is frequently detected initially when shaving. Otalgia is also observed with local extension affecting the glossopharyngeal nerve (CN IX). The overwhelming majority of laryngeal lesions are squamous cell carcinomas (94%), with the remaining tumors including verrucous carcinoma, adenocarcinoma, sarcoma, and rare metastasis (renal cell, breast, prostate, and melanoma).

Anatomically, the larynx is described as having three divisions (Fig. 26-8). The *supraglottis* extends from the tip of the epiglottis to the ventricular folds, located immediately superior to the vocal cords (Fig. 26-9). Extensive lymphatics from this area drain anteriorly to the preepiglottic space and bilaterally to level II to V lymph nodes. Metastasis to lymph nodes is present in 40% of patients at the time of diagnosis. Approximately 30% of all laryngeal cancers originate in the supraglottis. The *glottic portion* begins at the ventricular fold and extends 1 cm inferiorly to the vocal cord. Most laryngeal cancers (67%) arise in the glottis. These tumors are frequently detected early in the course of the disease due to hoarseness or airway compromise. Only 15% will have identifiable nodal metastasis at diagnosis. The *subglottis* extends from a point 1 cm below the vocal cords to the inferior border of the cricoid cartilage. Although the rarest of the laryngeal cancers (3%), these tumors carry a poor prognosis because patients develop symptoms late in the disease and extensive regional spread is common.

Staging of laryngeal carcinomas follows the American Joint Committee on Cancer criteria (Tumor-Node-Metastasis, or TNM). Tumors are evaluated on the basis of vocal cord function (fixed vs. mobile) and local extension to soft tissue and cartilage. Flexible fiberoptic laryngoscopy is used to assess cord position and mobility. Other diagnostic modalities include CT scans, which provide information on integrity of thyroid and cricoid cartilage, invasion of esophagus and laryngeal musculature, and lymph node status. Early carcinomas with limited nodal disease carry an excellent 5-year survival rate (more than 70%). More extensive disease (stages T3 and T4) carries a significantly poorer prognosis (20% to 40%). Treatments include surgical approaches, radiation, and chemotherapy. Extensive surgical resections (partial and total laryngectomy) carry the significant morbidity associated with voice loss. However, in recent years, voice-conservative procedures (such as supracricoid laryngectomy) have been described that preserve some level of phonation. Discrete mapping of tumor location allows for preservation of portions of the glottis that might have been resected previously. When performed in combination with radiation and chemotherapy protocols, survival rates are maintained and quality of life is improved. In instances where complete laryngectomy is performed, a tracheostomy is necessary for ventilation. Postoperative communication can be accomplished with the electrolarynx or via placement of a tracheoesophageal prosthesis, which diverts air through the esophagus and relies on the cricopharyngeus muscle and oral musculature for phonation.

TRAUMA

Otologic Trauma

The temporal bone is one of the hardest bones in the human body and fractures affecting this structure are rare. Those that do occur are typically the result of high-speed motor vehicle accidents, falls, or assault. Men have a higher incidence of injury due to their greater propensity to engage in high-risk behavior. Children account for 50% of all temporal bone injuries. Two principal classifications have been described with diagnosis made on the basis of temporal bone CT scans. Longitudinal fractures (70% to 90%) are caused by lateral trauma to the squamous portion of the temporal bone. The fracture line extends from the posterosuperior portion of the external canal, through the eardrum to the otic capsule and petrous apex. Delayed paresis of the facial nerve occurs in approximately 15% of cases and is due to edema. This weakness will typically resolve with time. Physical examination findings include mastoid hematoma (Battle sign), blood in the external auditory canal, and tympanic membrane perforation. Conductive hearing loss is common due to disruption of middle-ear ossicles at the incudostapedial joint and eardrum perforation. Vestibular symptoms and sensorineural hearing loss are unusual (20%) and are due to the concussive effect to the cochlea and inner ear.

Transverse fractures represent 20% of injuries and occur with trauma to either the posterior occiput or to the frontal area. Transverse fractures typically are associated with higher mortality secondary to severe head trauma. The fracture line extends across the petrous pyramid, through the foramen spinosum or foramen lacerum, and through the internal auditory canal. Facial nerve injury occurs in 50% and is due to crush or laceration of the nerve. Evidence of immediate facial nerve injury warrants middle-ear exploration to identify compressed or transected areas. Sensorineural loss is severe and is due to avulsion of the cochlear nerve. The eardrum is not torn, but blood is often present behind the tympanic membrane (hemotympanum). Bilateral periorbital ecchymosis (raccoon eyes) is often noted. Vestibular complaints including vertigo occur due to concussion of the semicircular canals. Cerebrospinal fluid (CSF) leak is much more common and is recognized by the presence of a satellite ring around a blood stain on the pillow. CSF leaks are usually managed conservatively with bed rest, head of bed elevation, and possible lumbar drain placement. Two weeks are allowed for spontaneous resolution prior to attempting surgical repair. Antibiotic coverage is initiated to decrease risk of meningitis although this issue is controversial and differences in management exist between both neurosurgeons and otorhinolaryngologists (Chapter 1).

Auditory complaints of hearing loss, aural fullness, and disequilibrium may be due to leakage of perilymphatic fluid from the cochlea via the oval window and round window. Etiologies of fistulae include skull trauma or more commonly barotrauma due to scuba diving. Conservative management includes observation and bed rest for 2 weeks before consideration of surgical repair. Options for management of temporal bone trauma depend on the nature of defects. As stated above, immediate facial nerve paralysis warrants explanation but is often delayed due to concomitant severe injuries. Sensorineural hearing loss is rarely reversible. Conductive hearing loss is due to tympanic membrane perforation, which repair spontaneously in 75% of cases. Ossicular fracture or joint discontinuity can be repaired several months following the original trauma.

Trauma can also be localized to the external ear and canal. Blunt trauma is common in athletes (wrestling and boxing). Typically, a subperichondral hematoma can develop between the cartilage and the anterior perichondrium (Fig. 26-10). The cartilage has no intrinsic blood supply. Therefore, if the hematoma is not drained, the cartilage is deprived of nutrition, which leads to necrosis and loss of helical shape (cauliflower ear, wrestler's ear). Treatment involves hematoma evacuation and placement of a bolster for 1 week. Additional injuries or laceration may expose cartilage to infection. Treatment involves surgical debridement of devitalized cartilage and repositioning of perichondrium and skin. Antibiotics are required. Animal bites can be closed primarily. Human bites carry a greater risk of infection and closure is delayed for several days. Again, antibiotics are required for a period of 7 to 10 days. The remaining common form of trauma to the ear is thermal injury. The crucial factor leading to complications include inadequate debridement of devitalized tissue. In addition, avoidance of pressure on burned ears and topical chemotherapeutic agents can control *Pseudomonas* infection.

Mandibular Trauma

The classification of mandibular fractures is based on location and tendency for displacement or distraction. Affected regions of the mandible include the body (36%), the angle (20%), the condylar head (35%), the ramus (3%), the coro-

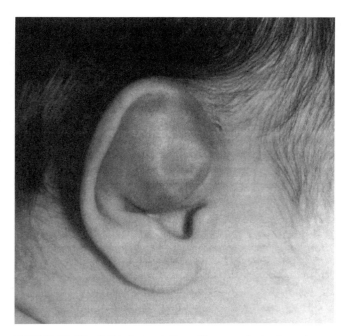

FIGURE 26-10. Child abuse victim with an auricular hematoma. (From Bailey BJ, ed. *Head and neck surgery: otolaryngology.* Philadelphia: JB Lippincott Co, 1993, with permission.)

noid process (2%), the symphysis (1%), and the parasymphysis (14%) regions, as well as the alveolus (3%). The sites of weakness that are predisposed to fracture include the third molar (particularly when impacted), the parasymphysial region at the mental foramen between the first and second bicuspid teeth, and the condylar neck. Thirty-two teeth are present in adults while twenty teeth are present in children. In the pediatric population, areas of uninterrupted teeth represent potential areas of fracture. Examination should determine degree of maxillomandibular occlusion. Normal class I occlusion has the mesiobuccal cusp of the maxillary first molar meeting the buccal groove of the first mandibular molar. This condition exists in 73% of the population. Class II occlusion (24%) suggests an overbite or mandibular retrognathism while class III occlusion (3%) is seen with mandibular prognathism. Presence of teeth on both sides of the fracture facilitates interdental wire fixation. An intact molar in the fracture line should be left untouched to maximize repositioning surface. A mobile tooth is usually removed. Trismus, or inability to open the mouth greater than 35 mm, suggests injury to the condyles. Unilateral subcondylar fractures produce a unilateral open-bite deformity while bilateral subcondylar fractures result in an anterior open-bite deformity (i.e., posterior mandibular and maxillary molars meet but anterior teeth do not). Condylar fractures may be associated with external auditory canal laceration or bloody otorrhea. Minimally displaced condylar fractures are treated with soft food diet and physiotherapy.

A simple fracture does not communicate with the oral cavity while a complex fracture is associated with violation of mucous membrane or skin and elevated risk of infection. A complex fracture is suggested by the presence of blood in the oral cavity. The panorex x-ray provides a complete view of the mandible and is optimal for diagnosing fractures. The reverse Towne film may be used for identifying fractures of the condylar neck.

Most fractures in the pediatric age group require closed reduction, rather than plating, to avoid injury to tooth roots and buds. If a fracture involves the tooth bud, then it should be left undisturbed (unless avulsed). Many fractures in the pediatric population are incomplete (greenstick fractures) and can be managed with rubber band fixation. Although isolated fractures occur in children, the overwhelming majority of fractures in adults are multiple. Favorability of fractures reflects the influence of forces exerted across the fracture lines by muscles that insert upon the mandible (Fig. 26-11). Favorable fractures (60%) can be treated with wire fixation and Erich Arch bars. Unfavorable fractures typically require open reduction and manipulating across the fracture line to stabilize the union. Bony fragments are either drawn together or distracted. Nine major muscle groups act on the mandible and potentially exert forces that favor or hinder fusion. The posterior muscle groups pull segments upward (elevate), forward (protrude), and medially and are responsible for mastication. These muscles include the medial and lateral pterygoids, the temporalis and the masseter. Anterior muscles pull the anterior segment of the mandible posteroinferiorly (i.e., open the mouth) and include the mylohyoid, geniohyoid, genioglossus, and anterior belly of the digastric. Of these, the mylohyoid is most important and exerts unfavorable forces upon fractures of the body, symphysis, and parasymphysis. Most angle fractures are horizontally unfavorable due to the action of the masseter, medial pterygoid, and temporalis muscles.

Additional factors influence healing and morbidity. The elderly, edentulous population or the indigent population with poor dentition will represent a greater challenge to fixation, due to the lack of repositioning surface area provided by the teeth. In certain cases, fixation can be performed with dentures in place to ensure adequate height of the mandibular ramus.

In general, any form of compression plating increases the risk of intraoperative damage to the inferior alveolar nerve. When plating is required, screws should be secured superior to the alveolar ridge to avoid trauma to the nerve, which runs in the mandibular canal and exits the mental foramen as the mental nerve. Screws directed superior to the oblique line (insertion of the mylohyoid muscle) can result in hypesthesia of the ipsilateral anterior chin and lower lip. It is important to document any injury of the inferior alveolar nerve prior to surgical fixation. There is a 7% to 13% risk of infection and 2% risk of osteomyelitis with mandibular fractures. Infections are commonly the result of inadequate fixation and hematoma at the fracture line or systemic factors (e.g., diabetes, immunocompromised state).

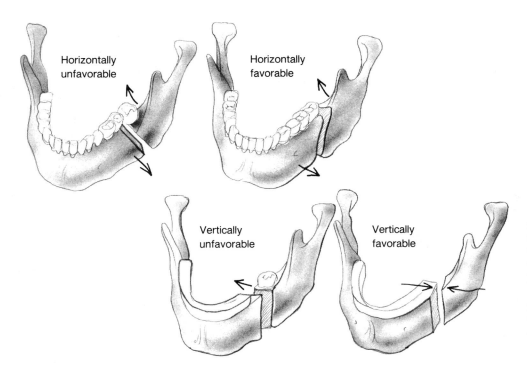

FIGURE 26-11. A horizontally unfavorable fracture of the angle exhibits displacement in a vertical direction due to the action of masticatory musculature. A vertically unfavorable body fracture is distracted horizontally by the mylohyoid. (From Bailey BJ, ed. *Head and neck surgery: otolaryngology.* Philadelphia: JB Lippincott Co, 1993, with permission.)

Emergencies resulting from mandibular fractures are rare. These include airway collapse due to bilateral body fractures or multisegment fractures. Management includes placement of the patient in the lateral decubitus position. An airway should be established with intubation or tracheostomy. If unable to intubate a patient with major facial fractures or suspected cervical spine injury, cricothyroidotomy is indicated, with subsequent formal tracheostomy performed in the operating room. Hemorrhage can occur secondary to laceration of the inferior alveolar artery within the mandibular canal. Tamponade is accomplished with fracture reduction. On a general note, the cricothyroidotomy procedure offers the advantage of rapid airway access with a decreased risk of thyroid hemorrhage. However, there is a greater likelihood of injury to the recurrent laryngeal nerve, which pierces the thyrohyoid membrane. In addition, there is an elevated risk of subglottic stenosis due to the proximity of the cricothyroid membrane to the vocal cords. Therefore, cricothyroidotomy should be considered only a temporizing measure until a revision tracheostomy can be performed.

Zygomatic, Maxillary, and Orbital Trauma

High-velocity blunt trauma to the head can result in fractures to the zygomatic arch, the maxilla, and the orbits. An understanding of management issues requires review of the structural support systems of the face. The middle one third of the facial skeleton consists of an intersecting system of buttresses that distribute forces generated through mastication. The vertical dimensions are maintained by the (i) nasomaxillary, (ii) zygomaticomaxillary, and (iii) pterygomaxillary buttresses. These vertical supports are interconnected via the lesser horizontal buttresses, which include the orbital rims, maxillary alveolus and palate, zygomatic process, greater wing of the sphenoid, and medial and lateral pterygoid plates. If sufficient force is directed at the anterior face, predictable patterns of structural collapse are observed.

In 1901, Rene Le Fort described these patterns, which bear his name (Fig. 26-12). Each of the three classifications involves a fracture of the pterygoid plates. The Le Fort I fracture line passes horizontally along the palate inward to the pterygoid plates. The Le Fort II fracture line incorporates the nasofrontal suture line, traverses the lamina papyracea (medial orbital wall) of the ethmoid bone, proceeds across the orbital floor, and proceeds inferiorly beneath the zygomatic arch to the palate. The Le Fort III fracture is the most serious and involves each of the three vertical buttresses, resulting in craniofacial dysjunction. The fracture line extends from the nasofrontal suture line posteriorly along the cribriform plate/anterior skull base, travels through the root of the zygoma, and disrupts the junction of pterygoid plates with skull base.

The classic finding indicative of a Le Fort fracture is a palate, which is mobile to traction. Le Fort II and III fractures are commonly associated with CSF rhinorrhea, profound epistaxis, visual loss, and upper airway obstruction necessitating tracheostomy. Nasal intubation is contraindicated secondary to risk of intracranial injury. Typically, trauma with force sufficient to produce facial fractures will

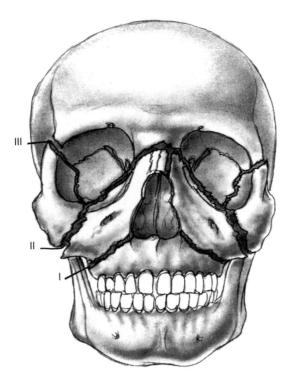

FIGURE 26-12. Le Fort fracture levels. (From Bailey BJ, ed. *Head and neck surgery: otolaryngology.* Philadelphia: JB Lippincott Co, 1993, with permission.)

result in extensive cerebral injury (52%). Most of these Le Fort fractures are managed in a delayed fashion (days) following stabilization of the patient. Poor candidates are those with Glasgow coma scale scores of less than 6, evidence of intracerebral hemorrhage, midline shift, intracerebral pressures of more than 15 mm Hg, and basal cistern effacement. Correction is directed at plating to reestablish vertical and horizontal buttresses. Common postoperative complications include malocclusion and less frequently facial asymmetry.

The *tripod fracture* is the most common fracture of the midface. The principal fracture sites include the frontozygomatic suture line, the zygomatic arch, and the maxilla extending from inferior orbital rim to palate. Posterior displacement of the complex produces a flattened appearance of the malar eminence. Compression of the infraorbital nerve produces hypesthesia in the CN V^2 distribution. The tripod fracture and isolated fractures of the zygomatic arch are easily identified with head CT scanning.

A difficult intubation occurring in the posttraumatic patient may be due to the inability to adequately open the mouth. In such instances, it is necessary to consider the possibility of a fracture to the zygomatic arch, entrapping the temporalis muscle and causing trismus. In such situations, tracheostomy or immediate reduction of the fracture is required. An incision is created posterior to the temporal hairline. The plane between the underside of the temporalis muscle and the deep temporal fascia is entered. Insertion of a Joseph elevator into this plane permits directed elevation along the medial surface of the zygomatic arch, without causing injury to the temporal branch of the facial nerve that courses directly over the zygomatic arch (Fig. 26-2). Surgical correction of the tripod fracture requires reapproximation and plating of the orbital rim, zygomatic arch, and maxilla. Stable fixation is achieved by methods that involve the use of at least one miniplate and that incorporate the frontozygomatic suture line as one of the points of fixation. Ideally, these procedures are performed within 7 to 10 days of the traumatic insult.

An additional group of facial fractures involves the orbit. The blowout fracture is caused by blunt trauma to the malar or frontal regions. Medially directed forces produce a fracture of the thin orbital floor along the infraorbital canal. Palpation along the inferior orbital rim will detect irregularity of contour, or "step off." Additional fractures are frequently observed in the medial orbital wall. Downward displacement of orbital contents into the maxilla results in enophthalmos and entrapment of the inferior rectus muscle. The extraocular muscle examination is remarkable for limitation of upward gaze. Diplopia on upward gaze is also noted. A CT scan directed at the orbits will reveal soft tissue extravasation into the maxillary or ethmoid sinus. Edema of ocular muscles due to trauma from bony spicules is also noted. The CT scan assists in identifying intraorbital free air, which suggests violation of the bony orbit. Surgical correction of orbital floor fractures requires repair, employing donor bone from anterior maxilla, with metal mesh, Teflon, or Silastic material, or with repositioned bone supported by gel film or cartilage. If orbital injury is suspected, an ophthalmology consultation is mandated to assess ocular entrapment, globe projection, and document visual acuity. Most fractures should be repaired between days 7 and 10 prior to bone fusion. However, optic nerve compression, nerve sheath hematoma, or suspected orbital hemorrhage are indications for emergent exploration. Unrecognized orbital floor fractures can result in late presentation (after 6 weeks) of enophthalmos and diplopia due to slow, inferior herniation of orbital contents. Delayed surgical correction is technically more complicated.

An additional facial injury requiring surgical repair involves the region located between the eyes, the naso-orbital-ethmoid region. The ethmoid sinus, located between the orbits, represents a delicate lattice of bones, which incorporate the medial orbital walls and floor of the anterior cranial fossa (cribriform plate). Collapse of this area can occur with posteriorly directed force applied to the bridge of the nose. Again, the CT scan is the preferred examination to assess integrity of the orbits and ethmoid sinus. Clinically, the patient has a flattened appearance of the nasal bridge. The distance between the canthi is increased (less than 35 mm is normal), as is the interpupil-

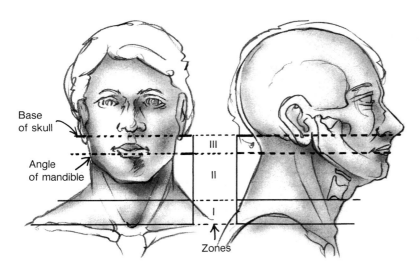

FIGURE 26-13. Anatomical zones of the neck for evaluation of penetrating trauma. (From Jurkovich GJ. The neck. In: Moore EE, ed. *Early care of the injured patient,* 4th ed. Toronto: Becker, 1990:126, with permission.)

lary distance. Telecanthus (more than 35 mm) is associated with diplopia and cosmetic defects that are extremely difficult to correct. Functionally, disruption of the attachment of the medial canthal tendons causes epiphora secondary to dysfunction of the lacrimal system. Tears normally drain via the nasolacrimal duct into the nose, where they exit beneath the anterior margin of the inferior turbinate at the valve of Hasner. If no obstruction is present, application of 2% fluorescein dye into the conjunctiva can be detected with nasal pledgets (positive Jones test results). If necessary, recanalization of the nasolacrimal duct with a Silastic stent can be performed at a later date.

Nasal Fracture

The most common trauma to facial bones involves the nose. The nasal bones are located at the insertion of the nose between the eyes. These small bones (less than 1 cm long) provide superior support for the nose. However, most structural support is provided by the bony septum, which extends from the maxilla to connect with the cartilaginous septum. Presenting symptoms may include epistaxis, which is typically self resolving. In certain instances, reduction of fractures is required for hemostasis. Simple fractures of the nasal bones are corrected by repositioning with an elevator and then placing an external nasal splint with internal nasal packs. In all cases of nasal trauma, an inspection of the nasal cavity is required to rule out septal hematoma. This bluish swelling of the midline septum represents dissection of blood between the mucoperichondrium and septal cartilage. As there is no intrinsic blood supply to the cartilage, the presence of hematoma predisposes to infection and cartilage necrosis. This combination results in delayed collapse of the nose and severe cosmetic defects. If identified, the hematoma should be evacuated and the patient placed on antibiotics. In rare instances, nasal trauma is associated with CSF rhinorrhea. In most of these patients, spontaneous resolution will occur in response to bed rest, head of bed elevation, and antibiotics.

Penetrating Trauma of the Pharynx

Penetrating trauma of the oropharynx is relatively rare in the adult population but not uncommon in the pediatric age group. Children who fall while an object is in the mouth sustain injury to the soft palate. Impalement is most dangerous when it occurs in the lateral soft palate near the course of the internal carotid artery. However, most such injuries are associated with a minimal amount of self-limited bleeding. A laceration can be sutured in the emergency room and the child can be sent home with antibiotics, if the caretaker is reliable. Altered mental status or neurological status require admission and angiography to rule out carotid injury. If the object is impaled in the oropharynx on presentation, it should not be removed. Rather, angiography followed by removal in the operating room is indicated. Rare, late sequela includes retropharyngeal hematoma particularly in patients taking aspirin or nonsteroidal antiinflammatory drugs (NSAIDS). Bleeding or infection in the area between the prevertebral fascia and the alar fascia (danger space) can extend inferiorly into the posterior mediastinum. For this reason, management includes antibiotics and cessation of medications that may inhibit hemostasis. Patients should be instructed to return to the emergency room if hoarseness, breathing difficulty, or symptoms of infection are noted.

Penetrating Trauma of the Neck

Penetrating wounds to the neck are classified according to location, and they frequently result from stab and gunshot trauma (Fig. 26-13). Three zones have been described. Zone I refers to the area from the sternal notch and clavicles inferiorly to the cricoid cartilage superiorly. At-risk structures include the great vessels, the trachea, and the lung. Zone II refers to the area between the cricoid cartilage and the angle of the mandible. It is the most commonly injured region, and at-risk structures include the carotid

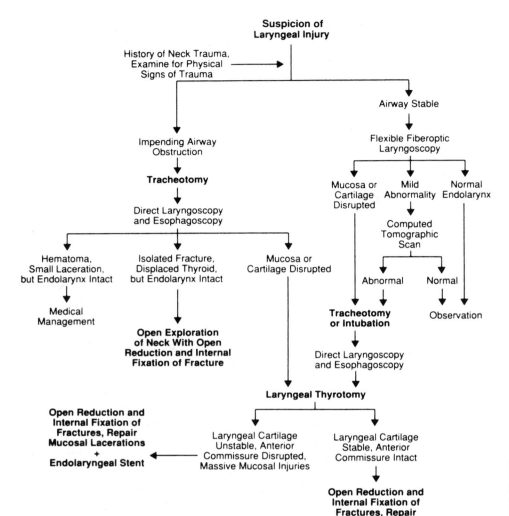

FIGURE 26-14. Management of an acute injury of the larynx. (From Schaefer SD. The treatment of acute external laryngeal injuries. *Arch Otolaryngol* 1991;117:35, with permission.)

and jugular vessels, the esophagus, and the larynx. Zone III refers to the area between the lower border of the mandible and skull base. Injury can occur to the distal carotid, pharynx, and salivary glands. Patients who present with injury to these regions should undergo physical examination, anterior-posterior (AP), chest x-ray, AP and lateral neck x-ray, and presumptive airway control test. Physical signs of injury may include bleeding/hematoma, dyspnea, hoarseness, stridor, subcutaneous emphysema, dysphagia or odynophagia, and hematemesis or neurological deficit.

Any hemodynamically or neurologically unstable patient with zone I, II, or III injury requires emergency operative control, which may include sternotomy and craniotomy. Management of the stable but symptomatic patient is dependent on the zone involved. Therefore, in the symptomatic but stable patient with penetrating injuries to zones I and III, angiography is indicated with formal surgical exploration if positive for vascular injury. Angiography possesses a diagnostic sensitivity of 97% and a specificity of 90% for vascular injury in these three regions. Zone II injury in the symptomatic but stable patient requires direct transport to the operating room for formal exploration. In the asymptomatic patient, zone II and III injuries can be observed. However, zone I injuries still require angiography. For zone I wounds on the left, excellent proximal control can be achieved with a left anterior thoracotomy. Aneurysm, arterial rupture, and thrombosis are the most common immediate complications of zone I to III vascular injuries. The most common delayed complication is formation of arteriovenous fistulae.

Additional considerations involve the management of the esophagus. In zone I to III traumas, the most commonly missed injuries are those to the esophagus. In patients with stable cervical spines, esophageal injury should be evaluated. Rigid esophagoscopy is 100% successful in identifying cervical esophageal injuries. Single-layer closure, external drainage, and prolonged *nil per os* status have been associated with minimal risk of esophageal leak. Modified barium swallow examination is recommended before initiation of oral intake in patients with suspected or documented esophageal injury.

Laryngeal Trauma

Laryngeal injury should be considered in all patients sustaining blunt or sharp trauma to the neck (Fig. 26-14). Signs of acute trauma include voice change, stridor, respiratory distress, dysphagia, odynophagia, and hemoptysis. Physical examination may reveal edema, subcutaneous emphysema, hematoma, ecchymosis, loss of thyroid cartilage prominence, or palpable thyroid fracture. Initial management consists of securing an adequate airway. When laryngeal or tracheal injury is apparent and airway compromise is imminent, a controlled tracheostomy should be performed. Ideally, the trachea is entered below the cricoid cartilage with a vertically oriented incision through tracheal rings 3 and 4. A cricothyroidotomy (access through the cricothyroid membrane) should not be used because of potential injury to the larynx and upper trachea. Oral endotracheal intubation is not recommended because additional iatrogenic trauma may result. The next steps in management by the acute trauma life support (ATLS) protocol include cardiopulmonary resuscitation, control of hemorrhage, stabilization of neural and spinal injuries, and systemic evaluation of injury to other organ systems.

In cases where trauma has occurred but the airway is stable, the mainstay of treatment includes flexible fiberoptic laryngoscopy to assess vocal cord motion, integrity of mucosa, and evidence for subglottic swelling, ecchymosis, or hematoma. In the absence of obvious injury, management should include elevation of the head of bed, humidified oxygen, and steroids. If there is evidence of mucosal or cartilage disruption, a tracheostomy is performed emergently, as the stable airway can be lost rapidly with progression of edema. Most mucosal lacerations can be expected to heal primarily. Tears of the anterior commissure (anterior junction of right and left true vocal cords) will require operative reapproximation. Following stabilization of the airway, a CT scan is obtained to identify fracture of the thyroid and cricoid cartilages. If a fracture is present, open exploration of the neck is performed with reduction and internal fixation, employing nonabsorbable suture, wires, or microplates. Small fragments of cartilage with no intact perichondrium should be removed to prevent subsequent chondritis. Endolaryngeal stents for 4 to 6 weeks may be required if the cricoid ring is unstable.

Facial Nerve Injury

Injury to CN VII frequently accompanies trauma to the head. The portion of the facial nerve proximal to the stylomastoid foramen is composed of motor, sensory, and autonomic fibers. The nerve is divided into the meatal, labyrinthine, tympanic, and mastoid segments. In addition, the extratemporal portion exists on the stylomastoid foramen and is composed almost entirely of motor fibers. The nerve courses posteriorly around the angle of the mandible and enters the parotid gland. There, the nerve divides into a superior and an inferior segment prior to dividing into five divisions referred to as the "pes anserinus": (i) temporal, (ii) zygomatic, (iii) buccal, (iv) marginal mandibular, and (v) cervical (Fig. 26-2). All head trauma patients should undergo full CN evaluation. With respect to the facial nerve, each subdivision should be evaluated.

Penetrating trauma to the face that results in loss of facial nerve function may be repaired surgically if the injury is proximal to the lateral canthus. Distal to this point, nerve fibers are too narrow to be surgically approximated. Extensive arborization between buccal and zygomatic branches

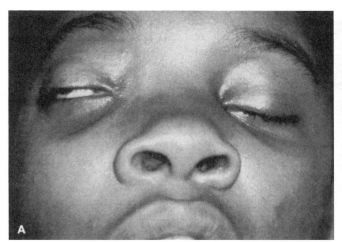
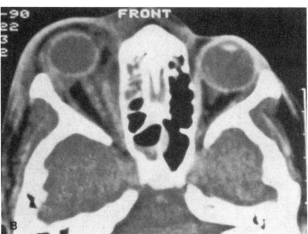

FIGURE 26-15. A: Patient with asymmetric proptosis secondary to a subperiosteal abscess. **B:** Axial computed tomography scan of the same patient. (From Bailey BJ, ed. *Head and neck surgery: otolaryngology.* Philadelphia: JB Lippincott Co, 1993, with permission.)

limits paresis affecting these divisions and regeneration will occur spontaneously within 4 months. Prior to wound closure, a nerve stimulator can be employed to test exposed nerve fibers. Intraoperative stimulation suggests that nerve recovery will occur, despite absence of volitional movement. After 72 hours, identification of segments distal to the transection point is more difficult because distal nerve branches are no longer able to be stimulated. If sections of the facial nerve are missing, exposed segments should be tagged with metal clips for later identification. Interposition grafting using the greater auricular nerve or sural nerve can be performed at the time of exploration or at a later date. If larger segments are absent, some innervation can be restored with the hypoglossal facial nerve anastomosis (XII to VII) or the cross-facial nerve (VII-to-VII) technique. Both procedures result in synkinesis and limited movement. However, tone is preserved and muscle atrophy avoided. Nerve recovery times are on the order of 6 to 18 months. Shorter times are required with injury to more distal segments.

Electromyography can detect asymmetry in the activation of right- and left-sided mimetic muscles. Additional information is gained from analysis of electrical activity patterns. The presence of fibrillation potentials indicates degeneration of the muscle nerve supply and diminished possibility of spontaneous nerve recovery while the presence of polyphasic motor units indicates that regenerative processes are occurring. Aside from cosmetic asymmetry, facial nerve paresis is concerning for potential corneal desiccation due to incomplete eye closure. This problem can be addressed with lubricants, surgical implantation of upper-lid gold weights to assist closure or lid-shortening procedures to prevent lagophthalmos. In cases of permanent nerve injury, additional surgical suspension procedures are available to address function of the oral commissure and closure of the eye.

Salivary Gland Trauma

Injury to the salivary gland may be blunt, lacerating, intraoral, or extraoral. Of the glands, the parotid is the most commonly injured. Lacerations of the face, posterior to the anterior margin of the masseter muscle, may injure the parotid (Stensen) duct. Unrecognized injury is associated with weakness of midface musculature and swelling secondary to sialocele. The injury site can be identified by cannulating the duct intraorally through the orifice located adjacent to the second upper molar. Edges can be reapproximated over the catheter, which remains in place for 2 weeks. Postoperative stenosis of the duct may require dilation with ophthalmic lacrimal probes. Similarly, lacerations to the Wharton duct of the submandibular gland can be repaired primarily. Smaller lacerations to salivary gland parenchyma can be repaired with careful closure of the gland capsule. The principal late complication of salivary gland trauma is the recurrent sialocele or salivary cyst. Management includes aspiration and in rare cases introduction of a scarifying agent. Persistent collections are best addressed by gland excision. Ample production of saliva by the remaining glands minimizes the impact of resection of any one gland.

ANATOMY OF THE NOSE AND SINUS

The external nose consists of a bony skeleton limited to the upper one third of the nose and a cartilaginous skeleton present in the lower two thirds. The internal nose is divided by the septum, which is composed of four structures, the perpendicular plate of the ethmoid, the vomer, the quadrilateral cartilage, and the membranous septum. The term *deviated septum* refers to folding or bending of the quadrilateral cartilage. An asymptomatic deviation is present in most individuals. In severe instances where unilateral nasal obstruction is present, the cartilage can be excised, trimmed, reshaped, and replaced to increase air flow. For cosmetic indications, manipulations of the upper and lower lateral cartilages form the basis of most rhinoplasty procedures.

Four paired sinus groups are continuous with the nasal cavity. All sinuses begin development *in utero,* however, adult dimensions are not attained until late adolescence. Each sinus produces mucus, which serves to warm and humidify inspired air, as well as to trap inspired allergens or fine particulate matter. The maxillary sinuses develop beneath the orbits, the frontal sinuses are anterosuperior to the orbits, and the sphenoid sinuses are midline and posterior to the orbits. The ethmoid sinuses consist of two groups of eight to twelve cells located between the orbits. The inferior, middle, and superior turbinates represent the terminal extensions of bony lamellae, which traverse the ethmoid region. These turbinates project into the right and left nasal cavities and direct air flow and mucus posteriorly into the nasopharynx. Beating of cilia directs mucus to natural openings (ostia) located in each sinus.

Paranasal Sinus Infections

Most complaints related to the nasal cavity concerns symptoms of sinus disease. In response to allergic challenge, immune-mediated edema of mucous membranes can develop. Patients report classic hay-fever symptoms, such as dry, itchy, or watery eyes. Obstruction of mucous drainage from the sinus produces the symptoms of "pressure headache." Prolonged stasis of mucus can lead to bacterial overgrowth, resulting in sinusitis with pain, fever, sinus tenderness, purulent exudate, and occasional facial cellulitis. Persistent sinus infections cause reactive polyp formation from mucosa, further exacerbating obstruction. Additional anatomical etiologies of obstruction include deviation of septum and enlarged or deviated turbinates. All of these anomalies can predispose an individual to develop sinus disease. First-line therapy involves topical nasal steroid spray, antihistamines, and antibiotics. In patients who have failed conservative management, endoscopic sinus surgery is performed to enlarge natural openings and to resect areas of obstructing bony overgrowth. In this manner, egress of mucus from the sinus is improved. Over 90% of patients with sinusitis report significant improvement following sinus surgery.

Sinoorbital Infections

The most serious complications of sinus infections involve spread to the orbits and potential for spread to the CNS. The ethmoid sinus are the most frequent source of these infections. Typically, an indolent sinus infection suddenly develops into a more serious process involving the orbits. For unknown reasons, teenage boys have the greatest risk for developing serious sinus infections progressing to orbital cellulitis (Fig. 26-15).

Five stages of orbital cellulitis have been described: (i) periorbital cellulitis (inflammation limited to the eyelids), (ii) subperiosteal abscess (collection between the bony wall of the orbit and periorbita, with proptosis and restricted extraocular muscle activity), (iii) orbital cellulitis (retrobulbar inflammation and decreased vision), (iv) orbital abscess (more severe proptosis and visual loss), and (v) cavernous sinus thrombosis (CN III, IV, and V palsies and meningitis). Patients with periorbital cellulitis can be managed with broad-spectrum intravenous antibiotics. More advanced stages with abscess formation require surgical drainage and opening of involved sinus. An ophthalmology consultation is required to document any progression of visual compromise or ocular muscle entrapment, which would prompt surgical intervention. Typically, the procedure involves resection of ethmoid contents to promote drainage. Either the endoscopic (internal) or external approach would be employed. In the presence of orbital abscesses, ethmoidectomy with partial resection of medial orbital wall is advised.

Epistaxis

Epistaxis represents a potentially serious medical emergency. Any individual called to manage the bleeding patient should have an algorithm for management. Initial questions should address hemodynamic stability of the patient. Airway safety should be established and suctioning equipment should be at the bedside, as aspiration of blood with subsequent clotting can cause obstruction. Information regarding prescription and nonprescription medications (Coumadin, aspirin, NSAIDs, cocaine), history of hypertension, constipation, myelodysplasias, known coagulopathy, hemodialysis, hepatic disease, prior bleeding episodes, and recent trauma should be elicited. Duration and quantity of bleeding, as well as unilateral versus bilateral nature should be determined. Most bleeding originates from one side. (However, after flowing posteriorly, blood may be regurgitated from the contralateral nares.) Pharmacologic control of blood pressure should be initiated in the hypertensive patient. Intravenous access should be established if there is evidence of significant epistaxis or hemodynamic instability. Laboratory studies including complete blood count and prothrombin time and partial thromboplastin time tests should be ordered. In the presence of significant bleeding with anemia, blood products should be available, particularly in the elderly patient.

Identification of the source of bleeding may require intranasal examination. The great majority of bleeding episodes (>90%) arise from a rich confluence of blood vessels located bilaterally at the anterior septum. Branches of the sphenopalatine artery, the descending palatine artery, the ophthalmic artery, and the facial artery anastomose to form Kiesselbach plexus (the area of Little). Posterior bleeds are seen in patients with significant history of arteriosclerosis. The sphenopalatine artery is the most frequent source of posterior bleeding.

In the absence of trauma, conservative hemostatic measures can be tried initially and include pressure and ice to the bridge of the nose, control of hypertension, and correction of coagulopathy. All clots should be evacuated from the nasal cavity. Endoscopic inspection may identify a superficial source of bleeding, which can be cauterized with silver nitrate. Alternatively, a posterior bleed can be addressed with a sphenopalatine block, which causes vasoconstriction of the sphenopalatine artery. With heavy bleeding, anterior packing may be required. Nonabsorbable packs are used in most patients and withdrawn in 72 hours. In the coagulopathic patient (leukemia or valve patient on heparin or Coumadin), an absorbable material should be considered to minimize trauma to mucosal surfaces. For more severe bleeding, a Foley catheter is inflated in the nasopharynx and drawn forward to occlude the choana. Packing is then placed in the anterior nasal cavity and secured.

In the extreme case, transnasal surgical ligation of the internal maxillary artery or surgical ligation of the anterior or posterior ethmoid arteries may be required. Preoperative angiography and embolization may be helpful in identifying and controlling bleeding. Patients with nasal packing should receive appropriate antibiotics for *S. aureus* to prevent toxic shock syndrome, which has been reported. Special consideration is required in the trauma patient. CT scans should be obtained to identify facial fractures, which can be distracted further with aggressive nasal packing.

SUGGESTED READING

Bailey BJ, ed. *Head and neck surgery: otolaryngology.* Philadelphia: JB Lippincott Co, 1993.
Cummings CW, ed. *Otolaryngology: head and neck surgery,* 3rd ed. St. Louis: Mosby–Year Book, 1997.
Lee KJ, ed. *Essential otolaryngology,* 6th ed. New York: Medical Examination Publishing Co, 1997.
Paparella MM, Shumrick DA, Gluckman JL, et al., eds. *Otolaryngology.* Philadelphia: WB Saunders, 1991.

27

ORTHOPEDIC SURGERY

GEROGE YEH AND JOHN L. ESTERHAI, JR.

The evaluation and treatment of the trauma patient demands a large amount of overlap between the role of the trauma surgeon and that of the orthopedic surgeon. Patients can present with multiple musculoskeletal injuries, and the rapid assessment, diagnosis, and provisional treatment by the trauma team can prevent permanent neuromuscular disability and even death. To fully understand the theories of orthopedic fracture management, it is essential to understand the biologic and biomechanical basis of bone formation, bone injury, and fracture repair. After a discussion of orthopedic basic science, this chapter will review the principles of emergency management of orthopedic trauma as well as the diagnosis and treatment of specific injuries.

ORTHOPEDIC SURGERY BASIC SCIENCE

Bone Structure and Formation

The long bone is divided into the epiphysis, metaphysis, and diaphysis (Fig. 27-1). Bone formation consists of a combination of two *microscopic forms,* lamellar and woven bone. *Woven bone* (primary bone) is most abundant in the newborn and in the metaphyses of growing bone. It is composed of a randomly distributed collagen matrix and has a high cell count. *Lamellar bone* (mature bone) largely replaces woven bone as a person matures and consists of a highly organized collagen matrix in which the fibers are commonly distributed parallel to the direction of force application.

The two main *gross structural patterns* of bone formation are trabecular and cortical bone. *Trabecular bone* (also known as "cancellous" or "spongy" bone) is most abundant in the epiphysis and metaphysis and consists of a branching lattice pattern (Fig. 27-1). Trabecular bone has a much higher turnover rate but is significantly less dense than cortical bone. Cortical bone is most common in the diaphysis (midshaft) of long bones and consists largely of lamellar bone that is well suited for the rotational and compressive forces most common in this area. Cortical bone is most commonly arranged in osteon units, which are comprised of haversian canals (vascular channels) surrounded by lamellar bone (Fig. 27-2).

The major cell types of bone are the osteoblasts, osteocytes, and osteoclasts. *Osteoblasts* are involved in the formation of bone and line trabecular bone as well as the Volkmann canals and canaliculi of cortical bone. Osteoblasts, which are derived from undifferentiated mesenchymal cells, are the primary responders to extracellular signals such as bone morphogenic protein (BMP), parathyroid hormone (PTH), $1,25(OH)_2D$, and glucocorticoids. Once bone is mineralized with hydroxyapatite crystals and osteoblasts are surrounded by bony matrix, the intracellular makeup of the osteoblast changes, and the cells are now termed "osteocytes." *Osteocytes,* which are embedded within the bone in lacunae and are arranged concentrically around the center of the osteon, are thought to be important in bone mineral exchange processes and in communicating messages to other cells through cell processes in the haversian canalicular system in response to strains and stresses on bone. *Osteoclasts,* which lie in bony pits known as Howship lacunae, are multinucleated giant cells derived from *hemopoietic* macrophage precursors. They are involved in bone resorption. Bone remodeling consists of a highly organized interaction of osteoblasts and osteoclasts (Fig. 27-3).

Bone is composed of 60% to 70% inorganic tissue, 5% to 8% water, and organic tissue. The inorganic tissue is largely *hydroxyapatite crystals,* which mainly consist of calcium phosphate salts. The organic bone matrix undergoes mineralization with these salts and provides extra strength and support to the bone structure. The organic phase of bone is composed chiefly of *type I collagen* and matrix proteins such as osteocalcin and osteonectin. The long linear collagen molecules associate in a staggered array to produce large collagen fibrils. As described earlier (Chapter 6), collagen is then organized into either the parallel fibers of lamellar bone or the random arrangement of woven bone.

The bone *blood supply* consists of three systems: diaphyseal, metaphyseal, and periosteal. The diaphysis is supplied by a variable number of nutrient arteries that enter the bone

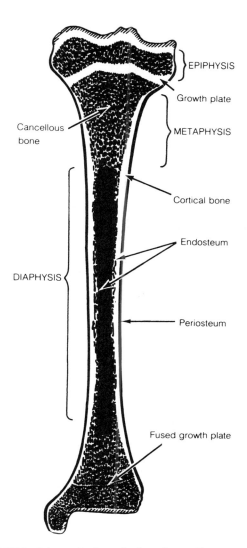

FIGURE 27-1. Schematic view of a long bone. The growth plate (physis) is present only in the growing child. (From Favus MJ, et al., eds. *Primer on the metabolic bone diseases and disorders of mineral metabolism,* 4th ed. Philadelphia: Lippincott Williams & Wilkins, 1999:3, with permission.)

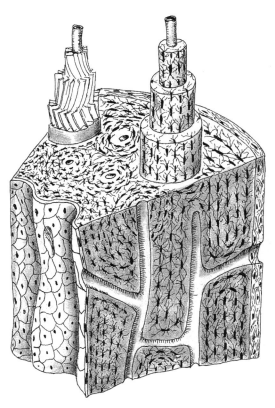

FIGURE 27-2. Cortical bone consists of cylindrical haversian systems oriented parallel along the shafts of long bones. (From Vigorita VJ. *Orthopaedic pathology.* Philadelphia: Lippincott Williams & Wilkins, 1999:37, with permission.)

through foramina and branch into a vast network of intraosseous arterioles. The metaphyseal regions are supplied by a periarticular or geniculate complex that penetrates the bone. Finally, the outer 15% to 20% of cortical bone, the periosteal tissue, and muscular attachments to the bone are supplied by a periosteal capillary system. These three systems are ultimately interconnected, and the intermediate watershed areas become very important in situations in which one vascular system is insufficient (such as when the bone is fractured).

Bone is formed by either *intramembranous ossification* or *endochondral ossification*. During intramembranous ossification, seen during the development of the skull, maxilla, mandible, and clavicle, the bony trabecula is laid down directly by the mesenchymal cells. In endochondral ossification, which is responsible for interstitial (lengthwise) growth of the bone, an initial cartilaginous framework is followed by bony deposition and cartilage resorption. Active growth occurs at the epiphysis, which is separated from the metaphysis by the cartilaginous growth plate (physis) in the growing child. Once the skeleton reaches maturity, the growth plate closes and the epiphysis fuses with the metaphysis (Fig. 27-1).

Bone formation is dependent on *calcium metabolism,* which is finely balanced by the kidney, osteoclasts, osteoblasts, PTH, vitamin D, and calcitonin. Calcium is absorbed from the duodenum (regulated by $1,25(OH)_2D$, which is activated in both the kidney and liver) and by passive diffusion through the jejunum. PTH, secreted by the chief cells of the parathyroid glands, stimulates an increase in serum calcium level by stimulating absorption and activation of vitamin D, promoting urinary excretion of phosphate and stimulating osteoclastic resorption of bone. Calcitonin, secreted by the parafollicular cells of the thyroid in response to elevated calcium levels, inhibits osteoclast resorption and thus lowers serum calcium levels.

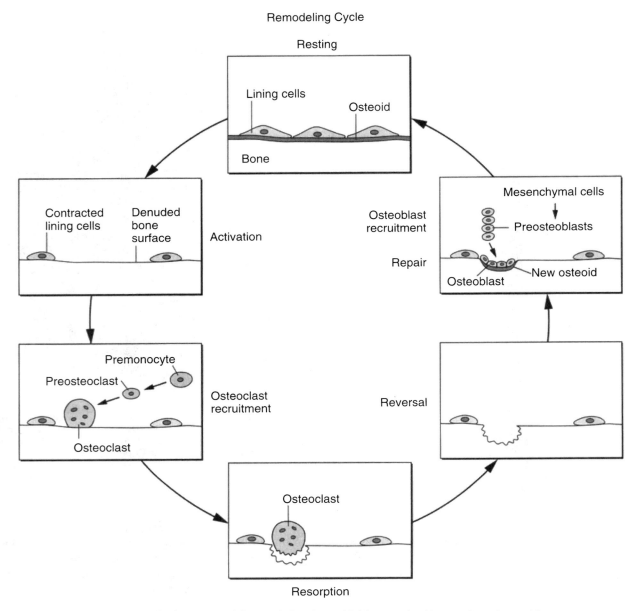

FIGURE 27-3. The bone remodeling cycle involves a highly organized interaction of osteoblasts and osteoclasts. (From Vigorita VJ. *Orthopaedic pathology.* Philadelphia: Lippincott Williams & Wilkins, 1999:32, with permission.)

Biomechanics and Patterns of Fractures

A bone fractures when it is overloaded, as a result of either abnormal stresses on normal bone or normal stresses on abnormal bone (which results in a pathologic fracture). As bone absorbs more kinetic energy (kinetic energy = $\frac{1}{2}$ mass × velocity^2) from a traumatic insult, it is forced to release the energy it can not sustain by undergoing structural change. Greater injury is consequently caused by objects or stresses with a higher mass or velocity. The fracture patterns will vary depending on the severity of the force, the direction of the force, and the age of the patient. The fracture can be simple (one fracture line) or comminuted (more than two fragments). Bending forces place tensile stresses on bone, which is poorly tolerated compared to compressive forces. Uneven bending forces can cause an oblique fracture while pure bending forces result in transverse fracture formation. Torsional and rotatory forces cause *spiral fractures* (Fig. 27-4), in which the oblique fracture line circles longitudinally along part of the length of the bone. A combination of bending and compressive forces can result in *butterfly fractures* (formation of three segments). Severely comminuted fractures, which involve destruction of bone

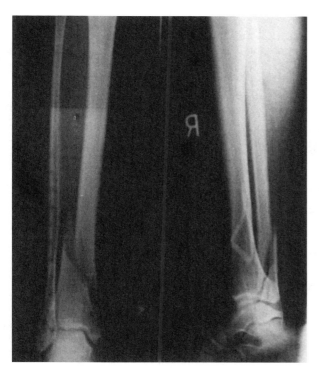

FIGURE 27-4. Spiral fracture of the distal tibia. Note the accompanying fibula fracture. (From Rockwood CA Jr, et al., eds. *Rockwood and Green's fractures in adults,* 4th ed. Philadelphia: Lippincott-Raven Publishers, 1996:2135, with permission.)

into multiple small pieces, can result from a severe crush injury by heavy machinery or high-velocity motor vehicle accident. *Compression fractures* occur in trabecular bone and are common in osteopenic vertebrae. In the *open fracture,* which usually signifies a higher energy injury, there is communication between the fracture and the outside environment. The size of the skin laceration can range from a pinprick-size puncture to a grossly contaminated degloving injury.

Repetitive trauma over time results in *stress fractures* of cortical bone such as a long-distance runner developing a stress fracture of the metatarsi. With increased load over time, the stiffness and strength of the bone decrease, and microfractures develop. Although microfractures do not easily progress to complete full-thickness fractures, with continued fatigue, they become so numerous that a complete fracture is inevitable.

Because of the thicker periosteum and the open growth plates, children are susceptible to two unique fracture patterns. In the *greenstick fracture,* there is an incomplete fracture because a significant portion of the thick periosteum usually remains intact on the concave (compression) side of the injury (Fig. 27-5). *Physeal injuries* occur when the fracture involves the epiphysis or the physis (growth plate). These injuries can be devastating if growth plate arrest occurs.

Bone and Fracture Healing

Fractures caused by increased energy generally heal with greater incidence of complications than fractures produced by less stress. Fracture healing is completed in five stages (Fig. 27-6): (i) *Induction* involves fracture hematoma development and proceeds with local bone necrosis and the release of factors that attract inflammatory cells. (ii) *Inflammation* involves the migration of polymorphonuclear neutrophils, macrophages, and other inflammatory cells to the fracture site and the eventual initiation of bone and cartilage formation with fibroblast recruitment. (iii) In the *soft callus stage,* which can be seen by 2 weeks, bone and cartilage formation continues until fracture motion is significantly limited and involves subperiosteal bone formation at the fracture ends. By 4 weeks, there is a significant increase in the stiffness of the healing bone. (iv) The *hard callus stage* involves conversion of the soft callus to hard woven bone by endochondral ossification. At this point, there is a gradual disappearance of the radiolucent line, signifying radiographic healing. (v) *Bone remodeling,* the final

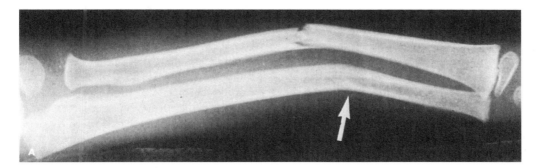

FIGURE 27-5. Greenstick fracture of the forearm in a child. Note that the radial cortex is completely fractured while the ulnar cortex is still intact. (From Rockwood CA Jr, et al., eds. *Rockwood and Green's fractures in children,* 4th ed. Philadelphia: Lippincott-Raven Publishers, 1996:28, with permission.)

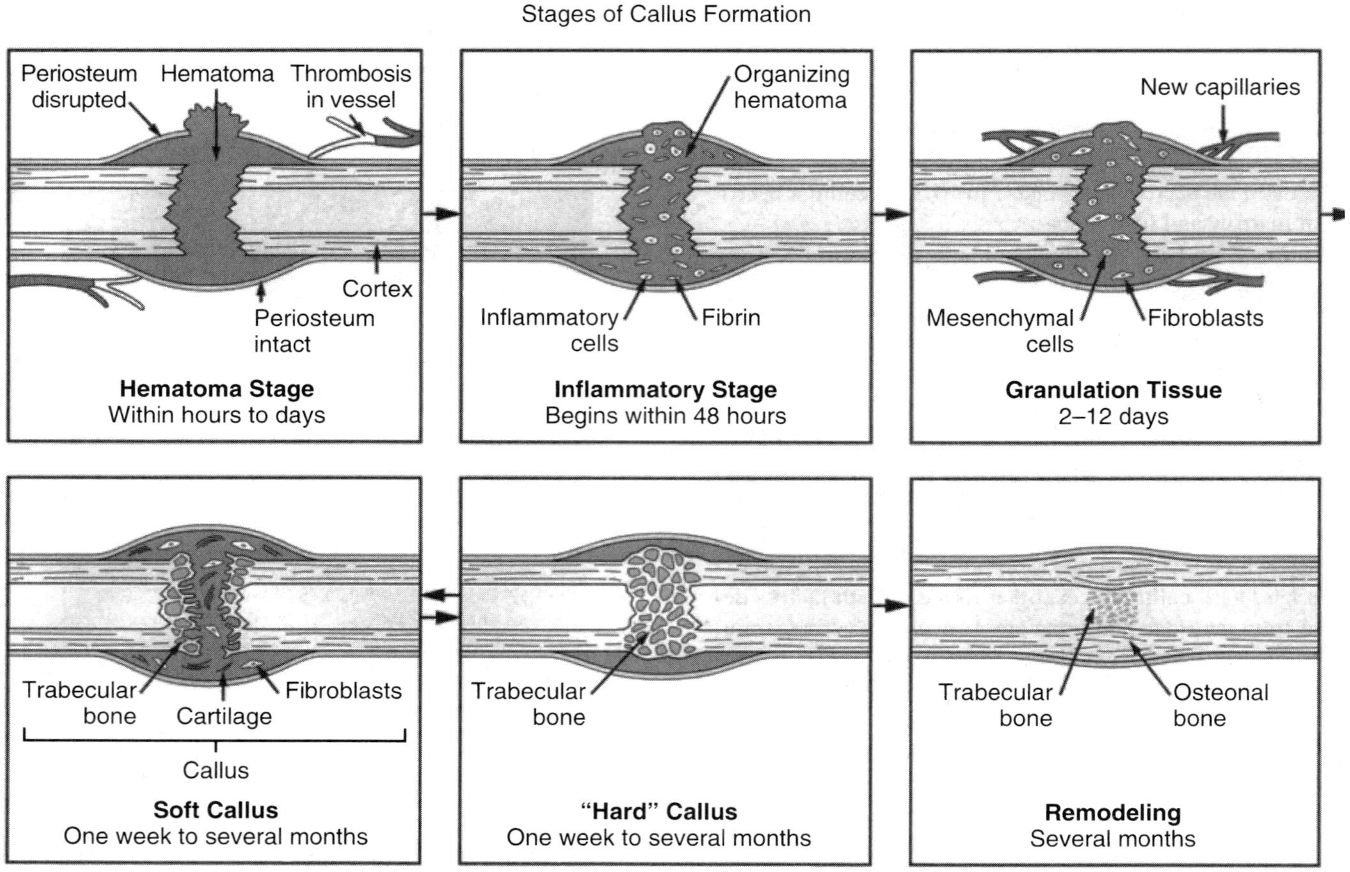

FIGURE 27-6. Stages of fracture healing. (From Vigorita VJ. *Orthopaedic pathology.* Philadelphia: Lippincott Williams & Wilkins, 1999:87, with permission.)

stage, refers to the eventual replacement of woven bone with structurally stronger lamellar bone and is guided by the *law of Wolff* (which states that bone formation and resorption is influenced by mechanical stresses on the bone). Remodeling can be fast and extensive in the child due to the higher osteogenic potential, but in the adult, it can take many years.

For the first several hours to days after the fracture, the vascular supply to the bone is decreased due to the initial trauma and to small vessel disruption. After this point, vascular supply increases to supernormal levels until approximately 12 weeks postfracture when it returns to prefracture levels. Disruption of the medullary blood supply by the insertion of an intramedullary rod or disruption of the periosteal blood supply by periosteal stripping during surgical fixation may delay bone healing.

Bone growth factors have recently been discovered to play an important role in normal fracture healing and therapy for poorly healing fractures. *BMP* has been shown to induce bone formation by causing transformation of mesenchymal cells into osteoblasts. BMP-3, which is also known as "osteogen," is particularly effective in promoting this transformation and is now being studied for potential therapeutic use. Other factors important in fracture as well as wound healing are insulinlike growth factor-I and -II, transforming growth factor-β, and platelet-derived growth factor (Chapter 6).

A *nonunion* is defined as a fracture that has not healed in a 6-month period. Several factors that increase the risk of nonunion fractures include systemic states such as poor nutritional status and tobacco use, as well as local determinants such as soft tissue trauma, bone loss, infection, vascular injury, and insufficient stabilization. Nonunion occurs in three varieties: (i) atrophic, characterized by little or no callus formation because of poor vascularity; (ii) hypertrophic, characterized by lack of union despite rich vascularity and the formation of a large amount of callus; and (iii) pseudoarthrosis, characterized by jointlike synovial tissue surrounding the unhealed ends.

Treatment of the nonunion fracture involves open resection of interposed fibrous or synovial tissue, reduction of the fracture, and rigid fixation. Autogenous iliac crest bone graft is often used, along with recombinant BMP in certain circumstances, to increase healing of nonunions. An alternative or adjunct to surgery is the use of electrical or ultrasound stimulation for healing of a nonunion fracture. The electrical current may function by stimulating cyclic adenosine monophosphate and angiogenesis while encouraging fibrocartilage calcification. It may also alter the ionic status of the bone.

Bone grafting promotes osteogenesis and structural support. The bone graft mainly serves as a framework for chondrocytes and angiogenic cells (*osteoconduction*). With osteoinduction by bone growth factors, the bone graft is eventually incorporated into native bone by the transformation of local mesenchymal cells to osteogenic cells and remodeling of the graft.

The bone graft can be harvested from either cortical or cancellous bone. Cortical grafts are used in situations in which structural support is needed. However, because significant resorption occurs before incorporation, osteogenesis, mineralization, and vascular supply are established, cortical bone grafts take longer to incorporate than cancellous grafts. Cancellous bone is commonly used for grafting nonunions and filling cavitary defects because it is quickly remodeled and incorporated due to the increased surface area of this bone.

Autograft, most commonly harvested from the iliac crest, is the gold standard because it is both osteoinductive and osteoconductive. Allograft can also be used, but processes such as freeze-drying decrease the osteoinductive factors. Allograft is often freeze-dried, stored at −70°C, and sterilized by gamma irradiation or ethanol. Protection against human immunodeficiency virus-1 (HIV-1) and hepatitis is effectively ensured by careful screening of donors. Fresh allografts, which are used mostly for replacement of damaged articular cartilage, must be used within 12 to 24 hours to preserve the viability of chondrocytes. Bone graft substitutes such as coral have been developed and primarily consist of ceramics, which serve in an osteoconductive role as a framework for new bone formation. They lack the osteoinductive factors that induce the transformation of mesenchymal cells to osteogenic cells. Recombinant BMP may soon be available commercially to provide the osteoinductive signaling that the bone graft substitutes lack.

Articular Cartilage

Composed of *hyaline cartilage,* articular cartilage provides joints with the characteristics of remarkably decreased friction, excellent lubrication, and shock absorption. It consists of chondrocytes (10% dry weight), proteoglycans (40% dry weight), collagen (50% dry weight), and water (65% to 80% of the wet weight of the cartilage). Chondrocytes are highly differentiated cells that maintain the extracellular matrix (ECM), and that respond to biochemical signaling and biomechanical forces to adapt cartilage structurally to the local and systemic environment. Chondrocytes are also responsible for producing collagen and proteoglycans.

The predominant type of collagen in articular cartilage is type II, which consists of three identical alpha chain proteins formed into a triple helix. These small type II helices interact and eventually form large fibrils that are the functional molecules of active cartilage. The collagen in cartilage is organized in a cross-linked network, which is thought to provide tensile strength to the articular cartilage.

Proteoglycans consist of a large protein core to which are attached 1 to 150 carbohydrate side chains known as "glycosaminoglycans" (GAGs). Most GAGs in articular cartilage are either chondroitin sulfates (most common) or keratan sulfates. Most of the proteoglycans in articular cartilage are long and complex, termed *aggrecans*, and as many as 200 of these are in turn linked to another carbohydrate molecule, hyaluronate, creating even larger proteoglycans (Chapter 6) The structure of the ECM is strongly dictated by the interactions between the large proteoglycan molecules. By interacting with collagen in a porous-permeable collagen-proteoglycan solid matrix, proteoglycans help to provide the articular cartilage with structural rigidity.

Blood vessels do not pass the *tide mark,* which is the area separating the articular cartilage from the subchondral bone. As a result of this arrangement, *articular cartilage* receives minimal to no blood supply. Cartilage receives its nutrients from the circulating milieu of synovial fluid that surrounds the joint space. Immobilization of a joint for an extended time results in decreased proteoglycan content of the ECM, causing increased fluid flow, deformation of the cartilage, and decreased load-carrying capacity. These changes probably result from decreased circulation of synovial fluid in an immobile joint.

A laceration of the cartilage above the tide mark does not result in the formation of a fibrin clot because there is no blood supply to the tissue. Because there are no mobile undifferentiated cells, minimal tissue replacement occurs by chondrocytes, and the nonhealing injury gap remains in the cartilage for the lifetime of the patient. In addition, softening of the cartilage around the injury creates more surface gaps, and intermittent sloughing of surrounding cartilage leads to the eventual complete wear down to subchondral bone. Lacerations extending into the subchondral bone beyond the tide mark results in bleeding into the cartilage and formation of a fibrin clot. This allows access of undifferentiated cells and materials necessary for healing. However, much of the new cartilage formation is fibrocartilage, instead of hyaline cartilage. Nevertheless, the repair of cartilage even after these injuries is rarely complete because collagen is not deposited in its original ordered configuration and the cartilage rapidly loses elasticity with abnormal increases in permeability.

Osteoarthritis (OA) is a disease that involves the destruction of articular cartilage and changes in bone structure. In OA, the cartilage undergoes a sequence of fibrillation, extreme fissuring of the tissue, and finally a total loss of cartilage with exposure of the subchondral bone. Underlying bony changes include the formation of bone cysts, sclerotic bone formation, extraosseous deposition of collagen, and osteophyte formation. Loss of cartilage from OA is associated with a substantially diminished amount of proteoglycans (particularly keratan sulfate), which is directly proportional to the severity of the disease. The poor healing capacity of the cartilage explains the high incidence of post-traumatic arthritis after intraarticular fractures.

Muscle

The most basic unit of muscle is the myofibril, which is composed of an organized matrix of actin and myosin. Several myofibrils associate to make up a multinucleated cell, the muscle fiber. The muscle fiber is enclosed by the connective tissue endomysium, and several fibers join to form the most basic unit of muscle visible to eye, the fascicle. Fascicles are surrounded by perimysium and are organized into various arrangements. They combine to form muscle, which is covered by a layer of epimysium (Fig. 27-7). Muscles originate in bone or cartilage and have tendinous insertions.

Each myofibril is made up of *actin thin filaments* and *myosin thick filaments* organized into the basic muscle unit, the sarcomere (Fig. 27-8). Actin is associated with tropomyosin and troponin molecules. Binding of calcium to troponin leads to the uncoupling of the troponin-tropomyosin complex from actin thin filaments and allows myosin cross bridges to interact with actin. Cleavage of phosphate from adenosine triphosphate attached to myosin results in conformational change of myosin cross bridges, which brings about sarcomere and associated fiber shortening. If enough fibers decrease in length, the entire muscle undergoes contraction.

The stimulus for muscle contraction is signaled by the nerve fibers that branch to supply several fibers. The combination of a nerve terminal and its muscle fiber is termed a "motor unit." In muscles used for fine movement, each

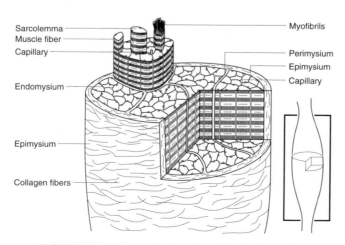

FIGURE 27-7. Schematic drawing of skeletal muscle.

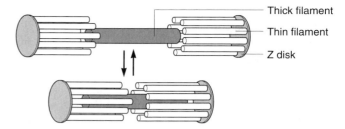

FIGURE 27-8. The sarcomere is made up of actin thin filaments and myosin thick filaments. When the muscle contracts, the actin and myosin filaments slide past one another.

axon innervates few fibers so that differential signals can be sent to several parts of the muscle for finely controlled movement. Few motor units are recruited at one time in the small muscles responsible for fine movements. In contrast, muscles used for gross movements, usually the larger muscles, have innervation of many motor units by several branches of one axon because differential control is unnecessary. In addition, near full recruitment of fibers is carried out for optimal force production.

Each nerve terminal releases acetylcholine upon stimulation by an action potential. The acetylcholine crosses the synaptic cleft and binds to acetylcholine receptors, which allows depolarizing currents to enter the cell. As an action potential is conducted down the muscle fiber cytoplasm (sarcoplasm), the sarcoplasmic reticulum is depolarized, resulting in intracellular calcium release from the sarcoplasmic reticulum. The calcium, which is integral in muscle contraction, binds to troponin, thus allowing myosin/actin interaction. Several pharmacological agents including tubocurarine (inhibitory agent) and succinylcholine (depolarizing agent) act on the acetylcholine receptor and induce paralysis (Chapter 8)

Muscle fiber types include type I, IIA, and IIB. Type I fibers (red fibers), which are more common in muscles with smaller motor units, are highly aerobic, less fatigable, and contract slowly. In contrast, type IIA fibers (white fibers) are fast contracting, more anaerobic, fatigable, and common in muscles with large motor units. Type IIB muscle fibers are the fastest contracting and have the quickest rate of fatigue. Recruitment of contracting muscle fibers is based on the size of the motor unit, with the smaller motor units activated first. Sprinting and heavy weigh lifting involve recruitment of larger motor units, most often type II fibers. It has been shown that sprinters hypertrophy largely type II fibers, and therefore, more of their muscle consists of fast and forceful contracting fibers. On the other hand, distance runners have improved perfusion to muscles with increased capillary density and mitochondria, which aids the highly aerobic, less fatigable type I fibers.

In an individual muscle, the force of muscle contraction is dependent on two factors: (i) the frequency of action potential stimulation within muscle fibers and (ii) the number of muscle fibers stimulated (recruited). The force a muscle is capable of generating is also related to its cross-sectional area. Another important concept governing muscle performance is the length/tension relationship. At short muscle lengths, the contractile force of muscle is relatively low. As the muscle is stretched to greater lengths, its contractile force increases to a peak amount. Increases in length beyond this ideal value once again lead to decreases in contractile forces with stimulation. Structurally, this phenomenon may be explained by the arrangement of the sarcomere. At an intermediate length, the myosin and actin of the sarcomere undergo maximal overlap, and therefore, their interaction can affect the greatest contractile force production. At lesser or greater sarcomere lengths, the overlap is no longer complete, and contractile force is decreased.

Muscle biomechanics is also better understood with knowledge of the relationship of force and velocity in muscle contraction. With minimal load applied to muscle, contraction results in shortening of muscle (decreasing muscle lengths) at a rate approaching maximal velocity (concentric contraction). If a load applied to the muscle is greater than the muscle contraction force, then the velocity of muscle lengthening slows, but increasing force is generated within the muscle during contraction (eccentric contraction). Therefore, the force and velocity of muscle contraction are inversely related. Because higher forces can be generated during eccentric loading, exercises using eccentric contraction are popular in many training regimens. However, muscle strain injuries also occur most often during eccentric muscle activity.

With muscle *disuse* and *immobilization,* structural changes that occur result in muscle weakness and dysfunction. Among the first changes is atrophy with a decrease in both fiber size and fiber number. Changes have also been demonstrated within the fibers as the organization of the sarcomere is disrupted and fiber metabolism is altered. The fatigability and weakness of the affected muscle is also increased.

Muscle laceration by a sharp object results in incomplete healing via scar tissue and fibrosis when the cut ends are reapproximated. Although fiber regeneration across the scar tissue is rare, much of the muscle function can return depending on the severity of injury. Contusion of a muscle by blunt force injury results in hematoma formation, inflammation, and muscle cell injury and death. Recovery is dependent on hematoma clearance and revascularization of the injured tissue. This process can be promoted by initial rest in flexion and early muscle movement and rehabilitation.

Indirect muscle injury occurs most often at the myotendinous junction. This refers to failure of muscle by excessive stress rather than by direct trauma and includes muscle strains and tears. The forces responsible for the tear are often eccentric contractions, as these contractions place more strain on involved muscle. Healing involves muscle cell necrosis followed by some muscle fiber regeneration and the reconstitution of the vascular supply. Decreasing inflammation and ensuring minimal vascular injury improves healing time.

Orthopedic Pathology

Neoplasms originating from tissues are grouped together and named accordingly. Benign tumors from osteoblasts include osteoblastomas, osteomas, and osteoid osteomas while malignant tumors are termed "osteosarcomas." Benign tumors of cartilage include enchondromas, osteochondromas, and chondroblastomas while malignant tumors of cartilage are "chondrosarcomas."

Diagnosis is often made on plain radiographs. In addition, magnetic resonance imaging (MRI) and computed tomography (CT) scans are necessary to evaluate the precise extent of the bony involvement as well as any soft tissue extension. Lesions can be sampled by percutaneous needle biopsy using fine needle aspiration, which provides samples for cytology or by using Tru-cut or large bore needles, both of which can provide samples for histology as well as cytology. However, the gold standard for definitive diagnosis of a bony lesion is the *open incision biopsy.* The open biopsy of a tumor must be carried out carefully to prevent seeding of the tumor by creating extra soft tissue or muscle planes. Immunohistochemical analysis is very useful in differentiating the various tumors. Neoplasms can have a similar clinical presentation as an infection, so it is important to send all specimens for pathologic as well as microbiologic analysis to prevent mistaking a neoplasm for a simple infection. Once the diagnosis is made, treatment is surgical resection. *Marginal excision* involves excision through the pseudocapsule of the tumor and is used for some benign tumors such as lipomas. In the *wide excision,* the pseudocapsule, as well as several more centimeters of the surrounding normal tissue, is removed. *Radical excision* (such as an amputation) involves the removal of the entire compartment or compartments that the tumor occupies and is used to treat tumors that have multiple local satellites or that are recurrent. The compartments refer to the fascia-separated anatomic compartments of the body (such as a group of muscles or the bone itself), and penetration through the fascia of a compartment is ominous because it signifies a more aggressive tumor. *Wide excision* (with or without salvage reconstruction) is used for most malignant tumors today. For active high-grade tumors, adjuvant chemotherapy or radiation therapy is often helpful.

The *most common benign lesions* are described in Table 27-1. Most of the lesions are latent and asymptomatic and require no treatment. Currettage and bone grafting is used for large lesions that are at risk for a pathologic fracture. Aggressive tumors such as the giant cell tumor may require earlier intervention in the form of currettage and cementation.

The *most common malignant neoplasms* affecting bone are metastatic tumors. After the lung and liver, bone is the third most common site of metastatic disease. Breast, prostate, lung, kidney, and thyroid tumors account for 80% of the metastasis. The most common bones affected are the spine (lumbar vertebrae), ribs, pelvis, and the proximal ends of

TABLE 27-1. BENIGN TUMORS OF BONE

Tumor	Age of onset	Location	Diagnosis	Treatment	Miscellaneous
Osteochondroma (exostosis) 40% of benign bone tumors	Childhood	Out-of bone lesion connected to metaphysis by trabecular stalk	Palpable mass; the stalk blends into metaphyseal trabecular bone; has cartilaginous cap	Marginal excision if symptomatic; e.g., nerve irritation, bursitis; no treatment if asymptomatic	Low rate of malignant transformation to chondrosarcoma; multiple osteochondromas in hereditary multiple exostoses with 1% risk of malignant transformation
Giant cell tumor 20% of benign bone tumors	Third and fourth decades	Metaphysis and epiphysis of long bones, most commonly around knee	Expansile and radiolucent lesions of bone; osteoclast-like giant cells on histology	Intralesional curettage with cementation or bone grafting; adjuvant cryotherapy reduces recurrence	Benign but aggressive lesion; can metastasize to the lungs
Unicameral bone cyst (simple bone cyst)	Childhood	Metaphysis, 90% in proximal humerus or femur	Cystic lesion that abuts but does not involve the growth plate; usually diagnosed after pathologic fracture through the cyst	Immobilization until fracture healing followed by steroid (methylprednisolone acetate) injection into the cyst or curettage and bone grafting	The fracture itself may stimulate the cyst to heal on its own
Nonossifying fibroma	Childhood	Metaphysis	Eccentric lucent lesions, sometimes multiloculated, bubbly, usually incidental plain film findings	Smaller lesions will heal, no treatment; large lesions, curettage and bone grafting to prevent pathologic fracture	
Enchondroma	Childhood and adulthood	Central metaphysis, 53% in phalanges	Well-circumscribed lucent lesion with punctate calcifications	Inactive enchondroma, no treatment; active enchondroma or low-grade chondrosarcoma, curettage with adjuvant cryotherapy	Chondrosarcoma can be distinguished from enchondroma by increased pain, variable lucency on plain films, and endosteal erosion

long bones. Metastasis to the facial bones and to the skeleton distal to the elbows and knees is rare.

The most common primary malignant tumors affecting bone are described in Table 27-2 and Fig. 27-9. Malignant bone tumors typically present with pain and a mass or swelling. Radiographic features often include either an osteolytic or osteosclerotic lesion, poorly demarcated borders (signifying the aggressive nature of the tumor), and periosteal reaction, which can form a triangular shape (Codman triangle). Ewing sarcoma is usually seen in the adolescent population while multiple myeloma, chondrosarcoma, and malignant fibrous histiocytoma are usually seen in middle-aged and elderly adults. Although osteosarcoma is usually a childhood malignancy, it can present in adults who have underlying bone diseases such as Paget disease, osteochondroma, or previous radiation exposure. Treatment of these malignant tumors is generally wide excision with limb salvage and adjuvant chemotherapy. Radical resection such as an amputation may be necessary for the most aggressive tumors.

GENERAL CLINICAL PRINCIPLES OF ORTHOPEDIC SURGERY

Evaluation and Treatment

Initial evaluation of the polytrauma patient should focus on stabilizing the patient according to ATLS guidelines. A coordinated team approach between the trauma team and the orthopedic surgeons is crucial. A complete history will offer invaluable clues about the nature of the injury. Knowledge of the mechanism of injury will help with clinical diagnosis, and familiarity with the patient's medical history and functional status will help dictate the treatment. While fractures or dislocations can be obvious on physical examination, nondisplaced fractures or massive

TABLE 27-2. PRIMARY MALIGNANT TUMORS OF BONE

Tumor	Age of Onset	Location	Diagnosis	Treatment	5-year Survival
Multiple myeloma (plasma cell tumor), most common	Adulthood after age 40	Spine (most common), ribs, skull, long bones; often presents with vertebral compression fractures	Multiple discrete lytic lesions; bone scan may be cold; monoclonal gammopathy on serum and immunoelectrophoresis; Bence-Jones proteinuria; sheets of plasma cells on histology	Chemotherapy is the mainstay of therapy; supportive orthopedic care (treat pathologic or impending pathologic fractures)	
Osteosarcoma, second most common bone tumor after myeloma	Adolescence 75% occurs at 10–30 y of age	56% involving the metaphysis of the distal femur or proximal tibial	Bone pain with palpable mass, increased alkaline phosphatase; radiodense lesion with bony destruction and soft tissue extension on radiographs	High grade tumor adjuvant preoperative and postoperative chemotherapy and wide resection with limb salvage reconstruction or amputation	>50%
Chondrosarcoma, 10%–20% of malignant bone tumors	Adulthood 50–70 y	Metaphysis of proximal femur or pelvis	May arise from preexisting enchondroma or osteochondroma; On x-ray, lucent lesion with punctate calcifications	Usually slow growing and low grade, so no chemotherapy or x-ray therapy; usually treated with wide surgical resection	Good
Ewing sarcoma (primitive neuroectodermal tumor), 5% of malignant bone tumors	Childhood 5–15 y	Pelvis and diaphysis-metaphysis of large long bones (lower extremity)	Radiologically destructive bone-forming lesion with raised periosteum (Codman triangle), soft tissue extension, and onion skinning; histologically, sheets of blue small round cells, which are derived from mesenchymal stem cell or neural crest origin; associated with 11:22 translocation	Often high grade with rapid growth; treat with neo-adjuvant chemotherapy, wide-resection with limb salvage (if possible), and possibly x-ray therapy; must not be confused with osteomyelitis	65%
Malignant fibrous histiocytoma	>50 y of age	Metaphysis or diaphysis of lower extremities	Predominantly lytic lesion; pleomorphic malignant cells on histology; commonly presents as a primary soft tissue tumor	Often high grade; treatment is wide surgical resection with adjuvant chemotherapy	60%

swelling can make the diagnosis more difficult. Localized pain and tenderness, swelling, shortening, deformity, loss of function of the affected extremity, and abnormal motion are indicative of a possible fracture or dislocation. It is important to examine carefully the joint above and joint below the fracture site. Neurovascular examination is also vital, particularly before performing a reduction maneuver. Routine radiographic evaluation must include at least two views of the injured area as well as the joints above and below the injury. A CT scan may be useful in evaluating a comminuted intraarticular fracture; an MRI is helpful to look at soft tissue structures such as ligaments; and bone scan and an MRI both may identify occult fractures not visible on plain radiographs.

The goal for the treatment of all orthopedic fractures is fracture union, early mobilization, and rapid return to baseline activity level. In the polytrauma patient, there is a special emphasis on rigid fixation of the fracture to facilitate earlier mobilization. In most cases, definitive treatment should be delayed until the patient has been medically stabilized. There are a few exceptions in which emergent operative intervention is required within 6 hours of the initial injury: open fractures, fractures with vascular injuries, amputations, and compartment syndromes. In cases in which soft tissue swelling can seriously compromise the wound healing (e.g., calcaneus fractures and tibial plateau fractures), waiting 1 to 2 weeks to allow the swelling and fracture blisters to resolve may be preferable.

The fracture or dislocation can be treated with either closed reduction, closed reduction with percutaneous internal fixation, or open reduction with internal fixation. For many fractures and dislocations, closed reduction will be successful if attempted acutely with adequate muscle relaxation. However, certain circumstances such as soft tissue

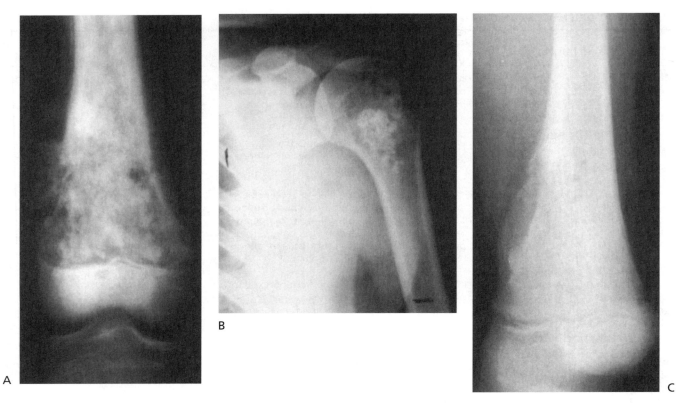

FIGURE 27-9. Common malignant tumors. **A:** Osteosarcoma of the distal femur showing osteosclerosis and bony destruction. **B:** Chondrosarcoma of the proximal humerus. Note the poorly defined margins and dense calcifications. **C:** Ewing sarcoma of the metaphysis-diaphysis of the distal tibia, showing a poorly defined lytic lesion with cortical destruction and periosteal new bone formation. (From Vigorita VJ. *Orthopaedic pathology*. Philadelphia: Lippincott Williams & Wilkins, 1999:328, 374, 442, with permission.)

interposition, comminuted fractures, and inadequate muscle relaxation will require open reduction.

There are four broad categories of *fixation methods* to hold the fracture: (i) splinting and casting, (ii) traction, (iii) external fixation, and (iv) internal fixation. The choice depends on many factors, including the inherent stability of the fracture. For the most part, the initial injury, particularly the amount of displacement and comminution, will determine the maximal degree of fracture instability. There are many fractures in which splinting or casting is the treatment of choice (e.g., clavicle, humerus, distal radius, and foot). In addition, most pediatric fractures can be treated successfully in a cast because of the incredible remodeling potential. When splinting or casting a fracture, the physician must immobilize the joints above and below the fracture site. The main disadvantages are the inability to rigidly hold a reduction, joint stiffness from prolonged immobilization, and ulcerations at bony prominences. Traction is more often used in the lower extremity, in which longitudinal traction is applied to a pin inserted either through the distal femur or through the proximal tibia (Fig. 27-10). It is generally used in patients with unstable fractures who cannot tolerate surgery. The main drawbacks are suboptimal fracture fixation (tendency for shortening and rotational malunion) and the need for prolonged immobilization, which can lead to sacral ulcers and joint stiffness. External fixation is indicated in fractures with segmental bone loss, associated vascular injuries, and massive soft tissue injuries with a high risk of infection. In addition, because of the speed in which it can be applied, external fixation is also indicated in the unstable patient with multiple extremity injuries and in the hemodynamically unstable patient with a pelvic fracture. The main complications are pin tract infection and less rigid fixation compared to complications of internal devices.

The five main types of internal fixation devices are pins (such as K wires), screws (such as lag screws), plates, intramedullary (IM) rods, and prosthetic replacements. Pins, which can be inserted percutaneously, are often used to hold fractures in the hand and foot and to supplement fixation elsewhere. Lag screws, which provide compression across a fracture site, are used to fix simple transverse or oblique fractures such as the femoral neck fracture. Plates such as the dynamic compression plate are useful in long-bone fractures and provide rigid fixation and compression across the fracture site. However, the extensive stripping

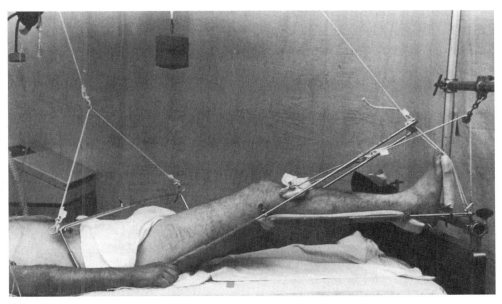

FIGURE 27-10. Skeletal traction for a tibia fracture using a tibial traction pin. (From Rockwood CA Jr, et al., eds. *Rockwood and Green's fractures in adults,* 4th ed. Philadelphia: Lippincott-Raven Publishers, 1996:45, with permission.)

required to secure the plate onto the bone can devitalize the fracture fragments, thus delaying healing and increasing the risk of infection. The IM rod, which is commonly used for femur and tibia fractures, also provides rigid fixation. The rod is inserted from one end of the bone down the intramedullary canal, thus transfixing the fracture site and providing translational and angular stability. Rotational motion is controlled by the interlocking screws at the proximal and distal ends. The smaller incision used to insert the IM rod avoids extensive soft tissue dissection and allows rapid healing and early return to function. Sometimes the intramedullary canal is reamed to allow for insertion of a larger (and hence, stiffer) rod. However, there have been reports of embolization of fat and marrow elements during IM reaming and rodding. Lastly, prosthetic replacement such as the hemiarthroplasty of the humeral head and femoral head is used in situations in which there is a high risk of avascular necrosis (AVN) or the comminution of the bone and cartilage is so severe that anatomic reduction can not be restored.

Complications and Associated Injuries

Posttraumatic arthritis is a common complication that occurs after an intraarticular fracture. Articular displacement of greater than 2 mm is associated with an increased risk of subsequent arthritis. Anatomic reduction and fixation of the fracture can help to minimize the risk.

Malunion results from inadequate fracture alignment or later loss of fixation. While children have the potential for a great deal of remodeling, very little spontaneous correction can be expected in the adult bone, and it is unlikely that the malunion will resolve without further intervention. There are many possible causes of *delayed union* and *nonunion*: (i) poor fixation leading to motion at the fracture site, (ii) large gap at the fracture site, (iii) infection, (iv) poor vascular supply, (v) soft tissue interposition, and (vi) significant bone loss. The tibia, ulna, scaphoid, and femoral neck are particularly susceptible to delayed unions or nonunions. Please refer to the basic science section for a complete discussion of nonunions.

Loss of fixation after either closed or open treatment can lead to malunions and nonunions and is related to several factors. Patient risk factors include obesity, noncompliance with the weight-bearing limitations, increased age, and medical conditions such as osteopenia. In addition, infection and inherent fracture instability due to fracture comminution can lead to a loss of fixation. Lastly, poor casting technique or inappropriate choice of internal fixation might also result in a loss of fixation.

Postoperative *wound infections* and *osteomyelitis* are usually related to high-energy injuries, which are associated with significant wound contamination and osseous devascularization. Other risk factors include prolonged open wound time, inadequate fixation, and extensive surgical dissection and periosteal stripping, which compromise blood flow to the wound. Leaving a skin bridge less than 7 cm wide will also compromise the vascular status of the soft tissue and increase the incidence of infection. *Staphylococcus aureus* is the most common offending organism (90% of cases). Treatment for osteomyelitis consists of incisional drainage followed by intravenous antibiotics. Temporary implantation of antibiotic-impregnated cement beads and hyperbaric oxygen can help with more resistant cases of infection.

Heterotopic ossification, the formation of ectopic (extra) bone adjacent to the fracture site and within the soft tissues, can be a debilitating complication because of pain and loss of motion that may occur if the ectopic bone crosses the joint. It is mainly associated with fractures of the elbow, acetabulum, and hip. Although the exact causes of heterotopic ossification are not known, risk factors include head trauma, burns, extensive surgery, immobilization, and passive range of motion. Use of indomethacin for 4 to 6 weeks can help reduce the chances of developing heterotopic ossification. In the trauma patients in whom indomethacin would be contraindicated, low-dose single-fraction limited field radiation (800 cGy) is another alternative. (Although long-term effects are not fully known, there is a theoretical risk of future radiation-induced sarcoma.) To be most effective, indomethacin or radiation treatment must be started within 5 days of the injury.

AVN (avascular necrosis), which is also known as "osteonecrosis" or "aseptic" necrosis, describes the death of bone cells due to impairment in circulation. Posttraumatic AVN occurs when the amount of displacement from the fracture or dislocation is severe enough to disrupt the blood supply to the bone. Sites that are more susceptible to AVN are the scaphoid, femoral head, talus, and odontoid. Other causes of AVN include (i) arterial and venous obstruction due to thrombosis, (ii) fat embolism, (iii) nitrogen gas (decompression sickness, Caisson disease), (iv) radiation therapy, (v) corticosteroid use, and (vi) ethanol abuse. Radiographic changes include sclerosis of the bone on x-ray and edema of the bone marrow on MRI.

Trabecular bone repair from necrosis involves formation and deposition of osteoid and mineral matrix on top of the existing structural framework, a process that increases the density of the cancellous bone. Cortical bone must be largely resorbed by osteoclasts before osteoblastic deposition of new cortical bone, a process that can take up to 2 years. During resorption of the cortical matrix, the necrotic bone becomes very susceptible to fracture because the bone framework is weakened. If osteonecrosis occurs under a region of articular cartilage, eventual fracture and permanent damage to the cartilage is likely. This phenomenon may be caused by an increased stress within the area, an inability to repair microfractures, or an increased vascularity in the area leading to more extensive resorption of necrotic bone. The end result of AVN is collapse of the articular surface, which leads to osteoarthritis.

Deep venous thrombosis (DVT) can occur in up to 58% of trauma patients and is most frequently seen in patients with spinal cord injury and fractures of the pelvis, femur, or tibia. Venography is the diagnostic gold standard, but Doppler ultrasound has been shown to be effective and reliable. While iodine-labeled fibrinogen is good for diagnosing thrombosis below the popliteal fossa, it is unreliable in detecting clots in the upper thigh or pelvis or in the vicinity of a deep wound. Prophylaxis against DVT and the potential sequelae of pulmonary embolism is important in all trauma patients. If there are no contraindications, subcutaneous heparin or low-dose warfarin can be used, along with compression or pneumatic stockings. In patients with contraindications to anticoagulation or with proximal venous thrombosis with major pelvic, acetabular, or femur fractures, vena cava filters should be placed.

In the polytrauma patient, *fat embolism* is an important cause of acute respiratory distress syndrome (ARDS) and a major source of morbidity and mortality. Fat embolism syndrome is clinically apparent in 10% of polytrauma patients, although the actual incidence rate (which includes subacute presentation) is probably much higher. The risk factors include trauma, long-bone (femur or tibia) fractures, myeloplastic disorders, collagen vascular disease, osteoporosis, and immobilization. Fat embolism has also been documented after intramedullary reaming and rodding and after prosthetic hemiarthroplasty of the hip. It may not appear until 2 to 3 days after the injury and may present as respiratory distress (shortness of breath and tachypnea), arterial hypoxemia, tachycardia, fevers, and a deterioration of neurological status (restlessness, confusion, or coma). In addition, petechiae (which may be short lived) can appear across the chest and axilla. Treatment consists of pulmonary support and early orthopedic care. Corticosteroids, heparin, and hypertonic glucose have also been used with variable amounts of success.

Compartment syndrome is a true orthopedic emergency because of the potential for irreversible muscular and neurological compromise within 6 hours of onset. Compartment syndrome after a closed injury can result from swelling of the extremity after a fracture or blow, severe crush injury, tight cast, and prolonged external compression of the extremity (e.g., being trapped in a wrecked car). Stab wounds resulting in arterial puncture or hemophiliac bleeding can also lead to compartment syndrome. The mechanism of compartment syndrome involves fluid exudation at the capillary level within a tight fascial space, leading to venous obstruction. Because the compliant venous system is obstructed before the arterial system, compartment syndrome perpetuates itself.

The most commonly involved extremities are the lower leg and the forearm. The lower leg contains four compartments (anterior, lateral, posterior, and deep posterior). The most frequently affected compartments are the anterior compartment (which contains the deep peroneal nerve and the ankle/toe dorsiflexors such as the tibialis anterior, extensor digitorum longus, and extensor hallucis longus) and the deep posterior compartment (which contains the posterior tibial nerve, posterior tibial artery, peroneal artery, and ankle/toe plantar flexors such as the tibialis posterior, flexor hallucis longus, and flexor digitorum longus).

Diagnosis is based on a high index of suspicion and a careful physical examination. The compartment may be hard and tense on palpation. The classic findings are pain, pulselessness, paralysis, pallor, and paresthesias. The earliest and most consistent sign is pain, particularly to passive range of motion, which is described as "pain out of proportion to the injury." It is also important to remember that pulses may continue to be palpable and strong despite the onset of compartment syndrome. Although the diagnosis of compartment syndrome should be made clinically, compartment pressure measurements may be helpful, particularly in the unconscious patient. Absolute compartment pressures of over 40 to 45 mm Hg have classically defined the criteria for compartment syndrome (normal pressures are about 0 mm Hg). However, comparing the compartment pressures with the systemic blood pressure is more accurate because hypotension can exacerbate ischemia, although hypertension can actually maintain tissue perfusion despite increased compartment pressures. Therefore, another criteria for compartment syndrome is a pressure rise in the extremity to within 30 mm Hg of the patient's diastolic blood pressure.

The treatment of compartment syndrome is a fasciotomy of all of the compartments (four in the lower leg and three in the forearm) along with thorough debridement of the involved muscles. The skin is closed secondarily, and a skin graft may be needed for the wound closure. Untreated compartment syndrome leads to muscular and neurological dysfunction, which results in loss of function of the extremity as well as contractures and clawing of the fingers (Volkmann ischemic contracture) or toes.

Open fractures and *open joint wounds* are significant because of the increased risk of infection, which can result from the grossly contaminated wound, extensive soft tissue and skeletal injury, and a delay in treatment. Open fractures are also at a greater risk of nonunion. The Gustilo open fracture classification reflects the severity of the soft tissue injury (Table 27-3). Treatment is surgical debridement within 6 hours of the injury. Repeated debridement in 48 hours and delayed primary closure when the wound is clean are recommended. Antibiotic coverage for grade I and II open fractures consists of 48 hours of intravenous cephalosporin to treat *S. aureus*. For grade III open fractures, an aminoglycoside is added to cover Gram-negative organisms. In open fractures with significant contamination such as a barnyard injury, penicillin is added to cover anaerobes such as *Clostridium perfringens*. Although external fixation is commonly used for severely contaminated fractures, internal fixation as well as external fixation can be used in most grade I, grade II, and grade IIIA fractures. Low-velocity gunshot wounds do not require formal irrigation and debridement of the deeper soft tissues. They can be treated with local wound care and immediate internal fixation. High-energy gunshot wounds (close-range shotgun or military rifle wounds) are more serious and should be managed as a grade IIIB open injury.

Because many of the major nerves run in close proximity to the bones, neurological injuries are commonly associated with fractures and dislocations. For example, radial nerve injuries are associated with humerus fractures, sciatic nerve injuries are associated with hip dislocations, and peroneal nerve injuries are associated with knee injuries. The initial treatment for acute neuropathy is gentle reduction of the fracture or dislocation. Because most nerve injuries sustained in fractures, dislocations, and gunshot wounds are a result of neuropraxia (contusion to the nerve), recovery over a few weeks or months often occurs spontaneously, and immediate surgical exploration is not indicated. However, in nerve injuries caused by sharp trauma such as a knife wound, surgical exploration and repair of the lacerated nerve is indicated.

To prevent irreversible muscle and nerve injury, the surgeon must treat *fractures associated with vascular injury* (Gustilo grade IIIC fractures) within 6 hours. Immediate reduction and stabilization of the fracture in the emergency room may alleviate any arterial compromise associated with a kinked or entrapped vessel. If the presence and location of the vascular injury is obvious based on the mechanism of injury, the patient should be brought directly to the operating room instead of going to interventional radiology for an

TABLE 27-3. CLASSIFICATION OF OPEN FRACTURES[a]

Type	Wound	Level of contamination	Soft tissue injury	Bone injury
I	<1 cm long	Clean	Minimal	Simple, minimal comminution
II	>1 cm long	Moderate	Moderate, some muscle damage	Moderate comminution
III[b]				
A	Usually >10 cm long	High	Severe with crushing	Usually comminuted; soft tissue coverage of bone possible
B	Usually >10 cm long	High	Very severe loss of coverage	Bone coverage poor; usually requires soft tissue reconstructive surgery
C	Usually >10 cm long	High	Very severe loss of coverage plus vascular injury requiring repair	Bone coverage poor; usually requires soft tissue reconstructive surgery

[a]From Chapman MW. The role of intramedullary fixation in open fractures. *Clin Orthop* 1986;212:27, with permission.
[b]Segmental fractures, farmyard injuries, fractures occurring in a highly contaminated environment shotgun wounds, or high-velocity gunshot wounds automatically result in classification as a type III open fracture.

angiogram. To avoid injury to the vascular repair, the surgeon must place a *temporary vascular shunt* to allow debridement and stabilization of the bone before definitive vascular repair. In addition, *fasciotomies should be routinely performed after reperfusion* of the ischemic limb to avoid a subsequent compartment syndrome.

With modern advances in microvascular surgery, the treatment of *traumatic amputations* has become more successful. Replantation is more commonly performed in the upper extremity. Because of the difficulties presented by an insensate foot and the good functional results of a lower extremity prosthesis, replantations are less frequently performed for lower extremity injuries. One of the most important determining factors for a successful replantation is the allowable ischemia time, which is inversely related to the volume of muscle in the amputated part. In general, acceptable ischemia times are 6 hours for warm ischemia and 10 to 12 hours for cool ischemia. Smaller parts such as a digit may be viable after a warm ischemia time of greater than 12 hours. Replantation after prolonged ischemia time may lead to acute renal failure secondary to muscle necrosis.

Initial care of an amputated extremity consists of loosely dressing the stump. A tourniquet should not be used if there is any possibility of microvascular repair. The amputated part should be wrapped in a moist gauze and placed in a sterile container or plastic bag, which in turn should be placed in ice water (4° to 10°C). Placing the amputated part directly on ice may lead to frostbite injury. The general sequence for replantation is skeletal fixation, tendon repair, arterial and nerve repair, and lastly venous reanastomosis. Immediate postoperative care includes elevation, keeping the room warm, and avoidance of nicotine and caffeine. Venous congestion can be relieved by the application of leaches. A compromise of arterial flow within 48 hours warrants reexploration. Aspirin, Persantine, low molecular weight dextran, heparin, and a sympathetic blockade may also prevent arterial thrombosis and spasm.

A complication unique to pediatric fractures is growth plate injury and arrest. If the injury or fracture involves the physis (growth plate), then there is a risk that the growth plate may be injured, leading to a partial or total arrest of growth. A partial arrest at the growth plate will lead to an imbalance in the rate of growth of the bone, leading to angular deformities. Depending on the child's age and growth remaining, a complete growth arrest may result in significant shortening and leg-length discrepancy.

INJURIES OF THE UPPER EXTREMITY

Sternoclavicular Dislocations

Injuries of the sternoclavicular (SC) joint are rare because of the strong ligamentous support of the SC joint. Because of the strong forces involved and the proximity of the SC joint to the great vessels and other mediastinal structures, SC dislocations can be very serious and potentially life threatening. The two most common causes of the traumatic SC injuries are motor vehicle accidents and athletic activities, particularly contact sports such as American football.

Anterior dislocations are more common (73% to 95% of dislocations) than posterior (retrosternal) dislocations. Clinical suspicion is the most important factor in diagnosing an SC injury, because this injury is often dismissed as a soft tissue injury or contusion because of equivocal deformity or a negative radiograph. Clinical findings may include swelling, prominence of the medial end of the clavicle in anterior dislocations, discoloration, and a severe boring pain that is exacerbated by movement of the arm and by deep breathing. Signs of potentially dangerous and life-threatening associated injuries to the trachea, esophagus, brachial plexus, and vascular structures include breathing difficulties, dysphagia, paresthesias, and vascular congestion in the upper extremity.

Because of the superimposed shadows of the clavicle and the manubrium, routine plain radiographs are extremely difficult to interpret. CT scan in the axial plane is the best study to visualize the SC joint (Fig. 27-11). It is also important to evaluate the remainder of the thorax for a pneumothorax, widened mediastinum, or other skeletal fractures. An angiogram or a venogram may be indicated if vascular injury is suspected.

Nonoperative management is the treatment of choice for most SC injuries. Conservative management, consisting of benign neglect and closed or percutaneous reduction and immobilization in a sling-and-swath dressing, which often produces good long-term results. Because of the potential for iatrogenic surgical injury to the underlying neurovascular structures, open reduction is reserved for cases in which the posterior displacement of the medial clavicle is associated with complications caused by mediastinal compression.

Due to the proximity of the SC joint to the important superior mediastinal structures, retrosternal dislocations are associated with much higher complication rates than anterior dislocations. *Intrathoracic injuries* involving the trachea, esophagus, brachial plexus, and great vessels occur in 30% of retrosternal dislocations.

Fractures of the Scapula

Fractures of the scapula (most commonly involving the scapular body) usually occur as a result of a direct high-energy impact to the scapular region. Scapular fractures are often seen incidentally on chest radiographs. However, one should be more suspicious of a scapular fracture in the polytrauma patient with complaints of shoulder pain and with associated rib or pulmonary injuries. In complex fractures, CT scans are particularly useful.

Fractures of the scapular body, even with severe displacement, usually do well with conservative care. Nonunion is rare. Displaced fracture of the scapular neck, spine, and glenoid have a high rate of associated disability because of shoul-

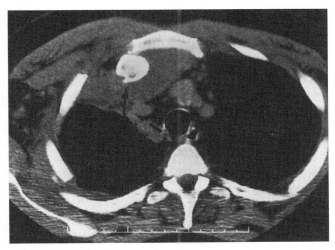

FIGURE 27-11. Computed tomography scan showing a right retrosternal sternoclavicular dislocation (*arrow*). (From Rockwood CA Jr, et al., eds. *Rockwood and Green's fractures in adults*, 4th ed. Philadelphia: Lippincott-Raven Publishers, 1996:1422, with permission.)

der abduction weakness, rotator cuff dysfunction, and subacromial pain. Surgical management may be warranted in these cases.

Because of the large amount of energy required to fracture the scapula, *associated injuries* are found in up to *96% of patients*. The most common associated injuries are upper thoracic rib fractures. Other associated injuries include pulmonary injuries (hemopneumothorax and pulmonary contusion), head injuries, ipsilateral clavicle fractures, cervical spine injuries, and brachial plexus injuries.

Fractures of the Clavicle

Clavicle fractures are common injuries in both adults and children and result from direct trauma or a fall on an outstretched arm. Because there is usually superior displacement of the fracture, the diagnosis is easily made both clinically and radiographically. Ecchymosis, swelling, and crepitus over the clavicle, as well as pain with use of the affected arm, will be present. However, because of the proximity of the underlying neurovascular structures, a complete neurovascular examination of the upper extremity is essential. On the radiograph, it is important to look for an associated injury such as a pneumothorax.

Because most fractures will heal with minimal treatment, *initial management* usually consists of immobilization in either a sling or a figure-eight harness. Delayed union and nonunion rates of between 0.1% and 23% have been reported.

While conservative management is usually the rule, there are some indications for acute surgical stabilization using plates or IM rods. An associated injury to the underlying vascular structures may require vascular repair, as well as fixation and stabilization of the clavicle. Open fractures will require operative incisional drainage, as well as immediate or delayed fixation. Tenting of the skin by sharp bone fragments may lead to skin necrosis and may warrant operative intervention. However, the initial management for an associated brachial plexus injury should be observation, because as many as 66% of these cases will resolve spontaneously.

Injuries of the Shoulder

Acromioclavicular (AC) sprains (also known as "shoulder separations") are commonly caused by a direct impact to the AC joint. Depending on the severity of the sprain, the AC joint capsule is disrupted, the coracoclavicular ligament may be partially or completely disrupted, and the distal end of the clavicle is displaced relative to the acromion. There is pain to direct palpation over the AC joint on physical examination. Diagnosis can be confirmed by an anterior-posterior (AP) stress radiograph of the AC joint (in which downward traction is applied to the affected arm in to accentuate the AC joint separation). In the absence of severe displacement (more than 100% displacement), the treatment is most often conservative, consisting of a sling and mobilization when comfortable.

Rotator cuff tears most commonly involve the supraspinatus and infraspinatus tendons. There is pain with overhead motion of the affected arm and weakness with shoulder abduction and external rotation. Diagnosis is confirmed by MRI. Treatment options are observation, physical therapy, or surgical repair.

Dislocations of the shoulder (glenohumeral joint) are common injuries that affect all age groups. They are caused by a direct blow to the shoulder or indirect trauma such as a fall onto an outstretched arm. The *most common direction for shoulder dislocations is anterior*. Less than 5% of dislocations are posterior, which can be associated with epileptic seizures.

On clinical examination, severe pain and deformity involving the affected shoulder and arm are present. In a thin person, the anteriorly dislocated humeral head is often noticeable and palpable, but in a heavier patient, the soft tissue and swelling may often obscure the humeral head and make the diagnosis less evident. A careful neurovascular examination to rule out associated brachial plexus injuries is also important.

Three views of the shoulder are essential for evaluation of the shoulder. While the anterior dislocation may be easily seen on the AP view and the lateral view (Y view of the scapula), the axillary view more reliably demonstrates a dislocation, particularly the posterior dislocation. It is also important to look for associated fractures of the proximal humerus, which may change the treatment protocol.

Urgent reduction of the acute dislocated shoulder under sedation or general anesthesia, followed by immobilization in a sling for 3 weeks, is the initial treatment of choice.

Open reduction may be necessary in an irreducible dislocation, such as in a shoulder that is chronically dislocated or that has an associated humerus fracture.

Because of the proximity of the brachial plexus, neurological injuries are relatively common. *Axillary nerve palsy* following shoulder dislocations is 10%. Another complication is chronic (recurrent) instability, which is more often seen in the younger patient who has sustained a high-energy trauma. Inability to abduct the arm should raise suspicions for an associated rotator cuff injury, which is particularly common in elderly patients. Lastly, a missed diagnosis, which is more commonly seen for the posterior dislocation, will result in a chronically dislocated shoulder.

Fractures of the Proximal Humerus

Fractures of the surgical neck of the humerus are commonly seen in the elderly osteoporotic patient and can occur following a simple fall. In the younger patient, it is usually seen following more serious trauma.

Evaluation and diagnosis of the proximal humerus fracture is similar to that of the shoulder dislocation. Again, it is important to look for associated injuries to the brachial plexus. In addition, in the severely displaced fracture, an expanding axillary hematoma or diminished or absent distal pulses requires immediate evaluation for axillary artery laceration.

The three radiographic views (AP, lateral, and axillary) will demonstrate the displacement and angulation of the fracture. The fracture may involve not only the surgical neck of the humerus, but also the greater tuberosity (attachment of the supraspinatus, infraspinatus, and teres minor muscles) and the lesser tuberosity (attachment of the subscapularis muscle). Displacement and angulation are considered significant if they are greater than 1 cm and 45 degrees, respectively. CT scans may also be helpful to evaluate the exact nature of the fracture.

In 80% of fractures, the fragments are relatively nondisplaced and nonangulated, and these fractures can be treated simply by *immobilization in a sling* and early motion exercises once the patient is comfortable. Early motion is essential to prevent stiffness, because loss of significant shoulder range of motion can lead to a very poor outcome.

In fractures with significant displacement or angulation, surgical intervention is usually necessary to help restore function. Surgical options include closed reduction and percutaneous pinning or open reduction and internal fixation. Surgical treatment for displaced fractures of the humeral head and severely comminuted proximal humerus fractures is prosthetic replacement of the humeral head because of the high risk of osteonecrosis of the head (Fig. 27-12A, B).

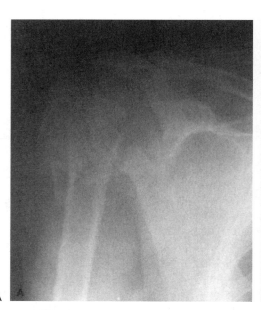 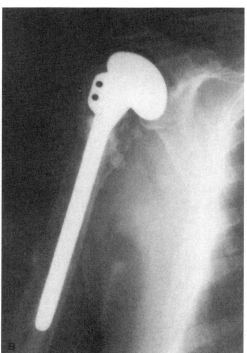

FIGURE 27-12. A: Comminuted fracture of the proximal humerus. **B:** Because of the high risk of avascular necrosis in comminuted proximal humerus fractures, the treatment is prosthetic replacement. (From Rockwood CA Jr, et al., eds. *Rockwood and Green's fractures in adults,* 4th ed. Philadelphia: Lippincott-Raven Publishers, 1996:1080, with permission.)

Fractures of the Humeral Shaft

Humeral shaft fractures are relatively simple fractures to diagnose and treat. Special attention must be taken to examine the function of the radial nerve, because it is the neurovascular structure that is most at risk as it courses in the spiral groove at the junction of the middle and distal third of the humerus. The inability to extend the wrist or thumb may indicate a *radial nerve palsy*.

In the isolated closed injury, the treatment of choice is nonsurgical management in a splint or brace because rigid fixation and perfect alignment are not necessary to achieve healing and good functional results (Fig. 27-13). There are some occasions when surgical intervention is preferable. *Absolute indications for surgery* are open fractures and fractures with associated vascular injuries. Relative indications include failure of closed treatment to achieve acceptable alignment, poor patient compliance, ipsilateral humeral shaft and forearm fractures (floating elbow), and fractures associated with brachial plexus injuries. In the polytrauma patient, rigid fixation of the fracture is important to facilitate earlier mobilization and prevent the secondary pulmonary complications caused by immobility. Surgical options are plating and IM rodding. External fixation is rarely used except in severe open fractures or when rapid stabilization is essential.

Uneventful healing is generally the outcome for simple humeral fractures treated nonsurgically. However, potential complications include nonunion and malunion, both of which can be treated with subsequent surgery. Radial nerve palsies (neuropraxia) have been reported in 2% to 24% of humeral shaft fractures and are commonly seen in transverse fractures of the middle third of the humerus. Spiral fractures of the distal third are more likely to cause laceration or entrapment of the nerve. The treatment for humerus fractures associated with radial nerve injury is controversial. Because spontaneous recovery of the nerve function within 6 to 12 months occurs in more than 70% of reported cases, closed treatment and observation may be preferable to surgical exploration.

Fractures of the Distal Humerus

Fractures of the distal humerus are complex injuries that include fractures of the supracondylar region of the elbow and the articular surface of the elbow. In more severe fractures, CT scans are helpful to evaluate articular comminution. Because this fracture is often a result of a high-energy injury, associated soft tissue injury is common.

Since closed reduction and casting or bracing is usually incapable of restoring the anatomy of the supracondylar humerus and the articular surface of the elbow, the only indication for nonoperative treatment is a nondisplaced distal humerus fracture. The treatment of choice for most distal humeral fractures is open reduction and plate fixation, followed by early mobilization. In grossly contaminated open fractures, an external fixator that spans the elbow joint may be used to temporarily stabilize the fracture.

Although fractures of the distal humerus account for only 2% of adult fractures, they account for a large number of poor outcomes and complications such as pain, deformity, instability, stiffness, nonunion, and malunion. *Ulnar nerve injury* is also a common complication, which can be caused by the injury itself or by impinging hardware. Ulnar neuropathy can be minimized by performing an ulnar nerve transposition during surgery. As with all elbow injuries, *heterotopic ossification* is another potential complication and is seen in 4% of distal humerus fractures.

Injuries of the Elbow

Injuries of the elbow are common and include elbow dislocations, olecranon fractures, and radial head fractures. Physical findings can be variable, ranging from a small effusion seen in a nondisplaced radial head fracture to gross deformity seen in an elbow dislocation. Radiographs may show an obvious fracture or dislocation. However, in the

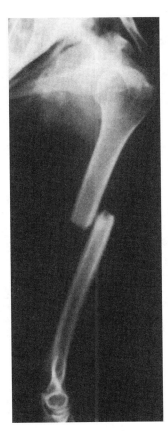

FIGURE 27-13. A simple transverse fracture of the humerus midshaft, which can be treated in a splint or brace. (From Rockwood CA Jr, et al., eds. *Rockwood and Green's fractures in adults*, 4th ed. Philadelphia: Lippincott-Raven Publishers, 1996:16, with permission.)

absence of an obvious finding, the presence of a posterior fat pad sign signifies an elbow effusion, suggesting an occult injury such as a nondisplaced radial head fracture.

The most common elbow dislocation is the posterior dislocation. Good anesthesia and traction usually allow easy closed reduction with minimal force. The elbow is then placed in a posterior splint at 90 degrees of elbow flexion for 7 to 10 days, followed by progressive mobilization. Nondisplaced fractures of the olecranon can be treated with casting or splinting. However, most olecranon fractures are displaced because of the pull of the triceps and require operative fixation with tension-band technique or plating.

Nondisplaced or minimally displaced fractures of the radial head are common injuries that can usually be treated by immobilization in a sling and early mobilization. In the displaced fracture, open reduction and internal fixation may be necessary, and in the severely comminuted radial head fracture, radial head excision may be necessary.

Neurovascular complications include ulnar and radial nerve injuries in elbow dislocations, ulnar nerve injuries in olecranon fractures, and radial nerve injury in radial head fractures. For all elbow fractures, stiffness (exacerbated by prolonged immobilization for more than 3 weeks) and *heterotopic bone formation* are other potential complications.

Fractures of the Forearm

Fractures of the radial and ulnar shafts are commonly caused by high-energy trauma from a direct blow (e.g., nightstick fracture of the ulna) or from a fall from a height. In evaluating the forearm fracture, it is particularly important to examine both the wrist and the elbow for an associated fracture. A common injury that may be missed is the Monteggia fracture, in which an ulna fracture is accompanied by a radial head dislocation (Fig. 27-14).

Because of the difficulty of maintaining anatomic alignment of the forearm fracture in a cast, there is a limited role for conservative care in forearm fractures. Isolated nondisplaced ulna fractures are usually treated in a cast, but most fractures of the radius, as well as combined radius and ulna fractures, are treated by open reduction and internal plate fixation. For comminuted fractures, additional bone grafting may be necessary.

Associated injuries include radial head dislocation (Monteggia fracture) and injuries to the distal radial ulnar joint (DRUJ). Both are easily seen on routine radiographs. In the elbow x-ray, the radial head should align with the capitellum in both the AP and lateral views. In the wrist x-ray, injury to the DRUJ results in widening of the joint space. Other complications include nerve injury to the posterior interosseus nerve (branch of the radial nerve), which can occur with radial head dislocations or with the surgical approach, compartment syndrome, and radioulnar synostosis, which can occur with plate fixation.

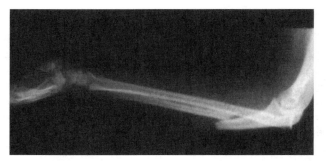

FIGURE 27-14. Monteggia fracture in which there is a radial head dislocation associated with an ulna fracture. Notice that the radial head lies posterior to the capitellum. (From Rockwood CA Jr, et al., eds. *Rockwood and Green's fractures in adults,* 4th ed. Philadelphia: Lippincott-Raven Publishers, 1996:916, with permission.)

Fractures of the Distal Radius

Fractures of the wrist are one of the most common orthopedic injuries (1 in 500 people). Although wrist fractures are mainly seen in young adolescents and in the elderly, it is becoming more common in young adults as a result of activities such as in-line skating.

In the common extraarticular distal radius fracture with a dorsally angulated distal fragment (also known as the "Colles fracture") (Fig. 27-15), closed reduction and cast immobilization is the treatment of choice. Unstable injuries with extensive comminution and open injuries are best treated surgically with external fixation. Open reduction and pinning or internal plating is also useful in unstable fractures and in intraarticular fractures.

The most common complication following the distal radius fracture is nerve injury. *Median nerve injury* is the most common, followed by ulnar neuropathy. Radial nerve injury is usually a result of external fixator pin placement. Acute neuropathy is usually caused by a contusion from the initial injury, but subsequent swelling and immobilization in excessive wrist flexion can also lead to neuropraxia. Initial treatment is reduction of the fracture, but if there is no improvement, then nerve decompression (such as a carpal tunnel release for median neuropathy) may be necessary. Scaphoid fractures are also associated with distal radius fractures. Other complications include compartment syndrome, reflex sympathetic dystrophy, arthritis, and tendon entrapment, adhesion, and late tendon rupture (most commonly involving the extensor pollicis longus).

Fractures of the Hand

Common fractures of the hand include scaphoid fractures, fractures of the base of the thumb metacarpal, fractures of the fifth metacarpal neck (boxer's fracture), and phalangeal fractures. It is particularly important to diagnose and treat

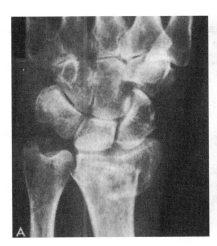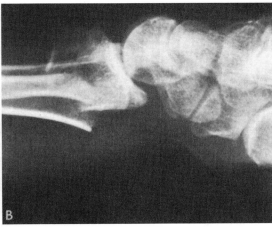

FIGURE 27-15. **A:** Anterior-posterior and **B:** lateral view of the wrist showing a Colles distal radius fracture with characteristic shortening and dorsal angulation of the distal fragment. (From Rockwood CA Jr, et al., eds. *Rockwood and Green's fractures in adults,* 4th ed. Philadelphia: Lippincott-Raven Publishers, 1996:776, with permission.)

the scaphoid fracture because of the high risk of nonunion and AVN. Pain to palpation over the anatomic snuffbox of the wrist, even in the absence of an apparent scaphoid fracture on the radiograph, is suggestive of a scaphoid fracture, and the wrist should be immobilized in a thumb spica cast. If there are any questions, a bone scan or MRI will definitively reveal a scaphoid fracture. For the fifth metacarpal neck fractures, it is important to look for tooth marks resulting from a punch to a mouth, because this may represent an open fracture requiring operative incisional drainage.

In general, most fractures of the hand can be treated by closed reduction and buddy taping, splinting, or casting. A scaphoid fracture is treated in a thumb spica cast. While residual angular deformity in the hand may be well tolerated (e.g., 45 degrees of angulation is acceptable in fifth metacarpal neck fractures), rotational deformity is never acceptable. Unsuccessful attempts at nonsurgical treatment necessitate operative intervention, usually in the form of closed reduction and percutaneous pinning. However, other techniques such as plating, screw fixation, or external fixation can be used in certain situations.

The risk of AVN in scaphoid fractures is related to the level of the fracture. Because the vascular supply enters the scaphoid distally, fractures involving the proximal pole have a higher incidence of AVN than fractures of the distal or middle third. AVN presents radiographically as sclerosis and fragmentation, typically at the proximal pole of the scaphoid.

Other complications of hand fractures include capsular or collateral ligament contractures (particularly in the metacarpophalangeal joint following immobilization in extension), decreased motion, and extensor and flexor tendon adhesions. Prolonged immobilization (more than 3 weeks) can aggravate the stiffness. Because of the abundant vascular supply of the hand, infections following open fractures in the hand are less common than those in other areas of the body.

Amputation and Injuries of the Hand

Although it is now possible to reattach most amputated parts of the hand with microvascular techniques, reattachment may not always lead to a better cosmetic or functional outcome. The nature of the injury, the level of the injury, and the age of the patient are important considerations. While sharp amputation is amenable to replantation, crush and avulsion injuries have a poor prognosis. Functional results are best with replantation at the level of the metacarpal and the wrist and worst at the level of proximal phalanx (poor flexor tendon function) and higher levels such as the forearm or upper arm. Also, results are better in children than in adults. Specific indications for replantation include (i) injury to multiple digits, (ii) amputations of the thumb, (iii) most amputations in children, and (iv) sharp amputations at the level of the hand, wrist, or distal forearm. Relative contraindications include (i) contaminated or severe crush or avulsion injury, (ii) single-digit amputations in adults, and (iii) a history of smoking. Absolute contraindications include (i) severe medical problems, (ii) multilevel injury of the amputated part, and (iii) a psychiatric patient with a self-inflicted injury.

Peripheral nerve injuries to the upper extremity are common and disabling injuries. The most important aspect of the diagnosis of the injury is the knowledge of the distribution and motor function of the major nerves (Table 27-4). The three major nerves in the upper extremity are the radial, median, and ulnar nerves. Both the median and the ulnar nerves innervate muscles in the

TABLE 27-4. NERVES OF THE WRIST AND HAND

	Radial nerve	Median nerve	Ulnar nerve
Location	Posterior compartment of the forearm, entering the wrist dorsally	Volar surface of the forearm between the FDP and FDS, entering the wrist through the carpal tunnel	Behind the medial epicondyle of the elbow, along the ulnar aspect of forearm between the FDP and FCU, entering the wrist through the Guyon canal (ulnar to the carpal tunnel) ulnar to the ulnar artery
Motor function	Wrist extension (ECRB, ECRL), thumb extension (EPL), extension of fingers at MCP joint (EDC)	*Extrinsic:* wrist flexion (FCR), finger and thumb flexion (FDS, FDP for index finger, FPL) *Intrinsic:* thumb abduction (APB) and opposition (OP), MCP flexion (radial lumbricals)	Extrinsic: wrist flexion (FCU), ring and little finger flexion (FDP for ring and little finger) Intrinsic: finger abduction/adduction (interosseous), intrinsic hand movements (hypothenar muscles, ulnar lumbricals)
Sensory innervation	See Figure 16	See Figure 16	See Figure 16
Specific areas of sensory innervation	First dorsal web space (between thumb and index finger)	Palmar aspect of the tip of the index finger	Palmar aspect of the tip of the little finger

forearm (extrinsic muscles) and in the hand (intrinsic muscles), although the radial nerve does not innervate any muscles in the hand (Fig. 27-16). The digital nerves, which supply sensation to the fingers, are terminal branches of these three nerves. Because most nerve injuries sustained in fractures, dislocations, crush injuries, and gunshot wounds result in neurapraxia, immediate surgical exploration is not indicated. However, in sharp trauma, surgical exploration and primary nerve repair or nerve grafting is the treatment of choice.

Flexor tendon lacerations will result in severe disability if not treated. Although extensor tendon lacerations may be repaired in the emergency room, flexor tendon injuries are best repaired in the operating room under more controlled circumstances. Repair within 1 to 2 weeks is acceptable and will not compromise the outcome.

FRACTURES OF THE PELVIS AND ACETABULUM

Pelvic Fractures

Fractures of the pelvic ring are life-threatening injuries that result from high-energy trauma such as a car accident or a fall from a height. The overall mortality rate is 8.6%, with hemorrhage accounting for 60% of the deaths. Open pelvic fractures have a mortality rate of up to 50%.

External clues to an underlying pelvic fracture are scrotal or labial swelling, ecchymosis, abnormal positioning of the lower extremity, unexplained hypotension, and instability and pain of the pelvis on examination. Rectal and perineal examination is essential to look for open communication with the vagina or rectum. Evaluation should include an abdominal CT scan or deep peritoneal lavage (DPL) to assess the sources of bleeding. For the DPL, the needle must be inserted supraumbilically to avoid inadvertent puncture and decompression of a large intrapelvic hematoma. Urogenital injuries will present as bleeding from the urethral meatus, a high-riding prostate, or difficulty with passing a urinary catheter into the bladder. If this occurs in the trauma bay, a retrograde urethrogram is indicated.

As with all multitrauma patients, the first priority is aggressive resuscitation and stabilization of the patient according to ATLS protocol. The orthopedic issues must be addressed concurrently: retroperitoneal hemorrhage, pelvic ring instability, and associated injury to the urogenital and gastrointestinal system. The most common

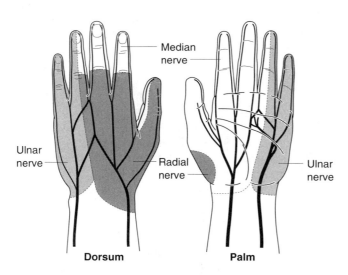

FIGURE 27-16. Sensory innervation of the hand.

sources of retroperitoneal bleeding are from low-pressure sources such as cancellous bone bleeding from the fracture site and retroperitoneal venous bleeding. Because only 15% of the hemorrhage-related deaths are a result of the high-pressure arterial bleeds (most commonly injured artery is the superior gluteal artery), emergent angiography before pelvic stabilization may not be helpful. In the hypotensive patient suspected of suffering from retroperitoneal bleeding, the pelvis must be immediately stabilized by application of an external fixator, pelvic clamp, military antishock trousers (pneumatic antishock garment), or even a sheet tied around the pelvis. A stabilized pelvis will help with tamponade of the retroperitoneal bleeding by reducing pelvic volume. For continued uncontrollable blood loss and a rapidly expanding or pulsatile retroperitoneal hematoma, emergent angiography with embolization is warranted. Pelvic fractures that communicate with the rectum or perineum are open fractures by definition and must be managed surgically with a *diverting colostomy*. Early treatment of a vaginal laceration can minimize formation of a pelvic abscess.

Definitive management of the unstable pelvic injury consists of surgical stabilization. Posterior instability (such as with disruption of the sacroiliac joint) is associated with increased patient mortality. Indications for external fixation include pelvic instability, hemodynamic instability, and associated pelvic soft tissue injuries. In certain situations, open reduction and internal fixation may be another option. Pubic symphysis disruptions (diastasis of more than 2.5 cm) can be plated through an anterior Pfannenstiel incision. Posterior sacroiliac joint injuries can be fixed with plates, sacral bars, or iliosacral lag screws. Pubic rami fractures generally do not need to be surgically repaired. Because of the complexity of the repair, the surgery should be delayed until the patient is stable and the entire surgical staff is fully prepared.

Associated injuries are common in patients with pelvic fractures: hemodynamic instability (20%), urogenital injury (12% to 20%), and injury to the lumbosacral plexus (8%). A very high risk of injury to the lumbosacral nerve roots is seen with associated sacral foraminal fractures. In addition, 60% to 85% of patients have other associated fractures. Lastly, the risk for DVT is also significant because of injury to the pelvic veins.

Acetabular Fractures

Most acetabular fractures result from high-energy blunt trauma, which may involve other significant life-threatening injuries. The diagnosis can be made on the plain radiograph (Fig. 27-17A, B), but the fracture can be best evaluated by the CT scan. Nondisplaced fractures can be treated with protected weight bearing. For fractures with a greater than 2-mm articular step off, open reduction and plate fixation is preferred to help decrease the likelihood of posttraumatic arthritis. Skeletal traction can be used as a temporary measure or as definitive treatment in the patient who cannot undergo surgery. Complications include het-

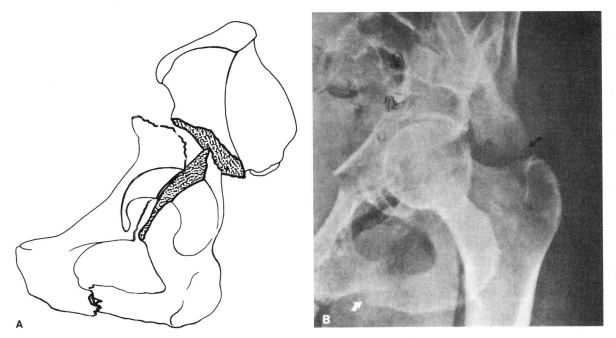

FIGURE 27-17. A, B: Fracture of the acetabulum. (From Rockwood CA Jr, et al., eds. *Rockwood and Green's fractures in adults,* 4th ed. Philadelphia: Lippincott-Raven Publishers, 1996:1632, with permission.)

erotopic ossification, sciatic nerve injury, and posttraumatic arthritis, as well as osteonecrosis of the femoral head if there is a concomitant posterior hip dislocation.

INJURIES OF THE LOWER EXTREMITY

Hip Dislocations

Because of the intrinsic stability of the hip joint, an isolated hip dislocation is an uncommon injury and is usually caused by a high-energy trauma such as in a motor vehicle accident in which the hip is driven posteriorly by the dashboard. In the classic clinical presentation of the more common posterior hip dislocation, the leg is adducted, internally rotated, and shortened (Fig. 27-18). Special attention must be paid to the neurological examination, particularly the sciatic nerve. The dislocation is usually evident in the standard AP pelvis and hip radiograph. In the posterior dislocation, the femoral head lies superiorly out of the acetabulum.

Prompt reduction within 24 hours (and preferably within 6 hours) is important to minimize the risk of AVN of the femoral head. Closed reduction may not be possible if there is entrapment of a tendon, a capsule, or a fracture fragment, and open reduction will be necessary. After reduction, the hip should be tested for stability. In addition, a CT scan may be useful to confirm a congruent reduction. When comfortable, the patient may begin ambulation with full weight bearing.

AVN of the femoral head, which usually presents 1 to 5 years after the injury, is a devastating complication and has been reported in up to 17% of patients. Prompt reduction has been shown to decrease the risk of AVN. The most frequent long-term complication is posttraumatic arthritis and is related to the severity of the injury. Because of the proximity of the sciatic nerve, sciatic nerve injuries (more commonly the peroneal branch) occur in 8% to 19% of posterior hip dislocations. However, 50% of the time, the patient eventually recovers full function.

Hip Fractures

Femoral Neck Fractures and Intertrochanteric Fractures

Femoral neck fractures are common injuries that result from low-energy trauma (such as a fall) in the elderly and high-energy trauma in young adults. Hip fractures are more common in women, and risk factors include poor balance and vision, smoking, lack of physical activity, medications such as sedatives, and neurological impairments. Osteoporosis has not been shown to be a risk factor for the femoral neck fracture. The femoral head is mainly supplied by the lateral epiphyseal artery (branch of the medial femoral circumflex artery), which can be disrupted in the femoral neck fracture. In the classic clinical presentation, the leg is abducted, externally rotated, and shortened (distinct from the hip dislocation). AP and cross-lateral radiographs of the hip are required for evaluation. In the patient who has negative findings on the radiograph but who has examination results suspicious for a hip fracture, a bone scan performed 48 hours after the injury or an MRI will be diagnostic.

Because early mobilization in patients with hip fractures can help prevent DVT and pneumonia, the *treatment of choice* is surgical stabilization. The technique is dictated by the amount of displacement of the fracture. Nondisplaced or minimally displaced fractures can be treated by closed or open reduction and fixation with multiple screws (Fig. 27-19A, B). Prosthetic replacement of the femoral head (hemiarthroplasty) is preferred in displaced fractures because of the higher risk of AVN of the femoral head. Patients with preexisting osteoarthritis and rheumatoid arthritis should be treated with a prosthetic total hip replacement. Although hip fractures do not need to be fixed emergently, fixation within 2 days has been shown to decrease the risk of mortality within the first year after the fracture.

In patients with femoral neck fractures, disruption of the blood supply to the femoral head is proportional to the amount of displacement. In nondisplaced or minimally displaced fractures, the *risk of AVN* is less than 10%, compared to a rate of 25% in displaced fractures. Other complications include nonunion and failure of fixation.

The evaluation and diagnosis of the intertrochanteric hip fracture is similar to that of the femoral neck fracture. Although isolated avulsion fractures of the greater or lesser trochanter can be managed by protected weight bearing, surgical stabilization in the form of a compression hip

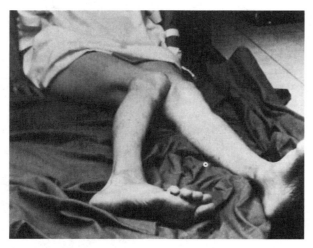

FIGURE 27-18. The classic appearance of a posterior dislocation of the right hip. (From Rockwood CA Jr, et al., eds. *Rockwood and Green's fractures in adults,* 4th ed. Philadelphia: Lippincott-Raven Publishers, 1996:1771, with permission.)

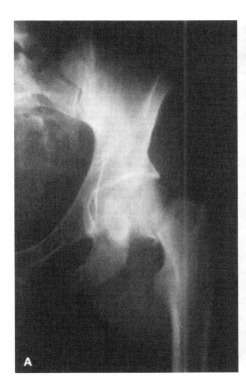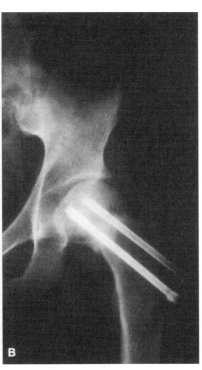

FIGURE 27-19. A: Fracture of the femoral neck with minimal displacement. **B:** The fracture has been fixed by lag screw fixation. The treatment for completely displaced fractures is prosthetic replacement of the femoral head. (From Rockwood CA Jr, et al., eds. *Rockwood and Green's fractures in adults,* 4th ed. Philadelphia: Lippincott-Raven Publishers, 1996:1698, with permission.)

screw and side plate is the treatment of choice for the intertrochanteric fracture. Prosthetic replacement is an option for comminuted fractures or pathologic fractures. In contrast to femoral neck fractures, there is no increased risk of AVN with the intertrochanteric hip fracture. The major complication is the loss of fixation.

Fractures of the Femur

Fractures of the femoral shaft and distal supracondylar femur are generally high-energy injuries that are easily diagnosed on physical examination because of the obvious swelling, shortening, deformity, and pain in the thigh. Radiographs should include views of the knee, hip, and pelvis. It is particularly important to look for an associated femoral neck fracture, which is often missed.

Immediate stabilization of femoral shaft fractures, particularly in a patient with multiple injuries, has been shown to decrease the incidence of pulmonary complications (such as ARDS) and the length of stay in the hospital. *IM rodding* is the treatment of choice for most femoral shaft fractures. Results are excellent, with a 99% union rate and only a 0.9% infection rate. Traction and external fixation can be used as a temporary measure in patients with open fractures, in patients awaiting medical stabilization, or in patients too ill to undergo surgery. Plate fixation is not optimal in most cases because of the extensive exposure required. In patients with gunshot wounds, IM rods can be inserted following local wound care.

Minimally displaced distal femur fractures can be treated nonoperatively in a knee immobilizer or a long leg cast. Displaced fractures and fractures with articular involvement are best treated surgically with devices such as an IM nail, condylar screws and plates, or lag screws and buttress plates.

Femoral neck fractures are found in 2.5% to 5% of femoral shaft fractures. However, because the femoral neck fracture is often nondisplaced and the femoral shaft fracture is so obvious, the femoral neck fracture is missed 30% of the time. In these cases, the femoral neck fracture is given priority over the femoral shaft fracture. Infections, nonunion, and malunion following IM nailing for femoral shaft fractures are rare. Compartment syndrome of the thigh is also rare. Heterotopic ossification can occur in 25% of patients following IM nailing, but the long-term negative impact is minimal. Complications following distal femur fractures include infection, nonunion, malunion, loss of fixation, knee stiffness, and posttraumatic arthritis.

Soft Tissue Injuries of the Knee

Isolated sprains and ruptures of the ligaments of the knee are common injuries and can be caused both by minor and major trauma. The anterior cruciate ligament (ACL) and the posterior cruciate ligament (PCL) provide anterior and posterior stability to the knee, respectively. The medial collateral ligament (MCL) and the lateral collateral ligament provide stability in the medial-lateral plane. ACL ruptures, which commonly occur as a low-velocity rotational noncontact sports injury, are often associated with MCL and medial meniscus injuries. The MRI is the radiographic study of choice to evaluate the status of the ligaments. Treatment of isolated injuries to any of the four ligaments is bracing. For the younger and more active patient, surgical reconstruction of the ACL or PCL may be recommended.

Meniscal tears are very common injuries and can be traumatic or degenerative in nature. Treatment is symptomatic unless there are mechanical symptoms such as knee catching or locking, in which case, arthroscopic partial meniscectomy may be indicated.

Knee Dislocations

Knee dislocations can be devastating injuries because of associated injuries to the neurovascular bundle as it passes posteriorly through the popliteal fossa. Anterior dislocations are usually caused by hyperextension, and posterior dislocations can be caused when the proximal tibia is driven posteriorly, such as when the proximal tibia strikes the dashboard during a car accident. Although knee dislocations are usually clearly seen on routine radiographs, it is important to remember that spontaneous reductions can sometimes occur. Injuries that involve a suspicious mechanism or multiligamentous instability should be treated as knee dislocations until proven otherwise. Evaluation of the neurovascular status of the involved extremity is particularly important. Although distal pulses may be present, they do not rule out vascular injury such as an intimal tear. Therefore, arteriography is recommended in all patients with a history of ischemia or diminished pulses. Status of the four major knee ligaments should be determined, and in most patients, the ACL and PCL are both ruptured.

Immediate closed reduction can restore the neurovascular status of the leg. The vascular surgery team should be consulted immediately, as increased rates of amputation are seen with delays in vascular repair after more than 6 hours. Reverse saphenous vein interposition graft is the treatment of choice for occlusive vascular injuries. Four-compartment fasciotomy for ischemia times greater than 4 hours is also recommended. Attention is then directed toward the associated ligamentous injuries. If there is a vascular injury, any associated ligamentous repair should be delayed a few weeks or should be performed without a tourniquet. Because the use of a tourniquet may aggravate an underlying vascular repair, arteriography should be performed before tourniquet use.

Associated injuries include vascular injury (30%), neurological injury typically involving the peroneal nerve (23%), open injury (5%), and fractures (10%). Meniscal injury is also common (40%), but compartment syndrome is rare. Knee stiffness is the most common complication, but surprisingly, instability is rarely a major complaint.

Fractures of the Tibial Plateau

Tibial plateau (proximal tibia) fractures are most commonly seen in high-energy trauma in middle-aged men and in osteopenic fractures in elderly women. The mechanisms of injury include falls, motor vehicle accidents, and pedestrian accidents (such as when the car bumper hits the lateral aspect of the pedestrian's knee). On physical examination, the status of soft tissue and skin and the neurovascular structures should be carefully documented. Although standard radiographs will show the fracture (most commonly involving the lateral tibial plateau), a CT scan or MRI will better delineate the comminution of the articular surface.

For nondisplaced fractures with minimally depressed articular fragments, the fracture can be treated with casting or bracing and early range of motion. In fractures with a significant amount of articular depression (5 to 10 mm) or with significant ligamentous laxity, surgical reduction and fixation with lag screws and buttress plates is preferred (Fig. 27-20A, B). External fixation can be used in markedly comminuted fractures or open fractures.

Meniscal tears and ligamentous injuries (particularly to the MCL) are commonly associated with tibial plateau fractures. In more severe injuries involving the medial or bilateral tibial plateaus, neurovascular injury such as peroneal nerve palsy (accompanied by fibular head fracture) and popliteal artery lesions can occur. The most common complications are posttraumatic arthritis (meniscal preservation is important to prevent arthritis) and knee stiffness (prevented by early mobilization). Surgical complications include infection and skin sloughing secondary to poor skin condition in high-energy traumas and extensive surgical dissections in complex fractures.

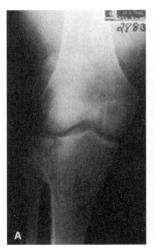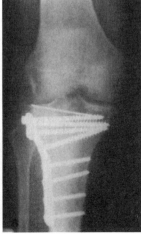

FIGURE 27-20. Intraarticular fracture of the **(A)** lateral tibial plateau, which has been stabilized by a **(B)** buttress plate. (From Rockwood CA Jr, et al., eds. *Rockwood and Green's fractures in adults*, 4th ed. Philadelphia: Lippincott-Raven Publishers, 1996:1933, with permission.)

Fractures of the Tibia

Fractures of the tibial shaft are the most common long-bone fractures. Because of the subcutaneous location of the tibia, the deformity is usually evident. Intraarticular fractures of the distal tibia (also known as a "tibial plafond fracture" or "pilon fracture") are usually high-energy injuries that result from axial loading and are accompanied by significant soft tissue swelling. Although radiographs are adequate in most cases, bone scan or MRI can be used to diagnose occult stress fractures in the tibial shaft.

For minimally displaced and angulated tibial shaft fractures (less than 10 degrees of angulation), cast immobilization is an acceptable treatment option. For unstable and comminuted fractures, surgical fixation in the form of IM rodding is the preferred treatment. External fixation is useful in grossly contaminated open injuries. In grade IIIC open tibial fractures, amputation may be preferable to leg salvage because of poor results following neurovascular repair.

Delayed unions and nonunions are relatively common complications of tibial shaft fractures. For nonsurgical treatment, the delayed union rate is 19% and the nonunion rate is 4%. Malunions are also more common with nonsurgical treatment. Complications specific to IM rodding include implant failures and anterior knee pain (because of the entrance point of the rod in the anterior knee). Pin tract infections can occur in up to 50% of patients treated with external fixation. Because compartment syndrome is also more common in the lower leg, close observation is essential.

The nondisplaced tibial plafond fracture is treated nonsurgically. Because the fracture usually involves comminution of the articular surface, surgical fixation is generally preferred. Due to the high risk of wound infection and sloughing, it may be prudent to wait 7 to 10 days to allow the swelling to subside before surgery is performed. Surgical options include plate fixation, although the potential for wound complications does make external fixation an attractive alternative. Because of the intraarticular injury in the pilon fracture, posttraumatic arthritis of the ankle joint is an expected complication. However, the most feared complication is wound infection and dehiscence.

Fractures of the Fibula

Because the fibula bears only a small percentage of the body weight as compared to the tibia, isolated fractures of the fibula are generally successfully managed conservatively. Symptomatic treatment and splinting for comfort are the mainstays of treatment. There usually are no long-term complications. Fractures of the proximal fibula near the level of the fibular head may result in peroneal nerve neuropraxia.

Achilles Tendon Ruptures

In the acute rupture of the Achilles tendon, pain is localized at the posterior calf and there is an absence of ankle plantar flexion with passive squeezing of the calf muscles (Thompson test). Nonsurgical treatment consists of casting with the ankle in plantar flexion. For the more active patient, open repair will allow for quicker return to activities and a lower rerupture rate when compared to nonsurgical treatment. However, because of the thin soft tissue envelope around the Achilles tendon, postsurgical wound infection is seen in up to 13% of open repairs.

Fractures of the Calcaneus

Fractures of the calcaneus are caused by a high-energy axial load, such as a fall from a height. A common presentation is a patient who has fallen from a building who presents with severe foot pain and deformity as well as lower back pain. Careful examination of the spine is essential because of the risk of associated compression fractures of the lumbar vertebrae. In addition to plain radiographs, CT scan of the calcaneus is useful in evaluating the integrity of the articular surface. Treatment is nonsurgical for extraarticular fractures (25% of fractures) and open reduction and internal fixation for intraarticular fractures. Because massive soft tissue swelling is usually present, surgical fixation is best performed in 7 to 10 days to allow the swelling to subside.

Complications are posttraumatic arthritis to the subtalar joint, which may cause significant pain. Compartment syndrome of the foot occurs in up to 10% of fractures. Wound infection and dehiscence and injury to the sural nerve are potential risks related to the surgical repair.

SUGGESTED READING

Rockwood CA Jr, Wilkins KE, Beaty JH, eds. *Fractures in children,* 4th ed. Philadelphia: Lippincott-Raven Publishers, 1996.

Rockwood CA Jr, Wilkins DP, Beaty RW, et al., eds. *Rockwood and Green's fractures in adults,* 4th ed. Philadelphia: Lippincott-Raven Publishers, 1996.

Simon SR. *Orthopaedic basic science.* Rosemont: American Academy of Orthopaedic Surgeons, 1994.

SECTION V

ENDOCRINE SYSTEM

28

THYROID, PARATHYROID, AND ADRENAL GLANDS

TODD W. BAUER, DAVID MARON, EUGENE A. CHOI, AND DOUGLAS L. FRAKER

THYROID

During the third week of gestation, the median thyroid anlage forms at the base of the tongue in the region of the foramen cecum. It is an *endodermal* pocket, which originates from the primitive alimentary tract, initially protruding between the first pair of pharyngeal pouches. It subsequently descends in the midline to reach its normal anatomic location developing into a bilobed organ. As the lateral lobes of the thyroid develop follicles can be noted. Iodine trapping occurs as thyroid hormones are first seen in the third month of gestation. Lateral anlagen develop from the fourth pharyngeal pouch and fuse with the median anlagen at about the seventh week of gestation. Ultimobranchial bodies, which originate from the fourth pharyngeal pouch, give rise to parafollicular or C cells. These cells, which are responsible for the secretion of calcitonin, originate from the neural crest and are of *ectodermal* origin. The original attachment of the thyroid mass to the buccal cavity is the thyroglossal duct, which is normally resorbed by the sixth week of gestation. The distal end of the duct may be retained as the pyramidal lobe of the gland in adults. Failure of the thyroid anlage to migrate can result in persistence of a functional *lingual thyroid gland*. Most lingual thyroids can be treated with thyroid-stimulating hormone (TSH) and exogenous thyroid hormone to decrease the size of the gland. Excision may result in hypothyroidism and is required only for airway obstruction, difficulty swallowing, or hemorrhage.

Failure of resorption of the *thyroglossal duct* results in a thyroglossal duct cyst or fistula. These are the most common developmental malformations of the thyroid gland that require surgery. Thyroglossal cysts are usually located at or near the midline between the base of the tongue and the suprasternal notch (Fig. 28-1). Seventy-five percent are located just inferior to the hyoid bone. A mass or infection of the cyst is what usually leads to medical evaluation. The wall of the cyst or fistula usually contains some thyroid tissue. Thyroglossal duct cysts may be the source of thyroid cancer, which is usually papillary in type. All thyroglossal duct cysts should be excised because of the potential for infection. It is important to excise the entire cyst or fistula up to the base of the tongue including a portion of the hyoid bone (*Sistrunk* procedure). Papillary cancer arising in a thyroglossal duct cyst or fistula is treated with excision of the cyst or tract if there are no lymph node metastases. Treatment with iodine-131 (^{131}I), followed by thyroid hormone replacement, is an alternative treatment. Overdescent of the thyroid can result in ectopic thyroid tissue, which may be found in the central compartment of the neck or anterior mediastinum. Thyroid nodules in the carotid sheath or lateral neck are not due to aberrant migration but typically represent metastases of well-differentiated thyroid cancer.

Anatomy

The normal adult thyroid gland weighs between 20 and 30 g. The thyroid lobes lie adjacent to the thyroid cartilage, anterior to the larynx and trachea. The two lobes are connected by the isthmus. In the midline pyramidal process, the distal remnant of the thyroglossal duct is present in approximately 40% to 50% of adults. It can extend cranially to the hyoid bone or rarely to the base of the tongue. The anterior aspect of the thyroid gland is covered by the infrahyoid muscles and their fasciae. These muscles include the sternohyoid, sternothyroid, thyrohyoid, and omohyoid. Posteriorly lies the trachea and posterolaterally lie the common carotid arteries, the internal jugular veins, and the vagus nerves.

The thyroid gland is enclosed in a true capsule that requires sharp dissection to remove it from the parenchyma. Exterior to the capsule, the thyroid gland is covered by a thin layer of connective tissue, the thyroid sheath, which is derived from the pretracheal fascia. Above the isthmus, this fascia forms the anterior suspensory ligament of the thyroid. Posteromedially, it attaches the gland to the upper two or three tracheal rings and the cricoid cartilage and is known as the "ligament of Berry." The recurrent laryngeal nerve usually runs just underneath or rarely over this liga-

---

Hospital of the University of Pennsylvania, Philadelphia, Pennsylvania

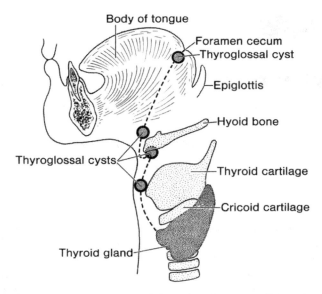

FIGURE 28-1. The location of thyroglossal cysts parallels embryological thyroid descent. These cysts are most frequently found in the thyroid region and are always located close to the midline. (From Sadler TW. *Langman's medical embryology,* 5th ed. Baltimore: Williams & Wilkins, 1985:294, with permission.)

ment before entering the larynx. Parathyroid glands can be occasionally enveloped by the thyroid sheath. They can usually be safely identified by dissecting the sheath from the thyroid capsule.

The thyroid gland is supplied by four main *arteries*: two superior thyroid arteries and two inferior thyroid arteries (Fig. 28-2). The superior thyroid artery is the first anterior branch of the external carotid artery. At the apex of the thyroid gland, the superior thyroid artery divides into an anterior branch that runs over the anterior surface of the gland and a posterior branch that forms an anastomosis with the ascending branch of the inferior thyroid artery. The superior thyroid artery lies adjacent to the external branch of the superior laryngeal nerve. The inferior thyroid artery arises from the thyrocervical trunk of the subclavian artery, travels behind the carotid sheath, then downward and medially, where it divides into ascending and descending branches before entering the middle portion of the thyroid gland. The inferior thyroid arteries, in addition to supplying the thyroid gland, are also the principal blood supply to all four parathyroid glands in 80% of individuals (Fig. 28-2). The inferior thyroid artery should therefore be ligated close to the thyroid gland to avoid ischemia to the parathyroid glands. Thyroidea ima arteries, which arise from the innominate artery or directly from the aorta, are encountered only infrequently. When present, they travel on the anterior surface of the trachea and enter the lower isthmus of the thyroid.

Venous blood drains from the thyroid gland via three pairs of veins: superior, lateral, and inferior thyroid veins. The superior thyroid veins travel with the superior thyroid arteries and drain into the internal jugular vein at the level

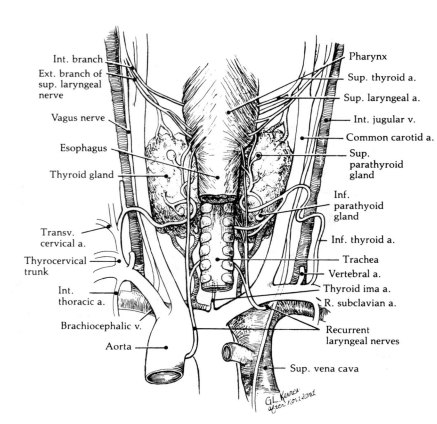

FIGURE 28-2. Posterior view of the larynx, trachea, thyroid, parathyroid glands, and the recurrent laryngeal nerve illustrates the anatomical relationship of these structures. (From Black S. Surgical anatomy of the thyroid gland. In: Nyhus LM, Baker RJ, eds. *Mastery of surgery,* 2nd ed. Little, Brown and Company, 1992:193, with permission.)

of the carotid bifurcation. The lateral thyroid veins originate from the anterolateral surface of the thyroid gland in the middle portion and also drain into the internal jugular veins. The inferior thyroid veins originate from the lower poles of the gland and empty into the brachiocephalic veins.

The thyroid gland has a rich *lymphatic drainage.* Intraglandular lymphatics are located beneath the capsule and travel through the isthmus to connect both lobes, which explains the relative frequency with which multifocal tumors are encountered in the thyroid. These intraglandular lymphatics also drain into perithyroidal lymphatics and lymph nodes. The closest regional nodes include the paraglandular nodes, pretracheal nodes, paratracheal nodes, and the recurrent laryngeal chain. The next lymphatic stations include anterosuperior mediastinal nodes, upper, middle, lower jugular nodes, and the retropharyngeal and esophageal nodes. In patients with advanced thyroid cancers, the lateral cervical nodes in the posterior triangle may be involved. Most patients with papillary or medullary carcinoma have lymph node metastases at the time of diagnosis. In these cases, the central compartment nodes must be dissected, which includes all lymph nodes from the level of the hyoid bone to the innominate artery and lateral to the jugular veins.

Detailed knowledge of the relation of the *recurrent laryngeal nerve* (RLN) to the thyroid gland is critical, as nerve damage may have grave consequences. Routine exposure of the nerve during thyroid operations has been recommended by many surgeons. It provides the motor fibers to all intrinsic muscles of the larynx, except the cricothyroid, and the sensory innervation to the mucous membranes below the vocal cords. Recurrent laryngeal nerve injury can result in paralysis of the vocal cord on the ipsilateral side. This may result in hoarseness or a weakened voice because the vocal cord remains in an abducted position. Shortness of breath may result in some patients because the airway may become narrowed. Bilateral RLN injury may result in complete loss of voice or complete airway obstruction, requiring emergent intubation or tracheostomy.

The endocrine surgeon needs to be aware of potential variations in the course of the RLN relative to the inferior thyroid artery and the ligament of Berry. The right RLN branches from the vagus nerve, loops under the right subclavian artery, and then ascends in the neck between the trachea and esophagus. It enters the larynx posterior to the thyroid gland at the level of the cricothyroid articulation. Due to an inconstant relationship between recurrent nerve and inferior thyroid artery, most endocrine surgeons prefer to identify the nerve inferior to the inferior thyroid artery and trace its course superiorly. The nerve may lie anterior or posterior to the artery or between branches of the inferior thyroid artery. The recurrent nerve is also at risk during ligation of the ligament of Berry and should always be identified. The nerve frequently branches there and may travel through the ligament. In this anatomical area, the nerve travels directly posterior to the lateral posterior extension of the thyroid lobe. The right laryngeal nerve has been reported to be nonrecurrent in less than 1% of patients, but rather coming directly off the vagus nerve in the neck. The left RLN branches from the vagus nerve lateral to the ligamentum arteriosum. After traveling underneath the aortic arch, it runs superiorly along the tracheoesophageal groove to the larynx. Nonrecurrent left laryngeal nerves are extremely rare.

The *superior laryngeal nerve* arises from the vagus nerve at the skull base and descends along the internal carotid artery, branching at the level of the hyoid bone. The larger internal branch penetrates the thyrohyoid membrane and provides sensory innervation to the larynx above the vocal cords. The smaller external branch travels adjacent to the superior thyroid artery. It supplies motor fibers to the cricothyroid muscle and the inferior constrictor muscle of the pharynx. To avoid injury to this nerve, the superior thyroid artery should be divided distal to the bifurcation on the thyroid capsule.

Physiology

The thyroid gland synthesizes and secretes hormones that are necessary for normal growth and development. *Iodine* in the form of dietary iodine is essential for the formation of thyroid hormone. The daily requirement of iodine is approximately 100 to 200 µg. Iodine in foods is converted to iodide and then absorbed in the upper gastrointestinal tract. It reaches the thyroid gland via the bloodstream, where it is trapped by the thyroid follicular cells through an adenosine 5'-triphosphate–dependent (ATP-dependent) transmembrane transport. Approximately 90% of the total body iodine is found in the thyroid gland in organic form. The thyroid/serum ratio of iodine is approximately 50:1 in healthy individuals.

The synthesis of *thyroid hormone* occurs at the apical border of the follicular cell and colloid. The predominant component of colloid is thyroglobulin, a glycoprotein. In the follicular cell, iodine is rapidly oxidized to a free radical form by thyroid peroxidases. This activated form of iodine binds to tyrosine in the thyroglobulin molecule, forming either monoiodotyrosine or diiodotyrosine. This step in the organification of iodine is inhibited by reducing substances such as propylthiouracil (PTU). The iodotyrosines then combine with each other to form triiodothyronine (T_3) or thyroxine (T_4). TSH, which is secreted by the anterior pituitary gland, regulates the function of the thyroid gland (Fig. 28-3). TSH mediates its action via the second messenger adenosine 3',5'-cyclic monophosphate (cyclic AMP). It regulates iodine trapping by the thyroid gland and stimulates the synthesis of iodothyronines. TSH also causes proteolytic separation of T_3 and T_4 from thyroglobulin. Under normal circumstances, thyroglobulin is too large to be transported across the follicular cell membrane. It thus stimulates the

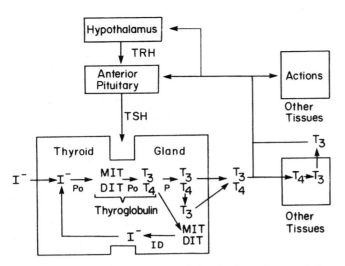

FIGURE 28-3. The regulation and feedback pathway of the hypothalamic/pituitary/thyroid system and intrathyroidal thyroid hormone synthesis and release. DIT, diiodotyrosine; I, inorganic iodide; ID, iodotyrosine deiodinase; MIT, monoiodotyrosine; P, proteolytic enzymes; Po, thyroid peroxidase; T_3, triiodothyronine; T_4, thyroxine; TRH, thyrotropin-releasing hormone; TSH, thyroid-stimulating hormone. (From Utiger RD. Disorders of the thyroid gland. In: Kelley WN, ed. *Textbook of internal medicine*, 3rd ed. Philadelphia: Lippincott-Raven Publishers, 1997:2205, with permission.)

release of thyroid hormones into the circulation. Secretion of TSH is stimulated by thyrotropin-releasing hormone (TRH), a tripeptide that is synthesized by the hypothalamus and carried to the anterior lobe of the hypophysis via the hypophyseal portal system. Increased plasma levels of free T_3 or T_4 decrease the secretion of TSH directly and also inhibit the action of TRH on the anterior hypophysis. Large amounts of ingested iodine can also decrease iodine trapping and thus hormone synthesis.

T_4 is the iodothyronine found in highest concentration in the plasma. Because there is no conversion of T_3 to T_4 in the periphery, T_4 arises exclusively from secretion from the thyroid gland. On the other hand, peripheral T_3 is largely derived by cleavage of the 5'-iodine from the outer ring of T_4 by 5'-monodeiodinase in the liver, muscle, and kidney. PTU decreases the activity of 5'-monodeiodinase and therefore inhibits the peripheral conversion from T_4 to T_3. If the 5'-iodine is removed from the inner ring of T_4, this results in reverse T_3, which is metabolically inactive. In healthy individuals, direct T_3 secretion from the thyroid gland accounts for approximately 20% of T_3 present in the periphery. However, in hyperthyroid conditions, such as Graves disease and toxic nodular goiter, the proportion of T_3 secreted by the thyroid gland may be greatly increased.

Only a small amount of thyroid hormone (less than 1%) circulates unbound in the plasma in a metabolically active form. While the plasma concentration of free T_4 is severalfold higher than that of T_3, T_3 is more potent. Iodothyronines are predominantly bound to carrier proteins to increase their solubility. Most thyroid hormones are bound to thyroxine-binding globulin (TBG) with the remainder bound to prealbumin and albumin. Pregnancy and oral contraceptives increase the levels of TBG and therefore the levels of total T_3 and T_4, but not the levels of free T_3 or free T_4. On the other hand, androgens and anabolic steroids decrease serum levels of TBG and T_4. Free thyroid hormone levels remain within normal limits and these patients are euthyroid.

The cellular effects of thyroid hormone are dependent on binding of thyroid hormone to an intracellular receptor, which migrates to the nucleus to regulate transcription and translation. An excess of thyroid hormone upregulates the activity and number of ATP-dependent sodium pumps, which increases basal metabolic rate and oxygen consumption of most cells. In addition, oxidative phosphorylation is upregulated by thyroid hormone. T_3 may increase or decrease fat formation depending on the caloric status of the individual. Overall, the lipolytic effect of thyroid hormones predominates, as evidenced by decreased triglyceride and cholesterol levels and elevated levels of free fatty acids and glycerol in hyperthyroid patients. Thyroid hormone induces heat production through the increased number of sodium pumps in the cellular membrane, new protein production in the nucleus, and mitochondrial oxidative phosphorylation.

Thyroid Function Tests

The *serum total* T_4 *concentration* is a most commonly used test of thyroid function. Because more than 99% of circulating T_4 is bound to carrier proteins and only the free T_4 is metabolically active, total T_4 levels alone may not necessarily reflect the thyroid functional status. Total T_4 levels change with alterations in serum levels of TBG, prealbumin, or albumin. These should therefore be measured along with total T_4. While total T_4 concentrations are elevated in most patients with hyperthyroidism, they can also be increased by elevated TBG levels during pregnancy or with estrogen use. Similarly, decreased levels of total T_4 can be due to hypothyroidism or low levels of carrier proteins, as can be the case with anabolic steroid use or nephrotic syndrome. Total T_4 levels in serum are measured by radioimmunoassay (RIA). *Free* T_4 is a direct measurement of the level of biologically available T_4 in the circulation and is more reliable than total T_4 levels at assessing thyroid function. However, this test is more expensive.

T_3 *resin uptake* measures the level of thyroid hormone–binding proteins. Radiolabeled T_3 is added to the patient's serum and then absorbed on a resin. The radiolabeled T_3 can bind the resin or binding proteins depending on the level of thyroid hormone and the level of TBG in the serum. T_3 resin uptake level will be elevated in hyperthyroidism because the elevated thyroid hormone is already bound to TBG and the added radiolabeled T_3 remains free in the serum. The resin uptake level will also be high when TBG levels are low. The resin uptake level will be low in hypothyroidism or in cases of TBG excess. Because pregnancy and oral contraceptive use result in excess TBG, total T_4 levels are elevated and T_3 resin uptake is decreased. The *free T_4 index* can be estimated by calculating the ratio of the patient's T_3 resin uptake and a mean T_3 resin uptake of a control population and then multiplying this ratio with the total serum T_4 concentration. *Total T_3* measures both free T_3 and protein-bound T_3. The test should not be used as a screening tool because it reflects peripheral metabolism of thyroid hormone, rather than thyroid function. It should be obtained in patients in whom hyperthyroidism is suspected but who have a normal T_4 level. The thyroid gland may produce more T_3 than T_4 in patients who suffer from hyperthyroid conditions.

Measurement of *serum TSH* levels, in combination with an estimate of a free T_4 index, has been recommended as the most efficient test combination of thyroid function. A normal TSH level in a healthy ambulatory patient essentially excludes the possibility of thyroid dysfunction. The test may be used to screen ambulatory patients with a risk of primary thyroid dysfunction such as those with autoimmune disorders, a family history of autoimmune thyroid disease, and the elderly. TSH levels are thought to be the most sensitive indicator of thyroid dysfunction during the early stages of disease. Unlike total T_4 or T_3 levels, TSH serum levels are independent of the concentration of carrier proteins in the circulation. TSH levels are also used to titrate thyroid hormone–replacement therapy; however, at least 4 to 8 weeks must be allowed between alteration of oral T_4 dosage and serum TSH measurement. Additionally, TSH measurement can be used to optimize hormone levels for suppressive therapy in benign and malignant disease. TSH levels are not reliable indicators of thyroid dysfunction in patients who suffer from neuropsychiatric disorders or diseases of the pituitary gland.

The *TRH stimulation test* determines the functional status of the anterior pituitary TSH secretion. It is performed by checking a baseline TSH level, then administering synthetic TRH intravenously (i.v.) and measuring TSH after 30 and 60 minutes. A normal response is a rise in TSH from the baseline. Patients who suffer from hypothyroidism have a blunted response or no rise in TSH at all. This test can also determine whether TSH secretion is decreased in patients with pituitary tumors. The role for the TRH stimulation test has diminished due to increased sensitivity of TSH assays. Serum levels of antithyroid microsomal antibodies are elevated in the vast majority of patients who suffer from Hashimoto autoimmune thyroiditis. Elevation of these autoantibodies in combination with elevated serum TSH levels in euthyroid patients indicate an increased risk of developing clinically overt hypothyroidism. Graves disease is generally associated with the presence of thyroid-stimulating immunoglobulins.

The *serum thyroglobulin* assay can be applied for the surveillance of patients with differentiated thyroid carcinoma following therapy to detect recurrent or metastatic disease. This test is complementary with ^{131}I scintiscanning for this purpose. In most cases, a high thyroglobulin level, even with negative thyroid scan results, indicates metastatic disease.

Thyroid Imaging

Radionuclide imaging allows a functional assessment of the thyroid gland. This imaging modality is good at evaluating whether a thyroid nodule is overactive or "hot" and suppresses activity in the remainder of the gland. It can localize thyroid tissue, and it allows for an estimate of the size of the thyroid gland. Furthermore, nuclear medicine studies can detect functional metastatic lesions from thyroid cancers. Several radioisotopes are in clinical use for scanning of the thyroid gland. Technetium-99m (^{99m}Tc) pertechnetate is the most commonly available radionuclide scan for the thyroid. After i.v. injection, ^{99m}Tc is rapidly trapped in the thyroid gland and the study can be completed in less than 1 hour. Unlike iodine, pertechnetate molecules are not organified and stored in the colloid. The radiation exposure from ^{99m}Tc is far less than with ^{131}I. In a normal thyroid gland, the tracer should be seen uniformly in both lobes on anteroposterior and oblique views. Any defect in tracer uptake represents a nonfunctional or hypofunctional (cold) nodule, whereas areas of increased tracer uptake represent functional (hot) nodules. Nuclear medicine scans are less reliable at diagnosing hypofunctional than autonomously hyperfunctional nodules. If the organification by the thyroid needs to be assessed in addition to trapping, then an iodine-123 (^{123}I) scan should be obtained because this radionuclide is trapped and organified by the thyroid gland. The study is more expensive and less convenient to obtain compared to ^{99m}Tc with imaging 4 hours and 24 hours after the oral administration of ^{123}I. ^{131}I results in much higher radiation exposure to the patient and the images obtained are inferior to those for ^{99m}Tc or ^{123}I. This is the study of choice, however, to assess the distribution of functioning metastatic thyroid tumors, which concentrates radioiodine and determines the potential effectiveness of cancer therapy with ^{131}I. Images are obtained at 24, 48, and 78 hours, at which point background levels of tracer are negligible compared to that in metastases.

Ultrasonography of the thyroid is a noninvasive and inexpensive technique to differentiate solid and cystic lesions. This technique is particularly useful for detection and fine needle aspiration (FNA) of nodules that can not be palpated and for tumor recurrences in the thyroid bed or regional lymph nodes. *Computed tomography* (CT) and *magnetic resonance imaging* (MRI) can detect subclinical cervical lymphadenopathy and substernal goiters. These studies can not differentiate benign from malignant thyroid lesions and have therefore only a limited role in the evaluation of thyroid nodules. These studies may be used preoperatively in patients with anaplastic tumors to assess involvement of adjacent structures. They can not be obtained before radionuclide imaging because the iodine in the contrast blocks the uptake of radionuclides by the thyroid for at least 6 weeks.

Benign Conditions of the Thyroid

Hyperthyroidism is a condition of thyroid hormone excess. The three causes that require surgical intervention are Graves disease (or toxic diffuse goiter), which accounts for over 80% of cases, toxic nodular goiter, and solitary toxic nodule. Thyroid glands trap iodine avidly in these conditions. Other causes that rarely require surgery are postpartum thyroiditis, iodine-induced hyperthyroidism, iatrogenic hyperthyroidism, struma ovarii, and functioning metastatic carcinoma.

Graves disease is an autoimmune disorder characterized by the presence of antibodies directed against the receptor of TSH on the follicular cell, which stimulates thyroid hormone production and secretion. It is generally believed that it is a family of antibodies that contributes to the pathology of Graves disease. Graves disease is six to seven times more common in women than in men. Genetic factors seem to play an important role. Clinical manifestations of Graves disease are generally due to increased effect of thyroid hormones on a wide variety of tissues. These can include fatigue, heat intolerance, weight loss, irritability, tremor, arrhythmias, hypertension, osteoporosis, amenorrhea, sweating, diarrhea, dermopathy such as pretibial myxedema and ophthalmopathy with periorbital edema, proptosis, and upper lid twitching. Clinically important involvement of the eyes is seen only in a minority of patients. Older patients may present with initial findings of atrial fibrillation or congestive heart failure. The thyroid gland is typically diffusely enlarged, symmetric, and smooth; however, it may also be irregular. Abnormal laboratory test results include elevated T_4 or T_3, or both, and a suppressed serum TSH level. Uptake of radioiodine is markedly elevated. Diffuse, increased uptake of ^{131}I within a symmetrically enlarged gland is diagnostic of Graves disease.

If Graves disease is left untreated, one third of patients with the disease will improve to euthyroid states or even develop hypothyroidism, one third will remain chronically hyperthyroid, and one third will progress to thyroid storm, a condition that can be fatal. Until the 1920s, the treatment for patients with Graves disease was rest. In the early 1920s, Plummer was the first to use iodine in the treatment of Graves disease. Today, there are three treatment options for Graves disease: medical therapy, radioactive iodine, and surgical intervention. The optimal treatment for a patient will be based on age, health, severity of disease, size of the gland, and the patient's preference. Antithyroid drugs are the first line of therapy in most patients with Graves disease. Thionamides such as PTU, methimazole, and carbimazole, which is converted *in vivo* to the active metabolite methimazole, block the incorporation of iodine into the tyrosine residues of thyroglobulin by inhibiting peroxidase enzymes, preventing the oxidation of iodide to iodine. PTU also blocks the peripheral conversion of T_4 to T_3. The most significant, although infrequent, risk with long-term thionamide therapy is agranulocytosis. Any patient with a rash, fever, or sore throat should be evaluated with a white blood cell count. Thionamide therapy must be continued for a prolonged time, with a long-term hope of spontaneous remission. However, recurrence rates up to 90% have been reported after medication was discontinued. The success rate of therapy correlates inversely with gland size: 75% for small to normal size glands and less than 30% for large goiters. Patients with a high T_3 level or high T_3/T_4 ratio have a lower success rate. Children and young adults are not likely to remain in remission following long-term thionamide therapy; however, it remains the first line of therapy in this patient population. The benefit of thionamide therapy is that there is no risk of hypothyroidism when the drug is dosed appropriately. β-blocking agents such as propranolol may be used in an adjuvant setting.

Radioiodine (^{131}I) is a therapy with lasting results in most patients, with very few side effects. The treatment delivers locally destructive beta particles to the thyroid gland. Following treatment, it usually takes several months for the hyperthyroidism to be controlled. Most patients can be treated with a single dose; however, a small percentage of patients will require a second or third dose. Once an initial response occurs, there is a less than 5% risk of recurrence. Hypothyroidism is an expected complication following effective therapy, which can be easily diagnosed and treated with lifelong replacement therapy. Radioiodine can also induce transient hyperthyroidism. Most adult patients in the United States receive ^{131}I as definitive therapy for Graves disease. There is no evidence that ^{131}I therapy results in chromosomal damage or oncogenesis. However, there is still reluctance to treat children with radioactive iodine. Women of childbearing age, patients with concomitant thyroid nodules, those with very large glands, and patients opposed to the radioactive drug are not treated with ^{131}I.

Due to the success of nonsurgical therapy, *operative intervention* is generally reserved for the following conditions: (i) noncompliance or intolerance of antithyroid drug therapy, (ii) contraindications to ^{131}I therapy such as pregnancy, (iii) failure of antithyroid drug therapy, and (iv) concurrent nodular disease with fine needle biopsy results warranting surgery. Patients less than 20 years of age with large goiters are unlikely to become euthyroid with drug therapy and often require thyroidectomy. It is controversial whether thyroidectomy decreases the risk of progressive eye disease in patients with ophthalmopathy. Risks of thyroidectomy include injury to the recurrent laryngeal nerve, transient or permanent hypoparathyroidism, and recurrent or persistent hyperthyroidism with subtotal thyroidectomy. An euthyroid state should be achieved medically in the preoperative phase to minimize the risk of intraoperative or postoperative thyroid storm. This also affords the patient a better nutritional status and allows for the normal homeostatic response to the stress of surgery. Administration of PTU in combination with propranolol should be initiated 4 to 8 weeks before surgery and continued during and after the surgery. Historically, Lugol solution (a combination of potassium iodide and iodine) was given to decrease the vascularity of the gland and make it firmer and easier to resect. Some surgeons believe that propranolol results in the same decrease in gland vascularity, making the use of Lugol solution unnecessary. The extent of thyroidectomy for Graves disease remains controversial. The traditional operation has been bilateral subtotal thyroidectomy, leaving small remnants of thyroid tissue either bilaterally or unilaterally. This approach does not completely eliminate the risk of postoperative thyrotoxicosis. An alternative is to perform total thyroidectomy. There is virtually no incidence of persistent hyperthyroidism; however, all patients must receive lifelong thyroid replacement. When performed by an experienced surgeon, there is no difference in rate of injury to the recurrent laryngeal nerve or rate of hypoparathyroidism with subtotal versus total thyroidectomy.

Autonomously functioning thyroid nodules are presumably independent of TSH for function and growth. They appear hot on radionuclide studies and the function of surrounding thyroid tissue is frequently suppressed with nodules that are large in size. Patients can have either solitary or multiple autonomously functioning nodules. Most patients with autonomously functioning nodules are euthyroid. However, untreated hot nodules may progress to toxicity. The risk of developing hyperthyroidism is increased with large nodules. Only about 20% of autonomous hot nodules enlarge enough to result in hyperthyroidism. Most of these nodules enlarge, develop central necrosis, and become nonfunctioning. The peak incidence of *solitary toxic nodules* is during the fifth decade and is much more common in women. Clinically or biochemically, toxic nodules are usually at least 3 cm in diameter. *Toxic multinodular goiter* (Plummer disease) accounts for approximately 20% of patients with hyperthyroidism and is usually seen in women over 50 years of age. Patients usually have a nodular goiter for some time before they develop symptoms of hyperthyroidism. Patients with a nodular goiter and subclinical hyperthyroidism may develop thyrotoxicosis following iodine-containing medication or after receiving an iodine-containing contrast media.

Treatment of solitary functional nodules is influenced by size and functional degree of the nodule, as well as by the patient's age and overall health. Toxic nodules that usually exceed 3 cm in diameter should be treated surgically with a thyroid lobectomy. Alternatively, radioiodine can be used. However, a prolonged treatment regimen may be required, as the nodule persists in approximately 20% of patients. Many surgeons recommend prophylactic excision of nontoxic large solitary nodules with secretory function in the upper range of normal in elderly patients. The standard treatment for toxic multinodular goiter is antithyroid drug therapy, followed by thyroidectomy. ^{131}I may be used as an alternative in poor-risk patients without airway compression. Although ^{131}I may correct the hyperthyroidism, it does not decrease the gland size and may cause acute enlargement from radiation-induced thyroiditis. Therefore, any patient with airway compression should not be considered a candidate for ^{131}I therapy. The standard surgical procedure has been bilateral subtotal thyroidectomy. The most important point is to remove all autonomous nodules. Remnant size is not important, because after subtotal thyroidectomy, patients are placed on thyroid hormone for thyroid suppression.

Thyroiditis is generally classified based on the rapidity of onset into acute, subacute, and chronic types. *Acute thyroiditis* is an infectious disorder, which is more common in women. Bacteria such as *Streptococcus pyogenes*, *Staphylococcus aureus*, and *Pneumococcus pneumoniae* account for most cases, which usually spread via lymphatics from local infectious foci. The risk of developing acute thyroiditis is increased in patients with nodular goiters or anatomical defects such as thyroglossal ducts. This condition presents with acute onset of neck pain and fever. Most patients are euthyroid. Patients should be treated with i.v. antibiotics and surgical drainage of the abscess.

Subacute thyroiditis (granulomatous thyroiditis or de Quervain thyroiditis) is a disease that occurs in middle-aged women within weeks of an upper respiratory or other viral infection. Symptoms may include weakness, depression, easy fatigability, anterior neck pain, or referred pain to the ear or angle of the jaw. On examination, the patient is usually febrile and the thyroid is firm and extremely tender to palpation. The thyroid is swollen unilaterally and the overlying skin is occasionally erythematous. Laboratory evaluation and biopsy are usually not necessary. Transient mild hyperthyroidism can be observed during the initial phase of the disease in about half of these patients. This is thought to be due to a release of preformed thyroid hormone from the inflamed gland into the circulation. The later course of disease can be complicated by hypothyroidism and some patients may require hormone replacement therapy. The disease is typically self limited and usually resolves within a few months. The discomfort can be managed with salicylates, nonsteroidal antiinflammatory drugs, or corticosteroids. Surgical therapy may be indicated only rarely if the disease is persistent despite several months of steroid therapy.

Hashimoto thyroiditis (also known as "chronic lymphocytic thyroiditis" or "struma lymphomatosa") is the most common inflammatory condition of the thyroid. It is a common cause of diffuse goiter and is the most frequent cause of spontaneous hypothyroidism. It can occur in any age group but is most common in middle-aged women. It is an *autoimmune disease* with apparent genetic predisposition, which is characterized by high levels of circulating antibodies against the microsomal fraction of the thyroid cell, thyroglobulin, T_3, T_4, and the TSH receptor. Hashimoto disease occurs more commonly in geographic areas with a high dietary iodine intake and is more common in patients who received radiation during infancy or childhood. Hashimoto disease results in impaired thyroid hormone synthesis, due to a lack of organification of trapped iodine. Low T_4 and T_3 levels cause increased TSH secretion, which results in a goiter. Although the thyroid gland is usually large, it may be small in some patients. During the acute phase of the disease, transient hyperthyroidism may be seen. Patients usually develop a diffuse, slow-growing goiter. Pain is not a common manifestation of Hashimoto thyroiditis. On palpation, the gland is usually firm and rubbery with a lobulated surface. An elevated antimicrosomal antibody titer, along with the clinical examination, is usually sufficient to make the diagnosis. Treatment with thyroid hormone usually causes regression of the goiter. In some patients, the gland continues to grow despite thyroid suppression therapy, and in these patients, partial thyroidectomy is indicated, particularly if symptoms of compression occur. If a solitary nodule is found in a patient with Hashimoto disease, it should be evaluated fully. Any rapid enlargement of the thyroid gland in a patient with a history of Hashimoto thyroiditis needs to be evaluated for the possibility of *lymphoma*. FNA and cytology should be performed if lymphoma is suspected.

A goiter where thyroid tissue has been replaced by fibrous tissue, which also involves the strap muscles and carotid sheaths, is referred to as "invasive fibrous thyroiditis," or Riedel struma. It is the rarest form of the inflammatory disorders of the thyroid gland. Similar to other forms of thyroiditis, Riedel struma is most commonly seen in middle-aged women. It involves both lobes of the thyroid gland and the isthmus. Riedel struma is associated with other fibrotic processes such as retroperitoneal fibrosis, mediastinal fibrosis, periorbital fibrosis, and sclerosing cholangitis. Patients with Riedel struma are generally euthyroid. An open biopsy should be obtained to rule out the presence of thyroid carcinoma or lymphoma. The goiter may result in considerable localized pain and compression of adjacent tissues. If airway compromise is present, surgical therapy with isthmectomy is indicated. If airway compression is not present, then treatment with steroids may be beneficial.

Thyroid Nodules

Clinically apparent thyroid nodules are more prevalent in women than in men. They are present in approximately 5% of the adult population. Previous exposure to radiation increases the risk of developing both benign and malignant thyroid nodules. Thyroid nodules have been reported in up to one third of individuals who have been exposed to radiation. The risk of malignancy in palpable solitary thyroid nodules in patients who have no history of neck irradiation is approximately 10%. Radiation exposure is associated with a severalfold increase in the risk of malignancy, with some studies reporting an up to 50% incidence of cancer in thyroid nodules from this patient population. Men and patients at the extremes of age are also at a higher risk for malignancy. A solitary nodule is more worrisome than a thyroid with multiple nodules. However, any nodule that increases in size in the setting of a multinodular goiter needs to be evaluated to exclude carcinoma. Except for the association of Hashimoto disease with lymphoma, other benign thyroid disorders do not seem to predispose to the development of thyroid carcinoma. The appearance of a new nodule, a rapid increase in the size of an existing nodule, and a painful nodule are worrisome for malignancy. New onset of hoarseness or the development of a Horner syndrome may indicate local invasion. On physical examination, the size, mobility, firmness, adherence to adjacent structures, and presence of adenopathy are all clues to the presence of carcinoma.

Very high serum levels of thyroglobulin in a patient with a small thyroid nodule may be suggestive of metastatic thyroid carcinoma. However, thyroid function tests generally don't play a role in differentiating benign from malignant nodules. Inhibition of TSH production with administration of thyroid hormone is based on the principle that benign lesions are less autonomous than malignant tumors and will therefore decrease in size over a period of several months of TSH suppression. However, due to issues such as patient compliance and lack of rigorously defined size criteria, this modality plays only a limited role in the diagnostic workup of thyroid nodules. Because most of both benign and malignant thyroid nodules are hypofunctional when compared to normal functioning thyroid tissue, the finding of a cold nodule on radionuclide scanning with ^{123}I or ^{99m}Tc is nonspecific. Ultrasonography is useful to determine the size of nodules, number of nodules, and character of nodules (solid vs. cystic), as well as to assist in FNA of nodules. Thyroid nodules that are greater than 3 cm in diameter, cystic/solid lesions, and cystic lesions that recur after three aspirations are more likely to be malignant and, therefore, should be biopsied.

FNA biopsy is safe, minimally invasive, inexpensive, and accurate in the diagnosis of thyroid nodules. It can be performed by direct palpation or with ultrasound guidance for nonpalpable nodules. It should be used to evaluate any new palpable thyroid nodule or any lesion greater than 1.5 cm identified by imaging. The four diagnostic categories of FNA are the following: (i) benign or negative, (ii) suspicious or indeterminate, (iii) malignant, and (iv) insufficient sample.

One of the main limitations of FNA is the difficulty in distinguishing benign follicular cell adenomas from follicular cell carcinomas. FNA biopsies of follicular neoplasms or those with extensive Hurthle cell changes are characterized as suspicious or indeterminate. Because 25% of these nodules are found to be malignant, they must be surgically resected. The false-negative rate of nodules with benign FNA biopsy results is less than 5%, and these patients can generally be followed medically. Nodules can be followed by physical examination or by ultrasonography, which is more precise at delineating changes in size. However, if a nodule is worrisome based on its clinical features (fixed, firm, painful), it should be resected despite "negative" FNA biopsy results.

Thyroid Carcinoma

Thyroid malignancies are derived from either follicular cells (papillary, follicular, Hurthle cell, and anaplastic carcinomas) or C cells (medullary carcinoma). These tumors can be grouped by their clinical aggressiveness as follows: well differentiated (papillary carcinoma, follicular carcinoma), intermediate differentiation (Hurthle cell carcinoma, some variants of papillary carcinoma, insular carcinoma, medullary carcinoma), and undifferentiated (anaplastic carcinoma).

Papillary and *follicular thyroid carcinoma* comprise the well-differentiated thyroid carcinomas. Papillary and follicular elements can be found in most well-differentiated thyroid carcinomas. All thyroid tumors with papillary elements are generally classified as papillary carcinomas, because pure papillary, mixed papillary, and follicular tumors have similar biology. Papillary carcinoma comprises about 80% to 85% of thyroid cancer in countries with sufficient dietary iodine intake. Most papillary carcinomas are intrathyroidal and are partially encapsulated. Cystic changes in these tumors are not uncommon. Histologically, approximately one half of papillary carcinomas have laminated calcific material, referred to as "psammoma bodies." They have distinctive nuclear features including large size, pale-staining appearance, and deep grooves. Papillary carcinomas spread through lymphatics to regional lymph nodes. Several variants of papillary cancer exist including the follicular, the tall cell variant, the columnar variant, and the diffuse sclerosis variant. The sclerosis variant has a 100% incidence of lymph node metastasis at the time of diagnosis. The RET oncogene translocation has been identified in approximately 25% of papillary thyroid cancers. Follicular carcinomas are defined as tumors with follicular elements only. Pure follicular thyroid carcinomas are rare, making up only 5% to 10% of thyroid malignancies in nonendemic goiter areas of the world. Follicular thyroid carcinomas are unifocal and thickly encapsulated, showing invasion of or through the capsule, frequently with vascular invasion. Because these carcinomas often invade veins and not lymphatics, lymph node involvement by follicular carcinoma is rare.

The female to male ratio for both types is about 2.5:1. *Radiation exposure* to the thyroid is the only factor that has been shown to increase the incidence of well-differentiated thyroid carcinoma. The latent period after exposure is at least 3 to 5 years and the majority of radiation-associated thyroid cancers have a papillary histology. However, previous radiation exposure accounts for only fewer than 10% of cases in the United States and most well-differentiated thyroid carcinomas are not clearly linked to specific etiologic factors. Both radiation-associated and nonradiation-associated papillary thyroid cancers have lymph node involvement at the time of diagnosis in one third of cases. Well-differentiated thyroid carcinoma usually presents as an asymptomatic thyroid nodule. Few patients present with palpable cervical lymphadenopathy without an identifiable thyroid primary. Other symptoms may include hoarseness, dyspnea, and dysphagia, reflecting local invasion of the recurrent laryngeal nerve, the trachea, and the esophagus, respectively. Most patients with well-differentiated thyroid carcinoma are euthyroid. It is a relatively indolent solid neoplasm with a favorable long-term survival rate. In contrast to other solid neoplasms, the presence of lymph node metastases has no strong correlation with overall survival in most series. At presentation, up to one half of patients with papillary thyroid carcinoma and 1% of patients with follicular thyroid carcinoma have involved cervical lymph node metastases. The overall 10-year survival rate for papillary cancer ranges from 74% to 93%, compared with 43% to 94% for follicular cancer.

The two dominant prognostic factors for well-differentiated thyroid cancer are age at diagnosis and the presence of distant metastases. Low-risk age categories have been defined as men less than 40 years of age and women less than 50 years of age. The Lahey Clinic developed the AMES (age, metastases, extent of primary cancer, and tumor size) criteria to place patients into different risk groups with different prognoses. With this system, low-risk patients have a long-term overall survival of 98%, compared with 54% for high-risk patients. The Mayo Clinic group devised a similar scoring system called the AGES (age, grade of tumor, extent of tumor, size of tumor) system. A recent modification of this system is MACIS (metastasis, age, completeness of resection, invasion, size). The survival rates for patients based on these prognostic factors are shown in Table 28-1.

The major decisions in the surgical management of thyroid nodules and thyroid cancers are who to operate on and how extensive of a resection to perform. The extent of resection for well-differentiated thyroid malignancies has been a point of controversy among endocrine surgeons. Acceptable procedures for a thyroid neoplasm include a thyroid lobectomy, subtotal thyroidectomy, near-total thyroidectomy, and total thyroidectomy. A subtotal thyroidectomy leaves a rim of 2 to 4 g of tissue in the region of the ligament of Berry of the contralateral lobe. This decreases the risk of injury to the recurrent laryngeal nerve in that area and helps preserve the blood supply to the upper parathyroid gland

TABLE 28-1. SURVIVAL RATES IN PATIENTS WITH WELL-DIFFERENTIATED THYROID CANCER BASED ON VARIOUS PROGNOSTIC CLASSIFICATION SCHEMES[a]

AMES risk group	Low	High		
Overall survival rate	98%	54%		
Disease-free survival rate	95%	45%		
DAMES risk group	Low	Intermediate	High	
Disease-free survival rate	92%	45%	0%	
AGES PS	<4	4–5	5–6	>6
20-year survival rate	99%	80%	33%	13%
MACIS PS	<6	6–7	7–8	>8
20-year survival rate	99%	89%	56%	24%

[a]AMES, age, metastases, extent of primary cancer, tumor size; DAMES, AMES system modified by DNA content; AGES, age, tumor grade, tumor extent, tumor size; PS, prognostic score; MACIS, metastasis, age, completeness of resection, invasion, size.

on that side. A near-total thyroidectomy leaves only 1 g of tissue adjacent to the ligament of Berry.

Some surgeons feel that patients with unilateral well-differentiated thyroid carcinoma defined as low-risk by AGES or AMES criteria can safely undergo an ipsilateral thyroidectomy and isthmectomy with careful medical surveillance of the contralateral lobe. Many surgeons prefer this procedure for patients with papillary tumors that are smaller than 1 cm and follicular cancers with minimal capsular invasion. Advantages of this procedure include a lower risk of postoperative complications such as permanent hypoparathyroidism. However, patients undergoing more radical procedures have lower recurrence rates. Indications for total thyroidectomy for well-differentiated thyroid carcinoma include a history of prior head or neck irradiation or invasion of the neoplasm through the thyroid capsule. Most experienced endocrine surgeons recommend thyroidectomy for all patients with a papillary carcinoma of larger than 1.5 cm in diameter. Proponents of total thyroidectomy for all well-differentiated thyroid tumors feel that this more radical approach is indicated because of the high incidence of occult tumors in the contralateral lobe, decreased survival rates with recurrent disease, and more accurate surveillance for tumor persistence and recurrence with serum thyroglobulin levels. As mentioned above, patients with FNA cytology that is read as suspicious should undergo surgical resection due to an incidence of follicular carcinoma of up to 25%. These patients should undergo thyroid lobectomy on the side of the nodule with further management based on the final pathology report. If the lesion is a follicular carcinoma with characteristics that place the patient at high risk, then a completion total or subtotal thyroidectomy should be done at a second operation.

Controversy exists over the surgical management of *cervical lymph node metastases from well-differentiated thyroid carcinoma*. Some surgeons perform selective resection only for grossly involved nodes while others advocate prophylactic modified radical neck dissections in an attempt to remove asymptomatic metastatic disease. Because lymph node involvement is a marker for more aggressive papillary carcinoma, a formal neck dissection is indicated in patients with macroscopically involved lymph nodes. If carcinoma is identified by frozen section of suspected lymph nodes at the time of thyroidectomy, then a complete dissection of lymph nodes in the central neck and the paratracheal region is indicated.

Radioiodine therapy with ^{131}I ablation is dependent on residual thyroid tissue concentrating iodine under the stimulation of elevated TSH levels. It has been recommended to ablate residual thyroid functional tissue after surgical resection for well-differentiated carcinomas and to aid in the detection of metastatic disease. Additionally, ^{131}I ablation eliminates thyroglobulin production by any remnants of normal thyroid, which allows this marker to be used to follow patients postoperatively. Patients with lymph node metastases should also be given ^{131}I ablation to decrease the risk of recurrence. However, there is debate over the efficacy of postoperative radioiodine therapy. Many studies have shown that ^{131}I ablation decreases cancer death, tumor recurrence, and the incidence of distant metastases while other studies have failed to demonstrate an effect. ^{131}I ablation is performed at 6 weeks after near-total or total thyroidectomy. Typically, a diagnostic scan is performed before ablation. Thyroid hormone replacement is discontinued 4 weeks and a low iodine diet is initiated 1 to 2 weeks before scanning, to optimize uptake and retention of ^{131}I by residual normal thyroid and thyroid cancer. A posttherapy whole-body scan is obtained at 5 to 7 days to determine the extent of disease, with follow-up scanning at 6- to 12-month intervals. Radioiodine treatment should be continued until there is no further ^{131}I uptake, until serum thyroglobulin is in the athyrotic range, or until complications of ^{131}I arise. Side effects of ^{131}I include sialadenitis, nausea, taste dysfunction, reversible impairment in spermatogenesis, temporary bone marrow suppression, and rarely vocal cord paralysis. There is a dose-dependent relationship between ^{131}I therapy and the development of leukemia. Furthermore, a low incidence of bladder carcinoma has been reported with high cumulative doses of ^{131}I. As mentioned above, *thyroglobulin* is the protein found in the thyroid follicles, which provides a matrix for thyroid hormone synthesis and is important for thyroid hormone storage within the gland. Following thyroidectomy and ^{131}I ablation, the thyroglobulin is in the athyrotic range. It serves as an important tumor marker in the follow-up of thyroid cancer patients who do not have residual normal thyroid tissue. Elevated serum thyroglobulin levels in patients who have undergone surgical resection and radioablation and received suppressive thyroid hormone replacement is an indicator of persistent or recurrent thyroid carcinoma.

The *intermediate differentiation tumors* of the thyroid include Hurthle cell carcinoma, insular carcinoma, and medullary thyroid carcinoma. *Hurthle cell tumors* account for less than 5% of all thyroid carcinomas. They are considered to be variants of follicular tumors and can not be classified as benign or malignant based on FNA. Compared to follicular tumors, Hurthle cell tumors are more often bilateral and multifocal and can spread to regional lymph nodes. Hurthle cell tumors do not take up radioiodine. Similar to the management of follicular tumors, patients who are found to have Hurthle cell neoplasm by FNA should undergo an ipsilateral lobectomy and isthmectomy. In addition, these patients should undergo an ipsilateral central neck dissection. Total completion thyroidectomy is indicated if the final pathology reveals a carcinoma. *Insular carcinomas* are considered an aggressive variety of thyroid cancer. They have a worse prognosis than differentiated thyroid carcinomas. Histologically, these tumors resemble pancreatic islets. They have small follicles and stain positively for thyroglobulin. Insular carcinomas invade lymphatics and veins and are commonly associated with nodal and distant metastases. Necrosis is common in the tumor and the only viable tumor may be near blood vessels. Treatment of insular carcinoma consists of surgical resection and radioablation.

Medullary thyroid cancer (MTC) arises from the parafollicular C cells, which produce calcitonin, which lowers serum calcium levels. MTC represents about 5% to 10% of thyroid cancers. MTC is not associated with radiation exposure. MTC is sporadic or nonfamilial in 60% to 70% of cases and is associated with a familial syndrome in the rest of the cases (either multiple endocrine neoplasia [MEN] 2A or 2B or non-MEN familial MTC). Sporadic tumors are usually unilateral and involve regional lymph nodes. Familial tumors are generally multifocal. Patients with non-MEN familial MTC have the least aggressive form of this tumor while MEN 2B is associated with the most aggressive variant. The characteristics of sporadic and familial forms of MTC are shown in Table 28-2. The C cells arise from the neural crest cells and have the typical characteristics of APUD cells (amine precursor uptake, decarboxylase) of high chromogranins and neuron-specific enolase content, as well as the ability to secrete various peptides. The C cells are located primarily in the upper and middle thirds of the thyroid lobes posteriorly. Similar to those of other neuroendocrine tumors, the nuclei of MTC are round and have a stippled "salt and pepper" chromatin and the tumor stroma is highly vascular. The stroma contains amyloid. Immunostains for calcitonin are typically required to make the diagnosis because of the various possible histologic patterns. Immunostaining also aids in prognosis, as tumors with less than 25% of cells staining for calcitonin typically metastasize early. MTC can secrete various peptide hormones

TABLE 28-2. CHARACTERISTICS OF SPORADIC AND VARIOUS FAMILIAL FORMS OF MEDULLARY THYROID CANCER[a]

	Sporadic	Familial		
		Non-MEN	MEN 2A	MEN 2B
Age at diagnosis (y)	42–45	43–45	24–27[b]	15–20
Gender	M = F	M = F	M = F	M = F
Associated diseases	None	None	(1) Pheochromocytoma (2) Hyperparathyroidism	(1) Pheochromocytoma (2) Marfanoid body habitus (3) Oral & eye mucosal neuromas (4) Gastrointestinal ganglioneuromas
Disease extent	Unilateral	Bilateral	Bilateral	Bilateral
Lymph nodes involved at diagnosis	40%–50%	10%–20%	14%	38%
Distant metastases at diagnosis	12%	0%	0%–3%	20%
Cured of MTC	14%–30%	70%–80%	56%–100%	0%
Dead due to MTC	30%	0%	0%–17%	50%
Mutations in RET on chromosome 10	MET 918 → Thr (33%) Glu 768 → Asp	Mutations in cysteines in extracellular domain near membrane	Mutations in cysteines in extracellular domain near membrane	Met 918 → Thr

[a]MTC, medullary thyroid cancer; MEN, multiple endocrine neoplasia.
[b]The age at diagnosis at centers doing genetic screening can be at or even before birth. Numbers reported reflect series based on biochemical screening of families at risk.

including adrenocorticotropic hormone (ACTH) and serotonin and can also produce mucin or melanin.

Patients with familial MTC who are identified by screening are identified before any macroscopic mass. Defects in the RET protooncogene have been found to be responsible for MEN and non-MEN familial forms of MTC. Gene carriers can be identified before development of overt disease and are candidates for prophylactic surgery. Patients with sporadic MTC typically present with a mass in the thyroid. Some patients present with advanced cases with local invasion and symptoms of hoarseness, dysphagia, or cough. Those with extremely high levels of calcitonin may have severe secretory diarrhea. The basal and stimulated *serum calcitonin test* is an important tool for confirming diagnosis, screening patients for familial MTC, and following patients after treatment. The test involves administering calcium gluconate and pentagastrin and measuring serum calcitonin before and at multiple times after stimulation. An increase to more than 1,000 pg/mL (normal serum level 250 to 300 pg/mL) is distinctly abnormal and pathognomonic for MTC. Elevation to between 300 and 1,000 pg/mL is borderline and warrants close observation with sequential retesting. Because MTC does not concentrate iodine, ^{131}I scans are of no use in MTC. Thallium and technetium scans have not proved to be beneficial. ^{131}I metaiodobenzylguanidine scans, which are useful in identifying pheochromocytomas and neuroblastomas, fail to identify a large proportion of MTCs. A strategy to regionally localize occult lesions is selected venous sampling for serum calcitonin after stimulation with calcium or pentagastrin.

Surgical therapy is the only effective therapy for MTC. Chemotherapy and external beam radiation are of no benefit. Patients who present with sporadic MTC should undergo total thyroidectomy and central node dissection. If there is evidence of metastatic spread in the central neck nodes, a formal modified radical neck dissection is performed. Total thyroidectomy and central neck dissection should be performed for all cases of familial MTC. There is a direct correlation between lesion size and incidence of nodal metastases, with lesions greater than 2 cm having a 60% incidence of lymph node metastases. Therefore, some surgeons advocate a modified radical neck dissection for all lesions greater than 2 cm. The incidence of distant metastases at the time of diagnosis is the lowest for familial non-MEN MTC and MEN 2A (less than 5%) and the highest for MEN 2B (20%). Recent series show a 5-year survival rate between 80% and 90% and a 10-year survival rate between 70% and 80% for all MTCs. The appropriate management of persistently elevated calcitonin levels following resection is close follow-up and reoperation only when clinically apparent disease is present.

Anaplastic thyroid cancer (ATC) accounts for 1% of thyroid cancers and is one of the most aggressive and lethal human malignancies. The median survival time is 4 to 5 months, with rare long-term survivors. Patients who are diagnosed with ATC are typically in their seventh decade of life. There is an equal gender distribution in patients with ATC. Patients with ATC commonly have a prior or concurrent diagnosis of well-differentiated thyroid cancer or benign thyroid disease. There is evidence that ATC can arise from the dedifferentiation of well-differentiated thyroid cancer. Iodine deficiency in endemic goiter regions of the world is associated with ATC. Most patients with ATC have not had prior radiation. Patients with ATC present with a palpable mass that is growing. The median tumor size is 8 to 9 cm, compared to 2 to 3 cm for well-differentiated thyroid cancer. Synchronous pulmonary metastases are observed in up to 50% of patients at the time of diagnosis. Most patients with ATC die from aggressive local-regional disease, mostly from upper airway obstruction. Therefore, aggressive local therapy is indicated whenever possible. Aggressive resection should include removal of the strap muscles and any other structures with local invasion and tracheostomy if needed. There is no role for ^{131}I therapy for ATC patients. External beam radiation has been used with limited success for recurrent ATC. Doxorubicin-based chemotherapy has also been shown to prolong survival.

Lymphoma of the thyroid represents only 1% of all lymphomas and 2% of extranodal non-Hodgkin lymphoma. It is usually seen in older women with Hashimoto thyroiditis. Patients virtually never have hyperthyroidism but frequently have hypothyroidism. The appropriate treatment of lymphoma of the thyroid is radiation therapy and chemotherapy. There is no role for surgical resection. Clinically apparent metastases to the thyroid from other sites account for less than 1% of all thyroid malignancies, although autopsy studies identify metastases to the thyroid in 2% to 26% of people. In these series, the most predominant primary sites are breast, lung, melanoma, renal cell carcinoma, and gastrointestinal tract malignancies. In patients with premortem detection of metastasis to the thyroid, renal cell carcinoma accounts for most of the cases. Some patients may need thyroidectomy for palliation of symptoms.

PARATHYROID GLANDS

The parathyroids are flat, ovoid, and red-brown to yellow glands that weigh between 30 and 50 mg each. Typically, there are four parathyroid glands: two superior glands and two inferior glands located on the right and left side of the neck. The superior glands usually lie embedded in the fat on the posterior surface of the upper thyroid lobe close to the site where the recurrent laryngeal nerve enters the larynx. The inferior glands are usually located more ventral and lie close to or within the superior portion of the thymus that extends from the inferior pole of the thyroid gland. Although these locations are typical, anatomical variations caused by differences in patterns of embryogenesis are common.

Embryologically, parathyroid tissue develops in the third and fourth pharyngeal pouches as early as the sixth week of gestation. The *superior glands* arise from the *fourth pharyngeal pouch* along with the lateral thyroid while the *inferior glands* arise from the *third pouch* along with the thymus (Fig. 28-4). The superior glands then descend a short distance and remain close to the upper pole of the thyroid. Variations in their descent may cause a gland to become completely embedded within thyroid tissue, or a gland may migrate caudally along the tracheoesophageal groove into the posterior mediastinum. The inferior glands descend with the thymus toward the inferior pole of the thyroid, but this migration is highly variable and glands can be found anywhere from the pharynx to the mediastinum. More than four glands can be identified in up to 15% of patients, most often in association with the thymus.

The arterial supply to both the superior and inferior parathyroids is usually from the inferior thyroid artery (Fig. 28-2), although it may arise from the superior thyroid artery. The inferior, middle, and superior thyroid veins drain the parathyroids into the internal jugular or the innominate vein. Histologically, normal adult glands are about half parenchymal cells and half stromal cells, including fat cells. The predominant cell is the chief cell, but with increasing age, acidophilic, mitochondria-rich oxyphil cells are present in increasing numbers and are intermixed with polygonal water-clear cells. The functional significance of the various cell types is not known.

Physiology

The parathyroid gland's primary physiologic role is the endocrine regulation of calcium and phosphate metabolism. Calcium is a critical ion for cellular homeostasis, participating in enzymatic reactions and mediating hormone metabolism. It is the major cation in bone and teeth, representing about 2% of the average body weight. The normal range of serum calcium is 9 to 10.5 mg/dL. About half of the total serum calcium is in an ionized, biologically active form. Forty percent is bound to serum protein (albumin) and the remaining 10% is complexed with citrate. Calcium is absorbed in its inorganic form from the duodenum and proximal jejunum, with absorption regulated based on body calcium status. Calcium reabsorption from the kidney under normal conditions is about 99% of the filtered load.

Phosphate is also an important component of many biological systems, including the pathways of glycolysis. It is the functional group of ATP, and it is the major anion in crystalline bone. The normal range of serum phosphate ranges from 2.5 to 4.3 mg/dL, and the level varies inversely with that of the serum calcium. Unlike that of calcium, phosphate absorption from the diet is relatively constant, and excretion provides the major mechanism for the regulation of phosphate balance.

The primary hormonal regulators of calcium and phosphate homeostasis are parathyroid hormone (PTH), vitamin D, and calcitonin. Regulation depends on three organ

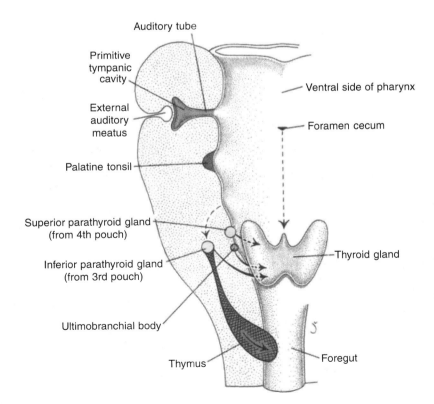

FIGURE 28-4. Schematic representation of the migration of the parathyroid glands. Although the inferior parathyroid gland arises from the third pharyngeal pouch, it migrates along with the thymus and ends its descent inferior to the superior parathyroid gland, which arises from the fourth pharyngeal pouch. (From Sadler TW. *Langman's medical embryology*, 5th ed. Baltimore: Williams & Wilkins, 1985:289, with permission.)

systems: the gastrointestinal tract, the skeleton, and the kidney.

PTH appears to be the most important regulator of calcium and phosphate metabolism. PTH is synthesized by the parathyroids as a precursor preproparathyroid hormone, which is then cleaved to form PTH. Secretion of PTH is regulated by plasma calcium levels through a negative feedback mechanism. Secreted PTH is then cleaved by the Kupffer cells of the liver into N- and C-terminal fragments. The N terminus contains most of the biological activity. In target tissues, PTH binds to membrane receptors, activating the cyclic AMP pathway to regulate intracellular enzymes. In bone, PTH stimulates osteoclasts and inhibits osteoblasts, thereby stimulating bone resorption with the release of calcium and phosphate. In the kidney, PTH increases the reabsorption of extracellular calcium throughout the nephron, but particularly in the distal nephron. PTH also increases renal phosphate excretion. PTH has no direct effects on the gastrointestinal tract, although it does stimulate hydroxylation of 25-hydroxy vitamin D to 1,25-dihydroxy vitamin D in the kidney (Fig. 9-3).

Vitamin D has two major sites of action. It increases intestinal absorption of calcium and phosphate, and it promotes mineralization and enhances PTH-mediated mobilization of calcium and phosphate from bone. Vitamin D_3 is produced normally by the action of sunlight on 7-dehydrocholesterol in the skin. It then binds to plasma proteins and is transported to the liver where 25-hydroxylation occurs. In turn, 25-hydroxy vitamin D_3 undergoes a second hydroxylation in the renal tubular epithelial cell to form the active 1,25-dihydroxy vitamin D_3.

Calcitonin is composed of 32 amino acid proteins and is secreted by the parafollicular cells of the thyroid gland. Calcitonin inhibits bone resorption and increases urinary calcium and phosphate excretion, both of which are mediated through cyclic AMP pathways. Total thyroidectomy, however, is well tolerated, and it has been concluded that calcitonin is not essential for normal control of calcium metabolism.

Pathophysiology

Symptoms of *hypercalcemia* are varied and nonspecific, but symptoms due to *primary hyperparathyroidism* typically can be remembered by the mnemonic "painful bones, renal stones, abdominal groans, and psychic moans." Abdominal groans can be due to various disorders, including peptic ulcer disease and pancreatitis. Psychic moans range from lethargy and confusion to depression and paranoia. Multiple causes of hypercalcemia exist and must be considered in the differential diagnosis of hyperparathyroidism (Table 28-3).

Hyperparathyroidism, a common cause of hypercalcemia, is typically organized into three categories: primary, secondary, and tertiary. When normal control of serum calcium is disturbed and there is increased autonomous production of PTH, this is referred to as "primary hyperparathyroidism." This category includes both benign single-gland and multiple-gland enlargements and parathyroid carcinoma. *Secondary hyperparathyroidism* occurs when there is a defect in the homeostasis that leads to a compensatory increase in parathyroid function. The most common example of this is renal failure. Long-standing secondary stimulation can sometimes lead to autonomously functioning parathyroid glands, which are no longer sensitive to elevated serum calcium levels. This state is referred to as *tertiary hyperparathyroidism* and develops most commonly after renal transplantation has corrected the defect in calcium homeostasis.

Hyperparathyroidism develops in about 50 to 100 people per 100,000 in the United States. It is more common in women than in men and typically occurs after the age of 40. The most common cause of parathyroid adenomas is a translocation of the PTH enhancer/promoter region to the cell cycle regulator, the so-called "prod1" oncogene. Genetic studies of MEN syndromes types 1 and 2A have defined other oncogenes that may be involved.

Pathologically, parathyroid *adenomas,* or *hyperplasia,* is extremely difficult to differentiate from normal parathyroid tissue; therefore, the most reliable index of abnormality is

TABLE 28-3. CAUSES OF HYPERCALCEMIA

- **Hyperparathyroidism.** Discussed in detail in the text. Typically patients have elevated serum calcium and parathyroid hormone (PTH) levels, normal or elevated urine calcium excretion, and low or normal plasma concentration of phosphate.
- **Hypercalcemia of malignancy.** Patients with solid tumors often have elevated serum calcium levels, including those with lung carcinoma, breast carcinoma, and squamous cell carcinoma of the head and neck. The hypercalcemia is thought to be caused by PTH related protein secreted by the tumor. Patients with hematologic malignancies may also have increased serum calcium levels, but this is thought to be due to cytokines causing increased osteoclastic activity in bone.
- **Excess vitamin D and vitamin A.** Patients will have normal or elevated serum phosphate levels associated with a low PTH level.
- **Thiazide Diuretics.** Thiazides may increase serum calcium level while serum phosphate may also be depressed.
- **Hyperthyroidism.** Hyperthyroidism may cause increased calcium by stimulating bone resorption. Serum calcium levels normalize when the patient becomes euthyroid.
- **Milk-alkali syndrome.** This syndrome typically occurs in patients suffering from peptic ulcer disease who consume large amounts of milk and absorbable antacids. PTH levels are low.
- **Sarcoidosis.** Granulomas are hypertensive to vitamin D, converting the inactive vitamin into its active form. PTH levels are low.
- **Paget disease (osteitis deformans).**
- **Adrenal insufficiency.**

the determination of gland size by visual inspection. A single enlarged gland is the most common finding (65%), but all four glands may be involved. Parathyroid *carcinoma* is also often difficult to diagnose histologically, but some pathologic criteria include thick, fibrous bands, pleomorphic cells in a trabecular pattern, and a high incidence of mitotic figures. In addition, parathyroid carcinoma may locally invade into adjacent structures such as the thyroid gland or strap muscles of the neck.

Signs and symptoms of hyperparathyroidism discussed previously primarily affect the skeletal, renal, and gastrointestinal systems and vary with the magnitude of plasma calcium elevation. Symptomatic patients can be divided into two groups. Patients in the first group have a slower onset of symptoms, generally have lower plasma calcium levels, and tend to develop renal complications. Members of the second group have a more rapid onset of symptoms, higher serum calcium levels, and significant bone disease. Renal complications develop because the hypercalcemia leads to increased urinary calcium excretion and because PTH increases the excretion of phosphate and causes urinary alkalosis; both predispose to stone formation. Five percent to fifteen percent of patients will present with significant symptoms of skeletal disease, including bone pain and pathological fractures. Characteristic radiological findings include subperiosteal resorption on the radial aspect of the middle phalanges, tufting of the distal phalanges, and bone cysts of the long bones and skull. Hypercalcemia also causes nonspecific gastrointestinal complaints (nausea, vomiting, and constipation), as well as the previously mentioned psychologic manifestations.

Except in patients with deformities of advanced bone disease, physical examination is usually not helpful. Diseased parathyroids are not frequently palpable, except in patients with parathyroid carcinoma. Hypercalcemia is the single most important diagnostic finding. Measurements of ionized calcium are more accurate because hypoalbuminemia produce normal total serum calcium levels. The demonstration of an elevated plasma PTH concentration in the setting of an inappropriately elevated serum calcium level is virtually diagnostic of hyperparathyroidism.

Several modalities exist that allow for *preoperative imaging* and *localization* of the parathyroid glands. Although the sensitivity of these imaging studies has improved over the past several years, the cure rate for hyperparathyroidism at the initial operation approaches 95% in the hands of an experienced surgeon. It is recommended, therefore, that these tests should be reserved for the patient undergoing reoperation after a failed initial procedure. Real-time ultrasonography is a rapid and relatively inexpensive technique that permits conformation by sonographically directed FNA for cytologic confirmation. CT scanning is more expensive but allows for identifying deeper structures and imaging of the retrosternal mediastinum. Nuclear medicine imaging modalities initially were the thallium-technetium subtraction scans and currently are the sestamibi scans. Thallium is taken up by both the thyroid and the parathyroid glands while technetium is selectively taken up by the thyroid. The technetium scan is then subtracted from the thallium scan, leaving only the parathyroid image. Sestamibi is a radionuclide that is taken up and retained by the parathyroids and allows visualization of the glands in three dimensions on delayed images. The sensitivity of all of these examinations is only about 60%, still significantly lower than the sensitivity of a neck exploration. Recent reports have demonstrated improved sensitivity with sestamibi scanning of 70% to 80%, making this the diagnostic test of choice for hyperparathyroidism.

Generally, the only practical therapeutic option is surgery. Nephrolithiasis, bone disease, and neuromuscular symptoms all respond well to surgical intervention. In contrast, surgery in patients with renal failure, hypertension, and psychiatric complaints is not as uniformly successful, although it benefits some patients and is indicated in all patients but those at highest risk. An increasing number of patients diagnosed with hyperparathyroidism are asymptomatic, and the appropriate treatment for these patients remains controversial. In 1990, the National Institutes of Health Consensus Development Conference released possible indications for surgery in asymptomatic patients. These included markedly elevated serum calcium (more than 12 mg/dL), history of an episode of life-threatening hypercalcemia, reduced creatinine clearance, elevated urinary calcium level (more than 400 mg per 24 hours), presence of one or more renal stones on x-ray, substantially reduced bone mass on bone density studies, and young age. Due to the uncertainty of the natural history of untreated disease, almost all patients should undergo operation, and those who do not must be closely followed.

Although in the past, some have advocated unilateral exploration if a single enlarged gland and one normal gland are found on the first side explored, most experienced endocrine surgeons now feel that both sides of the neck should be explored at the initial operation because of the possibility of multiple-gland disease. Intraoperative frozen sections, although unable to differentiate between normal and diseased tissue, can confirm the presence or absence of parathyroid tissue. The location of the superior glands is fairly constant; the inferior glands, however, may be located anywhere from well above the thyroid to the anterior mediastinum. If the inferior glands can not be localized, the thymic pedicle should be carefully examined and mobilized and a transcervical thymectomy should be performed. Parathyroid glands in the anterior mediastinum can sometimes be removed by mobilizing the thymus through the cervical incision. If this is unsuccessful in localizing the gland, the thyroid lobe on the side of the missing gland is mobilized and palpated. Intraoperative ultrasound may be helpful in visualizing an intrathyroid gland. As a last resort, blind excision of the lobe may be indicated. If all of these maneuvers are unsuccessful, most surgeons would favor terminating the operation.

The operative procedure performed is based on the number of enlarged glands identified. *Single-gland disease* should be treated by simple excision, whereas any combination of two- or three-gland disease is treated by resection of the diseased tissue and leaving the normal glands in place. Many investigators feel that "double adenomas" do not exist and are actually asymmetric hyperplasia. Patients with four-gland hyperplasia can be treated by subtotal parathyroidectomy (removing three and a half glands) or by total parathyroidectomy with autotransplantation of some parathyroid tissue into a forearm muscle bed. Both procedures carry about a 5% risk of permanent hypoparathyroidism. The high risk of recurrent hypercalcemia in patients with familial parathyroid hyperplasia (such as patients with MEN 1) makes the total parathyroidectomy with autotransplantation option preferable, as reoperation is greatly simplified. The advantage of a subtotal parathyroidectomy is that severe postoperative hypoparathyroidism is avoided. Patients with sporadic four-gland hyperplasia may be treated by either procedure.

Persistent hyperparathyroidism occurs in less than 5% of patients after exploration, most commonly due to a single diseased gland (missed adenoma) still remaining in the neck or in the mediastinum. Recurrent disease develops after an interval of normocalcemia and is most commonly due to unrecognized hyperplasia but may be the result of regrowth of a partially resected adenoma, implantation from a tumor broken at the initial procedure, or even recurrent parathyroid carcinoma. For reoperative parathyroid surgery, noninvasive localization studies should always be performed, and if these are unsuccessful, selective angiography and venous sampling for PTH should be done. Surgical exploration should be guided by these studies in virtually all cases, with no "blind exploration." Reexploration can be very difficult and there is an increased risk of complications, including a 5% to 10% incidence of unilateral recurrent laryngeal nerve injury and a 10% to 20% incidence of permanent hypoparathyroidism.

Parathyroid carcinoma accounts for less than 1% of all cases of hyperparathyroidism. Patients are typically older and the gender distribution is equal, which differs from benign parathyroid adenomas, which have a higher female predominance. Symptoms occur in up to 90% of cases, and serum calcium levels are typically much higher (15 to 16 mg/dL, as compared with 11 to 12 mg/dL seen with parathyroid adenomas). PTH levels are also consistently higher and patients may have an elevated human chorionic gonadotrophin level. Parathyroid carcinomas are typically larger in size, and the affected gland is palpable in about 50% of patients (palpable parathyroid adenomas are exceedingly rare). The only effective treatment of parathyroid carcinoma is surgical resection. Initial treatment should include radical resection of the involved gland, the ipsilateral thyroid lobe, and the regional lymph nodes. Neither chemotherapy nor radiation has shown any benefit. If the disease recurs, reresection should be attempted because, and if left untreated, these patients usually succumb to uncontrolled hypercalcemia.

Signs and symptoms of *hypocalcemia* are due to the reduction in plasma-ionized calcium, which causes an increase in neuromuscular excitability (Table 28-4). Symptoms include numbness and tingling in the circumoral area, fingers, and toes, and patients may become anxious, depressed, or confused. Tetany may develop, often characterized by carpopedal spasm. On physical examination, hypocalcemia may be detected by eliciting contraction of the facial muscles by tapping anterior to the facial nerve (*Chvostek sign*) or by the development of carpal spasm after occluding blood flow to the forearm with a blood pressure cuff for 3 minutes (*Trousseau sign*).

TABLE 28-4. CAUSES OF HYPOCALCEMIA

- **Postoperative hypoparathyroidism.** This most commonly occurs after total thyroidectomy for malignancy. The low calcium level probably represents contusion or temporary alteration of the blood supply to the parathyroids; the hypocalcemia is usually transient and is not treated unless significant symptoms develop. In patients with preoperative hyperparathyroidism and significant bone disease, removing the offending gland or glands may cause marked skeletal bone deposition ("**hungry bone**"), requiring calcium and vitamin D therapy.
- **Idiopathic hypoparathyroidism.** This occurs in both sporadic and familial forms and may have an autoimmune basis. **DiGeorge syndrome** is a congenital disorder involving the branchial pouches and produces agenesis of the thymus and parathyroids.
- **Vitamin D deficiency.** This may be due to dietary deficiency or lack of exposure to sunlight. There is a decrease in calcium absorption and an increased secretion of parathyroid hormone (PTH).
- **Pseudohypoparathyroidism.** A familial disease characterized by an unresponsiveness of the kidney to PTH. Elevated PTH levels cause bone resorption, but patients remain hypocalcemic and hyperphosphatemic.
- **Hypomagnesemia.** The defect appears to block the physical response to PTH as well as its release from the parathyroids.
- **Malabsorption.**
- **Pancreatitis.**

ADRENAL GLAND

The *adrenal cortex* is derived from *coelomic mesoderm*, adjacent to the urogenital ridge. Aberrant adrenocortical tissue may be found near the kidney or in the pelvis possibly along the bladder. The *adrenal medulla* is derived from the *neural crest*; consequently, the medulla and sympathetic nervous system develop together. During the fifth week of gestation, the neural crest cells migrate toward the adrenocortical cells and situate themselves within a capsule of mesodermal cortex. The chromaffin and neuronal cells are derived from the neural crest. This explains the development of two distinct tumors, pheochromocytomas and neuroblastomas, in the adrenal medulla.

Anatomy

The adrenal glands are bilateral retroperitoneal organs, located on the superior medial aspect of the upper portion of each kidney. Each gland weighs approximately 5 g. The right adrenal gland is situated between the inferior vena cava, the liver, and the right diaphragmatic crus. The left adrenal gland is situated near the aorta, the tail of the pancreas, and the spleen (Fig. 28-5). The glands receive blood from the inferior phrenic artery, the aorta, and the renal artery. A number of small vessels pass directly into the organ, running from the cortex (outer layers) to the medulla. Most of these vessels form cortical sinusoids that empty into the medullary sinusoids. The venous blood is emptied by a central vein into the inferior vena cava and the left renal vein on the right side and the left side, respectively. The left adrenal vein may also have branches directly into the inferior vena cava.

The adrenal cortex is organized into three distinct layers. The *zona glomerulosa* is the outer layer, situated beneath the outer capsule and making up 15% of the cortex. This layer is the location of aldosterone production. The *zona fasciculata* is the middle and largest layer (75%), consisting of cells in linear patterns arranged perpendicular to the surface of the gland. The middle layer is the source of carbohydrate-active steroid, cortisol, and sex steroids. The *zona reticularis* is the most inner layer of the cortex, surrounding the medulla and area for cholesterol storage used for steroid production, as well as cortisol, androgens, and estrogen secretion. The medullary cells appear as homogenous sheets and have abundant cytoplasm. Electron microscopy can demonstrate the secretory granules of epinephrine and norepinephrine in the cytoplasm that is transported to the cell membrane and released via exocytosis upon nerve stimulation.

Physiology

The adrenal cortex is the source of glucocorticoids, mineralocorticoids, and adrenal steroid production. All adrenal steroids have 19 or 21 total carbon molecules. They have a 17-carbon structure, made of three hexane rings and single pentane rings. Cortisol and aldosterone have an additional two-carbon side chain.

Cortisol regulates the intermediary metabolism of carbohydrate, protein, and lipids. It stimulates the release of glucagon and lactate from muscle and down-regulates the sensitivity of insulin. Muscle cells undergo proteolysis and adipocytes undergo lipolysis and the resulting amino acids and glycerol molecules are channeled to the liver for gluconeogenesis. Cortisol acts also directly on hepatic enzymes involved in gluconeogenesis. The combined effect of these processes is the production of a hyperglycemic state. It promotes an anabolic state in vital organs such as the brain and the liver at the expense of the lymphoid tissue, skin, muscle, and adipocytes, where a catabolic state predominates.

In addition to the effect on intermediate carbohydrate metabolism, cortisol regulates the intravascular volume and modulates the immune system. It has a positive chronotropic and inotropic effect on the heart. By stimulating angiotensin release and inhibiting prostaglandin I_2 (a potent vasodilator) synthesis, cortisol maintains blood pressure. To the detriment of surgery patients, the glucocorticoids retard wound healing by decreasing interleukin-2 production and release and lymphocyte activation, as well as making mononuclear cells less responsive and less efficient for chemotaxis and phagocytosis. Osteoblast cell development necessary for bone growth and strength and fibroblast activity for collagen formation are also adversely affected. Chronic corticosteroid excess can cause emotional and psychological disturbances.

Aldosterone regulates the fluid and electrolyte balance by stimulating sodium resorption and indirectly free water, as well as potassium and hydrogen ion excretion. An average individual secretes approximately 100 to 150 mg of aldosterone per day. The half-life of the mineralocorticoid is rela-

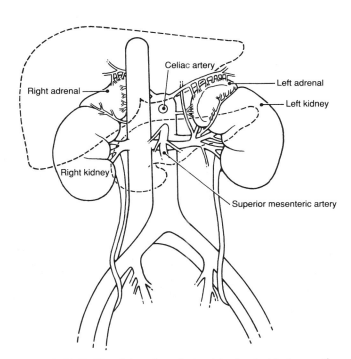

FIGURE 28-5. The right adrenal gland is situated between the inferior vena cava, the liver, and the right diaphragmatic crus. The left adrenal gland is situated near the aorta, the tail of the pancreas, and the spleen. (From Scott-Conner C, Dawson DL, eds. *Operative anatomy.* Philadelphia: JB Lippincott Co, 1993:499, with permission.)

tively short (15 minutes), and it is bound to transcortin and albumin much like cortisol. A majority (90%) of this steroid is cleared from the plasma after a single pass via the liver.

Cells of the adrenal medulla secrete *biologically active amines,* including dopamine, norepinephrine, and epinephrine in response to sympathetic nerve innervation. There are two general types of receptors, α and β, as well as subtypes α_1, α_2, β_1, and β_2, found in different concentrations in many groups of cells. The catecholamines that are released from secretory granules bind to receptors with different affinities that are based on the local concentration of each molecule and elicit different physiological responses. For example, β_1-receptor stimulation causes an increased chronotropic and inotropic effect on the heart and stimulation of lipolysis while β_2-receptor stimulation causes relaxation of smooth muscle. In contrast to steroids, catecholamines elicit physiological responses in minutes, using a secondary messenger molecule, cyclic AMP.

The major adrenal *androgens* are dehydroepiandrosterone, androstenedione, and testosterone. Estrogen is produced from androstenedione in the peripheral tissue. In adults, androgens promote the development of secondary sex characteristics such as deepening of the voice, producing a male hair distribution, coarsening of the skin, and promoting protein deposition in muscles. Estrogen has the opposite effects. In the fetus, the androgens stimulate Wolffian duct development, which results in male external genitalia. The lack of androgens in the female fetus allows the genital tubercle, labial folds, and urethral opening to remain in the normal female position. Adrenal androgen production and release is stimulated by ACTH and not by the gonadotropins.

Biosynthetic Pathways

The early steroid synthesis pathways are common to all adrenal hormones and steroids. It begins with cholesterol, which is converted to pregnenolone by a desmolase enzyme in the cell mitochondria (Fig. 28-6). Pregnenolone is shuttled via a pathway for the direct synthesis of testosterone and is also shuttled via a pathway for the conversion to progesterone, which is an intermediate substrate for cortisol, aldosterone, and additional testosterone synthesis. Testosterone and cortisol are made in the zona fasciculata and reticularis, and aldosterone is made in the zona glomerulosa.

The adrenal medulla is the area of catecholamine synthesis, storage, and release as well as reuptake of released steroids. Sympathetic stimulation of the chromaffin cells increases the activity of the tyrosine hydroxylase, which converts the amino acid tyrosine into dihydroxyphenylalanine (DOPA) and ultimately leads to the sequential production of dopamine, norepinephrine, and epinephrine.

Regulatory Mechanisms for Hormone Secretion

Various regulatory mechanisms control the release of glucocorticoids, mineralocorticoids, and catecholamines. The production of cortisol is regulated by the hypothalamus-pituitary axis (Fig. 28-7). The central and peripheral nervous systems signal the hypothalamus during periods of emotional and physical stress to release corticotrophin-releasing hormone (CRH). CRH is delivered to the anterior pituitary via a rich blood plexus and in response, the pituitary releases ACTH and the adrenal glands synthesize and release cortisol.

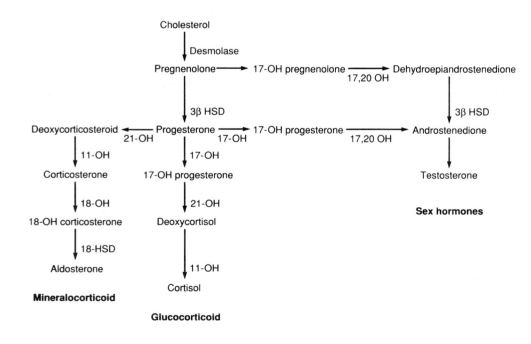

FIGURE 28-6. Steroidogenic pathways of the adrenal cortex includes sex hormones, as well as glucocorticoid and mineralocorticoid hormones. A deficiency of 21-hydroxylase is the most common cause of congenital adrenal hyperplasia. This condition results in decreased cortisol and aldosterone production as well as an excess of progesterone, which is shuttled to increase androgen production. (From Newsome HH. Adrenal glands. In: Greenfield LJ, Mulholand MW, Oldham KT, et al., eds. *Surgery:* scientific principles and practice, 2nd ed. Philadelphia: Lippincott-Raven Publishers, 1997:1334, with permission.)

The resulting high level of cortisol signals the hypothalamus and pituitary to stop secreting CRH and ACTH, respectively. This regulatory negative-feedback system, which includes a short and long loop, ensures tight regulation.

Aldosterone is a mineralocorticoid that controls intravascular volume by stimulating the distal convoluted tubules (DCTs) of the kidney to reabsorb sodium and indirectly free water, as well as to excrete potassium and hydrogen ion. Aldosterone secretion is regulated by multiple factors including the *renin/angiotensin system* and plasma sodium concentration. The juxtaglomerular apparatus of the kidney and the macula densa—a grouping of cells located near the afferent arteriole—detect decreased renal blood flow and low plasma sodium concentration (Fig. 28-8). In response, the juxtaglomerular apparatus releases renin that converts angiotensinogen to angiotensin I, a decapeptide derived from a large hepatic protein. Angiotensin I is converted to angiotensin II in the lung by an efficient carboxypeptidase. The newly formed protein signals aldosterone release. Conversely, a high sodium load, overhydration, and the supine position result in decreased renin and aldosterone production. Two other minor factors that affect aldosterone release are plasma potassium concentration and ACTH. This hormone signals the adrenal glands to convert cholesterol into steroid products that are common to the mineralocorticoid and glucocorticoid synthesis pathway, but it favors the latter.

Catecholamine release is controlled by the *sympathetic nervous system*. The adrenal medulla is derived from the neural crest and is supplied by preganglionic sympathetic nerves from the greater splanchnic nerve and the celiac ganglion. Stimulation of the chromaffin cells moves the secretory granules to the cell membrane for release via exocytosis. The released catecholamines can be taken up by the chromaffin cells, enter the systemic circulation or neuronal cells, and undergo degradation or be excreted in the urine. The neuronal cells metabolize epinephrine and norepinephrine into vanillylmandelic acid (VMA) with monamine oxidase. Another enzyme, carboxy-*O*-methyltransferase converts extraneuronal epinephrine and norepinephrine into metabolic products, metanephrine and norepinephrine, respectively. A small portion will bind to receptor and elicit a physiological response.

Pathophysiology

The production, release, and metabolism of the glucocorticoids and mineralocorticoids are tightly regulated to maintain body homeostasis. However, both benign and malignant adrenal and extraadrenal tumors, adrenal hyperplastic states, and congenital enzymatic deficiencies can cause the overproduction and insufficiency of glucocorticoids and mineralocorticoids and result in pathological conditions.

Cushing syndrome results from the excessive production of cortisol, and patients affected present with certain characteristic clinical features. These include central obesity, glucose intolerance, hypertension, plethora, hirsutism, osteoporosis, menstrual irregularity in women, and muscle weakness. There is also an increased incidence of peptic ulcer disease and pancreatitis. The incidence of Cushing syndrome is ten per one million. The most common cause is iatrogenic due to excessive and chronic administration of exogenous glucocorticoid steroids, which can produce similar clinical features. The most common cause of endogenous hypercortisolism is excessive pituitary ACTH (Cushing disease) secretion. Other causes include ectopic ACTH production, adrenal adenoma or carcinoma, micronodular pigmented hyperplasia, macronodular hyperplasia, and steroid-dependent adrenal hyperplasia. In children, the most common cause of hypercortisolism is adrenocortical neoplasms. Girls are affected three times more often than boys, and the predominant clinical presentation in children is obesity. Ectopic production of ACTH from malignant neoplasms is rare.

The *evaluation* and *diagnosis of hypercortisolism* is to first determine whether hypercortisolism is indeed present, second to determining whether the pathological state is pituitary dependent or pituitary independent, and finally to determine the exact cause using imaging studies such as CT and MRI. Hypercortisolism secondary to pituitary or non-

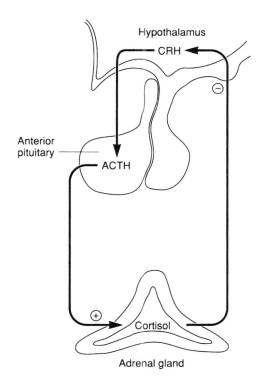

FIGURE 28-7. Feedback loop between the hypothalamus, the anterior pituitary, and the adrenal. (From Newsome HH. Adrenal glands. In: Greenfield LJ, Mulholand MW, Oldham KT, et al., eds. *Surgery: scientific principles and practice,* 2nd ed. Philadelphia: Lippincott-Raven Publishers, 1997:1334, with permission.)

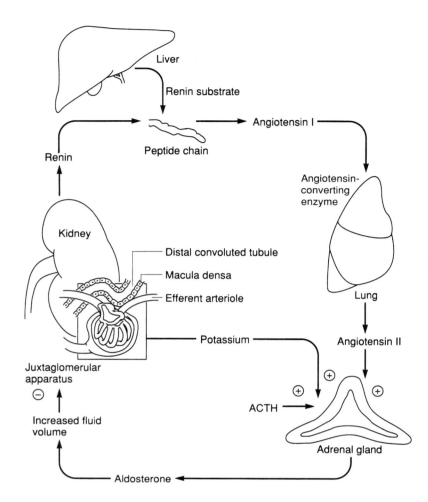

FIGURE 28-8. The renin/angiotensin/aldosterone system including their sites of production. (From Newsome HH. Adrenal glands. In: Greenfield LJ, Mulholand MW, Oldham KT, et al., eds. *Surgery: scientific principles and practice,* 2nd ed. Philadelphia: Lippincott-Raven Publishers, 1997:1335, with permission.)

pituitary pathology is associated with a loss in diurnal variation of serum cortisol levels. However, 24-hour urine collection for free cortisol or 17-hydroxysteroid is more sensitive in establishing a diagnosis of hypercortisolism. When the levels of cortisol are elevated, the binding proteins become saturated to a level that additional small increases in cortisol production result in exponential increases in urinary free cortisol. An overnight low-dose dexamethasone suppression test may be included in the diagnostic workup as well. The dexamethasone test involves a single dose of steroid the night (11 o'clock) before the morning (8 o'clock) measurement of cortisol levels in plasma and urine. In a healthy person, the single dose of steroid suppresses additional release and patients have levels less than 5 μg/dL in the morning. The disadvantage of the latter test is the percentage of false negatives and false positives; however, the combination of the 24-hour urine collection and dexamethasone test virtually excludes the diagnosis of hypercortisolism.

A patient may be given CRH to help determine whether the hypercortisolism is dependent on the pituitary. While patients with Cushing disease will have a rise in ACTH and cortisol levels in response to CRH, patients with adrenal or ectopic sources of cortisol production do not respond to the administration of CRH. Measurement of urinary 17-hydroxysteroid levels after administration of a high-dose of dexamethasone (8 mg per day) can also aid in determining the source of cortisol production. The urinary levels of 17-hydroxysteroid decrease significantly in patients with Cushing disease. On the other hand, there is no change in 17-hydroxysteroid levels in patients with adrenal or ectopic production of ACTH.

Lastly, imaging studies such as CT and MRI can help localize the exact cause of the cortisol production. When the CT and MRI results are normal with Cushing disease, petrosal sinus sampling may be performed to differentiate between a pituitary and an ectopic source of ACTH. This test involves bilateral sampling of the inferior petrosal sinus and peripheral veins for plasma ACTH levels before and after CRH administration. Among patients with primary sources of hypercortisolism, CT has great sensitivity (95%) and allows imaging of the primary tumor, as well as local invasion and distant metastases. However, this imaging study lacks specificity, which the MRI may add. T2-

weighted MRI may help differentiate a primary adrenal adenoma from metastatic disease, an adrenal carcinoma, or pheochromocytoma based on brightness. An additional scan using a labeled iodocholesterol may be performed to differentiate between an adenoma and carcinoma.

The treatment of the many causes of Cushing syndrome is surgical. In Cushing disease, transphenoidal resection of the pituitary adenoma is the treatment of choice. Radiation or medical therapy may be used if the symptoms persist or recur after surgery. Likewise, patients with adrenal adenoma or carcinoma require adrenalectomy. Patients with small adrenal adenomas may undergo laparoscopic adrenalectomy, which reduces the recovery time and the number of postoperative hospital days. However, adrenal carcinomas require an open laparotomy, either via bilateral subcostal or thoracoabdominal incision, which allows the thorough examination of the abdomen for local invasion or distant metastases. Lastly, for those patients with ectopic ACTH syndrome, the primary lesion must be surgically removed. Unresectable lesions or tumor recurrences may be debulked with or without bilateral adrenalectomy to provide palliation of symptoms. Drugs including metyrapone, aminoglutethimide, and mitotane can be used to suppress the production of cortisol. In the past, patients who underwent bilateral adrenalectomy for Cushing syndrome with an unknown cause developed a condition known as "Nelson syndrome," characterized by pituitary tumors with dark skin pigmentation, visual disturbances, and amenorrhea.

Hyperaldosteronism

Hypersecretion of mineralocorticoids can cause a syndrome of hypertension and hypokalemia. *Primary hyperaldosteronism* is generally due to autonomously functioning adrenal cortex tumors (Conn syndrome). *Secondary hyperaldosteronism* can be caused by an elevated level of renin in patients with renal artery stenosis, cirrhosis, congestive heart failure, and normal pregnancy. Treatment of the latter conditions usually corrects the hyperaldosteronism. In addition to moderate diastolic hypertension and hypokalemia, hyperaldosteronism can cause impaired insulin sensitivity and hyperglycemia. Potassium depletion can produce muscle weakness, fatigue, polyuria, and polydipsia. For a diagnosis of primary hyperaldosteronism, the patient must have diastolic hypertension without edema, hyposecretion of renin despite low intravascular volume, and hypersecretion of aldosterone. The patients have serum potassium levels of less than 3.5 mEq/L and a 24-hour urinary excretion of potassium that exceeds 30 mEq. The plasma aldosterone/renin ratio is more than 30. Captopril, an angiotensin-converting enzyme (ACE) inhibitor, may be given to the patient before measuring his or her aldosterone and renin levels. In normal patients, the ACE inhibitor decreases aldosterone production and increases renin production, thus lowering the aldosterone/renin ratio. However, a patient with primary hyperaldosteronism will have a continuous high level of aldosterone and a aldosterone/renin ratio of more than 50. Twenty-four-hour urinary aldosterone secretion of more than 14 µg following 5 days of high-sodium diet is highly suggestive of primary hyperaldosteronism. Measuring urinary sodium and aldosterone levels after i.v. saline infusion may also be helpful in the diagnosis of primary hyperaldosteronism. The next step in the workup is to determine whether the aldosterone production is due to a functional tumor or is the result of idiopathic adrenal cortical hyperplasia. CT scan can image approximately 75% to 95% of aldosterone-producing tumors, and the use of the iodocholesterol scan with 6β[^{131}I]-iodomethyl-19-norcholesterol can help differentiate between idiopathic adrenal cortical hyperplasia, which demonstrates bilateral uptake of the isotope, adenoma with localized uptake, and carcinoma with no uptake. The most definitive but invasive diagnostic test is to sample the adrenal veins for serum aldosterone and cortisol levels before and after ACTH administration. The lateralization of high serum levels of aldosterone suggests a functional adenoma on the positive side. The measurement of plasma aldosterone and renin levels in the supine position and 2 hours later in the standing position and the measurement of serum 18-hydroxycorticosterone are two additional tests that may be obtained. Patients with functional adenomas demonstrate suppression of renin and aldosterone levels when they move from a recumbent to a standing position and have elevated levels of 18-hydroxycorticosterone. Patients with primary hyperaldosteronism are treated with adrenalectomy. Those with idiopathic adrenal hyperplasia are managed medically with spironolactone and other potassium-sparing diuretics.

Pheochromocytoma

Pheochromocytoma, a tumor of the adrenal medulla or the neuroectodermal cells in certain extraadrenal sites, can produce a syndrome of hypertension that can be life threatening. It occurs in 0.05% to 0.1% of the population, affecting men and women equally. Ten percent of the tumors are bilateral, extraadrenal, familial, malignant, in children, or multicentric. The tumor is associated with individuals with MEN types 2A and 2B, von Recklinghausen neurofibromatosis, and von Hippel-Lindau disease. Patients may have sustained elevated blood pressure with no episodic elevations, normal blood pressure with paroxysmal hypertensive episodes, or sustained elevated blood pressure with acute episodes of blood pressure elevation, and develop anxiety attacks. The diagnosis of a pheochromocytoma can be made by performing 24-hour urine collections of catecholamines and metabolites including dopamine, VMA, and metanephrine and serum measurements of epinephrine and norepinephrine. Because of episodic secretion, repeated 24-hour urinary tests may be necessary. If the urinary and plasma measurements are equivocal for the diagnosis of pheochromocytoma, the patient may be given clonidine, a centrally acting antihypertensive. In normal patients, clonidine suppresses plasma concentrations of catecholamines.

Patients with pheochromocytomas require surgical excision of the tumor. However, the patients must be treated medically in preparation for the surgery. Patients are given phenoxybenzamine, an α-blocker, to reduce blood pressure and to restore intravascular volume. After adequate α-blockade has been achieved, a β-blocker may be added if the patient has evidence of tachycardia. β-blockers such as propranolol have negative inotropic and chronotropic effects and can produce a vasoconstrictor effect, which can precipitate malignant hypertension and cardiac failure in patients with pheochromocytomas who are not adequately α-receptor blocked. An alternative or additional preoperative medication is metyrapone, which blocks production of catecholamines in the tumor. This decreases blood pressure changes that occur with the manipulation of the tumor during operative resection.

Neuroblastoma

Neuroblastoma is another type of tumor of neural crest origin that occurs primarily in children. The tumors are associated with elevated levels of dopamine, but not epinephrine or norepinephrine or hypertension. Because the tumor is aggressive, distant metastases are a common accompaniment. The treatment of metastatic neuroblastoma is a combination chemotherapy regimen of cyclophosphamide, vincristine, and dacarbazine. The reported response rates have been as high as 80%.

Once the diagnosis is made, imaging studies with CT scan and MRI can be used to localize the tumor. Both tests are able to detect tumors approximately 1 cm in diameter. MRI has a higher specificity than the CT scan. MRI T2-weighted images can differentiate between pheochromocytomas and adenomas based on the brightness. A nuclear scan using labeled metaiodobenzylguanidine—a compound similar to epinephrine and concentrated in adrenergic tissue—may also help localize suspected pheochromocytomas. This scan has a sensitivity between 71% to 94% depending on the nature of the pheochromocytoma, as well as an overall specificity of 100%.

Adrenocortical Carcinoma

Excessive hormone production by the adrenal gland can be caused by adrenocortical carcinomas, which comprise only a small number of all cancers. Functional tumors can present with syndromes of hypercortisolism or virilization. There is a bimodal occurrence by age, in the first 4 years and then later in the fourth to fifth decade of life. Women develop functional adrenocortical carcinomas more commonly than men. The tumors usually are larger than 6 cm and weigh between 100 and 5,000 g. Like other aggressive forms of tumors, adrenocortical carcinomas have areas of necrosis, and microscopically, the cells have nuclear pleomorphism. They often metastasize and have a tendency to recur. Most carcinomas are discovered in stages III and IV, when the tumors have spread to the lymph nodes and distant organs. Several studies have demonstrated that metastasizing or recurring tumors are associated with high mitotic activity, nuclear DNA ploidy, and production of abnormal amounts of androgens and 11-deoxysteroids.

Congenital Adrenal Hyperplasia

In addition to functional tumors, enzyme deficiencies of the steroid synthesis pathway in the adrenal gland can result in overproduction of sex steroids. These enzymatic deficiencies result in a syndrome known as "congenital adrenal hyperplasia." It is the most common adrenal disorder of infancy and childhood. The syndrome results in decreased cortisol production and an accumulation of intermediate steroid metabolites that are shunted to androgen production. Peripheral tissues convert the androgen to testosterone, which can cause virilization. Prenatal congenital adrenal hyperplasia in girls produces ambiguous external genitalia (female pseudohermaphroditism), but the reproductive organs develop normally. Postnatal congenital adrenal hyperplasia can cause virilization of girls. Moreover, both sexes develop short stature, premature closure of bone epiphyses, and advanced bone age.

The most common cause of congenital adrenal hyperplasia is 21-hydroxylase deficiency (Fig. 28-6). This enzyme is responsible for the conversion of progesterone to 11-deoxycorticosterone, and subsequently to corticosterone and aldosterone. Without the enzyme, there is an accumulation of progesterone and delta-5-pregnenolone, which are converted to androgen by 17α-hydroxylase, as well as a decreased production of aldosterone that results in dehydration, hyponatremia, and hyperkalemia. The other less common causes of the hyperplasia are 11β-hydroxylase and 3β-hydroxydehydrogenase deficiencies. 3β-hydroxydehydrogenase deficiency results in early infant death secondary to significant salt wasting. The most severe form is congenital lipoid adrenal hyperplasia, which results from the deficiency of cholesterol desmolase. All the steroid synthesis pathways are inhibited, and as a result, all affected infants are phenotypic girls with several salt-wasting symptoms. The treatment of the deficiency is surgical correction of the external genitalia in girls, and medical treatment of the excess androgens.

Adrenal Insufficiency

The opposite condition of Cushing syndrome is primary or secondary adrenal failure, which is caused by a deficiency of cortisol with or without deficiency of aldosterone. Primary adrenal failure (*Addison disease*) is caused by an inherent disease of the adrenal gland, whereas secondary failure is caused by disorders of the pituitary or hypothalamus. The symptoms of low cortisol are nonspecific but can present as nausea, vomiting, weight loss, weakness, and lethargy. Rarely, hypocortisolism can produce a sudden episode of hypotension or shock (crisis) that is life threatening. Biochemically, the condition can produce hyponatremia and hyperkalemia. The causes of primary adrenal failure include autoimmune adrenalitis, infections including tuberculosis, histoplasmosis, and hemorrhagic adrenal infarction after surgery, during sepsis, and with hypercoagulable states. Secondary adrenal failure is due to chronic glucocorticoid therapy or inherent pituitary or hypothalamic disease. Exogenous steroid administration suppresses the hypothalamus/pituitary regulatory feedback mechanism. It may require up to 6 months before the regulatory mechanism functions properly.

A short cosyntropin stimulation test can be performed to make the diagnosis of primary and secondary adrenal failure. Cosyntropin (ACTH) (250 μ i.v. or intramuscular) is administered and plasma cortisol is measured 30 minutes later. Patients with adrenal failure will not demonstrate an increase in cortisol levels. An ACTH level can help distinguish between primary and secondary adrenal failure. In primary failure, patients will have elevated levels of ACTH but insufficient levels of glucocorticoids. Moreover, serum potassium and sodium levels may also be helpful in making the diagnosis.

The treatment of adrenal failure is exogenous glucocorticoids given twice daily with a higher morning dose. In primary failure, the treatment also includes the administration of a mineralocorticoid (Florinef) because all adrenal hormone synthesis is affected. The treatment of an Addisonian crisis is volume resuscitation with appropriate crystalloids and i.v. glucocorticoids. If the diagnosis of primary adrenal failure is known, the patients may be given hydrocortisone (100 mg i.v. every 8 hours), otherwise dexamethasone should be administered. Hydrocortisone is detected by the plasma cortisol assay and may cause confusion in making the diagnosis. Patients who use glucocorticoids or recently discontinued them require increased doses of the medication during illness, injury, or surgery, as well as in the postoperative period.

Incidentaloma

The prevalent use of imaging studies for diagnostic purposes has increased the detection of asymptomatic adrenal masses, or *incidentalomas,* most of which are benign cortical adenomas. Incidentalomas are seen in 0.6% of abdominal CT scans. Patients with positive CT scans for incidentalomas must undergo thorough physical examinations including measurement of blood pressure and histories that focus on signs and symptoms of functional tumors including weight loss, weakness, occult bleeding, and irregular menstruation. Twenty-four-hour collections of urine for cortisol, VMA, metanephrines, and catecholamines should be performed. Serum potassium levels should also be determined. If the potassium levels are low and the patient is hypertensive, serum aldosterone and renin levels should be collected.

The treatment for all functional tumors regardless of size and for all tumors greater than 5 cm is unilateral adrenalectomy. Masses that are less than 5 cm in size or are nonfunctional can be followed with repeated CT scans every 6 months. Size increase between observation periods warrants surgical resection. If a patient with a positive CT scan has a history of cancer and a negative biochemical workup, specifically urine that is negative for catecholamines, an FNA may be performed to help detect suspected metastatic disease to the adrenal or lymphoma. Otherwise, FNA should not be routinely performed, because it can not distinguish between benign and malignant tumors.

SUGGESTED READING

DeVita VT Jr, Hellman S, Roseberg SA, eds. *Cancer: principles and practice of oncology,* 5th ed. Philadelphia: Lippincott-Raven Publishers, 1997:1629–1652.

Parathyroid Disease. *Selected readings in general surgery.* University of Texas, Southwestern Medical Center of Dallas, Texas, Vol 23. No 4. 1996.

Adrenal. *Selected readings in general surgery.* University of Texas, Southwestern Medical Center of Dallas, Texas, Vol 26. No 7. 1999.

THE PANCREAS

PATRICK K. KIM AND ERNEST F. ROSATO

The pancreas is rightfully accorded a great deal of awe and respect by surgeons. The particulars of its anatomy and physiology make the treatment of pancreatic disease among the most challenging in surgery.

ANATOMY AND PHYSIOLOGY

The pancreas is situated in the retroperitoneum at the level of L-2, posterior to the stomach and anterior to the vertebrae and left kidney (Fig. 29-1). Its lateral relations are the second portion of the duodenum and the spleen. The head of the pancreas is the portion between the duodenum and the superior mesenteric vessels. The neck overlies the superior mesenteric vessels. The body of the pancreas begins lateral to the superior mesenteric vessels and extends to the splenic hilum. The portion of the head posterior to the superior mesenteric vessels is the uncinate process. Exocrine pancreatic secretions enter the duodenum via the main pancreatic duct (duct of Wirsung) or the accessory duct (duct of Santorini). The main pancreatic duct drains the tail, body, and most of the head of the pancreas. The lesser duct drains the superior portion of the pancreatic head into the second portion of the duodenum through the lesser papilla, approximately 2 cm proximal to the ampulla of Vater. The communication between the lesser duct and the main duct is typically patent, although several variations exist. The lesser duct may have a nonpatent communication with the main duct; it may communicate with the duodenum but not with the main duct; or it may communicate with the main duct but not with the duodenum. Also, the relationship of the common bile duct and main pancreatic duct is variable. The common bile duct and main pancreatic duct may join just at the ampulla of Vater, or they may have separate openings at the ampulla or a common channel may be present.

The pancreas is derived from the endoderm and begins development during the fifth week of life as two diverticula. The uncinate process and inferior head of the pancreas arise from the ventral bud while the body, tail, and superior portion of the pancreatic head arise from the dorsal bud (Fig. 29-2). The ventral bud rotates clockwise with respect to the long axis and fuses with the dorsal bud. The fusion of the ventral bud duct and the dorsal bud duct gives rise to the main pancreatic duct. The proximal duct of the dorsal bud becomes the lesser pancreatic duct.

Pancreas divisum is a condition in which the dorsal and ventral pancreatic ducts fail to fuse during embryonic development. Instead, the accessory duct, a derivative of the embryonic dorsal pancreatic duct, drains the entire pancreas (Fig. 29-3). If drainage is inadequate, chronic pain and pancreatitis may result. Pancreatic resection, longitudinal pancreatojejunostomy (Puestow procedure) or ductal sphincteroplasty may be indicated. Another developmental abnormality is *annular pancreas*, in which the ventral pancreatic bud fails to rotate normally, resulting in a pancreas that completely surrounds the second portion of the duodenum. In children, it is often associated with cardiac defects, malrotation, and mongoloid appearance. In adulthood, annular pancreas may cause upper gastrointestinal tract obstruction, chronic pancreatitis, and peptic ulcer. Treatment is enteroenteric bypass.

The pancreas is supplied *arterial blood* through branches of the celiac axis and superior mesenteric artery. The celiac trunk supplies blood to the pancreatic head via the gastroduodenal artery, a branch of the common hepatic artery. The gastroduodenal artery gives rise to two arcades, the anterosuperior pancreaticoduodenal artery and the posterosuperior pancreaticoduodenal artery, which anastomose with the anteroinferior pancreaticoduodenal artery and posteroinferior pancreaticoduodenal artery, respectively. The anteroinferior pancreaticoduodenal and posteroinferior pancreaticoduodenal arteries are branches of the superior mesenteric artery. The pancreaticoduodenal arteries supply both the duodenum and the head of the pancreas, necessitating duodenectomy if the head of the pancreas is removed. The pancreatic body and tail are supplied by the splenic artery and its branches, the dorsal pancreatic artery, great pancreatic artery, and caudal pancreatic artery. These collateralize with the inferior pancreatic artery, a branch of the superior mesenteric artery. Surgery involving the pan-

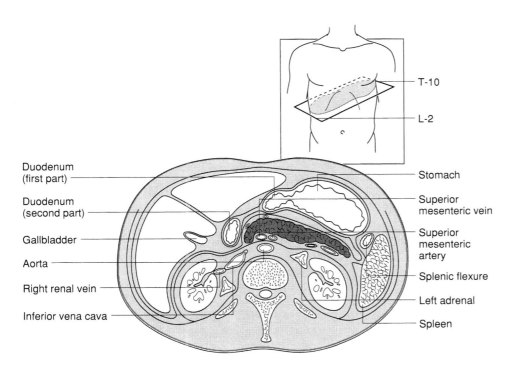

FIGURE 29-1. Relationship of the pancreas to other abdominal organs and viscera. (From Mackie CR, Moosa AR. Surgical anatomy of the pancreas. In: Moosa AR, ed. *Tumors of the pancreas.* Baltimore: Willimas & Wilkins, 1980, with permission.)

creatic head may potentially jeopardize hepatic blood flow, because at least 11% of patients have a replaced or accessory right hepatic artery arising from the superior mesenteric artery and coursing posterior to the head of the pancreas.

Venous drainage of the pancreas parallels the arterial supply. The head of the pancreas is drained by the anterosuperior and posterosuperior pancreaticoduodenal veins, which drain into the portal vein. The inferior aspect of the head of the pancreas is drained by the anteroinferior and posteroinferior pancreaticoduodenal veins, which unite to form the Henle trunk just prior to draining into the superior mesenteric vein. Of practical note, the relative paucity of vessels directly anterior to the portal vein makes this the preferred anteroposterior plane of division of the pancreas in pancreatoduodenectomy.

Lymphatic drainage is extensive throughout the retroperitoneum, explaining the frequent metastasis of pancreatic adenocarcinoma at the time of diagnosis. The celiac and superior mesenteric nodes drain the head of the pancreas. The tail and body are drained by the peripyloric and pancreaticolienal nodes. Other sites of lymphatic drainage are the splenic, transverse mesocolic, subpyloric, hepatic, lesser gastric omental, jejunal, and colonic nodes.

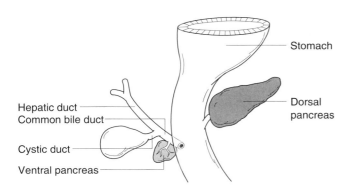

FIGURE 29-2. Relationship of the dorsal and ventral pancreas prior to rotation. (From Langman J. *Medical embryology,* 3rd ed. Baltimore: Williams & Wilkins, 1975:287, with permission.)

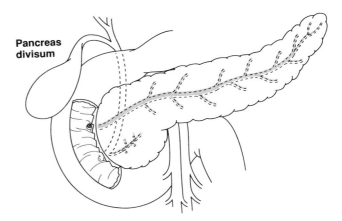

FIGURE 29-3. In pancreas divisum, there is no communication between the accessory duct of Santorini and the duct of Wirsung. Most of the pancreas is drained through the duct of Santorini and the accessory ampulla. This anatomy can be found in about 10% to 15% of normal children. (From Arnold G. Coran. Pediatric pancreas. In: Greenfield LJ, Mulholand MW, Oldham KT, et al., eds. *Surgery: scientific principles and practice,* 2nd ed. Philadelphia: Lippincott-Raven Publishers, 1997, with permission.)

Sympathetic innervation is supplied by the splanchnic nerves and parasympathetic innervation by the vagus nerve. Furthermore, peptidergic neurons secrete somatostatin, vasoactive intestinal peptide (VIP), calcitonin gene-related peptide, and galanin. While the experimental effects of these peptides have been characterized, their physiologic roles are not fully understood. The parasympathetic nerves stimulate exocrine and endocrine function while the sympathetic nerves inhibit these functions. A rich supply of afferent sensory fibers is present, explaining the pain associated with pancreatic carcinoma and chronic pancreatitis.

The *exocrine pancreas* accounts for over 80% of the mass of the pancreas. The functional unit of the exocrine pancreas is the acinus. The cells comprising an acinus secrete enzymes or proenzymes into a common intercalated duct (Fig. 17-6). Cells in the intercalated duct secrete alkaline fluid. From the intercalated ducts, exocrine secretions flow through interlobular ducts, secondary ducts, and finally, the main pancreatic or accessory duct.

The pancreas secretes 500 to 800 mL per day into the duodenum from centroacinar cells and epithelial cells of the pancreatic ducts. While the sodium and potassium concentrations equal that of plasma, the bicarbonate concentration varies from 20 to 150 mmol/L, depending on stimulation. Carbonic anhydrase in the fluid-secreting cells catalyzes the reaction of water and carbon dioxide to form bicarbonate and hydrogen ion. The major stimulant for bicarbonate secretion is the hormone *secretin,* secreted from duodenal mucosal S cells of the duodenal crypts of Lieberkuhn when the duodenal luminal pH level is less than 3. Cholecystokinin (CCK), gastrin, and acetylcholine are all weaker stimulants of bicarbonate secretion.

Pancreatic secretion of digestive enzymes is hormonally and neurally regulated. *CCK* and *acetylcholine* stimulate secretion. Secretin and VIP are weaker stimulants.

Amylase, lipase, ribonuclease, and deoxyribonuclease are secreted into the duodenum as active enzymes. The remainder of the pancreatic enzymes are secreted into the duodenum as *inactive proenzymes,* which are activated by other enzymes or by appropriate pH levels.

The *endocrine pancreas* consists of islets interspersed throughout the exocrine pancreas. Hormones secreted by pancreatic islets include insulin, glucagon, somatostatin, and VIP. *Insulin* is the principal hormone of the anabolic, or "fed" state. Insulin secretion is tightly coupled to plasma glucose concentration. Insulin stimulates uptake of glucose from the blood into all cell types except β cells, hepatocytes, and the central nervous system. Insulin inhibits glycogenolysis and fatty acid oxidation and stimulates protein synthesis. A significant reserve of insulin secretion is suggested by the fact that diabetes is not clinically apparent until over 80% of the islet cell mass is removed. Type I diabetes is characterized by an absolute deficiency of insulin secretion due to autoimmune destruction of β cells while type II diabetes is characterized by *insulin resistance* and adequate insulin synthesis.

Hormonal stimulants of insulin secretion include glucagon, gastric inhibitory peptide (GIP), and CCK. Hormonal inhibitors of insulin secretion include somatostatin, amylin, and pancreatin. Insulin secretion is stimulated by cholinergic and β-adrenergic input and inhibited by α-adrenergic input. Pharmacologically, sulfonylureas stimulate insulin secretion. The secretion of insulin is greater after orally administered glucose than after the same amount of glucose given intravenously (i.v.). This is due to the presence of an enteroinsular axis, which is likely mediated by the hormone GIP.

Glucagon is secreted by A cells of the pancreatic islets and is the principal hormone of the catabolic, or "stress," state. Glucagon stimulates glycogenolysis and gluconeogenesis. Nutrient stimulants of glucagon secretion include arginine and alanine. Insulin and somatostatin inhibit glucagon secretion.

Somatostatin inhibits secretion of virtually all gut peptides and inhibits gastric, pancreatic, and biliary secretion. It is secreted by the D cells of the islets. Somatostatin likely regulates pancreatic endocrine function in a paracrine manner. Pancreatic polypeptide is secreted by the F cells. Its role *in vivo* is unclear, but it has been shown to inhibit exocrine secretion, choleresis, and gallbladder emptying. VIP, galanin, and serotonin are neuropeptides that probably regulate islet cell secretion. Pancreatin has an unknown physiologic role, although it has been shown to inhibit insulin secretion.

TESTS OF PANCREATIC EXOCRINE FUNCTION

The pancreas has significant reserve exocrine function. Exocrine dysfunction is clinically apparent only after a significant portion of the pancreas is removed. When pancreatic exocrine insufficiency is suspected, various tests may confirm the diagnosis. Many of these tests are of physiologic interest but are not utilized in clinical evaluations. The *secretin test* measures pancreatic exocrine response to secretin stimulation. A tube is advanced into the duodenum. A baseline sample of duodenal fluid is obtained, and a total of four samples are obtained at 20-minute intervals after i.v. administration of secretin 2 U/kg. The samples are analyzed for total volume, bicarbonate concentration, and enzyme secretion.

The *dimethadione* (DMO) test also measures pancreatic exocrine function. Trimethadione (Tridione), an anticonvulsant, is metabolized to DMO by the pancreas and secreted in an exocrine manner. Trimethadione is administered orally for 3 days and the duodenum is intubated. Secretin is then administered i.v. and duodenal samples are collected and analyzed for DMO. The *Lundh test* assesses pancreatic enzyme secretion in response to a specific meal. The duodenum is intubated and a baseline sample of duodenal fluid is collected. The patient then consumes a meal of glucose, casein, and corn oil, and samples are collected every 30 minutes for 2 hours. The samples are analyzed for amylase, lipase, and trypsin. The *triolein breath test* is a noninvasive test of pancreatic exocrine function. In this test, the patient consumes corn oil radiolabeled with ^{14}C. This lipid is metabolized to $^{14}CO_2$, which is exhaled. Breath samples are collected 4 hours after ingestion, and radioactivity is measured. Low levels of radioactivity suggest abnormal fat digestion or absorption. If the test results remain abnormal after replacement of exocrine enzymes, then malabsorption is likely rather than exocrine insufficiency.

The *paraaminobenzoic acid* (PABA) *test* is another noninvasive test of exocrine function. Chymotrypsin hydrolyzes *N*-benzoyl-*L*-tyrosyl-*p*-aminobenzoic acid to PABA, which is absorbed and then excreted in the urine. Low urinary PABA level suggests exocrine insufficiency. The *test-meal pancreatic polypeptide* (PP) response measures pancreatic polypeptide levels after a meal of specific fat/carbohydrate/protein composition. Baseline and postprandial PP levels are measured. In pancreatic insufficiency, the baseline and/or postprandial peak level of PP is low. PP level may also be low in diabetic autonomic neuropathy or posttruncal vagotomy or antrectomy. The *fecal fat test* differentiates pancreatic and intestinal etiologies of steatorrhea. Lipase deficiency of greater than 90% results in steatorrhea with elevated fecal fat (more than 20 g per 24 hours). Intestinal dysfunction is suggested by steatorrhea with low levels of fecal fat.

TESTS OF PANCREATIC ENDOCRINE FUNCTION

The *oral glucose tolerance test* is an indirect measure of endocrine function. Serum glucose is measured before administration of oral glucose (40 g/m^2) and every 30 minutes for 2 hours afterward. Abnormally elevated serum glucose levels suggest diabetes. Although this test is primarily a measure of insulin function, it is affected by hormones of the enteroinsular axis, such as GIP, CCK, and glucagonlike peptide-1. The *i.v. glucose tolerance test* is similar to the oral glucose tolerance test. Serum glucose is measured before administration of i.v. glucose (0.5 g/kg) and every 10 minutes for 1 hour. The advantage of this test over the oral glucose tolerance test is that it eliminates the effects of the enteroinsular axis. The *i.v. arginine test* can be used to diagnose hormone-secreting tumors. Arginine stimulates endocrine secretion. Blood samples are obtained before administration of arginine (0.5 g/kg) and every 10 minutes afterward. Hormones are detected by radioimmunoassay. The *tolbutamide response test* is another method of diagnosing hormone-secreting tumors. Serum glucose in measured before administration of i.v. tolbutamide and for an hour afterward. Hormones are detected by radioimmunoassay.

Insulinoma is diagnosed by hypoglycemia with elevated levels of insulin. Somatostatinoma can also be diagnosed in this manner.

PANCREATIC PATHOLOGY

Acute pancreatitis is a disease of the exocrine pancreas with a broad range of clinical and pathological findings ranging from simple edematous pancreatitis to fulminant necrotizing pancreatitis with systemic inflammatory response syndrome (SIRS), multiple-organ dysfunction syndrome (MODS), or multiple organ failure (MOF). Acute pancreatitis has many etiologies. Most cases of acute pancreatitis are due to ethanol use or gallstone disease. In the United States, over 50% of cases of acute pancreatitis can be attributed to ethanol use. Gallstone pancreatitis accounts for an additional 30% of cases. Acute pancreatitis is most common in adults between 30 and 70 years. Older patients are more likely to have gallstone disease, and younger patients are more likely to have ethanol-induced disease. Furthermore, gallstone pancreatitis sufferers are more likely to be women, and ethanol-induced pancreatitis sufferers are more likely to be men. Eighty-five percent of patients with acute pancreatitis have uneventful recovery. Overall pancreatitis is a variable disease, ranging from mild edema of the gland to hemorrhagic pancreatitis defined by loss of parenchymal viability, gangrene, and necrosis. The overall mortality rate of acute necrotizing pancreatitis is 5% to 10%, mostly due to sepsis.

Acute pancreatitis begins with disruption of ordered secretion of pancreatic exocrine enzymes. Most pancreatic enzymes are secreted into the duodenum as inactive proenzymes and become activated in the duodenal lumen. Endogenous protease inhibitors present in plasma and pancreatic tissue prevent activation of pancreatic enzymes. Acinar cell injury results from intracellular activation of proteases and inappropriate discharge of acinar cell contents through the basolateral membrane (Fig. 29-4).

Experimental evidence suggests that ethanol has several detrimental effects on pancreatic exocrine function. Ethanol decreases protective trypsin inhibitor activity and decreases pancreatic microvascular blood flow, predisposing the acinar cells to hypoxic injury. Ethanol stimulates the formation of stone protein in the pancreatic ductules and increases pancreatic exocrine secretion by stimulation of gastrin secretion. Furthermore, ethanol increases tone of the sphincter of Oddi.

Gallstones induce acute pancreatitis by the obstruction of the ampulla of Vater. Obstruction of the ampulla causes ductal hypertension, and edema of the ampulla may cause sphincter of Oddi dysfunction, allowing free reflux of bile or duodenal contents into the pancreatic duodenal system. In patients with gallstone pancreatitis, the most common finding on ultrasound examination is simple cholelithiasis.

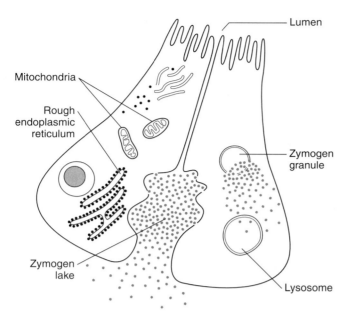

FIGURE 29-4. Acute pancreatitis begins with cytoplasmic activation of pancreatic enzymes, loss of acinar cell polarity, and inappropriate basolateral discharge. (From Guice KS. Acute pancreatitis. In: Greenfield LJ, Mulholand MW, Oldham KT, et al., eds. *Surgery: scientific principles and practice*, 2nd ed. Philadelphia: Lippincott-Raven Publishers, 1997, with permission.)

Cholecystitis and choledocholithiasis are less commonly noted during an ultrasound examination. Choledocholithiasis is rarely noted, because most obstruction is only transient.

Acute pancreatitis may also be induced by ischemia as a result of low-flow or microvascular thrombosis. Causes of ischemia include myocardial infarction, celiac artery stenosis, thromboembolic disease, ruptured abdominal aortic aneurysm, massive hemorrhage, and cardiopulmonary bypass. The incidence of postprocedural pancreatitis, such as acute pancreatitis after upper abdominal surgery or endoscopic retrograde cholangiopancreatography (ERCP), is approximately 1%. The incidence of acute pancreatitis after abdominal trauma (blunt or penetrating) is approximately 6%. Hyperparathyroidism, drugs, and tumors of the duodenum or pancreas are more uncommon etiologies of acute pancreatitis.

The *host inflammatory response* plays an important role in the pathophysiology of acute pancreatitis. The complement system is activated, and histamine and bradykinin release occurs, altering local (and sometimes systemic) vascular tone and permeability. Proinflammatory cytokines TNF-α, IL-1, and IL-6 are secreted from inflammatory cells. Activation of neutrophils, macrophages, monocytes, and lymphocytes occurs. Neutrophils produce oxygen-free radicals and secrete inflammatory mediators such as elastase, collagenase, cathepsins, phospholipases, DNAse, RNase, glycosidases, hydrolases, platelet-activating factor, and myeloperoxidase, all of which may injure acinar or endothelial tissue and contribute to microvascular permeability. Macrophages elaborate cytokines and perform phagocytosis. Lymphocytes also secrete cytokines. Systemic "spillover" of the inflammatory process results in the SIRS, characterized by fever (or hypothermia), tachycardia, tachypnea, and leukocytosis.

MODS, defined as the demonstrable organ dysfunction due to SIRS, most frequently affects the pulmonary system. Microvascular permeability results in pulmonary edema and infiltration of inflammatory cells, leading to hypoxemia. Respiratory function may be further compromised by abdominal distention, elevation of the diaphragm, and decreased surfactant lecithin due to increased lecithinase activity. Other susceptible organs in SIRS and MODS include the liver, kidney, and heart.

Acute pancreatitis causes striking alterations in metabolism. The production of both glucose and insulin increases, but target cells become resistant to insulin. This has been described as the "diabetes of injury." Furthermore, significant catabolism occurs, and the body undergoes a negative nitrogen balance. *Hypocalcemia* results from the binding of calcium to saponified peripancreatic fat. The degree of hypocalcemia has been shown to reflect severity of pancreatitis.

Acute pancreatitis may lead to shock by a variety of mechanisms. *Hypovolemic shock* may occur due to vomiting, lack of oral intake, and massive third space sequestration in the pancreas and the retroperitoneum. Acute pancreatitis with superinfection of the pancreatic bed may lead to sepsis and septic shock. SIRS may directly impair cardiac performance, potentially leading to *cardiogenic shock*.

Clinical features of acute pancreatitis include epigastric pain, nausea/vomiting, anorexia, ileus, fever, and palpable mass. The degree of pain is highly variable. Jaundice and hypotension may be present in severe pancreatitis. Rarely, pancreatic necrosis leads to retroperitoneal hemorrhage, which dissects to the subcutaneous tissues and becomes visible as ecchymoses of the flank, umbilicus, or inguinal ligament.

Elevation of serum amylase supports the diagnosis of acute pancreatitis when signs and symptoms are present. However, the degree of hyperamylasemia is a poor predictor of severity or prognosis. In transient duct obstruction, hyperamylasemia may resolve before presentation, because amylase has a short half-life. In chronic pancreatitis or necrotizing pancreatitis, acinar cell mass may be insufficient to produce enough amylase for systemic hyperamylasemia. Furthermore, not all amylase is of pancreatic origin. Extrapancreatic sources of amylase include salivary glands, fallopian tubes, and small bowel. Hyperamylasemia may accompany cholelithiasis, perforated peptic ulcer, small bowel obstruction, and mesenteric infarct. Lipase, like amylase, may confirm the diagnosis when suspected clinically, but hyperlipemia is also nonspecific.

Abdominal plain film findings suggestive of acute pancreatitis include adynamic ileus or the presence of a sentinel loop in the left upper quadrant. Chest radiograph may demonstrate left-sided pleural effusion. Either ultrasound or computed tomography (CT) with oral and i.v. contrast should be performed for evaluation of suspected pancreatitis. Suggestive findings on these studies include enlargement of the pancreas, irregular or indistinct contour, and presence of peripancreatic fluid. Gallstones, if present, can be visualized. Fluid collections are most commonly seen in the lesser sac or the left pararenal space. Pancreatic necrosis is suggested by the absence of enhancement on contrast CT. Ranson's criteria are clinical signs and symptoms that can help to stratify outcome of this highly variable disease. Five criteria are assessed on admission, and six criteria are assessed after 48 hours (Table 29-1). Morbidity and mortality correlate with the number of criteria present and the 20% risk of mortality associated with three or four Ranson's criteria increases close to 100% if seven or more criteria are met.

Therapy for sterile acute pancreatitis is supportive. In all cases, oral feedings should be discontinued and i.v. fluids initiated, with careful attention to urine output. Nasogastric suction is indicated to prevent vomiting and to manage ileus. Resuscitation with crystalloid should be aggressive, because fluid requirements may be enormous due to gastrointestinal tract losses, third space losses, fever, and tachypnea. Invasive hemodynamic monitoring is indicated in patients with cardiac or pulmonary disease. Supplemental oxygen should be administered. Respiratory failure may require mechanical ventilation. Renal dysfunction is typically a prerenal azotemia, underscoring the need for aggressive fluid resuscitation. Occasionally, acute renal failure will require transient dialysis. Electrolytes must be monitored closely and deficits corrected. Nutritional support should be instituted in an attempt to halt nitrogen loss due to catabolism. The route of nutrition support is open to debate. The advantages of parenteral hyperalimentation include minimization of pancreatic secretion and expansion of the intravascular volume. The advantages of enteral nutrition include cost, trophism of the gut mucosa, and a more "physiologic" route compared to parenteral nutrition. Jejunal tube feedings may be less stimulatory of pancreatic secretion than gastric or duodenal feedings. Antibiotics are indicated only for treatment of documented infection. Medical therapies intended to decrease pancreatic secretion (octreotide), inhibit protease activation (aprotinin), and correct coagulation disorders (heparin) have not been consistently shown to decrease the early morbidity of acute pancreatitis.

The few cases of acute pancreatitis associated with persistent choledocholithiasis should be treated early with endoscopic sphincterotomy. This procedure is highly successful if performed by a skilled endoscopist. Because of the high rate of recurrence of choledocholithiasis (50% within 6 weeks), elective cholecystectomy is indicated when the attack of acute pancreatitis resolves. Operative intervention is indicated for management of the complications of acute pancreatitis, for an anatomically correctable defect such as pancreas divisum, if deterioration occurs despite maximal supportive therapy or if infection is demonstrated in the tissues. Laparotomy and drainage, debridement, or resection has not been shown to improve outcome of routine sterile acute pancreatitis. In fact, early laparotomy and sump drainage may increase rates of septic and respiratory complications. Peritoneal lavage has been practiced with evidence of improved early survival. This involves placement of Silastic catheters via small laparotomy. Closed lavage is then performed for up to several days.

Complications of *acute pancreatitis* include formation of fluid collections, pancreatic ascites, pseudocyst, and pancreatic abscess. Sterile fluid collections typically resolve without intervention. *Pancreatic ascites* results from leakage of pancreatic fluid from the pancreatic duct and anterior leakage into the peritoneal cavity causes ascites. Posterior leaks may fill the mediastinum or pleural space. Typically the left pleural space is involved due to the proximity of the pancreatic tail to the left hemidiaphragm (Fig. 29-1). This fluid is typically rich in amylase. Surgery for pancreatic ductal compromise is indicated if nonoperative management fails. The location of the leak should be determined by preoperative ERCP or by operative pancreatic ductogram. Depending on the location of the leak, distal pancreatectomy or Roux-en-Y pancreatoenterostomy may be indicated.

Pancreatic abscess develops in 10% of patients with acute pancreatitis as a later complication. Signs and symptoms include persistent or new fever, abdominal distention, abdominal mass, and leukocytosis. On CT, the presence of gas in the peripancreatic tissues is pathognomonic for infection. During CT scan, aspiration and Gram stain of the aspirate may be obtained for diagnosis of infection. Bacter-

TABLE 29-1. RANSON'S PROGNOSTIC CRITERIA FOR ACUTE PANCREATITIS

Negative prognostic criteria upon admission	Negative prognostic criteria after 48 hours
Age above 55 years	A hematocrit decrease of 10% or greater
White blood cell count above 16,000/μL	Blood urea nitrogen increase of 5 mg/dL or greater
Serum glucose level above 200 mg/dL	Serum calcium level below 8 mg/dL
Serum lactate dehydrogenase above 350 IU/L	Pa_{O_2} below 60 mm Hg on room air
Serum glutamic-oxaloacetic transaminase level above 250 IU/L	Base deficit above 4 mEq/L
—	Fluid sequestration greater than 6 L

ial growth is typically polymicrobial in origin. Once an abscess has been diagnosed, immediate surgical therapy is indicated, because pancreatic abscess is almost uniformly fatal without surgery. The operation should consist of laparotomy, thorough exploration, debridement, and sump drainage. During exploration, the pancreas gland should be directly visualized and the lesser sac opened and inspected. Marsupialization treatment may be utilized as an adjunct to debridement. Debridement is performed and may be concluded by placement of gauze packs into the debrided pancreatic bed. The wound is left open to allow regular dressing changes. These are performed initially in the operating room under general anesthesia. As granulation tissue accumulates, dressing changes may be performed in the intensive care unit under sedation, and when the patient is sufficiently stable.

Pancreatic pseudocysts enclose collections of blood, pancreatic juice, and debris that arise from peripancreatic tissue after an attack of acute pancreatitis. They are so named because the walls, composed of adjacent pancreatic tissue, peritoneal surfaces, and serosa of adjacent bowel, have no true epithelial lining. The incidence of pseudocyst formation after acute pancreatitis is close to 40%, which is much higher than previously believed. Pseudocyst associated with acute pancreatitis may form anywhere from the thoracic cavity to the pelvis, although most are found in the lesser sac or anterior pararenal space. Pseudocysts associated with chronic pancreatitis are more commonly found in the pancreas gland itself. Pseudocyst should be suspected in patients with persistent symptoms of pancreatitis. An ultrasound or CT examination is indicated to investigate suspected pseudocyst. Angiography should be considered to rule out pseudoaneurysm, which may lead to hemorrhage. ERCP provides information regarding communication of the pseudocyst to the pancreatic duct and is therefore useful for planning surgical treatment of chronic pseudocysts.

Most pseudocysts resolve by reabsorption, decompression into the pancreatic duct, or erosion into an adjacent viscus. Factors that decrease the probability of spontaneous resolution include size greater than 6 cm (or progressive increase in size), multiplicity, and chronicity. Internal drainage is the procedure of choice for pseudocysts that are chronic (duration of greater than 6 weeks). Internal drainage is associated with decreased morbidity and mortality compared to external drainage. The location of the pseudocyst and its relation to the gastrointestinal tract determine the surgical procedure. Options include transgastric cystogastrostomy, transduodenal cystoduodenostomy, and simple cystojejunostomy or Roux-en-Y cystojejunostomy (Fig. 29-5). External drainage is generally reserved for emergent complications of pseudocyst formation, such as infection, bleeding, and free rupture into the peritoneum or thorax. External drainage is also indicated for the sterile, intact pseudocyst if the pseudocyst wall is found to be immature and incapable of holding suture (immature pseudocyst). The rate of recurrence or fistula formation after external drainage is 20% while the recurrence rate after internal drainage is 5%.

Chronic pancreatitis is characterized by a progressive loss of pancreatic exocrine tissue mass and function, fibrosis of the gland, and in many cases, clinically evident endocrine pancreas dysfunction. Seventy percent of chronic pancreatitis cases can be linked to alcohol use. Chronic pancreatitis may also be caused by obstruction of the main pancreatic duct by a congenital anomaly, prior inflammation, fibrosis of the ampulla, or a mass such as tumor. The fibrosis and atrophy of obstructive pancreatitis may reverse or at least stabilize with relief of the obstruction in contrast to the irreversible deterioration seen in alcoholic pancreatitis. Early alcoholic chronic pancreatitis is characterized histologically by patchy normal acini among abnormal lobules. Later, ductules become irregularly dilated. Proteinaceous deposits obstruct the ducts (Fig. 29-6). Finally fibrosis replaces exocrine tissue.

The most common presenting symptom is *dull pain* of the *epigastrium* radiating to the back. The pain worsens with food or alcohol intake. No routine laboratory test is diagnostic for chronic pancreatitis. Serum amylase level may be normal, elevated, or even decreased, depending on the amount of exocrine tissue present. Similarly serum levels of lipase and other exocrine enzymes do not improve reliability of diagnosis. Pancreatic endocrine insufficiency is common. The incidence of diabetes in patients with chronic pancreatitis is 40%. Other complications of chronic pancreatitis include pancreatic pseudocyst, splenic vein thrombosis, and pancreatic ascites.

Imaging studies useful for confirmation of chronic pancreatitis include abdominal plain film, ultrasound, CT, and ERCP. On abdominal plain film, calcifications of the pancreas are seen in 30% of patients with chronic pancreatitis. Ultrasound findings include pancreatic atrophy, reduced echogenicity, pancreatic ductal dilation of greater than 4 mm, and cystic lesions. CT findings include pancreatic atrophy, calcification, irregularity of pancreatic outline, and ductal dilation. ERCP is the most sensitive and specific imaging study for the diagnosis of chronic pancreatitis, with sensitivity and specificity of 90%. Findings may include irregularity of ducts and ductules, common bile duct stenosis, or pancreatic pseudocyst. In late chronic pancreatitis, alternating dilation and stenosis of pancreatic ducts may give rise to a "chain-of-lakes" appearance (Fig. 29-6).

Treatment of chronic pancreatitis begins with abstinence from alcohol. Pain may respond to nonsteroidal antiinflammatory agents, but most patients require narcotics. Malabsorption is treated with oral preparations of pancreatic enzymes. Surgery is indicated for pain that is intractable, and it substantially affects quality of life, impairs nutrition, or results in narcotic addiction. Surgical options include lateral pancreatojejunostomy or pancreatic resection. Lateral pancreatojejunostomy (Puestow procedure) involves longitudinal opening of the main pancreatic duct and creation of a side-to-side anastomosis with a loop of jejunum. Pain is eliminated or improved in 80% of patients, but fibrosis continues. A dilated duct is required for lateral pancreatojejunostomy. Pancreatic resection may be considered when the pancreatic duct is small in diameter, when disease is limited to one part of the pancreas, or when prior lateral pancreatojejunostomy fails. Postoperative exocrine insufficiency and diabetes are proportional to the extent of resection. The long-term results of pancreatic resection for chronic pancreatitis are unpredictable but frequently poor. Similarly, pancreatoduodenectomy may be considered for disease of the head of the pancreas or when prior lateral pancreatojejunostomy fails to drain the uncinate process.

Ten percent of patients with chronic pancreatitis have common bile duct stenosis. In contrast to malignant stricture of the common bile duct, biliary stricture of chronic pancreatitis is smooth and tapering and limited to the intrapancreatic portion of the duct. Cholangitis and biliary cirrhosis occur in 7% to 10% of patients with chronic pancreatitis. Indications for surgery of bile duct stricture are persistent jaundice, cholangitis, biliary cirrhosis, radiographic progression of stricture, persistent elevation of serum alkaline phosphatase of more than three times the normal level, and inability to exclude malignancy. Operative options include choledochoduodenostomy and choledochojejunostomy. Pain is not a symptom of chronic bile duct stricture. Relief of pain would not occur with relief of the obstruction of the bile duct alone.

The increased mortality of those with chronic pancreatitis is primarily due to extrapancreatic complications of alcoholism and include aerodigestive cancers, diabetes, and cirrhosis.

In late-stage chronic pancreatitis, malabsorption occurs due to insufficient exocrine tissue mass. Lipase deficiency causes steatorrhea, which in turn results in deficiencies of fat-soluble vitamins. Protease deficiency causes azoturia. Bicarbonate secretion is also impaired, altering duodenal pH level and therefore protease function.

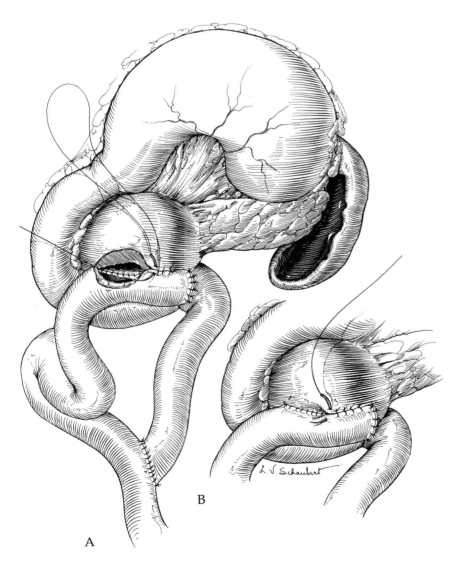

FIGURE 29-5. Roux-en-Y cystojejunostomy can be used to drain a pseudocyst at the head of the pancreas. (From Way LW. Roux-en-Y cystojejunostomy for pancreatic pseudocyst. In: Nyhas LM, Baker RJ, eds. *Mastery of surgery,* 2nd ed. Boston: Little, Brown and Company, 1992, with permission.)

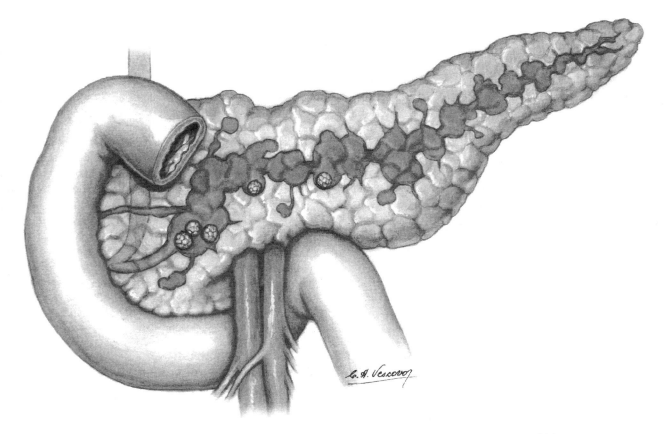

FIGURE 29-6. Main pancreatic duct in chronic pancreatitis can take on a "chain-of-lakes" appearance with proteinaceous deposits obstructing the ducts. (From Etala E. *Atlas of gastrointestinal surgery.* Philadelphia: Williams & Wilkins, 1997:527, with permission.)

TRAUMA

Pancreatic trauma is more commonly due to penetrating rather than blunt injury. Overall mortality rate is between 10% and 25% and associated injuries are the rule. Major vascular injury (aorta, vena cava, and portal vein) frequently accompanies penetrating pancreatic injury. The liver, spleen, and hollow viscera are most commonly associated with blunt pancreatic injury. Considering all traumatic pancreas injuries, vascular injuries are the most common cause of early death while sepsis, SIRS, and MOF are the most common causes of late death in these patients. For either blunt or penetrating trauma to the pancreas, conservative operative management is indicated. Nonoperative management is rare due to the frequency of associated injuries. If nonoperative management is chosen, close serial examination is necessary and the threshold for intervention should be low. Simple drainage is indicated for pancreatic parenchymal injury with sparing of the pancreatic duct. If the distal pancreatic duct is injured, distal pancreatectomy can be performed and a splenectomy should be considered. Management of proximal ductal injury is determined by the presence or absence of duodenal injury. If the duodenum is spared, the proximal duct may be ligated and a distal pancreatoenterostomy performed. In the situation of concomitant duodenal injury, pancreatoduodenectomy is indicated. Given the instability usually associated with such an injury, it is prudent to limit the initial operation to control of hemorrhage and contamination. This is followed by stabilization and resuscitation for 24 to 48 hours in the intensive care unit prior to formal pancreatoduodenectomy.

ENDOCRINE NEOPLASMS

Insulinoma is the most common endocrine neoplasm of the pancreas. The Whipple triad defines classic signs and symptoms of insulinoma and includes (i) symptoms of hypoglycemia while fasting, (ii) serum glucose level of less than 50 mg/dL while fasting, and (iii) relief of symptoms of hypoglycemia after administration of glucose. Signs and symptoms of hypoglycemia include confusion, seizure, obtundation, personality change, coma, palpitations, trembling, diaphoresis, and tachycardia. Insulinoma is diagnosed by the monitored fast test where serum glucose and insulin are measured periodically during fasting and when symptoms occur. In patients with insulinoma, serum insulin/glucose ratio is greater than 0.4 (normally less than 0.3). Furthermore, serum levels of proinsulin and insulin C-peptide are elevated, distinguishing insulinoma from surreptitious self-administration of insulin. After biochemical confirmation of insulinoma, imaging studies such as CT with contrast or endoscopic ultrasound are performed to identify primary tumor and rule out metastases. Visceral arteriography is now uncommonly employed. Insulinoma is found with equal frequency in the head, body, and tail of the pancreas. The most common finding is a solitary benign nodule, occurring in 90% of patients. Ten percent of insulinomas are malignant, and 10% of insulinomas are associated with multiple endocrine neoplasia 1 (MEN 1). Compared to sporadic insulinoma, MEN 1–associated insulinoma is usually multifocal, and recurrence rate after resection is higher. Enucleation is indicated for tumors less than 2 cm in diameter, unless the tumor is close to the main duct. Insulinomas close to the main duct or greater than 2 cm in diameter are treated by distal pancreatectomy or pancreatoduodenectomy. Common sites of metastases include the lymph nodes and liver. Tumor debulking is indicated for those with metastatic disease to improve hypoglycemic symptoms. Treatment of those with unresectable insulinoma includes dietary modification to prevent periods of hypoglycemia. Medical therapy may include diazoxide or octreotide to inhibit insulin release. Chemotherapy is sometimes effective.

Gastrinoma is the second most common neoplasm of the endocrine pancreas. Gastrinoma is responsible for about 1 in 1,000 cases of primary duodenal ulcer disease. Three fourths of gastrinomas are sporadic, and the remainder are associated with MEN 1 syndrome. Sixty percent of gastrinomas are malignant. The most common symptom of a gastrinoma is abdominal pain due to peptic ulcer. Other common symptoms include diarrhea and gastroesophageal reflux. Peptic ulceration, esophagitis, and gastroesophageal reflux are frequently confirmed by endoscopy. Fasting serum gastrin level greater than 200 pg/mL suggests gastrinoma, and serum gastrin level greater than 1,000 pg/mL is virtually diagnostic. Other disease states are associated with hypergastrinoma and may be classified into diseases of excess acid secretion (antral G-cell hyperplasia, gastric outlet obstruction, and retained excluded antrum) and diseases of normal or low acid secretion (atrophic gastritis, pernicious anemia, previous vagotomy, renal failure, and short-gut syndrome). Hypersecretion is defined as gastric acid production greater than 15 mEq per hour (or 5 mEq per hour in patients with prior vagotomy) or ratio of basal to maximal acid production of greater than 1.6.

After hypersecretory hypergastrinoma has been established, the diagnosis of gastrinoma is based on the *secretin stimulation test*. Serum gastrin levels are measured before and after i.v. administration of secretin. A rise in serum gastrin level greater than 200 pg/mL is diagnostic. If the secretin stimulation test results are positive, then antisecretory therapy (omeprazole) is initiated and imaging studies are performed to locate the primary tumor and rule out metastases. CT with contrast, visceral arteriography, and endoscopic ultrasound are commonly employed. Other modalities include the selective arterial secretin stimulation test and percutaneous transhepatic portal venous gastrin sampling.

Most gastrinomas are found to the right of the superior mesenteric vessels in the head of the pancreas or the duodenum, an area known as the "gastrinoma triangle" (Fig. 29-7). Enucleation is indicated for primary pancreatic gastrinomas of less than 2 cm in diameter or gastrinomas with a well-formed capsule. Distal pancreatectomy or pancreatoduodenectomy is indicated for other resectable pancreatic gastrinomas. Primary gastrinomas of the duodenal wall are excised with primary closure of the duodenum. If preoperative imaging studies demonstrate unresectable disease, the patient is maintained on omeprazole therapy. Total gastrectomy is reserved for rare patients who are unresponsive to medical therapy. Survival in patients with unresectable metastases has not been improved by chemotherapy or debulking surgery.

When treating patients with MEN 1–associated gastrinoma, surgery for parathyroid hyperplasia should precede gastrinoma surgery. Compared to sporadic gastrinoma, MEN 1–associated gastrinoma is more commonly multifocal, and surgical treatment has lower rates of cure.

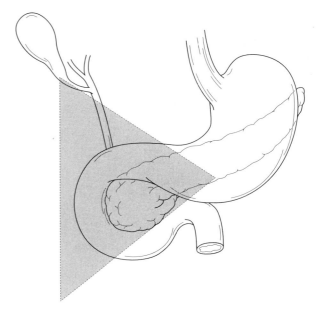

FIGURE 29-7. Most gastrinomas are found to the right of mesenteric vessels, in the head of the pancreas, or duodenum, an area known as "gastrinoma triangle." (From Stabile BE, Morrow DJ, Passaro E. *The gastrinoma triangle: operative implications. Am J Surg* 1984;147:26, with permission.)

VIPoma, a tumor secreting VIP, has several synonyms, including WDHA (watery diarrhea, hypokalemia, and achlorhydria) syndrome, pancreatic cholera, and Verner-Morrison syndrome. The predominant symptom is intermittent watery diarrhea. Other symptoms include weakness, lethargy, nausea, and cutaneous flushing. Hyperglycemia and hypercalcemia may be present. Multiple fasting VIP levels should be obtained, as secretion of VIP may be episodic. Abdominal CT with contrast is indicated to localize the primary tumor and rule out metastases. Chest CT is indicated if abdominal CT is negative for tumor, because 10% of patients with VIPomas have extrapancreatic tumors, usually in the retroperitoneum or chest. Most VIPomas are located in the tail of the pancreas and are treated with distal pancreatectomy. VIPomas may also be found in the adrenal glands, the liver, or the retroperitoneal lymph nodes, in which case palliative debulking is indicated. Before surgery for VIPoma, electrolyte and fluid abnormalities must be corrected aggressively. Preoperative octreotide is indicated to decrease diarrhea.

Glucagonoma is manifested by diabetes, stomatitis, necrolytic migratory erythema, anemia, and weight loss. Serum glucagon level is elevated, and hypoproteinemia may be present due to the catabolic effect of glucagon. CT with contrast usually localizes the tumor. Glucagonomas are typically large and solitary, located in the body or tail of the pancreas. Distal pancreatectomy is indicated for amenable lesions. Glucagonoma is usually metastatic, and debulking surgery should be performed if possible. For unresectable disease, octreotide has been used with some success. Chemotherapy is not particularly effective.

Somatostatinoma is extremely rare. Symptoms include steatorrhea, diabetes, hypochlorhydria, and cholelithiasis. Serum somatostatin levels are elevated. CT with contrast is indicated to localize the tumor. Somatostatinoma is typically a large tumor, most commonly located in the head of the pancreas or the periampullary region and frequently metastatic. Surgery should entail resection of the tumor and debulking of metastases. In all cases, cholecystectomy is indicated to prevent complications of cholelithiasis.

PERIAMPULARY TUMORS

Periampullary tumors are defined as neoplasms arising in close proximity to the ampulla of Vater. Although most of these neoplasms (85%) originate as adenocarcinoma of the pancreatic acinar cell, 10% represent ampullary carcinomas, 10% duodenal carcinomas, and 5% arise as carcinoma of the distal bile duct. Due to this anatomical location, the presentation of these tumors can be very similar and consists of jaundice, weight loss, and abdominal pain. Although similar in location and symptoms, the prognosis is based on the origin of the tumor and can be quite different. Resectable neoplasms arising from the duodenum, distal bile duct, and ampulla of Vater are associated with up to a 60% five-year survival. Only 5% to 25% of patients with resectable adenocarcinoma of pancreatic origin are alive 5 years later due to the high incidence of metastatic and micrometastatic disease upon presentation.

Pancreatic adenocarcinoma, a malignancy of the pancreatic acinar cells, is the most common periampullary tumor and the fourth most common cause of cancer death in the United States. Cigarette smoking is the only known risk factor, with a relative risk of 2 to 3 times that of non-smokers. The overall 1-year survival rate from the time of diagnosis is less than 10%, and the median survival time is 4 months. Early stage tumors have a markedly more favorable prognosis. However, pancreatic adenocarcinoma is frequently metastatic at the time of diagnosis because symptoms are vague or absent until jaundice occurs. The presentation has classically been described as "painless jaundice," although abdominal pain is often present. Jaundice occurs if the carcinoma arises from the pancreatic head and compresses the common bile duct. Pancreatic adenocarcinoma may arise from any part of the pancreas, but the pancreatic head is the most common location. A mutation of the p53 tumor suppressor gene has been implicated in the pathogenesis of pancreatic adenocarcinoma. The k-*ras* oncogene has also been implicated. Tumor metastasis is facilitated by the retroperitoneal location of the pancreas. The rich network of lymphatics in the retroperitoneum facilitates widespread metastasis of pancreatic adenocarcinoma. There is no definitive laboratory test for the diagnosis of pancreatic adenocarcinoma. Although the tumor marker CA 19-9 is elevated in many patients with pancreatic adenocarcinoma, sensitivity and specificity are low. It is more useful for follow-up after surgical therapy. Other tumor markers, including α-fetoprotein and carcinoembryonic antigen, suffer from the same lack of clinical usefulness.

CT is indicated to evaluate suspected pancreatic carcinoma. Contributory findings include pancreatic mass, dilated pancreatic duct or common bile duct, lymphadenopathy, and hepatic metastases. Surface ultrasound may provide similar information as CT with some advantage in cost and speed. Endoscopic ultrasound is emerging as a useful modality in evaluation and diagnosis of suspected pancreatic adenocarcinoma, particularly when located in the head of the pancreas. Endoscopic ultrasound can provide much more detailed anatomical information than surface ultrasound. Based on CT or ultrasound, criteria for resectability include the absence of distant metastasis and the absence of vascular invasion. Tumors larger than 3 cm have a poor prognosis. CT has 90% sensitivity in diagnosis of pancreatic adenocarcinoma and has a near 100% success in predicting unresectability.

A definitive tissue diagnosis may be obtained by brush biopsy as part of ERCP. However, if the lesion appears surgically resectable by imaging studies, the lack of a positive diagnosis should not preclude an attempted resection. Per-

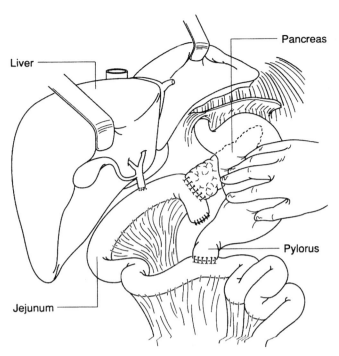

FIGURE 29-8. Pylorus-preserving pancreatoduodenectomy may decrease the incidence of postgastrectomy symptoms. (From Mullholand MW. Chronic Pancreatitis. In: Greenfield LJ, Mullholand MW, Oldham KT, et al., eds. *Surgery: scientific principles and practice*, 2nd ed. Philadelphia: Lippincott-Raven Publishers, 1997, with permission.)

cutaneous biopsy should be avoided except to secure a diagnosis in cases of unresectable carcinoma.

The pancreaticoduodenectomy (Whipple procedure) is the standard operation for adenocarcinoma of the head of the pancreas and other periampullary tumors. Advances in the technique and in postoperative care have resulted in a mortality rate of below 5%. Preoperative decompression of the biliary tree is probably not indicated, as it has not been shown to decrease postoperative morbidity. Coagulation abnormalities must be corrected. Pancreaticoduodenectomy involves resection of pancreatic head and duodenum with pancreaticoduodenectomy, choledochojejunostomy, and gastrojejunostomy. The operation has classically included resection of the pylorus and antrum with the duodenum, but currently the pylorus-preserving pancreatoduodenectomy is more commonly performed, having a lower incidence of both postgastrectomy symptoms and marginal ulceration (Fig. 29-8). However, the pylorus-preserving pancreaticoduodenectomy has a higher incidence of delayed gastric emptying, which is overall the most common complication of pancreaticoduodenectomy. The most morbid complication is an anastomotic leak of the pancreaticojejunostomy. Five-year survival after pancreaticoduodenectomy is between 19% and 24%. Favorable prognostic factors include tumor less than 3 cm in diameter, negative surgical margins, absence of tumor in lymph nodes, and diploid DNA in the specimen. Postoperative chemosensitized radiation therapy improves long-term outcomes.

Palliative bypass is indicated for metastatic or unresectable disease. Biliary bypass is indicated for treatment of jaundice and pruritus. Surgical options include cholecystojejunostomy or loop or Roux-en-Y choledochojejunostomy. If unresectability is established before surgery, transhepatic or endoscopic stent placement should be utilized instead of surgical bypass. Gastrojejunostomy with or without feeding jejunostomy or gastrostomy should also be considered at the time of surgery.

The role of laparoscopy in managing pancreatic adenocarcinoma is evolving. It is useful for confirming the absence of metastases before proceeding with major resection. If metastases are discovered, then an open procedure can be avoided. Surgery is currently the only potentially curative therapy for pancreatic adenocarcinoma, although adjuvant radiation therapy, combined with chemotherapy, may prolong survival.

30

THE BREAST

SUBHASIS CHATTERJEE AND LINDA S. CALLANS

EMBRYOLOGY

The breast develops in the thickened portion of the ectodermal tissue known as the "milk streak" coursing from the pubis to the axilla in early fetal life. By late in the first trimester, this becomes the nipple bud and the entire gland develops as a dermally derived organ. After birth, *in utero* exposure to maternal hormones may cause the infant breast to produce colostrum, or "witch's milk." Failure of proper regression of the milk streak leads to the most common congenital breast anomaly: accessory breast tissue that can be located anywhere from groin to axilla. An accessory nipple (*polythelia*) is encountered along the milk line in about 2% of patients and can be seen in either gender. Abnormal regression of the milk streak can lead to underdevelopment of the breasts (hypoplasia). Complete absence of the breast (*amastia*) is usually associated with hypoplasia of the ipsilateral pectoralis muscle and chest wall (*Poland syndrome*).

ANATOMY

The breast sits on the anterior chest wall, and in women, it extends from the sternocostal junction medially to the midaxillary line laterally. It spans from the second to the sixth rib in the midclavicular line. The breast extends into the axilla with the axillary tail of Spence. The areola has a variable location at the center of the breast mound and contains Montgomery tubercles on its surface, which lubricate the nipple during lactation. The fascia that envelops the breast abuts the fascia of the pectoralis major and serratus anterior muscles. The projections of this fascia course through the breast to the skin and create the supporting framework for the breast parenchyma. These fascial bands are known as the "suspensory ligament of Cooper" and are very well developed in the upper breast.

From a structural standpoint, the breast can be divided into lobular and ductal elements, each of which contains connective tissue, nerves, blood vessels, and lymphatic channels. The functional unit of the breast is the lobule.

Within each lobule, the alveoli are the terminal elongated tubular ductules. About 10 to 100 alveoli coalesce to form a larger duct that defines the lobular unit. Next, 20 to 40 lobular ducts join to form progressively larger ducts and ultimately form a large excretory duct. About 10 to 20 excretory ducts then dilate into a short excretory sinus just beneath the nipple (Fig. 30-1).

The arterial supply to the medial and central breast comes from perforating branches of the internal mammary artery. The lateral thoracic artery, branches of the thoracodorsal and subscapular arteries, and perforating branches of the intercostal arteries nourish the lateral breast.

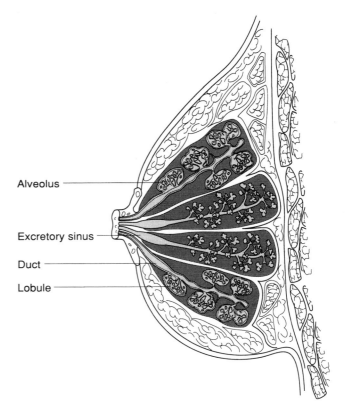

FIGURE 30-1. The basic lobular and ductal structure of the breast. (From August DA, Sondak VK. Breast. In: Greenfield LJ, Mulholland M, Oldham KT, et al., eds. *Surgery: scientific principles and practice*, 2nd ed. Philadelphia: Lippincott-Raven Publishers, 1997:1361, with permission.)

Hospital of the University of Pennsylvania, Philadelphia, Pennsylvania

The anatomy of the veins generally follows that of the arteries. There is also a connection with intercostal veins, which communicates with the venous vertebral system known as "Batson plexus." This route may be responsible for occasional rib or vertebral metastases without pulmonary involvement.

The lymphatic anatomy is important to understand because of the tendency of breast cancer to involve the regional lymph nodes. Most of the breast lymphatics drain to the axilla (as high as 97% by radiotracer studies) including those of the medial portion. Isolated lymph nodes can be found between the pectoralis major and minor (Rotter nodes), as well as within or alongside the lateral edge of the breast (intramammary nodes). The deep breast tissue drains to the submammary plexus of lymphatics lying superficial to the fascia overlying the pectoralis major. Consequently, removal of the fascia overlying the pectoralis major is required when performing a mastectomy.

The axillary nodes are found within an area bordered laterally by the latissimus dorsi, superiorly by the axillary vein, and medially by the chest wall. These nodes are divided into three levels based on their relation to the pectoralis minor muscle. Level I nodes are lateral to the pectoralis minor, level II are deep, and level III are medial to the pectoralis minor (Fig. 30-2).

The medial and lateral pectoral nerves originate from the medial and lateral cords of the brachial plexus. The medial pectoral nerve enters the deep surface of the pectoralis minor after supplying a branch to this muscle and then enters the pectoralis major and ends by supplying the lower costal fibers. If the pectoralis minor is removed during the operation, there is partial denervation of the pectoralis major. The lateral pectoral nerve penetrates the clavipectoral fascia (and hence is medial to the medial pectoral nerve) and enters the underside of the pectoralis major.

The thoracodorsal nerve is a motor nerve that supplies the latissimus dorsi and comes from the posterior cord of the brachial plexus. It runs down the posterior axillary wall behind the subscapular artery. Injury to this nerve results in slight weakness in abduction and internal rotation.

The long thoracic nerve of Bell is a motor nerve arising from the roots of the brachial plexus and innervates the serratus anterior and subscapularis. Transection of this nerve results in a winged scapula and is often accompanied by severe shoulder pain.

The intercostobrachial nerve is a sensory nerve, which arises from the second intercostal and supplies the skin of the axilla and the inner aspect of the arm. Transection of this nerve results in anesthesia of the denervated area, but paresthesias and hyperesthesias can occur with traumatic or intraoperative stretch injuries.

PHYSIOLOGY

Breast growth, development, and function are closely regulated by its hormonal milieu and the presence of growth factors. Mammary tissue is a target organ of trophic pituitary factors and circulating hormones including estrogens, progestins, prolactin, oxytocin, corticosteroids, thyroid hormone, and growth hormone. Cyclic changes associated with the menstrual cycle have a major influence on breast morphology and physiology. Breast engorgement and tenderness are at a minimum 5 to 7 days after menstruation. This is the point when the breast examination is most sensitive for detecting an abnormal mass and most comfortable for the patient. During this period, estrogen stimulates breast epithelial proliferation. As the luteal phase is entered, progesterone levels rise, resulting in mammary ductal dilation and differentiation of alveolar epithelial cells into secretory cells. Continued estrogen stimulation leads to increased blood flow and breast engorgement associated with the premenstrual phase. At the onset of menstruation, the rapid hormonal decline leads to breast involution. Since there is variability in proliferation and involution and the rates may be slightly different in different parts of the breast, all cycling women have some transient breast nodularity.

During pregnancy, there are marked changes in ductal, lobular, and alveolar growth under the influence of estrogen, progesterone, placental lactogen, prolactin, and chorionic gonadotropin. These changes prepare the breast for milk production at parturition.

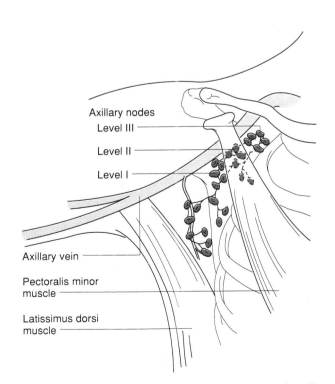

FIGURE 30-2. Axillary anatomy and distribution of axillary lymph nodes. (From August DA, Sondak VK. Breast. In: Greenfield LJ, Mulholland M, Oldham KT, et al., eds. *Surgery: scientific principles and practice*, 2nd ed. Philadelphia: Lippincott-Raven Publishers, 1997:1360, with permission.)

The abrupt withdrawal of placental lactogen and sex hormones upon delivery leaves the breasts predominantly under the influence of the pituitary-derived prolactin, resulting in the production of milk by alveolar cells. Initially, colostrum is secreted, and by day 4 or 5, milk is produced. Milk production and secretion is maintained during lactation by ongoing secretion of prolactin by the anterior pituitary. Oxytocin results from nipple/areolar stimulation causing the ductal myoepithelial breast cells to contract and eject milk.

Postlactational involution occurs about 3 months after weaning. This is characterized by regression of the extralobular stroma and glandular and ductal atrophy. In contrast, the mammary involution that occurs after menopause involves actual loss of glandular tissue. The postmenopausal breast consists primarily of fat, connective tissue, and mammary ducts.

BREAST EXAMINATION

The evaluation of the patient's breast is focused on detecting breast problems and identifying risk factors for the development of breast cancer. It also provides an opportunity to reassure anxious patients with normal examination results and offers a chance to formulate a diagnostic strategy if abnormal examination results are encountered.

The patient history should stress the nature of the presenting complaint and assess the cancer risk factors. It is important to elicit symptoms such as breast pain and tenderness, nipple discharge, or a self-palpated lump. The nature and duration of symptoms in relation to the menstrual cycle is revealing. In general, complaints that vary with the menstrual cycle are likely to be benign. A history of prior breast problems, age at menarche and/or menopause, last menstrual period, family history of breast cancer, hormone use (i.e., oral contraceptive use or hormone-replacement therapy), pregnancy history including age at birth of first child, and exposure to radiation should be sought.

The physical examination is easiest during the week after menses, when tenderness and engorgement are at a minimum. A proper breast and nodal examination is done sitting and supine and stresses inspection and palpation with comparison to the contralateral breast. It is also the time to discuss breast self-examination.

The proven breast imaging methods include mammography, ultrasonography, and ductography with an increasing role for breast magnetic resonance imaging (MRI). Technetium-99m sestamibi imaging is also used in some centers.

There are three modalities used to screen for breast cancer. These include monthly breast self-examination (BSE), annual clinical breast examination (CBE) by a health care professional, and mammography.

Screening mammography can detect a breast density, microcalcifications, or architectural distortion. There is evidence that in the 50- to 69-year-old age-group, screening mammography has led to approximately a 25% decrease in mortality from breast cancer evident after a 7- to 9-year follow-up. A review of screening mammography trials for women younger than 50 years showed a modest 18% reduction in breast cancer mortality after 12 years of follow-up. The 10-year survival rate for all cancers detected mammographically is 95%, suggesting the survival advantage with mammography is related to early detection.

Current screening mammography guidelines are listed in Table 30-1. However, 10% to 15% of all palpable masses are not detected on mammogram, underscoring the importance of combining physical examination with mammography for breast cancer screening. Moreover, 40% of all breast cancers are initially detected on BSE, emphasizing the important role of BSE in cancer detection.

In addition to screening, mammography is important in the evaluation of symptomatic breast disorders. It may help to establish a diagnosis in patients presenting with a dominant mass or other palpable abnormality. Moreover, bilateral mammography should be performed before biopsy in all women older than 30 years, to detect synchronous nonpalpable lesions. Although sensitive, the specificity is low and only 25% to 30% of lesions thought to be sufficiently suspicious to biopsy by mammography are carcinomas. Mammography is classified according to the The Breast-Imaging Reporting and Data System classification system according to six categories (Table 30-2).

Ultrasonography is most useful to distinguish between cystic and solid lesions. For solid lesions, factors such as shape, borders, echogenicity, and acoustic shadowing might suggest a benign versus malignant lesion. Ductography can be used in the evaluation of nipple discharge.

TABLE 30-1. SCREENING MAMMOGRAM GUIDELINES

Age 40	Screening mammogram
Age 41–50	Every other year (National Cancer Institute recommendation)
	Every year (American Cancer Society)
Age >51	Annual

TABLE 30-2. MAMMOGRAPHY INTERPRETATIONS AND THE BREAST IMAGING REPORTING AND DATA SYSTEM CLASSIFICATION WITH RECOMMENDATIONS

Category 0	Needs additional studies
Category 1	Negative; routine screening mammogram
Category 2	Benign finding; routine screening mammogram
Category 3	Probably a benign finding; repeated mammogram in 6 months
Category 4	Suspicious abnormality; biopsy
Category 5	Highly suggestive of malignancy; biopsy if palpable or needle localization biopsy if nonpalpable

EVALUATION OF SPECIFIC COMPLAINTS

The most common breast problems causing women to seek medical attention are nipple discharge, breast pain, and breast masses.

About 3% to 11% of patients with carcinoma have *nipple discharge*. Conversely, only about 10% of patients with bloody nipple discharge will have underlying carcinoma. The likelihood of nipple discharge being secondary to breast cancer increases with age. Most often, bloody nipple discharge in women under age 40 is benign, whereas one third of women older than 60 who present with nipple discharge have an underlying carcinoma. The first step in the evaluation of nipple discharge is to classify the discharge as physiologic or pathologic.

Physiologic discharge is usually nonspontaneous and bilateral, it can be expressed from multiple ducts. Its color is typically green, cream, or white. Galactorrhea, a bilateral milky discharge, may be secondary to a pituitary tumor (prolactinoma) or medications (oral contraceptives, phenothiazines, and some antihypertensives). The *most common benign causes of bloody discharge* are intraductal papilloma, mammary duct ectasia, and periductal fibrosis.

Pathologic nipple discharge is usually spontaneous and unilateral, and it arises reproducibly from a single duct. Watery and bloody discharge is more likely to be malignant than serous or serosanguineous discharge, although carcinoma can be found in patients presenting with any type of discharge. Discharge associated with a mass or mammographic abnormality or a new discharge in a postmenopausal woman is highly suspicious for carcinoma.

Spontaneous or inducible discharge that arises reproducibly from a single duct warrants further evaluation. The physical examination should identify the draining duct and trigger point, as well as any associated palpable mass. A nipple smear for cytology should be obtained. A galactogram may be useful to identify intraductal lesions and delineate ductal anatomy. The standard surgical technique for the diagnosis of a pathologic nipple discharge is a terminal duct excision with biopsy of the surrounding breast tissue focusing on the area of the trigger point.

Breast pain, or mastalgia, can occur in up to 70% of women. It is most commonly cyclic, occurring premenstrually. A careful history to establish its relationship to the menstrual cycle is necessary. Moreover, it is important to determine its chronicity and whether there are any associated skin changes or masses. The most common causes include fibrocystic changes, cysts, and infection. Breast pain is a rare presenting symptom for cancer. Women over the age of 35 should obtain a mammogram, and an ultrasound should be done for focal breast pain. The treatment consists of eliminating daily caffeine, minimizing dietary salt and fat intake, using nonsteroidal antiinflammatory drugs, primrose oil, vitamin B_6, and vitamin E. For severe cases, oral contraceptives, tamoxifen, danazol, and Elavil have been used.

A *palpable breast mass* often leads to a surgical evaluation. The initial step is to determine whether a true dominant mass is present or whether the area in question is part of the normal glandular nodularity of the breast. Dominant masses persist throughout the menstrual cycle and may be cystic or solid. Any dominant breast mass or asymmetric area within the breast should be evaluated and a definitive diagnosis reached. The important questions to answer concern the duration of the mass, any interval changes since first noticed, and its relation to the menstrual cycle.

The differential diagnosis of a solid mass includes a fibroadenoma, a broad range of lesions grouped under "fibrocystic changes," fat necrosis, or carcinoma. Suspicious masses tend to be hard or firm with indistinct irregular borders and may be attached to the skin or deep fascia. Benign masses tend to be more mobile with well-demarcated borders. Physical examination is 60% to 85% accurate for malignancy, but least accurate in young women.

Solid masses require further evaluation to establish a diagnosis. The appropriate workup should be tailored to the age and index of suspicion for the patient. For example, a solid mass in a woman in her 20s is more likely to be benign. A mammogram in this patient is unlikely to be revealing due to the dense glandularity of the breast, but an ultrasound will have high diagnostic utility.

Premenopausal women who present to the office with a palpable breast mass and no imaging studies should undergo fine needle aspiration (FNA) to determine whether the mass is a cyst. Although ultrasound also distinguishes solid from cystic lesions, the FNA is both diagnostic and therapeutic. Bloody cyst fluid should be sent for cytology. Surgical excision is indicated if the cyst fluid is bloody, the mass does not resolve completely with aspiration—suggesting a solid component—or it recurs multiple times in a short time. If an ultrasound was obtained, and its results reveal a simple cyst, then no further intervention is necessary unless it is painful, which is when cyst aspiration is appropriate to relieve symptoms. Routine cytology of cystic fluid is not indicated. A complex cyst should undergo ultrasound-guided cyst aspiration for cytology or excision.

Most dominant solid masses warrant definitive tissue diagnosis by either FNA, core needle biopsy (stereotactic core for a mammographically identified lesion), excision biopsy, or needle localization biopsy (for a nonpalpable mammographic abnormality). The relative advantages and disadvantages of the different biopsy techniques are noted in Table 30-3.

Although biopsy is the gold standard for palpable abnormalities, overall only 8% are positive for cancer. Combining the physical examination, mammogram, and FNA in the form of the "triple test" can help rationally guide the need for excision biopsy. Indications for excision biopsy include FNA results discordant with clinical or mammographic impression, cytologic atypia on needle biopsy, or the patient's wish to eliminate a source for concern. The triple test has a negative predictive value of almost 100% and a positive predictive value of about 75% and may prevent unnecessary surgery.

TABLE 30-3. COMPARISON OF VARIOUS BIOPSY TECHNIQUES

Technique	Advantages	Disadvantages
Fine needle aspiration	Rapid, painless, no incision, high diagnostic accuracy	Unable to distinguish *in situ* from invasive cancer, no histologic details, 5%–10% false negative, insufficient tissue in 25%–30%
Core biopsy	Same as above, tissue available for histology	Higher false-negative rate than fine needle aspiration
Stereotactic core needle biopsy	Limited incision, scarring, pain, no apparent disadvantage in specificity and sensitivity, minimally invasive for nonpalpable lesions	Questionable risk of seeding the needle tract with tumor cells
Excision biopsy	Complete histology before treatment decision	Expense, pain, incision
Needle localization for nonpalpable lesions	Avoids false negatives	Incision

BENIGN BREAST DISEASES

Simple *breast cysts* are fluid-filled epithelial-lined cavities. The lifetime incidence is 1:14, and ovarian hormones in a cyclic fashion influence their occurrence. They appear during the menstrual cycle, grow rapidly before menstruation, and spontaneously regress with completion of menses. There are no studies demonstrating an increased risk of cancer. In the absence of atypical pathologic findings, there is no increased risk of cancer. There are, however, factors that increase the suspicion for a cystic carcinoma including a bloody aspirate, an associated solid mass, an irregular cyst wall on ultrasound, or multiple recurrences after aspiration. Benign cysts are particularly common in the last decade of reproductive years. The treatment for simple breast cysts is reassurance. The indications for cyst aspiration are to confirm the diagnosis of a mass, relieve symptoms, and facilitate BSE by removing the lump. Complex cysts should be aspirated for cytology and recurrent cysts should be excised to rule out cystic carcinoma.

Fibroadenomas are benign tumors composed of both stromal and epithelial elements in the breast. They are the most common tumor in women under the age of 30 and the second most common tumor in all age-groups (after breast carcinoma). It may enlarge in pregnancy and usually involutes after menopause. Grossly, it is well encapsulated and mobile with smooth or slightly lobulated borders. It generally presents as a palpable painless mass and must be differentiated from cancer. The risk of cancer in a fibroadenoma, however, is exceedingly rare. Since the clinical diagnosis is incorrect in 25% to 30% of cases, it is important that any solid breast mass in a woman older than 30 be biopsied for a definitive diagnosis with an FNA, core needle biopsy, or excision biopsy. Observation is reasonable in a younger woman, as the lesion is likely to be a fibroadenoma.

The natural history of fibroadenomas is that 50% will resolve spontaneously, about 45% will remain stable without any change, and less than 5% will grow, at which time, they can be excised for pathologic confirmation. In 10% to 15% of cases, multiple adenomas are encountered. Although rare, cyclic changes with the menstrual cycle are possible. Because these occur in young women with very dense tissue mammographically, mammography has a limited role in the evaluation of a fibroadenoma. Ultrasound may be used to determine whether it is solid or cystic. The management is excision or core biopsy for diagnosis, followed by observation. Occasionally, a diagnosis may be made by FNA. If the lesion grows or is larger than 2 cm, excision is preferred.

A fibroadenoma is considered a *giant fibroadenoma* when its size exceeds 5 cm. This is most common in adolescents and young adults. Its rapid growth may lead to venous engorgement and the clinical appearance of an inflammatory carcinoma. The treatment is complete mass excision without mastectomy.

Mammary duct ectasia is an inflammatory condition causing distortion and dilation of the lactiferous sinus under the nipple. It frequently is responsible for nipple inversion in older women and can be associated with nipple discharge.

Mastitis is a generalized cellulitis of the breast, which can complicate lactation. The most common etiologic organism is *Staphylococcus*, with *Streptococcus* a close second. The treatment consists of heat/ice packs to the breast and oral antibiotics (first-generation cephalosporin or penicillin), and a breast pump if lactating. If complicated by an abscess, or the patient is diabetic or systemically ill, incision and drainage with intravenous antibiotics is required.

Mondor disease is a variant of thrombophlebitis involving the superficial veins of the anterior chest wall and breast. The patient presents with acute pain in the lateral half of the breast and anterior chest wall, as well as an associated tender cordlike structure corresponding to the thrombosed vein. The cause is usually unknown, but Mondor disease has been associated with repetitive exercise or with surgery. It is a benign self-limited disorder, not indicative of a neoplasm. If the clinical diagnosis is in doubt an excision biopsy can be performed. Treatment consists of warm compresses and antiinflammatory agents. If the condition is refractory to this treatment, then a complete excision of the involved vein can be performed.

Solitary intraductal papillomas are true polyps of epithelial-lined breast ducts. They are the most common cause of a bloody nipple discharge. Because they are usually 3 to 4 mm large, they are rarely palpable. Nipple smears may show papilloma cells. In most cases, the papillomas are located in the major duct under the areola and may be demonstrated by ductography. The treatment is excision of the draining duct via a circumareolar incision.

PHYLLODES TUMOR

Phyllodes tumor represents a spectrum of lesions ranging from benign to malignant and occurs as less than 1% of all breast cancers. It is the most common neoplasm of nonepithelial origin in the breast and is composed of epithelial and stromal elements. Cystosarcoma phylloides, the malignant tumor, usually presents as a large (more than 5 cm) painless breast mass, resembling a fibroadenoma in 30- to 40-year-old women. It is rarely associated with skin fixation, edema, or axillary adenopathy. Twenty-five percent to fifty percent are histologically malignant (high mitotic rate, stromal cellularity and overgrowth, and cellular atypia) while 6% to 22% have metastasized to distant sites by presentation. Axillary lymph node metastases generally do not occur. Regardless of their malignant potential, phyllodes tumors tend to have high local recurrence rates. Treatment involves wide excision of small benign-appearing lesions with a 2- to 3-cm margin of normal tissue or total mastectomy without axillary lymph node dissection for large or malignant lesions or recurrence.

BREAST CANCER

The annual incidence of breast cancer in the United States is estimated for the year 2000 to be 184,200 new cases, making it the number one cancer for women in America (Fig. 30-3). Approximately 1 in 8 women will be diagnosed

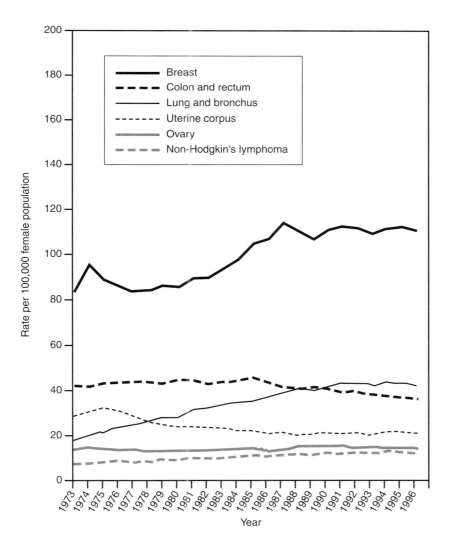

FIGURE 30-3. Age-adjusted cancer-related incidence rates in women in the United States by site: 1973 to 1996. (From Greenlee RT, Murray T, Bolden S, et al. *Cancer statistics, 2000. CA: a cancer journal for clinicians.* Vol 50. No 1. American Cancer Society/Lippincott Williams & Wilkins, Philadelphia, 2000:18, with permission.)

with breast cancer during their lives. Moreover, approximately 1,400 men are afflicted each year. About 41,200 women will die of breast cancer in 2000, making it the second leading cause of cancer death behind lung cancer in women and the leading cause of death in women aged 40 to 49. Although there was a slight increase in the absolute incidence of breast cancer during the twentieth century, there has been a decrease in the overall case-fatality rate.

The identification of patients at increased risk of developing breast cancer is essential for early detection. It also provides an opportunity to plan preventive and diagnostic strategies as well as to enhance the understanding of the disease. Risk factors can be classified as major and minor. Major risk factors include gender, since women make up 99% of breast cancer patients. Breast cancer risk increases with age, although the rate of increase slows after menopause. The annual risk for a 30-year-old woman to develop breast cancer is 1 in 6,000 women, compared to 1 in 300 women for an 80-year-old woman.

A *positive family history* of breast cancer is also a major risk factor with a twofold to threefold increase in risk if breast cancer is present in two first-degree relatives (mother, sister, or daughter). The patient's risk increases if the relative's cancer was bilateral or premenopausal. If there is a strong family history (i.e., at least two first-generation relatives with premenopausal breast cancer), the lifetime risk approaches 50%. Overall, however, only 10% to 15% of breast cancer is attributable to familial breast cancer, with about three fourths of this attributable to dominantly inherited susceptible genes.

Women with prior breast cancer are two to three times more likely to develop a second breast cancer than age-matched controls. Those who develop a primary breast cancer before the age of 45 are five to six times more likely to develop a second breast cancer. The annual risk of a second breast cancer can be 1% per year.

Nonproliferative breast diseases such as adenosis, fibroadenomas, apocrine changes, duct ectasia, and ductal hyperplasia without atypia carry no associated increased risk. There is a mildly increased risk with sclerosing adenosis (one and a half to two times). A moderately increased risk is conferred by atypical ductal or lobular hyperplasia (four to five times increased risk), and atypical hyperplasia with a positive family history increases the risk 11-fold. Figure 30-4 illustrates the long-term risk of breast cancer with various benign breast biopsy results.

The high-risk category also includes lobular carcinoma *in situ* (LCIS). Unlike ductal carcinoma *in situ* (DCIS), LCIS is not a true cancer but represents a marker of increased risk and arises from the lobular and terminal ducts of the breast. About 75% of cases occur in premenopausal women (significantly younger than in invasive carcinoma) and the incidence decreases after menopause. Usually LCIS is detected as an incidental finding at the time of biopsy for another lesion and is seen in about 10% of

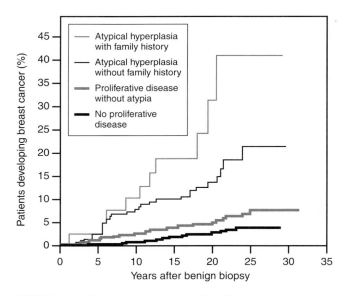

FIGURE 30-4. Risk of breast cancer with different benign breast biopsy results. (From August DA, Sondak VK. Breast. In: Greenfield LJ, Mulholland M, Oldham KT, et al., eds. *Surgery: scientific principles and practice*, 2nd ed. Philadelphia: Lippincott-Raven Publishers, 1997:1380, with permission.)

mammographically generated biopsies. About 70% are multicentric and 30% are multifocal.

Patients with LCIS carry an eightfold to tenfold increased risk of invasive carcinoma during their lifetime and a 1% per-year annual risk. The lifetime risk approaches 20% to 30% but increases to 50% if there is a previous family history of bilateral or premenopausal breast cancer. Furthermore, the risk of cancer is conferred to both breasts, not just the side involved with LCIS. Most cancers that develop are invasive ductal carcinomas, but there is a higher incidence of lobular carcinoma than in the general population.

Minor, or some controversial, *risk factors* for breast cancer include the pattern of endogenous and exogenous hormonal exposure. Greater exposure to uninterrupted hormonal (menstrual) cycles conveys a slight increase in the lifetime risk of breast cancer. Women with early menarche (before age 12) have a relative risk (RR) of one and a half and those with late menopause (after 55) have a relative risk of two for developing breast cancer. Similarly, there is an increased risk in nulliparous women or those whose first live-birth is after the age of 30.

Postmenopausal hormone-replacement therapy (HRT) has shown equivocal results, with some studies suggesting an increased risk with prolonged HRT. Women who undergo oophorectomy after the age of 35 and do not use hormone replacement reduce their risk by two thirds. The addition of HRT eliminates the beneficial effect of oophorectomy. A large 1991 metaanalysis of HRT showed the only increased risk of breast cancer was in those women with a positive family history and more than 15 years of HRT. Recent studies of estrogen combinations with progesterone show a lower risk of breast cancer. It is important to balance the beneficial effects of HRT on the cardiovascular system, bone density, and lipid profile against the patient's overall breast cancer risk. Most experts, however, would insist on stopping HRT once breast cancer has been diagnosed.

Prior *chest and neck radiation* is associated with a slightly increased risk of developing breast cancer with a 10- to 30-year latency period. Obesity has been associated with an increased incidence of postmenopausal breast cancer (by two times) and endometrial cancer. This is postulated to be related to increased peripheral conversion of androstenedione to estrogen by adipocytes. There is a small environmental association with alcohol use; on the other hand, rigorous exercise resulting in ovarian cycle disruption reduces the risk of breast cancer. Unlike other common cancers, breast cancer incidence is higher among women of upper, rather than lower, socioeconomic class. In the United States, rates are lowest among women of Asian ancestry and highest among white women, except below age 40, when the rate in African American women is the highest.

Inherited Breast Cancer Syndromes

A genetic cause of breast cancer is suggested if multiple relatives have breast cancer (more than three), particularly if the disease develops at a young age or in conjunction with other cancers such as an ovarian malignancy. It is important to identify individuals with such family backgrounds to assess the risk to the patient and proceed with patient and family counseling. Overall, inherited genetic factors contribute to about 10% of breast cancers but may be responsible for as many as 25% of those occurring in patients younger than 30 years.

Several known clinical syndromes exist. *Li-Fraumeni syndrome* is an autosomal-dominant disease with an underlying mutation of the p53 tumor suppressor gene and is associated with an increased incidence of breast cancer and various sarcomas. Recently, a mutation on the short arm of chromosome 2 (2p mutation) associated with faulty DNA repair has been identified that is responsible for a syndrome with both an increase in breast and colon cancers.

The BRCA-1 and BRCA-2 gene mutations account for about three fourths of all familial breast cancers, with BRCA-1 responsible for about 80% of these. The BRCA-1 gene is located on the long arm of chromosome 17. It is a tumor suppressor gene encoding a secreted protein in the granin family. Mutations in this gene are inherited in an autosomal-dominant fashion with high penetrance. About 1 in 300 women carry this gene, which is implicated in about only 4% of all breast cancers but in close to 25% of those diagnosed in patients younger than age 40. Patients with this mutation have an 85% lifetime risk of developing breast cancer, a 65% risk of developing a second breast cancer, and a 25% to 30% risk of developing ovarian cancer.

About 60% of patients will develop breast cancer by age 50. There is also an increased risk of male breast and prostate cancer.

BRCA-2 is located on the long arm of chromosome 13. The lifetime risk of developing breast cancer from this autosomal-dominant mutation approaches 70%, and there is a lower but still increased risk of ovarian cancer with BRCA-2 than with BRCA-1. Finally, most forms of familial male breast cancer are associated with BRCA-2.

Breast Cancer Prevention

In 1993 National Surgery Adjuvant Breast and Bowel Project (NSABP) P-1 prevention trial demonstrated an overall 49% reduction in the risk of invasive breast carcinoma in high-risk women who took tamoxifen for 5 years. Candidates for the trial included women with a significant family history of breast cancer, LCIS, atypical ductal hyperplasia, or multiple prior breast biopsies. Patients with LCIS had a 50% risk reduction while those with atypical ductal hyperplasia had an 80% risk reduction. Women identified as high risk for breast cancer should be counseled regarding their risk and potential risk-reduction strategies including tamoxifen.

Prophylactic mastectomy with immediate reconstruction can also be considered in women at high risk for developing breast cancer. This is particularly relevant in women testing positive for BRCA-1 or BRCA-2 with a 70% to 80% lifetime risk of breast cancer. Some patients with LCIS may consider prophylactic bilateral mastectomy because both breasts are equally at risk even with unilateral LCIS, particularly if there is an associated family history. Nevertheless, most recommend that these patients be observed with close follow-up consisting of annual mammograms, biannual CBE, and monthly BSE.

Pathology of Breast Cancer

Malignancies of the breast are broadly divided into epithelial tumors originating from cells lining ducts and lobules and nonepithelial malignancies arising from the surrounding stroma. A second distinction must be made between invasive and noninvasive cancers, which are confined within the basement membrane of the ducts or lobules. Histologically, it is important to analyze tumor type, size, hormone receptor status, and excisional margins, as well as the status of various prognostic indicators such as nuclear grade, angiolymphatic invasion, S phase, and ploidy.

Noninvasive (In Situ) Breast Carcinomas

DCIS, or intraductal carcinoma, is thought to arise from the duct epithelium in the region of the terminal lobular-ductal unit. Malignant ductal epithelial cells proliferate within and are confined to the mammary ducts and lobules

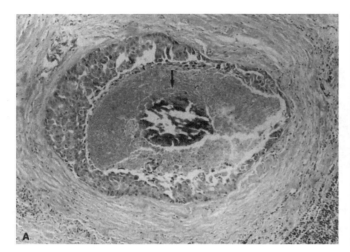 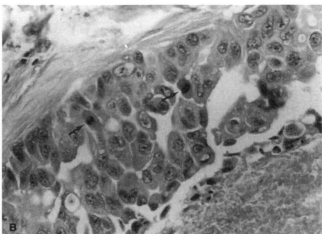

FIGURE 30-5. A: Comedo-type ductal carcinoma in situ with prominent central necrosis and dense calcification. **B:** Considerable nuclear atypia and pleomorphism is consistent with poorly differentiated ductal carcinoma in situ. (From Harris JR, Lippman ME, Morrow M, et al., eds. *Diseases of the breast*. Philadelphia: Lippincott Williams & Wilkins, 1996:356, with permission.)

without basement membrane invasion. It likely represents a phase in the continuum between atypical ductal hyperplasia and invasive ductal carcinoma. The common finding of an invasive carcinoma with DCIS suggests a progression from noninvasive to invasive disease. The histopathologic classification involves three types including (i) papillary (well differentiated, pleomorphic, best prognosis), (ii) cribriform (intermediate), and (iii) comedo (high grade with necrosis, architectural distortion, and worst prognosis). Figure 30-5 illustrates the histopathology of DCIS.

Prior to the advent of mammography, DCIS accounted for only 1% to 3% of all breast cancers. Today, DCIS makes up 15% of all breast cancers and 30% of all those discovered by mammography. DCIS usually presents as an abnormal mammogram with clustered, pleomorphic microcalcifications, and rarely as a palpable nodule. The incidence of DCIS has increased fivefold since the early 1970s, mostly due to widespread mammography testing and early detection. Nodal metastases are rare (1%) and are likely associated with unrecognized microinvasion. Multifocality is common, defined as separate foci of DCIS more than 5 mm from the original site but within the same quadrant. Multicentricity, separate foci of DCIS in another quadrant, occurs in 30% to 40% of patients. After complete excision of DCIS, 15% of patients will develop a recurrence with half being DCIS and half being invasive ductal carcinoma. Most recurrences are in the same quadrant as the original DCIS. Table 30-4 compares LCIS with DCIS.

Invasive Carcinomas

Invasive carcinomas are adenocarcinomas arising from the terminal duct. The most common breast malignancy (75%) is invasive or infiltrating ductal carcinoma. It presents either as a palpable mass or as a mammographic abnormality. On gross pathologic examination, it is a gray-white mass with irregular spiculated edges. Microscopically, it is an invasive adenocarcinoma of the ductal elements (Fig. 30-6), often associated with DCIS in the same specimen. Other less common variants include medullary carcinoma (6%),

TABLE 30-4. COMPARISON OF DUCTAL CARCINOMA IN SITU VERSUS LOBULAR CARCINOMA IN SITU

	Ductal carcinoma in situ	Lobular carcinoma in situ
Age distribution	<50% premenopausal (same as invasive ductal cancer)	75% premenopausal
Palpable mass	Rare	Never
Radiographic findings	Microcalcification	Usually none
Node involvement	≤1%[a]	None
Subsequent type of cancer	Invasive ductal cancer	Invasive ductal or lobular cancer
Location of subsequent cancer	Same breast, same quadrant	Either breast any quadrant

[a]Some early studies report up to 5% with palpable ductal carcinoma *in situ*.

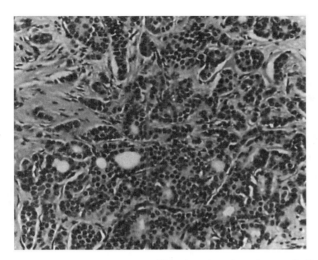
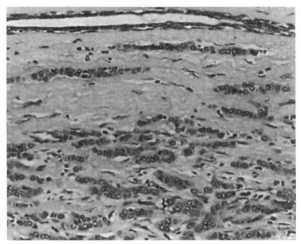

FIGURE 30-6. Infiltrating ductal carcinoma (*left*) and infiltrating lobular carcinoma (*right*). (From Harris JR, Lippman ME, Morrow M, et al., eds. *Diseases of the breast.* Philadelphia: Lippincott Williams & Wilkins, 1996:396, with permission.)

which typically grows into large (5 to 10 cm) well-circumscribed lesions with a marked lymphocytic infiltrate and anaplastic cells. Tubular carcinoma (2%) is characterized by a small (less then 1-cm) well-differentiated tumor with excellent prognosis. Because the incidence of nodal disease is low, a lymph node dissection is not indicated. Mucinous (colloid) carcinoma (1% to 2%) feels soft and gelatinous with extracellular mucin, and secretory (juvenile) carcinoma occurs in adolescents and can be mistaken for benign fibroadenoma. All of these variants carry a better prognosis than invasive ductal carcinoma.

Invasive lobular carcinoma makes up about 10% of all breast cancers. It is characterized by indistinct margins with extensive infiltration and the absence of microcalcifications, which make it much harder to detect mammographically. There is a significant incidence of multicentric disease and bilaterality, as well as an increased incidence in patients with a prior history of LCIS. On gross examination, lobular cancer appears as a tan rubberlike mass. Microscopically, it consists of tumor cells infiltrating single file, often growing concentrically around the ducts (Fig. 30-6).

Other histologic types accounting for the remaining 2% of breast cancers include metaplastic carcinoma, pure squamous carcinoma, apocrine carcinoma, adenoid cystic carcinoma, lymphomas, and sarcomas.

Breast Cancer Biology and Natural History

The biology of breast cancer reveals a strong suggestion of a carcinoma sequence. Normal breast tissue can develop mild hyperplasia and then hyperplasia with atypia, carcinoma *in situ,* and ultimately invasive carcinoma. This sequence is suggested by histology revealing severe atypical ductal hyperplasia adjacent to DCIS and also by demographic data. For example, the average age for LCIS is 45 while that for invasive lobular carcinoma it is 55.

Estrogen plays a crucial role in breast cancer with estrogen receptors (ER) mediating the estrogen-induced effects of breast tissue. ER expression is low in normal tissues but

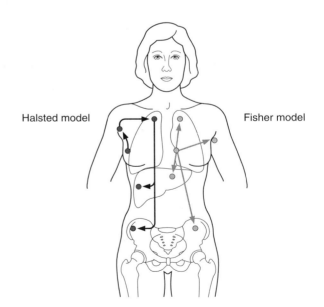

FIGURE 30-7. Halsted's local/reginal model of breast cancer spread compared to Fisher's systemic model of spread. (From August DA, Sondak VK. Breast. In: Greenfield LJ, Mulholland M, Oldham KT, et al., eds. *Surgery: scientific principles and practice,* 2nd ed. Philadelphia: Lippincott-Raven Publishers, 1997:1386, with permission.)

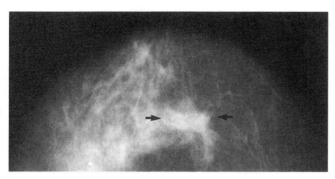

FIGURE 30-8. Typical mammographic appearance of a spiculated cancer. (From Harris JR, Lippman ME, Morrow M, et al., eds. *Diseases of the breast.* Philadelphia: Lippincott Williams & Wilkins, 1996:72, with permission.)

overexpressed in many cancers. Moreover, estrogen has been shown to stimulate global transcription in cells *in vitro*. Other proteins such as growth factors have been shown to stimulate breast cells, with as many as 70% of breast cancers demonstrating overexpression of TGF-α. The c-myc protooncogene has been shown to be amplified in many primary tumors and the HER-2/neu protooncogene is overexpressed in 40% of breast cancers. Finally, numerous genetic mutations have been identified in breast cancer.

Historically, there have been two opposing views concerning the natural history of breast cancer (Fig. 30-7). Halsted argued that breast cancer dissemination was orderly and predictable. He hypothesized that the local tumor spread first to lymph nodes and only then spread systemically with distant metastases. As a result of this theory, extensive local control was greatly emphasized. Recently, Fisher and others have proposed the systemic paradigm, emphasizing that dissemination was not orderly and not predictable. This theory proposes that local tumor simultaneously spreads by both lymphatic and hematogenous routes. It argues that breast cancer is a systemic disease at its inception and surgery has little impact on the systemic disease. Moreover, the systemic spread is simultaneous with the lymphatic metastasis because it has been found that overall 30% of node-negative patients will ultimately die of metastatic disease.

Clinical Presentation

In 60% to 85% of patients, breast cancer presents as a painless mass found during breast examination. Typically, the mass is an irregular, firm, and painless nodule. Occasionally, there may be protrusion, asymmetry of breast contour, skin dimpling, or nipple inversion. On mammography, the characteristic findings include stellate lesions, indistinct irregular densities, clusters of five or more microcalcifications, and architectural distortion (Fig. 30-8). Finally, bloody nipple discharge (7%) or breast pain are rare presenting symptoms for breast cancer.

Workup

Bilateral mammograms are essential even in patients with unilateral palpable lesions to assess for multicentric disease or extensive microcalcifications in the ipsilateral breast. Also, contralateral cancers may be present in as many as 10% of patients. The standard metastatic evaluation includes a chest x-ray, liver function tests, and a bone scan with subsequent studies pending those results. A bone scan is not necessary for clinical stage I disease unless symptoms of bone pain exist. If neurological symptoms or signs exist then a brain MRI is indicated.

Staging

Breast cancer staging provides for meaningful prognostic and therapeutic discussions. Tumor-Node-Metastasis (TNM) staging allows the grouping of breast tumors into clearly identifiable prognostic categories (Tables 30-5 and 30-6). For all patients who initially present with breast cancer, 40% to 50% will present with lymph node involvement and 10% to 15% with distant metastatic dis-

TABLE 30-5. TNM CLASSIFICATION OF BREAST CANCER (AMERICAN JOINT COMMITTEE ON CANCER)

TNM	Tumor Size	Nodal Status	Metastasis
	In situ	N0	N0
1	<2 cm	Movable axillary nodes (includes Rotter or interpectoral nodes)	Yes (includes supraclavicular nodes)
2	2–5 cm	Fixed axillary nodes	—
3	>5 cm	Internal mammary nodes	—
4	Any size plus involvement of skin (edema/*peau d'orange*, satellite skin nodules, ulcers) or chest wall; inflammatory cancer	—	—

TABLE 30-6. STAGING AND PROGNOSIS OF BREAST CANCER

Stage	TNM	5-year survival
0	Tis N0 M0	
I	T1 N0 M0	90%
IIA	T0-1 N1 M0	75%
	T2 N0 M0	
IIB	T2 N1 M0	65%
	T3 N0 M0	
IIIA	T0-1-2 N2 M0	40%–50%
	T3 N1-2 M0	
IIIB	T4 Any N M0	
	Any T N3 M0	
IV	Any T Any N M1	15%

TABLE 30-7. FIVE-YEAR RATES OF RECURRENCE AND SURVIVAL RELATED TO THE NUMBER OF PATHOLOGICALLY POSITIVE AXILLARY NODES[a]

Positive axillary nodes	Patients	Survival rate (%)	Recurrence rate (%)
0	12,299	72	19
1	2,012	63	33
2	1,338	62	40
3	842	59	43
4	615	52	44
5	478	47	54
6–10	1,261	41	63
11–15	562	29	72
16–20	301	29	75
≥21	225	22	82

[a]Nemoto T, Vana J, Bedwani R, et al. Management and survival of female breast cancer: results of a national survey by the American College of Surgeons. *Cancer* 1980;45:2917, with permission.

ease. The presence or absence of ipsilateral axillary node metastases predicts outcome after surgical treatment more precisely than any other prognostic factor. In addition, it is important to look for signs of locally advanced breast cancer (LABC). This includes evidence of T4 disease such as skin edema or peau d'orange due to invasion of the dermal lymphatics, skin ulceration, chest wall fixation, or N2 disease such as large (more than 2.5 cm), matted, or fixed axillary nodes. An even poorer prognosis is seen when breast edema involves more than one third of the breast or is associated with the presence of satellite tumor nodules, arm edema, or changes of inflammatory breast cancer (warm, red, or edematous).

Pathologic staging includes analysis of estrogen and progesterone receptor status, S-phase analysis reflecting cell proliferation activity, DNA index (a measure of ploidy), amplification of the HER/neu oncogene, and expression of cathepsin D made by the breast cancer cells.

Prognostic Factors

The status of the axillary lymph nodes is the most important prognostic factor. Table 30-7 reveals the direct relationship between the number of nodal metastases, recurrence, and survival. Tumor size correlates well with axillary lymph node involvement but also has independent prognostic significance for survival (Fig. 30-9). The median time to the development of metastases for a lesion less than 2.5 cm is 42 months, whereas a lesion greater than 8 cm develops metastatic disease in 4 months. Tumor location is a minor factor. Corrected for tumor size, lesions on the medial half of the breast do slightly worse than those on the lateral side due to a tendency to metastasize to the internal mammary nodes. Finally, the presence of vascular or lymphatic invasion worsens prognosis while the status of the estrogen and progesterone receptors predicts the response to subsequent hormonal therapy.

Flow cytometry has been used to identify aneuploid populations in the tumor. Tumors with a high DNA index have a significant aneuploid cell population and are more poorly differentiated with a worse prognosis. Also, the percentage of cells in the synthesis or S phase known as the S-phase fraction can be calculated. Cancers with high S phase have been associated with a worse prognosis.

Treatment

Surgery for Resectable Tumors

In women with breast cancer that is potentially curable (without evidence of distant metastasis), surgery is the treatment of choice. Goals of surgical treatment include providing optimal local control, staging the disease to identify patients at higher risk for recurrence, and providing the best chance for overall survival. The history of surgical treatment of breast cancer goes back 2,000 years. However, it was the radical mastectomy first reported by Halsted and Meyer in 1894 that demonstrated a landmark reduction in the rate of local recurrence from 50% to 6%. It was established as the definitive procedure for the next 75 years. The Halsted radical mastectomy involved primary resection of the breast and pectoralis major and minor muscles and an en bloc axillary lymph node dissection. The Meyer variation completed the axillary dissection first and then the breast and pectoral muscle followed. Both surgeons advocated complete axillary dissection of all nodal levels (level I, II, and III) from the latissimus dorsi laterally to the thoracic outlet medially. The long thoracic nerve and the thoracodorsal neurovascular bundle were routinely resected. Much of the initial criticism involved shoulder motion limitation (winged scapula) and lymphedema of the arm. Currently, efforts are made to spare the long thoracic and thoracodorsal

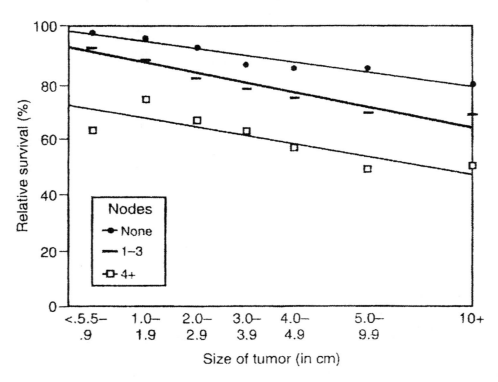

FIGURE 30-9. Five-year relative survival rates related to tumor size and positive nodes. (From Bland KI, Copeland EM. *The breast: comprehensive management of benign and malignant disease*, 2nd ed. Vol 1. Philadelphia: WB Saunders, 1998:421, with permission.)

nerves. Urban further developed the extended radical mastectomy, which added en bloc removal of the internal mammary nodes.

Patey in 1932 developed the modified radical mastectomy (MRM), sparing the pectoralis major and dividing the pectoralis minor to provide access to the medial lymph node chain. The operation also included a level I to III axillary lymph node dissection (ALND). Madden and Auchincloss further modified the MRM in 1936 to spare even the pectoralis minor and include only a level I and II ALND. This method of the MRM is currently the most common operation performed for breast resection; however, some surgeons still prefer to divide the pectoralis minor muscle and expose the axillary space permitting removal of level III lymph nodes. Avoiding the division of the pectoralis minor and limiting dissection to the level I and II lymph nodes decreases the risk of injury to the medial or lateral pectoral nerves and reduces post–axillary dissection lymphedema (Fig. 30-10).

A landmark trial that significantly changed the clinical practice of breast surgery include the NSABP protocols B-04. Results from NSABP B-04 trial replaced the radical mastectomy with the modified radical mastectomy as the standard of care. This trial occurred from 1971 to 1974 with 1765 patients randomized to radical mastectomy versus total mastectomy versus total mastectomy with radiation therapy. No differences were found in the overall disease-free survival in all three groups. This trial proved the equivalence of the modified mastectomy with the radical mastectomy in terms of survival with the lesser complications and disfigurement.

Breast Conservation

Breast conservation treatment (BCT) consists of a lumpectomy and an axillary lymph node dissection, followed by radiation therapy (4 to 5,000 cGy) for 6 weeks to the whole breast with a boost to the tumor bed. The NSABP protocol B-06 accrued 1,843 patients over 8 years who were randomized to total mastectomy versus lumpectomy versus lumpectomy with radiation therapy. No survival advantage was detected in either group. The incidence of local recurrence in the BCT group was higher (4% to 20% compared to 2% to 9%), but the 5-year survival rate was 70% to 80% in both groups. Six additional prospective randomized trials, some with follow-up of 15 years, have demonstrated no survival advantage to BCT versus MRM. Given an informed choice, 81% of women will choose breast conservation.

Less than 1% of women with stage I and 30% of those with stage II cancer will have a contraindication to BCT (Table 30-8). A critical aspect of local control in BCT is the radiation therapy to the breast mound after lumpectomy. When radiation therapy is added to local excision, the recurrence rate drops from 40% to less than 10%.

The final aspect of local treatment is the ALND. The Halsted concept of axillary nodes considers them a "filter," or a gateway, to distant metastasis. By the 1970s, however, it was realized that the ALND had limited impact on survival. The

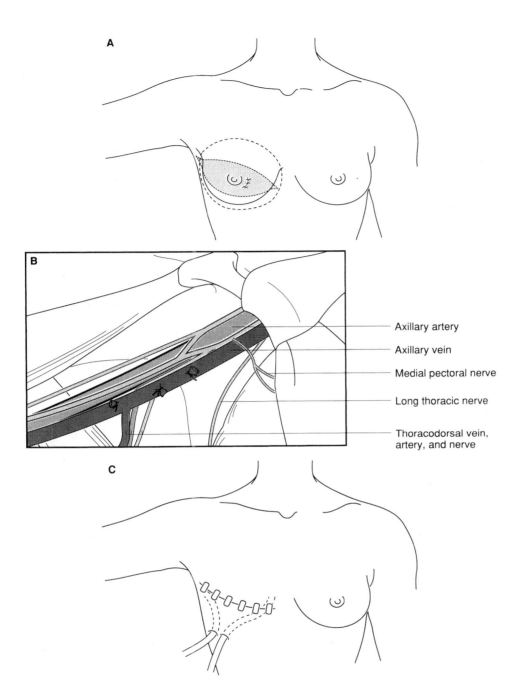

FIGURE 30-10. Technique of modified radical mastectomy. (From August DA, Sondak VK. Breast. In: Greenfield LJ, Mulholland M, Oldham KT, et al., eds. *Surgery: scientific principles and practice*, 2nd ed. Philadelphia: Lippincott-Raven Publishers, 1997:1393, with permission.)

principal rationale for the axillary dissection is the detection of lymph node metastases for use as a prognostic indicator of systemic disease. Tumor in the axillary lymph nodes might indicate concurrent systemic spread and systemic therapy is recommended. In the setting of large, palpable lymph nodes, ALND is indicated for local control. However, the clinical examination is notoriously unreliable for assessing axillary adenopathy with a sensitivity of about 29% (false negative in 27%) and a specificity of 94% (false positive in 6%).

Most surgeons recommend a level I and level II ALND. Although "skip metastases" can occur when level III nodes are involved without level I or II disease, this occurs in less than 2% of cases and the morbidity of a level III dissection rarely justifies its use. However, if level II nodes are grossly involved at the time of axillary exploration, then a level III dissection is advised for optimal local control. It is necessary to remove at least ten nodes to improve the detection of metastatic disease. The presence and number of positive

TABLE 30-8. CONTRAINDICATIONS TO BREAST CONSERVATION THERAPY

Absolute	Relative
First/second trimester pregnancy	Large tumor:breast ratio
Multicentric disease	Anticipated poor cosmetic result
Tumor sign >5 cm	Large breast size
Diffuse microcalcifications	Central tumor under the nipple requiring nipple excision
History of prior x-ray therapy	—
History of collagen vascular disease	—

axillary nodes is the single most reliable prognostic indicator for distant metastasis and survival. In early T1 and T2 tumors, if the nodes are positive, the recurrence rate approaches 25% to 30%; if the axillary lymph nodes are negative, the recurrence rate is 5% to 10%.

The technique of sentinel lymph node (SLN) mapping and biopsy has recently been applied to breast cancer. Using SLN biopsy, it may be possible to identify node-positive patients by removal of one or a few sentinel node(s) and limit the morbidity of a full ALND to selected patients. This technique assumes that the lymphatics draining the region of tumor drain first into one or a few sentinel lymph nodes. The sentinel nodes are identified by injection of a marker such as a vital blue dye or a radionuclide into the breast at the site of the tumor, which then tracks through the lymph channels to the first or sentinel nodes. The sentinel nodes are identified by either visual inspection or with a handheld gamma probe. By excising these nodes, an accurate assessment of nodal metastasis can be made.

The positive predictive value of a successful SLN biopsy approaches 100%, whereas its negative predictive value exceeds 95%. If the SLN biopsy results are negative, then an ALND and its 10% to 15% risk of lymphedema, neuropathies, and seromas are avoided. If the SLN biopsy results are positive, then a completion ALND for local control and to complete the axillary staging can be performed at another operation. Because of the 5% to 10% false-negative rate and the lack of long-term follow-up at this point, SLN biopsy is still considered experimental in the setting of breast cancer and should be carried out within clinical trials with close follow-up.

Management of Ductal Carcinoma *In Situ*

The management of DCIS is perhaps the most controversial area in the local therapy of breast cancer today. The options available include total mastectomy versus local excision alone versus local excision with adjuvant radiation therapy. Lymph node dissection is not performed because nodal metastases are detected in less than 1% of cases. Although total mastectomy offers a 98% cure, most feel breast conservation is appropriate in most cases. However, breast conservation is contraindicated with large (more than 5 cm) tumors or if diffuse microcalcifications or multicentric disease is present. The incidence of ipsilateral multicentric DCIS is 30% to 35%.

The value of adjuvant radiation therapy was demonstrated in NSABP-17 where the 3-year recurrence rate after excision alone was 20% but was decreased to 10% with the addition of radiation therapy. Nevertheless, there has been considerable effort to determine whether all patients need radiation therapy. The van Nuys Prognostic Index (VNPI) was developed to assess the risk of recurrence and stratifies DCIS patients according to three significant predictors of local recurrence: tumor size, width of surgical margins, and pathologic classification (nuclear grade and comedo necrosis). In one series of 333 DCIS patients assigned retrospectively to a VNPI score, the lowest risk patients (low-grade DCIS without comedo necrosis, tumors less than 2 cm and with margins of more than 1 cm) did not appear to benefit from radiation while those in the moderate and high-risk groups did. This has led to a belief in some circles that lumpectomy alone in the lowest risk groups is sufficient treatment without an increased incidence of local recurrence. A prospective randomized trial is underway to study this issue.

Management of Locally Advanced Breast Cancer

Stage III or LABC is characterized by large tumors (more than 5 cm) or by skin changes of edema and ulceration, chest wall fixation, or fixed axillary lymph nodes. About 10% to 15% of patients in the United States present with LABC while in developing countries, it can be as high as one third. Initially, radiation therapy plus surgery can reduce locoregional recurrence to 10% to 20%, but the 5 year disease-free survival rate is less than 30%. The best results are achieved with neoadjuvant chemotherapy. Up to two thirds of patients have a partial response of their primary tumor after chemotherapy. Surgery then follows with either BCT or MRM with adjuvant radiation as appropriate. Subsequent chemotherapy recommendations are based on pathology findings.

The management of inflammatory breast cancer consists of preoperative chemotherapy followed by MRM and chest wall radiation.

Follow-up

The overall relapse rate for breast cancer depends on the initial TNM stage of the tumor. The most common sites for metastatic recurrence are the bones (50%), lung/pleura (25%), followed by liver, brain, and spine. Table 30-9 lists

TABLE 30-9. SITES OF METASTASES FROM BREAST CANCER IN THREE COLLECTED SERIES[a]

Organ	160 cases (%)	43 cases (%)	100 cases (%)
Lung	59	65	69
Liver	58	56	65
Bone	44	—	71
Pleura	37	23	51
Adrenal glands	31	41	49
Kidneys	—	14	17
Spleen	14	23	17
Pancreas	—	11	17
Ovaries	9	16	20
Brain	—	9	22
Thyroid	—	—	24
Heart	—	—	11
Diaphragm	—	—	11
Pericardium	—	21	19
Intestine	—	—	18
Peritoneum	12	9	13
Uterus	—	—	15
Skin	39	7	30

[a](From Harris JR, Lippman ME, Morrow M, et al., eds. *Diseases of the breast.* Philadelphia: Lippincott Williams & Wilkins, 1996:388, with permission.)

the most common sites of recurrence found in three different series. The subsequent risk for the development of a contralateral breast cancer is 0.5% to 1.0% per year. There is also an increased risk of recurrence if the first tumor is diagnosed before the age of 50, if there is a positive family history, or if the tumor is multicentric or an invasive lobular carcinoma. It is recommended to have monthly BSE, annual mammograms, and CBE every 3 to 6 months depending on whether the patient had mastectomy or breast conservation and the time elapsed since surgery was performed.

Breast Reconstruction

To restore the aesthetic symmetry of the breast contour, reconstruction techniques are available. Reconstruction may be immediate, concurrent with the mastectomy, delayed, or performed as a separate procedure some time after the mastectomy. The advantage to an immediate reconstruction is exposure to a single anesthetic and operation for both physical and psychological reasons. The disadvantages include the theoretical incidence of local failure due to the delay in diagnosis as well as risks of complications from reconstruction, which can delay radiation or chemotherapy. Usually, reconstruction is delayed if radiation therapy is planned or in the setting of high-risk advanced disease; however, there is no need to wait if routine adjuvant chemotherapy is planned.

The options for reconstruction include a prosthetic or an autologous tissue flap. The transverse rectus abdominis muscle (TRAM) flap is the procedure of choice, particularly in the irradiated breast (Fig. 30-11). Other options include the latissimus dorsi musculocutaneous flap or a free TRAM flap. Prosthesis options include silicone or saline implants with or without a tissue expander. Comorbidities that have a negative impact on the success of immediate breast reconstruc-

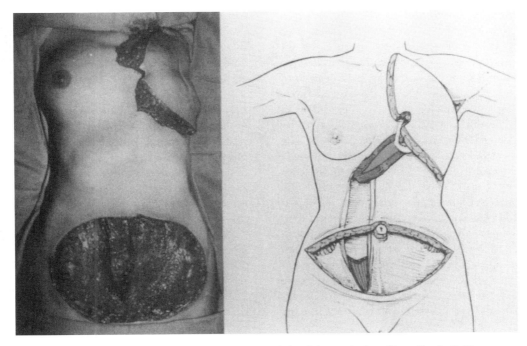

FIGURE 30-11. Illustration of the transverse rectus abdominis muscle flap. (From Harris JR, Lippman ME, Morrow M, et al., eds. *Diseases of the breast.* Philadelphia: Lippincott Williams & Wilkins, 1996:609, with permission.)

TABLE 30-10. GUIDELINES FOR ADJUVANT THERAPY IN STAGE I AND II BREAST CANCER

Tumor characteristics	Premenopausal estrogen receptor+	Premenopausal estrogen receptor−	Postmenopausal estrogen receptor+	Postmenopausal estrogen receptor−
<1-cm, −Nodes	No treatment/tamofixen	No treatment	No treatment	No treatment
>1-cm, −Nodes	Tamoxifen ± chemotherapy	Chemotherapy	Tamoxifen	NT ± chemotherapy[a]
+Nodes	Chemotherapy + tamofixen	Chemotherapy	Tamoxifen + chemotherapy	Chemotherapy

[a]Chemotherapy may be indicated depending on tumor size and other prognostic factors.

tion include diabetes mellitus, uncontrolled hypertension, cardiovascular disease, tobacco use, and morbid obesity.

Adjuvant Systemic Therapy

Although postmastectomy radiotherapy reduces the incidence of local and regional recurrence by 50% to 75%, in most randomized trials, this reduction was not accompanied by a survival benefit. For that reason and because of its potential for long-term adverse effects, radiation therapy after mastectomy is indicated only for women at high risk for local or regional recurrence. This includes patients with large tumors (more than 5 cm) or lesions that invade the skin or chest wall, positive surgical margins, or those with more than four positive axillary nodes.

Currently, because 30% of all node-negative patients recur and ultimately succumb to metastatic disease, adjuvant therapy is recommended. Current recommendations for adjuvant therapy in stage I and II breast cancer are based on patient age, tumor size, nodal and estrogen receptor status of the tumor, and the patient's menopausal status (Table 30-10). Other prognostic features of the tumor such as tumor grade, vascular lymphatic invasion, S phase, and DNA index are considered in making recommendations. Studies have shown a survival benefit in treating patients with tumors larger than 1.0 cm. Combination chemotherapy regimens are generally based on cyclophosphamide and/or doxorubicin and given for 4 to 6 months. The two most common regimens include cyclophosphamide/methotrexate/fluorouracil (CMF) or methotrexate/fluorouracil (MF) and adriamycin and cyclophosphamide (AC) with response rates of about 50%. Taxol is effective in breast cancer and is being used increasingly in the adjuvant setting in combination with AC in high-risk patients. In general, premenopausal node-negative patients are offered chemotherapy while postmenopausal, hormone-receptor positive, node-negative patients are usually offered tamoxifen alone. New trials suggest that simultaneous chemotherapy and radiation therapy may be possible.

Neoadjuvant or preoperative chemotherapy is administered in inflammatory breast cancer. However, for women with large operable tumors, preoperative chemotherapy may also have some advantages. The primary tumor may decrease in size, allowing breast conservation to be possible in patients who would otherwise have required a mastectomy. There is, however, no survival advantage to preoperative as opposed to postoperative chemotherapy.

Immunotherapy options include monoclonal antibodies directed against the extracellular domain of the HER-2/neu oncoprotein. The HER-2/neu oncogene is overexpressed in 30% of breast cancers and is a poor prognostic indicator. A recent randomized trial showed a survival advantage in patients treated with chemotherapy and monoclonal antibodies compared to those treated with chemotherapy alone.

Adjuvant Hormonal Therapy

Patients with tumors that are both estrogen and progesterone receptor positive (ER+/PR+) have a high likelihood (70%) of response to hormonal treatment. Tumors that are ER−/PR+ are hormone responsive but at a lower rate. Historically, hormone ablation therapies were used including oophorectomy, ovarian radiation, adrenalectomy, and hypophysectomy. With the addition of the medication tamoxifen, a pharmacologic antiestrogen, those therapies are currently rarely used.

Adjuvant tamoxifen leads to a prolonged disease-free survival in postmenopausal/ER+ women with positive nodes and both premenopausal and postmenopausal women with negative nodes. Overall, patients can expect a 50% reduction in risk of recurrence. The combination of tamoxifen (or ovarian ablation in premenopausal women) and chemotherapy is more effective than either one administered alone and is recommended for women with a high risk of recurrent disease.

NSABP B-24 compared the addition of tamoxifen to lumpectomy/radiation therapy against lumpectomy/radiation therapy alone in the prevention of invasive and noninvasive cancers in the ipsilateral and contralateral breast. This trial demonstrated an additional benefit of tamoxifen due mainly to a decrease in the rate of invasive cancer, particularly in the ipsilateral breast. Tamoxifen has also been reported in the setting of elderly patients (over 70 years old) with low-risk T1 and T2 ER+ tumors treated with lumpectomy alone with low local recurrence rates.

Since tamoxifen is a weak estrogen agonist/antagonist, there is a slightly increased risk of endometrial cancer (two and a half times) and thromboembolic events due to unopposed estrogen activity. There is some improvement in the cholesterol and lipid profile and on bone density in postmenopausal women taking tamoxifen.

The current recommendations for the use of tamoxifen in breast cancer are from the 1985 National Cancer Institute Consensus Conference but have been validated subsequently in recent randomized trials. Women with invasive ER+ or ER−/PR+ breast cancer should be treated with tamoxifen for 5 years. Various studies are examining the optimal duration of treatment, but studies to date have confirmed the 5-year recommendation.

Management of Recurrent Cancer

Overall, the local and distant recurrence rate for node-negative patients after adjuvant therapy is 20%, and it is 60% for node-positive patients. If a recurrence is detected in the ipsilateral breast after breast conservation surgery, a mastectomy is performed as a salvage operation after a metastatic evaluation is completed. It is difficult to distinguish between a local recurrence due to residual disease or multifocal disease from the initial cancer versus a new primary cancer. There is strong support for the view that most local recurrences (particularly in the first 3 to 4 years) actually represent residual disease. After mastectomy, chest wall recurrence is particularly ominous with a risk of distant disease of 30% and 60% at 2 and 10 years, respectively, in node-negative patients and 70% and 90% in node-positive patients. Radiation therapy is the best salvage option and is offered. There is usually little role for radical resection or chemotherapy for local control, but if the recurrent tumor is not fixed to the chest wall, then local excision is recommended.

Recurrence can also occur in the first draining group of nodes because of inadequate nodal dissection. Reexploration with more radical nodal dissection can target this disease, but if disease recurs with concurrently positive supraclavicular or cervical nodes, then radiation therapy is offered.

Widely metastatic disease usually indicates incurable disease and therapy is palliative only. The median survival is on the order of 2 years with worse prognosis if the tumor is ER− and/or associated with visceral metastases. Treatment options include hormonal therapy, chemotherapy, and bone/brain irradiation if needed. The rare patient with an isolated liver or lung metastasis might be considered for resection. Anti-neu antibody therapy (herceptin) can be offered to patients whose original tumor overexpressed this cell-surface protein. Peptide and autologous tumor vaccine protocols are also being developed.

PAGET'S DISEASE OF THE NIPPLE

Paget cells are large cells with pale cytoplasm and prominent nucleoli, which manifest with eczematous changes of the nipple, presenting with itching, erythema, and occasionally nipple discharge. It can be thought of as DCIS of the nipple and is usually associated with additional intraductal or invasive carcinoma of the underlying breast. Diagnosis is made by biopsy of the nipple skin with some underlying dermal tissue. The treatment is simple mastectomy or breast conservation with excision of the nipple areolar complex and breast radiation.

MALE BREAST CANCER

Male breast cancer represents about 1% of all breast cancers, which amounts to about 1,000 cases per year leading to 300 deaths. Approximately 30% of patients have a positive family history, Klinefelter disease, or a history of prior radiation therapy. It typically presents as a painless mass beneath the nipple areola complex. It is important to evaluate for gynecomastia due to cirrhosis or drugs. Unlike women, 80% of nipple discharge in men is associated with cancer. As in women, infiltrating ductal carcinoma (80%) is the most common pathologic subtype. The treatment is MRM with a radical mastectomy if the tumor extends into the pectoralis major. Stage for stage, the overall survival is similar to that of women, although men tend to present at a more advanced stage. Adjuvant therapy is also indicated with chemotherapy or tamoxifen.

SUGGESTED READING

Bland KI, Copeland EM, eds. *The breast: comprehensive management of benign and malignant disease.* Philadelphia: WB Saunders, 1996.

Greenfield LJ, Mullholland M, Oldham KT, et al., eds. *Surgery: scientific principles and practice,* 2nd ed. Philadelphia: Lippincott-Raven Publishers, 1997.

Harris JR, Lippman ME, Morrow M, et al., eds. *Diseases of the breast.* Philadelphia: Lippincott-Raven Publishers, 1996.

Jatii I, ed. *The surgical clinics of North America.* Vol 79. No 5. October 1999. Philadelphia: WB Saunders, 1999.

Kinne DW. *Multidisciplinary atlas of breast surgery.* Philadelphia: Lippincott-Raven Publishers, 1998.

INDEX

Page numbers followed by f indicate figures; page numbers followed by t indicate tables.

A

AA, 30
AAA. *See* Abdominal aortic aneurysms
Abciximab, 300
Abdominal aortic aneurysms (AAA), 347–349, 350f
   imaging of, 348
   pathophysiology of, 347
   risk factors for, 347
   symptoms of, 347–348
   treatment of, 348–349
Abdominal wall
   hernias of, 159–161, 160f
   layers of, 160t
ABI, 342
Absorption, 272–284
Acceptable upper limit (AUL), 182
Accessory nipples, 501
Acetabular fractures, 459–460, 459f
Achalasia, 189, 189f
Achilles tendon ruptures, 463
Acid, 193
Acid-base balance, 153–155
Acid-base disorders
   mixed, 155
Acid-base homeostasis, 387
Acidic fibroblast growth factors, 115–116
Acid load, 387
Acidosis, 153–154
Acinic cell carcinomas, 421
ACL, 461–462
Acoustic neuromas, 31
Acoustic schwannomas, 31
Acquired heart disease, 323–331
Acquired nevi, 91
Acquired valve disease, 324–328
Acral lentiginous melanoma, 92
Acromioclavicular sprains, 453
ACT, 300
Actin thin filaments, 444
Action potentials, 3
Activated clotting time (ACT), 300
Activated partial thromboplastin time (zPTT), 299
Active–specific immunotherapy, 89
Acute embolic occlusion, 350
Acute ischemia, 343
Acute lower extremity ischemia, 345–347
   etiology of, 345–346
   treatment of, 346–347
Acute pancreatitis, 492–495, 493f
   clinical features of, 492–493
   complications of, 494–495
   etiology of, 492
   pathophysiology of, 492
   with persistent choledocholithiasis, 494
   prognosis of, 493, 493t
   therapy of, 493–494
Acute renal failure, 387–388
Acute scrotal pain
   differential diagnosis of, 392
Acute thrombotic occlusion, 350–351
Acute thyroiditis, 470
Acute toxic megacolon, 239
Acute tubular necrosis, 50
ADCC, 40
Adenocarcinomas, 232–233, 232f, 421
Adenohypophysis, 9
Adenoid cystic carcinomas, 369, 421
Adenomas, 232, 241
   bronchial, 369
   Brunner gland, 232
   hepatocellular, 258
   parathyroid, 480
   pituitary, 32
   pleomorphic, 420
Adenoma–to–carcinoma sequence, 241, 241f
Adenosine, 49, 309
ADH, 149, 384
Adjuvant chemotherapy, 87
Adjuvant therapy
   for lymphatic spread, 95
Adnexal mass
   differential diagnosis of, 408
Adoptive immunotherapy, 89
Adrenal cortex, 481–482
   steroidogenic pathways of, 483, 483f
Adrenal glands, 381, 481–488
   anatomy of, 481, 482f
   pathophysiology of, 484–488
   physiology of, 481–484
Adrenal hyperplasia
   congenital, 487–488
Adrenal insufficiency, 488
Adrenocortical carcinoma, 487
Adrenocortical insufficiency, 158
Adult respiratory distress syndrome (ARDS), 156, 356, 450
Aflatoxin, 259
AFP, 76–78
Afterload, 308
AGES (age, grade of tumor, extent of tumor, size of tumor) system, 474
Air movement, 354–358
Airways, 354–355, 355f
Akinesia, 139
Alanine, 256, 289–290
Aldosterone, 148, 483–484
Alkali, 193
Alkaline reflux gastritis, 206
Alkalosis, 154
Alkylating agents, 86
Allopurinol, 49
Alpha error, 179
Alpha-fetoprotein (AFP), 76–78
Alternative hypothesis, 179–180
Alternative pathway, 40–41, 41f
Alveolar septum, 360, 360f
Amaurosis fugax, 28
Amebic abscesses
   of liver, 260
American Joint Committee on Cancer staging system, 93, 93t, 98t
Amine precursor uptake and decarboxylase (APUD), 214–215
Aminoglycosides, 64
Amoxicillin, 63–64
Amphotericin B, 65
Ampicillin, 63–64
Ampulla, 417
Anal canal, 236
Anal cancer, 253–254
Anal fistula
   classification of, 253f
Analysis of variance (ANOVA), 178
Anaplastic astrocytomas (AAs), 30
Anaplastic thyroid cancer (ATC), 477
Anatomical dead space, 354
Androgens, 483
Anencephaly, 18
Anergy, 46
Anesthesia, 139–147
   monitoring during, 140–142
   preoperative assessment for, 139–140, 140t
   techniques of, 140
Aneurysms, 347–352
   abdominal aortic. *See* Abdominal aortic aneurysms
   arch, 331
   ascending, 331
   cerebral, 26

Aneurysms *(contd.)*
  descending, 331
  fusiform atherosclerotic, 27
  mycotic, 27, 349
  of peripheral arteries, 349–350
  physiology of, 340
  surgical clipping of, 27
  traumatic, 27
ANF, 385
Angiogenesis, 115–116
Angiography, 14
  for GU trauma, 388
Angiomyolipoma, 393
Angiosarcomas, 259, 329
Angiotensin II, 156
Ankle-brachial index (ABI), 342
Annular pancreas, 489
Annulus fibrosis, 5
Anorectal line, 236
ANOVA, 178
ANS, 13
Anterior abdominal wall hernias, 168–171
Anterior cervical diskectomy, 15
Anterior cruciate ligament (ACL), 461–462
Anterior neuropores, 17
Anterior spinal artery syndrome, 24
Antibiotics, 86
Antibodies, 38
Antibody-dependent cell-mediated cytotoxicity (ADCC), 40
Antidiuretic hormone (ADH), 149, 385
Antifungals, 65
Antigen–presenting cells, 43, 43f
Antimetabolites, 86
Antimicrobial agents, 62–65
  classes of, 62–63, 63t
  topical
    for burn management, 134t
Antiseizure drugs, 21
Antral gland, 199
Anus
  coronal section of, 237f
  imperforate, 254
Aortic anastomosis, 56, 57f
Aortic arches
  embryology of, 303
Aortic dissection, 330–331, 330f
Aorticopulmonary septal defects, 316
Aortic regurgitation, 325–326
Aortic stenosis, 319, 324–325
Aortic valves, 305, 305f
Aortography
  for AAA, 348
Aortoiliac occlusive disease
  claudication resulting from, 341–342, 341f
  therapeutic intervention in, 344
APC, 71
Aphasia, 12
Apoprotein, 334
Apoptosis, 38
Appendicitis, 249
  during pregnancy, 414–415
Appendix, 235, 249–250
APUD, 214–215
Arachnoid cyst, 16

Arch aneurysms, 331
ARDS, 156, 356, 450
Area of enhancement, 14
Areflexia, 139
Arginine test, 492
Arnold-Chiari malformation, 17
Arrhythmia surgery, 328–329
Arterial hemodynamics, 337
Arterial insufficiency
  objective measurement of, 342–343
Arterial lines
  for anesthesia monitoring, 141, 141t
Arterial occlusive disease
  risk factors for, 333–334
Arterial stenoses, 339–340, 340f
Arteries, 332
Arteriosclerosis, 332
Arteriovenous malformations (AVMs), 14, 247
Articular cartilage, 443–444
Ascending aneurysms, 331
ASD, 311–312, 312f
Aseptic necrosis, 450
Aspartate transaminase, 256
Aspergillus flavus, 259
Aspiration biopsy, 80
Aspirin, 300
Assist-control (AC) ventilation, 362
Astrocytes, 3
ATC, 477
Atheromatous plaque, 334, 336f
Atherosclerosis, 332, 352
  pathogenesis of, 334–335, 335f
  theories of, 336–337
Atlanto–occipital dislocation, 22
Atlas, 5
Atresia
  congenital, 217
Atrial natriuretic factor (ANF), 385
Atrial septal defect (ASD), 313–314, 314f
Atrioventricular node, 308
Atrioventricular valves, 304–305
Attenuated polyposis coli (APC), 71
Auditory system, 12
  anatomy and physiology of, 416–417, 417f
AUL, 182
Auricular hematoma, 429, 430f
Autografts, 136, 443
Autoimmune disorders, 72
Autoimmune hemolytic anemia, 106
Autonomic nervous system (ANS), 13
Autonomously functioning thyroid nodules, 470
Avascular necrosis (AVN), 449–451, 457, 460
AVM, 14, 247
AVN, 449–451, 457, 460
A-V septal defects, 316–317
Axillary lymph nodes, 502, 502f
Axillary nerve palsy, 454
Axillopopliteal bypass, 345
Axis, 5
Axonotmesis, 24
Azathioprine, 48, 57, 239
Aztreonam, 64

B

Babinski sign, 35
Bacille Calmette–Guerin (BCG), 88
Bacteria, 61, 61f
Bacterial abscesses
  of liver, 260
Bacterial meningitis, 33
Bacteroides fragilis, 250
Balance, 417–419
Balloon embolectomy, 346, 347f
Balloon tamponade, 263–264
Barbiturates, 143
Barium esophagram, 188
Barrett esophagus, 191–192, 192f
Basal cisterns, 5
Basal energy expenditure (BEE), 284
Basal ganglia, 5
Basal metabolism, 284–288, 284t
Basic fibroblast growth factors, 115–116
Basilar skull fractures, 19
Bassini repair, 163
Battle sign, 19
BBB (blood brain barrier), 3
B-cell
  development of, 38
BCG, 88
BCT, 513, 515f
BEE, 284
Bell clapper deformity, 392
Benign bile–duct strictures, 270
Benign bone tumors, 445–446, 446t
Benign breast diseases, 505–506
Benign chest wall tumors, 370
Benign cystic teratomas, 408
Benign esophageal neoplasms, 193–194
Benign lung disease, 364
Benign lung tumors, 369
Benign lymphoepithelial lesion of Godwin, 420
Benign paroxysmal positional vertigo, 417
Benign pelvic masses, 407–408
Benign pleural disease, 371–372
Benign polyps, 194
Benign prostatic hypertrophy (BPH), 398–399
Benzodiazepines, 143–144
Bernstein test, 188
Berry aneurysms, 26
Beta–adrenergic receptors, 308
Beta error, 179
Beta-HCG, 79–80
Beta-lactam ring, 63–64, 64f
Bidirectional shunts, 320–323
Bile acids, 267–268, 268f, 278
Bile canaliculi, 278
Bile duct cancer, 271
Bile duct strictures
  benign, 270
Biliary atresia, 51–52
Biliary cancer, 271
Biliary system
  anatomy of, 266–271
Billroth II resection, 203, 204f
Billroth I resection, 203
Black pigment stones, 269

Bladder
  trauma of, 391
Bladder cancer
  staging of, 395t
Bleaches, 193
Bleeding disorders
  clinical testing of, 299
  preoperative screening of, 300
Bleeding time, 299
Blood flow
  principles of, 337–338
Blood products, 301–302
Blue toe syndrome, 341, 343
Blumer shelf, 210
Blunt cardiovascular trauma, 329–330
Blunt renal trauma
  staging of, 389, 389t, 390f
B lymphocytes, 38, 38f, 38t
Body fluid compartments, 148, 148f
Bone
  benign tumors of, 445–446, 446t
  formation of, 438–439, 439f
  grafts of, 443
  malignant neoplasms of, 445–446, 447t, 448f
  remodeling of, 440f
  structure of, 438–439, 439f
Bone window, 13
Boundary layer separation, 338–339, 340f
Bowen disease, 253
BPH, 398–399
Brachytherapy, 82–83, 99
Bradyarrhythmia, 328
Brain
  lateral surface of, 5f
  tumors of, 29–30
    metastatic, 32
  venous drainage of, 7f
  ventral surface of, 6f
  ventricular system of, 8f
Brain–dead, 22
Brain–gut axis, 214
Brainstem, 7, 8f
Brain Trauma Foundation, 20–21
Branchial cleft cysts, 425
BRCA-1, 508
BRCA-2, 508
Breast
  anatomy of, 501–502, 501f
  benign diseases of, 505–506
  cysts of, 505
  embryology of, 501
  evaluation of, 504
  examination of, 503
  masses of, 504
  pain of, 504
  physiology of, 502–503
  reconstruction of, 516–517, 516f
Breast cancer, 506–518
  adjuvant hormonal therapy of, 517–518
  adjuvant systemic therapy of, 517, 517t
  biology of, 510–511, 510f
  clinical presentation of, 511
  incidence of, 506–507, 506f
  and inherited syndromes, 507–508

invasive, 509–510, 510f
locally advanced
  management of, 515
male, 518
metastases from, 516t
natural history of, 511, 513f
noninvasive, 508–509
pathology of, 508–510
prevention of, 508
prognosis of, 512
recurrence of, 518
risk of, 507, 507f
staging of, 511–512, 511t, 512f
surgery of, 512–515
treatment of, 512–518
workup of, 511
Breast conservation treatment (BCT), 513, 515f
Breathy voice, 428
Broca aphasia, 12
Broca area, 12
Bronchial adenomas, 369
Bronchiectasis, 364
Bronchoscopy, 365
Brown pigment stones, 269
Brown-Sequard syndrome, 24
Brunner gland adenomas, 232
Bupivacaine, 146
Burn injury, 123–138
  classification of, 123–124, 124t
  fluid resuscitation in, 125–126
  gastrointestinal changes after, 126–127
  hematologic changes after, 129–130
  hemodynamic changes in, 125–126
  immunologic changes after, 129–130
  management of, 130–132
  metabolic energy expenditure after, 126t
  pathophysiology of, 123–124
  pulmonary changes in, 127
  renal system in, 129
  submersion
    pattern of, 133f
  triage for, 132, 132t
Burns, 290
  coverage of, 136–137, 136t
  management of, 133–135
Burn shock, 123
  resuscitation from, 125–130
Burn wound infection
  signs of, 135, 135t
Burr holes, 15
Butterfly fractures, 440–441
Butterfly gliomas, 30

C
CA 15-3, 79
CA 19-9, 79, 499
CA 125, 79
CABG
  indications for, 324, 324t
Calcaneal fractures, 463
Calcitonin, 479
Calcium
  absorption of, 282–283
  imbalance of, 151–153

metabolism of, 439
Calcium carbonate, 417
Call–Exner bodies, 413
Canadian Cardiovascular Society
  functional classification, 323, 323t
Canadian repair, 164, 164f
Canalicular bile, 266–267
Canalicular bile flow, 267–268, 268f
Cancer, 290. See also Malignant; Tumors
  cytoreductive surgery of, 82
  epidemiology of, 69
  familial influences on, 69–72
  hormonal factors in, 71–72
  mortality of, 69
  multimodal treatment of, 80–81
  palliative surgery of, 82
  prevention of, 82, 82t
  surgery of, 81–82
Cantlie line, 256
Capsid, 62
Carbohydrates, 285
  digestion of, 281f
Carbon monoxide poisoning, 128–129
Carcinoembryonic antigen (CEA), 75
Carcinogenesis
  multistep, 75, 75f
Carcinoid tumors, 216, 233, 369
Carcinoma in situ, 241
Cardia, 197
Cardiac action potentials, 307, 308f
Cardiac electrophysiology, 307–310
Cardiac glands, 198
Cardiac injury
  penetrating, 329
Cardiac neoplasms, 329
Cardiac physiology, 306–307
Cardiopulmonary bypass, 301, 311–312
Cardiovascular system
  embryology of, 303–304, 304f
Cardiovascular trauma, 329–330
  blunt, 329–330
Carotid-cavernous fistula (CC fistula), 27
Carotid endarterectomy, 29
Carpal tunnel syndrome, 25
Case-control studies, 174, 175f, 176f
Case report, 174
Case series, 174
Catecholamines, 483, 484
Categorical data, 177
Catheters
  central venous, 158
  infection of, 68
  pulmonary artery, 141, 141t
  urinary, 141–142
Cauda equina, 9
Cauda equina syndrome, 36
Caudal anesthesia, 140
Causalgia, 25
Caustic injury, 193
Cavernous transformation, 262
CC fistula, 27
CCK, 212, 215
CEA, 75
  in colonic cancer, 77t
Cecal bascule, 248

Cecum, 235
Cefotetan, 64
Ceftriaxone, 64
Cell cycle, 73
Cells, 296–299
   malignant
      characteristics of, 72–73
Cellular immune response, 38
Cellular immunodeficiencies, 59–60
Cell wall
   synthesis of
      inhibition of, 63–64, 64f
Central cord syndrome, 24
Central deletion, 46
Central nervous system (CNS)
   functional organization of, 10–13
   microscopic anatomy of, 3
Central venous catheters
   for hypovolemic shock, 158
Central venous lines
   for anesthesia monitoring, 141, 141t
Cephalosporins, 64
Cerebellum, 7
Cerebral aneurysms, 26
Cerebral perfusion pressure (CPP), 21
Cerebritis, 33
Cerebrovascular disease
   ischemic, 28
Cervical lymph node
   metastases from well-differentiated
      thyroid carcinoma, 475
Cervical malignancies, 410, 411t
Cervical spine
   fracture of, 234
Cervical spondylosis, 35
Cervical stenosis, 34–35
   management of, 35
Chance, 179–181
Chemical burns, 137
Chemical synapses, 4
Chemotherapy, 84
   administration of, 87
   adverse effects of, 88
   for breast cancer, 517
   combined with radiotherapy, 85–88
   induction, 87
Chest wall, 355
   injuries of, 379
   tumors of, 369–370
Chiari II malformation, 15, 17
Chiari I malformation, 17
Child abuse, 24, 132
CHILD B syndrome, 259
Children
   mandibular fractures in, 429–430
   small bowel diseases of, 218–223
Chi-square statistic, 178
Chitin, 61
Chloramphenicol, 64
Cholangiocarcinoma, 259, 271
Cholangitis, 270
Cholecystitis
   during pregnancy, 415
Cholecystokinin (CCK), 212, 215
Choledochal cysts, 270–271, 271f
Choledocholithiasis, 270

acute pancreatitis with, 494
Cholelithiasis, 268–270
Cholesteatoma, 418
Cholesterol, 269
   transport pathways for, 335f
Cholestyramine, 249
Chondromas, 370
Chondrosarcoma, 447t, 448f
Chorda tympani, 422
Choriocarcinoma, 413
Choroid plexus papillomas, 31
Chromosomal translocations, 74
Chronic lower extremity ischemia, 340–344
   noninvasive testing of, 343–344, 344f
Chronic lymphocytic thyroiditis, 470–471
Chronic mesenteric ischemia, 351–352
Chronic obstructive pulmonary diseases
     (COPD), 358
Chronic pancreatitis, 495–497, 496f
   with common bile duct stenosis, 496
   imaging of, 495
   mortality of, 496
   symptoms of, 495
   treatment of, 495–496, 496f
Chronic subdural hematoma, 19
Chronic venous insufficiency, 353
Chronic wound, 121
Chvostek sign, 481
Chyle, 372
Chylomicrons, 334
Chylothorax, 372
Cigarette smoking, 334
Circle of Willis, 6
Classical pathway, 40–41, 41f
Claudication, 341–342
Clavicular fractures, 453
Clinical economics, 182
Clopidogrel, 300
Closed fractures, 19
Closed loop obstruction, 225
Clostridial gangrene, 67
Clostridium difficile, 248–249
Clostridium perfringens, 451
Clostridium tetanii, 65–66
Clot generation, 295–297
Clotting cascade, 295, 296f
CMV, 46
CNS
   functional organization of, 10–13
   microscopic anatomy of, 3
Coagulation
   functional tests of, 299–301
Coagulation cascade
   drugs affecting, 300–301
   natural inhibitors of, 299
Coagulation pathway
   extrinsic, 296
   intrinsic, 296
Coarctation of the aorta, 320
Cohort studies, 175–176, 175f
Cold sepsis, 158
Collagen, 337
   distribution of, 117
   production of, 119t
   synthesis of, 117–118, 118f
   regulation of, 119, 119f

Colles fracture, 456, 456f
Colon, 283
   anatomy of, 235–237, 236f
   arterial supply to, 235, 236f
   motility of, 238
   pathology of, 238–240
   physiology of, 237–238
Colon cancer, 89
   CEA in, 77t
Colonic diverticula, 245f
Colonic lymphoma, 103
Colonic polyps, 240–242
Colonic volvulus, 247–248, 248f
Colorectal cancer, 82
   stages of, 242, 242t
Colorectal Crohn disease, 240
Comedo–type ductal carcinoma in situ, 509f
Comminuted fractures, 19
Compartment syndrome, 346, 450
Complement, 40–41
   activation of, 41f
Complex partial seizure, 30
Compound nevi, 92
Compression fractures, 441
Compressive cardiogenic shock, 155–156
Computed tomography (CT), 13, 188
   for AAA, 348
   for GU trauma, 386
   for lung cancer, 365
   of thyroid gland, 468–469
Concordant xenotransplantation, 46
Concussion, 18
Conduction aphasia, 12
Conductive hearing losses, 416
Confidence intervals, 180
Congenital adrenal hyperplasia, 487–488
Congenital atresia, 217
Congenital dermal sinus, 17–18
Congenital diaphragmatic hernias, 172–173, 172f
Congenital heart disease, 313–323
Congenital malformations, 17–18
Congenital nevi, 91
Contact activation system, 296
Continuous data, 177
Cooper ligament, 161
Cooper–ligaments repair, 164, 165f
COPD, 358
Cords of Billroth, 104
Core (needle) biopsy, 80
Corkscrew esophagus, 189, 189f
Coronary artery bypass grafting (CABG)
   indications for, 324, 324t
Coronary artery disease, 323–324
Coronary blood flow, 311
Coronary steel syndrome, 143
Corpectomy, 15
Corpus, 197
Corpus striatum, 6
Correlation, 178
Cortical bone, 439f
Corticosteroids, 47
Cortisol, 482
   secretion of, 483–484, 484f
Cor triatriatum, 314

Cost-benefit analysis, 182
Cost-effectiveness analysis, 182
Cost-minimization analysis, 182
Cost-utility analysis, 182
Cosyntropin, 488
Coumadin, 300–301
CPP, 21
Cranial dysraphism, 18
Craniectomy, 15
Craniotomy, 15
Critical stenosis, 339
Crohn's disease, 225f, 228–230
    colorectal, 240
    obstructions in, 229
Cryptorchidism, 82
Crypts, 211, 212f
C syndrome, 259
CT. *See* Computed tomography
CT angiography, 14
Cultured autologous keratinocytes, 136
Cultured epithelial autograft, 136
Cupulolithiasis, 417
Curling ulcer, 126, 209
Cushing disease, 209
Cushing syndrome, 484–486
Cushing triad, 22
Cutaneous allograft, 136–137
Cutaneous xenograft, 137
Cycling cells, 73
Cyclosporin, 47, 47f, 60, 239
Cylindromas, 369
Cysticercosis, 33
Cystic fibrosis, 354–355
Cystic medial necrosis, 330
Cystic teratomas
    benign, 408
Cystogram
    for GU trauma, 389
Cytokines, 39, 41–43, 42t, 113–114, 121
Cytomegalovirus (CMV), 46

D
DAI, 20
Dandy-Walker syndrome, 15
Data
    interpretation of, 176–177
DCIS, 508–509
    management of, 515
Deep inguinal ring, 160
Deep vein thrombosis (DVT), 353, 450
Delayed union, 449
Deletion, 46
Dendrites, 3, 89
Dens, 5
Depolarization, 3
De Quervain thyroiditis, 470
Dermal sinus
    congenital, 17–18
Dermatomes, 34, 34f
DES, 189, 189f
Descending aneurysms, 331
Descriptive statistics, 176
Descriptive studies, 174
Desflurane, 143
Desmoplastic melanoma, 93
Deviated septum, 436

Diabetes, 53–54, 150, 334
    and wound healing, 121–122
Diagnostic tests
    in epidemiology, 181, 181f, 181t
Diaphragma sellae, 9
Diaphragmatic hernias
    congenital, 172–173, 172f
Diaphragmatic injuries, 380
Diastatic fractures, 19
DIC, 301
Diencephalon, 7
Diffuse acute ischemia, 343
Diffuse axonal injury (DAI), 20
Diffuse esophageal spasm (DES), 189, 189f
Diffuse lymphoma, 376
Diffuse pedal ischemia, 343
Digestion, 272–284
Dimethadione (DMO) test, 491–492
Dipyridamole, 300
Dipyridamole thallium–201 scintigraphy (DTS), 323
Direct allorecognition, 45, 45f
Direct inguinal hernias, 161
Discrete data, 177
Disk
    herniation of, 35
    rupture of, 35
Disseminated intravascular coagulation (DIC), 301
Distal humerus
    fractures of, 455
Distal radius
    fractures of, 456, 456f
Distal splenorenal (Warren) shunt, 265, 266f
Diuretics, 388
Diverticular disease, 244–245, 245f
    of small bowel, 227
Diverticuli, 247
Diverticulitis, 244–245
    two–stage operation for, 246f
Diverticulosis, 244
Dix–Hallpike maneuvers, 417
DMO test, 491–492
DNA synthesis
    inhibitors of, 65
Dobutamine, 158
Donor cardiectomy, 56
Donor pancreatectomy, 54, 54f
Double inlet ventricle, 321–322
Double–lung transplantation, 58
Down syndrome, 218
DTS, 323
Ductal carcinoma in situ (DCIS), 508–509
    management of, 515
Dumping syndrome, 206
Duodenal atresia, 201, 218
Duodenal stenosis, 201
Duodenal ulcers, 201–206
    pathogenesis of, 201f, 202
    surgery of, 202–206
    treatment of, 202–206
Duodenum, 211, 211f
    anatomy of, 197–199, 212f
    physiology of, 199–201
Duplex imaging, 343–344

Duplication, 222
DVT, 353, 450
Dysgerminomas, 413
Dysmotility disorders, 188–190
Dysplastic nevus syndrome, 70, 92

E
Ear
    anatomy and physiology of, 416–417, 417f
    hematoma of, 429, 430f
    infection of, 418
Ebstein anomaly, 318
EBV, 46, 424
Echinococcosis, 33–34
Ec–IC bypass, 27
ECMO, 172–173
Ectopic pregnancy, 414
Edinger–Westphal nucleus, 11
EDRF, 333
Effective refractory periods, 307
EFTs, 188
Eisenmenger syndrome, 58, 319
Elastin, 337
Elbow injuries, 455–456
Elderly
    mandibular fractures in, 430
Elective lymph node dissection (ELND), 94
Electrical burns, 137
Electrolytes, 279–280, 280f
    balance of, 149
    imbalance of, 150–153
Electromagnetic radiation, 82
Electromyography (EMG), 25
Elliptocytosis
    hereditary, 106
ELND, 94
Embolic occlusion
    acute, 350
Emergency department
    and burn injury, 130–132
EMG, 25
Empyema, 372–373
Encephalocele, 18
Encephalopathy, 262
Enchondroma, 446t
Endoabdominal fascia, 160
Endocarditis, 327
Endochondral ossification, 439
Endocrine neoplasms, 497–499
Endocrine pancreas, 491
Endodermal sinus tumors, 413
Endolymph, 417
Endometrial cancer, 71, 408–409, 409t
Endometriosis, 407
Endoscopy, 188
Endothelial cells, 296–297, 297t
Endothelium–derived relaxing factor (EDRF), 333
Endotoxins, 62, 62f, 68
End-stage heart disease, 56
End-stage pulmonary parenchymal disorders, 58
End-to-end ileoanal anastomosis, 240, 240f
Enflurane, 143
Enteral nutrition, 127, 290–291

Enterobiliary fistula, 270
Enterochromaffin cells, 233
Enteroclysis, 225
Enterocutaneous fistula, 227–228
Enzymes, 79
   in collagen production, 119t
Ependymocytes, 3, 31
Ependymomas, 31
Epidemiology, 180
   diagnostic tests in, 181, 181f, 181t
Epidural abscess, 33
Epidural anesthesia, 140, 147
Epidural hematoma, 18–19, 20f
Epigastric hernias, 169
Epigastrium, 495
Epiphrenic diverticula, 191
Epistaxis, 437
Epithelial ovarian carcinoma, 412
Epstein-Barr virus (EBV), 46, 424
Equations
   for pulmonary physiology, 361t
ERV, 357
Erythropoietin, 387
Eschatory incisions, 131, 131f
Escherichia coli, 250
Esophageal diverticula, 190–191, 190f
Esophageal duplication cyst, 194
Esophageal function tests (EFTs), 188
Esophageal hemangiomas, 194
Esophageal manometry, 188
Esophageal neoplasms
   benign, 193–194
   malignant, 194–196, 195f, 196t
Esophageal perforation, 192–193
Esophageal varices, 265–266, 265t
Esophagus, 185–196, 273
   anatomy of, 185–186, 186f–187f
   arterial blood supply to, 186, 186f
   corkscrew, 189, 189f
   embryology of, 187, 187f
   innervation of, 185
   lymphatic drainage from, 186
   physiology of, 187–188
   venous blood supply from, 186
Estimated standard error of the mean, 178
Estrogen, 483
Ethmoid sinus, 436
Ewing sarcomas, 370, 447t, 448f
Excessive scar formation, 121
Excisional biopsy, 80
Excisional management
   of burn wounds, 133–134
Excitation contraction coupling, 310f
Exocrine pancreas, 491
Exotoxins, 62
Expectant management
   of burn wounds, 134–135, 134t
Expiratory reserve volume (ERV), 357
Explanatory studies, 174, 176
Exploratory studies, 174
Exposure odds ratio, 175, 176f
External hydrocephalus, 15
Extracellular fluid, 148
Extracellular matrix, 333
Extracorporeal membrane oxygenation
   (ECMO), 172–173

Extremities
   injuries of
      lower, 460–463
      upper, 452–458
Extremity soft tissue sarcoma, 97–100
   adjuvant therapy of, 98–100
   diagnosis of, 97
   radiologic imaging studies of, 97–98
   radiotherapy of, 98–99
   staging of, 97–98, 98f
   surgical treatment of, 98
Extrinsic coagulation pathway, 296

F

Fab, 38
Facial fractures, 431–433
Facial nerve injury, 435–436
Failed sclerotherapy, 264
Fallopian tubes, 402
   carcinoma of, 414
False localizing sign, 29
Falx cerebri, 5
Familial adenomatous polyposis (FAP), 71, 241–242
Familial (hereditary) breast cancer, 69–70
Familial hereditary nonpolyposis colon cancer (HNPCC), 70–71
Familial medullary thyroid carcinoma, 70
Familial melanoma, 70
FAP, 71, 241–242
Fasciotomy, 452
Fast cardiac action potentials, 307, 308f
Fat, 286
Fat embolism, 450
Fatty acid beta–oxidation, 286, 286f
Fecal fat test, 492
Female pelvis, 397, 397f–398f
Female pseudohermaphroditism, 487–488
Female reproductive system
   anatomy of, 400–404
   embryology of, 400, 401f
   lymphatic drainage of, 404
   pathology of, 406–414
Femoral artery aneurysms, 349
Femoral canal, 161
Femoral fractures, 460–461, 461f
Femoral hernias, 168
Femoral neck fractures, 460–461, 461f
Femoropopliteal tibial occlusive disease
   therapeutic intervention in, 344–345
Fentanyl, 144
Fetal wound healing, 120–121
FEV, 358
FGF, 333
Fibrin, 111, 112f
Fibrin–degradation products, 300
Fibrinolysis, 296
Fibroadenomas, 505
Fibroblast growth factor (FGF), 333
Fibroblasts
   migration of, 117
Fibromuscular dysplasia, 352
Fibronectin, 111, 112f
Fibronexi, 117
Fibroplasia, 116
Fibrosarcomas, 329

Fibrous dysplasia, 370
Fibrous histiocytoma
   malignant, 447t
Fibula
   fractures of, 463
Fifth–degree injury, 25
Finger–fracture technique, 262
First–degree injury, 25
Fisher exact test, 179
Fissure, 251–252, 252f
Fistula
   anal
      classification of, 253f
   enterobiliary, 270
   enterocutaneous, 227–228
   high–output, 227
Fistula in ano, 252–253
Flail chest, 379
Flank hematoma, 389
Flesh–eating bacteria, 67
Flexor tendon
   lacerations of, 458
Fluconazole, 65
Fluid balance, 279–280, 280f
Fluid energy, 337
Fluid energy losses, 338, 339f
Fluid pressure, 337
5-fluorouracil (5-FU), 244
FNH, 258
Focal nodular hyperplasia (FNH), 258
Folic acid synthesis
   inhibitors of, 64–65
Follicular thyroid carcinoma, 474
Foramen of Bochdalek hernia, 172, 172f
Foramen of Morgagni hernia, 172
Forced expiratory volume (FEV), 358
Forearm fractures, 456, 456f
Foreign bodies, 193
Fournier gangrene, 392–393
Fourth–degree injury, 25
Fractionation, 84
Fractures
   acetabular, 459–460, 459f
   associated with vascular injuries, 451–452
   basilar skull, 19
   biomechanics of, 440–441, 441f
   butterfly, 440–441
   clavicular, 453
   closed, 19
   comminuted, 19
   compression, 441
   diastatic, 19
   facial, 431–433
   femoral, 460–461, 461f
   femoral neck, 460–461, 461f
   fibula, 463
   forearm, 456, 456f
   greenstick, 440, 440f
   hand, 456–457
   healing of, 441–443, 442f
   hip, 460–461, 461f
   humeral shaft, 455, 455f
   linear, 19
   mandibular, 429–431
   odontoid, 22–23
   open, 451, 451t

pelvic, 458–459
proximal humerus, 454, 454f
scapular, 452–453
skull, 19
spinal, 23
spiral, 440, 441f
stellate, 19
sternal, 379
teardrop, 23
thoracolumbar spine, 23
tibia, 463
tibial plateau, 462, 462f
Frank-Starling relationship, 310
FRC, 355–357
Free radicals, 83
Free T4 index, 468
Frostbite, 137–138
5-FU, 244
Functional classification
    Canadian Cardiovascular Society, 323, 323t
    New York Heart Association, 323, 323t
Functional obstruction, 226
Functional residual capacity (FRC), 355–357
Fungal infection, 33
Fungi, 61
Funicular hernias, 161
Furosemide, 388
Fusiform atherosclerotic aneurysms, 27
Fusion, 15

G
GAGs, 114
Gallbladder, 267, 267f, 278–279
Gallbladder cancer, 271
Gallstone ileus, 226
Gallstones, 268–270
GALT, 213
Ganglioneuroblastomas, 378
Gangrene, 343
Gardner syndrome, 71, 97
Gardner-Wells tongs, 23
Gas exchange, 354, 360–362, 360f
Gastric cancer, 209–210
Gastric emptying, 275, 276f
Gastric inhibitory peptide (GIP), 275
Gastric mucosa-associated lymphoid tissue (MALT) lymphoma, 103
Gastric mucosal protection, 200, 200f
Gastric secretion, 275, 275f
Gastric ulcers, 206–207
    classification of, 206, 206f
Gastrin, 199, 215
Gastrinoma, 498–499, 498f
Gastroesophageal reflux disease (GERD), 191–192, 192f
Gastrointestinal bleeding
    lower, 247
Gastrointestinal lymphoma, 102–103, 103t
Gastroschisis, 173, 222–223
Gaussian distribution, 177
GBM, 30
Gene delivery systems, 89t
General anesthesia, 140
Generalized seizure, 30

Gene therapy, 89–90
Genetics
    of cancer, 69–72
Genitofemoral nerve, 161
Genitourinary system
    anatomy of, 381–383
Genitourinary trauma, 388–389
    radiographic studies of, 388–389
GERD, 191–192, 192f
Germ-cell tumors, 412–413
    malignant, 376
Gerota fascia, 381
Gestational trophoblastic disease (GTD), 414
GFR, 385
Giant cell tumors, 446t
GIP, 275
Glasgow coma scale, 18, 18t
Glenohumeral joint, 453
Glioblastoma multiforme (GBM), 30
Glioblastomas, 30
Glioma, 30
Gliosis, 3
Glisson capsule, 256
Global aphasia, 12
Glomerular filtration rate (GFR), 385
Glossopharyngeal nerve, 422
Glottis, 426–427
Glucagon, 216, 491
Glucagonoma, 499
Glucocorticoids, 21
Gluconeogenesis, 286
Glucose, 285
Glutamine, 127, 289–290
Glycine, 117, 117f
Glycolysis, 285, 285f
Glycosaminoglycans (GAGs), 114
GnRH, 405
Goblet cells, 211–212
Goiters, 473
Gold standard, 181
Gompertzian growth, 86
Gonadotropin-releasing hormone (GnRH), 405
Goodsall's rule, 252f, 253
Gram-negative bacterial sepsis, 67–68
Granulation tissue, 115
Granulomatous thyroiditis, 470
Granulosa theca cell tumors, 413
Graves disease, 469–470
Gray rami communicantes, 198
Gray scale, 13
Greater omentum, 197
Greenstick fractures, 440, 440f
Groin
    dissection of, 94, 94f
    hernias of, 161–168
Growth
    dysregulation of, 74
Growth factor receptor oncogenes, 74, 74f
Growth factors, 114
Growth fraction, 73
GTD, 414
Guidelines for the Management of Severe Head Injury, 20–21

Gut-associated lymphoid tissue (GALT), 213
Gut hormones, 214–216, 215f

H
HA, 115–116
Haemophilus influenzae, 109
Haemophilus influenzae type B, 60
Halogenated pyrimidines, 84
Halothane, 143
Halothane hepatitis, 143
Hand
    amputation of, 457–458
    fractures of, 456–457
    injuries of, 457–458
    nerves of, 457–458, 458f, 458t
Hangman's fracture, 22
Haplotype, 44
Haplotype matches, 44
Hartmann operation, 239
Hashimoto thyroiditis, 470–471
HCC, 258–259
HCG, 413
HDLs, 334
Head
    injuries of, 18–19
        critical pathways for, 21
        guidelines for, 20–21
        hyperventilation in, 21
        outcomes of, 21–22
    lymphatics of, 425–426, 426f
Head and neck neoplasms, 424–425
Hearing loss, 416–417
Heart
    anatomy of, 304–306
    electrophysiology of, 307–310
    embryology of, 303–304, 303f
    mechanics of, 310–311
    neoplasms of, 329
    penetrating injuries to, 329
    physiology of, 306–307
Heart disease
    acquired, 323–331
    congenital, 313–323
    end-stage, 56
Heart-lung transplantation, 58
Heart transplantation, 56–57, 57f
    contraindications for, 56
Heineke-Mikulicz pyloroplasty, 203, 204f
Helicobacter pylori, 201, 202t, 203, 206
Helper T cells, 39
Hemangioblastomas, 32
Hemangiomas, 232
Hematologic neoplasms, 105
Hematoma
    auricular, 429, 430f
    epidural, 18–19, 20f
    flank, 389
    intraparenchymal, 20
    subdural, 19, 20f
Hemobilia, 261–262
Hemodilution, 27
Hemophilia A, 301
Hemorrhoids, 250–251, 250f
Hemostasis, 295–303, 296f
Hemothorax, 372

Heparin, 301
Hepatic abscesses, 260
Hepatic allograft rejection, 53
Hepatic artery
 aneurysms of, 350
 thrombosis of, 53
Hepatic cysts, 260
Hepatic trauma, 260–262
Hepatitis
 halothane, 143
Hepatobiliary system, 256–278
Hepatoblastoma, 259
Hepatocellular adenoma, 258
Hepatocellular carcinoma (HCC), 258–259
Hepatocytes, 266–267, 267f
Hepatocyte–stimulating factor, 115
Hereditary elliptocytosis, 106
Hereditary (familial) breast cancer, 69–70
Hereditary nonpolyposis colorectal cancer, 242
Hereditary spherocytosis, 105–106
Hernias, 159–173
 anterior abdominal wall, 168–171
 congenital diaphragmatic, 172–173, 172f
 epigastric, 169
 femoral, 168
 funicular, 161
 groin, 161–168
 incisional, 169–171
 inguinal, 161, 168
 Littre, 161–162
 lumbar, 170f, 171
 obturator, 171
 pantaloon, 161
 pediatric developmental, 172–173, 172f
 pelvic, 171–172
 perineal, 171–172
 sciatic, 172
 sliding, 161, 162f
 spigelian, 169, 169f
 umbilical, 168
Herniorrhaphy
 laparoscopic, 166–167, 167f
Herpes simplex encephalitis, 33
Herpes simplex virus I
 in burn wounds, 135
Hesselbach triangle, 160
Heterotopic auxiliary heart transplantation, 56
Heterotopic ossification, 450, 455
High density lipoproteins (HDLs), 334
High–flow priapism, 392
High imperforate anus, 254
High–output fistula, 227
Hip
 dislocations of, 460, 460f
 fractures of, 460–461, 461f
Hirschsprung disease, 254
Histiocytosis X, 370
Histocompatibility, 43–44, 44f
Histoplasmosis, 375
HIV, 122
HLA, 44
Hodgkin disease, 106
Hodgkin lymphoma, 101–102, 102f, 376
Homeostasis, 385–386

Homonymous hemianopsia, 11
Hormone replacement therapy (HRT), 507–508
Hormones, 79–80, 86
 in cancer, 71–72
Host defenses, 59–60
 surgical breach of, 60
Hounsfield number scale, 13f
24–hour pH monitoring, 188
HRT, 507–508
Human chorionic gonadotropin (HCG), 413
Human immunodeficiency virus (HIV), 122
Human leukocyte antigen (HLA), 44
Human secretory IgA
 structure of, 213f
Humbry guarded knife, 133–134, 134f
Humeral shaft
 fractures, 455, 455f
Humoral immune response, 38
Hunt–Hess grading scale, 26–27
Hunting reaction, 138
Hurthle cell tumors, 476
Hyaline cartilage, 443
Hyaluronic acid (HA), 115–116
Hydatid cyst, 260
Hydatidiform moles, 414
Hydatidosis, 33–34
Hydrocephalus, 15, 16f
 causes of, 16
 external, 15
Hydrochloric acid, 200f
Hydrofluoric acid burn, 137
Hydrogen cyanide, 129
Hydromelia, 16
Hydroxyapatite crystals, 438
Hyperacute rejection, 45
Hyperaldosteronism, 486
Hyperbaric oxygenation, 67
Hypercalcemia, 479, 479t
Hypercortisolism, 484–486
Hyperdense, 14
Hyperintense, 14
Hyperkalemia, 137, 151
Hyperlipidemia, 333
Hypermagnesemia, 153
Hypernatremia, 150
Hyperparathyroidism, 479–480
Hyperplastic polyps, 240
Hyperpolarization, 4
Hyperprolactinemia, 32
Hypersplenism, 105
Hypertension, 27, 333–334
Hypertensive hemorrhage, 28
Hyperthermia
 malignant, 146
Hyperthyroidism, 469
Hypertrophic pyloric stenosis, 201
Hypertrophic scars, 121
Hyperventilation
 in head–injured patient, 21
Hypervolemia, 27
Hypocalcemia, 151–152, 152f, 481, 481t, 493
Hypodense, 13–14

Hypoglossal nerve, 422
Hypointense, 14
Hypokalemia, 150–151
Hypomagnesemia, 153
Hyponatremia, 150
Hypopharynx, 422
Hypophysis, 9
Hypoplastic left heart syndrome, 322
Hypothalamus-pituitary axis, 483–484, 484f
Hypothalamus-pituitary-ovarian axis
 endocrinology of, 405–406, 406f
Hypothermia, 49
Hypothesis testing, 179–181
Hypothyroidism, 469
Hypovolemia
 treatment of, 157–158
Hypovolemic shock, 155, 493
Hypoxemia, 127
Hypoxia, 361–362, 361t

I

IABP, 158, 312, 312t
IBD, 228
IC, 357
ICAM, 113
ICP monitor, 15
Idiopathic hypertrophic subaortic stenosis (IHSS), 326
Idiopathic thrombocytopenic purpura (ITP), 106
IDLs, 334
IgG, 38f
IHSS, 326
IL-1, 115
Ileoanal anastomosis, 239–240
Ileum, 211
Ileus, 127
Iliohypogastric nerve, 161
Ilioinguinal nerve, 161
Iliopubic tract, 161
ILP, 99
Imipenem, 64
Immune system, 37
 cells of, 38–48
Immunodeficiency, 72
Immunoglobulin
 abilities of, 38t
Immunological ignorance, 46
Immunomodulators, 88
Immunosuppression
 and wound healing, 122
Immunotherapy, 88
 adoptive, 89
 for breast cancer, 517
Imperforate anus, 254
Impotence, 349
IM rod, 449
IMV, 362
Incidentaloma, 488
Incisional biopsy, 80
Incisional hernias, 169–171
Indirect allorecognition, 45, 45f
Indirect inguinal hernias, 161
Induction chemotherapy, 87
Infection, 32–34

Infective endocarditis, 327
Inferential statistics, 176–179
Infiltrating ductal carcinoma, 509–510, 510f
Inflammatory abdominal aortic aneurysms (AAA), 349
Inflammatory bowel disease (IBD), 228
Inflammatory polyps, 240
Information bias, 174–175
Infrainguinal occlusive disease
    claudication resulting from, 342
Infratentorial herniation, 22
Infundibulum, 9
Inguinal canal, 160
Inguinal hernias
    diagnosis of, 162–163
    direct, 161
    etiology of, 162
    recurrent, 168
    surgery of, 163–168
    treatment of, 163
Inguinal herniorrhaphy, 163
Inguinal (Poupart) ligament, 159
Inhalational agents, 142–143, 142t
Inhalation injury, 127–128
Inherited breast cancer syndromes, 507–508
Injection sclerotherapy, 264
Injury
    metabolism in, 289–290, 289f
Inspiratory capacity (IC), 357
Inspiratory reserve volume (IRV), 357
Insulin, 491
Insulin-dependent diabetics, 53–54
Insulinoma, 497–498
Intercostobrachial nerve, 502
Intermediate density lipoproteins (IDLs), 334
Intermittent claudication, 342
Intermittent mandatory ventilation (IMV), 362
Internal data, 176
Internal fixation, 448–449
Internal hydrocephalus, 15
Internal oblique muscle, 160
Intervertebral foramen
    stenosis of, 34–35
Intestinal atresia, 201, 218–219, 219f
Intestinal epithelial cell, 213f
Intestinal obstructions
    classification of, 223t
Intestinal stenosis, 218–219, 219f
Intraabdominal chemotherapy, 87
Intraabdominal infection, 66–67
Intraaortic balloon pump (IABP), 158, 312, 312t
Intraarterial chemotherapy, 87
Intracellular adhesion molecule (ICAM), 113
Intracellular fluid, 148
Intradermal nevi, 92
Intraductal carcinoma, 508–509
Intramembranous ossification, 439
Intraparenchymal hematoma, 20
Intrarenal failure, 387
Intrathecal therapy, 87
Intravenous anesthesia, 143–145, 143t

Intrinsic coagulation pathway, 296
Intrinsic factor, 200
Intussusception, 219–220, 220f
Iodine, 466
Ionizing radiation, 82
Iron deficiency anemia, 206
IRV, 357
Ischemia
    acute, 343
Ischemic cerebrovascular disease, 28
Ischemic rest pain, 343
Ischemic ulcers, 343
Isointense, 14
Isolated limb perfusion (ILP), 99
ITP, 106
Ivor-Lewis operation, 194–195, 195f

J
Jefferson fracture, 22
Juvenile polyps, 240

K
Kaposi sarcoma, 72
Kasabach-Merritt syndrome, 257–258
Kehr sign, 107
Keloids, 121
Kerckring folds, 211
Ketamine, 144
Ketoconazole, 65
Kidneys
    anatomy of, 385, 386f
    physiology of, 385–388
    trauma of, 389–390
    vasculature of, 385–386, 386f
Kidney transplantation, 49–51, 50f
Killian triangle, 185
Knee
    dislocation of, 462
    soft tissue injuries of, 461–462
Krukenberg tumors, 210

L
Laboratory studies
    for preoperative workup, 139–140, 140t
Lacunar ligament, 159
Lag screws, 448–449
LAK cells, 89
Lamellar bone, 438
Laminectomy, 15
Laparoscopic herniorrhaphy, 166–167, 167f
Laparoscopic Nissen fundoplication, 191–192, 192f
Laparoscopic splenectomy, 108–109
Large intestine
    anatomy of, 235–237, 236f
Laryngeal carcinoma, 428–429
    staging of, 428
Laryngeal trauma, 434f, 435, 435f
Larynx, 426–429, 427f
Law of Wolff, 442
LCSG, 368
LDLs, 334
Lecithin, 269
Le Fort II fracture, 431–432, 432f
Left coronary artery, 305–306, 306f

    anomalous origin of from pulmonary artery, 320
Left gastric vena caval shunt, 226f
Left-to-right shunts, 313–317
Left ventricular end-diastolic volume (LVEDV), 141
Leiomyomas, 194, 231–232
Leiomyosarcomas, 233, 233f, 409–410
Lentigo maligna melanoma, 92
Leptomeninges, 5
LES, 187
Leukocytes
    recruitment of, 113f
Levamisole, 89, 244
Leydig cells, 385
Lichtenstein repair, 165, 166f
LICU, 507
Lidocaine, 145
Li-Fraumeni syndrome, 97, 508
Ligament of Berry, 464–466
Ligament of Treitz, 211
Ligaments
    of internal pelvic organs, 403
Limb-threatening ischemia, 342–343
Linear fractures, 19
Linear regression, 178
Lingual nerve, 422
Lingual thyroid gland, 464
Linitis plastica, 209–210
Lipids, 281, 286
    absorption of, 281, 282f
    metabolism of, 334, 335f
Lipomas, 232
Lipomyelomeningocele, 17
Lipopolysaccharide, 68
    chemical structure of, 62, 62f
Littre hernias, 161–162
Liver, 278–279
    abscesses of, 260
    allograft rejection, 53
    anatomy of, 256
    benign tumors of, 257–258
    cysts of, 260
    failure of
        Child's classification of, 265, 265t
    lobar anatomy of, 256, 256f
    malignant tumors of, 258–259
    metastases to, 82
    metastatic tumors of, 259–260
    studies of, 256–257
    trauma of, 260–262
Liver function tests, 256–257
Liver transplantation, 51–53, 52f
    contraindications for, 52
    postoperative complications of, 52–53
Living donor nephrectomy, 49–50
LMN, 11
Lobular carcinoma
    vs. ductal carcinoma, 509f
Lobular carcinoma in situ (LICU), 507
Local anesthetics, 145–146, 145t
Localizing sign
    false, 29
Locally advanced breast cancer
    management of, 515
Loop diuretics, 388

Low density lipoproteins (LDLs), 334
Lower esophageal sphincter (LES), 187
Lower extremities
   injuries of, 460–463
Lower extremity ischemia
   acute, 345–347
      etiology of, 345–346
      treatment of, 346–347
   chronic, 340–344
      noninvasive testing of, 343–344, 344f
Lower gastrointestinal bleeding, 247
Lower motor neuron (LMN), 11
Low–grade astrocytomas, 30
Ludwig angina, 374, 422, 423f
Lumbar hernias, 170f, 171
Lumbar spin stenosis, 36
Lumboperitoneal shunt, 16
Lumbosacral spine, 35
Lundh test, 491–492
Lung cancer, 365–369
   classification of, 366t
   epidemiology of, 365–366
   incidence of, 365–366
   molecular biology of, 365–366
   recurrence of, 368
   staging of, 367f
Lung Cancer Study Group (LCSG), 368
Lung disease
   benign, 364
Lungs
   compliance of, 356–357, 357f
   injuries of, 379–380
   vasculature of, 358–360
Lung transplantation, 57–58
Lung tumors
   benign, 369
Lung volumes, 357–358, 357f
Lung zones, 359f
LVEDV, 141
Lymphatics, 333
Lymphatic spread
   adjuvant therapy for, 95
   radiation therapy for, 95
Lymph nodes
   biopsy of, 95, 101
   dissection of, 81
      complications of, 95
Lymphocytic thyroiditis
   chronic, 470–471
Lymphoepithelial lesion of Godwin
   benign, 420
Lymphoid organs, 37, 37f
Lymphokine-activated killer cells (LAK cells), 89
Lymphokines, 43
Lymphoma, 101–103, 473
   diffuse, 376
   Hodgkin, 376
   non–Hodgkin, 10
   primary CNS, 31–32
   of thyroid, 477
Lynch syndrome, 70–71, 242
Lysine oxidase, 118
Lysis, 295–297

Lysyl hydroxylase, 117
Lytic agents, 373

M

MAC, 142
MACIS (metastasis, age, completeness of resection, invasion, size), 474
Macrolides, 64
Macrophages, 115
Macula, 417
Mafenide acetate, 135
Magnesium, 288
   imbalance of, 153
Magnetic resonance angiography (MRA), 14, 344
Magnetic resonance imaging (MRI), 14
   for AAA, 348
   for lung cancer, 365
   of thyroid gland, 468–469
Magnetic resonance venography (MRV), 14
Major ampullae of Vater, 211
Major histocompatibility class 1 antigens
   structure of, 44f
Major histocompatibility class II antigens
   structure of, 44f
Malaria, 105
Male breast cancer, 518
Malformations
   arteriovenous, 14, 247
   congenital, 17–18
Malignant cells
   characteristics of, 72–73
Malignant chest wall tumors, 370
Malignant esophageal neoplasms, 194–196, 195f, 196t
Malignant fibrous histiocytoma, 447t
Malignant germ-cell tumors, 376
Malignant hyperthermia, 146
Malignant mesothelioma, 373
Malignant mixed tumors, 421
Malignant nonseminomatous tumors, 376–377
Malignant otitis externa, 418
Malignant pleural disease, 373
Mallory-Weiss syndrome, 193
Malnutrition, 262, 284
Malrotation, 218
MALT, 37
MALT lymphoma, 103
Malunion, 449
Mammary duct ectasia, 505
Mammography, 503, 503t
Mandibular fractures, 429–431
Mandibular trauma, 429–431
Marfan syndrome, 330
Mastalgia, 504
Mastectomy
   modified radical, 513, 514f
Mastitis, 505
Maxillary sinus, 436
Maxillary trauma, 431–433
MCL, 461–462
McNemar test, 179
McVay repair, 164, 165f
Mdr, 86

Mean, 177, 177f
Mechanical cardiac assistance, 311–312
Mechanical ventilation, 362–363, 363f
Meckel diverticulum, 217, 220, 221f
Meconium ileus, 222
Meconium peritonitis, 222
Meconium plug syndrome, 222
Medial cruciate ligament (MCL), 461–462
Median, 177, 177f
Median nerve, 458t
Mediastinal carcinoma
   primary, 377
Mediastinal cysts, 377
Mediastinal disease, 374–378
Mediastinal germ-cell tumors, 376
Mediastinal masses, 375–376, 375t
Mediastinitis, 374
Mediastinoscopy
   for lung cancer, 365
Mediastinum
   structure of, 375t
Medulla, 7
Medullary thyroid cancer (MTC), 476–477, 476t
Medulloblastomas, 31
Melanoma, 91–95
   acral lentiginous, 92
   classification of, 92–93
   desmoplastic, 93
   differential diagnosis of, 91–92, 91f
   distant metastases of, 95–96
   familial, 70
   of head and neck, 95
   history and physical examination for, 92
   lentigo maligna, 92
   local recurrences of, 96
   mucosal, 93
   nodular, 92
   prognosis of, 96–97, 96f
   staging of, 93, 93f, 93t
   superficial spreading, 92
   surgical treatment of, 93–94
Meniere disease, 417–418
Meningeal carcinomatosis, 32
Meninges, 5
Meningiomas, 31
Meningocele, 17
Menstrual cycle, 405
MEN syndromes, 70, 71t
Meperidine, 144
Mepivacaine, 146
Mercaptopurine, 239
Mesenteric ischemia, 350–351, 350f–351f
   chronic, 351–352
Mesenteric venous thrombosis, 351
Mesocaval shunt, 265
Mesosalpinx, 403
Mesothelioma
   malignant, 373
Metabolic acidosis, 153–154
Metabolic alkalosis, 154
Metabolism, 284–290
   in starvation, 288–289
   in stress, 289–290
Metastasis, 75–76, 76f

surgery for, 81–82
Methotrexate, 48
Metronidazole, 240
Micelles, 281
Microbial flora, 59
Microdiskectomy, 15
Microglial cells, 3
Microvilli, 211
Midazolam, 143–144
Midbrain, 7
Migrating motor complex (MMC), 214
Milk streak, 501
Milrinone, 158
Minerals, 282–283, 287–288
Minimum alveolar concentration (MAC), 142
Minor ampulla of Santorini, 211
Mitotic inhibitors, 86
Mitral regurgitation, 326–327
Mitral stenosis, 319–320, 326
Mitral valve prolapse, 328, 328f
Mitral valves, 305, 305f
Mixed acid–base disorders, 155
Mixed tumors
 malignant, 421
MMC, 214
Mode, 177, 177f
Modified radical mastectomy, 513, 514f
MODS, 155, 493
Monckeberg medial calcific sclerosis, 332
Mondor disease, 505
Monoclonal antibodies, 48, 88
Monocytes, 299
Monokines, 43
Monro–Kellie hypothesis, 29
Monteggia fractures, 456, 456f
Morphine, 144
Motilin, 216
Motor homunculus, 10–11, 12f
Mouth, 284
MRA, 14, 344
MRI, 14
 for AAA, 348
 for lung cancer, 365
 of thyroid gland, 468–469
MRV, 14
MTC, 476–477, 476t
Mucoepidermoid carcinoma, 369, 421
Mucosa–associated lymphoid tissue (MALT), 37
Mucosal melanoma, 93
Mucosal villi, 211
Multimodal distribution, 177
Multiple endocrine neoplasia, 70, 71t
Multiple myeloma, 447t
Multiple–organ dysfunction syndrome (MODS), 155, 493
Muscle fibers, 444
Muscle relaxants, 144–145, 144t
Muscles, 444–445, 444f
 biomechanics of, 445
Muscular tetany, 152
Myasthenia gravis, 375–376
Mycobacterium tuberculosis, 364
Mycophenolate mofetil, 48, 57

Mycotic aneurysms, 27, 349
Myelin, 3–4
Myelography, 14
Myelomeningocele, 17
Myelopathy, 35
Myeloschisis, 17
Myocardial infarction, 324
Myofibrils, 444, 444f
Myoglobinuria, 137
Myosin thick filaments, 444
Myxomas, 329

N
NADPH, 115
Nasal fracture, 433
Nasoenteric tube, 290–291
Nasopharyngeal carcinoma, 424, 425f
Nasopharynx, 422, 425f
National Surgery Adjuvant Breast and Bowel Project (NSABP), 244, 508
Natural killer cells (NK cells), 89
NEC, 220–223, 221f
Neck
 fractures of, 22
 lymphatics of, 425–426, 426f
 neoplasms of, 424–425
 penetrating trauma of, 424–425, 433f
Necrotizing enterocolitis (NEC), 220–223, 221f
Necrotizing fasciitis, 67
Necrotizing soft tissue infection, 67
Needle (core) biopsy, 80
Negative predictive value, 181, 182f
Neisseria meningitidis, 109
Neoadjuvant therapy, 87
Nervous system
 anatomy of, 4–10
 functional organization of, 10–13
Neurapraxia, 24
Neuraxial blockade, 140
Neurenteric cysts, 17
Neurilemmomas, 378
Neuroblastomas, 378, 487
Neuroendocrine response, 289
Neurofibromatosis I, 97
Neurofibromatosis type II, 31
Neurogenic claudication, 36
Neurogenic dumbbell tumor, 377f
Neurogenic obstruction, 226
Neurogenic shock
 treatment of, 158
Neurogenic tumors, 377–378
Neuromas, 25, 418
Neuron, 3
Neuron–specific enolase (NSE), 79
Neuroradiology, 14–15
Neurotmesis, 25
Neurotransmitters, 4
Neutrophil products, 114t
Neutrophils, 114–115
Nevi
 acquired, 91
 congenital, 91
 intradermal, 92
New York Heart Association

 functional classification, 323, 323t
Nicotinamide adenine dinucleotide phosphate (NADPH), 115
Nipples
 accessory, 501
 discharge from, 504
 Paget's disease of, 518
Nissen fundoplication
 laparoscopic, 191–192, 192f
Nitric oxide, 295
Nitrous oxide, 142–143
NK cells, 40, 41f, 89
Nodes of Ranvier, 4
Nodular melanoma, 92
Nominal data, 176–177
Noncommunicating hydrocephalus, 15
Non–Hodgkin lymphoma, 10
Nonocclusive mesenteric ischemia, 351
Nonossifying fibroma, 446t
Nonparametric statistical tests, 178
Nonseminomatous germ cell tumors (NSGCTs), 396–397, 396t
 classification of, 396, 396t
Nonseminomatous tumors
 malignant, 376–377
Non–small cell lung cancer (NSCLC), 365–368
 adjuvant therapy of, 368
 resection of, 366–368
Nonspecific immunotherapy, 88
Nonunion, 449
Nonunion fracture, 442–443
Nose
 anatomy of, 436–437
 fracture of, 433
NSABP, 244, 508
NSAID–induced ulcers, 202, 206
NSCLC, 365–368
 adjuvant therapy of, 368
 resection of, 366–368
NSE, 79
NSGCTs, 396–397, 396t
 classification of, 396, 396t
Nuclear oncogenes, 74–75
Nucleus pulposus, 5
 herniation of, 34
Null hypothesis, 179–180
Nutcracker esophagus, 190
Nutrition, 284–290
Nutritional support, 290–291
Nystagmus, 418

O
Obliterative bronchiolitis, 58
Observational studies, 174–176
Obstructive cardiogenic shock, 155–156
Obstructive hydrocephalus, 15
Obturator hernias, 171
Occult spinal dysraphism, 17
Octreotide, 263
Odontoid fractures, 22–23
Odontoid process, 5
OER, 84
Ogilvie syndrome, 238
Oligodendrocytes, 3

534 Subject Index

Oligodendrogliomas, 30–31
Omeprazole, 203
Omphalocele, 173, 222–223
Oncocytomas, 393
Oncofetal antigens, 76–77
Oncofetal proteins, 77–78
Oncogenes, 74–75, 74f, 90
Open fractures, 451, 451t
Open incision biopsy, 445
Open nerve gliomas, 30
Open pneumothorax, 379
Open spinal dysraphism, 17
Opioids, 144
OPSI, 109
Oral cavity, 422–424
  malignant lesions of, 423–424, 424t
Oral glucose tolerance test, 492
Orbital cellulitis, 437
Orbital trauma, 431–433
Ordinal data, 176
Organ preservation, 48–49
Oropharynx, 422–424
Orthopedic pathology, 445–446
Orthopedic surgery, 438–446
  complications of, 449–452
  evaluation and treatment in, 446–449
Orthotopic heart transplantation, 56, 57f
Osmolality, 148–149, 149f
Osmotic diuretics, 388
Osteoarthritis, 443–444
Osteoblasts, 438
Osteochondromas, 370, 446t
Osteoclasts, 438
Osteocytes, 438
Osteogenic sarcomas, 370
Osteomyelitis, 32–33, 449
Osteonecrosis, 450
Osteophytes, 34
Osteosarcoma, 447t, 448f
Otitis externa
  malignant, 418
Otolithic organs, 417
Otologic infection, 418
Otologic neoplasms, 418–419
Otologic trauma, 429, 430f
Otomycosis, 418
Otorrhea, 418
Otosclerosis, 416
Ototoxic agents, 416
Outcome measures, 182
Ovaries
  arteries of, 404, 405f
  carcinoma of, 410–413, 412t
  metastasis to, 413
Overwhelming postsplenectomy infection (OPSI), 109
Oxygen, 83–84
Oxygen enhancement ratio (OER), 84
Oxyntic gland, 198, 199f

P
PABA test, 492
Pacemakers, 307–308, 328–329, 328t
Paget's disease of the nipple, 518
Paired t test, 178
Palliative chemotherapy, 87

Pancreas, 176–178, 176f
  anatomy and physiology of, 489–491, 490f
  arterial blood to, 489–490
  bladder drainage of, 54, 55f
  innervation of, 491
  lymphatic drainage from, 490
  pathology of, 492–497
  venous blood from, 490
Pancreas divisum, 489, 489f
Pancreas–kidney transplantation, 53
Pancreas transplantation, 53–55, 54f
  indications for, 53
Pancreatic abscess, 494–495
Pancreatic adenocarcinoma, 499–500
Pancreatic ascites, 494
Pancreatic duct
  in chronic pancreatitis, 497f
Pancreatic endocrine function
  tests of, 492
Pancreatic exocrine function
  tests of, 491–492
Pancreatic juice, 276–277, 277f
Pancreatic pseudocysts, 495
Pancreatic trauma, 497
Pancreatitis
  acute. See Acute pancreatitis
  chronic, 495–497, 496f
    with common bile duct stenosis, 496
    imaging of, 495
    mortality of, 496
    symptoms of, 495
    treatment of, 495–496, 496f
Pancreatoduodenectomy, 233, 233f, 500, 500f
Paneth cells, 212
Pantaloon hernias, 161
PAOP, 141
Papillary carcinoma, 464, 474
Papillary cystadenoma lymphomatosum, 420
Pap smear, 410
Paraaminobenzoic acid (PABA) test, 492
Parabronchial diverticula, 190
Paragangliomas, 418
Paranasal sinus infections, 436–437
Paraplegia, 349
Parasitic infection, 33
Parasympathetic nervous system, 13
Parasympathetic system, 309–310
Parathyroid carcinoma, 481
Parathyroid glands, 477–481, 478f
  pathophysiology of, 479–481
  physiology of, 478–479
Parathyroid hormone (PTH), 151, 479
Parenteral fluid, 149
Parenteral nutrition, 291
Parotid glands, 419
Parotid neoplasms, 421
Paroxysmal positional vertigo
  benign, 417
Partial seizure
  with secondary generalization, 30
Particulate radiation, 82
Patent ductus arteriosus (PDA), 315–316
Patent processus vaginalis, 162

PCL, 461–462
PDA, 315–316
PDGF, 112, 114, 333
PDT, 196
Pediatric developmental hernias, 172–173, 172f
PEEP, 362
Pelvic diaphragm, 171
Pelvic inflammatory disease (PID), 406–407, 407t
Pelvis
  autonomic nerves of, 404
  female, 397, 397f–398f
  fractures of, 458–459
  hernias of, 171–172
  masses of
    benign, 407–408
Penetrating cardiac injury, 329
Penicillin, 63
Penis, 387
  trauma of, 392
Pepsinogen, 200
Peptic ulcers, 201–208
  perforated, 207–208
Percutaneous transluminal angioplasty (PTA), 352–353
Perfusion, 354, 359
Periampulary tumors, 499–500
Perianal abscess, 252–253
Pericardial cysts, 377
Perineum
  coronal section of, 237f
  hernias of, 171–172
Period of normal excitability, 307
Peripheral arteries
  aneurysms of, 349–350
Peripheral nerve block, 140, 147
Peripheral nerve injuries, 24–26
Peripheral nerve stimulators, 142
Peripheral nervous system (PNS)
  microscopic anatomy of, 3
Peripheral vascular disease, 340–347
  therapeutic intervention in, 344–345
Peristalsis, 187–188
Peritonitis, 66–67
Peutz-Jeghers syndrome, 232
Pharynx, 284
  malignant lesions of, 423–424
  trauma to, 433
Pheochromocytomas, 378, 486–487
Phosphate, 49, 478–479
Phosphorous, 288
Photodynamic therapy (PDT), 196
Phyllodes tumor, 506
Physeal injuries, 441
Physical examination
  for preoperative workup, 139–140
PID, 406–407, 407t
Pigmented lesion, 91
  differential diagnosis of, 91, 92t
Pilocytic astrocytomas, 30
Pins, 448–449
Pituitary adenomas, 32
Pituitary hormones
  actions of, 9f
Placental hormone, 79–80

Plaque
 atheromatous, 334, 336f
Plasmacytomas, 370
Plasmin, 296
Platelet–derived growth factor (PDGF), 112, 114, 333
Platelets, 111, 297, 298f
 drugs affecting, 300
 products of, 113t
Plates, 448–449
Pleomorphic adenomas, 420
Pleural diseases, 371–373
 benign, 371–372
 malignant, 373
Pleural effusion, 371
Plummer disease, 470
PNETs, 31
Pneumatocele, 380
Pneumatosis, 221
Pneumonia, 127
Pneumothorax
 open, 379
PNS
 microscopic anatomy of, 3
Poland syndrome, 501
Polyclonal antibodies, 48
Polycythemia, 32
Polyhydramnios, 187
Polypoid carcinoma, 209–210
Polyps
 benign, 194
 colonic, 240–242
 hyperplastic, 240
 inflammatory, 240
 juvenile, 240
Polytetrafluoroethylene (PTFE), 344–345
Polythelia, 501
Pons, 7
Popliteal artery aneurysms, 349
Population, 176
Portacaval shunt, 265
Portal hypertension, 262–265, 263f
 collateralization of, 263f
Portal vein thrombosis, 262
Positive end–expiratory pressure (PEEP), 362
Positive predictive value, 181, 182f
Posterior cruciate ligament (PCL), 461–462
Posterior neuropores, 17
Postoperative graft
 surveillance of, 345
Postoperative ileus, 226
Postoperative radiation therapy, 85
Postoperative small bowel obstruction (SBO), 226
Postrenal failure, 387–388
Posttransplant lymphoproliferative disorder, 46
Posttraumatic arthritis, 449
Potassium, 148
 balance of, 387
 imbalance of, 150
Potassium–sparing diuretics, 388
Pouchitis, 240
Poupart (inguinal) ligament, 159
Power, 179

Pregnancy
 breast changes during, 502–503
 ectopic, 414
 surgical issues in, 414–415
Prehospital care
 of burn injury, 130
Preload, 310
Preoperative radiation therapy, 85
Preprogastrin, 199
Prerenal azotemia, 387
Prerenal failure, 387
Pressure control (PC) ventilation, 362
Pressure support (PS) ventilation, 362
Pressure–volume loops, 310, 311f
Priapism, 392
Primary CNS lymphomas, 31–32
Primary lymphoid organs, 37, 37f
Primary motor disorders, 188–190
Primary sclerosing cholangitis, 270
Primitive neural ectoderm tumors (PNETs), 31
Pringle maneuver, 261, 261f
Procollagen, 118
Proctitis, 227
Profundaplasty, 345
Proliferating cells, 73
Prolyl hydroxylase, 117
Propeptides, 118
 cleavage of, 118f
Propofol, 144
Prostacyclin, 297
Prostate cancer, 71, 397–398
 staging of, 397, 398t
Prostate gland, 387
Prostate–specific antigen (PSA), 76–77
Prostheses
 infection of, 68
Prosthetic ring annuloplasty, 328, 328f
Prosthetic valves, 327
Protein, 286–287, 287f
Proteoglycans, 115, 116f, 443
Prothrombin time (PT), 299
Proton pump inhibitors, 203
Protooncogenes, 74
Provisional matrix, 111
Proximal humerus
 fractures of, 454, 454f
Pruning, 351
PSA, 76–77
Pseudoaneurysm, 349
Pseudocholelithiasis, 64
Pseudohermaphroditism
 female, 487–488
Pseudohyponatremia, 150
Pseudomembranous colitis, 248–249
PT, 299
PTA, 352–353
PTFE, 344–345
PTH, 151, 479
Puborectalis muscle, 236
Pulmonary artery catheters
 for anesthesia monitoring, 141, 141t
Pulmonary artery occlusion pressure (PAOP), 141
Pulmonary atresia, 318–319
Pulmonary circulation, 306–307

Pulmonary embolism, 353
Pulmonary function tests, 357–358, 357f
 for lung cancer, 365–366
Pulmonary metastases, 82
 resection of, 368–369
Pulmonary parenchymal disorders
 end–stage, 58
Pulmonary parenchymal injuries, 379–380
Pulmonary physiology
 equations for, 361t
Pulmonary tuberculosis, 364
Pulmonary valves, 305, 327
Pulmonary valve stenosis (PVS), 318
Pulmonary vasculature, 358–360
Pulse volume recordings (PVRs), 343, 344f
Pulsion diverticula, 190
PVRs, 343, 344f
PVS, 318
Pylorus, 197
 obstruction of, 208
Pyrimidines
 halogenated, 84

Q

QALYs, 182
Quality–adjusted life–years (QALYs), 182
Quinsy tonsillectomy, 422–423

R

Radial nerve, 458t
Radial nerve palsy, 455
Radiation
 combined with chemotherapy, 85–88
 combined with surgery, 85
 complications of, 85
 pharmacologic modifiers of, 84
 techniques of, 82–83
 types of, 82
Radiation biology, 83
Radiation enteritis, 226–227
Radiation oncology, 82–88
Radiation survival curve, 83, 83f
Radiation therapy, 85
 for breast cancer, 517
 for lymphatic spread, 95
Radical oxygen intermediates, 49
Radicular symptoms, 35
Radioiodine therapy, 475–476
Radionuclide imaging
 of thyroid gland, 468
Raffinose, 49
Ramsay Hunt syndrome, 418
Randomization, 176
Randomized clinical trial, 176
Range, 177
Ranson's criteria
 for acute pancreatitis, 494, 494t
Rapamycin, 48
Ratio data, 176
RBF, 387–388
Reaction to injury hypothesis
 theory of atherosclerosis, 336–337, 336f
Recall bias, 174
Recipient operation, 50

Rectum
  anatomy of, 236–237, 237f
  coronal section of, 237f
  prolapse of, 251, 251f
Recurrences
  local, 96
Recurrent inguinal hernias, 168
Recurrent laryngeal nerve (RLN), 466
REE, 284
Reflex sympathetic dystrophy, 25–26
Refractory periods, 307
Regional anesthesia, 140, 146–147
Regional enteritis, 228–230
Regional lymph nodes, 94
Rejection, 44–45, 45f
Relative refractory periods, 307
Relaxing incision, 163
Renal artery stenosis, 352–353
Renal blood flow (RBF), 387–388
Renal cell carcinoma, 393–394
Renal failure
  acute, 387–388
Renal masses, 393
Renal pelvis, 381
Renal plasma flow (RPF), 388
Renal systemic renin index (RSRI), 352
Renal transplantation, 49–51, 50f
  postoperative complications of, 50–51
Renal trauma, 389–390
  blunt
    staging of, 389, 389t, 390f
Renin/angiotensin/aldosterone series, 388
Renin/angiotensin system, 484
Renin–dependent hypertension, 352
Renovascular hypertension, 352
Reoxygenation, 84
Repopulation, 83
Reproductive system
  female
    anatomy of, 400–404
    embryology of, 400, 401f
    lymphatic drainage of, 404
    pathology of, 406–414
Resection margin
  guidelines for, 93–94
Residual volume (RV), 357
Respiratory acidosis, 154
Respiratory alkalosis, 154–155
Resting energy expenditure (REE), 284
Resting membrane potential, 3
RET oncogene, 70
Retrograde urethrogram
  for GU trauma, 389
Retroperitoneal lymph node dissection, 396–397
Retroperitoneal soft tissue sarcoma, 100–101
  diagnosis of, 100
  treatment of, 100–101, 100f
Revascularization
  indications for, 324, 324t
Reversible ischemic neurological deficit (RIND), 28
Rhabdomyosarcomas, 329, 395
Ribosomal protein synthesis
  inhibitors of, 64

Richter hernia, 157, 157f
Riedel struma, 473
Right coronary artery, 306, 306f
Right–to–left shunts, 317–319
RIND, 28
Ring-enhancing lesion, 33
RLN, 471
Rotator cuff tears, 453
Roux-en-Y cystojejunostomy, 496f
RPF, 388
RSRI, 352
Ruptured arteriovenous malformations (AVMs), 27–28
RV, 357

S
Sacromere, 444, 444f
Saddle anesthesia, 36
SAH, 14
Salivary glands
  anatomy of, 419f
  malignant tumors of, 420–422
  pathophysiology of, 419–422
  trauma to, 436
Salivary secretion, 273f
Sample, 176
Sample selection process, 176
Sarcomas, 81, 409–410
  extremity soft tissue. See Extremity soft tissue sarcoma
SBO, 223–236, 224f
  symptoms of, 223, 225
  treatment of, 225–226
SBS, 230–231
Scalp, 4
  laceration of, 18–19
Scapular fractures, 452–453
Scar formation
  excessive, 121
Schwann cells, 3
Sciatica, 36
Sciatic hernias, 172
SCLC, 368
Scleroderma, 190
Scrotal pain
  acute
    differential diagnosis of, 392
Scrotum, 387
  trauma of, 392
Secondary hyperparathyroidism, 51
Secondary lymphoid organs, 37, 37f
Second–degree injury, 25
Secretin, 215, 216
Secretin stimulation test, 498
Segmental colonic resection, 243f
Selective portosystemic shunt, 265–266, 266f
Sella turcica, 9
Semilunar aortic valves, 305
Seminomas, 376
  classification of, 396, 397t
Semustine, 244
Sengstaken–Blakemore tube, 263–264
Sensitivity, 181
Sensorineural hearing loss, 416–417
Sensory homunculus, 10–11, 12f

Sentinel bleed, 26
Sentinel nodes, 81
Sepsis
  metabolism in, 289–290
Septic shock, 67–68
  treatment of, 158
Septum, 436
Sequestration, 66
Serotherapy, 88
Serotonin, 216
Serous cystadenomas, 408
Sertoli cells, 387
Sertoli-Leydig tumors, 413
Serum glutamic–oxaloacetic transaminase, 256
Serum glutamic–pyruvic transaminase, 256
Serum total T4 concentration, 467
Sevoflurane, 143
Sex cord stromal tumors, 413
Shear rate, 338
Shear stress, 338
Shock, 155–156, 155t
  cardiovascular response to, 156
  diagnosis of, 157
  management of, 157
  pathophysiology of, 156
  physiologic characteristics of, 157t
  pulmonary response to, 156–157
  renal response to, 157
Short-bowel syndrome (SBS), 230–231
Short-gut syndrome, 230–231
Shoulder
  dislocations of, 453
  injuries of, 453–454
  separations of, 453
Shouldice repair, 164, 164f
Shunt, 361–362
SIADH, 150
Sialolithiasis, 419–420
Sickle cell disease, 106
Sigmoid colon ischemia, 349
Sigmoid volvulus, 248, 248f
Signal transduction oncogenes, 74
Silvadene, 135
Silver sulfadiazine, 135
Simple partial seizure, 30
SIMV, 362
Sinoatrial node, 308
Sinoorbital infections, 435f, 437
Sinus
  anatomy of, 436–437
SIRS, 156
Sistrunk procedure, 464
Sjogren syndrome, 419–420, 420f
Skin-sparing effect, 82
Skipper's law, 85–86
Skull, 4
  fractures of, 19
Sliding hernias, 161, 162f
Slow cardiac action potential, 309f
SMA, 211
Small bowel, 211–234
  anatomy of, 211–212
  benign diseases of, 223–231
  diseases of
    in children, 218–223

diverticular disease of, 227
embryology of, 216–217, 217f
immunity of, 213–214, 213f
motility of, 214
physiology of, 212–213
transplantation of, 55, 56f
tumors of, 231–234
Small bowel–liver transplantation, 55
Small bowel obstruction (SBO), 223–236, 224f
   symptoms of, 223, 225
   treatment of, 225–226
Small cell lung cancer (SCLC), 368
Small intestine, 279–283, 284f
Smoke, 128
Smoking, 334
Smooth muscle cells, 333, 337
Sodium, 148
   balance of, 388
   imbalance of, 150
Soft disk, 34
Soft tissue sarcomas, 97–100, 370
   etiology of, 97
   of extremities. *See* Extremity soft tissue sarcoma
   extremity, 97–100
   retroperitoneal, 100–101
Solitary intraductal papillomas, 506
Solitary toxic nodules, 470
Somatostatin, 215–216, 491
Somatostatinoma, 499
Spermatic cord, 160–161, 160t
Spherocytosis
   hereditary, 105–106
Spiculated cancer, 511f
Spigelian hernias, 169, 169f
Spina bifida, 17
Spina bifida aperta, 17
Spina bifida cystica, 17
Spina bifida occulta, 17
Spinal anesthesia, 140
Spinal cord, 4–5, 4f
   anatomy of, 9–10
   arterial blood supply of, 10, 10f
   injuries of, 23–24
Spinal dysraphism, 17
Spine
   degenerative disease of, 31–36
   fracture of, 234
   fractures of, 23
Spiral fractures, 440, 441f
Spirometry, 357, 357f
Splanchnic artery aneurysms, 350
Spleen, 103–105
   anatomy of, 103–104, 104f
   rupture of, 106
Splenectomy, 60, 105–109, 108f
   complications of, 109
   laparoscopic, 108–109
   technical considerations of, 107–108
Splenomegaly, 105, 262–263
Split cord malformation, 17
Spondylolisthesis, 36
Spondyiosis
   cervical, 35
Spontaneous pneumothorax, 371–372

Squamous cell carcinoma, 194, 395, 424t
Staging laparotomy, 101, 102f
Standard deviation, 177
Starvation
   metabolism in, 288–289
Statistical methods, 176–177
Statistical significance, 180
Statistical tests
   selection of, 179
Steal syndrome, 27
Stellate fractures, 19
Stereotactic biopsy, 15
Stereotactic radiosurgery, 32
Sternoclavicular dislocations, 452, 453f
Sternum
   fractures of, 379
Steroid synthesis
   pathways of, 483, 483f
Stewart-Treves syndrome, 97
Stomach, 274–276, 274f
   anatomy of, 197–199
   cancer of, 209–210
   parts of, 197, 198f
   physiology of, 199–201
   venous drainage of, 197, 198f
Straight-leg raising test, 35–36
Stress
   metabolism in, 289–290
Stress ulcers, 209
Stria vascularis, 417
Stricturoplasty, 225f, 229
Stroke, 28–29
Stroke volume (SV), 156
Struma thyroiditis, 470–471
Studies
   design of, 174–176
Subacute subdural hematoma, 19
Subacute thyroiditis, 470
Subarachnoid hemorrhage (SAH), 14
Subdiaphragmatic diverticula, 191
Subdural abscess, 33
Subdural hematoma, 19, 20f
   chronic, 19
Subdural window, 13
Subfalcine herniation, 22
Subgaleal abscess, 32
Subglottis, 426–427
Submandibular glands, 419
Submersion injury
   pattern of, 133f
Substance P, 216
Substantia nigra, 7
Succinylcholine, 145, 145t
Sucking chest wound, 379
Sucralfate, 203, 209
Sugiura operation, 264, 264f
Suicide gene therapy, 90
Sulfamylon, 135
Sulfasalazine, 239
Superficial inguinal ring, 159–160
Superficial spreading carcinoma, 209–210
Superficial spreading melanoma, 92
Superior laryngeal nerve, 471
Superior mesenteric artery (SMA), 211
Supraglottis, 426–427
Supranormal period, 307

Supratentorial brain herniation, 22
Surgery
   combined with radiation, 85
   prophylaxis for, 65–66
Surgical infection
   pathogenesis of, 60–61, 61t
   therapy guidelines of, 66
Surgical patients
   impaired host defenses in, 59–60
Suspensory ligament of Cooper, 501
SV, 156
Swallowing, 187, 273, 273f
Swedish Melanoma Study Group trial, 93
Sympathectomy, 26
Sympathetic nervous system, 13, 311, 484
Sympathetic tone, 388
Synchronized intermittent mandatory ventilation (SIMV), 362
Syndrome of inappropriate antidiuretic hormone secretion (SIADH), 150
Syringomyelia, 16
Systemic inflammatory response syndrome (SIRS), 156

T

Tacrolimus, 47–48, 57
Tamoxifen, 517–518
Tapeworm, 34
TAPP repair, 167
TAPVC, 322
Tardy ulnar palsy, 25
TBSA, 123, 131–132, 132f
TBW, 148
T-cell
   activation of, 40f
   two-signal model of, 43f
T-cell precursors, 39f
T-cell receptor, 39, 39f
Teardrop fractures, 23
Technetium–99m pertechnetate, 468
Tectospinal tract, 11
TEE, 142
Teletherapy, 83
Tension pneumothorax, 380
TEP repair, 167
Teratomas, 376
Terminal bronchioles, 354
Terminal ileum, 228–229
Testes, 387
Testicular cancer, 395–396
Testicular torsion, 392
Test-meal pancreatic polypeptide (PP) response, 492
Tethered cord, 18
Tetracaine, 146
Tetralogy of Fallot, 317, 317f
TGF-beta, 112
Thalamus, 7
Thalassemia major, 106
Therapeutic range, 84
Thermal injury, 290
Thiazides, 388
Third-degree injury, 25
Thoracic aorta
   aneurysms of, 331
Thoracic nerve of Bell, 502

Thoracic outlet syndrome (TOS), 373–374, 374f
Thoracic spine, 35
Thoracic trauma, 378–380
Thoracodorsal nerve, 502
Thoracolumbar spine
 fractures at, 23
 three–column model of, 23, 23f
Thrombin time (TT), 299–300
Thrombosis, 295–303
Thrombotic occlusion
 acute, 350–351
Thrombotic thrombocytopenic purpura (TTP), 106
Thymomas, 375
Thyroglossal duct, 464
Thyroid carcinoma, 71–72, 477–480, 478t
 cervical lymph node metastases from, 477
Thyroid function tests, 472–473
Thyroid gland, 469–480
 anatomy of, 469–471, 470f
 arterial supply to, 470, 470f
 benign conditions of, 474–476
 imaging of, 473–474
 lymphatic drainage of, 471
 physiology of, 471–472
 venous blood supply from, 470–471
Thyroid hormone, 471–472, 472f
Thyroiditis, 475
 acute, 475
Thyroid nodules, 476–477
Thyroplasty, 424
TIA, 28
Tibial fractures, 465
 traction for, 449f
Tibial plateau
 fractures of, 464, 464f
Tibial traction pin, 449f
Ticlopidine, 300
TILs, 89
TIPS, 264
Tissue hypoperfusion, 156
Tissue thromboplastin, 111
TLC, 357
T lymphocytes, 38–39, 39f
TNF, 115
TOA, 407
Tolbutamide response test, 492
Tolerance, 46
Topical antimicrobial agents
 for burn management, 134t
Topical silver nitrate, 135
TOS, 373–374, 374f
Total anomalous pulmonary venous connection (TAPVC), 322
Total body surface area (TBSA), 131–132, 132f
Total body water (TBW), 148
Total lung capacity (TLC), 357
Totally extraperitoneal (TEP) repair, 167
Total proctocolectomy, 239
Toxic megacolon
 acute, 239
Toxic multinodular goiter, 470
Toxins, 62
Trabecular bone, 438

Trace elements, 288, 288t
Tracheobronchial injuries, 380
Tracheomalacia, 355
Traction diverticula, 190–191, 190f
Traction morphogenesis, 117
Transabdominal properitoneal (TAPP) repair, 167
Transependymal flow, 16
Transesophageal echocardiography (TEE), 142
Transformation zone, 410
Transforming growth factor beta (TGF–beta), 112
Transfusion therapy, 301–302
Transient ischemic attack (TIA), 28
Transitional cell carcinoma, 394–395
Transjugular intrahepatic portosystemic shunt (TIPS), 264
Transplant recipients, 72
Transposition of the great arteries, 321, 321f
Transurethral resection of the prostate (TURP), 399
Transversalis fascia, 160
Transverse rectus abdominis muscle flap, 516, 516f
Transversus abdominis, 160
Trauma, 18–24, 254–255
 during pregnancy, 415
Traumatic amputations, 452
Traumatic aneurysms, 27
Traumatic shock
 treatment of, 158
Traumatic subdural hematoma, 20
T3 resin uptake, 467–468
TRH stimulation test, 468
Tricuspid atresia, 317–318, 317f
Tricuspid valves, 305, 327
Trimethadione, 491–492
Triolein breath test, 492
Tripod fracture, 432
Tropocollagen, 118, 118f
Trousseau sign, 481
True–negative rate, 181
True–positive rate, 181
Truncal vagotomy, 203–205, 205f, 205t
Truncus arteriosus, 321
TT, 299–300
T test, 178
TTP, 106
Tuberculosis, 364
Tuberous sclerosis, 393
Tuboovarian abscess (TOA), 407
Tubular necrosis
 acute, 50
Tumor antigens, 76–78
Tumor–associated antigens, 76–79
Tumor cachexia, 115
Tumor–infiltrating lymphocytes (TILs), 89
Tumor markers, 76–77
Tumor necrosis factor (TNF), 115
Tumors, 29–30
 mixed
  malignant, 421
 proliferation of, 73–74, 73f
 radiobiology of, 84–85, 84f
Tumor suppressor genes, 90

Tumor vaccines, 89
Tunica adventitia, 332
Tunica media, 332
Turbulence, 338
Turcot syndrome, 71
TURP, 399
Type I collagen, 438
Type II collagen, 443

U

UES, 187
Ulcerating carcinoma, 209–210
Ulcerative colitis, 82, 238–240
Ulnar nerve, 458t
 injuries of, 455
Ultrasonography
 for GU trauma, 388–389
 of thyroid gland, 468–469
Umbilical hernias, 168
UMN, 10–11
Unicameral bone cysts, 446t
University of Wisconsin (UW) solution, 49
Unruptured arteriovenous malformations (AVMs), 27–28
Upper esophageal sphincter (UES), 187
Upper extremities
 injuries of, 452–458
Upper gastrointestinal bleeding, 207, 247
Upper motor neuron (UMN), 10–11
Ureteroneocystostomy, 50
Ureters, 381–382, 403, 404f
 trauma of, 391
Urethra
 male, 383
 trauma of, 391
Urinary bladder, 382–383
Urinary catheters
 for anesthesia monitoring, 141–142
Urinary tract infection, 68
Urokinase, 296
Urologic emergencies, 392–393
Urologic neoplasms, 393–399
Uterus, 402
 malignancies of, 408–411
Utility of the outcome, 182
Utricle, 417
UW solution, 49

V

Vagina, 402
 carcinoma of, 413
Vagus nerve, 197, 199f, 427
Valve disease
 acquired, 324–328
Valve prosthesis, 327
Valve repair, 327–328
Valvulae conniventes, 211
Vancomycin, 64
Variance, 177
Varicose veins, 353
Vascular claudication, 36
Vascular disorders, 26–29
Vascular endothelium, 113, 311, 333
Vascular injuries
 fractures associated with, 451–452
Vasoactive intestinal polypeptide (VIP), 216

Vasoactive shock, 156
Vasodilation, 113
Vasogenic shock, 156
Vasospasm, 27
VC, 357
Veins, 333
Venal caval filters, 353
Venous anatomy, 6
Venous disorders, 353
Venous insufficiency
  chronic, 353
Ventilation, 354, 359
  mechanics of, 355–356
Ventilation–perfusion (V/Q) mismatch, 362
Ventricles, 6, 306–307
Ventricular arrhythmias, 328
Ventricular assist device, 312, 312t
Ventricular outflow obstruction, 319–320
Ventricular septal defect (VSD), 314–315, 315f
Ventriculoperitoneal shunt, 15, 16
Ventriculostomy, 15, 16
Vermis, 7
Vertebrae, 4–5, 4f
Vertebrobasilar junction, 26
Very low density lipoproteins (VLDLs), 334
Vessel wall, 333f
Vestibular neuritis, 417
Vestibular system, 417–419
Viewer bias, 174
Vincristine, 244
VIP, 216
VIPoma, 499

Viral encephalitis, 33
Viral hepatitis, 260
Viruses, 61–62
Viscosity, 338
Visual deficits, 12f
Visual input, 11
Vital capacity (VC), 357
Vitamin A, 122
Vitamin D, 479
Vitamins, 282, 287–288, 287f
VLDLs, 334
Voice
  breathy, 428
  chronic changes in, 428
Volume–dependent hypertension, 352
Von Hippel Lindau disease, 32
Von Recklinghausen disease, 97
V/Q mismatch, 362
VSD, 314–315, 315f
Vulva, 400
  carcinoma of, 413

W

Wallerian degeneration, 24
Warren shunt, 265, 266f
Warthin tumors, 420, 421f
Water, 149
Water balance, 384–385
Wernicke aphasia, 12
Wernicke area, 12
Whipple procedure, 234, 500, 500f
Whipple triad, 497–498
White blood coagulation, 299

White matter, 3
Wound healing, 110–122
  clinical implications of, 121–122
  fetal, 120–121
  stages of, 110–120, 111t
Wound infections, 66
  postoperative, 449
Wounds
  chronic, 121
  classification of, 66
  contraction of, 120
  reepithelialization of, 120
Woven bone, 438
Wrist
  nerves of, 457–458, 458t

X

Xanthochromatic, 26
Xenotransplantation, 46

Y

Yolk sac tumors, 413

Z

Zenker diverticulum, 185, 190–191, 191f
ZES, 215
Zollinger–Ellison syndrome (ZES), 215
Zona fasciculata, 482
Zona glomerulosa, 482
ZPTT, 299
Zygomatic trauma, 431–433